W9-DGJ-008

Treatment of
Advanced Heart Disease

Fundamental and Clinical Cardiology

1. Drug Treatment of Hyperlipidemia, *edited by Basil M. Rifkind*
2. Cardiotonic Drugs: A Clinical Review, Second Edition, Revised and Expanded, *edited by Carl V. Leier*
3. Complications of Coronary Angioplasty, *edited by Alexander J. R. Black, H. Vernon Anderson, and Stephen G. Ellis*
4. Unstable Angina, *edited by John D. Rutherford*
5. Beta-Blockers and Cardiac Arrhythmias, *edited by Prakash C. Deedwania*
6. Exercise and the Heart in Health and Disease, *edited by Roy J. Shephard and Henry S. Miller, Jr.*
7. Cardiopulmonary Physiology in Critical Care, *edited by Steven M. Scharf*
8. Atherosclerotic Cardiovascular Disease, Hemostasis, and Endothelial Function, *edited by Robert Boyer Francis, Jr.*
9. Coronary Heart Disease Prevention, *edited by Frank G. Yanowitz*
10. Thrombolysis and Adjunctive Therapy for Acute Myocardial Infarction, *edited by Eric R. Bates*
11. Stunned Myocardium: Properties, Mechanisms, and Clinical Manifestations, *edited by Robert A. Kloner and Karin Przyklenk*
12. Prevention of Venous Thromboembolism, *edited by Samuel Z. Goldhaber*
13. Silent Myocardial Ischemia and Infarction: Third Edition, *Peter F. Cohn*
14. Congestive Cardiac Failure: Pathophysiology and Treatment, *edited by David B. Barnett, Hubert Pouleur and Gary S. Francis*
15. Heart Failure: Basic Science and Clinical Aspects, *edited by Judith K. Gwathmey, G. Maurice Briggs, and Paul D. Allen*
16. Coronary Thrombolysis in Perspective: Principles Underlying Conjunctive and Adjunctive Therapy, *edited by Burton E. Sobel and Desire Collen*
17. Cardiovascular Disease in the Elderly Patient, *edited by Donald D. Tresch and Wilbert S. Aronow*
18. Systemic Cardiac Embolism, *edited by Michael D. Ezekowitz*
19. Low-Molecular-Weight Heparins in Prophylaxis and Therapy of Thromboembolic Diseases, *edited by Henri Bounameaux*
20. Valvular Heart Diseases, *edited by Muayed Al Zaibag and Carlos M. G. Duran*
21. Implantable Cardioverter-Defibrillators: A Comprehensive Textbook, *edited by N. A. Mark Estes, Antonis S. Manolis, and Paul J. Wang*
22. Individualized Therapy of Hypertension, *edited by Norman M. Kaplan and C. Venkata S. Ram*
23. Atlas of Coronary Balloon Angioplasty, *Bernhard Meier and Vivek K. Mehan*

24. Lowering Cholesterol in High-Risk Individuals and Populations, *edited by Basil M. Rifkind*
25. Interventional Cardiology: New Techniques and Strategies for Diagnosis and Treatment, *edited by Christopher J. White and Stephen Ramee*
26. Molecular Genetics and Gene Therapy of Cardiovascular Diseases, *edited by Stephen C. Mockrin*
27. The Pericardium: A Comprehensive Textbook, *David H. Spodick*
28. Coronary Restenosis: From Genetics to Therapeutics, *edited by Giora Z. Feuerstein*
29. The Endothelium in Clinical Practice: Source and Target of Novel Therapies, *edited by Gabor M. Rubanyi and Victor J. Dzau*
30. Molecular Biology of Cardiovascular Disease, *edited by Andrew R. Marks and Mark B. Taubman*
31. Practical Critical Care in Cardiology, *edited by Zab Mohsenifar and P. K. Shah*
32. Intravascular Ultrasound Imaging in Coronary Artery Disease, *edited by Robert J. Siegel*
33. Saphenous Vein Bypass Graft Disease, *edited by Eric R. Bates and David R. Holmes, Jr.*
34. Exercise and the Heart in Health and Disease: Second Edition, Revised and Expanded, *edited by Roy J. Shephard and Henry S. Miller, Jr*
35. Cardiovascular Drug Development: Protocol Design and Methodology, *edited by Jeffrey S. Borer and John C. Somberg*
36. Cardiovascular Disease in the Elderly Patient: Second Edition, Revised and Expanded, *edited by Donald D. Tresch and Wilbert S. Aronow*
37. Clinical Neurocardiology, Louis R. Caplan, *J. Willis Hurst, and Mark Chimowitz*
38. Cardiac Rehabilitation: A Guide to Practice in the 21st Century, *edited by Nanette K. Wenger, L. Kent Smith, Erika Sivarajan Froelicher, and Patricia McCall Comoss*
39. Heparin-Induced Thrombocytopenia, *edited by Theodore E. Warkentin and Andreas Greinacher*
40. Silent Myocardial Ischemia and Infarction: Fourth Edition, *Peter F. Cohn*
41. Foundations of Cardiac Arrhythmias: Basic Concepts and Clinical Approaches, *edited by Peter M. Spooner and Michael R. Rosen*
42. Interpreting Electrocardiograms: Using Basic Principles and Vector Concepts, *J. Willis Hurst*
43. Heparin-Induced Thrombocytopenia: Second Edition, *edited by Theodore E. Warkentin and Andreas Greinacher*
44. Thrombosis and Thromboembolism, *edited by Samuel Z. Goldhaber and Paul M. Ridker*
45. Cardiovascular Plaque Rupture, *edited by David L. Brown*
46. New Therapeutic Agents in Thrombosis and Thrombolysis: Second Edition, Revised and Expanded, *edited by Arthur A. Sasahara and Joseph Loscalzo*
47. Heparin-Induced Thrombocytopenia: Third Edition, *edited by Theodore E. Warkentin and Andreas Greinacher*
48. Cardiovascular Disease in the Elderly, Third Edition, *edited by Wilbert Aronow and Jerome Fleg*
49. Atrial Fibrillation, *edited by Peter Kowey and Gerald Naccarelli*
50. Heart Failure: A Comprehensive Guide to Diagnosis and Treatment, *edited by G. William Dec*

51. Phamacoinvasive Therapy in Acute Myocardial Infarction, *edited by Harold L. Dauerman and Burton E. Sobel*
52. Clinical, Interventional, and Investigational Thrombocardiology, *edited by Richard Becker and Robert A. Harrington*
53. Pediatric Heart Failure, *Robert Shaddy and Gil Wernovsky*
54. Cardiac Remodeling: Mechanisms and Treatment, *edited by Barry Greenberg*
55. Acute Coronary Syndromes, Third Edition, *edited by Eric Topol*
56. Treatment of Advanced Heart Disease, *edited by Kenneth L. Baughman and William A. Baumgartner*
57. Prevention of High-Risk Cardiovascular Disease, *edited by Antonio Gotto and Peter P. Toth*
58. Obesity and Cardiovascular Disease, *edited by Malcolm K. Robinson and Abraham Thomas*

Treatment of
Advanced Heart Disease

Edited by

Kenneth L. Baughman
Brigham and Women's Hospital
Boston, Massachusetts, U.S.A.

William A. Baumgartner
The Johns Hopkins Hospital
Baltimore, Maryland, U.S.A.

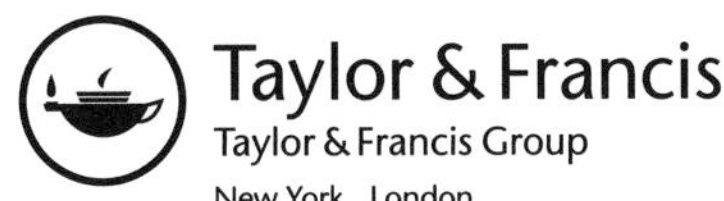
Taylor & Francis
Taylor & Francis Group
New York London

Published in 2006 by
Taylor & Francis Group
270 Madison Avenue
New York, NY 10016

Printed in the United States of America on acid-free paper
10 9 8 7 6 5 4 3 2 1

International Standard Book Number-10: 0-8493-3826-3 (Hardcover)
International Standard Book Number-13: 978-0-8493-3826-7 (Hardcover)
Library of Congress Card Number 2005046655

Library of Congress Cataloging-in-Publication Data

Treatment of advanced heart disease / edited by Kenneth L. Baughman, William A. Baumgartner.
p. ; cm. -- (Fundamental and clinical cardiology ; 56)
Includes bibliographical references and index.
ISBN-13: 978-0-8493-3826-7 (alk. paper)
ISBN-10: 0-8493-3826-3 (alk. paper)
1. Heart--Diseases--Treatment. I. Baughman, Kenneth L. II. Baumgartner, William A. III. Fundamental and clinical cardiology ; v. 56.
[DNLM: 1. Heart Diseases--therapy. WG 166 T784 2006]

RC683.8.T74 2006
616.1'206--dc22 2005046655

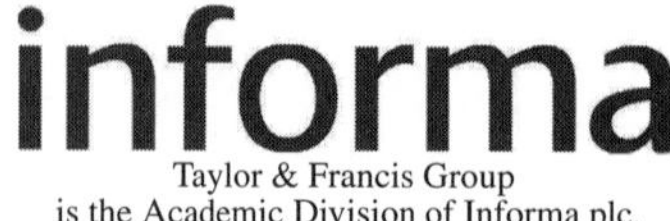

Taylor & Francis Group
is the Academic Division of Informa plc.

Visit the Taylor & Francis Web site at
http://www.taylorandfrancis.com

Series Introduction

Taylor & Francis Group has focused on the development of various series of beautifully produced books in different branches of medicine. These series have facilitated the integration of rapidly advancing information for both the clinical specialist and the researcher.

My goal as editor-in-chief of the Fundamental and Clinical Cardiology Series is to assemble the talents of world-renowned authorities to discuss virtually every area of cardiovascular medicine. In the current monograph, Drs. Baughman and Baumgartner have edited a much-needed and timely book that focuses on the cardiovasular pandemic of advanced heart failure. Future contributions to this series will include books on molecular biology, interventional cardiology, and clinical management of such problems as coronary artery disease and ventricular arrhythmias.

Samuel Z. Goldhaber, MD
Professor of Medicine
Harvard Medical School
Boston, Massachusetts, U.S.A.

Foreword

The incidence of congestive heart failure, an increasingly prevalent condition due to our aging population and myocardial-salvaging therapy, will rise dramatically over the next several decades. Recognition and treatment of this disorder has become more complicated. Much like interventional cardiology and electrophysiology, heart failure and heart transplantation have evolved into a distinct sub-discipline of cardiovascular medicine.

As with any rapidly advancing field of investigation and care, preparation of a definitive text that outlines the scope of the problem and reviews medical, device, and surgical management for both the adult and pediatric population presents a considerable challenge. Nonetheless, *Treatment of Advanced Heart Disease*, edited by Dr. Kenneth L. Baughman and Dr. William A. Baumgartner, accomplishes this mission. The book provides its audience with currently available and near-term future therapies for treatment of heart failure. Contributors include leading experts in their fields, many current members or former faculty and trainees of the cardiovascular sections of the Brigham and Women's Hospital, The Johns Hopkins Hospital, and Massachusetts General Hospital.

Treatment of Advanced Heart Disease represents a welcome addition to the medical literature as a single-source compilation. Given its focus on the growing population of individuals with advanced stages of heart failure and its emphasis on practical clinical management issues, this volume provides practitioners with a ready guide for their daily practices. The editors and authors merit congratulations for their successful efforts to provide this timely reference.

Peter Libby, MD
Mallinckrodt Professor of Medicine and
Chief, Cardiovascular Division
Brigham and Women's Hospital
Boston, Massachusetts, U.S.A.

Preface

Congestive heart failure affects approximately five million people in the United States, with over 500,000 new cases per year, and is the most common diagnosis-related group for hospitalizations of patients over 65 years of age. As the population ages, and as thrombolitic therapy and other interventions prolong the lives of patients with heart disease, the number of patients with congestive heart failure is increasing dramatically.

As patients' heart dysfunction advances, they require a proportionate response, including increased medical therapy, insertion of devices, and occasionally surgical therapy, in their management.

As a result, the number of physicians caring for this group of patients will also expand beyond the capability of heart failure specialists and cardiologists. Additional physicians, nurse practitioners, and physicians assistants will be needed to care for this population, including those in general internal medicine, general practitioners, general pediatricians, and surgical specialties who will be responsible for these patients intermittently before and after surgical intervention. Physicians caring for the patients will need a compendium of current management options and some sense of the new and experimental therapies soon to be available.

This book is meant to serve as a single-source guide to the care of patients with heart failure. The text begins with an overview of the current heart failure population and anticipated growth in the future. The authors guide the clinician through a consideration of the causes of advanced heart disease, in particular an algorithm for newly diagnosed patients to guide the assessment of potentially reversible etiologies. Medical management is considered from the most fundamental of interventions, including diet and exercise, to a consideration of the appropriate use of diuretics, afterload reduction therapy, and beta-blockers. The use of statin therapy in ischemic and nonischemic dilated cardiomyopathy is considered. The appropriate treatment of both superventricular and ventricular arrhythmias is addressed. Intravenous inotropes are considered as a bridge to more definitive therapy with careful assessment of the risks and benefits of this form of treatment.

The appropriate use of biventricular pacing and selection of candidates for implantable cardioverter defibrillators are addressed utilizing the most recently published data. Less frequently considered but equally important device therapies, including external and internal counterpulsation and treatment of sleep-disordered breathing, are considered to complete the evaluation of currently available device therapy.

No text on the management of advanced heart disease would be complete without consideration of surgical therapy, particularly heart transplantation. In view of the limited number of patients who will receive heart transplantation in the United States, all other surgical options are considered. These include high-risk revascularization, valve replacement or repair, ventricular reconstruction, and laser therapy. In addition, bridge and destination utilization of all forms of ventricular assist devices and total artificial hearts receive consideration in this comprehensive yet easy-to-understand book.

In addition to cutting-edge application of currently available therapy, the text explores the potential therapies of the future. These include cell therapy, gene therapy, genetics and heart failure, new drugs, new devices, and new surgical approaches. These sections will place the reader in the advantageous position of having awareness of therapies that will be introduced in the next three to five years. Unique to this text is the attention given to the management of the pediatric patient, including medical, device, and surgical therapies in patients less than 18 years of age.

Of special importance are sections dealing with the education and counseling of patients with heart failure and their families. This includes appropriate determination of prognosis and end-of-life issues.

The book provides readers with exposure to all of the currently available and near-term future therapies for patients with progressive heart failure. Readers have not only currently available therapy, but also a practical algorithm of management options and when each form of therapy is utilized in the care of an individual patient. Although all inclusive, the text is succinct, organized, readable, and provides the consumer with a single source for complete management of the most straightforward to the most difficult patients.

This book was written to have appeal to internists, cardiologists, cardiology fellows, general practitioners, cardiac surgery residents, cardiac surgery attendees, and pediatric cardiovascular specialists. As noted above, the book is also of interest to an expanded group of physicians who will have initial or intermittent responsibility for this patient population, including general practitioners, general pediatricians, and non-cardiovascular surgeons.

Kenneth L. Baughman
William A. Baumgartner

Contents

Series Introduction Samuel Z. Goldhaber . . . . *iii*
Foreword Peter Libby . . . . *v*
Preface . . . . *vii*
Contributors . . . . *xxi*

PART I: ETIOLOGY AND EPIDEMIOLOGY

1. Epidemiology and Prognosis in Chronic Heart Failure ***1***
G. William Dec
Introduction 1
Asymptomatic Left Ventricular Dysfunction 1
Risk Factors for Heart Failure Development 3
Multivariate Risk Prediction of Heart Failure 8
Special Populations 9
Establishing the Diagnosis of Heart Failure 10
Prognostic Features 11
Prognosis in Chronic Heart Failure 15
References 16

2. Causes and Evaluation for Reversible Etiologies ***23***
Edward K. Kasper
Introduction 23
Evaluation of Patients with Advanced Heart Failure 23
Causes of Cardiomyopathy 27
Reversible Causes of Cardiomyopathy 28
References 33

PART II: MEDICAL MANAGEMENT

3. Diet, Metabolic Syndrome, and Obesity ***37***
Michael M. Givertz
Introduction 37
Weight Gain and Loss 37

Diet 40
Metabolic Syndrome 41
Obesity 43
Transplant Considerations 51
References 52

4. Exercise and Heart Failure ***59***
Daniel E. Forman
Introduction 59
Heart Function and Functional Capacity 59
Exercise Training in HF 61
Safety of Exercise Training in HF 63
Exercise Training Modalities 63
Heart Failure with Normal Ejection Fraction 66
Exercise Adherence 67
References 67

5. Diuretics ***71***
Ilan S. Wittstein
Introduction 71
Effect of Diuretics on Heart Failure Symptoms 71
Hemodynamic Effects of Diuretics 72
Neurohormonal Effects of Loop Diuretics 73
Effect of Diuretics on Cardiac Remodeling 76
Effect of Diuretics on Mortality 77
Diuretic Pharmacology 78
Diuretic Use for the Treatment of Congestive Heart Failure 83
Diuretic-Related Side Effects 87
Other "Diuretic" Agents 89
Conclusion 91
References 91

6. Vasodilators in the Management of Heart Failure ***99***
David W. Markham and G. Michael Felker
Vasoconstriction in Heart Failure: Rationale for Vasodilator Therapy 99
Vasodilator Therapy in Acute Decompensated Heart Failure 101
Vasodilator Therapy in Chronic Heart Failure 105
Conclusions 109
References 109

7. Beta-Blockers in Heart Failure ***113***
Emily J. Tsai and Thomas P. Cappola
Introduction 113
β-Adrenergic Signaling in the Cardiovascular System 114

Evidence for the Role of Beta-Blockade 118
Clinical Guidelines 125
Future Directions 129
References 129

8. Inotropic Therapy in Heart Failure Management *137*
Lisa M. Mielniczuk and Anju Nohria
Introduction 137
The Cardiac Contractile Apparatus 137
Mechanism of Action of Inotropic Therapy 139
Mechanisms of Harm 143
Inotrope Therapy in Acute Decompensated HF 143
Inotrope Use in Chronic HF 145
Future Directions of Inotropic Therapy 149
Conclusions and Recommendations 150
References 151

9. Statins, Inflammation, and Cardiomyopathy: Old Pathways, New Targets *155*
Charles J. Lowenstein and Munekazu Yamakuchi
Introduction 155
The Discovery of Statins: From Microbes to Lipids 155
Anti-cholesterol Effects of Statins: The Most Decorated Molecule in Biology 156
Clinical Trials of Statins and LDL Cholesterol: The Lower the Better 157
Clinical Studies of Statins and Inflammation: Lowering LDL, Inflammation, or Both? 157
Statins Block Integrins and Leukocyte Trafficking 158
Statins Decrease Isoprenylation of Signaling Proteins: Rho 159
Statins Improve Endothelial Function: Nitric Oxide 159
Statins Decrease Vascular Inflammation: Blockade of Exocytosis 160
Statins and Cardiomyopathy 161
Conclusions: The True Significance of Statin Anti-inflammatory Effects 162
References 162

10. Atrial Arrhythmia *167*
Aamir Cheema and Hugh Calkins
Introduction 167
Atrial Fibrillation 167
Rhythm Control 169
Rate Control 172
Atrial Flutter 174

Other Supraventricular Tachycardias 176
Conclusion 176
References 177

11. Management of Ventricular Arrhythmias in Heart Failure *183*
Usha B. Tedrow and William G. Stevenson
Introduction 183
Ventricular Arrhythmias and Sudden Cardiac Death 183
Antiarrhythmic Drugs 192
Summary and Conclusions 195
References 196

12. Acute Heart Failure *203*
Stuart D. Russell
Introduction 203
Clinical Context 203
Assessment 205
Studies 210
Therapy 212
Pre-discharge Goals 220
Summary 222
References 222

13. Diastolic Heart Failure *227*
Michael M. Givertz and James C. Fang
Definitions and Classification 227
Epidemiology 229
Pathophysiology 231
Clinical Assessment 234
Treatment 238
New Directions 242
References 243

14. Diagnosis and Management of Secondary Pulmonary Hypertension *247*
Anna R. Hemnes and Hunter C. Champion
Introduction 247
Pathophysiology 247
Pathology and Basic Science 248
Epidemiology and Clinical Evaluation 249
Management 251
References 256

PART III: DEVICE THERAPY

15. Cardiac Resynchronization Therapy *259*
Michael O. Sweeney
A Heart Failure Epidemic 259

Abnormal Electrical Timing in Heart Failure Associated with DCM 259
Cardiac Resynchronization Therapy (CRT) 263
Implementation of CRT 266
CRT Pacing Systems 275
Programming Considerations in CRT 279
CRT Pacemaker Electrocardiography/Determining LV and RV Capture 284
Patient Selection for CRT 287
Clinical Trials of CRT 292
Clinical Trials of CRT/Defibrillation (CRTD) 292
Contak CD, Miracle ICD, and Companion 295
References 296

16. Device Therapy for Advanced Heart Disease: The Role of Implantable Defibrillators *301*
Akshay S. Desai and Bruce A. Koplan
Background: Sudden Cardiac Death 301
Predicting Sudden Death in Patients with Heart Failure 302
Selection of Heart Failure Patients for Defibrillator Therapy 304
Conclusions 318
References 321

17. Device Therapy for Heart Failure *325*
James C. Fang
Intra-aortic Balloon Counterpulsation (IABP) 325
Enhanced External Counterpulsation (EECP) 329
Continuous Positive Airway Pressure (CPAP) 334
References 339

PART IV: SURGICAL THERAPY

18. Revascularization *345*
Prem S. Shekar and Gregory S. Couper
Introduction and Epidemiology of Advanced Ischemic Heart Disease 345
The Concepts of Normal Myocardium, Stunned Hibernating Myocardium, and Scar 345
Coronary Disease, Left Ventricular Dysfunction, and Survival 346
Investigational Modalities 346
Tests to Determine Myocardial Viability 347
Selection of Patients for Surgical Revascularization 349
Principles of Surgical Revascularization 349

Technical Considerations 350
CABG, PCI, or Medical Management in Ischemic Cardiomyopathy 353
The Benefits of CABG in LV Dysfunction—Who and When 354
References 354

19. Valvular Surgery in Cardiomyopathy *357*
Frederick Y. Chen and Lawrence H. Cohn
Introduction 357
Valvular Repair or Replacement in Cardiomyopathy 358
Mitral Valve Surgery in Cardiomyopathy: A Problem of Regurgitation 359
Aortic Valve Surgery in Cardiomyopathy: Aortic Stenosis and Aortic Regurgitation 361
Conclusions 363
References 363

20. Surgical Ventricular Remodeling *367*
John V. Conte
Introduction 367
History 368
Indications for Surgery 369
Surgical Approaches 369
Dor Procedure (Endoventricular Circular Patch Plasty) 371
Linear Closure with Septoplasty 374
Multiple Purse String or Cerclage Technique 375
Septoplasty Technique 375
Outcomes 375
References 379

21. Transmyocardial Laser Revascularization *383*
Keith A. Horvath
Introduction 383
TMR as Sole Therapy 384
Results 387
TMR as an Adjunct to CABG 391
Results 391
Mechanisms 392
Percutaneous Myocardial Laser Revascularization 394
Future Uses of TMR 395
Summary 395
References 395

22. Percutaneous Left Ventricular Assist Devices *401*
Piotr Sobieszczyk and Andrew C. Eisenhauer
Introduction 401

Left Ventricular Assist Devices: Pulsatile and Non-pulsatile Flow 402
Historical Perspective 403
Contemporary Percutaneous Left Ventricular Assist Devices 407
Conclusion 414
References 414

23. Selecting Patients for Durable Support with Ventricular Assist Devices ***419***
Lynne Warner Stevenson
The Current Picture 419
Beyond "Optimal" Medical Therapy 419
Benefit of VAD for Durable Support 422
Contraindications for Current VADs 426
References 430

24. Ventricular Assist Devices ***433***
Jason A. Williams and John V. Conte
History of Mechanical Ventricular Assistance 433
Overview of Ventricular Assist Devices 434
Patient Selection 435
Patient Management 437
Device Selection 440
Bridge to Recovery Devices 440
Bridge to Bridge Devices 445
Bridge to Transplant and Destination Therapy 445
Devices in Development (Third Generation Devices) 452
Outcomes 453
The Future of Ventricular Assist Devices 455
References 455

25. Total Artificial Heart (AbioCor™) ***459***
Laman A. Gray Jr.
Background 459
Device Description 459
Preoperative Considerations 461
Operative Technique 462
Clinical Trial 464
New Devices 470
References 470

26. The SynCardia CardioWest™ Total Artificial Heart ***473***
Marvin J. Slepian, Richard G. Smith, and Jack G. Copeland
Introduction 473
Rationale for the Total Artificial Heart 474
Historical Overview of Artificial Heart Technology 475

Technical and Operational Details of the CardioWest™ TAH 478
Indications for Use of the CardioWest™ TAH 483
Clinical Experience with the CardioWest™ TAH 483
Future Applications of the CardioWest™ TAH 487
Conclusion 487
References 489

27. Selection and Management of Cardiac Transplantation Candidates *491*
Christopher Newton-Cheh and Marc J. Semigran
Introduction 491
General Indications for Cardiac Transplantation 491
Evaluation of Severity and Prognosis of Chronic HF: Is This Patient's Prognosis Poor Enough to Require Transplantation? 493
Timing of Referral to Transplant Center 497
Contraindications to Cardiac Transplantation 497
Implications of the System for Organ Allocation 503
Outcomes on Waitlist for Transplant 504
Management Prior to Transplant 505
Conclusion 505
Appendix A: Donor Identification and Management 505
References 506

PART V: PSYCHOSOCIAL ISSUES

28. Education, Psychosocial Issues, and Sociodemographic Barriers in Heart Failure Disease Management *511*
Aileen Aponte, Norma Osborn, Joanne R. Weintraub, and Michelle A. Young
Introduction 511
Patient Education 511
Challenges in Health Education 512
Outpatient Heart Failure Disease Management 515
Depression in Heart Failure Patients 518
Anxiety in Heart Failure Patients 519
Sociodemographic Barriers to Care 520
References 525

29. Prognosis Assessment and End of Life Issues *531*
Eldrin F. Lewis and Carol M. Flavell
Introduction 531
Clinical Use of Prognostic Factors 532
Targets of Therapy 536
Clinical Issues in End of Life Care of Heart Failure 538
References 543

PART VI: RESEARCH

30. Regenerative Medicine: The Promise of Cellular Cardiomyoplasty *547*
Anastasios P. Saliaris, Luciano C. Amado, Karl H. Schuleri, and Joshua M. Hare
Introduction 547
Repair Mechanisms 548
Cell Types Involved in Cardiac Regeneration and Repair 550
Delivery Routes 555
Homing and Migration of Stem Cells 556
Human Trials 557
Potential Complications 561
Conclusion 562
References 562

31. Gene Therapy for Heart Failure *573*
Shi Yin Foo and Anthony Rosenzweig
Introduction 573
Vectors for Cardiac Gene Transfer 574
Delivery Systems 577
Biological Targets in Heart Failure 578
Summary and Conclusions 583
References 583

32. Genetics and Heart Failure: Hypertrophic Cardiomyopathy *589*
Carolyn Y. Ho and Christine E. Seidman
Introduction 589
Hypertrophic Cardiomyopathy 589
Phenotype and Natural History 591
Genetic Aspects 594
New Paradigms of Inherited Cardiac Hypertrophy 598
Contemporary Diagnosis of HCM 600
References 603

33. Genetics and Heart Failure: Dilated, Restrictive, and Right Ventricular Cardiomyopathies *607*
Nicole M. Johnson and Daniel P. Judge
Introduction 607
Familial Dilated Cardiomyopathy 607
Familial Restrictive Cardiomyopathy 613
Right Ventricular Cardiomyopathy 614
Clinical Implications 616
References 617

34. New Drugs for Heart Failure: Emerging Role of Oxidative Stress as a Target *623*
Tania Chao and Wilson S. Colucci
New Therapeutic Targets in Heart Failure 623
Myocyte Death and Dysfunction in Heart Failure 623
Oxidative Stress in Heart Failure 624
Regulation of Reactive Species in the Myocardium 624
Oxidative Stress in Myocardial Failure 625
Myocyte Loss and Dysfunction in Heart Failure 625
Oxypurinol: An Antioxidant for the Therapy for Chronic Heart Failure 626
New Therapeutic Targets in Acute Decompensated Heart Failure 627
Cardioprotection via Activation of ATP-Dependent Potassium Channels 627
Levosimendan: A New Agent for the Treatment of Decompensated Heart Failure 628
Clinical Effects of Levosimendan 629
References 629

35. New Surgery for Congestive Heart Failure *633*
David D. Yuh
Introduction 633
Robot-Assisted, Minimally Invasive Coronary Revascularization 634
Geometric Mitral Reconstruction 637
Minimally Invasive Mitral Valve Repair 637
Minimally Invasive, Robot-Assisted Biventricular Pacemaker Lead Placement 640
Minimally Invasive, Robot-Assisted Transmyocardial Revascularization 642
Surgical Treatment of Atrial Fibrillation 643
Cardiac Restraint Devices: The Acorn CorCap® Device 648
References 650

PART VII: PEDIATRIC THERAPY

36. Device and Alternative Therapies in Pediatric Heart Failure *653*
Leslie B. Smoot, Jane E. Crosson, and Ravi Thiagarajan
Introduction 653
Unique Aspects of Pediatric Heart Failure and Device Use 653
Electrophysiology: Catheter Ablation and Device Therapy 654
Therapeutic Circulatory Support Modalities 657

Psychosocial Aspects of Advanced Heart Disease in
Pediatrics 660
References 660

37. Surgical Management of Pediatric Heart Failure *663*
Luca A. Vricella and Duke E. Cameron
Introduction 663
Heart Failure in Children: Surgical Indications for
Device Implantation 664
Choice of Ventricular Assist Device 666
Specific Ventricular Assist Devices 666
Conclusions 676
References 676

Index 681

Contributors

Luciano C. Amado Institute for Cell Engineering and Cardiology Division, Department of Medicine, Johns Hopkins University School of Medicine, Baltimore, Maryland, U.S.A.

Aileen Aponte Advanced Heart Disease Section, Cardiovascular Division, Brigham and Women's Hospital, Boston, Massachusetts, U.S.A.

Hugh Calkins Division of Cardiology, Department of Medicine, Johns Hopkins University School of Medicine, Baltimore, Maryland, U.S.A.

Duke E. Cameron Division of Cardiac Surgery, The Johns Hopkins Hospital, Baltimore, Maryland, U.S.A.

Thomas P. Cappola University of Pennsylvania School of Medicine, Philadelphia, Pennsylvania, U.S.A.

Hunter C. Champion Divisions of Cardiology and Pulmonary and Critical Care Medicine, Department of Medicine, Johns Hopkins University School of Medicine, Baltimore, Maryland, U.S.A.

Tania Chao Cardiovascular Section, Department of Medicine, Boston University Medical Center, Boston University School of Medicine, Boston, Massachusetts, U.S.A.

Aamir Cheema Division of Cardiology, Department of Medicine, Johns Hopkins University School of Medicine, Baltimore, Maryland, U.S.A.

Frederick Y. Chen Division of Cardiac Surgery, Brigham and Women's Hospital, Harvard Medical School, Boston, Massachusetts, U.S.A.

Lawrence H. Cohn Division of Cardiac Surgery, Brigham and Women's Hospital, Harvard Medical School, Boston, Massachusetts, U.S.A.

Wilson S. Colucci Cardiovascular Section, Department of Medicine, Boston University Medical Center, Boston University School of Medicine, Boston, Massachusetts, U.S.A.

John V. Conte Division of Cardiac Surgery, The Johns Hopkins Hospital, Baltimore, Maryland, U.S.A.

Jack G. Copeland Department of Cardiothoracic Surgery, University of Arizona Sarver Heart Center, Tucson, Arizona, U.S.A.

Gregory S. Couper Division of Cardiac Surgery, Brigham and Women's Hospital, Harvard Medical School, Boston, Massachusetts, U.S.A.

Jane E. Crosson Pediatric Cardiology, The Johns Hopkins Hospital, Baltimore, Maryland, U.S.A.

G. William Dec Cardiology Division, Massachusetts General Hospital, Boston, Massachusetts, U.S.A.

Akshay S. Desai Advanced Heart Disease Section, Division of Cardiovascular Medicine, Department of Medicine, Brigham and Women's Hospital, Harvard Medical School, Boston, Massachusetts, U.S.A.

Andrew C. Eisenhauer Cardiovascular Division and Cardiac Catheterization Laboratory, Brigham and Women's Hospital, Harvard Medical School, Boston, Massachusetts, U.S.A.

James C. Fang Advanced Heart Disease Section, Cardiovascular Division, Department of Medicine, Brigham and Women's Hospital, Harvard Medical School, Boston, Massachusetts, U.S.A.

G. Michael Felker Duke University School of Medicine and Duke Clinical Research Institute, Durham, North Carolina, U.S.A.

Carol M. Flavell Advanced Heart Disease Section, Cardiovascular Division, Brigham and Women's Hospital, Boston, Massachusetts, U.S.A.

Shi Yin Foo Program in Cardiovascular Gene Therapy, Cardiovascular Research Center and Cardiology Division, Massachusetts General Hospital, Harvard Medical School, Boston, Massachusetts, U.S.A.

Daniel E. Forman Divisions of Cardiovascular Medicine and Aging, Brigham and Women's Hospital, VAMC of Boston, Harvard Medical School, Boston, Massachusetts, U.S.A.

Michael M. Givertz Cardiovascular Division, Brigham and Women's Hospital, Harvard Medical School, Boston, Massachusetts, U.S.A.

Laman A. Gray Jr. Division of Thoracic and Cardiovascular Surgery, Department of Surgery, University of Louisville, Louisville, Kentucky, U.S.A.

Joshua M. Hare Institute for Cell Engineering and Cardiology Division, Department of Medicine, Johns Hopkins University School of Medicine, Baltimore, Maryland, U.S.A.

Anna R. Hemnes Divisions of Cardiology and Pulmonary and Critical Care Medicine, Department of Medicine, Johns Hopkins University School of Medicine, Baltimore, Maryland, U.S.A.

Carolyn Y. Ho Cardiovascular Division, Brigham and Women's Hospital, Harvard Medical School, Boston, Massachusetts, U.S.A.

Keith A. Horvath Cardiothoracic Surgery Branch, NHLBI, National Institutes of Health, Bethesda, Maryland, U.S.A.

Nicole M. Johnson Division of Cardiology, Johns Hopkins University School of Medicine, Baltimore, Maryland, U.S.A.

Daniel P. Judge Division of Cardiology, Johns Hopkins University School of Medicine, Baltimore, Maryland, U.S.A.

Edward K. Kasper Division of Cardiology, Johns Hopkins Bayview Medical Center, Baltimore, Maryland, U.S.A.

Bruce A. Koplan Cardiovascular Division, Brigham and Women's Hospital, Harvard Medical School, Boston, Massachusetts, U.S.A.

Eldrin F. Lewis Advanced Heart Disease Section, Cardiovascular Division, Brigham and Women's Hospital, Harvard Medical School, Boston, Massachusetts, U.S.A.

Charles J. Lowenstein Department of Medicine, Johns Hopkins University School of Medicine, Baltimore, Maryland, U.S.A.

David W. Markham University of Texas Southwestern Medical Center at Dallas, Dallas, Texas, U.S.A.

Lisa M. Mielniczuk Division of Cardiology, Department of Medicine, Brigham and Women's Hospital, Boston, Massachusetts, U.S.A.

Christopher Newton-Cheh Heart Failure and Transplantation Section, Massachusetts General Hospital, Harvard Medical School, Boston, Massachusetts, U.S.A.

Anju Nohria Advanced Heart Disease Section, Division of Cardiovascular Medicine, Department of Medicine, Brigham and Women's Hospital, Harvard Medical School, Boston, Massachusetts, U.S.A.

Norma Osborn Advanced Heart Disease Section, Cardiovascular Division, Brigham and Women's Hospital, Boston, Massachusetts, U.S.A.

Anthony Rosenzweig Program in Cardiovascular Gene Therapy, Cardiovascular Research Center and Cardiology Division, Massachusetts General Hospital, Harvard Medical School, Boston, Massachusetts, U.S.A.

Stuart D. Russell Division of Cardiology, Department of Internal Medicine, The Johns Hopkins Hospital, Baltimore, Maryland, U.S.A.

Anastasios P. Saliaris Institute for Cell Engineering and Cardiology Division, Department of Medicine, Johns Hopkins University School of Medicine, Baltimore, Maryland, U.S.A.

Karl H. Schuleri Institute for Cell Engineering and Cardiology Division, Department of Medicine, Johns Hopkins University School of Medicine, Baltimore, Maryland, U.S.A.

Christine E. Seidman Cardiovascular Division, Brigham and Women's Hospital, Harvard Medical School, Boston, Massachusetts, U.S.A.

Marc J. Semigran Heart Failure and Transplantation Section, Massachusetts General Hospital, Harvard Medical School, Boston, Massachusetts, U.S.A.

Prem S. Shekar Division of Cardiac Surgery, Brigham and Women's Hospital, Harvard Medical School, Boston, Massachusetts, U.S.A.

Marvin J. Slepian Department of Medicine (Cardiology), University of Arizona Sarver Heart Center, Tucson, Arizona, U.S.A.

Richard G. Smith Artificial Heart Program, University Medical Center–Tucson, Tucson, Arizona, U.S.A.

Leslie B. Smoot Department of Cardiology, Harvard Medical School, Children's Hospital, Boston, Massachusetts, U.S.A.

Piotr Sobieszczyk Cardiovascular Division and Cardiac Catheterization Laboratory, Brigham and Women's Hospital, Harvard Medical School, Boston, Massachusetts, U.S.A.

Lynne Warner Stevenson Cardiovascular Division, Brigham and Women's Hospital, Harvard Medical School, Boston, Massachusetts, U.S.A.

William G. Stevenson Cardiovascular Division, Brigham and Women's Hospital, Harvard Medical School, Boston, Massachusetts, U.S.A.

Michael O. Sweeney CRM Research and Cardiac Arrhythmia Service, Brigham and Women's Hospital, Harvard Medical School, Boston, Massachusetts, U.S.A.

Usha B. Tedrow Cardiovascular Division, Brigham and Women's Hospital, Harvard Medical School, Boston, Massachusetts, U.S.A.

Ravi Thiagarajan Department of Cardiology, Harvard Medical School, Children's Hospital, Boston, Massachusetts, U.S.A.

Emily J. Tsai Division of Cardiology, Department of Medicine, Johns Hopkins University School of Medicine, Baltimore, Maryland, U.S.A.

Luca A. Vricella Division of Cardiac Surgery, The Johns Hopkins Hospital, Baltimore, Maryland, U.S.A.

Joanne R. Weintraub Advanced Heart Disease Section, Cardiovascular Division, Brigham and Women's Hospital, Boston, Massachusetts, U.S.A.

Jason A. Williams Division of Cardiac Surgery, The Johns Hopkins Hospital, Baltimore, Maryland, U.S.A.

Ilan S. Wittstein Division of Cardiology, Department of Medicine, Johns Hopkins University School of Medicine, Baltimore, Maryland, U.S.A.

Munekazu Yamakuchi Department of Medicine, Johns Hopkins University School of Medicine, Baltimore, Maryland, U.S.A.

Michelle A. Young Advanced Heart Disease Section, Cardiovascular Division, Brigham and Women's Hospital, Boston, Massachusetts, U.S.A.

David D. Yuh Division of Cardiac Surgery, The Johns Hopkins Hospital, Baltimore, Maryland, U.S.A.

PART I: ETIOLOGY AND EPIDEMIOLOGY

1 Epidemiology and Prognosis in Chronic Heart Failure

G. William Dec
Cardiology Division, Massachusetts General Hospital, Boston, Massachusetts, U.S.A.

INTRODUCTION

Heart failure is the only common cardiovascular disease in the United States that has a rising incidence and prevalence (Fig. 1) (1–3). The latest statistics from the American Heart Association estimate that approximately 4.9 million Americans have this disorder (1). The current incidence of disease is estimated to exceed 400,000 new symptomatic cases per year, directly accounting for over 250,000 deaths annually (Fig. 2) (1,4). Between 1.5% and 2% of the U.S. population has symptomatic heart failure and its prevalence is estimated to be 6%–10% over the age of 65 yr (5). Using the Framingham Heart Study cohort, Lloyd-Jones et al. determined the life-time risk of developing heart failure for men and women free of overt disease at age 40 yr to approximate 20% (Fig. 3) (6). There is a marked age-dependence in heart failure incidence and prevalence with elderly patients being disproportionately affected by the disease (Fig. 4) (7–9). The increased ability to identify asymptomatic left ventricular dysfunction and its progressive nature recently led to a "redefinition" of heart failure by the American College of Cardiology/American Heart Association consensus guidelines (4). The new ACC/AHA re-classification emphasizes the large number of "at risk" patients and encourages physicians to implement treatment strategies similar to those utilized for asymptomatic patients with risk factors for coronary artery disease. Patients in stage A (high risk for heart failure but without structural heart disease) and stage B (structural heart disease without overt heart failure symptoms) are an increasingly important focus for identification and treatment (Fig. 5). A variety of studies have demonstrated that the prevalence of asymptomatic left ventricular dysfunction in the community setting ranges from 1% to 2.4% (Table 1) (10–11).

ASYMPTOMATIC LEFT VENTRICULAR DYSFUNCTION

The new treatment paradigm emphasizes the pharmacologic management of stage B disease. Impaired left ventricular contractile function leads to early activation of both sympathetic and neurohormonal systems that promote adverse ventricular remodeling (Fig. 6) (12). The process of remodeling alters ventricular geometry as well as myocyte and extracellular matrix composition and contractile function. As compensatory

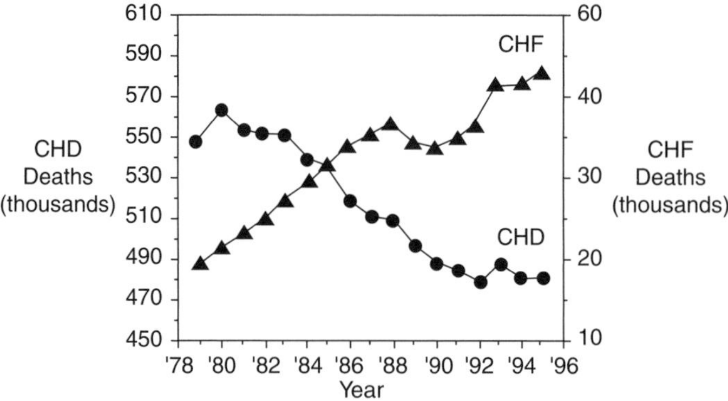

Figure 1 Evolving profile of deaths resulting from coronary heart disease and chronic heart failure in the United States from 1978 to 1996. *Source*: Adapted from Ref. 3.

mechanisms fail, the disease progresses and mortality ensues. Additional data from the Framingham Heart Study cohort demonstrate the lethal nature of asymptomatic LV dysfunction over time (Fig. 7) (10). Overall, 10-yr survival following initial diagnosis was surprisingly poor at 35% for asymptomatic patients whose LV ejection fractions fell between 40% and 50%; survival averaged only 25% when LVEF was below 40%. Hence, future reductions in heart failure mortality and morbidity will rest heavily upon the early identification of impaired cardiac function and the implementation of life-long preventive strategies before symptoms and signs of heart failure develop (12–15).

The clinical significance of asymptomatic diastolic dysfunction is just beginning to be recognized. Using echocardiographic screening techniques that focus upon transmitral Doppler flow patterns, several community-based studies have reported a prevalence of 20% with diastolic dysfunction among the general population.(11,16) As with asymptomatic LV systolic dysfunction, asymptomatic diastolic dysfunction also portends a worse prognosis (Fig. 8) (11). However, given the difficulties of screening large populations of asymptomatic individuals and the load-dependent nature of most

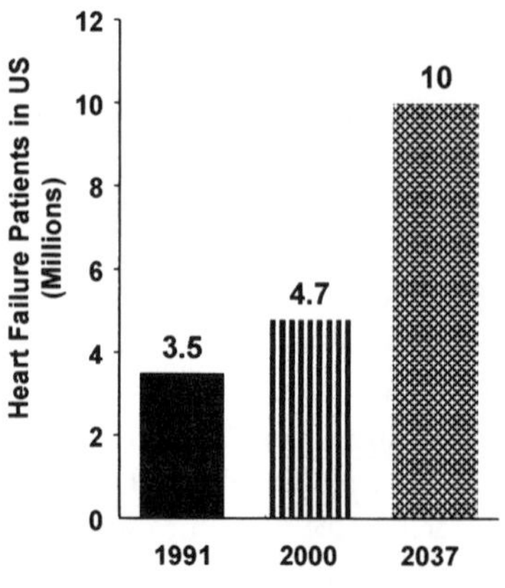

- More deaths from heart failure than from all forms of cancer combined
- 4.7 million symptomatic patients; estimated 10 million in 2037
- Incidence: About 550,000 new cases/year
- Prevalence is 1% between the ages of 50 and 59 years, progressively increasing to >10% over age 80 years

Figure 2 Epidemiology of chronic heart failure in the United States. *Source*: Adapted from Ref. 1.

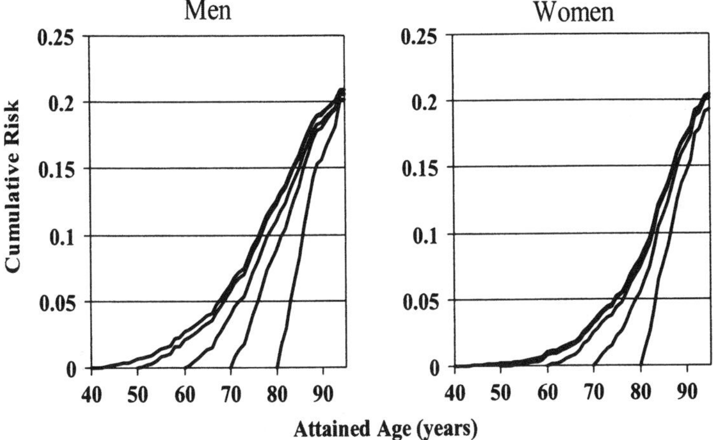

Figure 3 Cumulative risk of heart failure at selected index ages for men and women. Lifetime risk of heart failure for a given index age is cumulative risk through age 94. *Source*: Adapted from Ref. 6.

echocardiographic measures of diastolic dysfunction, it is not yet clinically advisable to consider general population screening for this disorder.

RISK FACTORS FOR HEART FAILURE DEVELOPMENT

Hypertension

Data from the Framingham Heart Study have stressed the very strong association between hypertension and heart failure. Levy et al. recently examined the progression from hypertension to heart failure using data from Framingham subjects between 1970 and 1988 (17). In this study, 91% of subjects who developed overt heart failure had antecedent hypertension. Adjusting for age and other known risk factors, multivariate analysis revealed the hazard ratio for heart failure development was two-fold greater in

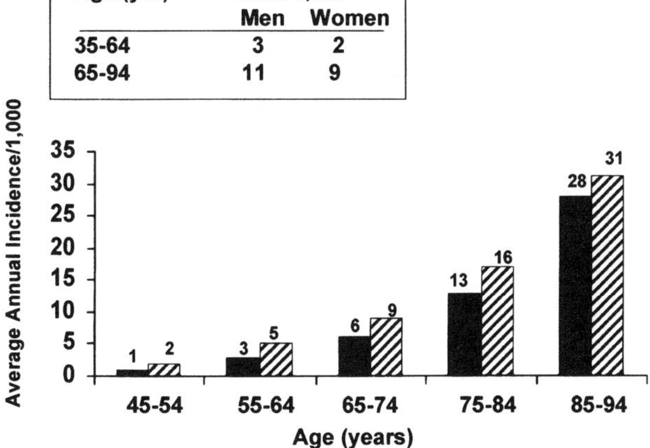

Figure 4 Incidence of heart failure by age and sex: 36-yr follow-up of the Framingham Study. *Source*: Adapted from Ref. 9.

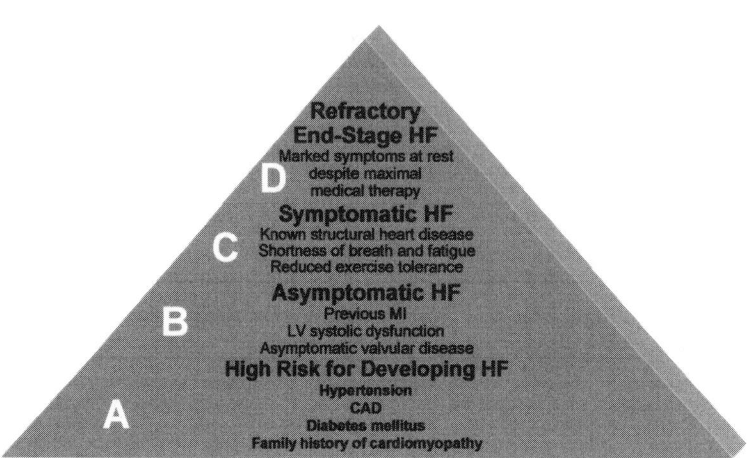

Figure 5 Staging system for heart failure as proposed by American College of Cardiology and American Heart Association guidelines on heart evaluation and management. *Source*: Adapted from Ref. 4.

hypertensive men and three-fold greater in hypertensive women compared with their normotensive (BP < 140/90 mm/Hg and not receiving any hypertensive therapy) counterparts. Simply analyzing hypertension using a static model does not account for progression from a normotensive state to a hypertensive one prior to the development of overt heart failure. When time-dependent dynamic models were utilized, which allowed re-classification of hypertension and other risk factors at periodic examinations prior to the development of heart failure, the hazard ratio for heart failure increased to almost three-fold for men and six-fold for women (17). It is important to note that heart failure risk is largely associated with systolic hypertension; diastolic blood pressure elevation contributes little (18). Ongoing studies are examining the role of pulse pressure as an independent risk factor for heart failure development.

A useful concept is the population-attributable risk (PAR), which indicates the proportion of cases in a population that may be attributed to the presence of a given risk factor (7). The PAR takes into account both the relative risk of disease conferred by the factor itself and the prevalence of that factor. Therefore, risk factors with very high relative risk for disease may have a low PAR value if they are rarely encountered in the population. Conversely, risk factors with only moderately elevated relative risk can have a very high PAR value if they are commonly observed. The latter case holds for hypertension: although the age- and risk factor-adjusted hazard ratio for heart failure with hypertension is 2.07

Table 1 Prevalence of Asymptomatic Left Ventricular Systolic Dysfunction in the Community

Author	Prevalence	Age range
McDonagh et al.	1.0%	25–74 yr
Mosterd et al.	2.2%	>55 yr
Deveaux et al.	2.1%	45–74 yr
Davies et al.	0.9%	>45 yr
Gottdiener et al.	2.4%	>55 yr
Levy et al.	2.2%	mean 69 yr
Redfield et al.	1.1%	>44 yr

Left ventricular ejection fraction < 40%.

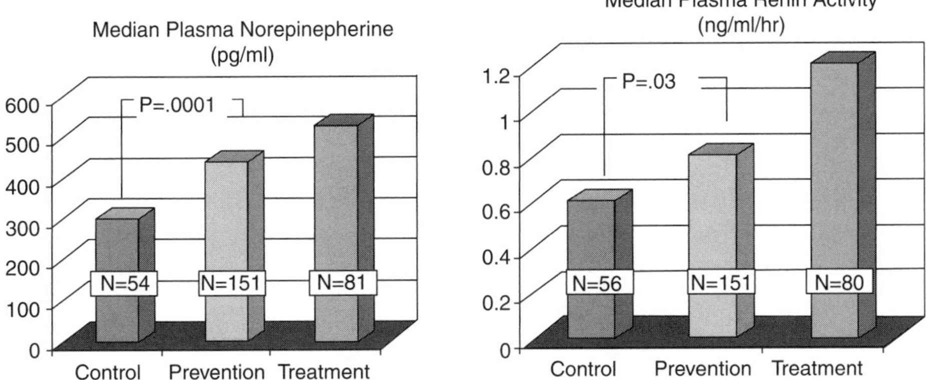

Figure 6 Neurohormonal activation in asymptomatic and symptomatic heart failure. Data are obtained from the Studies of Left Ventricular Dysfunction (SOLVD) Prevention (asymptomatic cohort) and Treatment (symptomatic cohort) trials. *Source*: Adapted from Ref. 64.

(95% CI, 1.34–3.20) for men and 3.35 (95% CI, 1.67–6.73) for women, the PAR value of heart failure associated with hypertension is 39% for men and 59% for women (17). These PAR values are higher than those for any other risk factor for heart failure, which is largely due to the high prevalence of hypertension in the population (Fig. 9).

Coronary Heart Disease

Myocardial infarction confers the highest relative risk of any predisposing factor for the development of symptomatic heart failure, with multivariate-adjusted hazard ratios of 6.34 (95% CI, 4.61–8.72) for men and 6.01 (95% CI, 4.37–8.28) for women (7,17).

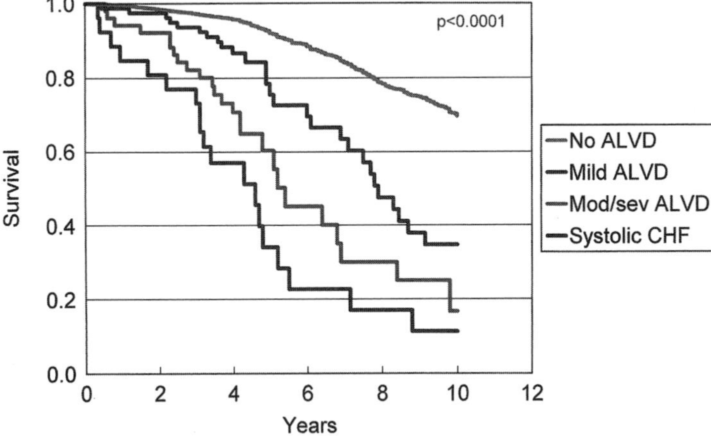

Figure 7 Kaplan–Meier curves for survival. Referent group consists of subjects with normal left ventricular systolic function (LVEF > 50%) and no history of heart failure. Mild ALVD indicates asymptomatic left ventricular dysfunction (EF 40% to 50%). Moderate/severe ALVD consists of asymptomatic subjects with LVEF < 40%. Systolic CHF, overt heart failure with LVEF < 50%. *Source*: Adapted from Ref. 10. *Abbreviations*: ALVD, asymptomatic left ventricular dysfunction; CHF, chronic heart failure; LVEF, left ventricular ejection fraction.

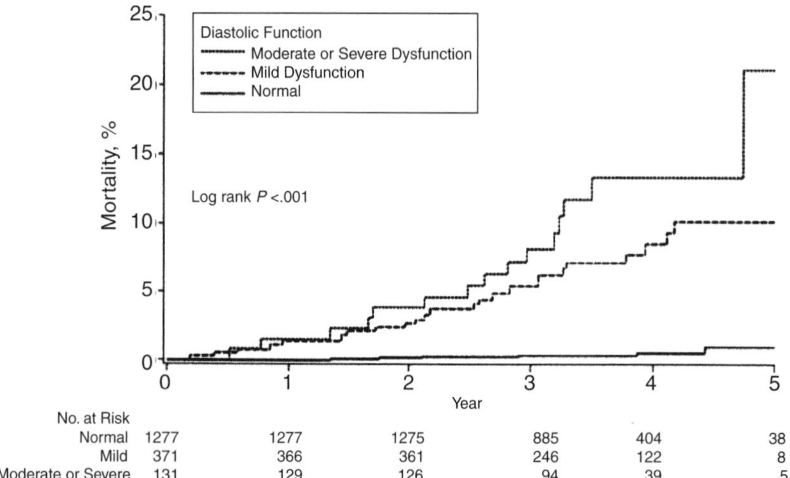

Figure 8 Mortality associated with varying degrees of diastolic dysfunction in the community. Extent of diastolic dysfunction is based upon transmitral Doppler filling patterns. Patients are stratified by normal, mild, or moderate/severe filling pattern. *Source*: Adapted from Ref. 11.

Nonetheless, because of its lower prevalence compared with hypertension in the community, myocardial infarction carries a lower PAR value for heart failure, at 34% in men and 13% in women. When angina pectoris in the absence of myocardial infarction is also included, the PAR values for these combined manifestations of ischemic heart disease increase to 39% and 18% for men and women, respectively (17), still lower than the PAR values for hypertension alone.

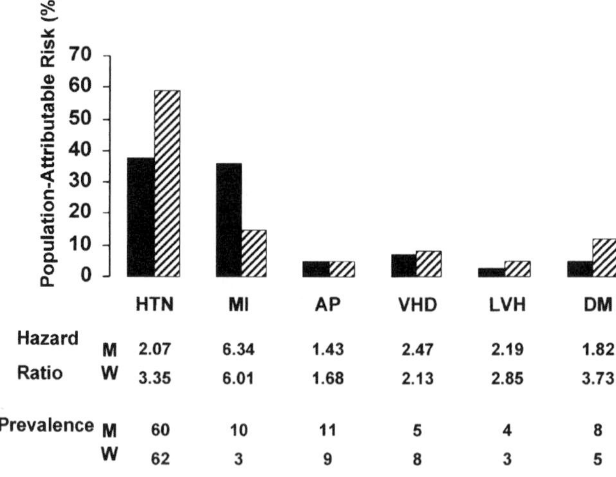

Figure 9 Population-attributable risk (PAR) of heart failure for selected risk factors in men (*black*) and women (*cross-hatched*). The multivariate-adjusted hazard ratios for the development of heart failure over 18 yr of serial follow-up and the prevalence of each risk factor at the baseline examination are also shown. *Abbreviations*: AP, angina pectoris (in the absence of myocardial infarction); DM, diabetes mellitus; HTN, hypertension; LVH, left ventricular hypertrophy; MI, myocardial infarction; VHD, valvular heart disease; M, men; W, women. *Source*: Adapted from Ref. 17.

Table 2 Common Causes of Left Ventricular Systolic Heart Failure

Coronary artery disease
Hypertension
Valvular heart disease
Familial/genetic cardiomyopathy
Myocarditis
Toxins (alcohol, chemotherapy, cocaine)
Collagen vascular disease
Metabolic disorders (hypocalcemia, hypophosphatemia)
Endocrine disorders (diabetes mellitus, hypo- and hyperthryroidsm)
Acidosis
Sepsis
Hypoxia
Peripartum disease

In contrast to these population-based findings, more recent data derived largely from clinical trials suggest that ischemic heart disease is the most common contemporary cause of heart failure (Table 2) (3). Data from the Studies of Left Ventricular Dysfunction (SOLVD) registry determined that 69% of patients had ischemic heart disease as the primary cause of heart failure (18). In this study, a history of hypertension was only observed in 43% of patients. As summarized by Gheorghiade and Bonow, numerous mechanisms account for the important role of coronary artery disease in the promulgation of heart failure (19). Differences in patient populations and follow-up methods between the Framingham Heart Study and the SOLVD registry probably account for these discrepant findings. SOLVD registry patients were typically identified from hospital records which potentially favored ischemic heart disease as a cause. Conversely, serial observations and direct determination of blood pressure in the Framingham cohort may have increased the likelihood of detecting hypertension, especially when compared with a clinical trial population. Finally the association between hypertension and increased risk of coronary heart disease are well known. Thus, hypertension is likely to remain an important precursor of heart failure, either as a sole factor or in conjunction with coronary artery disease (3).

Valvular Heart Disease

Valvular heart disease (particularly aortic stenosis and mitral regurgitation) confer a greater than two-fold adjusted risk for developing heart failure, and a PAR of 7%–8% (17). Mitral valve prolapse does not appear to confer an increased risk of heart failure development (7).

Left Ventricular Hypertrophy and Dilatation

Left ventricular hypertrophy is a common sequelae of longstanding hypertension, valvular heart disease, and inherited forms of hypertrophic cardiomyopathy. Even after controlling for hypertension and other risk factors, electrocardiographic evidence of LVH is associated with a greater than two-fold risk of heart failure, and a PAR value of approximately 5% in men and women (17).

Left ventricular dilatation is also associated with an increased risk of developing symptomatic heart failure. Cardiomegaly on chest film has been shown by multivariate risk modeling to increase the risk of heart failure by two-fold in men and women (20).

Vasan et al. confirmed this observation using echocardiographic measurements (21). Over an eleven year follow-up period, the risk-adjusted hazard ratio for heart failure was 1.47 (95% CI, 1.25–1.73) for each increment of one standard deviation in the left ventricular end-diastolic dimension indexed for height (21). A nearly identical hazard ratio was observed for end-systolic dimension. Even without evidence of a prior myocardial infarction, asymptomatic ventricular dilatation remained a significant predictor of heart failure risk.

Diabetes Mellitus

Diabetes mellitus has consistently been associated with increased risk of heart failure development in Framingham subjects (7). Diabetes has been associated with a population-attributable risk for heart failure of 6% in men and 12% in women (17). It may lead to heart failure because it is also a risk factor for premature coronary heart disease and because of its strong association with hypertension, obesity, and the metabolic syndrome. However, there may be an independent role for diabetes in the pathogenesis of heart failure as well.

Age

Age is consistently among the strongest risk factors for heart failure, leading to the clear-cut observation that this is a syndrome of the elderly. Ho et al. demonstrated a dramatic increase in the incidence and prevalence of heart failure with age (5). The annual incidence increased from 3/1000 in men aged 50–59 yr to 27/1,000 in men aged 80–89 yr. In women, the annual incidence increased from 2/1000 to 22/1000 across the same age groups (5). Overall, the risk of heart failure appears to increase by approximately 37% per decade of age in men and 24% per decade of age in women (20). Unfortunately, age remains an unmodifiable risk factor.

The burden of heart failure and its public health implications are greatest in the elderly population. Its prevalence exceeds 10% for subjects over 80 yr of age (1). Among patients hospitalized with decompensated heart failure, 80% are >65 yr of age (4). Further, in the Acute Decompensated Heart Failure Registry (ADHERE), the median age of 27,000 patients admitted to 250 U.S. hospitals for heart failure was 75 yr (22). In-hospital mortality for all participants was 4% but was substantially higher in the cohort over 75 yr of age (22). The mortality rate attributable to heart failure hospitalization is highest in the elderly and approximates that of acute myocardial infarction (22). Potential explanations for the high prevalence of heart failure in the elderly include a high prevalence of hypertension, ventricular remodeling following prior myocardial infarction, loss of functional myocytes (which averages 5%/yr in patients beyond the age of 65 yr), and increased extracellular matrix that contributes to alterations in left ventricular compliance. Several of these features combine to create a ventricular phenotype of "heart failure with preserved systolic function" (16). Thus, 40%–50% of heart failure admissions in the elderly occur in the setting of preserved systolic function but carry the same in-hospital risk of mortality (22).

MULTIVARIATE RISK PREDICTION OF HEART FAILURE

Kannel et al. recently devised a multivariate risk equation for estimating the four-year risk of developing overt heart failure (20). Regression coefficients were calculated using routinely available office-based diagnostic testing and a point score assigned for each risk factor.

In the simplest model for men, age (0–9 points), systolic blood pressure (0–5 points), resting heart rate (0–5 points), electrocardiographic evidence of LVH (4 points), coronary heart disease (8 points), valvular heart disease (5 points), and diabetes mellitus (1 point) were variables used to predict the four-year risk of heart failure. Similar variables plus body mass index (0–3 points) were included for women. Figure 10 illustrates the risk of heart failure based on the cumulative number of points. Using this model, 60% of heart failure episodes in men and 73% in women occurred in subjects in the top quintile of risk scores (20). This predictive rule may be of use for clinicians to identify those patients with predisposing factors for heart failure who are at intermediate risk (stage A or B disease) and who may benefit from preventive measures.

SPECIAL POPULATIONS

Major epidemiologic studies show that the overall prevalence rate of heart failure is similar in men and women (Fig. 2). This balance reflects a much lower prevalence in women below the age of 75 yr and a higher prevalence in older women than older men (1,17,23,24). Although age-adjusted rates for both sexes have decreased from 1988–1995, rates for women have fallen less than those for men (25).

Risk factors for heart failure appear markedly different between the sexes. As described above, the population-attributable risk of hypertension is greater in women (59%) then men (39%) (17). The higher prevalence of hypertension in women exists for both blacks and whites. The SOLVD trials reported coronary heart disease and, in particular, prior myocardial infarction to be less frequently identified as etiologic agents for heart failure in women (26). Further, although white women admitted with heart failure have less coronary artery disease than their white male counterparts, black women appear to have more coronary disease than black men (27). While the incidence of myocardial infarction is lower in women than men, those women who do sustain an MI are more likely to develop heart failure symptoms (28,29).

Diabetes mellitus is also a stronger risk factor in women than men, especially in younger women. Several studies, including the SOLVD trial (30,31), have reported that women with symptomatic heart failure are more likely to be diabetic than men (49.3% women versus 37.2% men, $p<0.02$) (31). Although both diabetic young women and men

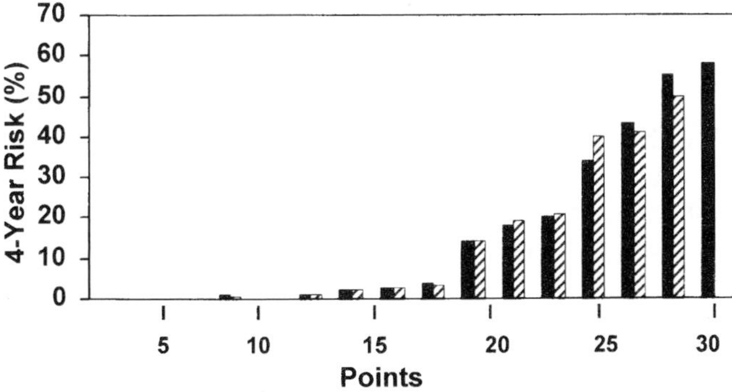

Figure 10 Probability of developing heart failure within 4 yr for men (*black columns*) and women (*cross-hatched columns*) according to a point score assigned by clinical predictor rule of Kannel et al. *Source*: Adapted from Ref. 7.

in the Framingham cohort had a greater incidence of heart failure than age-matched controls, the effect was substantially greater in women (an 8-fold versus a 4-fold increase).

While obesity is an independent risk factor for heart failure in both sexes, it carries greater predictive risk in women (32). Women have a markedly lower prevalence of idiopathic dilated cardiomyopathy (IDCM) in most studies (male: female ratio, 1.9–4.3:1), perhaps because men have a greater prevalence of alcohol use and/or asymptomatic coronary artery disease (25,33). Women who do develop IDCM, however, have a greater degree of ventricular enlargement and shorter exercise duration (34).

Ethnic Minorities

Heart failure incidence in the African American population is 50% higher than other racial groups (3% versus 2%) (35). The SOLVD Prevention trial confirmed that African Americans develop heart failure at a statistically higher rate than other races (36). Symptoms at presentation are generally associated with a more advanced stage of left ventricular dysfunction. Hypertension as a lone etiology for left ventricular dysfunction is far more likely to occur in this population than in non–African American populations (34). Conversely, the proportion of nonischemic disease is much higher in African Americans with heart failure. Both morbidity and mortality outcomes appear higher in the black population (37,38).

As socioeconomic factors appear insufficient to account for observed differences in outcome and clinical presentation, pathophysiologic differences may exist between races. Hypertension is known to be a more malignant vascular process in African Americans and associated with a markedly increased risk of left ventricular hypertrophy, a ten-fold increase of end-stage renal disease, and a higher incidence of stroke (39). In addition, single nucleotide polymorphisms (SNPs) that affect protein expression may contribute to an accelerated disease process. Transforming growth factor (TGF)-β_1, a cytokine stimulated by angiotensin II production, promotes collagen turnover, stimulates endothelin mRNA production, and is associated with ventricular hypertrophy. TGF-β_1 levels have been shown to be markedly elevated in hypertensive African Americans and associated with a polymorphism at codon 10 in this population (40). Recently, a unique combination of polymorphisms of the β_1-adrenergic receptor plus the α- receptor has been shown to be associated with a striking incidence of heart failure only among African Americans with this genotype (41). Differences in outcome and response to pharmacologic therapy may partially reflect these unique genotypic features.

ESTABLISHING THE DIAGNOSIS OF HEART FAILURE

Epidemiologic studies have been based on the identification of patients with clinical signs and symptoms of heart failure but generally do not distinguish between systolic and diastolic dysfunction. It should be remembered that heart failure is a syndrome comprised of symptoms and signs, confirmed by diagnostic modalities such as echocardiography, assessment of diastolic function, and exercise testing. In most observational studies, the symptoms most sensitive for diagnosing heart failure include exertional dyspnea, orthopnea, and paroxysmal nocturnal dyspnea (42,43). Orthopnea and paroxysmal nocturnal dyspnea remain the most specific symptoms. Table 3 summarizes the sensitivity and specificity of common symptoms and signs of heart failure. As is readily evident, the sensitivity of common symptoms ranges from 23% to 66% and the specificity from 52% to 81% (42). Heart failure signs are also inherently nonspecific (44). Rales are

Table 3 Sensitivity, Specificity, and Predictive Value of Symptoms and Physical Signs for Diagnosing Chronic Heart Failure

Symptom/sign	Sensitivity (%)	Specificity (%)	Predictive accuracy (%)
Exertional dyspnea	66	52	23
Orthopnea	21	81	2
Paroxysmal nocturnal dyspnea	33	76	26
History of edema	23	80	22
Heart rate > 100/min	7	99	6
Rales	13	91	21
Third heart sound	31	95	61
Jugular venous distension	10	97	2
Edema (on exam)	10	93	3

Source: Adapted from Ref. 42.

absent in up to 80% of patients with chronic heart failure due to enhanced pulmonary lymphatic drainage. Likewise, peripheral edema is evident in only 25% of patients under 70 yr of age with chronic heart failure (44). Evidence of right-sided heart failure is absent in up to 50% of patients at the time of diagnosis. In advanced heart failure, positive hepatojugular reflux and Valsalva square wave signs may provide ancillary evidence of elevated filling pressures (44). In a retrospective multivariate analysis of over 2500 participants in the SOLVD Treatment trial, the presence of an elevated jugular venous pressure and a third heart sound were both independently associated with an increased risk of hospitalization for heart failure, death or hospitalization for heart failure, and death due to progressive left ventricular dysfunction (45). However, only fair interobserver agreement between clinicians exists for assessment of jugular venous pressure (kappa statistic 0.3–0.65) (46–48). Accurate differentiation of heart failure due to systolic versus diastolic dysfunction is not possible based on physical findings, electrocardiographic findings, or chest film (49,50). Given the differences in prognosis and treatment, echocardiographic evaluation of all patients with suspected heart failure to differentiate underlying pathophysiology should be considered.

PROGNOSTIC FEATURES

Heart failure deaths are typically either sudden or due to progressive hemodynamic deterioration (i.e., pump failure). In mild heart failure, the proportion of deaths that occur suddenly is higher than in advanced heart failure but the absolute risk of death is only 5% per year (51). As heart failure severity increases, the absolute risk of sudden death increases but it accounts for a lower percentage of overall deaths as pump failure mortality increases dramatically. Approximately one-third of all heart failure patients will die suddenly. During the past 20 yr, over 50 variables have been examined in univariate and multivariate models and shown to predict mortality in heart failure populations (Table 4). Unfortunately, no single study has assessed all, or even most, of these predictors simultaneously in a multivariate fashion. Thus, it is impossible to rank prognostic factors strictly on their order of importance. Nonetheless, several factors appear repeatedly in the published literature. In his recent comprehensive review, Eichhorn identified norepinephrine levels, B-type natriuretic peptide levels, left ventricular ejection fraction (LVEF), peak oxygen uptake on cardiopulmonary exercise testing, advanced age, and a

Table 4 Predictors of Prognosis in Chronic Heart Failure

Demographics	Advanced age, sex, etiology
Symptoms	NYHA class IV, syncope
Signs	Chronic S3, right heart failure
Laboratory	Na^+, creatinine, anemia, CTR, LVEDD
ECG	QRS or QTc prolongation, NSVT, VT
Hemodynamic	LVEF, PCW, CI
Exercise	6-min walk distance, peak VO_2
Neurohormonal	PNE, ANP, BNP

Abbreviations: CTR, cardiothoracic ratio on chest film; LVEDD, left ventricular end-diastolic dimension on echocardiogram; NSVT, non-sustained ventricular tachycardia; VT, ventricular tachycardia; LVEF, left ventricular ejection fraction; PCW, pulmonary capillary wedge pressure; CI, cardiac index; VO_2, oxygen consumption on cardiopulmonary exercise testing; PNE, plasma norepinepherine; ANP, atrial natriuretic peptide; BNP, B-type natriuretic peptide.

history of symptomatic ventricular arrhythmias or sudden death as the most important predictors of outcome in chronic heart failure (52).

New York heart functional classification is easy to assess and remains a useful predictor of overall mortality. One-year mortality rates stratified by NYHA class are: Class I: 4%–5%; Class II: 5%–15%; Class III: 15%–30%; and Class IV: 30%–70%, depending upon response to therapy and degree of compensation (53).

Demographic features are also predictive. Advanced age remains a strong predictor of outcome in the Framingham study (54). In this cohort, mortality increased with advancing age in both sexes (hazard ratio for men: 1.27/decade of age; hazard ratio for women: 1.61/decade of age). Gender is also predictive of long-term outcome; women typically have lower mortality rates than men (54). As mentioned earlier, African Americans also appear to have less favorable outcomes than other racial groups.

Findings on physical examination also may predict prognosis. The presence of a chronic 3rd heart sound and elevation in jugular venous pressure have been shown to predict long-term mortality (45). Moderate-to-severe mitral or tricuspid regurgitation are both associated with increased morbidity and mortality (55–57).

One of the most consistent predictors of outcome is LVEF (52). In patients with moderate heart failure symptoms and a wide range of systolic dysfunction, LVEF has extraordinarily predictive power (58). LVEF is particularly useful at values below 35% (58). In fact, its clinical utility may be greatest in patients with few or no symptoms of heart failure (stage B disease) (Fig. 7) (10). LVEF appears to lose much of its predictive accuracy in patients with advanced symptoms (59) or among patients whose LVEF exceeds 45% (60). Thus, in a heterogeneous population of patients whose LVEF ranges from 10%–45%, it has high discriminatory power. However, among a homogenous population of patients with advanced heart failure, whose LVEF variation is small (i.e., 15%–25%), it has little independent predictive power (52).

Right ventricular function reflects right ventricular involvement in any ongoing myocardial process as well as inter-ventricular interaction and the effect of pulmonary hypertension. Thus, right ventricular ejection fraction (RVEF) has been shown, both at rest and with exercise, to be a useful predictor of outcome (61). Difficulties in its measurement have limited its routine usefulness. Left ventricular volumes reflect the extent of the remodeling process. Thus, left ventricular end-diastolic dimension and end-systolic dimension by echocardiography have prognostic significance (62).

A growing list of biomarkers have been shown to be elevated in asymptomatic and symptomatic heart failure. Plasma norepinephrine levels have been shown in a variety of trials to be a powerful predictor of outcome, independent of ejection fraction, mean arterial pressure, heart rate, serum sodium, and measured hemodynamics (63,64). In the Veterans Administration Heart Failure trials (V-HeFT I and II), one year mortality was approximately 7% for patients whose levels fell below 600 pg/mL, 15% for levels between 600–900 pg/mL, and over 25% for levels >900 pg/mL (63,64). Markers of activation of the renin-angiotensin system such as plasma renin activity, angiotensin II, aldosterone, and serum sodium have also been shown to predict prognosis but not as strongly as plasma norepinephrine. The natriuretic peptides are released by the atrium (ANP) and ventricular myocardium (BNP), respectively, in response to myocardial injury or increased wall stretch (65). In one small trial that directly compared the prognostic value of the two natriuretic peptides, BNP appeared to be a stronger predictor of overall outcome than ANP or norepinephrine (65). A growing number of observational studies and clinical trials are underway designed to assess the predictive value of alterations of B-type natriuretic peptide in response to therapy on all-cause mortality. The cytokines, tumor necrosis factor alpha (TNF-α) and interleukin-6, are elevated in heart failure and may play a role in its pathophysiology (52). To date, these cytokines have not been shown to have a strong correlation with clinical outcome. Endothelin-1 is a potent vasoconstrictor and is elevated in direct proportion to heart failure severity (66). One multivariate analysis has demonstrated endothelin-1 to be a more powerful predictor of outcome than plasma norepinephrine, NYHA functional class, age, or peak oxygen uptake (66). However, these findings need to be replicated in larger populations. It should be noted that the vast majority of studies that look at the prognostic significance of neurohormones loose their predictive ability in the presence of ACE inhibitor therapy (52). Because the majority of patients with moderate to advanced heart failure (>90%) are currently taking an ACE inhibitor, the utility of measuring neurohormones (with the exception of BNP) in patients who are receiving neurohormonal antagonists remains questionable.

Impaired exercise capacity is one of the principal hallmarks of chronic heart failure. A variety of mechanisms account for this impairment including exertional increases in pulmonary capillary wedge pressure, reduced skeletal muscle perfusion and/or conditioning, altered skeletal muscle metabolic function, and ventilatory muscle fatigue (67). Metabolic exercise testing as reflected by peak oxygen uptake (MVO_{2max}) has been shown in multiple studies to strongly predict outcome in patients with moderate and advanced heart faliure (52,58,68–70). Peak oxygen uptake is generally recognized as the strongest multivariate predictor of outcome when pulmonary capillary wedge pressure, LVEF, and cardiac index are included in modeling (68). Cohn et al. have reported that the combination of peak VO_2 and LVEF can provide additional prognostic information (58). Other less predictive exercise parameters include exercise duration, anaerobic threshold, and the ratio of ventilation to CO_2 production (VE/VCO_2) (70,71). Submaximal exercise protocols, particularly the 6 min walk test, have also been found to have predictive value but are generally less accurate than studies performed with gas exchange (71).

Ventricular arrhythmias are extremely common in heart failure patients and have been reported in up to 90% of patients (52,58). Patients with symptomatic ventricular arrhythmias (i.e., episodes of pre-syncope, syncope, or sudden death) are at increased risk for sudden death and all-cause mortality (52,58). The frequency of asymptomatic nonsustained runs of ventricular tachycardia increases as the disease severity worsens. Ventricular tachycardia was observed in over 50% of patients with NYHA Class II and III heart failure enrolled in the V-HeFT trial (58). The presence of ventricular couplets or nonsustained ventricular tachycardia has been reported to predict increased all-cause mortality in a number of studies (52). Its significance in predicting sudden death risk remains debated with some trials suggesting a moderate predictive value and others not finding such a correlation (58,72,73). Suppression of ventricular arrhythmias on Holter monitoring does not lower the risk of sudden death. It has been suggested that asymptomatic ventricular ectopy serves as a useful marker for disease severity rather than a specific marker for sudden cardiac death risk (73,74). The presence of atrial fibrillation/flutter has been reported to be associated with both an increased risk in all-cause mortality and sudden cardiac death risk (75–79). However, not all studies have found the presence of atrial arrhythmias to be an independent predictor of outcome when other prognostic variables are considered (51,76). Whether or not atrial fibrillation worsens survival, its occurrence often will exacerbate symptoms and, if poorly controlled, may further worsen ventricular systolic dysfunction.

Renal dysfunction has recently been recognized as an important predictor of heart failure outcome. It is well known that renal disease, either chronic renal insufficiency or end-stage renal failure, are strongly associated with both heart disease and heart failure (80). Deterioration in renal function in patients with chronic heart failure may result from diminished cardiac output and a corresponding reduction in glomerular filtration rate, alterations in the distribution of cardiac output, intra-renal vasoregulation, alterations in circulatory volume, intense neurohormonal activation, and the nephrotoxic effects of medications (80). Even mild degrees of renal insufficiency have been shown to be associated with increased mortality in both asymptomatic and symptomatic ambulatory heart failure patients (Fig. 11) (81–85). The presence of chronic renal insufficiency, defined as a serum creatinine >1.4 mg/dL for women and 1.5 mg/dL for men, has been shown to be associated with an increased relative risk (RR = 1.43) of death (84). Approximately 25% of hospitalized patients with decompensated heart failure will exhibit a deterioration in renal function despite appropriate medical therapy (86). In these hospitalized patients, a rise in serum creatinine of only 0.1–0.5 mg/dL is associated with a longer length of hospital stay and increased in-hospital mortality (87). This constellation of poorly understood physiologic mechanisms and unpredictable clinical responses to appropriate pharmacologic therapies has been termed the "cardiorenal syndrome"; its optimal management remains to be defined.

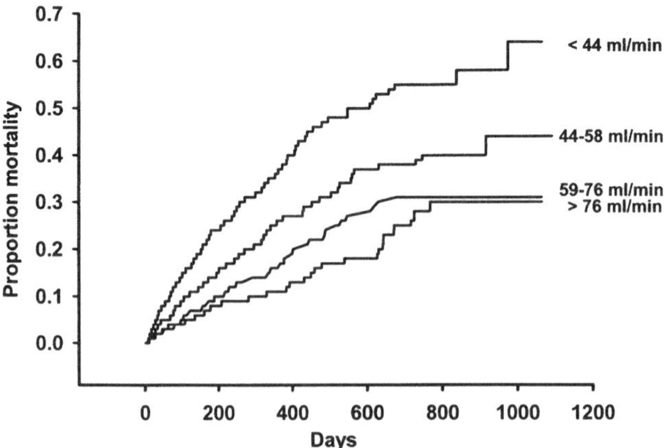

Figure 11 Influence of renal function on survival in chronic heart failure. Kaplan–Meier survival mortality curves for patients stratified by quartile of glomerular filtration rate corrected for age and body weight (GFRc). *Source*: Adapted from Ref. 80.

Anemia has also recently been identified as an independent predictor of adverse outcome in chronic heart failure. The Canadian Cohort Study of Chronic Renal Disease has demonstrated that for every 0.5 gm/dL hemoglobin decrease, the odds ratio for left ventricular hypertrophy increased by 32% (88). Each 1.0 gm/dL decline in hemoglobin was associated with an odds ratio for left ventricular dilatation of 1.46 (89). Anemia is common in heart failure and its prevalence is closely related to heart failure severity (88,90). It has been demonstrated to be linked to greater impairment in functional capacity, symptoms, and increased mortality in both moderate and severe heart failure (90–93). Its recognition as an important contributor to morbidity and mortality suggests that it may be an appropriate therapeutic target for chronic heart failure management.

PROGNOSIS IN CHRONIC HEART FAILURE

Older studies from the Framingham Heart Study have reported 5-yr mortality rates that exceed 50% for patients with symptomatic heart failure; importantly, no difference in survival was noted among patients diagnosed in the era of 1948–1974 compared to patients diagnosed between 1975–1988 (54). After adjustment for age, survival following initial diagnosis of heart failure remained better in women than men, with a hazard ratio of 0.64 (95% CI, 0.54–0.77). In men, heart failure secondary to known valvular heart disease conferred a particularly poor prognosis (hazard ratio: 1.68, 95% CI, 1.15–2.46) compared to heart failure secondary to coronary artery disease. In women, there were no significant differences in prognosis based on disease etiology. However, women with diabetes (hazard ratio: 1.7, 95% CI, 1.21–2.38) or prior evidence of LVH (hazard ratio: 1.63, 95% CI, 1.08–2.45) were at substantially increased risk of all-cause mortality (54). Fortunately, more recent data from the same group has noted reductions in 30-day, one year, and 5-yr age adjusted mortality rates in heterogeneous cohorts of both men (from 12%, 30%, and 70% to 11%, 28%, and 59%, respectively) and women (from 18%, 28%, and 57% to 10%, 24%, and 45%, respectively) comparing the periods of 1950–1969 to 1990–1999 (Fig. 12) (94).

The Resource utilization Among Congestive Heart failure study (REACH) provided a 10-yr epidemiologic survey of heart failure among 29,686 patients using ICD-9 codes to probe incidence, prevalence, and mortality (95). While the incidence of heart failure in the

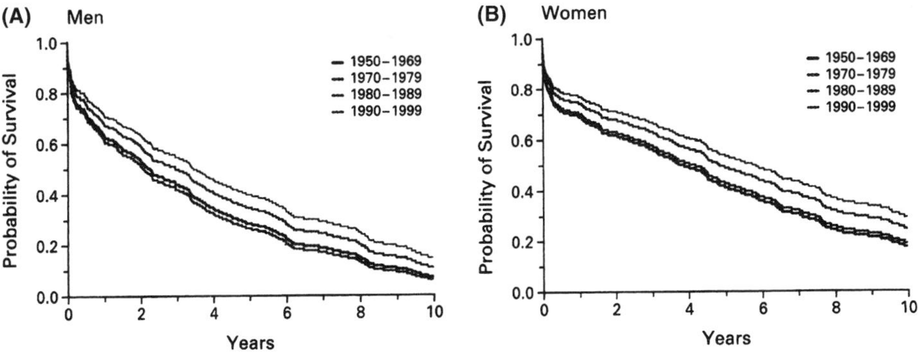

Figure 12 Temporal trends in age-adjusted survival after the onset of heart failure among men (**A**) and women (**B**). Values are adjusted for age (<55, 55 to 64, 65 to 74, 75 to 84, and ≥ 85 yr). Estimates are shown for subjects who were 65 to 74 yr of age. *Source*: Adapted from Ref. 2.

Framingham cohort was 4.7 cases/1000 for women and 7.2/1000 for men, the REACH study reported an incidence of 5.3/1000 for men and 5.5/1000 for women. The median survival in the REACH population was 4.5 yr for women compared to 3.7 yr for men (95).

Observational studies from several academic medical centers have also reported improved survival in patients with IDCM (96) and advanced heart failure (97). An important large observational study from Scotland noted improved survival in patients hospitalized between 1986 and 1995 (98). Case fatality rates declined in men and women by 26% and 17%, respectively, at 30 days and by 18% and 15%, respectively, at 12 mo (98). It is interesting that no temporal change in overall survival was noted in the initial Framingham cohort study from 1948 to 1988 (5,54). However, angiotensin-converting enzyme inhibitors and beta-blockers were not widely prescribed during the 1980s. Thus, the favorable effects on survival noted in more recent studies may largely derive from widespread use of neurohormonal antagonists. Finally, an observational study of community-dwelling elderly patients (mean age 74 yr) found a close relationship between symptoms, extent of systolic dysfunction, and heart failure mortality (99). The adjusted mortality hazard ratios were 1.48 (95% CI, 1.2–1.8) for patients with heart failure and normal left ventricular function, 2.4 (95% CI, 1.2–4.6) for patients with heart failure and borderline left ventricular systolic dysfunction, and 1.88 (1.0–3.4) for patients with overt heart failure and impaired systolic function (99). Importantly, more deaths occurred among patients with normal systolic function in this study because left ventricular function was more often normal than impaired in the elderly population (99). In a population-based observational study of over 38,000 consecutive unselected patients hospitalized for heart failure decompensation between 1994 and 1997, the crude 30-day and one-year case fatality rates after first admission for heart failure were 11.6% and 33.1%, respectively (100). These survival figures confirm the highly lethal nature of symptomatic heart failure from its time of onset. This diagnosis carries a greater 5-yr risk of death than that associated with acute myocardial infarction, breast cancer, or colon cancer. Aggressive strategies to detect left ventricular dysfunction before overt heart failure ensues and to target appropriate pharmacologic interventions should continue to improve its natural history in the decade ahead.

REFERENCES

1. American Heart Association. 2002 Heart and Stroke Statistical Update. Dallas, TX: American Heart Association, 2001.
2. Levy D, Kenchaiah S, Larson MG, et al. Long-term trends with the incidence and survival with heart failure. NEJM 2002; 347:1397–1402.
3. Adams KF. New epidemiologic perspectives concerning mild-to-moderate heart failure. Am J Med 2001; 110:6S–13S.
4. Hunt SA, Baker DW, Chin MH, et al. ACC/AHA guidelines for the evaluation and management of chronic heart failure in the adult: executive summary: a report of the American College of Cardiology/American Heart Association Task Force on practice guidelines (committee to revise the 1995 guidelines for the evaluation and management of heart failure). Circulation 2001; 104:2996–3007.
5. Ho KKL, Pinsky JL, Kannel WB, Levy D. The epidemiology of heart failure: the Framingham study. J Am Coll Cardiol 1993; 22:6A–13A.
6. Lloyd-Jones DM, Larson MG, Leip EP, et al. Life-time risk for developing heart failure. The Framingham heart study. Circulation 2002; 106:3068–3072.

7. Lloyd-Jones DM. The risk of congestive heart failure: sobering lessons from the Framingham heart study. Curr Cardiol Reports 2001; 3:184–190.
8. Rich MW. Epidemiology, pathophysiology, and etiology of congestive heart failure in older adults. J Am Geriat Soc 1997; 45:968–974.
9. Kannel WB, Ho KKL, Thom T. Changing epidemiologic features of cardiac failure. Br Heart J 1994; 72:3–9.
10. Wang TJ, Evans JC, Benjamin EJ, Levy D, LeRoy EC, Vasan RS. Natural history of asymptomatic left ventricular systolic dysfunction in the community. Circulation 2003; 108:977–982.
11. Redfield MM, Jacobsen SJ, Burnett JC, Mahoney DW, Bailey KR, Rodeheffer RJ. Burden of systolic and diastolic ventricular dysfunction in the community: appreciating the scope of the heart failure epidemic. JAMA 2003; 289:194–202.
12. Francis GH, McDonald KM, Cohn JN. Neurohumoral activation in preclinical heart failure: remodeling and the potential for intervention. Circulation 1993; 71:3C–11C.
13. SOLVD Investigators. The effect of enalapril on mortality and the development of heart failure in asymptomatic patients with reduced left ventricular ejection fractions. NEJM 1992; 327:685–691.
14. McDonagh TA, Morrison CE, Lawrence A, et al. Symptomatic and asymptomatic left-ventricular systolic dysfunction in an urban population. Lancet 1997; 350:829–833.
15. Davies M, Hobbs F, Davis R, et al. Prevalence of left-ventricular systolic dysfunction and heart failure in the echocardiographic heart of England screening study: a population based study. Lancet 2001; 358:439–444.
16. Vasan RS, Larson MG, Benjamin EJ, Evans JC, Reiss CK, Levy D. Congestive heart failure in subjects with normal versus reduced left ventricular ejection fraction: prevalence and mortality in a population-based cohort. J Am Coll Cardiol 1999; 33:1948–1955.
17. Levy D, Larson MG, Vasan RS, Kannel WB, Ho KKL. Progression from hypertension to congestive heart failure. JAMA 1996; 275:1557–1562.
18. Bourassa MG, Gurne O, Bangidiwala SI, for the Studies of Left Ventricular Dysfunction (SOLVD) Investigators. Natural history and patterns of current practice in heart failure. J Am Coll Cardiol 1993; 22:14A–19A.
19. Gheorghiade M, Bonow RO. Chronic heart failure in the United States: a manifestation of coronary artery disease. Circulation 1998; 97:282–289.
20. Kannel WB, D'Agostino RB, Silbershatz H, Belanger AJ, Wilson PWF, Levy D. Profile for estimating the risk of heart failure. Arch Int Med 1999; 159:1197–1204.
21. Vasan RS, Larson MG, Benjamin E, Evans JC, Levy D. Left ventricular dilation and the risk of congestive heart failure in people without myocardial infarction. NEJM 1997; 336:1350–1355.
22. Fonarow GC, for the ADHERE scientific advisory committee. The acute decompensated heart failure national registry (ADHERE): opportunities to improve care of patients hospitalized with acute decompensated heart failure. Reviews in Cardiovasc Med 2003; 4:S21–S30.
23. Massie BM, Shah NB. Evolving trends in the epidemiological factors of heart failure: rationale for preventive strategies and comprehensive disease management. Am Heart J 1997; 133:703–712.
24. Petrie MC, Dawson NF, Murdoch DR, Davie AP, McMurray JJV. Failure of women's hearts. Circulation 1999; 99:2334–2341.
25. Philbin EF, DiSalvo TG. Influence of race and gender on care process, resource use, and outcomes in congestive heart failure. Haldeman GA 1998; 82:76–81.
26. Johnstone D, Limacher M, Bousseau M, et al. Clinical characteristics of patients in studies of left ventricular dysfunction. Am J Cardiol 1992; 70:894–900.
27. Haldeman GA, Rashidee A, Horswell R. Changes in mortality from heart failure—United States. JAMA 1998; 280:874–875.

28. Tofler GH, Stone PH, Mueller JE, et al. Effects of gender and race on prognosis after myocardial infarction: adverse prognosis from women, particularly black women. J Am Coll Cardiol 1987; 9:473–482.
29. Kimmelsiel CD, Goldberg RJ. Congestive heart failure in women: focus on heart failure due to coronary artery disease and diabetes. Cardiology 1990; 77:71–79.
30. Croft JB, Giles WH, Polcard RA, Casper ML, Anda RF, Livengood JR. National trends in the initial hospitalization for heart failure. Am J Public Health 1997; 87:643–648.
31. Shindler DM, Kostis JB, Yusuf S. Diabetes mellitus: a predictor of morbidity and mortality in the studies of left ventricular dysfunction (SOLVD) trials and registry. Am J Cardiol 1996; 77:1017–1020.
32. Kannel WB, Belanger AJ. Epidemiology of heart failure. Am Heart J 1991; 121:951–957.
33. Codd MB, Sugrue DD, Gersh BJ, Melton J. Epidemiology of idiopathic and hypertrophic cardiomyopathy. Circulation 1989; 80:564–572.
34. DeMaria R, Gavazzi A, Recalcati F, Baroldi G, DeVita G, Camerini F. For the Italian multicentre cardiomyopathy study (SPIC): comparison of the clinical findings in idiopathic dilated cardiomyopathy in women versus men. Am J Cardiol 1993; 72:580–585.
35. Yancy CW. Heart failure in African Americans: a cardiovascular enigma. J Card Failure 2000; 6:183–186.
36. Dries DL, Strong MH, Cooper RS, Drazner M. Efficacy of angiotensin-converting enzyme inhibition in reducing progression form asymptomatic left ventricular dysfunction to symptomatic heart failure in black and white patients. J Am Coll Cardiol 2002; 40:311–317.
37. Dries DL, Exner DV, Gersh BJ, Cooper HA, Carson RE, Domanski MJ. Racial differences in the outcome of left ventricular dysfunction. NEJM 1999; 340:609–616.
38. Saunders E. Hypertension in minorities: blacks. Am J Hyperten 1995; 8:115S–119S.
39. Yancy CW. Heart failure in blacks: etiology and epidemiological differences. Curr Cardiol Rep 2001; 3:191–197.
40. Suthanthiran M, Li B, Song JO, et al. Transforming growth factor-beta1 hyperexpression in African–American hypertensives: a novel mediator of hypertension and/or target organ damage.. Proc Natl Acad Sci USA 2000; 97:3479–3484.
41. Small KM, Wagoner LE, Levin AM, Kardia SLR, Liggett SB. Synergistic polymorphisms of beta-1 and alpha 2C adrenergic receptors and the risk of congestive heart failure. NEJM 2002; 347:1135–1142.
42. Harlan WR, Oberman A, Grimm R, Rosati RA. Chronic congestive heart failure in coronary artery disease: clinical criteria. Ann Intern Med 1997; 86:133–138.
43. Marantz PR, Tobin JN, Wassertheil-Smoller S, et al. The relationship between left ventricular systolic function and congestive heart failure diagnosed by clinical criteria. Circulation 1988; 77:607–612.
44. Stevenson LW, Perloff JK. Limited reliability of physical signs for estimating hemodynamics in chronic heart failure. JAMA 1989; 261:884–888.
45. Drazen MH, Rame JE, Stevenson LW, Dries DL. Prognostic importance of elevated jugular venous pressure and a third heart sound in patients with heart failure. NEJM 2001; 345:574–581.
46. McGee SR. Physical examination of venous pressure: a critical review. Am Heart J 1998; 136:10–18.
47. Ishmail AA, Wing S, Ferguson J, Hutchinson TA, Magder S, Flegel KM. Interobserver agreement by auscultation in the presence of a third heart sound in patients with congestive heart failure. Chest 1987; 91:870–873.
48. Badgett RG, Lucey CR, Mulrow CD. Can the clinical examination diagnose left-sided heart failure in adults? JAMA 1997; 277:1712–1719.
49. Thomas JT, Kelly RF, Thomas SJ, et al. Utility of history, physical examination, electrocardiogram, and chest radiograph for differentiating normal from decreased systolic function in patients with heart failure. Am J Med 2002; 112:437–445.

50. Cheitlin MD. Can clinical evaluation differentiate diastolic from systolic heart failure? If so, is it important? Am J Med 2002; 112:496–497.
51. MERIT-HF Study Group. Effect of metoprolol CR/XL in chronic heart failure: metoprolol CR/XL randomized intervention trial in congestive heart failure (MERIT-HF). Lancet 1999; 353:2001–2007.
52. Eichhorn EJ. Prognosis determination in heart failure. Am J Med 2001; 110:14S–35S.
53. Exner DV, Dries DL, Waclawiw MA, Shelton B, Domanski MJ. Beta-adrenergic blocking agent use and mortality in patients with asymptomatic and symptomatic left ventricular systolic dysfunction: a post hoc analysis of the studies of left ventricular dysfunction. J Am Coll Cardiol 1999; 33:916–923.
54. Ho KKL, Anderson KM, Kannel WB, Grossman W, Levy D. Survival after the onset of congestive heart failure in Framingham heart study subjects. Circulation 1993; 88:107–115.
55. Robbins JD, Maniar PB, Cotts W, Parker MA, Bonow RO, Gheorghiade M. Prevalence and severity of mitral regurgitation in chronic systolic heart failure. Am J Cardiol 2003; 91:360–362.
56. Trichon BH, Felker GM, Shaw LK, Cabell CH, O'Connor CM. Relation of frequency and severity of mitral regurgitation to survival among patients with left ventricular systolic dysfunction and heart failure. Am J Cardiol 2003; 91:538–543.
57. Koelling TM, Aaronson KD, Cody RJ, Bach DS, Armstrong WF. Prognostic significance of mitral regurgitation and tricuspid regurgitation in patients with left ventricular systolic dysfunction. Am Heart J 2002; 144:373–376.
58. Cohn JN, Johnson GR, Shabetai R, et al. Ejection fraction, peak exercise oxygen consumption, cardiothoracic ratio, ventricular arrhythmias, and plasma norepinephrine as determinants of prognosis in heart failure. The V-HeFT veterans' administration cooperative studies group. Circulation 1993; 87:IV5–IV16.
59. Kao W, Costanzo MR. Prognostic determination in patients with advanced heart failure. J Heart Lung Transplant 1997; 16:82–86.
60. Curtis JP, Sokol SI, Wang Y, et al. The association of left ventricular ejection fraction, mortality, and cause of death in stable outpatients with heart failure. J Am Coll Cardiol 2003; 42:756–762.
61. Di Salvo TG, Mathier M, Semigran MJ, Dec GW. Preserved right ventricular ejection fraction predicts exercise capacity and survival in advanced heart failure. J Am Coll Cardiol 1995; 25:1143–1153.
62. Lee TH, Hamilton MA, Stevenson LW, et al. Impact of left ventricular cavity size on survival in advanced heart failure. Am J Cardiol 1993; 72:672–676.
63. Cohn JN, Levine TB, Olivari MT, et al. Plasma norepinephrine as a guide to prognosis in patients with chronic congestive heart failure. N Engl J Med 1984; 311:819–823.
64. Francis GS, Benedict C, Johnstone DE, et al, for the studies of left ventricular dysfunction (SOLVD) investigators. Comparison of neuroendocrine activation in patients with left ventricular dysfunction with and without congestive heart failure. Circulation 1990; 82:1724–1729.
65. Tsutamoto T, Wada A, Maeda K, et al. Endogenous cardiac natriuretic peptide system in chronic heart failure: prognostic role of plasma brain natriuretic peptide concentration in patients with chronic symptomatic left ventricular dysfunction. Circulation 1997; 96:509–516.
66. Pousset F, Isnard R, Lechat P, et al. Prognostic value of plasma endothelin-1 in patients with chronic heart failure. Eur Heart J 1997; 18:254–258.
67. Kao W, Costanzo WR. Prognostic determination in patients with advanced heart failure. J Heart Lung Transplant 1997; 16:52–56.
68. Mancini DM, Eisen H, Kussmaul W, Mull R, Edmunds LE, Wilson JR. Value of peak exercise oxygen consumption for optimal timing of cardiac transplantation in ambulatory patients with heart failure. Circulation 1991; 83:778–786.

69. Kao W, Winkel EM, Johnson MR, Piccione W, Lichenberg R, Costanzo MR. Role of maximum oxygen consumption in establishment of heart transplant candidacy for heart failure patients with intermediate exercise tolerance. Am J Cardiol 1997; 79:1124–1127.
70. MacGowan GA, Janosko K, Cecchetti A, Murali S. Exercise-related ventilatory abnormalities and survival in congestive heart failure. Am J Cardiol 1997; 79:1264–1266.
71. Bittner V, Weiner DH, Yusuf S, for the SOLVD Investigators. Prediction of mortality and morbidity with a 6-min walk test in patients with left ventricular dysfunction. JAMA 1993; 270:1702–1707.
72. Teerlink JR, Jalaluddin M, Anderson S, on behalf of the PROMISE Investigators, et al. Ambulatory ventricular arrhythmias in patients with heart failure do not specifically predict an increased risk of sudden death.. Circulation 2000; 101:40–46.
73. Stevenson WG, Stevenson LW. Predicting sudden death risk for heart failure patients in the implantable defibrillator age. Circulation 2003; 107:514–516.
74. Huikuri HV, Makikallio RH, Raathkainen P, Perkiomaki J, Castellanos A, Myerburg RJ. Prediction of sudden cardiac death. Appraisal of studies and methods assessing the risk of sudden arrhythmic death. Circulation 2003; 108:110–115.
75. Wang TJ, Larson MG, Levy D, et al. Temporal relations of atrial fibrillation and congestive heart failure and their joint influence on mortality: the Framingham heart study. Circulation 2003; 107:2920–2925.
76. Dries DL, Exner DV, Gersh BJ, Domanski MJ, Waclawiw MY, Stevenson LW. Atrial fibrillation is associated with an increased risk for mortality and heart failure progression in patients with asymptomatic and symptomatic left ventricular systolic dysfunction: a retrospective analysis of the SOLVD trials. J Am Coll Cardiol 1998; 32:695–703.
77. Maisel WH, Stevenson LW. Atrial fibrillation in heart failure: epidemiology, pathophysiology, and rationale for treatment. Am J Cardiol 2003; 91:2D–8D.
78. Cleland JG. Prevalence and incidence of arrhythmias and sudden death in heart failure. Heart Fail Rev 2002; 7:229–242.
79. Grazybowski K, Bilinska LT, Ruzyllo W. Determinants of prognosis in nonishemic dilated cardiomyopathy. J Cardiac Fail 1996; 2:77–85.
80. Hillege HL, Girbes AR, de Kam PJ, et al. Renal function, neurohormonal activation and survival in patients with chronic heart failure. Circulation 2000; 102:203–210.
81. Dries DL, Exner DV, Domanski MJ, Greenberg B, Stevenson LW. The prognostic implications of renal insufficiency in asymptomatic and symptomatic patients with left ventricular dysfunction. J Am Coll Cardiol 2000; 35:681–689.
82. Mahan NG, Blackstone EH, Francis GS, Starling RC, Young JB, Lauer MS. The prognostic value of estimated creatinine clearance alongside functional capacity in ambulatory patients with chronic congestive heart failure. J Am Coll Cardiol 2002; 40:1106–1113.
83. McAlister FA, Exekowitz J, Tonelli M, Armstrong PW. Renal insufficiency and heart failure: prognosis and therapeutic implications from a prospective cohort study. Circulation 2004; 109:1004–1009.
84. McClellan WM, Flanders WD, Langston RD, Jurkovitz C, Presley R. Anemia and renal insufficiency are independent risk factors for death among patients with congestive heart failure admitted to community hospitals; a population-based study. J Am Soc Nephrol 2002; 13:1928–1936.
85. Culleton BF, Larson MG, Wilson PMF, Evans JC, Parfrey PS, Levy D. Cardiovascular disease and mortality in a community-based cohort with mild renal insufficiency. Kidney Intern 1999; 56:2214–2219.
86. Weinfield MS, Chertow GM, Stevenson LW. Aggravated renal dysfunction during intensive therapy for advanced chronic heart failure. Am Heart J 1999; 138:285–290.
87. Gottlieb SS, Abraham W, Butler J, Krumholz HM, et al. The prognostic importance of different definitions of worsening renal function in congestive heart failure. J Cardiac Fail 2002; 8:136–141.

88. Ezekowitz JA, McAlister FA, Armstrong PW. Anemia is common in heart failure and is associated with poor outcomes: insights from a cohort of 12,065 patients with new-onset heart failure. Circulation 2003; 107:223–225.
89. Levin A, Thompson CR, Ethier J, et al. Left ventricular mass index increases in early renal disease: impact of decline in hemoglobin. Am J Kid Dis 1999; 34:125–134.
90. Horwich TB, Fonarow GC, Hamilton MA, MacLellan WR, Borenstein J. Anemia is associated with worse symptoms, greater impairment in functional capacity and a significant increased in mortality in patients with advanced heart failure. J Am Coll Cardiol 2002; 39:1780–1786.
91. Mozaffarian D, Nye R, Levy WC. Anemia predicts mortality in severe heart failure: the prospective randomized amlodipine survival evaluation (PRAISE). J Am Coll Cardiol 2003; 41:1933–1939.
92. Kosiborod M, Smith GL, Radford MJ, Foody JM, Krumholz HM. The prognostic importance of anemia in patients with heart failure. Am J Med 2003; 114:112–119.
93. Felker GM, Adams KF, Gattis WA, O'Connor CM. Anemia as a risk factor and therapeutic target in heart failure. J Am Coll Cardiol 2004; 44:959–966.
94. Levy D, Kenchaiah S, Larson MG, et al. Long-term trends in the incidence of and survival with heart failure. NEJM 2002; 347:1397–1402.
95. McCullough PA, Philbin EF, Spertus JA, Kaatz S, Sandberg KR, Weaver WD. Confirmation of a heart failure epidemic: findings from the resource utilization among congestive heart failure (REACH) study. J Am Coll Cardiol 2002; 39:60–69.
96. DiLenarda A, Secoli G, Perkan A, et al, the Heart Muscle Study Group. Changing mortality in dilated cardiomyopathy. Br Heart J 1994; 72:S46–S51.
97. Stevenson WG, Stevenson LW, Middlekauff HR, et al. Improving survival for patients with advanced heart failure. J Am Coll Cardiol 1995; 26:1417–1423.
98. MacIntyre K, Capewell S, Stewart S, et al. Evidence of improving prognosis in heart failure: trends in case fatality in 66,547 patients hospitalized between 1986 and 1995. Circulation 2000; 102:1126–1131.
99. Gottdeiner JS, McClelland RL, Marshall R, et al. Outcome of congestive heart failure in elderly persons: influence of left ventricular systolic function the cardiovascular health study. Ann Intern Med 2002; 137:631–639.
100. Jong P, Vowinckel E, Liu PP, Gong Y, Tu JV. Prognosis and determinants of survival in patients newly hospitalized for heart failure. Arch Intern Med 2002; 62:1689–1694.

2

Causes and Evaluation for Reversible Etiologies

Edward K. Kasper
Division of Cardiology, Johns Hopkins Bayview Medical Center, Baltimore, Maryland, U.S.A.

INTRODUCTION

This chapter will cover the evaluation of patients with advanced heart failure. Emphasis is placed upon reversible etiologies and exacerbating factors. There are many causes of heart failure such as valvular heart disease, pericardial disease, acute myocardial infarction, restrictive cardiomyopathy, and hypertrophic cardiomyopathy. We will concentrate on the dilated cardiomyopathies. Patients with advanced heart failure due to a dilated cardiomyopathy will often present to the hospital with florid symptoms of fluid retention. However, such symptoms may have been misinterpreted as bronchitis or asthma for a prolonged period of time prior to the incident presentation. Once recognized, evaluation and treatment for heart failure must occur rapidly and simultaneously.

EVALUATION OF PATIENTS WITH ADVANCED HEART FAILURE

History

As with any disorder, the foundation of evaluation is a complete history and physical examination. The evaluation may need to be performed once the patient is stabilized and more comfortable if the patient presents with advanced symptoms. The initial focus of the history should be on the presenting symptoms and the time course of their development. Is this something that truly did present within days or, upon retrospection, had the patient been feeling poorly for months prior to presentation? Fulminant myocarditis presents suddenly, while other forms of cardiomyopathy develop over months not days. Was there truly a preceding viral illness with fever, or did the patient simply have a cough, often a sign of incipient heart failure? Many patients with heart failure will cough especially when supine for months before the cause is recognized. Unexplained weight gain is a clue to fluid retention. Some patients will be able to pinpoint when their weight started to increase. Asking the patient when he or she last felt completely well is important. Knowing the time course of development helps both to narrow potential etiologies and focus the evaluation.

Since the majority of patients in the developed world will have coronary disease as the proximate cause of their cardiomyopathy, questions regarding prior cardiovascular history and coronary risk factors are critical. A history of hypertension, diabetes, hyperlipidemia, tobacco abuse, prior infarction, or coronary intervention are important and point towards coronary disease as the etiology. A sense of how well the hypertension and diabetes are controlled and whether intermittent ischemia might be present is crucial as these diseases may exacerbate heart failure regardless of the etiology.

It is important to inquire about other cardiovascular disorders such as valvular heart disease, prior episodes of pericarditis, or rheumatic fever. Therapy for other disorders may impact the heart. Chest irradiation and the use of cardiotoxic agents usually in the therapy of cancer should be investigated. Cocaine, alcohol, and amphetamine use should be documented. The possibility of infection with human immunodeficiency virus should be considered in those with multiple prior blood transfusions or risky personal habits. A history of exposure to ticks suggests the possibility of Lyme disease.

Finally, consideration should be given to systemic disorders known to involve the heart. This should include infiltrative disorders such as sarcoidosis, hemochromatosis, and amyloidosis. The infiltrative cardiomyopathies may initially present as a restrictive cardiomyopathy. Many will progress to a picture of dilated cardiomyopathy with unusually thick myocardial walls. A variety of collagen vascular diseases should be considered, although it should be remembered that most patients with a collagen vascular disease present with a cardiomyopathy late in the course of their disease. It is rare for advanced heart failure to be the presenting syndrome of an undiagnosed collagen vascular disease. Symptoms of heart failure, on the other hand, may be the presenting syndrome for thyroid disease and, very rarely, pheochromocytoma. Neuromuscular disorders, such as Becker's muscular dystrophy, may present with heart failure and should be considered.

A family history of cardiomyopathy, sudden death, heart failure, conduction disorder, or muscular dystrophy is important to note. A fair percentage of patients thought to have idiopathic cardiomyopathy may indeed have an unrecognized familial cardiomyopathy (1). This is important not only to the patient, but to their first-degree family members who should be screened for the same process with both echocardiography and an ECG.

Physical Examination

Along with an assessment of fluid retention, clues suggesting a systemic disorder should be sought. Macroglossia, nonpalpable purpura of the eyelids, hepatosplenomegaly, carpal tunnel syndrome or peripheral neuropathy could indicate amyloidosis. Eye findings, such as uveitis or conjunctivitis, erythema nodosum, a seventh cranial nerve palsy, or lymphadenopathy should suggest sarcoidosis. Fever should suggest either an infectious cause or a collagen vascular disease. Watching the patient walk or rise from a seated position may suggest a muscular dystrophy or polymyositis. A bronze-tan skin discoloration, splenomegaly, articular changes of the second metacarpophalangeal joint, and testicular atrophy suggest hemochromatosis. The findings of the patient's history and physical examination help to focus further laboratory evaluation.

Routine Laboratory Testing and Imaging

Routine Laboratory Testing

Laboratory testing is used to find disorders that can exacerbate heart failure or cause dilated cardiomyopathy (2). A typical laboratory evaluation for a patient presenting with heart failure would include serum electrolytes, calcium, magnesium, renal function, hepatic function, complete blood count, urinalysis, and lipid profile. Thyroid function tests are suggested, since both hyperthyroidism and hypothyroidism may cause cardiomyopathy and present with nonspecific findings, especially in the elderly. An ECG is done to evaluate for the possibility of ongoing ischemia, remote infarction, or arrhythmia. A chest radiograph may suggest sarcoidosis or another cause. An increase in cardiothoracic ratio and the presence of pulmonary congestion would be common in patients presenting in heart failure. The remainder of the laboratory evaluation should be tailored to those etiologies considered most likely based upon the history and physical examination. Many disorders may cause cardiomyopathy (Table 1). It is not cost effective to blindly evaluate all patients for every potential cause of cardiomyopathy.

Cardiac Imaging

Echocardiography is the imaging modality of choice (2). It is noninvasive, painless, quickly performed, and relatively inexpensive. Two-dimensional echocardiography with Doppler evaluation provides information on pericardial, myocardial, and valvular causes of heart failure. Assessment of chamber dimension, geometry, and function as well as wall thickness and regional wall motion can all be performed. The division of heart failure due to either systolic or non-systolic ventricular dysfunction is most often based on echocardiography.

Magnetic resonance imaging and computed tomography are playing an ever-increasing role in the evaluation of cardiovascular disease. Both imaging modalities can provide information on coronary anatomy, ventricular function and mass, as well as pericardial disease. In addition, quantification may be more precise than that provided by echocardiography. However, neither cardiac magnetic resonance imaging nor computed tomography is as widely available or as easy to perform as echocardiography. Magnetic resonance imaging with gadolinium perfusion may help in the evaluation of infiltrative disorders. Radionuclide ventriculography provides excellent quantification of ventricular function but is unable to assess wall thickness or valvular function. Because of these limitations, echocardiography remains the imaging modality of choice.

Evaluation of Coronary Disease

The evaluation of coronary disease is important because in the majority of patients with heart failure, coronary disease will be the underlying etiology (3). Noninvasive coronary evaluation, such as stress testing, is difficult in patients with dilated cardiomyopathy and heart failure. Baseline bundle-branch block, segmental wall motion abnormalities, and inhomogeneous resting nuclear images make stress testing with imaging difficult. Both computed tomography and magnetic resonance imaging of the coronaries hold potential, but remain unproven in this population. Many physicians will, therefore, go directly to cardiac catheterization. I tend to do cardiac catheterization once the acute heart failure has resolved in patients with risk factors for coronary disease. Right heart catheterization, at the same time, provides a measure of how well the patient has responded to therapy. In addition, there is little reason to perform cardiac catheterization if revascularization would not be considered due to patient preferences or comorbidities. Finally, cardiac catheterization does not need to be repeated unless there is a belief that coronary disease has developed and revascularization would be a possibility.

Patients with coronary disease and angina with a moderately reduced ejection fraction were shown to benefit from coronary artery bypass surgery (4). The issue of whether or not coronary bypass surgery provides benefit to patients with heart failure, poor

Table 1 Causes of Dilated Cardiomyopathy

Idiopathic
Familial
Myocarditis
  Infections[a]
    Viral—Coxsackie virus, echovirus, poliovirus, influenza, vaccinia, cytomegalovirus, adenovirus, parvovirus, herpes simplex, respiratory syncytial virus, Epstein–Barr virus, hepatitis, varicella zoster, human immunodeficiency virus
    Bacterial—*Streptococcus pyogenes*, *Staphylococcus aureus*, *Salmonella*, *Leptospira*, *Borellia burgdoferi*, *Mycoplasma pneumoniae*, *Chlamydia*, *Rickettsia*
    Fungi—Aspergillus, Candida
    Parasites—*Trypanosoma cruzii*, *Toxoplasma*
  Noninfectious[a]
    Drugs—multiple including a variety of antibiotics—ampicillin, sulfamethoxizole; anticonvulsants—carbamazepine, smallpox vaccination; diuretics—furosemide, hydrochlorothiazide
    Systemic diseases—a variety of collagen vascular disorders, peripartum cardiomyopathy
  Giant cell
  Cardiac rejection
Drug toxicity[a]
  Alcohol
  Amphotericin B
  Antidepressants
  Catecholamines
  Chinese herbal medicine
  Cocaine
  Doxorubicin
  Interferon alpha
  Interleukin 2
  Ipecac
  Lithium
  Prednisone
  Trastuzumab
  Multiple others
Metabolic[a]
  Acromegaly
  Addison's disease
  Carcinoid
  Diabetes mellitus
  Hypocalcemia
  Hypophosphatemia
  Thyroid disease
  Pheochromocytoma
Infiltrative disease
  Amyloid
  Hemochromatosis[a]
  Sarcoidosis[a]
  Storage diseases
Nutritional[a]
  Beriberi
  Carnitine
  Pellagra
  Scurvy
  Selenium

(Continued)

Table 1 Causes of Dilated Cardiomyopathy *(Continued)*

Connective-tissue disease[a]
Ankylosing spondylitis
Cryoglobulinemia
Churg-Strauss
Dermatomyositis/polymyositis
Polyarteritis nodosa
Relapsing polychondritis
Rheumatoid arthritis
Scleroderma
Systemic lupus erythematosus
Wegener's granulomatosis
Muscular dystrophies and neuromuscular disorders
Heat stroke[a]
Hypertension[a]
Morbid obesity
Peripartum[a]
Poisoning[a]
Carbon monoxide
Carbon tetrachloride
Cobalt
Heavy metals
Scorpion, spider and snake bites
Radiation
Sepsis/critical illness[a]
Tachycardia[a]
Uremia[a]

This is a relatively complete list.
[a]Possibly reversible.

ejection fraction, and no angina remains controversial. Some guidelines recommend bypass for such patients with left main stenosis and in patients with large areas of hibernating myocardium (5). How best to identify such patients is unknown.

Endomyocardial Biopsy

The ACC/AHA guidelines for the evaluation and management of chronic heart failure in the adult propose a limited role for endomyocardial biopsy and that it should not be performed as part of the routine evaluation of cardiomyopathy (2). In experienced hands, endomyocardial biopsy is safe with a mortality rate of about 0.5% (6). Tissue sampling is used to make the diagnosis of amyloidosis, hemochromatosis, myocarditis (including giant cell myocarditis), and endocardial fibroelastosis. Sarcoidosis is a patchy disorder but when granulomas are found on endomyocardial biopsy, the diagnosis is confirmed. Endomyocardial biopsy may also be used to evaluate the risk of continued anthracycline therapy (7). Therefore, endomyocardial biopsy is used to answer specific questions and use should be tailored to the specific patient.

CAUSES OF CARDIOMYOPATHY

Most patients with dilated cardiomyopathy but without coronary disease will not have an identifiable cause and will thus be labeled "idiopathic" (8–10). A large proportion of these patients may have an underlying genetic cause (1). This is important as it suggests that first-degree relatives of patients with idiopathic cardiomyopathy should be screened for asymptomatic left ventricular dysfunction. Otherwise, a wide variety of conditions may result in dilated cardiomyopathy. These are listed in Table 1. In an extensive evaluation of 1230 patients with initially unexplained dilated cardiomyopathy, we discovered a variety of diagnoses (8). These are listed in Table 2. This cohort of patients was drawn from a tertiary care institution and likely does not reflect the most common etiologies in a primary population where coronary disease and hypertension play a larger role. In addition, the underlying cause of cardiomyopathy had prognostic value. Patients with peripartum cardiomyopathy had a better prognosis than patients with other forms of cardiomyopathy. Patients with cardiomyopathy due to inflitrative myocardial diseases, HIV infection, or doxorubicin therapy had a worse prognosis (Fig. 1). In patients with infiltrative disease, those with sarcoidosis had a better prognosis than those with either amyloidosis or hemochromatosis.

REVERSIBLE CAUSES OF CARDIOMYOPATHY

The evaluation of dilated cardiomyopathy should be directed towards reversible or treatable causes of cardiomyopathy listed in Table 1. Many patients with left ventricular dysfunction will have an improvement in their ejection fraction with standard heart failure therapy including beta-blockers and angiotensin converting enzyme inhibitors. The term "reversible causes of cardiomyopathy" is used to refer to causes of dilated cardiomyopathy that will improve spontaneously or with a specific treatment. Several deserve comment.

Myocarditis

Myocarditis is an lymphocytic, inflammatory disease of the myocardium, which can lead to a dilated cardiomyopathy. A number of viruses have been identified in association with myocarditis (Table 1). Polymerase chain reaction (PCR) was used to identify viral genome in 38% of 624 patients with myocarditis and only 1.4% of control samples (11). The most commonly identified viral genome was adenovirus followed by enterovirus, cytomegalovirus, parvovirus, influenza A, herpes simplex virus, Epstein Barr virus, and respiratory syncitial virus. There were 26 patients infected with 2 different viruses. Other viruses that have been described as causes of myocarditis include human immunodeficiency virus and hepatitis C. In addition, myocarditis has been confirmed following smallpox vaccination in United States military personnel (12,13). A variety of other infectious agents have been shown to cause myocarditis including bacterial, fungal and parasitic organisms (Table 1).

Almost any drug may cause a hypersensitivity myocarditis, which may or may not get better with discontinuation of the offending drug (14). Myocarditis may also be associated with a systemic disorder such as a variety of autoimmune collagen vascular disorders, exposure to various drugs, and in peripartum cardiomyopathy. In cases of secondary myocarditis, prognosis appears to be more closely related to the underlying systemic disorder rather than the presence of myocarditis (15).

Natural History and Clinical Course

Four clinicopathologic forms of myocarditis have been described based upon both clinical presentation and findings on endomyocardial biopsy (16). Diagnosis is largely based upon

Table 2 Final Diagnoses in 1230 Patients with Initially Unexplained Cardiomyopathy

Diagnosis	Number (%)
Idiopathic cardiomyopathy	616 (50)
Myocarditis	111 (9)
Ischemic heart disease	91 (7)
Infiltrative disease	59 (5)
Amyloid	36
Sarcoidosis	14
Hemochromatosis	9
Peripartum cardiomyopathy	51 (4)
Hypertension	49 (4)
HIV	45 (4)
Connective-tissue disease	39 (3)
Scleroderma	12
Systemic lupus erythematosus	9
Marfan's syndrome	3
Polyarteritis nodosa	3
Dermatomyositis or polymyositis	3
Nonspecific connective-tissue disease	3
Ankylosing spondylitis	2
Rheumatoid arthritis	1
Relapsing polychondritis	1
Wegener's granulomatosis	1
Mixed connective-tissue disease	1
Substance abuse	37 (3)
Alcohol	28
Cocaine	9
Doxorubicin therapy	15 (1)
Other causes	117 (10)
Restrictive cardiomyopathy	28
Familial	25
Valvular heart disease	19
Endocrine dysfunction	
Thyroid disease	7
Carcinoid	2
Pheochromocytoma	1
Acromegaly	1
Neuromuscular disease	7
Neoplastic heart disease	6
Congenital heart disease	4
Complication of coronary bypass surgery	4
Radiation	3
Sepsis/critical illness	3
Endomyocardial fibroelastosis	1
Thrombotic thrombocytopenic purpura	1
Rheumatic carditis	1
Drug therapy (not including doxorubicin)	
Leukotrienes	2
Lithium	1
Prednisone	1
Total	1230 (100)

Source: Adapted from Ref. 8.

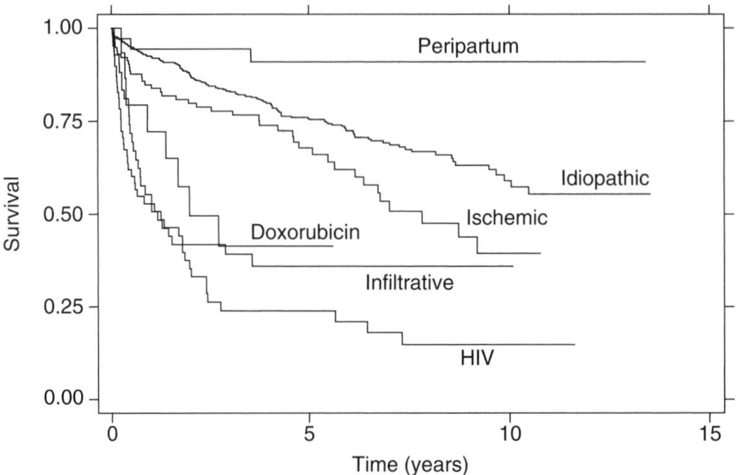

Figure 1 Kaplan–Meier estimates of survival according to underlying cause of cardiomyopathy. *Source:* From Ref. 8.

the findings at endomyocardial biopsy. Fulminant myocarditis is most commonly seen in young adults and presents abruptly with severe heart failure and cardiogenic shock following a viral illness. Patients present with poor left ventricular function but without left ventricular dilation. The ventricular walls are thick, likely due to a combination of intense inflammatory lymphocytic infiltrate with myocyte necrosis and edema (17). Patients will spontaneously recover completely or die of cardiogenic shock or ventricular arrhythmias (18). Standard immunosuppression with corticosteroids likely does not help. Aggressive supportive care with a mechanical assist device may be required until left ventricular function improves.

Acute myocarditis has an indistinct onset of symptoms, presents with dilated cardiomyopathy, and shows an inflammatory lymphocytic infiltrate with or without myocyte necrosis on endomyocardial biopsy. Some cases will respond to immunosuppression while others will not (16). Chronic active myocarditis has an indistinct onset and results in a restrictive cardiomyopathy. Endomyocardial biopsy shows inflammation and severe fibrosis. Chronic active myocarditis does not respond to immunosuppression (16). Chronic persistent myocarditis presents with atypical chest pain or ventricular arrhythmias. Left ventricular function is normal even though inflammation is seen on endomyocardial biopsy (16).

A fifth form of myocarditis, which does not fit nicely within the above schema, is giant cell myocarditis. While similar to chronic active myocarditis, giant-cell myocarditis shows a diffuse, lymphocytic infiltrate with myocyte necrosis and the presence of giant cells without well-formed granuloma on endomyocardial biopsy. Prognosis is poor with a median survival of 5.5 months after the development of symptoms (19). Patients often have a previous autoimmune disease and tend to be in their 40s. It has recurred in a transplanted heart. Heart transplantation, however, is the only therapy to offer a significant survival advantage (19). Immunosuppressive therapy increases survival in some patients.

Treatment remains controversial. The largest trial of immunosuppressive therapy for myocarditis showed no significant difference in survival (20). Patients with fulminant presentation will not need immunosuppression (18). Patients with chronic active myocarditis and chronic persistent myocarditis will often not respond to immunosuppression (16). Giant-cell myocarditis is often treated with immunosuppression, but this is rarely effective (19). There may be ways to tailor therapy to the particular disease. In a trial of 22 patients with PCR-proven enteroviral or adenoviral genomes and left ventricular dysfunction, treatment with Interferon-beta for 6 months resulted in the elimination of viral genome in all patients and improvement in left ventricular function in 15 of 22 patients (21). In another study of 112 patients with myocarditis, patients with circulating cardiac autoantibodies and no viral genome were most likely to respond to immunosuppression (22).

Peripartum Cardiomyopathy

Peripartum cardiomyopathy, defined by a National Institutes of Health Consensus Conference, is heart failure due to left ventricular systolic dysfunction developing in the final month of pregnancy or within 5 months after delivery in the absence of pre-existing heart disease or other cause of cardiomyopathy (23). The etiology is unknown but myocarditis due to either a viral infection or an autoimmune process has been postulated to be the proximate cause. In the United States, this occurs in one of every 3000 to 4000 live births (23). Risk factors reported in the literature include black race, high parity, old age, multiple gestation, and the use of tocolytics (23). In our experience, 62% of patients had myocarditis on endomyocardial biopsy but the presence or absence of myocarditis did not alter survival (24). Recovery of left ventricular function occurred in the majority of patients resulting in an excellent prognosis whether or not myocardits was present.

Treatment is usually supportive care and standard heart failure therapy. If left ventricular function at rest fails to normalize, standard heart failure therapy is continued indefinitely. In most patients, left ventricular function will normalize. Continued therapy may then be discontinued, especially if left ventricular function augments appropriately with exercise. We have argued that women with normal resting cardiac function who fail to augment left ventricular function with exercise should be continued on a beta-blocker and an angiotensin converting enzyme inhibitor (25). Heart failure symptoms and left ventricular dysfunction may return with subsequent pregnancies. In one study, 21% of patients redeveloped symptoms of heart failure out of 28 women whose left ventricular function had returned to normal. None of these patients died. However, in 16 women whose heart function had failed to normalize, death occurred in 19% while 44% of the women developed heart failure (26). These data are helpful in counseling women regarding future pregnancies.

Stress Cardiomyopathy

Reversible, severe left ventricular dysfunction has been described following sudden emotional stress, a variety of neurologic injuries, and other forms of non-emotional stress (27). The majority of patients are women. Chest pain and dyspnea are typical presenting complaints, and prolongation of the QT interval is common within the first 48 hours associated with widespread, deep, symmetrical T wave inversions. Echocardiography shows severe apical akinesis or dyskinesis with preservation of function at the base of the left ventricle. Marked improvement in left ventricular function is seen within a week and normalization of function within 3 weeks. Plasma catecholamine levels are massively elevated (27) and may play a major role in the etiology of this disorder resulting in myocardial stunning. Therapy is supportive care and standard heart failure therapy, which may be discontinued following normalization of left ventricular function. Given the massively elevated plasma catecholamine levels, pressors are avoided in favor of mechanical circulatory support with an intra-aortic balloon pump.

A reversible cardiomyopathy is often seen in critical-illness such as sepsis, pancreatitis, anaphylaxis, burn injuries, and a variety of other injuries and disorders (28,29). Whether or not this should be thought of as separate from stress cardiomyopathy is unclear. In sepsis and perhaps pancreatitis, circulating inflammatory mediators, such as tumor necrosis factor and interleukin-6, appear to play an etiologic role in the transient cardiomyopathy (29,30), while in stress cardiomyopathy, catecholamines play a more important role. This would suggest that either pro-inflammatory cytokines or catecholamines might cause a reversible cardiomyopathy.

Tachycardia-Induced Cardiomyopathy

Incessant or chronic ventricular or supraventricular tachycardias may cause a dilated cardiomyopathy (31). The incidence of this is unknown and it may occur at any age. It may also aggravate other causes of systolic dysfunction. The most frequent causes are atrial fibrillation and flutter with a rapid ventricular response (32). Normalization of heart rate by either rate or rhythm control results in an improvement in left ventricular function. In heart failure patients with atrial fibrillation, however, rhythm control using a catheter ablation technique, without the use of antiarrhythmic drugs, was associated with a significant improvement in left ventricular function as well as symptoms (33). If the arrhythmia recurs or the ventricular response is poorly controlled, the cardiomyopathy may return and is associated with a more rapid decline in left ventricular function (32). This entity is something to be considered in all patients with persistent arrhythmias and left ventricular dysfunction.

Sarcoid Cardiomyopathy

Sarcoidosis is a multisystem granulomatosis of unknown etiology. Cardiac sarcoidosis occurs in upwards of 70% of autopsy series (34). In clinical series, it is recognized less often because it is difficult to detect minimal disease clinically (35). Extracardiac symptoms are usually present but this is not always the case and sarcoidosis may present with a cardiomyopathy or sudden death (36). Noncaseating granulomas with giant cells are the hallmark pathologic feature. Arrhythmias are common and sudden death may be the initial presentation (36–38). The granulomas and fibrosis may result in a variety of conduction abnormalities, and dilated cardiomyopathy is not unusual (34,36,37).

Diagnosis is based upon the ECG, echocardiogram, and often biopsy of another organ or lymph node. Due to the scattered nature of the granulomas endomyocardial biopsy, while specific, is not sensitive. The most common areas of myocardial involvement are the left ventricular free wall particularly near the base of the papillary muscles and the base of the septum (36). These areas are not easily accessible to endomyocardial biopsy. Patchy thallium defects that do not correspond to coronary artery territories occur. Magnetic resonance imaging with gadolinium may also show evidence of infiltration (39).

Immunosuppression with corticosteroids may result in improvement (40). There has not been, however, a controlled study of the use of immunosuppression in patients with cardiac sarcoidosis. Despite this, corticosteroids are usually recommended and patients may require a prolonged course of treatment. A low threshold for an internal cardioverter defibrillator is suggested as the incidence of sudden cardiac death is high (36).

While both disorders have giant cells on histologic evaluation, cardiac sarcoidosis is clinically different from giant cell myocarditis (41). The granulomas in cardiac sarcoidosis are well formed, while in giant cell myocarditis they are not. The prognosis of cardiac sarcoidosis is relatively good compared to giant cell myocarditis. Finally, patients with cardiac sarcoidosis may respond to corticosteroids, while patients with giant cell myocarditis often will not.

Drug-Induced Cardiomyopathy

Some drugs are associated with a hypersensitivity myocarditis, which resolves with discontinuation of the offending drug. Patients are often prescribed and take multiple drugs so identification of the agent causing the myocarditis may be difficult. An incomplete list of drugs that have been shown to cause myocarditis is found in Table 1. Penicillins, sulfamethoxizole, and methyldopa are more commonly implicated. Other drugs have a direct toxic effect, such as catecholamines. A reversible cardiomyopathy has been associated with cocaine use and epinephrine overdose (42,43). Other direct toxins include heavy metals and carbon monoxide. Alcohol may cause a reversible cardiomyopathy, although the amount of alcohol needed to cause the cardiomyopathy is unknown and likely varies depending on a host of factors, including genetic susceptibility (44). It is likely that at least 5 years of daily alcohol consumption is necessary to produce left ventricular dysfunction (44). Some drugs used in the treatment of cancer, such as cyclophosphamide, trastuzumab, and and doxorubicin, may cause dilated cardiomyopathy. Prognosis in doxorubicin-induced cardiomyopathy is poor (8) but it is unclear if this is due to doxorubicin or the underlying cancer for which the drug was prescribed.

REFERENCES

1. Michels VV, Moll PP, Miller FA, et al. The frequency of Familial Dilated Cardiomyopathy in a series of patients with Idiopathic Dilated Cardiomyopathy. N Engl J Med 1992; 326:77–82.
2. Hunt SA, Baker DW, Chin MH, et al. ACC/AHA Guidelines for the Evaluation and Management of Chronic Heart Failure in the Adult: Executive Summary–A Report of the American College of Cardiology/American Heart Association Task Force on Practice Guidelines (Committee to Revise the 1995 Guidelines for the Evaluation and Management of Heart Failure): Developed in Collaboration With the International Society for Heart and Lung Transplantation; Endorsed by the heart Failure Society of America. Circulation 2001; 104:2996–3007.
3. Gheorghiade M, Bonow RO. Chronic heart failure in the United States: a manifestation of coronary artery disease. Circulation 1998; 97:282–289.
4. Alderman EL, Fisher LD, Litwin P, et al. Results of coronary artery surgery in patients with poor left ventricular function (CASS). Circulation 1983; 68:785–795.
5. Eagle KA, Guyton RA, Davidoff R, et al. ACC/AHA Guidelines for Coronary Artery Bypass Graft Surgery: A Report of the American College of Cardiology/American Heart Association Task Force on Practice Guidelines (Committee to Revise the 1991 Guidelines for Coronary Artery Bypass Graft Surgery). American College of Cardiology/American Heart Association. J Am Coll Cardiol 1999; 34:1262–1347.
6. Deckers JW, Hare JM, Baughman KL. Complications of transvenous right ventricular endomyocardial biopsy in adult patients with cardiomyopathy: a seven-year survey of 546 consecutive diagnostic procedures in a tertiary referral center. J Am Coll Cardiol 1992; 19:43–47.

7. Billingham ME, Mason JW, Bristow MR, Daniels JR. Anthracycline cardiomyopathy monitored by morphologic changes. Cancer Treat Rep 1978; 62:865–872.
8. Felker GM, Thompson RE, Hare JM, et al. Underlying causes and long-term survival in patients with initially unexplained cardiomyopathy. N Engl J Med 2000; 342:1077–1084.
9. Felker GM, Hu W, Hare JM. The spectrum of dilated cardiomyopathy. The Johns Hopkins experience with 1,278 patients. Medicine (Baltimore) 1999; 78:270–283.
10. Kasper EK, Agema WR, Hutchins GM, et al. The causes of dilated cardiomyopathy: a clinicopathologic review of 673 consecutive patients. J Am Coll Cardiol 1994; 23:586–590.
11. Bowles NE, Ni J, Kearney DL, et al. Detection of viruses in myocardial tissues by polymerase chain reaction. Evidence of adenovirus as a common cause of myocarditis in children and adults. J Am Coll Cardiol 2003; 42:466–472.
12. Murphy JG, Wright RS, Bruce GK, et al. Eosinophilic-lymphocytic myocarditis after smallpox vaccination. Lancet 2003; 362:1378–1380.
13. Halsell JS, Riddle JR, Atwood JE, et al. Myopericarditis following smallpox vaccination among vaccinia-naive US military personnel. JAMA 2003; 289:3283–3289.
14. Ansari A, Maron BJ, Berntson DG. Drug-induced toxic myocarditis. Tex Heart Inst J 2003; 30:76–79.
15. Pulerwitz TC, Cappola TP, Felker GM, et al. Mortality in primary and secondary myocarditis. Am Heart J 2004; 147:746–750.
16. Lieberman EB, Herskowitz A, Rose NR, Baughman KL. A clinicopathologic description of myocarditis. Clin Immunol Immunopathol 1993; 68:191–196.
17. Felker GM, Boehmer JP, Hruban RH, et al. Echocardiographic findings in fulminant and acute myocarditis. J Am Coll Cardiol 2000; 36:227–232.
18. McCarthy RE, III, Boehmer JP, Hruban RH, et al. Long-term outcome of fulminant myocarditis as compared with acute (nonfulminant) myocarditis. N Engl J Med 2000; 342:690–695.
19. Cooper LT, Jr., Berry GJ, Shabetai R. Idiopathic giant-cell myocarditis—natural history and treatment. Multicenter Giant Cell Myocarditis Study Group Investigators. N Engl J Med 1997; 336:1860–1866.
20. Mason JW, O'Connell JB, Herskowitz A, et al. A clinical trial of immunosuppressive therapy for myocarditis. The Myocarditis Treatment Trial Investigators. N Engl J Med 1995; 333:269–275.
21. Kuhl U, Pauschinger M, Schwimmbeck PL, et al. Interferon-beta treatment eliminates cardiotropic viruses and improves left ventricular function in patients with myocardial persistence of viral genomes and left ventricular dysfunction. Circulation 2003; 107:2793–2798.
22. Frustaci A, Chimenti C, Calabrese F, et al. Immunosuppressive therapy for active lymphocytic myocarditis: virological and immunologic profile of responders versus nonresponders. Circulation 2003; 107:857–863.
23. Pearson GD, Veille JC, Rahimtoola S, et al. Peripartum cardiomyopathy: National Heart, Lung, and Blood Institute and Office of Rare Diseases (National Institutes of Health) workshop recommendations and review. JAMA 2000; 283:1183–1188.
24. Felker GM, Jaeger CJ, Klodas E, et al. Myocarditis and long-term survival in peripartum cardiomyopathy. Am Heart J 2000; 140:785–791.
25. Ardehali H, Kasper EK, Baughman KL. Peripartum cardiomyopathy. Minerva Cardioangiol 2003; 51:41–48.
26. Elkayam U, Tummala PP, Rao K, et al. Maternal and fetal outcomes of subsequent pregnancies in women with peripartum cardiomyopathy. N Engl J Med 2001; 344:1567–1571.
27. Wittstein IS, Thiemann DR, Lima JA, et al. Neurohumoral features of myocardial stunning due to sudden emotional stress. N Engl J Med 2005; 352:539–548.
28. Parrillo JE, Burch C, Shelhamer JH, et al. A circulating myocardial depressant substance in humans with septic shock. Septic shock patients with a reduced ejection fraction have a circulating factor that depresses in vitro myocardial cell performance. J Clin Invest 1985; 76:1539–1553.

29. Ruiz BM. Reversible myocardial dysfunction in critically ill, noncardiac patients: a review. Crit Care Med 2002; 30:1280–1290.
30. Kan H, Finkel MS. Inflammatory mediators and reversible myocardial dysfunction. J Cell Physiol 2003; 195:1–11.
31. Umana E, Solares CA, Alpert MA. Tachycardia-induced cardiomyopathy. Am J Med 2003; 114:51–55.
32. Nerheim P, Birger-Botkin S, Piracha L, Olshansky B. Heart failure and sudden death in patients with tachycardia-induced cardiomyopathy and recurrent tachycardia. Circulation 2004; 110:247–252.
33. Hsu LF, Jais P, Sanders P, et al. Catheter ablation for atrial fibrillation in congestive heart failure. N Engl J Med 2004; 351:2373–2383.
34. Iwai K, Takemura T, Kitaichi M, et al. Pathological studies on sarcoidosis autopsy. II. Early change, mode of progression and death pattern. Acta Pathol Jpn 1993; 43:377–385.
35. Pisani B, Taylor DO, Mason JW. Inflammatory myocardial diseases and cardiomyopathies. Am J Med 1997; 102:459–469.
36. Roberts WC, McAllister HA, Jr., Ferrans VJ. Sarcoidosis of the heart. A clinicopathologic study of 35 necropsy patients (group 1) and review of 78 previously described necropsy patients (group 11). Am J Med 1977; 63:86–108.
37. Silverman KJ, Hutchins GM, Bulkley BH. Cardiac sarcoid: a clinicopathologic study of 84 unselected patients with systemic sarcoidosis. Circulation 1978; 58:1204–1211.
38. Perry A, Vuitch F. Causes of death in patients with sarcoidosis. A morphologic study of 38 autopsies with clinicopathologic correlations. Arch Pathol Lab Med 1995; 119:167–172.
39. Mana J. Magnetic resonance imaging and nuclear imaging in sarcoidosis. Curr Opin Pulm Med 2002; 8:457–463.
40. Chiu CZ, Nakatani S, Zhang G, et al. Prevention of left ventricular remodeling by long-term corticosteroid therapy in patients with cardiac sarcoidosis. Am J Cardiol 2005; 95:143–146.
41. Okura Y, Dec GW, Hare JM, et al. A clinical and histopathologic comparison of cardiac sarcoidosis and idiopathic giant cell myocarditis. J Am Coll Cardiol 2003; 41:322–329.
42. Budhwani N, Bonaparte KL, Cuyjet AB, Saric M. Severe reversible left ventricular systolic and diastolic dysfunction due to accidental iatrogenic epinephrine overdose. Rev Cardiovasc Med 2004; 5:130–133.
43. Chokshi SK, Moore R, Pandian NG, Isner JM. Reversible cardiomyopathy associated with cocaine intoxication. Ann Intern Med 1989; 111:1039–1040.
44. Piano MR. Alcoholic cardiomyopathy: incidence, clinical characteristics, and pathophysiology. Chest 2002; 121:1638–1650.

3
Diet, Metabolic Syndrome, and Obesity

Michael M. Givertz
Cardiovascular Division, Brigham and Women's Hospital, Harvard Medical School, Boston, Massachusetts, U.S.A.

INTRODUCTION

Clinically important changes in body weight are common in heart failure and impact daily patient management. Overweight and obesity, insulin resistance, and metabolic syndrome are increasing in prevalence and contribute directly to the development and progression of left ventricular dysfunction. At the same time, improved treatment of chronic heart failure has resulted in increasing numbers of patients with advanced disease and cardiac cachexia. Mechanisms underlying weight gain and loss in heart failure are complex, and an evolving understanding of pathophysiology has suggested novel targets of therapy. Standard pharmacologic strategies include titration of neurohormonal antagonists and diuretics while recognizing the limited reliability of the clinical evaluation. Sodium and fluid restriction, moderation of alcohol use, and exercise are equally important components of care for the majority of patients with heart failure, regardless of body weight. For obese patients, marked weight loss may contribute to reverse ventricular remodeling.

WEIGHT GAIN AND LOSS

The most common cause of weight gain in heart failure is an expanded extracellular volume. Increased volume is manifest on exam as elevated jugular venous pressure, pulmonary congestion, peripheral edema and ascites, and by symptoms such as ankle swelling, dyspnea on exertion, and orthopnea. Volume overload is related in part to avid sodium retention by the kidney, which is caused by a complex interaction between decreased cardiac output, neurohormonal activation, and impaired renal blood flow. The complex pathophysiology of the expansion of extracellular volume in heart failure has been reviewed in detail elsewhere (1). Importantly, unrecognized hypervolemia is frequently present in nonedematous patients with heart failure and is associated with increased cardiac filling pressures and worse outcomes (2). As discussed below, weight gain due to overweight or obesity is also common in heart failure and may be associated with improved outcomes (3).

Weight loss in patients with heart failure most commonly occurs following initiation or titration of diuretics. In the Framingham Heart Study, weight loss of greater than 4.5 kg in 5 days in response to treatment is a minor criterion for the diagnosis of heart failure (4). More typically, weight loss is used to assess response to therapy (see Chapter 5). Unexplained weight loss can also occur in heart failure, and may be related to an increase in resting metabolic rate of up to 70%, gastrointestinal malabsorption, and/or a general shift towards catabolism. Mechanisms underlying a catabolic shift in heart failure include an increased ratio of catabolic to anabolic steroids, resistance to insulin and growth hormone (5), and elaboration of proinflammatory cytokines such as tumor necrosis factor-alpha and interleukin-1 beta (6). There is also evidence that inflammatory cytokines may depress myocardial contractility, and contribute to ventricular remodeling by stimulating myocyte apoptosis and turnover of the extracellular matrix (7,8). Long-standing, severe heart failure, particularly right ventricular failure, may lead to anorexia as a consequence of hepatic and intestinal congestion, and mesenteric hypoperfusion.

The combination of reduced caloric intake and increased caloric expenditure may lead to a reduction of tissue mass and, in severe cases, to cardiac cachexia. In some patients, the loss of lean body mass may be masked by the accumulation of edema. Hippocrates described this presentation in 400 B.C. as follows: "The flesh is consumed and becomes water…the abdomen fills with water, the feet and legs swell, the shoulders, clavicles, chest and thighs melt away." Cardiac cachexia may occur in up to 15% of patients with chronic heart failure, and is an independent risk factor for mortality (Fig. 1) (9).

In addition to weight loss, there is evidence that vitamin and micronutrient deficiency may contribute to disease progression in heart failure (Table 1) (10). Selective deficiency of selenium, calcium, and thiamine can directly lead to heart

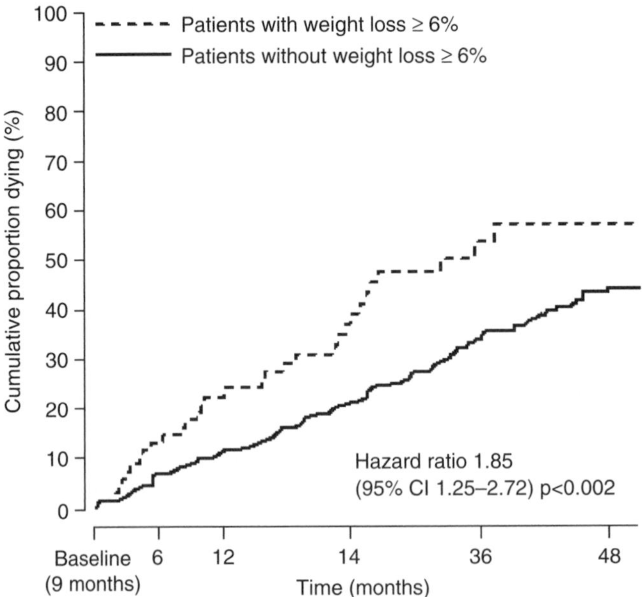

Figure 1 Cumulative risk of death in 619 patients with chronic heart failure in the V-HeFT II study stratified by change in weight at nine months of follow-up. Patients with weight loss greater than or equal to 6% *(dashed line)* had impaired long-term survival compared with patients without weight loss *(solid line),* independent of age, New York Heart Association (NYHA) class, or ejection fraction. *Source*: From Ref. 9.

Table 1 Vitamin and Micronutrient Deficiency in Heart Failure

Deficiency	Clinicopathological manifestations
Micronutrients	
Calcium	QT prolongation, myocardial dysfunction
Magnesium	Proarrhythmia, muscle fatigue, hypokalemia
Zinc	Myocardial oxidative stress, contractile dysfunction
Copper	Mitochondrial impairment, lipoprotein peroxidation
Selenium	Keshan disease, peripartum cardiomyopathy
Vitamins	
A	Increased risk of acute myocardial infarction
B_1	High output heart failure
B_6	Increased risk of CAD and cerebrovascular disease
C	LDL oxidation, endothelial dysfunction
E	Oxidative stress, platelet aggregation

Abbreviations: CAD, coronary artery disease; LDL, low-density lipoprotein.

failure, while deficiency of magnesium, zinc, and copper may contribute to myocardial dysfunction and proarrhythmia. Deficiency of antioxidant vitamins such as ascorbic acid and alpha-tocopherol has been linked experimentally and clinically to myocardial oxidative stress, platelet aggregation, and endothelial dysfunction. Vitamin B_6 deficiency with an associated elevation in homocysteine levels increases the risk for vascular disease, and vitamin A deficiency may increase the risk of acute myocardial infarction. Despite epidemiological data linking vitamin and micronutrient deficiency to cardiovascular disease in general and heart failure in particular, there is no proven role for supplementation.

A related nutraceutical that has received much attention in recent years is co-enzyme Q_{10}. Co-enzyme Q_{10} is an electron carrier in ATP synthesis and is found in high concentrations in myocyte mitochondria. Experimental data suggest that co-enzyme Q_{10} is a powerful antioxidant, and reduced levels in heart failure have been associated with increased mortality. While anecdotal reports and uncontrolled studies (11) of co-enzyme Q_{10} supplementation suggested beneficial effects on exercise tolerance and symptoms in heart failure, randomized, placebo-controlled trials have shown only mild (12) or no (13,14) benefits of co-enzyme Q_{10} on objective measures of cardiac structure and function (Fig. 2).

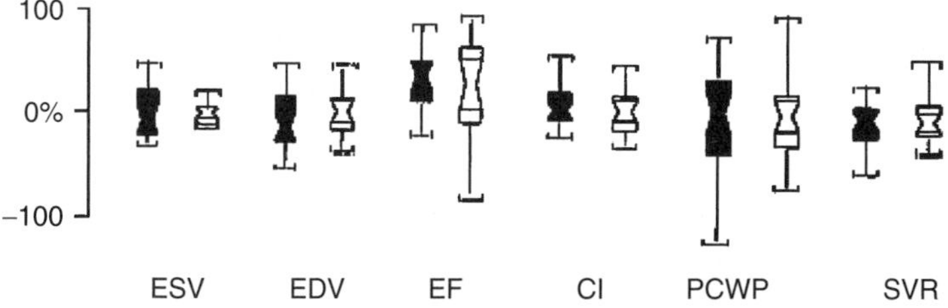

Figure 2 Box and whisker plots showing percent changes from baseline in left ventricular end systolic volume (ESV), end diastolic volume (EDV), ejection fraction (EF), cardiac index (CI), pulmonary capillary wedge pressure (PCWP), and systemic vascular resistance (SVR) during three months of treatment with co-enzyme Q_{10} (*black boxes*) or placebo (*open boxes*) in 30 patients with chronic heart failure. *Source*: From Ref. 14.

DIET

Sodium and Fluid Restriction

Restriction of dietary sodium intake is universally recommended for patients with heart failure. The failure to correctly implement a sodium-restricted diet may diminish the effectiveness of diuretics, aggravate potassium loss, and contribute to acute decompensation in up to 50% of patients. Cody et al. (15) studied 10 patients with severe heart failure who were monitored in a clinical research center on a very low sodium (approximately 200 mg/day) or moderately low sodium (approximately 2000 mg/day) diet. The very low sodium diet was associated with a significant reduction in weight, mean pulmonary artery pressure and mean pulmonary capillary wedge pressure. Other studies have shown that in patients with mild heart failure a high salt diet increases left ventricular volumes, exacerbates the rise in plasma natriuretic peptide levels and decreases daily sodium excretion (16). Additional studies performed in patients with hypertension clearly demonstrate that the level of sodium intake in the diet can have an important effect on hemodynamics and clinical status (17).

The recommended level of sodium restriction is generally based on the severity of heart failure and individual tendency to retain fluid. In patients with asymptomatic left ventricular dysfunction, a judicious restriction of sodium intake to no more than 3500 mg per day is probably useful, although there is no data on the long-term effects of this recommendation. Patients with mild heart failure typically require sodium restriction to less than 3000 mg per day, while those with moderate or severe heart failure will obtain clinical stability only when sodium intake is reduced to less than 2000 mg per day.

Maintaining compliance with sodium restriction can be enhanced by ongoing education and support from a nutritionist or heart failure nurse specialist (see Chapter 28). In addition, patient-oriented reading materials (18) and websites (19) can help reinforce important steps to maintaining a low-sodium diet. Several general principles should be followed. Since a single teaspoon of salt contains approximately 2300 mg of sodium, removing the saltshaker from the dining table and eliminating salt from cooking are important first steps. Patients are encouraged to experiment with no-salt herbs, spices, and seasoning mixes, and to marinate meat, chicken, or fish ahead of time. Second, it is important to recognize that most foods contain sodium naturally, so that it is impossible (nor recommended) to eliminate sodium entirely from the diet. Rather, patients should be taught to adapt preferred foods to low-sodium versions (e.g., low-salt cheese or yogurt), and pick foods naturally low in sodium (e.g., fresh fruits and vegetables, dried beans, or rice). Patients must also learn to read food labels carefully and recognize that total sodium intake can accumulate when eating large quantities of foods with relatively low sodium content. Building in some flexibility and encouraging the patient to take responsibility for this aspect of care can improve compliance.

As with restriction of sodium intake, recommendations regarding fluid restriction should be based on the severity of the underlying disease and tendency to retain fluid. Patients with mild heart failure generally require a fluid restriction of less than 2.5 L per day, while those with more advanced disease should limit fluid intake to less than 2 L per day. Practical suggestions that help with compliance include measuring fluids in a cup before drinking them, using one container such as a water bottle to drink from throughout the day, quenching thirst with gum or sugar free candies, and chilling drinks to make them more refreshing. Patients are taught that if a food melts at room temperature (e.g., ice cream), it should be considered fluid. Free water restriction is strongly recommended for patients with hyponatremia.

Since standard pharmacological therapy for heart failure includes both potassium-sparing [angiotensin-converting enzyme (ACE) inhibitors, aldosterone-receptor blockers] and potassium-wasting (diuretics) agents, careful attention must also be paid to potassium in the diet. Foods high in potassium include avocados, bananas, broccoli, cantaloupe, dried fruits, nuts, potatoes, and tomatoes. In addition, many of the no-salt seasoning substitutes contain significant quantities of potassium.

Alcohol

Recent surveys of U.S. adults suggest that approximately two-thirds of men and one-half of women drink alcohol at least once per month, and that up to 5% of the general population is dependent on alcohol (20). In the Studies of Left Ventricular Dysfunction (SOLVD), 45% of patients with mild-moderate heart failure reported consuming 1 to 14 drinks per week (21); and in the Survival and Ventricular Enlargement (SAVE) study, the baseline prevalence of light-moderate and heavy drinking was 32% and 11%, respectively (22). Despite data from the SOVLD study that demonstrates lower mortality rates among light-to-moderate drinkers compared to nondrinkers, national heart failure guidelines strongly recommend against the use of alcohol (23). These recommendations are based on concerns about the adverse effects of alcohol on cardiac structure and function.

Acute alcohol exposure has been known to cause adverse cardiovascular effects that can exacerbate heart failure (24). Both animal and human studies demonstrate that alcohol exerts negative inotropic effects that are mild and transient, and may be offset by a reduction in afterload. In patients following myocardial infarction, 2 oz of whiskey caused acute reductions in ejection fraction (58% to 56%) and cardiac output (4.5 to 3.8 L/min), while there were no changes in cardiac function in healthy controls (25). Greenberg et al. (26) studied the acute hemodynamic effects of 80 proof vodka (0.9 gm/kg body weight) in patients with advanced heart failure and demonstrated reductions in mean arterial, pulmonary artery and pulmonary capillary wedge pressures and systemic vascular resistance without a change in cardiac index or stroke work index. Chronic exposure to alcohol results in variable reductions in ejection fraction, and, in cases of prolonged heavy use, alcohol may cause a reversible, dilated cardiomyopathy (27).

Despite the known adverse effects of alcohol on cardiac structure and function, retrospective and prospective data suggest that alcohol may have neutral or beneficial effects on long-term outcomes. In a study of 5358 physicians following myocardial infarction, two to six drinks per week was associated with decreased total and cardiovascular mortality (28); and light-to-moderate alcohol use decreased the risk of sudden death in healthy adult men (29). Analysis of the SAVE study demonstrated that the risk of developing heart failure was similar among non-drinkers, light-to-moderate drinkers and heavy drinkers (22). For patients with alcoholic cardiomyopathy, an improvement in ejection fraction may be seen with either abstinence or controlled drinking of up to four drinks per day (Fig. 3) (30). These data have led some heart failure experts to recommend moderation of drinking rather than complete alcohol cessation for patients with symptomatic left ventricular dysfunction (31).

METABOLIC SYNDROME

The Adult Treatment Program III of the National Cholesterol Education Program has defined the metabolic syndrome as the presence of three or more traits that impact on subsequent cardiovascular risk (Table 2) (32,33). A recent national survey found that 22% of adult Americans meet criteria for the metabolic syndrome, and this prevalence has increased over the past five years, particularly in women (34). Major risk factors include

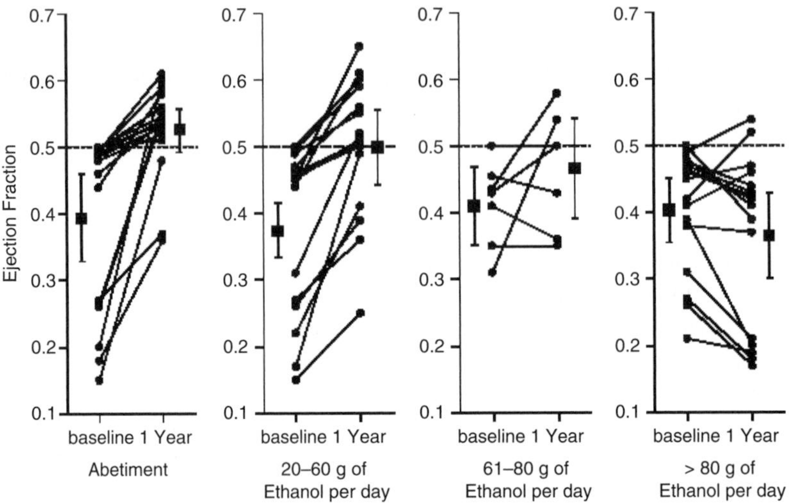

Figure 3 Changes in left ventricular ejection fraction in 55 men with alcoholic cardiomyopathy according to daily ethanol intake during the first year of observation in a prospective cohort study. Patients who abstained from alcohol or drank 20 to 60 g of ethanol per day showed a comparable improvement (0.39 to 0.53 and 0.37 to 0.50, respectively). *Source*: From Ref. 30.

old age, Mexican American race, and increased body weight; smoking and physical inactivity have also been linked to the metabolic syndrome. From a pathophysiological standpoint, the metabolic syndrome is considered a proinflammatory, prothrombotic state that independently predicts the development of diabetes and cardiovascular disease.

Several large, clinical studies have defined an evolving relationship between the metabolic syndrome and heart failure. In a prospective study of patients with acute myocardial infarction, the metabolic syndrome was present in 46%, and was a strong independent predictor of severe heart failure (35). In the Women's Ischemia Syndrome Evaluation study, 25% of women referred for coronary angiography met criteria for the metabolic syndrome; and in patients with angiographically significant CAD, the metabolic syndrome was associated with reduced four-year survival and higher rates of major adverse cardiac events including stroke and heart failure (36). In addition, insulin resistance, which is a major component of the metabolic syndrome, predicts the development of heart failure independent of hypertension or ischemic heart disease (37). Insulin resistance is also common in ambulatory patients with systolic heart failure (38), correlates with disease severity and may be mediated by neurohormonal activation,

Table 2 Criteria for the Metabolic Syndrome

Trait	Diagnostic criteria
Abdominal girth	>35 inches in women, >40 inches in men
HDL cholesterol	<50 mg/dL in women, <40 mg/dL in men
Triglycerides (fasting)	>150 mg/dL
Blood pressure	>130/85 mm Hg
Fasting glucose	≥110 mg/dL

Source: Adapted from Ref. 32.

skeletal myopathy, or endothelial dysfunction (39). Relevant to obese, diabetic patients with heart failure, the metabolic syndrome is associated with the development of chronic kidney disease and sleep-disordered breathing.

Treatment of the metabolic syndrome in heart failure should be directed towards weight loss, lipid management (see chapter 9), and blood pressure control (see chapter 6). For patients who are overweight (body mass index 25 to 30 kg per m^2), a balanced-caloric diet of 1500 to 2000 calories per day is an important first step towards healthy weight loss. For obese patients, a low-calorie liquid diet (500 to 1200 calories per day) may lead to significant and rapid weight loss but requires physician supervision and is relatively contraindicated in patients with moderate to severe heart failure due to fluid and electrolyte shifts. Long-term maintenance of dietary weight loss is enhanced with behavioral modification and exercise. Appetite suppressants are generally contraindicated in patients with heart failure due to adverse effects of excess adrenergic stimulation. An exception to this may be rimonabant, a cannabanoid-receptor antagonist without cardiac toxicity that causes sustained weight loss, improves lipid parameters, and may reverse the metabolic syndrome (40). Preliminary data also shows that rimonabant reduces body weight and improves glycemic control in patients with type II diabetes. Orlistat, an inhibitor of gastrointestinal lipase, may induce weight loss and improve symptoms in heart failure patients but is limited by side effects such as flatulence and oily stools (41). The role of bariatric surgery is discussed below.

OBESITY

Epidemiology and Prognosis

Recent estimates of obesity prevalence among US adults suggest that one in two Americans is overweight or obese as defined by a body mass index (BMI) ≥ 25 kg per m^2 (42). In addition, obesity incidence continues to rise such that the prevalence of marked obesity (BMI ≥ 40 kg per m^2) has nearly tripled between 1990 and 2000. As these trends in obesity continue, cardiovascular specialists will encounter a rising rate of obesity-related cardiovascular disorders, including hypertension, left ventricular hypertrophy, and heart failure (43). Several cross-sectional studies have shown that measures of body size and adiposity are independently associated with left ventricular mass (44–47), and that an increase in left ventricular mass in youth predicts a greater likelihood of subsequent cardiovascular disease (48).

Despite these observations, it remains uncertain whether obesity is an independent risk factor for heart failure among the majority of adults who have other comorbidities associated with left ventricular dysfunction. In the Framingham Heart Study, approximately 6000 patients were followed for the development of heart failure over a mean follow-up period of 14 years (49). Multivariate analyses demonstrated an overall two-fold increase in incident heart failure cases among participants with a BMI ≥ 30 kg per m^2 versus individuals with a normal BMI independent of other cardiovascular risk factors (Fig. 4). The estimated risk increase associated with a 1-kg per m^2 increment in BMI was 7% and 5% in women and men, respectively.

Although obesity is a risk factor for the development of heart failure, obese patients appear to have a better prognosis than non-obese patients with symptomatic left ventricular dysfunction (so-called "obesity paradox") (Fig. 5) (3). To assess the influence of body weight on survival in heart failure, Davos et al. (50) divided 589 non-cachectic heart failure patients into quintiles of BMI. Survival was greatest in the fourth quintile, with a relative risk of death of 0.91. Horwich et al. (51) also evaluated obesity and

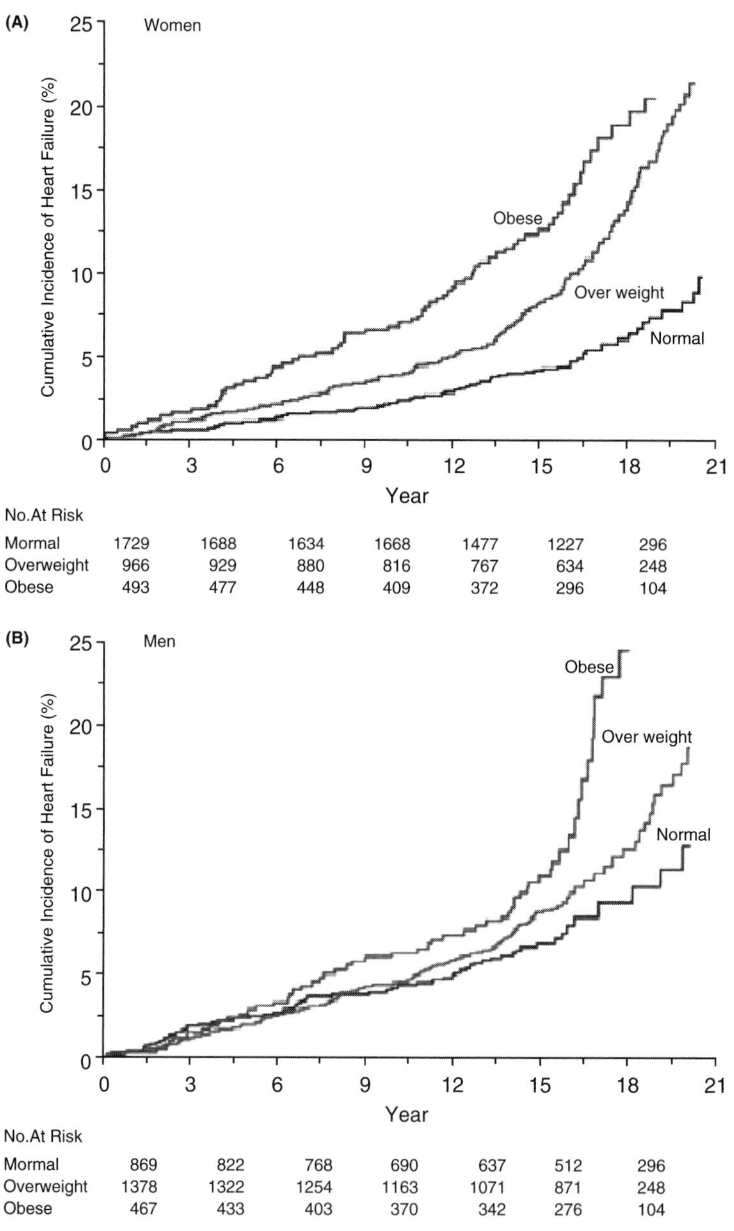

Figure 4 Cumulative incidence of heart failure according to category of body mass index (BMI) at baseline examination in the Framingham Heart Study. The BMI was 18.5 to 24.0 in normal subjects, 25.0 to 29.9 in overweight subjects, and 30.0 or more in obese subjects. *Source*: From Ref. 49.

mortality in 1200 patients with advanced heart failure divided into quartiles by weight. While the obese and overweight groups had higher rates of hypertension and diabetes, there was no difference in survival rates for the four BMI groups. Rather, a higher BMI was associated with a trend towards improved survival. In a study of less symptomatic patients, Lavie et al. (52) demonstrated that subjects with subsequent events had significantly lower body weight compared with event-free survivors.

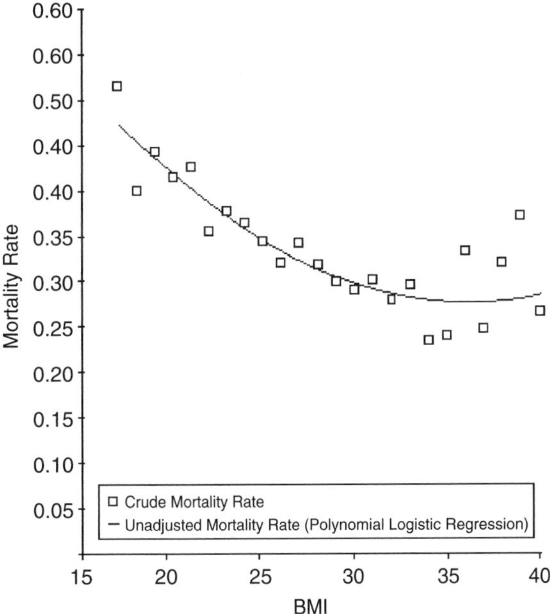

Figure 5 Association between body mass index (BMI) as a continuous variable and unadjusted all-cause mortality in 7767 patients with stable heart failure enrolled in the Digitalis Investigative Group trial. Each point represents the mortality rate associated with a BMI integer. *Source*: From Ref. 3.

The mechanisms underlying the "obesity paradox" in heart failure remain unclear, and recommendations for weight loss derived from the general population may not be appropriate in patients with heart failure. Lower body weight may represent a relative catabolic state in which an increase in proinflammatory cytokines causes myocardial depression and ventricular remodeling (7). In addition, obese patients may have less neurohormonal activation and increased nutritional or metabolic reserves compared with non-obese patients. An alternative explanation is that increased cardiac output and metabolic demands may lead to earlier diagnosis of heart failure in obese patients (e.g., lead-time bias) or that obese patients have less severe myocardial dysfunction than non-obese controls.

Pathophysiology

Clinical Factors

The pathophysiology of heart failure in obesity is complex and involves several hemodynamic, neurohormonal and clinicopathologic features (Fig. 6). Hemodynamic studies of morbidly obese subjects demonstrate relative volume expansion with increased total circulating blood volume, stroke volume, and cardiac output but typically normal cardiac index after taking into account increased body surface area (53,54). In a right heart catheterization study of 10 obese subjects without heart failure or confounding risk factors, such as diabetes and hypertension, de Divitiis et al. (53) demonstrated increased cardiac output and stroke volume. Ventricular end-diastolic pressures and atrial pressures ranged from normal to high and correlated with body weight. Measures of left ventricular

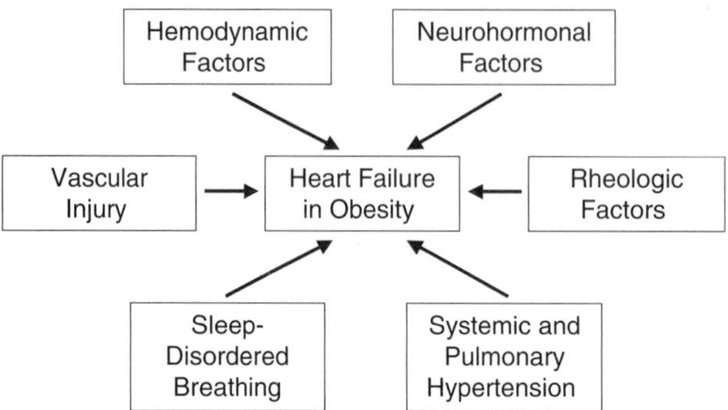

Figure 6 Clinical and pathophysiologic factors contributing to the development of heart failure in obesity.

function, such as the ratio of stroke work index to left ventricular end-diastolic pressure, were reduced and correlated inversely with the degree of obesity. A study using radionuclide angiography showed similar results: compared with lean subjects, overweight and moderately obese individuals had increased cardiac output, stroke volume, end-systolic volume, total blood volume, and total plasma volume with decreased ejection fraction (55).

Non-invasive studies have also explored the relationship among obesity, left ventricular mass, and hemodynamics. In the Hypertension Genetic Epidemiology Network Study, 1577 non-diabetic hypertensive subjects underwent assessment of cardiac structure and function by echocardiography and free-fat mass by bioimpadance (56). Free-fat mass increased in relation to weight, and correlated positively with stroke volume and cardiac output and inversely with total peripheral resistance. In addition, increased free-fat mass was directly related to left ventricular mass. In the Framingham Heart Study, BMI was a strong independent predictor of left ventricular chamber dilation (57) and hypertrophy (58) in both men and women, with hypertension having an additive effect on ventricular remodeling.

Neurohormonal factors may also play an important role linking obesity to heart failure. Activation of the sympathetic nervous and renin-angiotensin-aldosterone systems are characteristic of obese hypertensive patients and play an important role in ventricular and vascular remodeling in heart failure (59). Alterations in blood rheology due to neurohormonal activation, including increased blood viscosity, hematocrit, and fibrinogen may exert additional stress on the myocardium (60,61). Other contributors to left ventricular dysfunction include vascular injury potentiated by an atherogenic lipid profile and coronary arteriopathy (62), and insulin resistance, which may stimulate myocardial hypertrophy through activation of insulin-like growth factor-1 receptors (63).

In the United States the most common etiology of dilated cardiomyopathy is ischemic heart disease, and obesity is a well-recognized risk factor for coronary atherosclerosis (64). Obesity is also associated with known risk factors for ischemic heart disease including hypertension, dyslipidemia, and diabetes. In patients without atherosclerosis, hypertension and diabetes are independent risk factors for the development of dilated cardiomyopathy. In particular, elevated glucose levels may cause accumulation of advanced glycosylation end products, LDL oxidation, endothelial dysfunction, and myocardial oxidative stress (65). Echocardiographic assessment of children and adolescents with type I diabetes demonstrates sub-clinical abnormalities in cardiac structure and function, including left ventricular dilation and impaired relaxation (66). In adult studies, glucose intolerance is directly related to the development of left ventricular hypertrophy (67) and the risk of new onset heart failure (68). Other clinical features linking obesity and the development or progression of heart failure include increased dietary sodium intake (69) and obstructive sleep apnea (70).

Pathologic studies have also demonstrated an adverse effect of obesity on ventricular size and coronary anatomy. In a postmortem study of 12 patients weighing more than 300 pounds, the heart weight and right ventricular size were increased in all subjects, and the left ventricle was enlarged in 11 of 12 (71). Although only two patients had one or more coronary arteries narrowed by greater than 75%, virtually all patients had some degree of early arteriosclerosis. With regard to the existence of a distinct cardiomyopathy of obesity, additional evidence derives from a clinicopathological study of 43 markedly obese patients with heart failure (72). Compared to 409 non-obese patients with heart failure, obese subjects had higher filling pressures and cardiac output, and were more likely to have a final diagnosis of idiopathic dilated cardiomyopathy. Mild myocyte hypertrophy was the most common finding on endomyocardial biopsy.

Basic Mechanisms

Obesity is associated with increased plasma levels of leptin, and hyperleptinemia has been linked with the development and/or progression of heart failure (73). In vitro studies using isolated myocytes (74) or perfused hearts (75) demonstrate that acute leptin exposure exerts growth-promoting effects on the myocardium and causes mechanoenergetic uncoupling. Chronic exposure of myocytes to leptin impairs basal and stimulated contractile function and slows relaxation (76). Intact animal studies also support a pathophysiologic link between hyperleptinemia and heart failure that is mediated in part by activation of the sympathetic nervous system (77). The mechanisms underlying the direct myocardial depressant effects of leptin remain unclear, although increased production of myocardial nitric oxide synthase (78,79) and activation of cardiac fatty acid oxidation may play important roles.

Experimental models of hypertension and diabetes also provide evidence linking obesity and heart failure. Isolated myocytes from hypertensive (80) or pre-diabetic (81) rats with obesity demonstrate impaired contractile function and prolonged relaxation. Furthermore, mouse models of diabetic cardiomyopathy are characterized by increased myocardial fatty acid oxidation, decreased glucose uptake and oxidation (82), activation of apoptosis, and accumulation of intramyocyte lipid (83). Genetic markers of hypertrophic growth and cardiac remodeling are turned on in these models.

Clinical clues linking obesity and cardiomyopathy have also been described. In non-obese subjects, elevated plasma leptin levels are associated with increased sympathetic tone and abnormal baroreceptor function (84). In hypertensive patients, hyperleptinemia is associated with increased heart rate (85) and blood pressure (86), left ventricular hypertrophy (87) and impaired relaxation (88). While the stimuli for increased leptin production in obesity remain unclear, endothelin-1 has been implicated. Plasma endothelin-1 levels are elevated in patients with heart failure in relation to disease severity, and have been shown to stimulate leptin secretion by adipose tissue (89).

Diagnostic Considerations

The clinical evaluation of heart failure is difficult in the obese patient due to body habitus and the presence of comorbidities. Symptoms such as fatigue and weakness are frequently present but are non-specific and may be due to obesity rather than to decreased cardiac output. Symptoms of left-sided congestion such as shortness of breath are also difficult to sort out in the obese patient. Exertional dyspnea is a common complaint, and orthopnea and paroxysmal nocturnal dyspnea may be due to chronic obstructive pulmonary disease, gastroesophageal reflux, or sleep apnea. Right-sided congestive symptoms such as bloating, right upper quadrant pain and lower extremity edema are common in obesity. Jugular venous distention may be difficult to visualize in patients with short, thick necks, while assessment of hepatomegaly may be limited by body habitus. Venous stasis or prior episodes of thrombophlebitis may complicate the assessment of lower extremity edema, while truncal obesity may limit palpation of the cardiac impulse and auscultation for gallops and murmurs. Similarly, examination of the lungs is relatively insensitive due to hypoventilation and excess soft tissue.

While B-type natriuretic peptide levels have been proposed as a surrogate marker for volume status in heart failure (90), they are lower in obese patients (Fig. 7) and may be falsely normal in severely obese patients with marked volume overload (91,92).

Given the limited reliability of the history and physical examination for assessing heart failure in obesity, clinicians must rely on non-invasive imaging for patient management. The chest x-ray may support the diagnosis of heart failure when there is cardiomegaly, evidence of pulmonary venous hypertension, or both. Pleural effusions may be differentiated from atelectasis or elevated diaphragms, while non-cardiac causes of dyspnea such as chronic obstructive pulmonary disease may be ruled out. Enlargement of the main pulmonary artery and right ventricle with tapering of the peripheral pulmonary vasculature may suggest pulmonary hypertension secondary to chronic left ventricular failure, sleep apnea, or hypoventilation.

The echocardiogram is a relatively sensitive and specific tool to evaluate heart failure in obese subjects. Transthoracic echocardiography can define chamber size and function, identify abnormal valvular structure and function, and estimate pulmonary artery systolic pressure. Newer techniques such as tissue Doppler or strain rate imaging can be used to assess diastolic function and estimate left ventricular filling pressure (93). For obese patients in whom acoustic windows are limited, transesophageal echocardiography may be performed to assess cardiac structure and function, although respiratory status must be

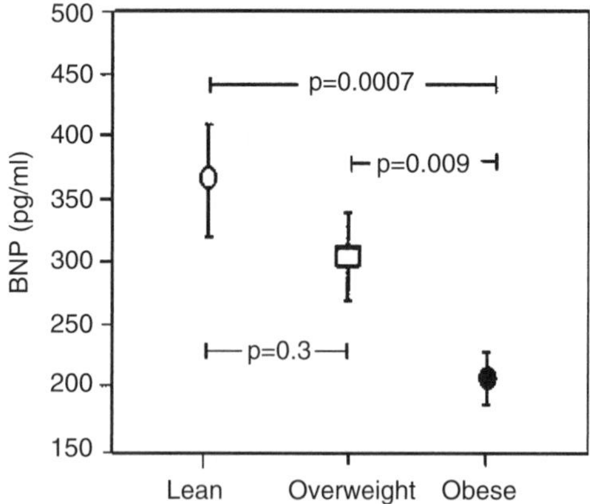

Figure 7 B-type natriuretic peptide levels in 318 patients with heart failure were significantly lower in obese patients (BMI ≥ 30 kg per m^2) compared to overweight (BMI ≥ 25 to 29 kg per m^2) or lean (BMI < 25 kg per m^2) patients. *Abbreviation*: BNP, B-type natriuretic peptide. *Source*: From Ref. 92.

monitored closely. Alternative imaging techniques include cardiac magnetic resonance (MRI) and positron emission tomography, assuming that the patient meets the weight limits of the exam table and, in the case of MRI, does not have an implantable device.

Treatment of Obesity

Several studies suggest that weight loss may be an important intervention for regression of left ventricular hypertrophy and prevention of heart failure in obesity. Case reports of extreme weight loss induced by biliopancreatic diversion have demonstrated near normalization of cardiac structure and function (94,95). Alpert et al. (96) performed echocardiograms on obese patients before and following bariatric surgery and found that weight loss was associated with reductions in left ventricular chamber size, wall stress, and mass, and with an improvement in diastolic function. In an observational study of patients undergoing gastroplasty compared with controls treated with diet alone, weight loss following surgery correlated with LVH regression independent of reduction in blood pressure (97). Conventional weight reduction through intensive diet and exercise has also been shown to reduce left ventricular mass (98).

While LVH regression is associated with improved outcomes in hypertensive patients (99), there are no data demonstrating reduced cardiovascular events with sustained weight loss in obese patients with LVH. This may be due to the difficulty in maintaining weight loss in this population or the lack of long-term outcomes data among obese patients undergoing bariatric surgery. In addition, there are serious risks associated with bariatric surgery, including pulmonary embolism and respiratory failure, which may be increased in obese patients with LVH, heart failure, or both (100).

Treatment of Heart Failure

Patients with obesity and heart failure should be treated with pharmacologic therapy as recommended by American College of Cardiology/American Heart Association guidelines (23). If clinical evaluation suggests fluid retention, standard loop diuretics should be administered to decrease intra- and extravascular volume (see chapter 5) (101). Given the limitations of the physical exam and chest x-ray for assessing volume status in obese patients, endpoints for therapy include the development of prerenal azotemia or other evidence of excess diuresis such as lightheadedness, postural hypotension, or excessive thirst. Careful attention should be given to electrolyte repletion and adjustment of vasodilators as dictated by orthostatic vital signs. Potassium-sparing diuretics may be added to loop diuretics to lessen the need for potassium repletion and decrease the risk of arrhythmia. In addition, aldosterone receptor blockade has been shown to reduce morbidity and mortality in patients with post-myocardial infarction left ventricular dysfunction or advanced heart failure (102,103).

Both ACE inhibitors and angiotensin receptor blockers (ARBs) improve the prognosis of patients with heart failure and reduced ejection fraction (31,104). While current guidelines state that ACE inhibitors should be used over ARBs, unless the patient is intolerant due to cough or angioedema, recent data from the Candesartan in Heart Failure Reduction in Mortality (CHARM) (104) and Valsartan in Acute Myocardial Infarction (VALIANT) (105) studies suggest equal efficacy of ACE inhibitors and ARBs in reducing morbidity and mortality in heart failure. Further reduction in events, heart failure hospitalizations in particular, may be gained by adding an ARB on top of an ACE inhibitor (106,107). Antagonists of the renin-angiotensin-aldosterone system should be titrated to doses demonstrated to be clinically effective in randomized controlled trials (108). However, achieving target doses may be limited by the development of hypotension, worsening renal function and/or hyperkalemia (109).

The combination of hydralazine and isosorbide dinatrate is indicated as alternative vasodilator therapy in patients who are intolerant to ACE inhibition or angiotensin receptor blockade. In the African-American Heart Failure Trial (A-HeFT), hydralazine and nitrates improved survival in black patients with advanced heart failure when added to standard therapy with neurohormonal antagonists (110).

Beta-blockers reverse ventricular remodeling, decrease the risk of sudden death and heart failure hospitalizations, and prolong survival in heart failure (see chapter 7) (111). Carvedilol and metoprolol CR/XL are currently approved for the treatment of heart failure and have similar beneficial effects on outcomes (112,113). The choice of an agent should be individualized. Metoprolol CR/XL, a beta-1-selective blocker, is dosed once daily and may be preferable in patients with reactive airways disease or for improved compliance. Alternatively, due to its favorable effects on insulin sensitivity and lipid metabolism, treatment with carvedilol, a non-selective beta-blocker with alpha-blocking properties may be preferred among insulin resistant patients with dyslipidemia (114,115). In a large study of patients with type II diabetes and hypertension, treatment with carvedilol was associated with stable hemoglobin A1c, improved insulin sensitivity and decreased progression to microalbuminuria compared to metoprolol (116).

Digitalis is approved as adjunctive therapy for patients who remain symptomatic despite ACE inhibitor, beta-blocker, and diuretic therapy (see chapter 8). In the Digitalis Investigation Group (DIG) trial, digoxin had no effect on survival but reduced the rate of hospitalization both overall and for worsening heart failure (117). However, a subsequent analysis from the DIG trial demonstrated that increased serum digoxin levels may have an adverse effect on survival (118). In obese patients, digoxin doses less than or equal to 0.25 mg per day should be administered with a target serum digoxin level range of 0.5 to 0.8 ng/mL. Decreased doses should be used in the setting of worsening renal function or following the addition of amiodarone.

Treatment of Comorbidities

Diabetes

Obesity is a strong, independent risk factor for the development of diabetes in children (119) and adults (120), and important considerations must be given to the treatment of diabetes in overweight and obese patients with heart failure. Diet and exercise are important non-pharmacologic measures to improve insulin sensitivity in type II diabetes, and exert beneficial effects in heart failure. Thiazolidinediones (TZDs) have important ancillary effects on lipid metabolism, endothelial function, and inflammatory cytokines (121), but should be used cautiously as they increase intravascular volume by 6%–7%. Edema is usually peripheral rather than central, is exacerbated by concomitant administration of insulin, and usually resolves upon drug withdrawal (122). While concerns about exacerbating heart failure have led to United States Food and Drug Administration warnings against the use of TZDs in patients with NYHA class III or IV heart failure, preliminary data in diabetic patients show that rosiglitazone had no adverse effect on cardiac structure or function over one year (123). Metformin, another popular insulin sensitizer, is associated with a low risk of life-threatening lactic acidosis and is contraindicated in patients with "heart failure requiring pharmacologic therapy." Despite cautionary alerts, nearly one-fourth of Medicare beneficiaries with heart failure are treated with either a TZD or metformin (124).

Dyslipidemia

Dyslipidemia is common in patients with obesity and heart failure, and all patients should be managed according to the National Cholesterol Education Program Adult Treatment Panel III guidelines (125). For patients with ischemic heart disease and elevated low-density lipoprotein levels, statins represent first-line therapy (see chapter 9). Retrospective data suggests that statins improve survival in patients with ischemic and non-ischemic heart failure regardless of the presence of obesity (126). In patients with the metabolic syndrome, it is important to remember that statins will not necessarily correct abnormalities of high-densitiy lipoprotein and triglycerides. Hypothyroidism should be ruled out, and the addition of niacin or fibric acid should be considered. A diet low in saturated fat and cholesterol and regular exercise (see chapter 4) are additional components of lipid management in heart failure patients with the metabolic syndrome.

Sleep Apnea

Recent studies suggest that at least 50% of patients with heart failure have sleep apnea (see chapter 17) (70), and screening is therefore strongly recommended in obese patients. Obstructive sleep apnea (OSA) occurs in the setting of fat accumulation in the pharynx and luminal narrowing that results in hypoventilation (70). Among heart failure patients, the prevalence of OSA ranges from 11% to 37% (127,128). Central sleep apnea (CSA) develops as a consequence of heart failure where pulmonary congestion and periodic arousals stimulate hyperventilation and hypocapnea triggering a central apnea (129). Sleep apnea may also contribute to heart failure progression through hypoxia, adrenergic stimulation, and loss of vagal tone. Treatment of OSA with nocturnal continuous airway pressure (CPAP) improves sleep architecture, reduces daytime blood pressure, and enhances cardiac function (130). The role of CPAP in CSA remains unclear, although a Canadian trial failed to demonstrate reduced morbidity and mortality (131).

Venous Thromboembolism

Obesity and heart failure are significant risk factors for deep venous thrombosis (DVT) and pulmonary embolism (PE) (132). Screening for DVT/PE is indicated when patients present with unilateral or asymmetric bilateral lower extremity edema, pleuritic chest pain, increased shortness of breath, and/or presyncope. Diagnostic studies include plasma D-dimer levels, lower extremity venous ultrasound, and high-resolution chest CT (133). Transthoracic echocardiograph and B-type natriuretic peptide levels may be used for risk stratification of acute PE (134). Obese patients with dyspnea on exertion out of proportion to findings of heart failure should be evaluated for chronic recurrent pulmonary emboli. Hospitalized patients should be prophylaxed against thromboembolic complications with low-molecular-weight heparin.

TRANSPLANT CONSIDERATIONS

Pre-transplant cachexia and morbid obesity predict worse outcomes after cardiac transplant. In an analysis of 4515 patients in the Cardiac Transplant Research Database, percent ideal body weight $<80\%$ or $>140\%$ was a risk factor for increased mortality post-transplant (135). In men and women under age 55, obesity was also associated with infection but not with acute rejection or cardiac allograft vasculopath. In a retrospective, single-center study of 474 transplant patients, morbidly obese (BMI >30 kg per m^2) and cachectic (BMI <20 kg per m^2) recipients had 30-day mortality rates of 12.7% and 17.7%, respectively, compared with 7.6% in normal or overweight patients (136). The development of cardiac cachexia while awaiting cardiac transplant, particularly in patients who are inotrope-dependent, is a relative indication for mechanical cardiac assist. Nutritional status should be followed closely with daily calorie counts and serial measurement of serum pre-albumin levels.

Obese patients with heart failure are often followed for longer periods of time before they are considered suitable candidates for cardiac transplant. This delay is due in part to the difficulty in distinguishing signs and symptoms of heart failure from those related to obesity, as well as, to concerns related to impaired post-transplant survival. Cardiopulmonary exercise testing and right heart catheterization can be used to risk stratify potential transplant candidates by providing objective measures of peak functional capacity and hemodynamics, respectively. Once listed for transplant, obese patients may have trouble finding a suitable donor matched for body weight. For patients who develop progressive cardiac failure despite inotropic support, mechanical cardiac assist has been used successfully as a bridge to cardiac transplant (see chapter 23). While obesity, is not associated with impaired survival in ventricular assist device patients, the risk of reoperation and renal dysfunction is higher (137).

In addition to impaired survival, retrospective studies demonstrate that transplant recipients who are obese experience decreased quality of life (138) after heart transplant. Problems related to obesity, including sleep apnea (139) and diabetes, are further exacerbated by additional weight gain due to corticosteroid use.

REFERENCES

1. Schrier RW, Abraham WT. Hormones and hemodynamics in heart failure. N Engl J Med 1999; 341:577–585.
2. Androne AS, Hryniewicz K, Hudaihed A, et al. Relation of unrecognized hypervolemia in chronic heart failure to clinical status, hemodynamics, and patient outcomes. Am J Cardiol 2004; 93:1254–1259.
3. Curtis JP, Selter JG, Wang Y, et al. The obesity paradox: body mass index and outcomes in patients with heart failure. Arch Intern Med 2005; 165:55–61.
4. Ho KK, Pinsky JL, Kannel WB, et al. The epidemiology of heart failure: the Framingham Study. J Am Coll Cardiol 1993; 22:6A–13A.
5. Anker SD, Chua TP, Ponikowski P, et al. Hormonal changes and catabolic/anabolic imbalance in chronic heart failure and their importance for cardiac cachexia. Circulation 1997; 96:526–534.
6. Torre-Amione G, Kapadia S, Benedict C, et al. Proinflammatory cytokine levels in patients with depressed left ventricular ejection fraction: a report from the studies of left ventricular dysfunction (SOLVD). J Am Coll Cardiol 1996; 27:1201–1206.
7. Feldman AM, Combes A, Wagner D, et al. The role of tumor necrosis factor in the pathophysiology of heart failure. J Am Coll Cardiol 2000; 35:537–544.
8. Mann DL, Spinale FG. Activation of matrix metalloproteinases in the failing human heart: breaking the tie that binds. Circulation 1998; 98:1699–1702.
9. Anker SD, Negassa A, Coats AJ, et al. Prognostic importance of weight loss in chronic heart failure and the effect of treatment with angiotensin-converting-enzyme inhibitors: an observational study. Lancet 2003; 361:1077–1083.

10. Witte KK, Clark AL, Cleland JG. Chronic heart failure and micronutrients. J Am Coll Cardiol 2001; 37:1765–1774.
11. Langsjoen PH, Folkers K. Long-term efficacy and safety of coenzyme Q10 therapy for idiopathic dilated cardiomyopathy. Am J Cardiol 1990; 65:521–523.
12. Hofman-Bang C, Rehnqvist N, Swedberg K, et al. Coenzyme Q10 as an adjunctive in the treatment of chronic congestive heart failure. The Q10 Study Group. J Card Fail 1995; 1:101–107.
13. Khatta M, Alexander BS, Krichten CM, et al. The effect of coenzyme Q10 in patients with congestive heart failure. Ann Intern Med 2000; 132:636–640.
14. Watson PS, Scalia GM, Galbraith A, et al. Lack of effect of coenzyme Q on left ventricular function in patients with congestive heart failure. J Am Coll Cardiol 1999; 33:1549–1552.
15. Cody RJ, Covit AB, Schaer GL, et al. Sodium and water balance in chronic congestive heart failure. J Clin Invest 1986; 77:1441–1452.
16. Volpe M, Tritto C, DeLuca N, et al. Abnormalities of sodium handling and of cardiovascular adaptations during high salt diet in patients with mild heart failure. Circulation 1993; 88:1620–1627.
17. Muntzel M, Drueke T. A comprehensive review of the salt and blood pressure relationship. Am J Hypertens 1992; 5:1S–42S.
18. Gazzaniga DA, Fowler MB. The No-Salt, Lowest-Sodium Cookbook: Hundreds of Creative Recipes Created to Combat Congestive Heart Failure and Dangerous Hypertension. Irvine: Griffin, 2002.
19. www.hfsa.org 2006.
20. Grant BF, Dawson DA, Stinson FS, et al. The 12-month prevalence and trends in DSM-IV alcohol abuse and dependence: United States, 1991–1992 and 2001–2002. Drug Alcohol Depend 2004; 74:223–234.
21. Cooper HA, Exner DV, Domanski MJ. Light-to-moderate alcohol consumption and prognosis in patients with left ventricular systolic dysfunction. J Am Coll Cardiol 2000; 35:1753–1759.
22. Aguilar D, Skali H, Moye LA, et al. Alcohol consumption and prognosis in patients with left ventricular systolic dysfunction after a myocardial infarction. J Am Coll Cardiol 2004; 43:2015–2021.
23. Hunt SA, Abraham WT, Chin MH, et al. ACC/AHA 2005 guideline update for the diagnosis and management of chronic heart failure in the adult: a report of the American College of Cardiology/American Heart Association Task Force on Practice Guidelines (Writing Committee to Update the 2001 Guidelines for the Evaluation and Management of Heart Failure): developed in collaboration with the American College of Chest Physicians and the International Society for Heart and Lung Transplation, endorsed by the Heart Rhythm Society. Circulation 2005; 104:e154–e235.
24. Piano MR. Alcohol and heart failure. J Card Fail 2002; 8:239–246.
25. Gould L, Gopalaswamy C, Yang D, et al. Effect of oral alcohol on left ventricular ejection fraction, volumes, and segmental wall motion in normals and in patients with recent myocardial infarction. Clin Cardiol 1985; 8:576–582.
26. Greenberg BH, Schutz R, Grunkemeier GL, et al. Acute effects of alcohol in patients with congestive heart failure. Ann Intern Med 1982; 97:171–175.
27. Urbano-Marquez A, Estruch R, Navarro-Lopez F, et al. The effects of alcoholism on skeletal and cardiac muscle. N Engl J Med 1989; 320:409–415.
28. Muntwyler J, Hennekens CH, Buring JE, et al. Mortality and light to moderate alcohol consumption after myocardial infarction. Lancet 1998; 352:1882–1885.
29. Albert CM, Manson JE, Cook NR, et al. Moderate alcohol consumption and the risk of sudden cardiac death among US male physicians. Circulation 1999; 100:944–950.
30. Nicolas JM, Fernandez-Sola J, Estruch R, et al. The effect of controlled drinking in alcoholic cardiomyopathy. Ann Intern Med 2002; 136:192–200.
31. Jessup M, Brozena S. Heart failure. N Engl J Med 2003; 348:2007–2018.

32. Wilson PW, Grundy SM. The metabolic syndrome: practical guide to origins and treatment: part I. Circulation 2003; 108:1422–1424.
33. Wilson PW, Grundy SM. The metabolic syndrome: a practical guide to origins and treatment: part II. Circulation 2003; 108:1537–1540.
34. Ford ES, Giles WH, Dietz WH. Prevalence of the metabolic syndrome among US adults: findings from the third National Health and Nutrition Examination Survey. JAMA 2002; 287:356–359.
35. Zeller M, Steg PG, Ravisy J, et al. Prevalence and impact of metabolic syndrome on hospital outcomes in acute myocardial infarction. Arch Intern Med 2005; 165:1192–1198.
36. Marroquin OC, Kip KE, Kelley DE, et al. Metabolic syndrome modifies the cardiovascular risk associated with angiographic coronary artery disease in women: a report from the Women's Ischemia Syndrome Evaluation. Circulation 2004; 109:714–721.
37. Arnlov J, Lind L, Zethelius B, et al. Several factors associated with the insulin resistance syndrome are predictors of left ventricular systolic dysfunction in a male population after 20 years of follow-up. Am Heart J 2001; 142:720–724.
38. Swan JW, Anker SD, Walton C, et al. Insulin resistance in chronic heart failure: relation to severity and etiology of heart failure. J Am Coll Cardiol 1997; 30:527–532.
39. Coats AJ, Anker SD. Insulin resistance in chronic heart failure. J Cardiovasc Pharmacol 2000; 35:S9–S14.
40. Poirier B, Bidouard JP, Cadrouvele C, et al. The anti-obesity effect of rimonabant is associated with an improved serum lipid profile. Diabetes Obes Metab 2005; 7:65–72.
41. Beck-da-Silva L, Higginson L, Fraser M, et al. Effect of orlistat in obese patients with heart failure: a pilot study. Congest Heart Fail 2005; 11:118–123.
42. Freedman DS, Khan LK, Serdula MK, et al. Trends and correlates of class 3 obesity in the United States from 1990 through 2000. JAMA 2002; 288:1758–1761.
43. Olshansky SJ, Passaro DJ, Hershow RC, et al. A potential decline in life expectancy in the United States in the 21st century. N Engl J Med 2005; 352:1138–1145.
44. Verhaaren HA, Schieken RM, Mosteller M, et al. Bivariate genetic analysis of left ventricular mass and weight in pubertal twins (the Medical College of Virginia twin study). Am J Cardiol 1991; 68:661–668.
45. Goble MM, Mosteller M, Moskowitz WB, et al. Sex differences in the determinants of left ventricular mass in childhood. The Medical College of Virginia Twin Study. Circulation 1992; 85:1661–1665.
46. Malcolm DD, Burns TL, Mahoney LT, et al. Factors affecting left ventricular mass in childhood: the Muscatine Study. Pediatrics 1993; 92:703–709.
47. Daniels SR, Meyer RA, Liang YC, et al. Echocardiographically determined left ventricular mass index in normal children, adolescents and young adults. J Am Coll Cardiol 1988; 12:703–708.
48. Mahoney LT, Schieken RM, Clarke WR, et al. Left ventricular mass and exercise responses predict future blood pressure. The Muscatine Study. Hypertension 1988; 12:206–213.
49. Kenchaiah S, Evans JC, Levy D, et al. Obesity and the risk of heart failure. N Engl J Med 2002; 347:305–313.
50. Davos CH, Doehner W, Rauchhaus M, et al. Body mass and survival in patients with chronic heart failure without cachexia: the importance of obesity. J Card Fail 2003; 9:29–35.
51. Horwich TB, Fonarow GC, Hamilton MA, et al. The relationship between obesity and mortality in patients with heart failure. J Am Coll Cardiol 2001; 38:789–795.
52. Lavie CJ, Osman AF, Milani RV, et al. Body composition and prognosis in chronic systolic heart failure: the obesity paradox. Am J Cardiol 2003; 91:891–894.
53. de Divitiis O, Fazio S, Petitto M, et al. Obesity and cardiac function. Circulation 1981; 64:477–482.
54. Kaltman AJ, Goldring RM. Role of circulatory congestion in the cardiorespiratory failure of obesity. Am J Med 1976; 60:645–653.
55. Licata G, Scaglione R, Barbagallo M, et al. Effect of obesity on left ventricular function studied by radionuclide angiocardiography. Int J Obes 1991; 15:295–302.

56. Palmieri V, de Simone G, Arnett DK, et al. Relation of various degrees of body mass index in patients with systemic hypertension to left ventricular mass, cardiac output, and peripheral resistance (The Hypertension Genetic Epidemiology Network Study). Am J Cardiol 2001; 88:1163–1168.
57. Lauer MS, Anderson KM, Levy D. Separate and joint influences of obesity and mild hypertension on left ventricular mass and geometry: the Framingham Heart Study. J Am Coll Cardiol 1992; 19:130–134.
58. Lauer MS, Anderson KM, Levy D. Influence of contemporary versus 30-year blood pressure levels on left ventricular mass and geometry: the Framingham Heart Study. J Am Coll Cardiol 1991; 18:1287–1294.
59. Ward KD, Sparrow D, Landsberg L, et al. Influence of insulin, sympathetic nervous system activity, and obesity on blood pressure: the Normative Aging Study. J Hypertens 1996; 14:301–308.
60. Carroll S, Cooke CB, Butterly RJ. Plasma viscosity, fibrinogen and the metabolic syndrome: effect of obesity and cardiorespiratory fitness. Blood Coagul Fibrinolysis 2000; 11:71–78.
61. Solerte SB, Fioravanti M, Pezza N, et al. Hyperviscosity and microproteinuria in central obesity: relevance to cardiovascular risk. Int J Obes Relat Metab Disord 1997; 21:417–423.
62. Ziccardi P, Nappo F, Giugliano G, et al. Reduction of inflammatory cytokine concentrations and improvement of endothelial functions in obese women after weight loss over one year. Circulation 2002; 105:804–809.
63. Ito H, Hiroe M, Hirata Y, et al. Insulin-like growth factor-I induces hypertrophy with enhanced expression of muscle specific genes in cultured rat cardiomyocytes. Circulation 1993; 87:1715–1721.
64. Manson JE, Colditz GA, Stampfer MJ, et al. A prospective study of obesity and risk of coronary heart disease in women. N Engl J Med 1990; 322:882–889.
65. Yoon YS, Uchida S, Masuo O, et al. Progressive attenuation of myocardial vascular endothelial growth factor expression is a seminal event in diabetic cardiomyopathy: restoration of microvascular homeostasis and recovery of cardiac function in diabetic cardiomyopathy after replenishment of local vascular endothelial growth factor. Circulation 2005; 111:2073–2085.
66. Suys BE, Katier N, Rooman RP, et al. Female children and adolescents with type 1 diabetes have more pronounced early echocardiographic signs of diabetic cardiomyopathy. Diabetes Care 2004; 27:1947–1953.
67. Rutter MK, Parise H, Benjamin EJ, et al. Impact of glucose intolerance and insulin resistance on cardiac structure and function: sex-related differences in the Framingham Heart Study. Circulation 2003; 107:448–454.
68. Iribarren C, Karter AJ, Go AS, et al. Glycemic control and heart failure among adult patients with diabetes. Circulation 2001; 103:2668–2673.
69. He J, Ogden LG, Bazzano LA, et al. Dietary sodium intake and incidence of congestive heart failure in overweight US men and women: first National Health and Nutrition Examination Survey Epidemiologic Follow-up Study. Arch Intern Med 2002; 162:1619–1624.
70. Bradley TD, Floras JS. Sleep apnea and heart failure: part I: obstructive sleep apnea. Circulation 2003; 107:1671–1678.
71. Warnes CA, Roberts WC. The heart in massive (more than 300 pounds or 136 kilograms) obesity: analysis of 12 patients studied at necropsy. Am J Cardiol 1984; 54:1087–1091.
72. Kasper EK, Hruban RH, Baughman KL. Cardiomyopathy of obesity: a clinicopathologic evaluation of 43 obese patients with heart failure. Am J Cardiol 1992; 70:921–924.
73. Leyva F, Anker SD, Egerer K, et al. Hyperleptinaemia in chronic heart failure. Relationships with insulin. Eur Heart J 1998; 19:1547–1551.
74. Rajapurohitam V, Gan XT, Kirshenbaum LA, et al. The obesity-associated peptide leptin induces hypertrophy in neonatal rat ventricular myocytes. Circ Res 2003; 93:277–279.
75. Atkinson LL, Fischer MA, Lopaschuk GD. Leptin activates cardiac fatty acid oxidation independent of changes in the AMP-activated protein kinase-acetyl-CoA carboxylase-malonyl-CoA axis. J Biol Chem 2002; 277:29424–29430.

76. Illiano G, Naviglio S, Pagano M, et al. Leptin affects adenylate cyclase activity in H9c2 cardiac cell line: effects of short- and long-term exposure. Am J Hypertens 2002; 15:638–643.
77. Haynes WG, Morgan DA, Walsh SA, et al. Receptor-mediated regional sympathetic nerve activation by leptin. J Clin Invest 1997; 100:270–278.
78. Wold LE, Relling DP, Duan J, et al. Abrogated leptin-induced cardiac contractile response in ventricular myocytes under spontaneous hypertension: role of Jak/STAT pathway. Hypertension 2002; 39:69–74.
79. Nickola MW, Wold LE, Colligan PB, et al. Leptin attenuates cardiac contraction in rat ventricular myocytes. Role of NO. Hypertension 2000; 36:501–505.
80. Hohl CM, Hu B, Fertel RH, et al. Effects of obesity and hypertension on ventricular myocytes: comparison of cells from adult SHHF/Mcc-cp and JCR:LA-cp rats. Cardiovasc Res 1993; 27:238–242.
81. Hintz KK, Aberle NS, Ren J. Insulin resistance induces hyperleptinemia, cardiac contractile dysfunction but not cardiac leptin resistance in ventricular myocytes. Int J Obes Relat Metab Disord 2003; 27:1196–1203.
82. Finck BN, Lehman JJ, Leone TC, et al. The cardiac phenotype induced by PPARalpha overexpression mimics that caused by diabetes mellitus. J Clin Invest 2002; 109:121–130.
83. Yokoyama M, Yagyu H, Hu Y, et al. Apolipoprotein B production reduces lipotoxic cardiomyopathy: studies in heart specific lipoprotein lipase transgenic mouse. J Biol Chem 2003.
84. Paolisso G, Manzella D, Montano N, et al. Plasma leptin concentrations and cardiac autonomic nervous system in healthy subjects with different body weights. J Clin Endocrinol Metab 2000; 85:1810–1814.
85. Narkiewicz K, Somers VK, Mos L, et al. An independent relationship between plasma leptin and heart rate in untreated patients with essential hypertension. J Hypertens 1999; 17:245–249.
86. Kazumi T, Kawaguchi A, Katoh J, et al. Fasting insulin and leptin serum levels are associated with systolic blood pressure independent of percentage body fat and body mass index. J Hypertens 1999; 17:1451–1455.
87. Paolisso G, Tagliamonte MR, Galderisi M, et al. Plasma leptin level is associated with myocardial wall thickness in hypertensive insulin-resistant men. Hypertension 1999; 34:1047–1052.
88. Galderisi M, Tagliamonte MR, D'Errico A, et al. Independent association of plasma leptin levels and left ventricular isovolumic relaxation in uncomplicated hypertension. Am J Hypertens 2001; 14:1019–1024.
89. Xiong Y, Tanaka H, Richardson JA, et al. Endothelin-1 stimulates leptin production in adipocytes. J Biol Chem 2001; 276:28471–28477.
90. Maisel AS, McCord J, Nowak RM, et al. Bedside B-Type natriuretic peptide in the emergency diagnosis of heart failure with reduced or preserved ejection fraction. Results from the Breathing Not Properly Multinational Study. J Am Coll Cardiol 2003; 41:2010–2017.
91. Wang TJ, Larson MG, Levy D, et al. Impact of obesity on plasma natriuretic peptide levels. Circulation 2004; 109:594–600.
92. Mehra MR, Uber PA, Park MH, et al. Obesity and suppressed B-type natriuretic peptide levels in heart failure. J Am Coll Cardiol 2004; 43:1590–1595.
93. Sanders GP, Mendes LA, Colucci WS, et al. Noninvasive methods for detecting elevated left-sided cardiac filling pressure. J Card Fail 2000; 6:157–164.
94. Zuber M, Kaeslin T, Studer T, et al. Weight loss of 146 kg with diet and reversal of severe congestive heart failure in a young, morbidly obese patient. Am J Cardiol 1999; 84:955–956.
95. Taylor TV, Bozkurt B, Shayani P, et al. End-stage cardiac failure in a morbidly obese patient treated by biliopancreatic diversion and cardiac transplantation. Obes Surg 2002; 12:416–418.
96. Alpert MA, Terry BE, Mulekar M, et al. Cardiac morphology and left ventricular function in normotensive morbidly obese patients with and without congestive heart failure, and effect of weight loss. Am J Cardiol 1997; 80:736–740.

97. Karason K, Wallentin I, Larsson B, et al. Effects of obesity and weight loss on left ventricular mass and relative wall thickness: survey and intervention study. BMJ 1997; 315:912–916.
98. MacMahon SW, Wilcken DE, Macdonald GJ. The effect of weight reduction on left ventricular mass. A randomized controlled trial in young, overweight hypertensive patients. N Engl J Med 1986; 314:334–339.
99. Levy D, Garrison RJ, Savage DD, et al. Prognostic implications of echocardiographically determined left ventricular mass in the Framingham Heart Study. N Engl J Med 1990; 322:1561–1566.
100. Steinbrook R. Surgery for severe obesity. N Engl J Med 2004; 350:1075–1079.
101. Brater DC. Diuretic therapy. N Engl J Med 1998; 339:387–395.
102. Pitt B, Zannad F, Remme WJ, et al. The effect of spironolactone on morbidity and mortality in patients with severe heart failure. Randomized Aldactone Evaluation Study Investigators. N Engl J Med 1999; 341:709–717.
103. Pitt B, Remme W, Zannad F, et al. Eplerenone, a selective aldosterone blocker, in patients with left ventricular dysfunction after myocardial infarction. N Engl J Med 2003; 348:1309–1321.
104. Pfeffer MA, Swedberg K, Granger CB, et al. Effects of candesartan on mortality and morbidity in patients with chronic heart failure: the CHARM-Overall programme. Lancet 2003; 362:759–766.
105. Pfeffer MA, McMurray JJ, Velazquez EJ, et al. Valsartan, captopril, or both in myocardial infarction complicated by heart failure, left ventricular dysfunction, or both. N Engl J Med 2003; 349:1893–1906.
106. Cohn JN, Tognoni G. A randomized trial of the angiotensin-receptor blocker valsartan in chronic heart failure. N Engl J Med 2001; 345:1667–1675.
107. McMurray JJ, Ostergren J, Swedberg K, et al. Effects of candesartan in patients with chronic heart failure and reduced left-ventricular systolic function taking angiotensin-converting-enzyme inhibitors: the CHARM-Added trial. Lancet 2003; 362:767–771.
108. Givertz MM. Manipulation of the renin–angiotensin system. Circulation 2001; 104:e14–e18.
109. Kittleson M, Hurwitz S, Shah MR, et al. Development of circulatory-renal limitations to angiotensin-converting enzyme inhibitors identifies patients with severe heart failure and early mortality. J Am Coll Cardiol 2003; 41:2029–2035.
110. Taylor AL, Ziesche S, Yancy C, et al. Combination of isosorbide dinitrate and hydralazine in blacks with heart failure. N Engl J Med 2004; 351:2049–2057.
111. Bristow MR. Beta-adrenergic receptor blockade in chronic heart failure. Circulation 2000; 101:558–569.
112. Packer M, Coats AJ, Fowler MB, et al. Effect of carvedilol on survival in severe chronic heart failure. N Engl J Med 2001; 344:1651–1658.
113. MERIT-HF Study Group. Effect of metoprolol CR/XL in chronic heart failure: Metoprolol CR/XL Randomised Intervention Trial in Congestive Heart Failure (MERIT-HF). Lancet 1999; 353:2001–2007.
114. Jacob S, Rett K, Wicklmayr M, et al. Differential effect of chronic treatment with two beta-blocking agents on insulin sensitivity: the carvedilol–metoprolol study. J Hypertens 1996; 14:489–494.
115. Giugliano D, Acampora R, Marfella R, et al. Metabolic and cardiovascular effects of carvedilol and atenolol in non-insulin-dependent diabetes mellitus and hypertension. A randomized, controlled trial. Ann Intern Med 1997; 126:955–959.
116. Bakris GL, Fonseca V, Katholi RE, et al. Metabolic effects of carvedilol vs metoprolol in patients with type 2 diabetes mellitus and hypertension: a randomized controlled trial. JAMA 2004; 292:2227–2236.
117. The Digitalis Investigation Group. The effect of digoxin on mortality and morbidity in patients with heart failure. N Engl J Med 1997; 336:525–533.
118. Rathore SS, Curtis JP, Wang Y, et al. Association of serum digoxin concentration and outcomes in patients with heart failure. JAMA 2003; 289:871–878.

119. Boney CM, Verma A, Tucker R, et al. Metabolic syndrome in childhood: association with birth weight, maternal obesity, and gestational diabetes mellitus. Pediatrics 2005; 115:e290–e296.
120. Mokdad AH, Ford ES, Bowman BA, et al. Prevalence of obesity, diabetes, and obesity-related health risk factors, 2001. JAMA 2003; 289:76–79.
121. Inzucchi SE. Oral antihyperglycemic therapy for type 2 diabetes: scientific review. JAMA 2002; 287:360–372.
122. Tang WH, Francis GS, Hoogwerf BJ, et al. Fluid retention after initiation of thiazolidinedione therapy in diabetic patients with established chronic heart failure. J Am Coll Cardiol 2003; 41:1394–1398.
123. Wilding J, Dargie H, Hildebrandt P, et al. Rosiglitazone (RSG) administered to patients with type 2 diabetes (T2DM) and class I/II congestive heart failure (CHF) does not adversely affect echocardiographic structure or function parameters. Diabetes 2005; 54:1.
124. Masoudi FA, Wang Y, Inzucchi SE, et al. Metformin and thiazolidinedione use in Medicare patients with heart failure. JAMA 2003; 290:81–85.
125. Akosah KO, Schaper A, Cogbill C, et al. Preventing myocardial infarction in the young adult in the first place: how do the National Cholesterol Education Panel III guidelines perform? J Am Coll Cardiol 2003; 41:1475–1479.
126. Horwich TB, MacLellan WR, Fonarow GC. Statin therapy is associated with improved survival in ischemic and non-ischemic heart failure. J Am Coll Cardiol 2004; 43:642–648.
127. Javaheri S, Parker TJ, Liming JD, et al. Sleep apnea in 81 ambulatory male patients with stable heart failure. Types and their prevalences, consequences, and presentations. Circulation 1998; 97:2154–2159.
128. Sin DD, Fitzgerald F, Parker JD, et al. Risk factors for central and obstructive sleep apnea in 450 men and women with congestive heart failure. Am J Respir Crit Care Med 1999; 160:1101–1106.
129. Bradley TD, Floras JS. Sleep apnea and heart failure: part II: central sleep apnea. Circulation 2003; 107:1822–1826.
130. Kaneko Y, Floras JS, Usui K, et al. Cardiovascular effects of continuous positive airway pressure in patients with heart failure and obstructive sleep apnea. N Engl J Med 2003; 348:1233–1241.
131. Bradley TD, Logan AG, Kimoff RJ, et al. Continuous positive airway pressure for heart central sleep apnea and heart failure. N Engl J Med 2005; 353:2070–2073.
132. Koniaris LS, Goldhaber SZ. Anticoagulation in dilated cardiomyopathy. J Am Coll Cardiol 1998; 31:745–748.
133. Goldhaber SZ, Elliott CG. Acute pulmonary embolism: part I: epidemiology, pathophysiology, and diagnosis. Circulation 2003; 108:2726–2729.
134. Kucher N, Goldhaber SZ. Cardiac biomarkers for risk stratification of patients with acute pulmonary embolism. Circulation 2003; 108:2191–2194.
135. Grady KL, White-Williams C, Naftel D, et al. Are preoperative obesity and cachexia risk factors for post heart transplant morbidity and mortality: a multi-institutional study of preoperative weight-height indices. Cardiac Transplant Research Database (CTRD) Group. J Heart Lung Transplant 1999; 18:750–763.
136. Lietz K, John R, Burke EA, et al. Pretransplant cachexia and morbid obesity are predictors of increased mortality after heart transplantation. Transplantation 2001; 72:277–283.
137. Butler J, Howser R, Portner PM, et al. Body mass index and outcomes after left ventricular assist device placement. Ann Thorac Surg 2005; 79:66–73.
138. Butler J, McCoin NS, Feurer ID, et al. Modeling the effects of functional performance and post-transplant comorbidities on health-related quality of life after heart transplantation. J Heart Lung Transplant 2003; 22:1149–1156.
139. Javaheri S, Abraham WT, Brown C, et al. Prevalence of obstructive sleep apnoea and periodic limb movement in 45 subjects with heart transplantation. Eur Heart J 2004; 25:260–266.

4
Exercise and Heart Failure

Daniel E. Forman
Divisions of Cardiovascular Medicine and Aging, Brigham and Women's Hospital, VAMC of Boston, Harvard Medical School, Boston, Massachusetts, U.S.A.

INTRODUCTION

Heart failure (HF) is a complex clinical syndrome with a multipart pathophysiology involving a wide variety of cells, tissues, organs, and organ systems. Whereas systolic HF remains commonly conceptualized in terms of impaired heart pumping function, i.e., a heart that is unable to pump to meet the body's needs with normal intracardiac chamber pressures, this textbook has accentuated the contrasting principle that HF pathophysiology extends well beyond the heart, including a constellation of peripheral effects that are integral to HF's notorious course (Fig. 1). Whereas resting pump function relates poorly to exercise capacity, a variety of extra-cardiac HF effects have significant bearing on functional limits. Given that exercise training modifies many tissues and organ systems, there is compelling rationale for its use to modify the systemic nature of HF. Consistently, exercise training has been demonstrated to modify many peripheral manifestations of HF with associated functional improvements. In this chapter, we will, therefore, review salient aspects of peripheral HF pathophysiology as a perspective from which benefits of exercise training can be highlighted. We will then review some of the trial data demonstrating utility of exercise training for systolic HF, and clarify related details regarding training strategies and safety.

HEART FUNCTION AND FUNCTIONAL CAPACITY

Reduced cardiac output is a critical component of systolic HF. A wide range of circumstances can lead to initial cardiac weakening but, irrespective of etiology, the fall in cardiac output triggers a subsequent cascade of physiological sequelae that tends to be fairly homogeneous. Cardiac dilation is common as myocytes stretch to facilitate the increased preload due to neurohormonal stimulation and volume retention. However, continued heart dilation ultimately results in deterioration of contraction along with worsening valvular regurgitation and arrhythmia (1).

While systolic HF management emphasizes medications that modify the pattern of progressive cardiac changes, such therapy does not always correlate with functional

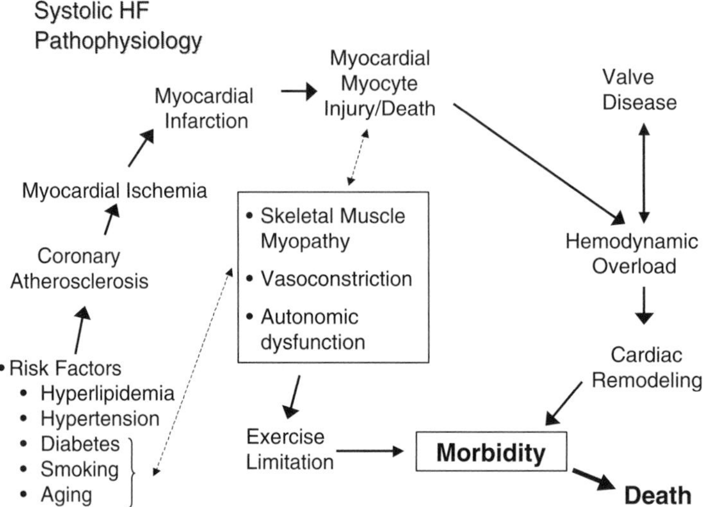

Figure 1 Central and peripheral physiologic abnormalities that are integral to systolic heart failure.

improvements (2,3). In fact, even among patients taking all recommended cardiac medications, functional capacity often erodes, and the resulting exercise intolerance is associated with increasing mortality and morbidity, as well as reduced quality of life (QOL) (4,5). Given the risks associated with functional decline, it seems key to broaden therapeutic goals to include (and prioritize) strategies that enhance functional capacity.

Although resting heart function does not predict exercise capacity, the ability of cardiac output to increase in association with exercise corresponds to maximal functional capacity (6). Therefore, increased vascular resistance, greater mitral regurgitation, and reduced maximal heart rate are among the pathophysiological factors in HF that can diminish exercise tolerance. Whereas treatment of angiotensin II, noradrenaline, and other neurohormones is often emphasized in terms of goals to modify their adverse impact on cardiac structure and function (e.g., remodeling, arrhythmia, and LV ejection fraction), these neurohormones also increase vasoconstriction, vascular resistance, and ventricular afterload, i.e., burdens that limit maximal cardiac output and tissue perfusion, and which induce exercise limitations (7). Similarly, diminished endothelial nitric oxide from HF (aka endothelium-derived relaxing factor) (8–10) exacerbates afterload stresses, especially during exercise, adding to functional limitations. Nitric oxide-mediated endothelial dysfunction also limits coronary artery flow reserve, which predisposes to constrained maximal cardiac output (11) (i.e., ischemia provoking inotropic and lucitropic dysfunction, reducing stroke volume and cardiac output). Autonomic dysfunction from HF also worsens functional limitations through vasoconstriction (excessive α-stimulation) and diminished chronotropic reserve (reduced maximal heart rate) (12).

Related to elevated neurohormones is a pervasive HF proinflamatory state that impacts functional capacity (13). Elevated TNF-α, IL-1β, and iNOS are typical, along with reduced IGF-1 and high oxidative stresses. In skeletal muscle, inflammatory stimuli trigger altered cell signaling patterns and abnormal metabolism, and bring about a typical HF myopathy, i.e., intrinsic skeletal muscle changes that are independent of flow. Muscle fatigability is commonly increased since reduced muscle oxygen uptake, increased lactate build-up, and lower pH are among the many myopathic features associated with exercise limitations (14). Muscle wasting is also associated with HF as part of the inflammatory process, but functional decline typically precedes muscle loss, with muscle atrophy then exacerbating antecedent functional decline.

Phenotypic changes in HF skeletal muscle myopathy include reduced type I aerobic fibers (slow twitch) and increases in less aerobic type II fibers (fast twitch). Histopathology analyses also show decreased fiber sizes (both type I and II) as well as reduced number and altered structure of mitochondria (15). More fundamentally, studies demonstrate altered skeletal muscle physiology, including shifts in aerobic enzyme distribution from myosin heavy chain 1 (MHC1) slow oxidative towards myosin heavy chain 2a (MHC2a) fast oxidative and myosin heavy chain 2b (MHC2b) fast glycolytic isoforms (16), decreased levels of mitochondrial creatine kinase (17), as well as downregulation of the sarcoplasmatic reticulum Ca-ATPase 1 (SERCA-1) (18).

Symptoms of exercise intolerance and dyspnea in HF also relate to skeletal muscle changes in the diaphragm (19). Dyspnea is commonly disproportionate to exercise load, with excessive increases in minute ventilation and significantly steeper slopes of minute ventilation by carbon dioxide output (20,21). Furthermore, increased ventilatory dead space also leads to ventilation–perfusion mismatch (21) and breathing limitations.

EXERCISE TRAINING IN HF

Rationale for exercise training for HF was first explored as part of a broader study of cardiac rehabilitation for coronary artery disease (CAD) patients who had suffered MI or undergone bypass surgery (22). In small, seminal, nonrandomized studies of cardiac rehabilitation in post-MI patients with LV dysfunction, exercise training improved work capacity and peak oxygen consumption. Furthermore, these trials began to illuminate the peripheral physiological benefits derived from exercise training that facilitated functional gains (23).

Since 1990, there have been multiple prospective, randomized, controlled studies specifically evaluating exercise training in HF patients (24–31) (Table 1). Most of these studies have been small trails, involving patients with both ischemic and non-ischemic cardiomyopathy, and typically NYHA class II or III HF. Training regimens varied but most studies used bicycle ergometers or walking at 50% to 70% peak VO_2, 3 to 7 times per week. Some of the training programs involved supervised exercise sessions, others involved independent exercise at home, or training combinations. All of the studies were single-center and were underpowered to meaningfully evaluate morbidity and mortality.

Most of these investigations focused on exercise capacity before and after training as the primary outcome. Peak oxygen utilization (VO_2) or oxygen utilization at ventilatory threshold is commonly used as the most objective and reliable measurements of functional capacity while duration of exercise and/or distance walked in a fixed time are also commonly used indices of exercise performance. Trial data consistently substantiate significant gains from exercise training (4).

Improved endothelial performance is a key benefit underlying functional gains from exercise training. After training, exercise-mediated endothelial nitric oxide release significantly increases among HF patients, (9,10,32), with reduced afterload stress and improved coronary perfusion. Vasoconstricting neurohormones also decrease after exercise training, with reduced afterload stress (33).

Some investigators have attributed functional improvements after exercise training in part to central cardiac training benefits (24), citing improved ventricular filling (34) and even enhanced cardiac perfusion (30). However, all such benefits may also be attributable to improved vascular flow responses, i.e., central cardiac changes resulting secondarily from improved coronary artery flow and reduced afterload pressures (35).

Table 1 Selected Exercise Training Trials

Authors	Training intensity	Training duration (min)	Training mode	Training frequency (d/wk)	Peak VO_2 (mL kg^{-1} min^{-1}) (before/after)
Roveda et al. (25)	HR at anaerobic threshold	25–40	Bike	3	T: 14.8/20.6; C: 16.6/17.5
Hambrecht et al. (15)	70% of peak VO_2	$\geq$40	Bike	7	T: 17.5/23.3; C: 17.9/17.9
Keteyian et al. (26)	60% initial, then 70-80% of peak VO_2	33	Bike, walk, row	3	T: 16.1/18.4; C:14.6/15.3
Linke et al. (27)	70% of peak VO_2	60	Bike ergometer	6	T: 16.0/19.4; C: 16.9/16.3
McKelvie et al. (28)	60-70% peak HR	30	Bike, arm ergometer, resistance training	3	T: 14.2; C:13.8
Keteyian et al. (29)	50-60% initial, then 70-80% of peak VO_2	30	Bike, walk, row	3	T:16.3/18.6; C: –/–
Belardinelli et al. (30)	60% of peak VO_2	40	Bike	2–3	T:15.7/19.9; C: 15.2/16.0
Giannuzzi et al. (31)	60% of peak VO_2	30–60	Bike, walk	3–7	T: 13.8/16.2; C: 13.8/13.7

Abbreviations: HR, heart rate; VO_2, volume of oxygen consumed; T, treatment, before/after training; C, control, before/after training.

A significant body of literature has also explored skeletal muscle changes in HF patients undergoing exercise training (15,36,37). Hambrecht et al. showed improved metabolism, with increased surface density of cytochrome c oxidase-positive mitochondria as the result of a training program, with these mitochondrial changes correlating closely to peak VO_2. Likewise, exercise training induced a re-shift from fast-twitch type II fibers to slow-twitch type I fibers (15). Investigations have also emphasized that most skeletal muscle morphological and metabolic training-related improvements among exercising HF patients are independent of vascular flow.

On an even more basic level, exercise training has been demonstrated to modify HF inflammation. Gielen et al. showed that expression of IL-1β and TNF-α decreased in the quadriceps muscle after longterm exercise training in HF patients (38). Reduced iNOS and increased IGF-1 also occurred (39).

Among the other benefits of exercise training for HF patients autonomic function is improved. Training is associated with decreased resting plasma norepinephrine (40,41), improved heart rate variability (HRV) (42), and reduced sympathetic peroneal nerve activity (25). A body of medical literature also describes a reduced ergoreflex among HF patients who exercise. The ergoreflex involves stimulation of skeletal muscle afferent fibers (particularly in an acidotic milieu) that provoke excessive sympathetic stimuli and tachypea (43). In particular, Peipoli et al. has demonstrated utility of exercise training to modify this HF pathophysiology (44).

Improved ventilatory responses after exercise training have also been reported (45). This may relate to improved skeletal muscle performance (including diminished lactate production that triggers tachypnea) and strengthening of the diaphragm, as well as to diminished ergoreflex and improved ventilation/perfusion matching in the lung (21).

SAFETY OF EXERCISE TRAINING IN HF

Even as studies have touted the benefits of exercise training for HF, its safety has been controversial. Whereas major cardiovascular complications are typically reported as only one in 60,000 participant hours for cardiac patients participating in outpatient exercise programs, concerns have been disproportionate regarding exercise training for HF patients. This is in part because ventricular enlargement and dysfunction predispose to added arrhythmia and hemodynamic risks (46). Furthermore, ischemic HF patients who often have more extensive underlying CAD, may also have particular vulnerability to new cardiac ischemic events. Concerns about exercise-induced cardiac remodeling are also high, especially in the weeks and months following MI (and/or other acute triggers of cardiac weakening). A small trial by Jugdutt et al. in 1988 seriously heightened clinical concerns about exercise training when he reported worsening LV asynergy in post-MI HF patients enrolled in a nonrandomized, controlled study (47). In that study, average LVEF also dropped from 43% to 30% after 12 weeks of exercise training.

In response to the Jugdutt trial multiple randomized controlled trials of moderate- to high-intensity exercise training have subsequently been completed. Investigators have used rigorous echocardiographic and MRI techniques to more definitively explore for the possibility of detrimental exacerbation of post-MI remodeling in HF patients as well as remodeling in general among patients with non-ischemic cardiomyopathy (48,49,50). Not only have these studies consistently refuted Jugdutt, they even demonstrated intrinsic cardiac benefits from exercise, i.e., exercise training led to smaller heart sizes and improved systolic function (31).

Likewise, apprehensions regarding arrhythmia, CAD, and other instabilities have been carefully assessed. In 1999, Belardinelli et al. (30) conducted a one-year trial involving 99 subjects that showed a 67% decrease in subsequent risk for deaths and hospitalizations with exercise training. In their more recent AHA-consensus scientific statement, Pina et al. reported on the careful evaluation of 21 exercise training studies conducted in a total of 467 patients with chronic HF, and described low adverse event rates (24). They described the most common sequelae as post-exercise hypotension, atrial and ventricular arrhythmias, and worsening HF symptoms—risks which the scientific statement asserts can be modified by careful patient selection and follow-up.

Currently, a multi-site, randomized clinical trial is underway to evaluate the clinical effectiveness and safety of exercise training in patients with chronic HF. HF—*A* *C*ontrolled *T*rial *I*nvestigating *O*utcomes of Exercise Trai*N*ing (HF-ACTION) will report its findings in 2008. HF-ACTION evaluates whether regular, supervised exercise that is then followed by home-based exercise training influences clinical outcomes and quality of life (QOL), and whether it does so in a safe and cost effective manner. Another particular advantage of the trial includes the fact that it is large and conducted in many institutions—features that respond to concerns regarding the limited generalizabity of the smaller single-center trials that have heretofore dominated this field.

EXERCISE TRAINING MODALITIES

Given the safety concerns pertaining to HF patients and the notorious reductions in exercise tolerance associated with HF, one might expect that exercise training modalities and exercise prescription would be specialized and refined. However, based on available data, exercise modalities remain similar to those used in people with normal systolic function. Moreover, as stated in the AHA-consensus scientific statement, "agreement on a universal exercise prescription for this population does not exist" (24). All one can ascertain about the training regimens from published reports is that any one of a variety of aerobic training modalities and intensities have led to functional gains in NYHA class II or III HF patients primarily through peripheral physiological changes. Studies also show that training in isolated muscle groups can yield systemic benefits, implicitly justifying training regimens limited to one part of the body (51). This is a useful consideration in formulating a realistic training regimen for patients who often lack stamina or stability for complex and/or lengthy exercise regimens. However, studies indicate that injury risk increases if any particular joint is subjected to excessive biomechanical impact, giving rationale for a training regimen that blends a variety of gentle maneuvers and that assiduously avoids overstressing any particular joint (52). Published data also demonstrate the value of ACE inhibitors and beta-adrenergic blockers during exercise training as the best means to stabilize both the heart as well as peripheral physiology during exercise training (53–55).

Prior to exercise training, all HF patients should be evaluated by a physician or physician extender to screen for any cardiac or non-cardiac contraindications to exercise (Table 2). Exercise should be initiated only for patients who have been in stable clinical condition for at least 2–4 weeks. Clinical stability is defined as no change in symptoms, weight, drug regimen, or NYHA class over this period. Safety concerns are highest in patients who are sedentary at baseline, as exercise morbidity is greatest among those who are beginning new exercise routines. Key clinical cues to consider during examination include hemodynamic instability, brady or tachy arrhythmia, weight gain, JVD, tachypnea, new gallops or murmurs, excessive ectopy, angina or ischemia on ECG. Pre-exercise screening assessment with stress testing helps to detect patients most susceptible to exercise-provoked instability, providing an opportunity to detect arrhythmia, hemodynamic compromise, and ischemia. Not only can such detection be useful in prompting additional medical interventions, it may also help identify patients who might particularly benefit from direct supervision during their training sessions and/or ECG monitoring during exercise. Stress testing also provides a useful means to formulate an exercise training prescription, i.e., basing training intensity on a percent of VO_2 or maximum heart rate (see below).

Table 2 Contraindications to Exercise Training for Heart Failure Patients

Relative contraindications	Absolute contraindications
Increasing weight over previous several days	Signs or symptoms of congestion
Abnormal increase or decrease of blood pressure with exercise	Severe blood pressure changes, early ischemic changes, or life-threatening arrhythmia
Complex ventricular arrhythmia at rest or appearing with exertion	Uncontrolled metabolic disorder (e.g., hypothyroidism, diabetes)
Resting tachycardia or excessive bradycardia (unresponsive to exercise)	Acute systemic illness or fever
Implantable cardiac defibrillator with heart rate limit set below the target heart rate for training	Recent embolism or thrombophlebitis
New ECG abnormalities, worsening LVEF by echo	Active pericarditis or myocarditis
New York Heart Association Functional Class IV	Second (type II) or third-degree heart block without pacemaker

Exercise training should typically include an adequate warm-up, usually 10-15 min, with warm-up longest in the most debilitated patients. Exercise duration is then usually 20-30 min, with cool-down thereafter. Most studies have used regimens of three to five times a week, adding rest days particularly if patients are excessively fatigued. To avoid musculoskeletal injury, low-impact exercise that avoids excessive stress on joints and bones is preferable.

The benefit of ECG monitoring during exercise remains controversial. Whereas the American Association of Cardiovascular and Pulmonary Rehabilitation recommends ECG monitoring for patients with advanced HF (56), many published trials show safety of home programs without such monitoring. However, more advanced HF patients and/or those with the highest arrhythmic risks were excluded from published trials. Some of these clinical concerns are modified by growing use of AICDs in HF management. These have been demonstrated to be safe and advantageous among patients participating in an exercise training regimen (57). Nonetheless, it raises the additional concern that training intensity be carefully targeted to avoid heart rates that may inadvertently trigger the defibrillator mechanism.

Benefits of exercise supervision are also debatable. Costs and logistics are notorious impediments to exercise training in a cardiac rehabilitation-like setting, yet adherence, training effects, and safety are more reliable in supervised settings. A supervised program also affords opportunity for education, including advice on symptom recognition, nutrition, understanding of the disease, medications, and compliance. If patients are to exercise at home, they should be encouraged to exercise with someone else. This partnering has been demonstrated to enhance both compliance and safety.

Table 1 summarizes some aspects of the modality, frequency, intensity, and duration of exercise used in selected randomized trials. Based on trial data, it is reasonable to assume that exercise should include a gross motor modality such as walking or biking, performed for 30-40 min, three to five days per week, at an intensity that falls in the range of 60% to 80% of peak VO_2 or heart rate reserve. Since agreement on a universal exercise prescription does not exist, an individualized training regimen that is sensitive to each person's needs, idiosyncrasies, and musculo-skeletal limitations is recommended. Although exercise guidelines provide a training target, it is often necessary and/or prudent to start patients at a lower level, e.g., 60% VO_2 peak, particularly those that are deconditioned at the onset. Furthermore, for all patients, higher intensities at the onset of a training program might feel overwhelming and/or provoke injury, and serve to undermine adherence. Interval training has also been demonstrated to be effective; frail patients often do best with interval training that includes periods of rest. Whatever the initial regimen, progression of exercise intensity is critical if functional capacity is to grow, especially as the patient becomes better conditioned.

Coupled to exercise testing, air–gas exchange measurements (i.e., cardiopulmonary stress testing) offer an objective assessment of functional capacity (at baseline or in response to therapy)—one that assesses function in a way that incorporates physiology of the heart, muscles, vasculature, lungs, and autonomic function in a provocative test (58,59). Cardiopulmonary testing also provides an optimal gauge for exercise prescription (a percentage of the VO_2 peak or relative to the VO_2 at the anaerobic threshold, aka ventilatory threshold). Whereas some patients find the use of a snorkel or facemask in cardiopulmonary testing to be somewhat cumbersome and unpleasant, new technologies are making air-gas equipment easier for patients to tolerate. For stress testing HF patients, it is important to select gentle exercise protocols that optimize accuracy of functional assessment but do not overwhelm patients who are often frail and debilitated. Progressive ramp protocols may offer some advantages over protocols that incrementally increase workloads in significant fixed stages. Although exercise testing on a treadmill is usually better able provoke peak VO_2 than exercise testing on a bicycle (since walking/running exercise involves largest muscle mass), use of a cycle ergometer for a stress test may still have advantages in patients for whom there are concerns regarding hemodynamic, arrhythmic, and other destabilizing risks.

Some clinicians still use HR-derived exercise prescriptions as a primary means to prescribe and guide exercise intensity. However, growing use of beta-blockers for HF patients confounds these measures. The Borg scale is a convenient alternative (exertion rated 6–20). Patients are encouraged to exercise at Rate of Perceived Exertion (RPE) levels 12–13 (ventilatory threshold is typically associated with a Borg scale 13–15).

Although the majority of trials conducted to date have used aerobic activities to improve function and exercise tolerance, some studies have studied and asserted value for resistance training (aka strength training) (60,61) or regimens combining aerobic and resistance training modalities (62). Rationale for resistance training is particularly compelling in a disease that is associated with skeletal muscle myopathy, i.e. skeletal muscle may be more efficiently modified by the direct muscle stimulation of resistance training. Furthermore, initial strength training in a frail patient can often help him/her to develop sufficient strength to tolerate an aerobic training component (63).

Based on the few published trials, resistance training intensity should be set at 50% to 60% of one-repetition maximum, with the patient starting with one set of 10 to 12 reps and then progressing to one set of 15 repetitions. Ideally, the exercises should include all major muscle groups, including the upper body, which will likely augment capacities in activities of daily living. This goal should be modified if any particular joint or muscle is sprained or encumbered by arthritic limitations. As patients improve, lift load is typically increased 5% to 10%. Further study of optimal strategy and safety of resistance training is warranted in larger trials.

Resistance training for HF patients has been particularly controversial as many have raised concerns regarding the potential for associated afterload pressures to provoke instability. Ironically, resistance training in isolated muscle groups has been found to be relatively well-tolerated and safe, and afterload stresses have not been found to be excessive. Furthermore, elevated heart rate responses and arrhythmias are less likely than with aerobic training modalities.

HEART FAILURE WITH NORMAL EJECTION FRACTION

With growing recognition of the widespread prevalence, morbidity, and mortality of HF with normal ejection fraction (HFNEF), the value of exercise training for this type of HF deserves consideration. While no definitive trial has yet studied benefits of exercise training for HFNEF, diastolic filling abnormalities are usually a consequence of aging, hypertrophy, ischemia, or some combination of these factors (64). For each factor, exercise training is known to exert favorable effects (i.e., lowering blood pressure, reducing LVH, and modifying age-related ventricular filling changes), with improved diastolic filling among exercising adults. Furthermore, given that HFNEF is a disease that is most common among older adults, exercise training may have particular benefit in modifying the frailty that results when HFNEF occurs in a deconditioned elder (65). Perhaps most important, it is now clear that many of the systemic effects of systolic HF also occur with HFNEF. As such, there is strong rationale to promote exercise training as a means to modify neurohormones, nitric oxide, inflammation, and other pathophysiological mechanisms that are inherent to HF, no matter what the ejection fraction.

EXERCISE ADHERENCE

While exercise benefits are reliably detected in patients participating in a regular exercise program, benefits are not sustained after exercise is terminated. While multiple training studies tout benefits of high intensity training for maximal physiological gains, adherence to high intensity training is usually poor. Furthermore, musculoskeletal injuries are greatest among those using high intensity regimens. Therefore, a key goal of exercise training for HF patients is to establish exercise behavior that can be sustained in a lifelong pattern (66).

REFERENCES

1. Jessup M, Brozena S. Heart failure. N Engl J Med 2003; 348:2007–2018.
2. Franciosa JA, Park M, Levine TB. Lack of correlation between exercise capacity and indexes of resting left ventricular performance in heart failure. Am J Cardiol 1981; 47:33–39.
3. Sullivan MJ, Hawthorne MH. Exercise intolerance in patients with chronic heart failure. Prog Cardiovasc Dis 1995; 38:1–22.
4. Rees K, Taylor RS, Singh S, Coats AJ, Ebrahim S. Exercise based rehabilitation for heart failure. Cochrane Database Syst Rev 2004;CD003331.
5. Coats AJ. Exercise and heart failure. Cardiol Clin 2001; 19:517–524 see also pp. xii–xiii.
6. Sullivan MJ, Higginbotham MB, Cobb FR. Exercise training in patients with chronic heart failure delays ventilatory anaerobic threshold and improves submaximal exercise performance. Circulation 1989; 79:324–329.
7. Drexler H. Reduced exercise tolerance in chronic heart failure and its relationship to neurohumoral factors. Eur Heart J 1991; 12:21–28.
8. Kubo SH, Rector TS, Bank AJ, Williams RE, Heifetz SM. Endothelium-dependent vasodilation is attenuated in patients with heart failure. Circulation 1991; 84:1589–1596.
9. Hornig B, Maier V, Drexler H. Physical training improves endothelial function in patients with chronic heart failure. Circulation 1996; 93:210–214.
10. Hambrecht R, Fiehn E, Weigl C, et al. Regular physical exercise corrects endothelial dysfunction and improves exercise capacity in patients with chronic heart failure. Circulation 1998; 98:2709–2715.
11. Treasure CB, Vita JA, Cox DA, et al. Endothelium-dependent dilation of the coronary microvasculature is impaired in dilated cardiomyopathy. Circulation 1990; 81:772–779.
12. Zelis R, Flaim SF, Liedike AJ, Nellis SH. Cardiocirculatory dynamics in the normal and failing heart. Annu Rev Physiol 1981; 43:455–476.
13. Mann DL. Inflammatory mediators and the failing heart: past, present, and the foreseeable future. Circ Res 2002; 91:988–998.
14. Wilson JR, Mancini DM, Dunkman WB. Exertional fatigue due to skeletal muscle dysfunction in patients with heart failure. Circulation 1993; 87:470–475.
15. Hambrecht R, Niebauer J, Fiehn E, et al. Physical training in patients with stable chronic heart failure: effects on cardiorespiratory fitness and ultrastructural abnormalities of leg muscles. J Am Coll Cardiol 1995; 25:1239–1249.
16. Sullivan MJ, Green HJ, Cobb FR. Skeletal muscle biochemistry and histology in ambulatory patients with long-term heart failure. Circulation 1990; 81:518–527.
17. Massie BM, Simonini A, Sahgal P, Wells L, Dudley GA. Relation of systemic and local muscle exercise capacity to skeletal muscle characteristics in men with congestive heart failure. J Am Coll Cardiol 1996; 27:140–145.
18. Spangenburg EE, Lees SJ, Otis JS, Musch TI, Talmadge RJ, Williams JH. Effects of moderate heart failure and functional overload on rat plantaris muscle. J Appl Physiol 2002; 92:18–24.

19. Tikunov B, Levine S, Mancini D. Chronic congestive heart failure elicits adaptations of endurance exercise in diaphragmatic muscle. Circulation 1997; 95:910–916.
20. Sullivan MJ, Hawthorne MH. Exercise intolerance in patients with chronic heart failure. Prog Cardiovasc Dis 1995; 38:1–22.
21. Myers J, Salleh A, Buchanan N, et al. Ventilatory mechanisms of exercise intolerance in chronic heart failure. Am Heart J 1992; 124:710–719.
22. Varnauskas E, Bergman H, Houk P, Bjorntorp P. Haemodynamic effects of physical training in coronary patients. Lancet 1966; 2:8–12.
23. Sullivan MJ, Higginbotham MB, Cobb FR. Exercise training in patients with severe left ventricular dysfunction. Hemodynamic and metabolic effects. Circulation 1988; 78:506–515.
24. Pina IL, Apstein CS, Balady GJ, et al. American Heart Association Committee on exercise, rehabilitation, and prevention. Exercise and heart failure: a statement from the American Heart Association Committee on exercise, rehabilitation, and prevention. Circulation 2003; 107:1210–1225.
25. Roveda F, Middlekauff HR, Rondon MUPB, et al. The effects of exercise training on sympathetic neural activation in advanced heart failure. J Am Coll Cardiol 2003; 42:854–860.
26. Keteyian SJ, Brawner CA, Schairer JR, et al. Effects of exercise training on chronotropic incompetence in patients with heart failure. Am Heart J 1999; 138:233–240.
27. Linke A, Schoene N, Gielen S, et al. Endothelial dysfunction in patients with chronic heart failure: systemic effects of lower-limb exercise training. J Am Coll Cardiol 2001; 37:392–397.
28. McKelvie RS, Teo KK, Roberts R, et al. Effects of exercise training in patients with heart failure: The Exercise Rehabilitation Trial (EXERT). Am Heart J 2002; 144:23–30.
29. Keteyian SJ, Duscha BD, Brawner CA, et al. Differential effects of exercise training in men and women with chronic heart failure. Am Heart J 2003; 145:912–918.
30. Belardinelli R, Georgiou D, Pucaro A. Randomized, controlled trial of long-term moderate exercise training in chronic heart failure. Circulation 1999; 99:1173–1182.
31. Giannuzzi P, Temporelli PL, Corra U, Tavazzi L. Antiremodeling effect of long-term exercise training in patients with stable chronic heart failure. Circulation 2003; 108:554–559.
32. Hambrecht R, Fiehn E, Weigl C, et al. Regular physical exercise corrects endothelial dysfunction and improves exercise capacity in patients with chronic heart failure. Circulation 1998; 98:2709–2715.
33. Braith RW, Edwards DG. Neurohormonal abnormalities in heart failure: impact of exercise training. Congest Heart Fail 2003; 9:70–76.
34. Todaka K, Wang J, Yi GH, et al. Impact of exercise training on ventricular properties in a canine model of congestive heart failure. Am J Physiol 1997; 272:H1382–H1390.
35. Hambrecht R, Gielen S, Linke A, et al. Effects of exercise training on left ventricular function and peripheral resistance in patients with chronic heart failure: a randomized trial. JAMA 2000; 283:3095–3101.
36. Harrington D, Anker SD, Chua TP, et al. Skeletal muscle function and its relation to exercise tolerance in chronic heart failure. J Am Coll Cardiol 1997; 30:1758–1764.
37. Tyni-Lenne R, Gordon A, Jansson E, Bermann G, Sylven C. Skeletal muscle endurance training improves peripheral oxidative capacity, exercise tolerance, and health-related quality of life in women with chronic congestive heart failure secondary to either ischemic cardiomyopathy or idiopathic dilated cardiomyopathy. Am J Cardiol 1997; 80:1025–1029.
38. Gielen S, Adams V, Mobius-Winkler S, et al. Anti-inflammatory effects of exercise training in the skeletal muscle of patients with chronic heart failure. J Am Coll Cardiol 2003; 42:861–868.
39. Schulze PC, Gielen S, Schuler G, Hambrecht R. Chronic heart failure and skeletal muscle catabolism: effects of exercise training. Int J Cardiol 2002; 85:141–149.
40. Coats AJ, Adamopoulos S, Radaelli A, et al. Controlled trial of physical training in chronic heart failure. Exercise performance, hemodynamics, ventilation, and autonomic function. Circulation 1992; 85:2119–2131.
41. Malfatto G, Branzi G, Riva B, Sala L, Leonetti G, Facchini M. Recovery of cardiac autonomic responsiveness with low-intensity physical training in patients with chronic heart failure. Eur J Heart Fail 2002; 4:159–166.

42. Adamopoulos S, Piepoli M, McCance A, et al. Comparison of different methods for assessing sympathovagal balance in chronic congestive heart failure secondary to coronary artery disease. Am J Cardiol 1992; 70:1576–1582.
43. Scott AC, Wensel R, Davos CH, et al. Skeletal muscle reflex in heart failure patients: role of hydrogen. Circulation 2003; 107:300–306.
44. Piepoli M, Clark AL, Volterrani M, Adamopoulos S, Sleight P, Coats AJ. Contribution of muscle afferents to the hemodynamic, autonomic, and ventilatory responses to exercise in patients with chronic heart failure: effects of physical training. Circulation 1996; 93:940–952.
45. Mancini DM, Henson D, La Manca J, Donchez L, Levine S. Benefit of selective respiratory muscle training on exercise capacity in patients with chronic congestive heart failure. Circulation 1995; 91:320–329.
46. Franklin BA, Bonzheim K, Gordon S, et al. Safety of medically supervised outpatient cardiac rehabilitation exercise therapy: a 15-year follow-up. Chest 1998; 114:902–906.
47. Jugdutt BI, Michorowski BL, Kappagoda CT. Exercise training after anterior Q wave myocardial infarction: importance of regional left ventricular function and topography. J Am Coll Cardiol 1988; 12:362–372.
48. Dubach P, Myers J, Dziekan G, et al. Effect of exercise training on myocardial remodeling in patients with reduced left ventricular function after myocardial infarction: application of magnetic resonance imaging. Circulation 1997; 95:2060–2067.
49. Myers J, Goebbels U, Dzeikan G, et al. Exercise training and myocardial remodeling in patients with reduced ventricular function: one-year follow-up with magnetic resonance imaging. Am Heart J 2000; 139:252–261.
50. Giannuzzi P, Tavazzi L, Temporelli PL, et al. Long-term physical training and left ventricular remodeling after anterior myocardial infarction: results of the Exercise in Anterior Myocardial Infarction (EAMI) trial. EAMI Study Group. J Am Coll Cardiol 1993; 22:1821–1829.
51. Lenne R, Gordon A, Jensen-Urstad M, Dencker K, Jansson E, Sylven C. Aerobic training involving a minor muscle mass shows greater efficiency than training involving a major muscle mass in chronic heart failure patients. J Card Fail 1999; 5:300–307.
52. Fletcher GF, Balady GJ, Amsterdam EA, et al. Exercise standards for testing and training: a statement for healthcare professionals from the American Heart Association. Circulation 2001; 104:1694–1740.
53. Dalla Libera L, Ravara B, Gobbo V, et al. Skeletal muscle myofibrillar protein oxidation in heart failure and the protective effect of Carvedilol. J Mol Cell Cardiol 2005; 38:803–807.
54. De Matos LD, Gardenghi G, Rondon MU, et al. Impact of 6 months of therapy with carvedilol on muscle sympathetic nerve activity in heart failure patients. J Card Fail 2004; 10:496–502.
55. Vescovo G, Dalla Libera L, Serafini F, et al. Improved exercise tolerance after losartan and enalapril in heart failure: correlation with changes in skeletal muscle myosin heavy chain composition. Circulation 1998; 98:1742–1749.
56. American Association of Cardiovascular and Pulmonary Rehabilitation. Guidelines for Cardiac Rehabilitation and Secondary Prevention Programs. Champaign, IL: Human Kinetics Publishers, 2004.
57. Olsson LG, Swedberg K, Clark AL, Witte KK, Cleland JG. Six minute corridor walk test as an outcome measure for the assessment of treatment in randomized, blinded intervention trials of chronic heart failure: a systematic review. Eur Heart J 2005; 26:778–793.
58. Myers J. Applications of cardiopulmonary exercise testing in the management of cardiovascular and pulmonary disease. Int J Sports Med 2005; 26:S49–S55.
59. Corra U, Mezzani A, Bosimini E, Giannuzzi P. Cardiopulmonary exercise testing prognosis in chronic heart failure: a prognosticating algorithm for the individual patient. Chest 2004; 126:942–950.
60. Pu CT, Johnson MT, Forman DE, et al. Randomized trial of progressive resistance training to counteract the myopathy of chronic heart failure. J Appl Physiol 2001; 90:2341–2350.
61. Selig SE, Carey MF, Menzies DG, et al. Moderate-intensity resistance exercise training in patients with chronic heart failure improves strength, endurance, heart rate variability, and forearm blood flow. J Card Fail 2004; 10:21–30.

62. Delagardelle C, Feiereisen P, Autier P, Shita R, Krecke R, Beissel J. Strength/endurance training versus endurance training in congestive heart failure. Med Sci Sports Exerc 2002; 34:1868–1872.
63. Fiatarune MA, O'Neill EF, Ryan ND, et al. Exercise training and nutritional supplementation for physical frailty in very elderly people. N Engl J Med 1994; 330:1769–1775.
64. Zile MR, Baicu CF, Gaasch WH. Diastolic heart failure—abnormalities in active relaxation and passive stiffness of the left ventricle. N Engl J Med 2004; 350:1953–1959.
65. Gigli G, Vallebona A. Physical training in the elderly with heart failure. Ital Heart J 2004; 5:69S–73S.
66. Corvera-Tindel T, Doering LV, Gomez T, Dracup K. Predictors of noncompliance to exercise training in heart failure. J Cardiovasc Nurs 2004; 19:269–277.

5
Diuretics

Ilan S. Wittstein
Division of Cardiology, Department of Medicine, Johns Hopkins University School of Medicine, Baltimore, Maryland, U.S.A.

INTRODUCTION

Diuretics play an essential role in the management of patients with congestive heart failure. Neurohormonal activation in patients with heart failure results in salt and water retention that frequently leads to symptoms of dyspnea and edema. By inhibiting the kidney's ability to reabsorb sodium, diuretics reduce extracellular fluid volume and are effective at rapidly reducing symptoms of congestion. The ability to relieve symptoms and improve functional capacity has made diuretics first line agents in the treatment of heart failure for the past several decades. Yet despite their universal acceptance, there are data suggesting that diuretics may have detrimental vascular, hemodynamic, and neurohormonal effects, and with the exception of the potassium sparing class, the impact of diuretics on mortality in patients with heart failure remains unknown. Because diuretics were introduced prior to the advent of rigorous clinical trials with mortality endpoints, they have escaped the scrutiny that other heart failure drugs have been subjected to. Randomized clinical trials involving diuretics in the modern era would be considered by many to be impractical if not unethical, and most heart failure trials performed today require that patients already be on a stable dose of diuretic. As a result, the direct influence of diuretics on cardiac performance, hemodynamic profile, ventricular remodeling, neurohormonal activation, and long term survival in patients with heart failure remains controversial and incompletely studied. This chapter will review the limited available data, highlighting both the beneficial and potentially deleterious effects of diuretics in the treatment of heart failure. Treatment strategies based on diuretic mechanisms of action and pharmacokinetic properties will be presented, and therapeutic options for treating patients with diuretic resistance will be discussed.

EFFECT OF DIURETICS ON HEART FAILURE SYMPTOMS

There is significant evidence that diuretics improve symptoms of heart failure and quality of life (1) but only a few trials have compared diuretics with other drugs as monotherapy. In one study of patients with moderate heart failure, increasing the dose of furosemide was more effective in relieving symptoms and improving exercise tolerance than adding captopril (2). Furosemide was also more effective in relieving symptoms and improving exercise tolerance when compared to the dopamine agonist ibopamine in a double-blind crossover study (3). In an important study by Haerer et al., subjects with ischemic cardiomyopathy and heart failure were randomized to either the loop diuretic piretanide or placebo (4). Subjects receiving diuretic experienced significant improvement in subjective symptoms, exercise tolerance, and pulmonary capillary wedge pressure compared to controls. In a meta-analysis of randomized controlled trials, diuretics improved heart failure symptoms and significantly increased exercise capacity when compared to other agents (e.g., ACE inhibitors, digoxin, ibopamine) (5). There is also evidence that some diuretics are more effective than others at relieving symptoms. In an open label study of furosemide versus torsemide in 234 patients with chronic heart failure, those randomized to torsemide had less dyspnea and fatigue and had significantly fewer hospital days for decompensated heart failure (6). The observed differences may have been related to torsemide's superior bioavailability.

Exacerbation of heart failure symptoms has also been observed in studies where diuretics were withdrawn. In a study by Grinstead et al., heart failure patients were taken off a stable dose of diuretic and randomized to either lisinopril or placebo (7). After a median of 15 days, 71% of the patients had to be restarted on diuretics due to worsening symptoms of heart failure, irrespective of their randomization arm. A history of hypertension, a baseline furosemide dose of greater than 40 mg/day, and a left ventricular ejection fraction <27% were independent predictors of diuretic re-initiation. In a separate small double-blind randomized crossover trial, well compensated patients developed pulmonary congestion when switched from a diuretic to an ACE inhibitor (8). Finally, Braunschweig et al. used an implantable cardiac monitor to demonstrate the relationship between clinical and hemodynamic deterioration in a small group of patients taken off furosemide (9).

HEMODYNAMIC EFFECTS OF DIURETICS

There are conflicting data regarding the direct effects of diuretics on myocyte contractility. Bumetanide, but not furosemide or torsemide, produced concentration-dependent increases in cell shortening and velocity of cell shortening in isolated rabbit ventricular myocytes (10). In contrast, furosemide had a direct inhibitory effect on contractility in the isolated perfused rabbit heart (11). In a separate study, furosemide had no effect on the action potential, potassium exchange, or mechanical function of isolated rabbit myocardium (12). In humans, diuretics have not been shown to have inotropic properties but they influence cardiac performance primarily through their effects on the vasculature and cardiac load (13). In patients with heart failure, the acute vascular effects of furosemide have been studied most extensively and are discussed below.

Furosemide-Induced Venodilation

As early as 1967, it was observed that following furosemide administration, relief of heart failure symptoms occurred prior to the onset of diuresis (14). This apparent extrarenal mechanism of action was illucidated by Dikshit et al. in a group of patients with pulmonary congestion following acute infarction (15). Within 5 min of furosemide administration, there was a significant decrease in pulmonary capillary wedge pressure, which corresponded with increased calf venous capacitance, increased calf blood flow, and a decrease in limb vascular resistance. All of these observations preceded peak diuresis and natriuresis by several minutes, suggesting that the early effects of furosemide were due to venodilation. Similar effects have been observed in healthy controls on sodium restricted diets (16,17). It is unknown if the venodilatory effects of furosemide are direct or indirect but the majority of evidence suggests that the mechanism may be prostaglandin mediated (16–18). Increased angiotensin II following furosemide administration may induce venous endothelial cell prostaglandin synthesis via the AT2 receptor. This hypothesis is supported by the observation that the venodilator response to furosemide is attenuated by cyclooxygenase inhibitors(17,19) and ACE inhibitors (20). Other diuretics have been studied less extensively but both thiazide diuretics(21) and carbonic anhydrase inhibitors (22) may exert direct vasodilatory effects through vascular potassium channel activation.

Furosemide-Induced Vasoconstriction

In contrast to the venodilation seen in patients with acute congestive heart failure, furosemide infusion results in arterial vasoconstriction in patients with chronic heart failure. Francis et al. demonstrated increased left ventricular filling pressure, mean arterial pressure, and systemic vascular resistance, and decreased stroke volume in the first 20 min after furosemide administration (23). Diuretic induced neurohormonal activation may have accounted for these adverse hemodynamic effects since there was an associated increase in plasma renin activity, norepinephrine, and arginine vasopressin (AVP). Similarly, in a group of healthy volunteers, furosemide administration increased plasma renin and pulmonary vascular resistance, and augmented the pulmonary vasoconstrictive response to hypoxemia (24). The observation that the pressor response to furosemide can be attenuated by ACE inhibitors in patients with heart failure suggests that these hemodynamic effects are angiotensin II mediated(25).

NEUROHORMONAL EFFECTS OF LOOP DIURETICS

Renin–Angiotensin–Aldosterone System

Several studies have shown that prior to the initiation of diuretic therapy, the renin–angiotensin–aldosterone system (RAAS) is not significantly stimulated in patients with heart failure (26–29). Following the administration of diuretic, however, there is marked RAAS activation (26,27,29–32). This occurs primarily due to volume contraction and subsequent stimulation of baroreceptors and the macula densa. Both acute and chronic diuretic administration can result in RAAS activation. An increase in plasma renin activity has been observed within a few min of intravenous furosemide infusion (23,33). The associated increase in systemic vascular resistance and decrease in cardiac output suggests that the acute vasoconstrictor response to furosemide may be RAAS mediated. Elevations in plasma renin activity, angiotensin II, and aldosterone have also been observed following chronic oral furosemide use over days to weeks (26,27,29,30). Baylis et al. showed that untreated patients with heart failure had normal renin and aldosterone levels both at rest and following exercise. While exercise tolerance improved following a month of treatment with furosemide and amiloride, there was also a significant increase in plasma renin and aldosterone (26). In a substudy of the Studies of Left Ventricular Dysfunction (SOLVD), elevated plasma renin activity was associated with chronic diuretic use (28). While RAAS activation may have long-term deleterious effects due to increased vasoconstriction, sodium and water retention, and aldosterone mediated myocardial fibrosis (34), it is not known whether loop diuretics potentiate these effects and thus lead to increased morbidity and mortality.

Sympathetic Nervous System

An elevated plasma norepinephrine concentration is a marker of enhanced sympathetic neural activity and correlates with worsening clinical status (35) and increased mortality (36) in patients with heart failure. Numerous studies have shown that in contrast to the RAAS, sympathetic nervous system (SNS) activity is increased prior to the initiation of diuretics (26–28,37). In patients with heart failure and other critical illnesses, the acute administration of furosemide causes a further rise in plasma norepinephrine that is accompanied by an increase in systemic vascular resistance and a reduction in cardiac output (23,33). In experimental animal models, vasoconstriction and increased plasma norepinephrine in response to acute furosemide administration are attenuated by intravertebral arterial infusion of angiotensin II antagonists (38) and the presynaptic α-2 receptor agonist clonidine (39). These agents do not inhibit the pressor response to furosemide when given intravenously, suggesting that the acute vasoconstrictor effects of furosemide are mediated by central sympathetic neural activation.

In contrast to the increase in plasma norepinephrine seen with acute diuretic administration, most studies have demonstrated a decrease in SNS activity following chronic diuretic use (26,27,37). Broqvist et al. showed a significant reduction in both plasma epinephrine and norepinephrine concentrations within one day of receiving furosemide, an effect that was maintained throughout the eight-day study period (27). Baylis et al. demonstrated that a month of diuretic therapy in previously untreated heart failure patients resulted in a decrease in plasma norepinephrine and an increase in exercise tolerance (26). In New York Heart Association (NYHA) class IV patients treated with diuretics and vasodilators, decreases in pulmonary capillary wedge pressure and systemic vascular resistance were associated with a decline in plasma norepinephrine concentration (37). There is also evidence that SNS activity can be influenced by the type of diuretic used. In a study comparing the effects of the short-acting loop diuretic furosemide to the long-acting loop diuretic azosemide, azosemide treatment was associated with lower plasma norepinephrine and renin concentrations, and with an improvement in quality of life (40). Because sympathetic neural activation can contribute to heart failure progression through a variety of mechanisms that include peripheral vasoconstriction, arrhythmias, induction of apoptosis (41), and cardiac remodeling (42), reduction of SNS activity with chronic diuretic therapy may impact favorably on myocardial function and survival.

Arginine Vasopressin

Few studies have examined the direct effects of diuretics on AVP in patients with heart failure. Francis et al. observed an increase in AVP concentration within 10 min of intravenous furosemide infusion. The concentration peaked at 30 min and returned to baseline at one hour (23). In contrast, Broqvist et al. demonstrated a gradual and sustained decline in AVP concentration when diuretics were administered over several days to heart failure patients with congestion (27). In a substudy of the SOLVD, subjects with left ventricular dysfunction had elevated plasma AVP concentrations compared to controls, but AVP concentrations were unaffected by the use of a diuretic (28). It is therefore unclear from the limited available data whether diuretics have a direct effect on AVP regulation. It is possible, however, that diuretics affect AVP indirectly by impacting on other neurohormonal systems. For example, diuretics may impact on AVP regulation through increased RAAS activation since angiotensin II is known to be an acute stimulus of AVP release (43).

Prostaglandins

Administration of furosemide in vivo causes an acute increase in venous capacitance that can be attenuated by cyclooxygenase inhibitors. This supports the idea that early venodilation in response to furosemide is prostaglandin mediated. This has been observed in salt restricted healthy adults (17), patients with acute heart failure following myocardial infarction (15), and patients with chronic heart failure (19). In a study by Liguori et al., plasma levels of the prostaglandin prostacyclin (PGI2) were measured in heart failure patients treated either with furosemide or torsemide (44). While both drugs increased PGI2 levels within a few minutes, levels were significantly higher in response to torsemide, and only furosemide stimulated the release of the PGI2 antagonist thromboxane. In the same study, cultured human endothelial and renal epithelial cells demonstrated enhanced PGI2 release after being treated with loop diuretics. The PGI2 release was detected within 5 min and was maximal by 15 min, a time course consistent with the venodilation seen in response to furosemide in vivo. In patients with heart failure being treated with diuretics, the increased prostaglandin release may help to preserve renal blood flow by countering enhanced RAAS activation. This may explain in part why the combination of diuretics and nonsteroidal anti-inflammatory drugs can have deleterious effects in patients with heart failure (45).

Natriuretic Peptides

Atrial natriuretic peptide (ANP) and brain natriuretic peptide (BNP) are secreted primarily in response to the atrial and ventricular stretch that occurs with volume overload (46–48). Diuretics would therefore be expected to decrease natriuretic peptide secretion by reducing preload and cardiac volumes. In normal subjects, plasma ANP levels increase following infusion of hypertonic saline and then fall significantly in response to furosemide administration (49,50). Furosemide also lowers plasma BNP levels in patients with refractory congestive heart failure (51). When patients with acute decompensated heart failure are treated with diuretics and vasodilators, both ANP and BNP levels decrease (37), and the fall in plasma BNP concentration correlates with the decline in pulmonary capillary wedge pressure (52). Natriuretic peptide production may also be affected by non-loop diuretics. Heart failure patients treated with spironolactone have a reduction in plasma ANP and BNP (53). The associated decrease in plasma procollagen type III aminoterminal peptide (a marker of fibrosis) and in left ventricular volume and mass suggests that the influence of spironolactone on natriuretic peptide secretion may be related to its effect on cardiac remodeling. It should be noted, however, that not all heart failure patients treated with diuretics and vasodilators have a reduction in natriuretic peptide levels (52,54). In the SOLVD substudy, patients in the treatment group receiving diuretics did not have lower ANP levels than patients from whom diuretics were withheld (28). Heart failure patients who do not manifest a decrease in

BNP concentration following diuretic and vasodilator therapy appear to be at increased risk of hospitalization and death (55,56).

EFFECT OF DIURETICS ON CARDIAC REMODELING

Loop Diuretics

In experimental animal models, loop diuretics do little to improve ventricular remodeling and may, in fact, be deleterious. In a post-infarct rat heart failure model, ramipril reduced fibrosis by enhanced interstitial collagenase expression, while furosemide had no beneficial effect on remodeling (57). In a tachycardia-induced porcine heart failure model, the administration of furosemide accelerated left ventricular systolic dysfunction, increased serum aldosterone levels, and resulted in impaired calcium handling (58). In humans, there is little data to support that loop diuretics improve ventricular remodeling following acute myocardial infarction or in patients with chronic heart failure. In a randomized, double-blind study, Sharpe et al. compared the effects of captopril and furosemide on ventricular remodeling following acute transmural myocardial infarction (59). Patients receiving captopril had a reduction in left ventricular cavity size and improvement in ejection fraction over a 12 mo follow-up period. Similar beneficial effects were not observed with furosemide, and patients in this group had a mild increase in cavity size and reduction in ejection fraction. A more recent study has suggested that loop diuretics may have an impact on myocardial fibrosis in patients with chronic heart failure (60). Right ventricular endomyocardial biopsies were obtained to quantify collagen volume fraction (CVF), and serum measurements were made of carboxy-terminal peptide of procollagen type I (PIP), a marker of collagen type I synthesis. Patients treated with torsemide had a reduction in CVF and PIP but these indexes did not change in patients treated with furosemide. These results suggest that torsemide may reduce myocardial fibrosis by inhibiting the extracellular synthesis of collagen type I. It is not known whether these apparent anti-fibrotic effects contribute to the lower mortality seen in heart failure patients treated with torsemide compared to furosemide (61).

Aldosterone Receptor Antagonists

Aldosterone plays an important role in cardiac remodeling (62) and aldosterone antagonists such as eplerenone have been shown to attenuate experimental myocardial fibrosis (63). In humans with heart failure, spironolactone decreases collagen formation (64) and improves left ventricular size and systolic function (65). There is indirect evidence from a substudy of the Randomized Aldactone Evaluation Study (RALES) that the mortality benefit seen with spironolactone in patients with chronic heart failure may in part be due to its anti-fibrotic effect (66). Elevated serum levels of procollagen types I and III, markers of collagen synthesis, were strong predictors of mortality. Reduction of these markers was associated with improved survival in patients treated with spironolactone. Aldosterone antagonists also improve remodeling in post-infarct patients. In a small randomized trial, the aldosterone antagonist canrenoate, when given in the post-infarct period, resulted in reduction of ventricular volumes and collagen formation (67). Similarly, spironolactone reduced collagen synthesis and improved cardiac function when given immediately after myocardial infarction (68). These data suggest that a beneficial effect on cardiac remodeling is a potential mechanism for the improved survival seen in patients receiving the aldosterone antagonist eplerenone following myocardial infarction (69).

EFFECT OF DIURETICS ON MORTALITY

Loop Diuretics

Because loop diuretics are so effective at relieving symptoms in patients with congestive heart failure, no placebo controlled trials have ever been done to study their effects on survival. Faris et al. conducted a meta-analysis of randomized controlled trials that used diuretics (e.g., furosemide, furosemide-hydrochlorothiazide) for the treatment of heart failure (5). Three placebo-controlled trials (N = 221) showed an absolute risk reduction of 8% in patients treated with diuretics, but all trials were small and lacked statistical power needed to demonstrate mortality reduction. There is evidence to support that loop diuretics may increase mortality risk. Preliminary data from the Acute Decompensated Heart Failure National Registry (ADHERE) database suggest that chronic diuretic therapy increases in-hospital mortality in patients admitted with decompensated heart failure, particularly those patients with renal dysfunction (54). In a retrospective analysis of the SOLVD trial, there was an increased risk of death in patients taking non-potassium-sparing diuretics compared to those taking potassium-sparing diuretics (70). Further, compared with patients taking no diuretics, those being treated with non-potassium-sparing diuretics had an increased risk of hospitalization or death due to worsening heart failure (relative risk = 1.31, 95% confidence interval 1.09–1.57). In another retrospective study of SOLVD patients, baseline use of a non-potassium-sparing diuretic was associated with an increased risk of arrhythmic death (relative risk = 1.33, 95% confidence interval 1.05–1.69) (71). High diuretic doses were also found to be independently associated with mortality, sudden death, and death due to pump failure in a retrospective study of 1153 heart failure patients enrolled in the Prospective Randomized Amlodipine Survival Evaluation (PRAISE) trial (72). It is not possible to discern from this study whether high diuretic doses were themselves harmful, or whether the need for higher doses identified a sicker population with poorer outcome. The effects of different loop diuretics on morbidity and mortality have also been compared. The Torasemide in Congestive Heart Failure Study (TORIC) looked at the safety and efficacy of torsemide versus furosemide and other diuretics in 1377 patients with mild to moderate heart failure. Though not designed to be a mortality study, mortality was found to be significantly lower in the torsemide group (2.2% vs. 4.5%, $p < 0.05$) (61). This suggests that the pharmacokinetic differences of the various loop diuretics may have an impact on long term survival.

Aldosterone Receptor Antagonists

The potassium-sparing aldosterone receptor antagonists are the only diuretics that have been shown to reduce mortality in patients with left ventricular dysfunction and congestive heart failure. The RALES study examined the effect of spironolactone on mortality in patients with NYHA class IV symptoms with an ejection fraction $\leq$35% who were already being treated with an ACE inhibitor and a loop diuretic (73). Patients receiving spironolactone had improvement in functional class, a 35% decrease in the frequency of hospitalization, and a 30% reduction in risk of death. A survival benefit was also observed in post-infarct patients with left ventricular dysfunction and heart failure in the Eplerenone Post-Acute Myocardial Infarction Heart Failure Efficacy and Survival Study (EPHESUS) (69). Compared to placebo, patients receiving the aldosterone antagonist eplerenone had a decrease in overall mortality (relative risk = 0.85), cardiovascular mortality (relative risk = 0.83), and sudden death from cardiac causes (relative risk = 0.79).

DIURETIC PHARMACOLOGY

Diuretic Classification and Mechanism of Action

Diuretics are commonly classified by their specific sites of action within the tubule, which also determine their maximal natriuretic effects (Table 1). The majority of filtered sodium (~60–70%) is reabsorbed at the proximal tubule. This is facilitated primarily by carbonic anhydrase which catalyzes the hydration of bicarbonate, resulting in the reabsorption of both sodium and bicarbonate (74). Carbonic anhydrase inhibitors such as acetazolamide interfere with proximal tubule sodium reabsorption (Fig. 1A). While one might expect a proximally acting agent to produce a profound natriuresis, the carbonic anhydrase inhibitors have limited efficacy for two reasons. First, most of the sodium escaping reabsorption at the proximal tubule is reabsorbed downstream at the thick ascending limb of the loop of Henle (74). Second, the inhibitory effect of these agents is diminished by the metabolic acidosis that results from urinary bicarbonate loss (75). For these reasons, carbonic anhydrase inhibitors are rarely used to treat patients with congestive heart failure.

Loop diuretics inhibit the $Na^+2Cl^-K^+$ cotransporter at the thick ascending limb of the loop of Henle (Fig. 1B). They are the most effective diuretics available and are capable of blocking the reabsorption of essentially all of the sodium that is delivered to this part of the tubule (20–30% of the total filtered sodium load). Because calcium is reabsorbed in parallel with sodium at the thick ascending limb, loop diuretics can also cause a calciuresis and can be used to treat hypercalcemia (74). The thiazide diuretics inhibit sodium

Table 1 Diuretic Types Listed by Sites and Mechanisms of Action

Diuretic type	Examples	Maximum effect (% of filtered Na^+ load)	Site of action	Mechanism of action
CA inhibitors	Acetazolamide	3–5	Proximal tubule	Inhibit CA
Loop diuretics	Furosemide; bumetanide; torsemide; ethacrynic acid	20–25	Thick ascending limb of the loop of Henle	Inhibit $Na^+2Cl^-K^+$ co-transporter
Thiazide diuretics	Chlorothiazide; chlorthialidone hydrochlorothiazide; metolazone	5–8	Early distal tubule	Inhibit the Na^+Cl^- co-transporter
Potassium-sparing diuretics	Amiloride; triamterene; spironolactone	2–3	Late distal tubule and collecting duct	Inhibit Na^+ reabsorption by blocking aldosterone or epithelial Na^+ channel

Abbreviations: CA, carbonic anhydrase; Cl^-, chloride; K^+, potassium; Na^+, sodium.
Source: Modified from Brater DC. Diuretics. In: Munson PL, Mueller RA, Breese GR, eds. Principles of Pharmacology. Basic Concepts and Clinical Application. New York; Chapman and Hall, 1995:658.

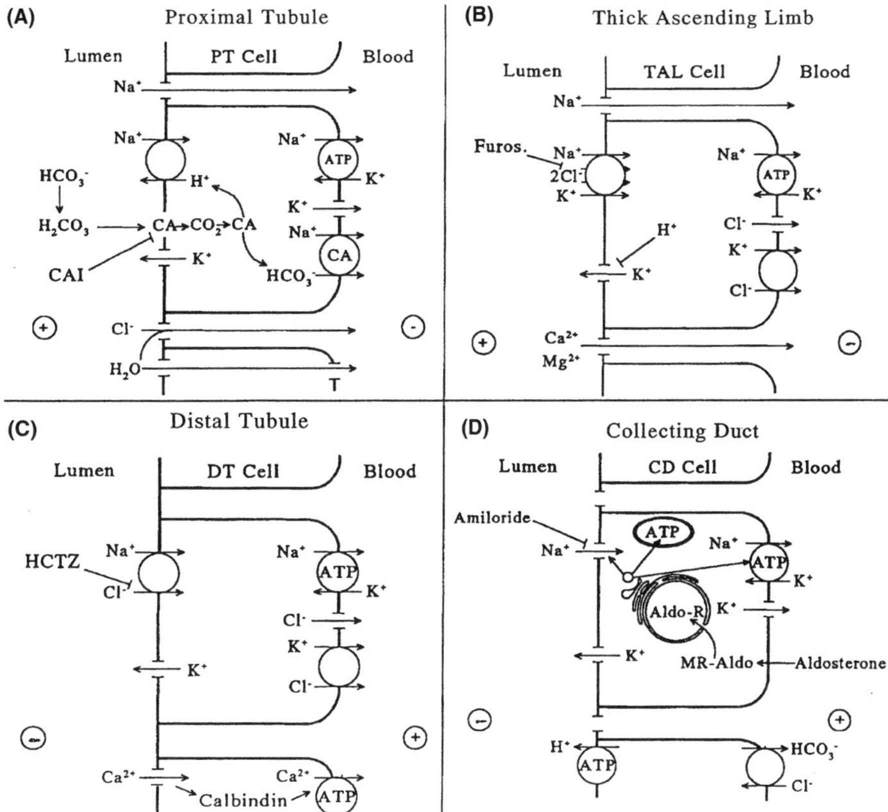

Figure 1 Schematic representation of the mechanism of sodium uptake inhibition by different diuretics at their specific sites of action. Carbonic anhydrase inhibitors (CAI) interfere with luminal sodium uptake in the proximal tubule (PT) through inhibition of carbonic anhydrase (CA) (**A**). Loop diuretics block the $Na^+2Cl^-K^+$ cotransporter at the thick ascending limb (TAL) of the loop of Henle (**B**), and thiazide diuretics inhibit the Na^+Cl^-cotransporter in the early distal tubule (DT) (**C**). Potassium-sparing diuretics inhibit sodium uptake in the late distal tubule and collecting duct (CD) by directly blocking the epithelial sodium channel (e.g., amiloride) or by blocking the aldosterone receptor (e.g., spironolatone) (**D**). Circles represent carrier systems, circles with ATP represent energy requiring transporters, and arrows are ion channels/conductances. *Abbreviations*: Aldo, aldosterone; Furos, furosemide; HCTZ, hydrochlorothiazide; R and MR, mineralocorticoid receptor. *Source*: From Gregef R. New insights into the molecular mechanism of the action of diuretics. Nephrol Dial Transplant 1999; 14:537.

reabsorption by blocking the Na^+Cl^-cotransporter in the distal convoluted tubule (Fig. 1C). Because only 5% of filtered sodium is reabsorbed in the distal tubule, these agents have limited efficacy. When used in combination with loop diuretics, however, they can induce significant natriuresis and diuresis (74).

In the principle cells of the collecting duct, the mineralocorticoid aldosterone stimulates the synthesis of the epithelial sodium channel (ENaC) through which sodium is reabsorbed in exchange for potassium and hydrogen ions (75). Potassium-sparing diuretics inhibit sodium reabsorption by directly blocking ENaC (amiloride and triamterene) or the aldosterone receptor (spironolactone; Fig. 1D). These agents have relatively weak natriuretic and diuretic effects but are frequently used in combination with other diuretic classes to help reduce kaliuresis. Spironolactone is also the only diuretic known to improve survival in patients with NYHA class IV symptoms of congestive heart failure (73).

Diuretic Pharmacokinetics

General Concepts

The pharmacokinetic properties of some of the commonly used diuretics are shown in Table 2. With the exception of spironolactone, all diuretics must reach the lumen of the renal tubule in order to be effective. Once absorbed into the bloodstream, diuretics have a high degree of protein binding (>95%), which limits glomerular filtration and keeps them in the vascular space. This ensures their delivery to the proximal tubule cells where they are taken up across the basolateral membrane by either an anion exchanger (loop diuretics, thiazides) or a cation exchanger (amiloride, triamterene), and then actively secreted into the lumen (75). The pharmacokinetic properties of a diuretic (i.e., availability of the drug at its specific site of action) are therefore determined by many factors including dose, absorption (if given orally), drug half-life, delivery of the drug

Table 2 Dosage and Pharmacokinetic Properties of Commonly Used Diuretics, Listed According to Site of Action

			Onset of action(%)		Action duration			
Diuretic	Dosage (mg/day)	Oral bio-availability	Oral (hr)	IV (min)	Oral (hr)	IV (hr)	Peak oral effect (hr)	Elimination half-life (hr)
Proximal tubule								
Acetazolamide	250–375	ND	1	30–60	8	3–4	2–4	ND
TAL of Henle								
Furosemide	40–400	10–100	1	5	6	2–3	1–3	1.5–2
Bumetanide	1–5	80–100	0.5	5	6	2–3	1–3	1
Torsemide	10–200	80–100	1	10	6–8	6–8	1–3	3–4
Ethacrynic acid	50–100	~100	0.5	5	6–8	3	2	1
Early distal tubule								
Chlorothiazide	500–1000	30–50	1	15–30	8	–	4	1.5
Chlorthalidone	25–200	64	2	–	24–48	–	6	24–55
Hydrochloro-thiazide	25–100	65–75	2	–	12	–	4	6–9
Metolazone	2.5–20	40–65	1	–	12–24	–	2–4	14
Late distal tubule								
Spironolactone	50–400	Conflicting data	48–72	–	48–72	–	24–48	1.5
Triamterene	75–300	>80	2	–	12–16	–	6–8	2–5
Amiloride	5–10	Conflicting data	2	–	24	–	6–16	17–26

Abbreviations: hr, hour; IV, intravenous; mg, milligram; min, minute; ND, not determined; TAL, thick ascending loop.

Source: Modified from Gottlieb SS: Diuretics. In: Hosenpud JD, Greenberg B, eds. Congestive Heart Failure: Pathophysiology, Diagnosis, and Comprehensive Approach to Management. Springer-Verlag New York Inc. 1994:348. Data also from Ref. 76.

to the proximal tubule, and the capability of the proximal tubule cell to secrete the drug into the tubule lumen.

Absorption

The bioavailability of furosemide (i.e., the amount of an oral dose that reaches the bloodstream) is approximately 50% but it can range from 10% to 100% (76). This widely variable bioavailability makes it difficult to predict how much drug will be absorbed in a given individual. In contrast, bumetanide and torsemide have absorptions that range from 80% to 100%. When switching from intravenous to oral administration, therefore, the dose of bumetanide and torsemide can remain the same while that of furosemide should be doubled. In addition, food decreases the absorption of furosemide and bumetanide but not torsemide (74).

It is a common misperception that oral loop diuretics are less effective in patients with congestive heart failure due to "gut edema" and decreased absorption. In actuality, gut edema does not decrease the *amount* of diuretic absorbed (bioavailability is normal in both compensated and decompensated patients) (77,78). Gut edema, however, may contribute to the decreased *rate* of diuretic absorption seen in patients with congestive heart failure. This slower absorption results in delayed peak concentrations and lower serum concentrations, particularly in patients who are decompensated (Table 3) (78). For this reason, higher oral doses may be needed in order to deliver a high enough concentration to the urinary active site to reach the steep portion of the dose-response curve. Since the rate of diuretic absorption improves in many patients once they are no longer decompensated, it is reasonable to use intravenous diuretics initially, and then resume oral diuretics once a euvolemic state has been achieved.

Plasma Half-Life and Metabolism

The frequency of diuretic administration is determined by its plasma half-life (Table 2). About 50% of a dose of furosemide is conjugated in the kidneys to glucuronic acid while 50% is excreted unchanged into the urine (76). The half-life of furosemide is therefore prolonged in patients with renal insufficiency. In contrast, bumetanide and torsemide are largely metabolized by the liver and have longer half-lives in patients with liver disease. The half-lives of the loop diuretics are also frequently prolonged in patients with congestive heart failure since many have renal insufficiency and hepatic congestion (Table 3). Even when prolonged, however, the half-lives of the loop diuretics are relatively short, and their effects tend to decline before the next dose is administered. During the period in between doses, there is enhanced sodium reabsorption by the nephron which may

Table 3 Altered Pharmacokinetics of Loop Diuretics in Patients with Congestive Heart Failure

	Normal subjects		Congestive heart failure patients	
Loop diuretic	Time to peak (min)	Half-life (hr)	Time to peak (min)	Half-life (hr)
Furosemide	108	1.5	180	2.7
Bumetanide	72	1	180	1.3
Torsemide	52	3–4	66	6

Abbreviations: hr, hour; min, minute.

Source: Modified from Brater DC. Diuretic Pharmacokinetics and Pharmacodynamics. In: Seldin D, Giebisch G, eds. Diuretic Agents: Clinical Physiology and Pharmacology. San Diego: Academic Press, 1997:200.

nullify the prior natriuresis (76,79). This explains why patients with heart failure must restrict their dietary sodium and must take loop diuretics more frequently in order to maintain a negative sodium balance.

Renal Clearance of Diuretic

Diuretic pharmacokinetics are also affected by impaired secretion of drug by the proximal tubular cells into the lumen. This is frequently seen in patients with chronic renal disease. In patients with heart failure who have preserved renal function, the amount and rate of diuretic excretion into the urine is similar to that seen in healthy people (80). When patients with heart failure have renal dysfunction, proximal tubule cell secretion of diuretic into the lumen is impaired, and patients must be given higher diuretic doses in order for a sufficient amount of the drug to reach the urinary site of action. For example, heart failure patients with renal insufficiency may require at least 120 mg of IV furosemide or 2–3 mg of IV bumetanide in order to achieve a maximal natriuretic response. Renal clearance of diuretics can also be affected by other drugs. Organic acids such as probenecid can decrease proximal tubule secretion of loop and thiazide diuretics by competing for the anion exchanger. Similarly, organic bases such as trimethoprim can compete for the cation exchanger and impair secretion of amiloride and triamterene (76).

Diuretic Pharmacodynamics

The relationship between diuretic delivery to its active site and natriuretic response determines the pharmacodynamics of the drug. This relationship is characterized graphically by a sigmoidally shaped curve (Fig. 2) and applies to both loop and thiazide diuretics (76,81). This sigmoidal dose response curve illustrates that in order to illicit a natriuretic response, a threshold quantity of drug must be delivered to its active site. For each individual, the diuretic must be titrated in order to determine the dose necessary to

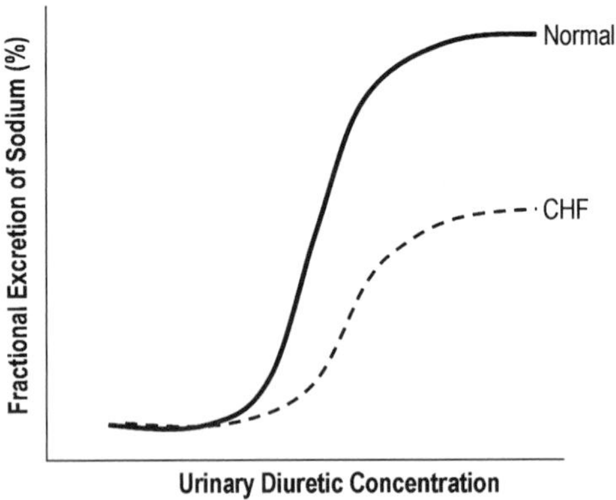

Figure 2 Dose-response curve of a loop diuretic in a normal subject (*solid line*) and in a patient with heart failure (*dashed line*). The relationship between the amount of diuretic reaching the active site and the amount of sodium excreted is represented by a sigmoid curve. Diuresis will not occur until a threshold amount of diuretic reaches the active site, and no further diuresis will occur above the ceiling dose. In patients with heart failure, diuretic resistance is reflected by a downward and rightward shift in the curve, primarily due to increased sodium reabsorption at other nephron sites. *Source*: Modified from Ellison DH. Diuretic therapy and resistance in congestive heart failure. Cardiology 2001; 96:132.

reach the steep portion of the curve (i.e., the effective dose). The sigmoidal curve also illustrates that diuretics have a ceiling dose above which no further natriuresis will occur. In healthy individuals, an intravenous dose of 40 mg of furosemide, 20 mg of torsemide, and 1 mg of bumetanide elicits a maximal natriuretic response (76). Therefore, while the potency varies between these three loop diuretics, their efficacy (maximal response) is the same and amounts to a fractional excretion rate of sodium of 20–25% in healthy individuals.

In patients with congestive heart failure, the dose-response curve is shifted downward and to the right (Fig. 2) (82). On average, the maximal fractional excretion of sodium that can be achieved in these patients is only 10% to 15%. The natriuretic response does not increase with higher diuretic doses, and these patients instead must be given effective doses more regularly. The precise mechanism of this abnormal dose response in patients with heart failure is unknown, but it likely involves several factors, including decreased diuretic delivery to the kidney due to reduced renal blood flow, increased sodium absorption in the proximal tubule due to activation of the RAAS and SNS (83), and increased distal tubule sodium absorption resulting from adaptive changes that are discussed further below (82,84).

Diuretic Resistance

Diuretic resistance can occur both acutely and with chronic diuretic administration. With acute resistance, the magnitude of natriuresis declines following each successive dose of diuretic. This 'braking phenomenon' seems to be dependent on a reduction in intravascular volume and may serve as a protective mechanism against dehydration (76,84). Indeed, when extracellular fluid volume remains constant, the natriuretic response to diuretics does not decrease (79). While activation of the RAAS and the SNS has been proposed as a potential mechanism of acute diuretic resistance, ACE inhibition and adrenergic blockade do not consistently prevent it (85,86).

With chronic administration of loop diuretics, there is increased solute delivery to the distal nephron. This results in several important changes in the epithelial cells of the distal nephron including hypertrophy and hyperplasia (84), increased Na-K-ATPase activity (87), and an increased number of thiazide sensitive Na-Cl cotransporters (88). Thus with chronic loop diuretic use, there is a decline in natriuresis due to the enhanced ability of the distal nephron cells to reabsorb sodium. This explains in part why the addition of a thiazide diuretic can significantly increase natriuresis and diuresis in patients resistant to a loop diuretic alone (89).

DIURETIC USE FOR THE TREATMENT OF CONGESTIVE HEART FAILURE

Treatment of Patients Responsive to Loop Diuretics

Patients with left ventricular dysfunction who have no signs or symptoms of congestion should be treated with ACE inhibitors and beta blockers but do not require diuretics (90). Diuretics should be reserved for symptomatic patients with clinical evidence of volume overload. Thiazide diuretics can be successfully used in some patients with mild heart failure but they are usually insufficient in patients with moderate to severe heart failure and ineffective in patients with renal failure (76). Most patients with moderate to severe volume overload will require a loop diuretic, and the minimum dose necessary to produce an effective diuresis should be determined. The usual starting dose is 20mg to 40 mg of furosemide or its equivalent. If the diuretic response is not adequate, the dose should be increased until the "effective dose" is determined. Because renal responsiveness to loop diuretics may be decreased in patients with heart failure, moderate doses may need to be given more frequently. The frequency of loop diuretic administration will also be influenced by dietary sodium intake. Because there is avid sodium reabsorption by the kidney in the hours following the drug-induced natriuresis, increased dietary sodium intake will necessitate more frequent diuretic administration in order to maintain a negative sodium balance (76,83).

Patients with renal insufficiency secrete less diuretic into the tubule lumen and therefore require higher doses to achieve a maximal natriuretic effect. Due to the sigmoidal nature of the dose response curve, maximal doses have been identified for all of the commonly used loop diuretics in heart failure patients both with and without renal insufficiency (76) (Table 4). Doses higher than these will not increase sodium excretion, and maximal doses may need to be given more frequently if further natriuresis is required. Because the absorption of loop diuretics is delayed in patients with heart failure, these drugs should be given intravenously to patients with more severe signs and symptoms of volume overload.

Though potassium-sparing agents are fairly weak natriuretics, they are frequently added to prevent the hypokalemia that can be seen with the more proximally acting diuretics. Patients on potassium-sparing agents should be monitored closely for hyperkalemia, particularly since many will have renal insufficiency and most will be taking ACE inhibitors or angiotensin receptor blockers. Because spironolactone has been shown to reduce mortality in patients with heart failure (73), it is frequently the agent of choice for treating hypokalemia. When hypokalemia is not a problem and aldosterone antagonists are used purely for mortality benefit, however, they should be reserved for patients who fulfill criteria for RALES (73) (NYHA class IV heart failure, preserved renal function, and normal or low serum potassium) or EPHESUS (69) (recent myocardial infarction, ejection fraction $\leq$40%, symptomatic heart failure, and/or diabetes).

Table 4 Doses of Loop Diuretics Required to Produce a Maximal Natriuretic Response in Heart Failure Patients Both with and Without Renal Insufficiency

	Maximal intravenous dose of loop diuretic (mg)		
	Congestive heart failure and preserved renal function[a]	Congestive heart failure and moderate renal insufficiency[b]	Congestive heart failure and severe renal insufficiency[c]
Furosemide	40–80	80–160	160–200
Bumetanide	1–2	4–8	8–10
Torsemide	10–20	20–50	50–100

[a]Creatinine clearance >75 ml per min.
[b]Creatinine clearance 25–75 ml per min.
[c]Creatinine clearance <25 ml per min.
Source: From Brater DC. Diuretic therapy. N Engl J Med 1998; 339:387–395.

Treatment Options for Patients with Loop Diuretic Resistance

Combination Diuretic Therapy

For patients demonstrating a suboptimal response to maximal doses of loop diuretics, the addition of other diuretic classes can result in substantial natriuresis due to "sequential blockade" of the various sodium reabsorption sites (91). The dose-response curve of a loop diuretic is not altered by other diuretic classes, so the effective loop diuretic dose should not be decreased when a second agent is added. A wide variety of diuretic regimens have been used (92), the most common being the combination of thiazide and loop diuretics. These diuretic classes are synergistic and produce a more potent diuresis when administered together than when either class is used alone (93). A common practice is to add the thiazide-like diuretic metolazone to a loop diuretic. Metolazone has slower absorption and is frequently given 30 to 60 min prior to the loop diuretic in an effort to maximize the synergistic effect. Because metolazone has a long duration of action and prevents sodium reabsorption at both distal and proximal tubule sites, it can induce significant sodium and volume loss when used in combination with a loop diuretic. For these reasons, patients often do best when metolazone is given just two to three times a week and at relatively low doses (e.g., 2.5 mg). For patients requiring intravenous therapy, the distal tubule inhibitor chlorothiazide is frequently used. Agents that selectively block at other nephron sites have also been used. Both the proximal tubule inhibitor acetazolamide (94) and the collecting duct inhibitor spironolactone (95) improve natriuresis in heart failure patients refractory to high dose loop diuretics. The addition of a potassium-sparing diuretic is particularly effective at improving natriuresis in those patients with decreased urinary sodium and increased urinary potassium (76). Options for combination diuretic therapy are listed in Table 5. Patients receiving any of these combined regimens should be followed closely for electrolyte abnormalities and signs of dehydration.

Continuous Diuretic Infusion

Another option for hospitalized patients with diuretic resistance is continuous intravenous diuretic infusion. When loop diuretics are given orally or in bolus infusion, their short half-lives result in periods of post-diuretic sodium retention that may minimize the negative sodium balance. By giving the diuretic in a continuous infusion, constant serum levels are

Table 5 Options for Combination Diuretic Therapy

If a patient is not responding to a ceiling dose of loop diuretic (Table 4), add one of the following[a]:	
Thiazide diuretic	Metolazone 2.5–10 mg po daily
	Hydrochlorothiazide 25–100 mg po daily
	Chlorothiazide 500–1000 mg iv daily
Potassium-sparing diuretic	Spironolactone 100–200 mg po daily
	Triamterene 75–300 mg po daily
	Amiloride 5–10 mg po daily
Carbonic-anhydrase inhibitor	Acetazolamide 250–375 mg po daily (and up to 500 mg iv daily)

[a] If adding more than one diuretic from the list above is required, the diuretics should be from different classes to maximize the synergistic effects.

Abbreviations: po, per os; iv, intravenous.

Source: Modified from Ellison DH. Diuretic therapy and resistance in congestive heart failure. Cardiology 2001; 96:139.

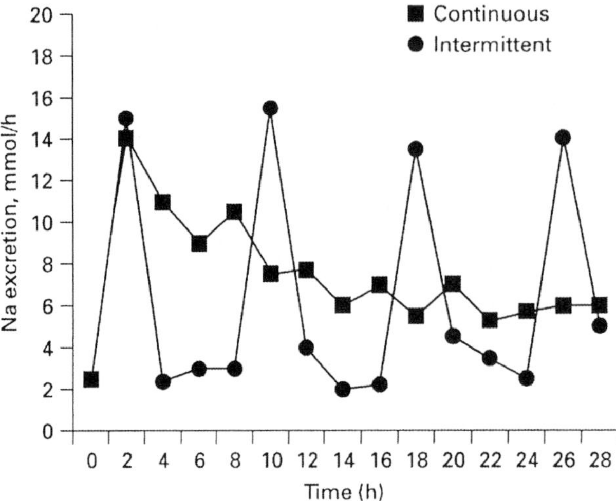

Figure 3 Comparison of the natriuretic response to continuous infusion (*squares*) versus bolus administration (*circles*) of furosemide in patients with congestive heart failure. With bolus administration, sodium excretion is low for several hours in between doses due to the drug's short half-life and the increased sodium reabsorption that occurs following diuretic administration. In contrast, continuous infusion delivers a more consistent effective dose to the urinary site of action, resulting in an 18.5% higher total urine output compared with bolus administration. *Source*: Reproduced from Ellison DH. Diuretic therapy and resistance in congestive heart failure. Cardiology 2001; 96:141. Original data from Ref. 97.

maintained, effective drug doses are delivered continuously to the urinary site of action, and periods of sodium retention are reduced. Studies have demonstrated that a continuous infusion of loop diuretic results in increased urine output and sodium excretion compared to bolus infusion in both patients with chronic renal failure (96) and congestive heart failure (Fig. 3) (97–100). Other potential advantages of continuous infusion include decreased activation of the RAAS and SNS, ease of titration in critically ill patients, and fewer side effects (84,99). Continuous diuretic infusions are typically started following an initial loading dose with rates adjusted according to renal function (Table 6) (76).

Table 6 Doses for Continuous Intravenous Infusion of Loop Diuretics

		Infusion rate (mg/hr)		
Loop diuretic	Intravenous loading dose (mg)	Creatinine clearance <25 ml/min	Creatinine clearance 25–75 ml/min	Creatinine clearance >75 ml/min
Furosemide	40	20 then 40	10 then 20	10
Bumetanide	1	1 then 2	0.5 then 1	0.5
Torsemide	20	10 then 20	5 then 10	5

Abbreviations: hr, hour; min, minute; mg, milligram; ml, milliliter.
Source: Reproduced from Brater DC. Diuretic therapy. N Engl J Med 1998; 339:387–395.

Ultrafiltration

Ultrafiltration may be an option for certain patients with diuretic resistance and refractory congestive heart failure. In patients with moderate congestive heart failure, ultrafiltration rapidly lowers right atrial and pulmonary capillary wedge pressures and results in sustained improvement in exercise tolerance and maximal oxygen consumption over a six month follow-up period (101). Marenzi et al. also demonstrated that ultrafiltration could be used to rapidly remove large fluid volumes in patients with refractory congestive heart failure without hemodynamic compromise (102). On the contrary, patients in this study demonstrated improvement in cardiac filling pressures, cardiac output, and systemic vascular resistance. In addition to its ability to remove volume from patients resistant to diuretic therapy, mechanical ultrafiltration may also offer a neurohormonal advantage. In contrast to loop diuretics, ultrafiltration does not stimulate the macula densa mechanism and may have less impact on RAAS activation (84). In one study, ultrafiltration significantly reduced plasma renin, aldosterone, and norepinephrine in volume overloaded patients refractory to diuretics (103). These favorable neurohormonal and hemodynamic changes may explain in part why some patients with refractory congestive heart failure demonstrate improved diuretic responsiveness following mechanical ultrafiltration (102,103).

DIURETIC-RELATED SIDE EFFECTS

Electrolyte Abnormalities

Hypokalemia is frequently observed in patients receiving loop and thiazide diuretics. These diuretics increase sodium delivery to the distal nephron where it is reabsorbed in exchange for potassium. Patients with congestive heart failure may be particularly sensitive to diuretic induced hypokalemia due to RAAS activation and increased aldosterone production. The primary concern in patients with left ventricular dysfunction is that hypokalemia increases ventricular arrhythmias and sudden cardiac death. While direct causality has not been established, this concern is supported by the observation that patients with left ventricular dysfunction taking non-potassium-sparing diuretics have an increased risk of arrhythmic death, while those on potassium-sparing diuretics do not (71). In contrast to the hypokalemic effects of thiazide and loop diuretics, hyperkalemia can be a serious side effect of the potassium-sparing diuretics. Their use has increased due to the mortality benefit observed with the aldosterone antagonists (69,73). The problem is compounded in patients with heart failure due to the concomitant use of ACE inhibitors or angiotensin receptor blockers, and to the high prevalence of renal insufficiency.

Hyponatremia is another complication of diuretic therapy. While it can occur with loop diuretics, it is most commonly observed with thiazide diuretics which increase sodium excretion and impair maximal urinary dilution. Elderly women appear to be most susceptible to thiazide related hyponatremia (104). It is important to remember, however, that because diuresis is typically isoosmotic, diuretic induced hyponatremia is relatively uncommon. In patients with heart failure, hyponatremia is most often a result of total body fluid overload and not sodium depletion. In this situation, loop diuretics may actually correct the hyponatremia by inhibiting urinary concentrating ability (104).

Thiazide and loop diuretics increase urinary magnesium excretion and reduce plasma magnesium concentrations by about 5%–10%. This effect is diminished in part by the potassium-sparing diuretics. Hypomagnesemia is seen most commonly in elderly patients receiving high doses of loop diuretic, and the extent of electrolyte depletion appears to be related to the duration of therapy (104). Serum magnesium levels are unreliable measures of intracellular stores, and the serum level can be normal in the setting of total body magnesium deficiency (105). An association between hypomagnesemia and arrhythmias has been suggested by some studies (106) but not by others (107). To date, there have been no large prospective studies evaluating the effect of hypomagnesemia or magnesium repletion on mortality in patients with heart failure.

Calcium is affected differently by the various diuretic classes. Loop diuretics increase calcium excretion and can be used to treat hypercalcemia. Thiazide diuretics decrease urinary calcium excretion and can exacerbate hypercalcemic states. It is unknown whether altered calcium balance due to diuretic therapy has an impact on cardiac function in patients with heart failure.

Acid–Base Abnormalities

Both thiazide and loop diuretics can cause a mild metabolic alkalosis. A more severe contraction alkalosis may be seen when thiazide and loop diuretics are used in combination. Metabolic alkalosis can decrease the natriuretic response to loop diuretics and may contribute to the diuretic resistance seen in some patients with heart failure (108). If treatment of the metabolic alkalosis is necessary, options include administration of potassium chloride, a distal potassium sparing diuretic, or a carbonic anhydrase inhibitor (109). In contrast, potassium-sparing diuretics and carbonic anhydrase inhibitors can cause a metabolic acidosis. A potentially dangerous hyperkalemic metabolic acidosis can occur with potassium sparing agents such as spironolactone, particularly in elderly patients with renal insufficiency (109).

Hyperuricemia

Thiazide diuretics decrease renal clearance of urate and increase serum urate levels by as much as 35% (104). Thiazides interfere with urate tubular secretion by competing for the same organic anion transporter (104). Both thiazide and loop diuretics can precipitate gout, particularly in patients who are prone to gout, have high baseline serum urate concentrations, and who are severely volume contracted.

Metabolic Abnormalities

Prolonged use of thiazide diuretics can cause glucose intolerance (110) and should be used cautiously in patients with diabetes. This does not mean, however, that thiazides are contraindicated in diabetic patients. Thiazides have been shown to decrease cardiovascular events in hypertensive diabetic patients (111). Further, in a recent large prospective study, patients taking thiazides for hypertension were not found to be at increased risk for developing diabetes mellitus (112). Short term thiazide use also increases plasma concentrations of total cholesterol, low density lipoprotein (LDL) cholesterol, and triglycerides, and it decreases high density lipoprotein (HDL) cholesterol in a dose-dependent fashion (109,113). This negative effect on lipid profile occurs following initiation of thiazide diuretics, but when combined with exercise, cholesterol levels return to baseline over the course of several months and may even improve following several years of diuretic therapy (114).

Allergic Reactions

Allergic drug reactions are possible with all of the diuretic classes. With the exception of ethacrynic acid, cross sensitivity with sulfonamide drugs can occur with all diuretics (104). Allergic reactions can range in severity from mild dermatitis and photosensitivity, to interstitial nephritis, necrotizing vasculitis and life threatening necrotizing pancreatitis. Ethacrynic acid has a different chemical makeup from the other loop diuretics and can therefore be used safely in patients who have had any of these allergic reactions (109).

Ototoxicity

The human middle ear contains a $Na^{+}2Cl^{-}K^{+}$ cotransporter that responds to loop diuretics. Hearing loss has been associated with all of the loop diuretics, particularly ethacrynic acid and furosemide. The risk of ototoxicity increases with higher diuretic doses, increased intravenous infusion rates, and co-administration of other ototoxic agents such as aminoglycocides (104,109).

Adverse Drug Interactions

Life threatening hyperkalemia can occur when potassium-sparing diuretics are used in combination with a variety of other drugs including potassium supplements, ACE inhibitors, angiotensin receptor blockers, ketoconazole, and trimethoprim. This is particularly the case in patients with renal insufficiency, diabetes, or type IV renal tubular acidosis (109). Loop diuretics can increase both the nephrotoxicity and ototoxicity seen with aminoglycocides, and can increase the risk of digitalis toxicity (115). Both thiazide (116) and loop diuretics (117) can increase plasma lithium concentrations and risk of toxicity. Nonsteroidal anti-inflammatory drugs can result in renal vasoconstriction and decreased GFR and can precipitate renal failure in patients being treated with diuretics (118).

OTHER "DIURETIC" AGENTS

Dopamine

Dopamine at low doses (<5 μg/kg/min) stimulates renal vasodilation, increases renal plasma blood flow, and increases sodium excretion (119). While it has been used as a natriuretic and diuretic agent for over 40 yr (120), studies are inconclusive regarding its efficacy in the management of congestive heart failure. In one study, patients were randomized to intravenous bumetanide alone versus the combination of bumetanide and low dose dopamine (121). Patients receiving dopamine had an increase in creatinine clearance, while the group treated with bumetanide alone had no improvement in renal function. In a separate study, however, dopamine failed to increase the rate of furosemide-induced urinary sodium excretion (122). Other dopaminergic agents that have been studied in patients with heart failure include the DA-1 receptor agonist ibopamine. This caused an increase in renal plasma flow, GFR, and diuresis in one small study (123) but was associated with increased mortality in a large randomized study of patients with advanced heart failure (124). The benefit of low-dose dopamine has also not been proven in patients with poor renal function, and it may even be harmful in critically ill patients (125).

Natriuretic Peptides

The natriuretic peptides are hemodynamically active agents that cause vasodilation and reduction in cardiac filling pressures. ANP has been approved in Japan since 1995 for the treatment of acute decompensated heart failure, while synthetic BNP (nesiritide) has been approved for the same indication in the United States since 2001. There are conflicting data, however, concerning the effects of the natriuretic peptides on renal function. Both ANP (126,127) and BNP (128–130) have been shown to increase natriuresis, diuresis, and GFR in individuals with normal left ventricular function. The natriuretic effects result not only from direct inhibition of distal nephron sodium reabsorption, (129–131) but also from suppression of RAAS activation (126,129,131–133). In contrast to loop diuretics, the ability to induce natriuresis in the absence of RAAS activation suggests one mechanism in which the natriuretic peptides may help to preserve renal function. In an experimental heart failure model, co-administration of BNP and furosemide increased natriuresis, diuresis, and GFR without aldosterone activation (134). In humans with congestive heart failure, however, some studies have demonstrated increased natriuresis and urine volume with BNP infusion (135–137), while others have concluded that BNP has no effect on sodium excretion, urine output, GFR, or effective renal plasma flow (138–140). More recently, it has even been suggested that BNP may have harmful renal effects. In a meta-analysis of randomized clinical trials comparing nesiritide with either placebo or active control for acute decompensated heart failure, nesiritide significantly increased the risk of worsening renal function (141). Larger clinical trials will therefore be needed to clarify the effects of these agents on renal function and to establish their role in the treatment of acute and chronic heart failure.

Vasopressin Antagonists

Vasopressin regulates the body's blood pressure and water content by influencing the rate of water excretion from the kidney. The two principle vasopressin receptors are located in vascular smooth muscle cells (V_{1A}) and in the renal collecting duct (V_2), and result in vasoconstriction and free water reabsorption, respectively (142). Several small studies have looked at the effects of vasopressin antagonists in patients with heart failure. The predominantly V_{1A} receptor antagonist conivaptan was administered intravenously to 142 patients with NYHA class III or IV heart failure in a randomized, double-blind placebo-controlled trial (143). Conivaptan reduced right atrial and pulmonary capillary wedge pressures and caused a significant dose-dependent increase in urine output. Similarly, an increase in urine output and urinary sodium excretion and a decrease in body weight were observed in heart failure patients randomized to the V_2 receptor antagonist tolvaptan (144,145). The long-term effects of these agents on renal function, functional capacity, and mortality in patients with heart failure are currently being studied in large multi-center trials (146,147).

Adenosine Antagonists

Adenosine has an important influence on renal function and sodium balance. Following an acute increase in sodium concentration in the proximal tubule, adenosine stimulates afferent arteriolar vasoconstriction via the A_1 receptor. This mechanism is referred to as tubuloglomerular feedback and results in decreased glomerular filtration and diuresis (148). Patients with heart failure have elevated plasma levels of adenosine (149), and small studies have been performed in these patients to examine the diuretic effects of selective

A_1 receptor blockade. In a study of 12 patients with heart failure, the A_1 receptor blocker BG9719 increased natriuresis and diuresis; in contrast to furosemide, there was no associated decrease in GFR (150). In a randomized, double-blind crossover study of 63 patients with heart failure, BG9719 increased sodium and water excretion and had an additive effect when given with furosemide (151). Additionally, co-administration of the A_1 receptor blocker with furosemide prevented the decrease in GFR observed with the loop diuretic alone.

CONCLUSION

Diuretics represent a therapeutic paradox in the treatment of congestive heart failure. On the one hand, there is considerable evidence that diuretics can have deleterious effects that include neurohormonal activation, systemic vasoconstriction, potentially life threatening electrolyte abnormalities, decreased renal blood flow and GFR, and increased mortality. On the other hand, no drugs are more effective at rapidly relieving symptoms of congestion and edema, or improving functional capacity and quality of life. Diuretics, therefore, remain first-line agents for the treatment of patients with heart failure, and a thorough understanding of their mechanisms of action and pharmacokinetic properties is essential for the optimal management of patients with severe volume overload and diuretic resistance. Newer agents such as the natriuretic peptides and adenosine antagonists can enhance natriuresis when used in conjunction with diuretics, but the long-term effects of these agents on quality of life, renal function, and mortality are still being investigated.

REFERENCES

1. Silke B. Diuretic induced changes in symptoms and quality of life. Br Heart J 1994; 72:S57–S62.
2. Cowley AJ, Stainer K, Wynne RD, et al. Symptomatic assessment of patients with heart failure: double-blind comparison of increasing doses of diuretics and captopril in moderate heart failure. Lancet 1986; 2:770–772.
3. Andrews R, Charlesworth A, Evans A, et al. A double-blind, cross-over comparison of the effects of a loop diuretic and a dopamine receptor agonist as first line therapy in patients with mild congestive heart failure. Eur Heart J 1997; 18:852–857.
4. Haerer W, Bauer U, Sultan N, et al. Acute and chronic effects of a diuretic monotherapy with piretanide in congestive heart failure—a placebo-controlled trial. Cardiovasc Drugs Ther 1990; 4:515–521.
5. Faris R, Flather M, Purcell H, et al. Current evidence supporting the role of diuretics in heart failure: a meta analysis of randomised controlled trials. Int J Cardiol 2002; 82:149–158.
6. Murray MD, Deer MM, Ferguson JA, et al. Open-label randomized trial of torsemide compared with furosemide therapy for patients with heart failure. Am J Med 2001; 111:513–520.
7. Grinstead WC, Francis MJ, Marks GF, et al. Discontinuation of chronic diuretic therapy in stable congestive heart failure secondary to coronary artery disease or to idiopathic dilated cardiomyopathy. Am J Cardiol 1994; 73:881–886.
8. Richardson A, Bayliss J, Scriven AJ, et al. Double-blind comparison of captopril alone against frusemide plus amiloride in mild heart failure. Lancet 1987; 2:709–711.
9. Braunschweig F, Linde C, Eriksson MJ, et al. Continuous haemodynamic monitoring during withdrawal of diuretics in patients with congestive heart failure. Eur Heart J 2002; 23:59–69.

10. Kelso E, McDermott B, Silke B, et al. Positive effect of bumetanide on contractile activity of ventricular cardiomyocytes. Eur J Pharmacol 2000; 400:43–50.
11. Feldman AM, Levine MA, Gerstenblith G, et al. Negative inotropic effects of furosemide in the isolated rabbit heart: a prostaglandin-mediated event. J Cardiovasc Pharmacol 1987; 9:493–499.
12. Poole-Wilson PA, Cobbe SM, Fry CH. Acute effects of diuretics on potassium exchange, mechanical function and the action potential in rabbit myocardium. Clin Sci Mol Med 1978; 55:555–559.
13. Dormans TP, Pickkers P, Russel FG, et al. Vascular effects of loop diuretics. Cardiovasc Res 1996; 32:988–997.
14. Biagi RW, Bapat BN. Frusemide in acute pulmonary oedema. Lancet 1967; 1:849.
15. Dikshit K, Vyden JK, Forrester JS, et al. Renal and extrarenal hemodynamic effects of furosemide in congestive heart failure after acute myocardial infarction. N Engl J Med 1973; 288:1087–1090.
16. Jhund PS, McMurray JJ, Davie AP. The acute vascular effects of frusemide in heart failure. Br J Clin Pharmacol 2000; 50:9–13.
17. Johnston GD, Hiatt WR, Nies AS, et al. Factors modifying the early nondiuretic vascular effects of furosemide in man. The possible role of renal prostaglandins. Circ Res 1983; 53:630–635.
18. Mackay IG, Muir AL, Watson ML. Contribution of prostaglandins to the systemic and renal vascular response to frusemide in normal man. Br J Clin Pharmacol 1984; 17:513–519.
19. Jhund PS, Davie AP, McMurray JJ. Aspirin inhibits the acute venodilator response to furosemide in patients with chronic heart failure. J Am Coll Cardiol 2001; 37:1234–1238.
20. Johnston GD, Nicholls DP, Leahey WJ, et al. The effects of captopril on the acute vascular responses to frusemide in man. Clin Sci (Lond) 1983; 65:359–363.
21. Pickkers P, Hughes AD, Russel FG, et al. Thiazide-induced vasodilation in humans is mediated by potassium channel activation. Hypertension 1998; 32:1071–1076.
22. Pickkers P, Hughes AD, Russel FG, et al. In vivo evidence for K(Ca) channel opening properties of acetazolamide in the human vasculature. Br J Pharmacol 2001; 132:443–450.
23. Francis GS, Siegel RM, Goldsmith SR, et al. Acute vasoconstrictor response to intravenous furosemide in patients with chronic congestive heart failure. Activation of the neurohumoral axis. Ann Intern Med 1985; 103:1–6.
24. Kiely DG, Cargill RI, Lipworth BJ. Effects of frusemide and hypoxia on the pulmonary vascular bed in man. Br J Clin Pharmacol 1997; 43:309–313.
25. Goldsmith SR, Francis G, Cohn JN. Attenuation of the pressor response to intravenous furosemide by angiotensin converting enzyme inhibition in congestive heart failure. Am J Cardiol 1989; 64:1382–1385.
26. Bayliss J, Norell M, Canepa-Anson R, et al. Untreated heart failure: clinical and neuroendocrine effects of introducing diuretics. Br Heart J 1987; 57:17–22.
27. Broqvist M, Dahlstrom U, Karlberg BE, et al. Neuroendocrine response in acute heart failure and the influence of treatment. Eur Heart J 1989; 10:1075–1083.
28. Francis GS, Benedict C, Johnstone DE, et al. Comparison of neuroendocrine activation in patients with left ventricular dysfunction with and without congestive heart failure. A substudy of the Studies of Left Ventricular Dysfunction (SOLVD). Circulation 1990; 82:1724–1729.
29. Kubo SH, Clark M, Laragh JH, et al. Identification of normal neurohormonal activity in mild congestive heart failure and stimulating effect of upright posture and diuretics. Am J Cardiol 1987; 60:1322–1328.
30. Ikram H, Chan W, Espiner EA, et al. Haemodynamic and hormone responses to acute and chronic frusemide therapy in congestive heart failure. Clin Sci (Lond) 1980; 59:443–449.
31. Nicholls MG, Espiner EA, Donald RA, et al. Aldosterone and its regulation during diuresis in patients with gross congestive heart failure. Clin Sci Mol Med 1974; 47:301–315.

32. Knight RK, Miall PA, Hawkins LA, et al. Relation of plasma aldosterone concentration to diuretic treatment in patients with severe heart disease. Br Heart J 1979; 42:316–325.
33. Yetman AT, Singh NC, Parbtani A, et al. Acute hemodynamic and neurohoromonal effects of furosemide in critically ill pediatrics patients. Crit Care Med 1996; 24:398–402.
34. Brilla CG, Matsubara LS, Weber KT. Anti-aldosterone treatment and the prevention of myocardial fibrosis in primary and secondary hyperaldosteronism. J Mol Cell Cardiol 1993; 25:563–575.
35. Kao W, Gheorghiade M, Hall V, et al. Relation between plasma norepinephrine and response to medical therapy in men with congestive heart failure secondary to coronary artery disease or idiopathic dilated cardiomyopathy. Am J Cardiol 1989; 64:609–613.
36. Cohn JN, Levine TB, Olivari MT, et al. Plasma norepinephrine as a guide to prognosis in patients with chronic congestive heart failure. N Engl J Med 1984; 311:819–823.
37. Johnson W, Omland T, Hall C, et al. Neurohormonal activation rapidly decreases after intravenous therapy with diuretics and vasodilators for class IV heart failure. J Am Coll Cardiol 2002; 39:1623–1629.
38. Ueno Y, Arita M, Suruda H, et al. Central actions of circulating angiotensin II on the sympathetic nervous system and blood pressure control. Jpn Heart J 1985; 26:105–112.
39. Ueno Y, Arita M, Suruda H, et al. Contributions of central sympathetic neural activity to furosemide-induced increases in plasma renin activity and noradrenaline. Jpn Heart J 1983; 24:259–267.
40. Tsutsui T, Tsutamoto T, Maeda K, et al. Comparison of neurohumoral effects of short-acting and long-acting loop diuretics in patients with chronic congestive heart failure. J Cardiovasc Pharmacol 2001; 38:S81–S85.
41. Singh K, Xiao L, Remondino A, et al. Adrenergic regulation of cardiac myocyte apoptosis. J Cell Physiol 2001; 189:257–265.
42. Dorn GW. Adrenergic pathways and left ventricular remodeling. J Card Fail 2002; 8:S370–S373.
43. Share L. Interrelations between vasopressin and the renin–angiotensin system. Fed Proc 1979; 38:2267–2271.
44. Liguori A, Casini A, Di Loreto M, et al. Loop diuretics enhance the secretion of prostacyclin in vitro, in healthy persons, and in patients with chronic heart failure. Eur J Clin Pharmacol 1999; 55:117–124.
45. Heerdink ER, Leufkens HG, Herings RM, et al. NSAIDs associated with increased risk of congestive heart failure in elderly patients taking diuretics. Arch Intern Med 1998; 158:1108–1112.
46. Dietz JR. Mechanisms of atrial natriuretic peptide secretion from the atrium. Cardiovasc Res 2005.
47. Kinnunen P, Vuolteenaho O, Ruskoaho H. Mechanisms of atrial and brain natriuretic peptide release from rat ventricular myocardium: effect of stretching. Endocrinology 1993; 132:1961–1970.
48. Clerico A, Iervasi G, Mariani G. Pathophysiologic relevance of measuring the plasma levels of cardiac natriuretic peptide hormones in humans. Horm Metab Res 1999; 31:487–498.
49. Kimura T, Abe K, Ota K, et al. Effects of acute water load, hypertonic saline infusion, and furosemide administration on atrial natriuretic peptide and vasopressin release in humans. J Clin Endocrinol Metab 1986; 62:1003–1010.
50. Yamasaki Y, Nishiuchi T, Kojima A, et al. Effects of an oral water load and intravenous administration of isotonic glucose, hypertonic saline, mannitol and furosemide on the release of atrial natriuretic peptide in men. Acta Endocrinol(Copenh.) 1988; 119:269–276.
51. Paterna S, Di Pasquale P, Parrinello G, et al. Changes in brain natriuretic peptide levels and bioelectrical impedance measurements after treatment with high-dose furosemide and hypertonic saline solution versus high-dose furosemide alone in refractory congestive heart failure: a double-blind study. J Am Coll Cardiol 2005; 45:1997–2003.

52. Kazanegra R, Cheng V, Garcia A, et al. A rapid test for B-type natriuretic peptide correlates with falling wedge pressures in patients treated for decompensated heart failure: a pilot study. J Card Fail 2001; 7:21–29.
53. Tsutamoto T, Wada A, Maeda K, et al. Effect of spironolactone on plasma brain natriuretic peptide and left ventricular remodeling in patients with congestive heart failure. J Am Coll Cardiol 2001; 37:1228–1233.
54. Silver MA, Maisel A, Yancy CW, et al. BNP Consensus Panel : A clinical approach for the diagnostic, prognostic, screening, treatment monitoring, and therapeutic roles of natriuretic peptides in cardiovascular diseases. Congest Heart Fail 2004; 10:1–30.
55. Bettencourt P, Azevedo A, Pimenta J, et al. N-terminal-pro-brain natriuretic peptide predicts outcome after hospital discharge in heart failure patients. Circulation 2004; 110:2168–2174.
56. Logeart D, Thabut G, Jourdain P, et al. Predischarge B-type natriuretic peptide assay for identifying patients at high risk of re-admission after decompensated heart failure. J Am Coll Cardiol 2004; 43:635–641.
57. Seeland U, Kouchi I, Zolk O, et al. Effect of ramipril and furosemide treatment on interstitial remodeling in post-infarction heart failure rat hearts. J Mol Cell Cardiol 2002; 34:151–163.
58. McCurley JM, Hanlon SU, Wei SK, et al. Furosemide and the progression of left ventricular dysfunction in experimental heart failure. J Am Coll Cardiol 2004; 44:1301–1307.
59. Sharpe N, Murphy J, Smith H, et al. Treatment of patients with symptomless left ventricular dysfunction after myocardial infarction. Lancet 1988; 1:255–259.
60. Lopez B, Querejeta R, Gonzalez A, et al. Effects of loop diuretics on myocardial fibrosis and collagen type I turnover in chronic heart failure. J Am Coll Cardiol 2004; 43:2028–2035.
61. Cosin J, Diez J. Torasemide in chronic heart failure: results of the TORIC study. Eur J Heart Fail 2002; 4:507–513.
62. Delcayre C, Swynghedauw B. Molecular mechanisms of myocardial remodeling. The role of aldosterone. J Mol Cell Cardiol 2002; 34:1577–1584.
63. Wahed MI, Watanabe K, Ma M, et al. Effects of eplerenone, a selective aldosterone blocker, on the progression of left ventricular dysfunction and remodeling in rats with dilated cardiomyopathy. Pharmacology 2005; 73:81–88.
64. MacFadyen RJ, Barr CS, Struthers AD. Aldosterone blockade reduces vascular collagen turnover, improves heart rate variability and reduces early morning rise in heart rate in heart failure patients. Cardiovasc Res 1997; 35:30–34.
65. Tsutamoto T, Wada A, Maeda K, et al. Effect of spironolactone on plasma brain natriuretic peptide and left ventricular remodeling in patients with congestive heart failure. J Am Coll Cardiol 2001; 37:1228–1233.
66. Zannad F, Alla F, Dousset B, et al. Limitation of excessive extracellular matrix turnover may contribute to survival benefit of spironolactone therapy in patients with congestive heart failure: insights from the randomized aldactone evaluation study (RALES). Rales Investigators. Circulation 2000; 102:2700–2706.
67. Modena MG, Aveta P, Menozzi A, et al. Aldosterone inhibition limits collagen synthesis and progressive left ventricular enlargement after anterior myocardial infarction. Am Heart J 2001; 141:41–46.
68. Hayashi M, Tsutamoto T, Wada A, et al. Immediate administration of mineralocorticoid receptor antagonist spironolactone prevents post-infarct left ventricular remodeling associated with suppression of a marker of myocardial collagen synthesis in patients with first anterior acute myocardial infarction. Circulation 2003; 107:2559–2565.
69. Pitt B, Remme W, Zannad F, et al. Eplerenone, a selective aldosterone blocker, in patients with left ventricular dysfunction after myocardial infarction. N Engl J Med 2003; 348:1309–1321.
70. Domanski M, Norman J, Pitt B, et al. Diuretic use, progressive heart failure, and death in patients in the Studies Of Left Ventricular Dysfunction (SOLVD). J Am Coll Cardiol 2003; 42:705–708.
71. Cooper HA, Dries DL, Davis CE, et al. Diuretics and risk of arrhythmic death in patients with left ventricular dysfunction. Circulation 1999; 100:1311–1315.

72. Neuberg GW, Miller AB, O'Connor CM, et al. Diuretic resistance predicts mortality in patients with advanced heart failure. Am Heart J 2002; 144:31–38.
73. Pitt B, Zannad F, Remme WJ, et al. The effect of spironolactone on morbidity and mortality in patients with severe heart failure. Randomized Aldactone Evaluation Study Investigators. N Engl J Med 1999; 341:709–717.
74. Brater DC. Pharmacology of diuretics. Am J Med Sci 2000; 319:38–50.
75. Greger R. New insights into the molecular mechanism of the action of diuretics. Nephrol Dial Transplant 1999; 14:536–540.
76. Brater DC. Diuretic therapy. N Engl J Med 1998; 339:387–395.
77. Greither A, Goldman S, Edelen JS, et al. Pharmacokinetics of furosemide in patients with congestive heart failure. Pharmacology 1979; 19:121–131.
78. Vasko MR, Cartwright DB, Knochel JP, et al. Furosemide absorption altered in decompensated congestive heart failure. Ann Intern Med 1985; 102:314–318.
79. Wilcox CS, Mitch WE, Kelly RA, et al. Response of the kidney to furosemide. I. Effects of salt intake and renal compensation. J Lab Clin Med 1983; 102:450–458.
80. Brater DC, Seiwell R, Anderson S, et al. Absorption and disposition of furosemide in congestive heart failure. Kidney Int 1982; 22:171–176.
81. Shankar SS, Brater DC. Loop diuretics: from the Na-K-2Cl transporter to clinical use. Am J Physiol Renal Physiol 2003; 284:F11–F21.
82. Brater DC. Pharmacokinetics of loop diuretics in congestive heart failure. Br Heart J 1994; 72:S40–S43.
83. Kramer BK, Schweda F, Riegger GA. Diuretic treatment and diuretic resistance in heart failure. Am J Med 1999; 106:90–96.
84. Ellison DH. Diuretic therapy and resistance in congestive heart failure. Cardiology 2001; 96:132–143.
85. Kelly RA, Wilcox CS, Mitch WE, et al. Response of the kidney to furosemide. II. Effect of captopril on sodium balance. Kidney Int 1983; 24:233–239.
86. Wilcox CS, Guzman NJ, Mitch WE, et al. Na+, K+, and BP homeostasis in man during furosemide: effects of prazosin and captopril. Kidney Int 1987; 31:135–141.
87. Scherzer P, Wald H, Popovtzer MM. Enhanced glomerular filtration and Na+-K+-ATPase with furosemide administration. Am J Physiol 1987; 252:F910–F915.
88. Abdallah JG, Schrier RW, Edelstein C, et al. Loop diuretic infusion increases thiazide-sensitive Na(+)/Cl(−)-cotransporter abundance: role of aldosterone. J Am Soc Nephrol 2001; 12:1335–1341.
89. Oster JR, Epstein M, Smoller S. Combined therapy with thiazide-type and loop diuretic agents for resistant sodium retention. Ann Intern Med 1983; 99:405–406.
90. Hunt SA, Baker DW, Chin MH, et al. ACC/AHA Guidelines for the Evaluation and Management of Chronic Heart Failure in the Adult: Executive Summary A Report of the American College of Cardiology/American Heart Association Task Force on Practice Guidelines (Committee to Revise the 1995 Guidelines for the Evaluation and Management of Heart Failure): Developed in Collaboration with the International Society for Heart and Lung Transplantation; Endorsed by the Heart Failure Society of America. Circulation 2001; 104:2996–3007.
91. Shah SU, Anjum S, Littler WA. Use of diuretics in cardiovascular diseases: (1) heart failure. Postgrad Med J 2004; 80:201–205.
92. Sica DA, Gehr T. Diuretics in congestive heart failure. Cardiol Clin 1989; 7:87–97.
93. Dormans TP, Gerlag PG. Combination of high-dose furosemide and hydrochlorothiazide in the treatment of refractory congestive heart failure. Eur Heart J 1996; 17:1867–1874.
94. Knauf H, Mutschler E. Sequential nephron blockade breaks resistance to diuretics in edematous states. J Cardiovasc Pharmacol 1997; 29:367–372.
95. van Vliet AA, Donker AJ, Nauta JJ, et al. Spironolactone in congestive heart failure refractory to high-dose loop diuretic and low-dose angiotensin-converting enzyme inhibitor. Am J Cardiol 1993; 71:21A–28A.

96. Rudy DW, Voelker JR, Greene PK, et al. Loop diuretics for chronic renal insufficiency: a continuous infusion is more efficacious than bolus therapy. Ann Intern Med 1991; 115:360–366.
97. Lahav M, Regev A, Ra'anani P, et al. Intermittent administration of furosemide vs continuous infusion preceded by a loading dose for congestive heart failure. Chest 1992; 102:725–731.
98. van Meyel JJ, Smits P, Dormans T, et al. Continuous infusion of furosemide in the treatment of patients with congestive heart failure and diuretic resistance. J Intern Med 1994; 235:329–334.
99. Dormans TP, van Meyel JJ, Gerlag PG, et al. Diuretic efficacy of high dose furosemide in severe heart failure: bolus injection versus continuous infusion. J Am Coll Cardiol 1996; 28:376–382.
100. Salvador DR, Rey NR, Ramos GC, et al. Continuous infusion versus bolus injection of loop diuretics in congestive heart ailure. Cochrane Database Syst Rev 2004; 1:CD003178.pub2, doi:10.1002/14651858.CD003178.pub2.
101. Agostoni PG, Marenzi GC, Pepi M, et al. Isolated ultrafiltration in moderate congestive heart failure. J Am Coll Cardiol 1993; 21:424–431.
102. Marenzi G, Lauri G, Grazi M, et al. Circulatory response to fluid overload removal by extracorporeal ultrafiltration in refractory congestive heart failure. J Am Coll Cardiol 2001; 38:963–968.
103. Marenzi G, Grazi S, Giraldi F, et al. Interrelation of humoral factors, hemodynamics, and fluid and salt metabolism in congestive heart failure: effects of extracorporeal ultrafiltration. Am J Med 1993; 94:49–56.
104. Sica DA. Diuretic-related side effects: development and treatment. J Clin Hypertens 2004; 6:532–540.
105. Reinhart RA. Magnesium metabolism. A review with special reference to the relationship between intracellular content and serum levels. Arch Intern Med 1988; 148:2415–2420.
106. Gottlieb SS, Baruch L, Kukin ML, et al. Prognostic importance of the serum magnesium concentration in patients with congestive heart failure. J Am Coll Cardiol 1990; 16:827–831.
107. Ralston MA, Murnane MR, Unverferth DV, et al. Serum and tissue magnesium concentrations in patients with heart failure and serious ventricular arrhythmias. Ann Intern Med 1990; 113:841–846.
108. Loon NR, Wilcox CS. Mild metabolic alkalosis impairs the natriuretic response to bumetanide in normal human subjects. Clin Sci 1998; 94:287–292.
109. Wilcox CS. Metabolic and adverse effects of diuretics. Semin Nephrol 1999; 19:557–568.
110. Furman BL. Impairment of glucose tolerance produced by diuretics and other drugs. Pharmacol Ther 1981; 12:613–649.
111. Curb JD, Pressel SL, Cutler JA, et al. Effect of diuretic-based antihypertensive treatment on cardiovascular disease risk in older diabetic patients with isolated systolic hypertension. Systolic Hypertension in the Elderly Program Cooperative Research Group. JAMA 1996; 276:1886–1892.
112. Gress TW, Nieto FJ, Shahar E, et al. Hypertension and antihypertensive therapy as risk factors for type 2 diabetes mellitus. Atherosclerosis Risk in Communities Study. N Engl J Med 2000; 342:905–912.
113. Kasiske BL, Ma JZ, Kalil RS, et al. Effects of antihypertensive therapy on serum lipids. Ann Intern Med 1995; 122:133–141.
114. Grimm RHJ, Flack JM, Grandits GA, et al. Long-term effects on plasma lipids of diet and drugs to treat hypertension. Treatment of Mild Hypertension Study (TOMHS) Research Group. JAMA 1996; 275:1549–1556.
115. Shapiro S, Slone D, Lewis GP, et al. The epidemiology of digoxin. A study in three Boston hospitals. J Chronic Dis 1969; 22:361–371.
116. Petersen V, Hvidt S, Thomsen K, et al. Effect of prolonged thiazide treatment on renal lithium clearance. Br Med J 1974; 3:143–145.

117. Juurlink DN, Mamdani MM, Kopp A, et al. Drug-induced lithium toxicity in the elderly: a population-based study. J Am Geriatr Soc 2004; 52:794–798.
118. Favre L, Glasson P, Vallotton MB. Reversible acute renal failure from combined triamterene and indomethacin: a study in healthy subjects. Ann Intern Med 1982; 96:317–320.
119. McDonald RHJ, Goldberg LI, McNay JL, et al. Effect of dopamine in man: Augmentation of sodium excretion, glomerular filtration rate, and renal plasma flow. J Clin Invest 1964; 43:1116–1124.
120. Goldberg LI, McDonald RHJ, Zimmerman AM. Sodium diuresis produced by dopamine in patients with congestive heart failure. N Engl J Med 1963; 269:1060–1064.
121. Varriale P, Mossavi A. The benefit of low-dose dopamine during vigorous diuresis for congestive heart failure associated with renal insufficiency: does it protect renal function? Clin Cardiol 1997; 20:627–630.
122. Vargo DL, Brater DC, Rudy DW, et al. Dopamine does not enhance furosemide-induced natriuresis in patients with congestive heart failure. J Am Soc Nephrol 1996; 7:1032–1037.
123. Lieverse AG, van Veldhuisen DJ, Smit AJ, et al. Renal and systemic hemodynamic effects of ibopamine in patients with mild to moderate congestive heart failure. J Cardiovasc Pharmacol 1995; 25:361–367.
124. Hampton JR, van Veldhuisen DJ, Kleber FX, et al. Randomised study of effect of ibopamine on survival in patients with advanced severe heart failure. Second Prospective Randomised Study of Ibopamine on Mortality and Efficacy (PRIME II) Investigators. Lancet 1997; 349:971–977.
125. Holmes CL, Walley KR. Bad medicine: low-dose dopamine in the ICU. Chest 2003; 123:1266–1275.
126. Conte G, Bellizzi V, Cianciaruso B, et al. Physiologic role and diuretic efficacy of atrial natriuretic peptide in health and chronic renal disease. Kidney Int 1997; 59:S28–S32.
127. La Villa G, Lazzeri C, Pascale A, et al. Cardiovascular and renal effects of low-dose atrial natriuretic peptide in compensated cirrhosis. Am J Gastroenterol 1997; 92:852–857.
128. van der Zander K, Houben AJ, Hofstra L, et al. Hemodynamic and renal effects of low-dose brain natriuretic peptide infusion in humans: a randomized, placebo-controlled crossover study. Am J Physiol Heart Circ Physiol 2003; 285:H1206–H1212.
129. Jensen KT, Carstens J, Pedersen EB. Effect of BNP on renal hemodynamics, tubular function and vasoactive hormones in humans. Am J Physiol 1998; 274:F63–F72.
130. La Villa G, Fronzaroli C, Lazzeri C, et al. Cardiovascular and renal effects of low dose brain natriuretic peptide infusion in man. J Clin Endocrinol Metab 1994; 78:1166–1171.
131. Costello-Boerrigter LC, Boerrigter G, Burnett JCJ. Revisiting salt and water retention: new diuretics, aquaretics, and natriuretics. Med Clin North Am 2003; 87:475–491.
132. Richards AM, Crozier IG, Holmes SJ, et al. Brain natriuretic peptide: natriuretic and endocrine effects in essential hypertension. J Hypertens 1993; 11:163–170.
133. Holmes SJ, Espiner EA, Richards AM, et al. Renal, endocrine, and hemodynamic effects of human brain natriuretic peptide in normal man. J Clin Endocrinol Metab 1993; 76:91–96.
134. Cataliotti A, Boerrigter G, Costello-Boerrigter LC, et al. Brain natriuretic peptide enhances renal actions of furosemide and suppresses furosemide-induced aldosterone activation in experimental heart failure. Circulation 2004; 109:1680–1685.
135. Marcus LS, Hart D, Packer M, et al. Hemodynamic and renal excretory effects of human brain natriuretic peptide infusion in patients with congestive heart failure. A double-blind, placebo-controlled, randomized crossover trial. Circulation 1996; 94:3184–3189.
136. Yoshimura M, Yasue H, Morita E, et al. Hemodynamic, renal, and hormonal responses to brain natriuretic peptide infusion in patients with congestive heart failure. Circulation 1991; 84:1581–1588.
137. Jensen KT, Eiskjaer H, Carstens J, et al. Renal effects of brain natriuretic peptide in patients with congestive heart failure. Clin Sci 1999; 96:5–15.

138. Abraham WT, Lowes BD, Ferguson DA, et al. Systemic hemodynamic, neurohormonal, and renal effects of a steady-state infusion of human brain natriuretic peptide in patients with hemodynamically decompensated heart failure. J Card Fail 1998; 4:37–44.
139. Wang DJ, Dowling TC, Meadows D, et al. Nesiritide does not improve renal function in patients with chronic heart failure and worsening serum creatinine. Circulation 2004; 110:1620–1625.
140. Lainchbury JG, Richards AM, Nicholls MG, et al. The effects of pathophysiological increments in brain natriuretic peptide in left ventricular systolic dysfunction. Hypertension 1997; 30:398–404.
141. Sackner-Bernstein JD, Skopicki HA, Aaronson KD. Risk of worsening renal function with nesiritide in patients with acutely decompensated heart failure. Circulation 2005; 111:1487–1491.
142. Sanghi P, Uretsky BF, Schwarz ER. Vasopressin antagonism: a future treatment option in heart failure. Eur Heart J 2005; 26:538–543.
143. Udelson JE, Smith WB, Hendrix GH, et al. Acute hemodynamic effects of conivaptan, a dual V(1A) and V(2) vasopressin receptor antagonist, in patients with advanced heart failure. Circulation 2001; 104:2417–2423.
144. Gheorghiade M, Niazi I, Ouyang J, et al. Vasopressin V2-receptor blockade with tolvaptan in patients with chronic heart failure: results from a double-blind, randomized trial. Circulation 2003; 107:2690–2696.
145. Gheorghiade M, Gattis WA, O'Connor CM, et al. Effects of tolvaptan, a vasopressin antagonist, in patients hospitalized with worsening heart failure: a randomized controlled trial. JAMA 2004; 291:1963–1971.
146. Russell SD, Selaru P, Pyne DA, et al. Rationale for use of an exercise end point and design for the ADVANCE (A Dose evaluation of a Vasopressin ANtagonist in CHF patients undergoing Exercise) trial. Am Heart J 2003; 145:179–186.
147. Gheorghiade M, Gattis WA, Barbagelata A, et al. Rationale and study design for a multicenter, randomized, double-blind, placebo-controlled study of the effects of tolvaptan on the acute and chronic outcomes of patients hospitalized with worsening congestive heart failure. Am Heart J 2003; 145:S51–S54.
148. Osswald H, Muhlbauer B, Vallon V. Adenosine and tubuloglomerular feedback. Blood Purif 1997; 15:243–252.
149. Funaya H, Kitakaze M, Node K, et al. Plasma adenosine levels increase in patients with chronic heart failure. Circulation 1997; 95:1363–1365.
150. Gottlieb SS, Skettino SL, Wolff A, et al. Effects of BG9719 (CVT-124), an A1-adenosine receptor antagonist, and furosemide on glomerular filtration rate and natriuresis in patients with congestive heart failure. J Am Coll Cardiol 2000; 35:56–59.
151. Gottlieb SS, Brater DC, Thomas I, et al. BG9719 (CVT-124), an A1 adenosine receptor antagonist, protects against the decline in renal function observed with diuretic therapy. Circulation 2002; 105:1348–1353.

6
Vasodilators in the Management of Heart Failure

David W. Markham
University of Texas Southwestern Medical Center at Dallas, Dallas, Texas, U.S.A.

G. Michael Felker
Duke University School of Medicine and Duke Clinical Research Institute, Durham, North Carolina, U.S.A.

VASOCONSTRICTION IN HEART FAILURE: RATIONALE FOR VASODILATOR THERAPY

Heart failure is a heterogeneous clinical syndrome but is fundamentally characterized by a decrease in myocardial performance with a resultant decrease in cardiac output. As cardiac output declines, a variety of compensatory mechanisms are activated, with both beneficial and harmful acute and long-term effects. Peripheral vasoconstriction, a physiologic response designed to maintain systemic perfusion pressure in response to a drop in cardiac output, is a hallmark of the heart failure syndrome. Regulation of vascular tone is controlled by complex neurohormonal and hemodynamic processes, including the sympathetic nervous system, the renin–angiotensin system, and multiple endogenous vasoconstrictive/vasodilatory factors. Vasoconstriction is functionally important in the setting of trauma, severe hemorrhage, or short term decrease in cardiac performance, acting to maintain arterial pressure and perfusion of the brain and other vital organs. However, in the setting of heart failure, chronic vasoconstriction leads to reduced cardiac output, increased myocardial oxygen consumption, decreased coronary perfusion, and increased cell death (Fig. 1). This fundamental observation establishes the rationale for the use of vasodilator agents in heart failure, a heterogeneous class of drugs that have become mainstays in the management of acute and chronic heart failure.

Mechanisms Regulating Vascular Resistance

It is important to understand the mechanisms that produce vasoconstriction in order to understand the mechanism of action of various vasodilator agents. The sympathetic nervous system is known to be activated in heart failure, leading to an increase in circulating levels of norepinephrine (1,2). This response is adaptive in acute situations when the vasculature must react quickly. Norepinephrine activates arteriolar smooth

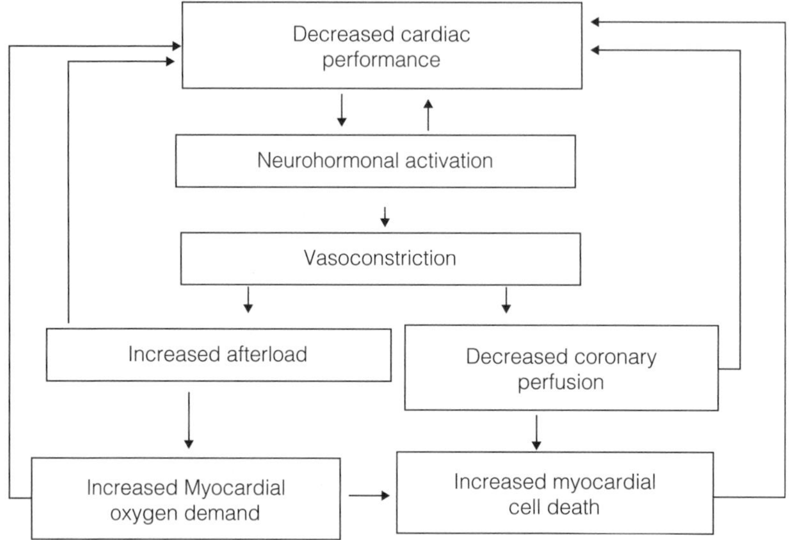

Figure 1 Role of vasoconstriction in the progression of heart failure.

muscle peripheral alpha1-adrenergic receptors causing vasoconstriction (3). Central, preganglionic alpha2-adrenergic receptors also bind norepinephrine and promote a counter-regulatory response by inhibiting sympathetic outflow. The renin–angiotensin system is adaptive for the long-term needs of increasing blood volume through salt retention, and produces vasoconstriction by the conversion of angiotensin I to angiotensin II. Clinicians in the late 19th century noted that extracts from the kidney increased blood pressure when injected into patients. Since this initial study of the substance that became known as renin, much has been elucidated about this pathway, such as the production of angiotensin I from angiotensinogen and the cleavage of angiotensin I to angiotensin II by angiotensin converting enzyme (ACE). Angiotensin II subsequently binds to the angiotensin receptor. In heart failure, the chronic effects of angiotensin II are maladaptive, producing vasoconstriction, fibrosis, and cardiomyocyte hypertrophy (4,5).

Other endogenous vasoconstricting/vasodilating factors include endothelin (ET), vasopressin, nitric oxide (NO), natriuretic peptides, bradykinins, and prostaglandins. ET is a potent vasoconstrictor that exists in three isoforms (endothelins 1, 2, and 4). ET1 is the most important isoform in the cardiovascular system, and it causes a vasoconstrictor response when bound to ET-A receptors on vascular smooth muscle. ET-B receptors on endothelial cells produce an inhibitory response by releasing vasodilators like NO and prostacyclin (6). ET1 levels are increased in patients with heart failure (7,8). Arginine vasopressin, or antidiuretic hormone, is an octapeptide produced in the hypothalamus and released from the posterior pituitary in response to increased plasma osmolarity and decreased blood volume. Like renin, it was discovered in the late 19th century when posterior pituitary extracts were injected into laboratory animals resulting in elevated blood pressure. The major physiologic action of vasopressin on the cardiovascular system involves vasoconstriction through activation of the V1 receptor. In patients with heart failure, the physiologic control mechanisms for vasopressin are altered, especially following the administration of diuretics; these maladaptive responses can lead to inappropriate vasopressin release leading to vasoconstriction and hyponatremia.

NO is produced by the endothelium from the conversion of L-arginine to L-citrulline by nitric oxide synthase (NOS). NO causes vasodilation and affects vascular permeability, oxidative phosphorylation, and platelet aggregation (9,10). NO is also intimately involved with inflammation and cytokine release. In heart failure, the vasculature is less responsive to NO mainly due to an attenuation of the vasodilatory response rather than reduced production of NO (11). It is known that reduced eNOS expression, particularly in aortic endothelial cells, is closely related to pulsatile flow and shear stress (12,13). Another potentially important feature of NO in heart failure is the inactivation of NO by superoxide anions. This mechanism is not entirely understood but there is evidence that increased oxygen free radicals subsequently lead to NO degradation and endothelial dysfunction (14).

Recent discovery of the natriuretic peptide system established the heart as an endocrine organ. This discovery came from the finding that atrial extracts induced a profound natriuretic response (15). Atrial natriuretic peptide (ANP) was later identified and found to have a counter-regulatory effect that inhibits salt and water retention and produces vasodilation. Natriuretic peptide levels are elevated in heart failure in response to ventricular wall stress, and are increasingly used as a diagnostic and prognostic marker in patients with ventricular dysfunction (16–18).

Bradykinins are produced in the vasculature through the breakdown of kininogens by proteolytic enzymes called kallikreins. Bradykinins bind the B2 kinin receptor and promote the release of NO, prostaglandins, and cyclic AMP (which causes smooth muscle relaxation). Bradykinin is a substrate for ACE. Thus, ACE inhibitors inhibit the breakdown of bradykinin, allowing reduced vasoconstriction not only through the decreased production of angiotensin II but also through increased bradykinin.

Prostaglandins include vasodilators (prostacyclin and prostaglandin E2) and vasoconstrictors (thromboxane). They are produced from polyunsaturated fatty acid derivatives by cyclo-oxygenase enzymes. Full discussion of this system is beyond the scope of this chapter, but these compounds are active in inflammation, platelet activation, and renal blood flow. Full elucidation of this system in the setting of heart failure, especially with regard to clinical targeting, remains a difficult task. Many non-steroidal anti-inflammatory drugs inhibit prostaglandins and cause fluid retention by altering renal perfusion. The endogenous mediators of vasoconstriction and vasodilation are summarized in Table 1.

VASODILATOR THERAPY IN ACUTE DECOMPENSATED HEART FAILURE

Hemodynamically, heart failure decompensation is characterized by some combination of elevated filling pressures, decreased cardiac output, and altered systemic vascular resistance (SVR). These variables have been used to create "hemodynamic profiles," which form a conceptual model for the selection of therapies in patients with acute heart failure (19).

Table 1 Endogenous Mediators of Peripheral Vascular Tone

Vasoconstrictors	Vasodilators
Norepinephrine	Natriuretic peptides (ANP, BNP, CNP)
Epinephrine	Nitric oxide
Renin	Bradykinins
Arginine vasopressin	Prostacyclin
Endothelin	Prostaglandin E2
Angiontensin II	

The concept of targeting excessive vasoconstriction in the setting of heart failure came from observations that cardiac biomechanics can be improved by appropriately matching afterload to inotropy (20). It was determined that in the patient with increased SVR, reducing afterload results in increased cardiac output, increased contractility, decreased myocardial energy expenditure, and decreased myocardial cell death.

The hemodynamic goal of acute therapy is to restore the patient's profile to a setting with adequate perfusion pressure and decreased volume overload (i.e., warm and dry). The use of invasive hemodynamic monitoring via a pulmonary artery catheter to obtain these hemodynamic goals has been termed "tailored therapy" and has been shown to result in improved freedom from congestion and repeat hospitalization in patients presenting with acute heart failure (21,22). Vasodilator therapy plays an important and often overlooked role in obtaining these goals. The recently completed Evaluation Study of Congestive Heart Failure and Pulmonary Artery Catheter Effectiveness (ESCAPE) trial evaluated the role of a hemodynamically guided approach using right heart catheterization versus standard care in patients with decompensated heart failure (23). Preliminary data from ESCAPE suggest no significant difference in outcomes between those patients randomized to hemodynamically guided therapy compared to those treated using clinical judgment alone. Ongoing analysis of these data may provide further insights into which patients are most likely to benefit from a tailored therapy approach.

In general, available vasodilators affect the venous system, the arterial system, or both (so called "balanced vasodilators"). Vasodilators with significant effects on the venous system such as nitroglycerin can lower preload and reduce ventricular filling pressures, particularly in conjunction with diuretics. Elevated filling pressures are not only important contributors to atrioventricular valvular regurgitation but also lead to cellular apoptosis, neurohumoral activation, increased automaticity, chronic remodeling, pulmonary hypertension, and right ventricular dysfunction. Each of these features contributes to mortality in heart failure.

Most patients with acute decompensated heart failure present with elevated SVR; administration of arterial vasodilators (such as sodium nitroprusside or hydralazine) results in reduction of SVR with a concomitant rise in cardiac output and a decrease in filling pressures (24–26). Although vasodilators may result in hypotension, in most cases the increase in cardiac output is sufficient to balance the decrease in SVR so that systemic blood pressure remains adequate. Given that most patients with decompensated heart failure present with both elevated filling pressures (preload) and elevated SVR (afterload), a balance of arterial and venous vasodilator therapy often achieves optimal hemodynamic results. The beneficial hemodynamic effects of vasodilators must be balanced against the possibility that excessive vasodilation may increase neurohormonal activation in some settings, mediated by baroreceptors that are sensitive to rapid drops in afterload or diminished ventricular filling (27). Other data suggest that neurohormonal activation can be avoided by the careful use of vasodilators as part of a tailored therapy strategy (28).

Below, we discuss specific agents, their mechanism of action, and the data supporting their use in acute and chronic heart failure therapy. Although some inotropic agents such as milrinone have important vasodilator properties, these agents are covered elsewhere in this textbook and will not be discussed here. A list of commonly used vasodilators and their hemodynamic effects is shown in Table 2.

Sodium Nitroprusside

Nitroprusside is an intravenous, vasodilatory agent that affects both arterial and venous smooth muscle. Nitroprusside was the first vasodilator shown to increase cardiac

Table 2 Commonly Used Vasodilators and Their Hemodynamic Effects

Agent	Form	Hemodynamic effects			Side effects	Mortality benefit
		Preload	SVR	CO		
Nitroglycerin	IV/PO/top	+++	+	+	Headache	No
Hydralazine	IV/PO	0	+++	++	Lupus-like syndrome, reflex tachycardia	No
Sodium nitro-prusside	IV	+	+++	+++	Cyanide toxicity	No
Nesiritide	IV	++	++	++	? Adverse renal effects	No
ACE inhibitors	IV/PO	+	++	++	Cough, hyperkalemia, renal insufficiency	Yes
ARBs	PO	+	++	++	Hyperkalemia, renal insufficiency	Yes if ACE intolerant
Amlodipine	PO	+	++	++	Peripheral edema	No

output (26). It is commonly used in the clinical situations of decompensated heart failure and hypertensive crisis. It has a rapid onset of action, and its circulatory half-life is only 2 min. Thus, the hypotensive effects last only 1–10 min following cessation of IV infusion. As with other nitrate compounds, this agent promotes the production of NO, which activates the enzyme guanylate cyclase and stimulates the production of cyclic GMP. Through the action of this important second messenger, myosin light chains in smooth muscle cells undergo dephosphorylation. The end result is muscle cell relaxation, reduced afterload, reduced preload, and decreased blood pressure. Myocardial contractility is not directly affected. Nitroprusside is only used for short durations because of the possibility of thiocyanate toxicity, which inhibits cellular respiration and can lead to cell death. This rare side effect is much more common in patients with preexisting renal insufficiency.

Nitrates

Nitroglycerin is produced in a variety of formulations: a tablet or spray for sublingual administration, an ointment for transdermal delivery, and an intravenous form. The mechanism of vasodilation is the same as that of nitroprusside. Intravenous nitroglycerin has been a mainstay of the treatment of acute heart failure for decades. Hemodynamically, the use of intravenous nitroglycerin results in a decrease in filling pressures and reduction in functional mitral regurgitation, although high doses may be required to achieve substantial hemodynamic effects (29). Additionally, its use is limited by the rapid development of nitrate tolerance and the subsequent diminution of its effects (30).

Hydralazine

Hydralazine was one of the earliest anti-hypertensive agents available in the United States (approved by the FDA in 1952). As a peripheral vasodilator, however, the mechanism of action is still incompletely understood, but its effect on vascular smooth muscle occurs in a manner that may be similar to nitrates. Hydralazine is selective for arterioles and is available in oral and IV forms. Hydralazine is frequently combined with nitrates to provide a balance of arterial and venous vasodilatation, and the concomitant use of hydralazine appears to ameliorate the problem of nitrate tolerance with long term nitrate therapy (31). When used chronically, hydralazine may rarely be associated with the development of a lupus-like syndrome.

Nesiritide

Nesiritide is an intravenous, recombinant preparation of human B-type natriuretic peptide. Administration of nesiritide augments the normal physiologic action of endogenous BNP, which includes arterial and venous vasodilation as well as lusitropic and anti-fibrotic effects. The mechanism of action of nesiritide is reminiscent of nitrates since it functions by activating gaunylate cyclase receptors that increases cGMP. The result depends on the cell-type. BNP action on the collecting duct results in natriuresis, and the effect on endothelial cells and vascular smooth muscle cells is vasodilation. Thus, infusion of nesiritide typically results in decreased arterial pressure, pulmonary capillary wedge pressure, SVR, and a resultant increase in cardiac index (24).

The pivotal trial in the development of nesiritide was the Vasodilation in the Management of Acute Congestive Heart Failure Trial (VMAC) (25). The VMAC study randomized 489 patients with acute decompensated heart failure to intravenous nesiritide, intravenous nitroglycerin, or placebo for 3 hr. After 3 hr, patients in the placebo arm were randomized to receive either nesiritide or nitroglycerin for up to 48 hr. The primary endpoint of VMAC was self evaluation of dyspnea at 3 hr. In a subset of patients with invasive hemodynamic monitoring, the change in pulmonary capillary wedge pressure (PCWP) at 3 hr was also considered a primary endpoint. In VMAC, nesiritide resulted in a small but statistically significant decrease in PCWP at 3 hr (5.8 mmHg decrease) compared to nitroglycerin (3.8 mmHg) or placebo (2 mmHg). The dyspnea score in all patients at 3 hr was reduced compared to placebo by both nesiritide and nitroglycerin, with no difference in dyspnea score between the two active agents. Based on the results of VMAC, the FDA approved nesiritide for the treatment of acute decompensated heart failure in 2001, the first new agent approved for this indication in over 10 yr. In clinical use, nesiritide has potential advantages over nitroglyerin, including a lower rate of headache and less development of tolerance. Recently, two controversial meta-analyses of available data have suggested the possibility that the use of nesiritide may be associated with increased risks of renal failure or death in patients with acute heart failure (32,33). These analyses were retrospective but do suggest caution in the use of this agent. Larger prospective trials with hard clinical endpoints will be required to more accurately define the risks and benefits of nesiritide in patients with acute decompensated heart failure.

Novel Agents

Tezosentan, an dual ET1 receptor antagonist, is a potent vasodilator that has been shown to decrease filling pressures and raise cardiac index in patients with decompensated heart failure (34). Despite its promising hemodynamic profile, large clinical trials (RITZ and VERITAS studies) in a variety of acute heart failure populations have failed to demonstrate significant clinical benefit with this agent (35–38). Clinical development of this agent and other similar drugs continues, although it is unknown whether ET antagonists will eventually have a role in the heart failure armamentarium.

VASODILATOR THERAPY IN CHRONIC HEART FAILURE

The pathophysiologic rationale and the favorable acute hemodynamic effects of short-term vasodilator therapy in heart failure have resulted in significant interest in the therapeutic use of chronic, oral vasodilators in heart failure. A variety of oral agents with differing mechanisms possess vasodilator properties and have been studied in chronic heart failure. The varying efficacy of these agents underscores the point that all vasodilators are not equally efficacious, and that varying mechanisms of action may be important in determining the clinical benefits. A variety of agents have shown neutral or negative effects when studied as chronic heart failure therapy, including minoxidil (39), nifedipine (40), flosequinan (41), prazosin (42), ibopamine (43), prostacyclin (44), and mibefradil (45). Below, we summarize the data on those chronic vasodilators that have demonstrated efficacy in heart failure.

ACE Inhibitors

ACE inhibitors are a mainstay of therapy across the clinical spectrum of heart failure, from patients with asymptomatic left ventricular dysfunction to those with advanced heart failure symptoms. Hemodynamically, these agents are balanced arterial and venous vasodilators. Additionally, ACE inhibitors appear to have a plethora of non-hemodynamic effects on vascular endothelium and the cardiac myocyte, which may account for some or all of their salutary effects. CONSENUS was the first study to demonstrate the efficacy of these agents in heart failure in a large scale clinical trial (46). Subsequently, the results of VHeFT-II (described in greater detail below) and the Studies of Left Ventricular Dysfunction (SOLVD) trials established the ACE inhibitor enalapril as an effective therapy to reduce mortality in patients with systolic dysfunction, with or without symptoms of heart failure (47–49). A meta-analysis of over 12,000 patients reported a 26% reduction in mortality with ACE inhibitor therapy that was consistent across studies (50). Based on these data, ACE inhibitors are the oral vasodilator of choice when transitioning patients from "tailored therapy" to chronic oral therapy or beginning therapy in stable patients.

Although usually well tolerated, ACE inhibitors do cause a drop in glomerular filtration rate in many heart failure patients. ACE inhibitors impair the ability of the kidney to regulate glomerular filling pressure through an effect on efferent arterial tone. A small, reversible rise in serum creatinine is typically seen at the time of initiation of therapy and is not sufficient reason to discontinue these highly efficacious agents. Selected patients, particularly those with renal arterial disease or very marginal cardiac output, may develop more severe renal insufficiency and require discontinuation of ACE inhibitor therapy. Additionally, ACE inhibitors may cause significant cough in a small percentage of patients, which is thought to be related to an increase in circulating bradykinins. The recent development of angiotensin receptor blockers (ARBs) provides an alternative to ACE inhibitor therapy in patients intolerant of this therapy.

Angiotensin Receptor Blockers

Angiotensin receptor blockers (ARBs) antagonize the angiotensin II receptor and therefore block the effects of angiotensin II. In patients treated chronically with ACE inhibitors, angiotensin II levels may increase over time due to the conversion of angiotensin I to angiotensin II by non-specific chymases, bypassing the ACE system (often termed "ACE escape") (51). ARBs therefore provide more complete blockade of the effects of angiotensin II, leading to speculation that these agents could be superior to ACE inhibitors as chronic therapy for chronic heart failure. Two large recent studies, the VAL-HeFT study and the CHARM Program, have evaluated the role of these agents in patients with chronic heart failure.

The VAL-HeFT study evaluated the efficacy of adding the ARB valsartan to standard therapy (including ACE-inhibitors in >90% of patients) in 5010 patients with NYHA class II-IV heart failure (52). This study showed no benefit from the addition of valsartan on all cause mortality but did demonstrate a 13% reduction in the primary endpoint of mortality or cardiovascular morbidity. Subgroup analysis of VAL-HeFT suggested the possibility of an adverse effect when valsartan was combined with beta-blockers and ACE-inhibitors, although this finding has not been confirmed by subsequent studies and may be due to chance alone (53,54).

The CHARM Program evaluated the role of the ARB candesartan in a variety of populations with chronic heart failure. The primary endpoint of CHARM was cardiovascular death or heart failure hospitalization. The CHARM program was made up of three constituent trials evaluating candesartan in patients intolerant of ACE inhibitors (CHARM-alternate), patients already taking ACE inhibitors (CHARM-added), and patients with heart failure in the setting of preserved systolic function (CHARM-preserved) (54–57). The CHARM-alternate trial demonstrated that candesartan was superior to placebo in patients who were intolerant to ACE-inhibitors, with a 23% reduction in the primary endpoint (Fig. 2) (55). This finding was confirmed in a subgroup analysis of the VAL-HeFT study (58). When candesartan was added to patients already taking an ACE inhibitor, there was a modest but statistically significant 15% decrease in the rate of the primary endpoint (54). Importantly, the CHARM program was the first large study to evaluate the role of an ARB in the important subgroup of patients with heart failure and preserved systolic function, in which candesartan treatment showed no improvement in mortality and only a small decrease in heart failure hospitalizations (57). Taken together, the results of CHARM and VAL-HeFT suggest that ARBs are well tolerated and indicated as first line therapy in heart failure patients intolerant of ACE-inhibitors. In patients already taking ACE inhibitors, these agents appear to have modest effects on morbidity endpoints, such as heart failure hospitalizations. ARBs may be better tolerated that ACE inhibitors with regard to cough but appear to have similar incidence of hyperkalemia, renal insufficiency, and hypotension. Based on the demonstrated long term benefits of ACE-inhibitors in multiple studies, it appears that these agents will remain the mainstay of oral vasodilator therapy for heart failure patients who tolerate them for the foreseeable future.

Nitrates and Hydralazine

When used chronically in combination, nitrates and hyrdalazine provide balanced venous and arterial vasodilatation with hemodynamic effects similar to that of sodium nitroprusside or ACE-inhibitors. The original Veterans Administration Cooperative Vasodilator Heart Failure Trial (V-HeFT I), published in 1986, represented a significant advance in the treatment of chronic heart failure. V-HeFT I was the first phase III trial to demonstrate improved survival with a pharmacologic intervention in patients with chronic heart failure. This study randomized 642 men with mild to moderate heart failure who were taking digoxin and diuretics to either placebo, the alpha-blocker prazosin, or a combination of isosorbide dinitrate and hyrdalazine. Patients were followed for an average of 2.3 yr, with a primary study endpoint of all cause mortality (42). Two year mortality in

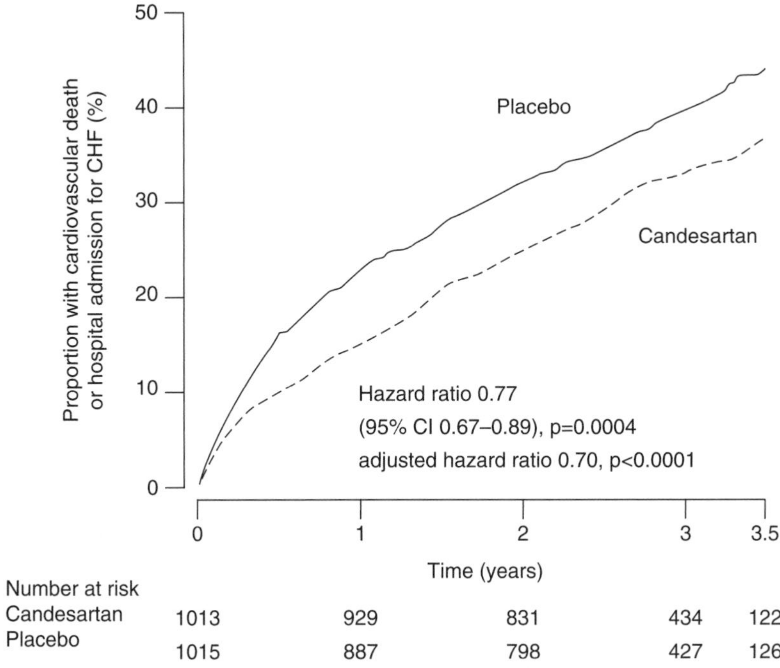

Figure 2 Improved survival with angiotensin receptor blockers in ACE inhibitor–intolerant patients in the Candesartan in Heart Failure: Assessment of Reduction in Mortality and Morbidity (CHARM) Alternate trial. *Source*: From Ref. 55.

the isosorbide dinitrate-hydralazine arm was 25.6% compared to 34.3% in the placebo group (p = 0.03). Prazosin was found to be no better than placebo with regard to mortality.

The results of V-HeFT I led to a follow-up study comparing the combination of isosorbide dinitrate and hyrdalazine to enalapril in a similar population with mild to moderate heart failure (49). V-HeFT II showed lower mortality at two years in the enalapril arm (18%) when compared to isosorbide dinitrate and hydralazine combination (25%). Notably, the isosorbide dinitrate/hydralazine arm had a larger improvement in maximal exercise capacity (as measured by maximal oxygen consumption) and ejection fraction than did enalapril, suggesting that the added benefits of enalapril on mortality may be mediated through mechanisms beyond vasodilatation alone. A subsequent analysis of the V-HeFT data demonstrated a significant interaction between drug effect and race, which suggested that the combination of isosorbide dinitrate and hydralazine might be particularly efficacious in African American patients compared to Caucasians (59).

The recently published African American Heart Failure Trial (AHeFT) represents a major advance in the medical management of this disease, demonstrating a highly significant mortality benefit in African American patients with advanced systolic heart failure (60). AHeFT was a multi-center, double-blind, placebo-controlled, randomized clinical trial of a fixed dose combination isosorbide dinitrate and hydralazine compared to placebo in self identified African American patients with heart failure. Study patients were treated with standard heart failure therapy, with high utilization of ACE inhibitors (69%), beta-blockers (74%), and ARBs (17%). AHeFT utilized a unique composite endpoint— a composite score that incorporated death, first hospitalization for heart failure, and quality of life assessment. Possible scores could range from +2 (a patient who survived, was not hospitalized, and had a > 10 unit improvement in their quality of life score) to -6 (patient who had a heart failure hospitalization, a decrement in quality of life, and subsequently died). AHeFT was terminated early by the Data Safety Monitoring Board for evidence of a highly significant mortality advantage with drug treatment (43% reduction in all cause mortality) (Fig. 3). The composite score (which could range from a worst score of -6 to a best score of $+2$) was -0.1 in the treatment group compared to -0.5 in the control group ($p=0.01$). The rate of first hospitalization for heart failure was also reduced by 33% compared to the placebo group (16.4% vs. 24.4%, $p=0.001$). AHeFT is significant due to the remarkable efficacy of the tested therapy in a group of patients with advanced systolic heart failure, a group that was already well treated with contemporary pharmacotherapy. Such a dramatic benefit (43% reduction in all cause mortality) represents a major step forward at a time when many investigators felt that a ceiling of benefit had been reached with current therapeutic approaches.

Several unanswered questions remain regarding the results of the AHeFT study. The regimen of isosorbide dinitrate and hydralazine used in AHeFT was associated with a significant risk of headache (48% vs. 19% for placebo, $p<0.001$) and dizziness (29% vs. 12% for placebo, $p<0.001$). No data have yet been provided about the proportion of patients who discontinued the active treatment due to intolerance of side effects. Among the most important unanswered questions regarding the AHeFT results is whether these benefits can be extended to a wider population of patients with heart failure than African Americans alone. The mechanistic considerations that led this trial to focus on African American patients (lower bioavailability of NO) also raise questions about whether this therapy will be as efficacious in other patient populations (61,62). Additionally, the same subgroup analyses supporting efficacy of this therapy in African American patients suggest a lack of efficacy in Caucasians. Future research will

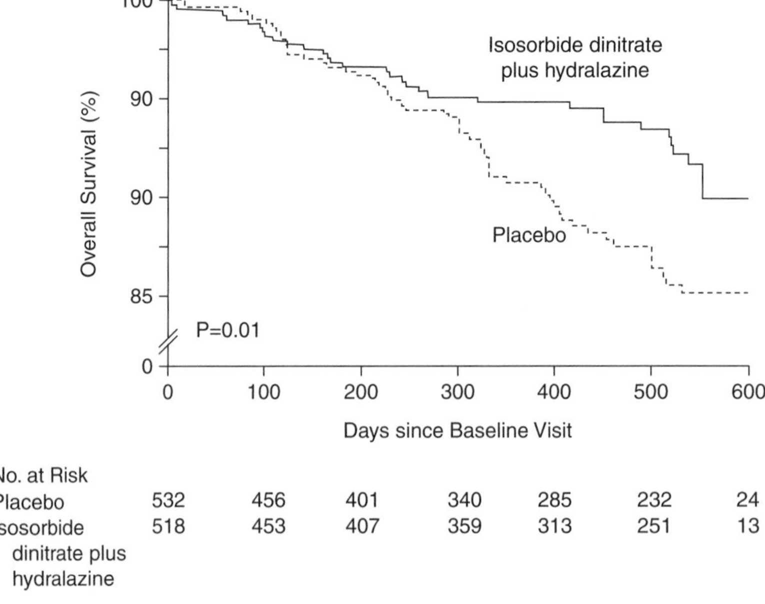

No. at Risk							
Placebo	532	456	401	340	285	232	24
Isosorbide dinitrate plus hydralazine	518	453	407	359	313	251	13

Figure 3 Improved survival in African American patients treated with isosorbide dinitrate plus hydralazine in the African–American Heart Failure Trial (A-HeFT). *Source:* From Ref. 60.

be required to identify markers of likely responsiveness to this therapy beyond racial classifications.

Amlodipine

Dihyrdopyridine calcium channel antagonists have hemodynamic vasodilator properties. The calcium channel blocker amlodipine was studied in the Prospective Randomized Amlodipine Survival Evaluation (PRAISE), a double-blind, placebo-controlled trial in patients with severe heart failure (NYHA class IIIb or IV) (63). PRAISE demonstrated no significant difference in mortality or cardiovascular morbidity between amlodipine and placebo added to the regimen of digoxin, diuretics, and ACE inhibitors. Secondary analysis of the data revealed a differential effect based on etiology, with non-ischemic patients deriving significant benefit from amlodipine compared to placebo. This finding led to the PRAISE 2 study, which compared amlodipine to placebo in patients with non-ischemic cardiomyopathy. In this follow-up study, no benefit was seen with amlodipine, suggesting that the subgroup analysis of PRAISE 1 may have been due to chance alone. Taken in total, the PRAISE trials suggest that amlodipine appears to be a relatively safe agent to use for ischemic or hypertension in the context of heart failure, but that it is not an efficacious treatment for heart failure itself.

CONCLUSIONS

Vasodilator drugs address one of the fundamental abnormalities of the heart failure syndrome-excessive vasoconstriction. A variety of agents are available for both acute and chronic use, each with varying hemodynamic effects, efficacy, and side effects. Clearly, all classes of vasodilators, even those with similar hemodynamic effects, do not have the same effects on outcomes in heart failure. Factors related to the class of drugs (such as mechanism of action) and to the individual patient (such as race) have an important impact on the choice of therapy. In chronic heart failure, ACE inhibitors remain the vasodilator of choice for patients with heart failure.

In patients intolerant of ACE inhibitors, ARBs appear to be an efficacious alternative, and these agents may provide morbidity benefit when added to ACE inhibitor therapy. Recent data suggest that African Americans may benefit uniquely from a combination of nitrates and hydralazine when added to standard therapy. In acute decompensated heart failure, the search for the optimal, safe, balanced vasodilator continues. Nesiritide shows some promise in this regard, but recent concerns about its long term safety will require adequately powered clinical trials to provide definitive data on its safety and efficacy. Ongoing research will continue to refine the role of these agents in the management of acute and chronic heart failure.

REFERENCES

1. Cohn JN, Levine TB, Olivari MT, et al. Plasma norepinephrine as a guide to prognosis in patients with chronic congestive heart failure. N Engl J Med 1984; 311:819–823.
2. Leimbach WN, Jr., Wallin BG, Victor RG, et al. Direct evidence from intraneural recordings for increased central sympathetic outflow in patients with heart failure. Circulation 1986; 73:913–919.

3. Creager MA, Faxon DP, Cutler SS, et al. Contribution of vasopressin to vasoconstriction in patients with congestive heart failure: comparison with the renin–angiotensin system and the sympathetic nervous system. J Am Coll Cardiol 1986; 7:758–765.
4. McEwan PE, Gray GA, Sherry L, et al. Differential effects of angiotensin II on cardiac cell proliferation and intramyocardial perivascular fibrosis in vivo. Circulation 1998; 98:2765–2773.
5. Timmermans PB, Wong PC, Chiu AT, et al. Angiotensin II receptors and angiotensin II receptor antagonists. Pharmacol Rev 1993; 45:205–251.
6. de Nucci G, Thomas R, D'Orleans-Juste P, et al. Pressor effects of circulating endothelin are limited by its removal in the pulmonary circulation and by the release of prostacyclin and endothelium-derived relaxing factor. Proc Natl Acad Sci USA 1988; 85:9797–9800.
7. Love MP, Haynes WG, Gray GA, et al. Vasodilator effects of endothelin-converting enzyme inhibition and endothelin ETA receptor blockade in chronic heart failure patients treated with ACE inhibitors. Circulation 1996; 94:2131–2137.
8. McMurray JJ, Ray SG, Abdullah I, et al. Plasma endothelin in chronic heart failure. Circulation 1992; 85:1374–1379.
9. Kelly RA, Han X. Nitrovasodilators have (small) direct effects on cardiac contractility: is this important? Circulation 1997; 96:2493–2495.
10. Kelly RA, Balligand JL, Smith TW. Nitric oxide and cardiac function. Circ Res 1996; 879:363–380.
11. Kubo SH, Rector TS, Bank AJ, et al. Endothelium-dependent vasodilation is attenuated in patients with heart failure. Circulation 1991; 84:1589–1596.
12. Rubanyi GM, Romero JC, Vanhoutte PM. Flow-induced release of endothelium-derived relaxing factor. Am J Physiol 1986; 250:H1145–H1149.
13. Smith CJ, Sun D, Hoegler C, et al. Reduced gene expression of vascular endothelial NO synthase and cyclooxygenase-1 in heart failure. Circ Res 1996; 78:58–64.
14. Belch JJ, Bridges AB, Scott N, et al. Oxygen free radicals and congestive heart failure. Br Heart J 1991; 65:245–248.
15. Baines AD, DeBold AJ, Sonnenberg H. Natriuretic effect of atrial extract on isolated perfused rat kidney. Can J Physiol Pharmacol 1983; 61:1462–1466.
16. Dao Q, Krishnaswamy P, Kazanegra R, et al. Utility of B-type natriuretic peptide in the diagnosis of congestive heart failure in an urgent-care setting. J Am Coll Cardiol 2001; 37:379–385.
17. Maeda K, Tsutamoto T, Wada A, et al. Plasma brain natriuretic peptide as a biochemical marker of high left ventricular end-diastolic pressure in patients with symptomatic left ventricular dysfunction. Am Heart J 1998; 135:825–832.
18. Maisel AS, Krishnaswamy P, Nowak RM, et al. Rapid measurement of B-Type natriuretic peptide in the emergency diagnosis of heart failure. N Eng J Med 2002; 347:161–167.
19. Nohria A, Tsang SW, Fang JC, et al. Clinical assessment identifies hemodynamic profiles that predict outcomes in patients admitted with heart failure. J Am Coll Cardiol 2003; 41:1797–1804.
20. Cohn JN, Franciosa JA. Vasodilator therapy of cardiac failure. N Engl J Med 1977; 297:27–31.
21. Steimle AE, Stevenson LW, Chelimsky-Fallick C, et al. Sustained hemodynamic efficacy of therapy tailored to reduce filling pressures in survivors with advanced heart failure. Circulation 1997; 96:1165–1172.
22. Stevenson LW. Tailored therapy to hemodynamic goals for advanced heart failure. Eur J Heart Fail 1999; 1:251–257.
23. Shah MR, O'Connor CM, Sopko G, et al. Evaluation Study of Congestive Heart Failure and Pulmonary Artery Catheterization Effectiveness (ESCAPE): design and rationale. Am Heart J 2001; 141:528–535.
24. Colucci WS, Elkayam U, Horton DP, et al. Intravenous nesiritide, a natriuretic peptide, in the treatment of decompensated congestive heart failure. N Engl J Med 2000; 343:246–253.

25. The VMAC Investigators. Intravenous nesiritide vs nitroglycerin for treatment of decompensated congestive heart failure: a randomized controlled trial. JAMA 2002; 287:1531–1540.
26. Guiha NH, Cohn JN, Mikulic E, et al. Treatment of refractory heart failure with infusion of nitroprusside. N Engl J Med 1974; 291:587–592.
27. Schrier RW, Abraham WT. Mechanisms of disease—hormones and hemodynamics in heart failure. N Engl J Med 1999; 341:577–585.
28. Johnson W, Omland T, Hall C, et al. Neurohormonal activation rapidly decreases after intravenous therapy with diuretics and vasodilators for class IV heart failure. J Am Coll Cardiol 2002; 39:1623–1629.
29. Loh E, Elkayam U, Cody R, et al. A randomized multicenter study comparing the efficacy and safety of intravenous milrinone and intravenous nitroglycerin in patients with advanced heart failure. J Card Fail 2001; 7:114–121.
30. Elkayam U, Kulick D, Mcintosh N, et al. Incidence of early tolerance to hemodynamic effects of continuous infusion of nitroglycerin in patients with coronary artery disease and heart failure. Circulation 1987; 76:577–584.
31. Gogia H, Mehra A, Parikh S, et al. Prevention of tolerance to hemodynamic effects of nitrates with concomitant use of hydralazine in patients with chronic heart failure. J Am Coll Cardiol 1995; 26:1575–1580.
32. Sackner-Bernstein JD, Kowalski M, Fox M, et al. Short-term risk of death after treatment with nesiritide for decompensated heart failure: a pooled analysis of randomized controlled trials. JAMA 2005; 293:1900–1905.
33. Sackner-Bernstein JD, Skopicki HA, Aaronson KD. Risk of worsening renal function with nesiritide in patients with acutely decompensated heart failure. Circulation 2005; 111:1487–1491.
34. Torre-Amione G, Young JB, Durand JB, et al. Hemodynamic effects of tezosentan, an intravenous dual endothelin receptor antagonist, in patients with class III to IV congestive heart failure. Circulation 2001; 103:973–980.
35. Louis A, Cleland JG, Crabbe S, et al. Clinical trials update: CAPRICORN, COPERNICUS, MIRACLE, STAF, RITZ-2, RECOVER and RENAISSANCE and cachexia and cholesterol in heart failure. Highlights of the scientific sessions of the American College of Cardiology. Eur J Heart Fail 2001; 3:381–387.
36. Coletta AP, Cleland JG. Clinical trials update: highlights of the scientific sessions of the XXIII Congress of the European Society of Cardiology—WARIS II, ESCAMI, PAFAC, RITZ-1 and TIME. Eur J Heart Fail 2001; 3:747–750.
37. Kaluski E, Kobrin I, Zimlichman R, et al. RITZ-5: randomized intravenous tezosentan (an endothelin-A/B antagonist) for the treatment of pulmonary edema: a prospective, multicenter, double-blind, placebo-controlled study. J Am Coll Cardiol 2003; 41:204–210.
38. O'Connor CM, Gattis WA, Adams KF, Jr., et al. Tezosentan in patients with acute heart failure and acute coronary syndromes: results of the Randomized Intravenous TeZosentan Study (RITZ-4). J Am Coll Cardiol 2003; 41:1452–1457.
39. Franciosa JA, Cohn JN. Effects of minoxidil on hemodynamics in patients with congestive heart failure. Circulation 1981; 63:652–657.
40. Elkayam U, Amin J, Mehra A, et al. A prospective, randomized, double-blind, crossover study to compare the efficacy and safety of chronic nifedipine therapy with that of isosorbide dinitrate and their combination in the treatment of chronic congestive heart failure. Circulation 1990; 82:1954–1961.
41. Massie BM, Berk MR, Brozena SC, et al. Can further benefit be achieved by adding flosequinan to patients with congestive heart failure who remain symptomatic on diuretic, digoxin, and an angiotensin converting enzyme inhibitor? Results of the Flosequinan-ACE inhibitor Trial (FACET) Circulation 1993; 88:492–501.
42. Cohn JN, Archibald DG, Ziesche S, et al. Effect of vasodilator therapy on mortality in chronic congestive heart failure. Results of a veterans administration cooperative study. N Engl J Med 1986; 314:1547–1552.
43. Hampton JR, Van Veldhusisen DJ, Kleber FX, et al. Randomized study of effect of ibopamine on survival in patients with advanced heart failure. Lancet 1997; 349:971–977.

44. Califf RM, Adams KF, McKenna WJ, et al. A randomized controlled trial of epoprostenol therapy for severe congestive heart failure: The Flolan International Randomized Survival Trial (FIRST). Am Heart J 1997; 134:44–54.
45. Levine TB, Bernink PJ, Caspi A, et al. Effect of mibefradil, a T-type calcium channel blocker, on morbidity and mortality in moderate to severe congestive heart failure: the MACH-1 study. Mortality assessment in congestive heart failure trial. Circulation 2000; 101:758–764.
46. The CONSENSUS Trial Study Group. Effects of enalapril on mortality in severe congestive heart failure. Results of the Cooperative North Scandinavian Enalapril Survival Study (CONSENSUS). N Engl J Med 1987; 316:1429–1435.
47. The SOLVD Investigators. Effect of enalapril on mortality and the development of heart failure in asymptomatic patients with reduced left ventricular ejection fractions. N Engl J Med 1992; 327:685–691.
48. The SOLVD Investigators. Effect of enalapril on survival in patients with reduced left ventricular ejection fractions and congestive heart failure. N Engl J Med 1991; 325:293–302.
49. Cohn JN, Johnson G, Ziesche S, et al. A comparison of enalapril with hydralazine-isosorbide dinitrate in the treatment of chronic congestive heart failure. N Engl J Med 1991; 325:303–310.
50. Flather MD, Yusuf S, Kober L, et al. Long-term ACE-inhibitor therapy in patients with heart failure or left-ventricular dysfunction: a systematic overview of data from individual patients. Lancet 2000; 355:1575–1581.
51. Jorde UP, Ennezat PV, Lisker J, et al. Maximally recommended doses of Angiotensin-Converting Enzyme (ACE) inhibitors do not completely prevent ACE-Mediated formation of angiotensin II in chronic heart failure. Circulation 2000; 101:844–846.
52. Cohn JN, Tognoni G, for the Valsartan Heart Failure Trial investigators. A randomized trial of the angiotensin receptor blocker valsartan in chronic heart failure. N Engl J Med 2001; 341:1675.
53. Pfeffer MA, McMurray JJV, Velazquez EJ, et al. Valsartan, captopril, or both in myocardial infarction complicated by heart failure, left ventricular dysfunction, or both. N Eng J Med 2003; 349:1893–1906.
54. McMurray JJV, Ostergren J, Swedberg K, et al. Effects of candesartan in patients with chronic heart failure and reduced left-ventricular systolic function taking angiotensin-converting-enzyme inhibitors: the CHARM-Added trial. Lancet 2003; 362:767–771.
55. Granger CB, McMurray JJ, Yusuf S, et al. Effects of candesartan in patients with chronic heart failure and reduced left-ventricular systolic function intolerant to angiotensin-converting-enzyme inhibitors: the CHARM-Alternative trial. Lancet 2003; 362:772–776.
56. Pfeffer MA, Swedberg K, Granger CB, et al. Effects of candesartan on mortality and morbidity in patients with chronic heart failure: the CHARM-Overall programme. Lancet 2003; 362:759–766.
57. Yusuf S, Pfeffer MA, Swedberg K, et al. Effects of candesartan in patients with chronic heart failure and preserved left-ventricular ejection fraction: the CHARM-Preserved trial. Lancet 2003; 362:777–781.
58. Maggioni AP, Anand I, Gottlieb SO, et al. Effects of valsartan on morbidity and mortality in patients with heart failure not receiving angiotensin-converting enzyme inhibitors. J Am Coll Cardiol 2002; 40:1414–1421.
59. Carson P, Ziesche S, Johnson G, et al. Racial differences in response to therapy for heart failure: analysis of the vasodilator-heart failure trials. Vasodilator-Heart Failure Trial Study Group. J Card Fail 1999; 5:178–187.
60. Taylor AL, Ziesche S, Yancy C, et al. Combination of isosorbide dinitrate and hydralazine in blacks with heart failure. N Engl J Med 2004; 351:2049–2057.
61. Kalinowski L, Dobrucki IT, Malinski T. Race-Specific differences in endothelial function: predisposition of African Americans to vascular diseases. Circulation 2004; 109:2511–2517.
62. Cardillo C, Kilcoyne CM, Cannon RO, et al. Racial differences in nitric oxide-mediated vasodilator response to mental stress in the forearm circulation. Hypertension 1998; 31:1235–1239.
63. Packer M, O'Connor CM, Ghali JK, et al. Effect of amlodipine on morbidity and mortality in severe chronic heart failure. N Engl J Med 1996; 335:1107–1114.

7
Beta-Blockers in Heart Failure

Emily J. Tsai
Division of Cardiology, Department of Medicine, Johns Hopkins University School of Medicine, Baltimore, Maryland, U.S.A.

Thomas P. Cappola
University of Pennsylvania School of Medicine, Philadelphia, Pennsylvania, U.S.A.

INTRODUCTION

Activation of the sympathetic nervous system in congestive heart failure was initially described in 1962 by Chidsey et al. who found that heart failure patients had augmented norepinephrine responses at rest and during exercise (1). The significance of the sympathetic nervous system in the pathophysiology of heart failure became increasingly more apparent as circulating catecholamine levels were found to correlate with disease severity and mortality in heart failure patients (2,3). While sympathoadrenergic activation initially improves and maintains cardiac function, the compensatory response eventually turns pathologic and maladaptive. The mechanisms by which sustained sympathoadrenergic activation leads to declining cardiac function are complex, involving deleterious alterations in the β-adrenergic receptor signaling pathway as well as direct cardiotoxic effects of norepinephrine. That β-adrenergic receptor antagonists, β-blockers, would have a role in the treatment for heart failure may now seem rudimentary. However, early paradigms of heart failure focused primarily on reduced systolic function and regarded negative inotropes such as β-blockers as intuitively contraindicated. It is only after nearly half a century of basic science investigations establishing biological rationale, mechanistic studies showing physiologic effects, and large randomized clinical trials (4–12) demonstrating morbidity and mortality benefits that β-blockers are now accepted as a weapon in the standard armamentarium against heart failure.

This chapter reviews the biology of the β-adrenergic signaling pathway in the cardiovascular system, the pathologic effects of chronic sympathoadrenergic activation, the pre-clinical evidence for β-blockade in heart failure, and the major clinical trials of β-blockers in heart failure management. It also offers an overview of clinical guidelines for β-blocker use in the management of congestive heart failure and addresses issues relevant to clinical practice.

Table 1 Classes of Adrenoceptors

Type	Typical location	Tissue	Effect of ligand binding	Action
α_1	Postsynaptic	Vascular smooth muscle	↑IP_3 and DAG, ↑Ca^{2+}	Contraction
		Cardiac muscle		Increases contractility
α_2	Presynaptic	Platelets	Inhibit AC, ↓cAMP	Aggregation
		Some vascular smooth muscle		Contraction
		Lipocytes		Inhibition of lipolysis
β_1	Postsynaptic	Cardiac muscle	Stimulate AC, ↑cAMP	Increases contractility Increases chronotropy Increases lusitropy
β_2	Postsynaptic	Vascular smooth muscle	Stimulate AC, ↑cAMP	Relaxation
		Skeletal muscle		Promotes potassium uptake
		Hepatocytes		Activates glycogenolysis
β_3	Postsynaptic	Lipocytes	Stimulate AC, ↑cAMP	Activates lipolysis

Source: Adapted from Ref. 13.

β-ADRENERGIC SIGNALING IN THE CARDIOVASCULAR SYSTEM

Contraction and relaxation of cardiac myocytes and vascular smooth muscle is mediated by a complex system of myofilament proteins, transmembrane ion channels, cell surface receptors, and signal transduction proteins. The sympathetic nervous system is an important regulator of this molecular machinery, especially in responses to stress. The ultimate effects of sympathetic stimulation are mediated by epinephrine and norepinephrine, which respectively act upon α- and β-adrenoceptors that are distributed throughout the cardiovascular system (Table 1, Figure 1). These two principal types of catecholamine receptors are differentiated by their potency profiles. Alpha-receptors are many times more potently activated by epinephrine and norepinephrine than isoproterenol, whereas β-receptors are more potently activated by isoproterenol. These major receptor groups are further classified into subtypes and are coupled by G proteins to various effector proteins. The various G proteins involved in adrenoceptor function include G_s, the stimulatory G protein of adenylyl cyclase (AC); G_i, the inhibitory G protein of AC; and G_q, the protein that couples α-receptors to phospholipase C (PLC).

Alpha Receptors

Typically, α_1 receptors stimulate polyphosphoinositide hydrolysis, leading to the formation of inositol 1,4,5-trisphosphate (IP_3) and diacylglycerol (DAG). In certain smooth muscle cells, the activation of the IP_3-DAG pathway results in the release of sequestered calcium ions from intracellular stores, thereby increasing cytoplasmic concentration of free Ca^{2+} and activating various calcium-dependent protein kinases. By controlling calcium influx in vascular smooth muscle cells, the α_1 adrenergic pathway regulates vascular tone and, indirectly, blood pressure. Other signal transduction pathways activated by α_1-receptors include those implicated in cell growth, mitogen-activated kinase (MAP kinase) and polyphosphoinositol-3-kinase (PI-3-kinase) pathways. Coupled to the inhibitory regulator protein G_i, α_2 receptors inhibit AC activity and cause intracellular cyclic adenosine monophosphate (cAMP) levels to decrease. Some of the effects of α_2 adrenoceptors are independent of AC inhibition, such as the activation of potassium channels and closing of calcium channels. Furthermore, G_q, which mediates interaction between some α receptors with PLC, may be involved in myocyte hypertrophy and apoptotic signaling (14).

Beta Receptors

All three subtypes of β receptors activate AC and, via the stimulatory coupling protein G_s, increase conversion of ATP to cAMP. Cardiac β receptors are primarily of the β_1 subtype, whereas most non–cardiac β receptors are β_2. However, there is evidence that myocardium contains both β_1 and β_2 adrenoceptors (15,16). β_1-receptor activation results in increased intracellular calcium concentrations and enhanced calcium cycling within cardiac myocytes, leading to positive chronotropic, lusitropic, and inotropic effects. While similarly increasing intracellular cAMP concentrations via G_s and AC activation, β_2 adrenergic stimulation relaxes peripheral vascular smooth muscle.

Adrenergic Activation as Acute Compensation

Early in heart failure, the diminished cardiac output is sensed by baroreceptors as a fall in blood pressure, thereby triggering a reflexive increase in sympathetic outflow. This central sympathoadrenergic stimulation leads to increased release and decreased uptake of norepinephrine. Elevated norepinephrine levels mediate arteriole constriction, increase venous return to the heart via constriction of capacitance vessels, and directly stimulate the heart by increasing ventricular contractility and heart rate. Adrenergic activation thus effectively increases peripheral vascular resistance and cardiac output. While this initially serves to raise cardiac output and heart rate, sustained adrenergic activation increases myocardial oxygen demand, ischemia, and oxidative stress. The progressive worsening of ventricular function eventually overwhelms any acute compensation offered by adrenergic activation. Negative feedback mechanisms render myocytes less responsive to adrenergic stimuli, further diminishing cardiac contractile function. Moreover, chronic adrenergic activation has other deleterious effects on the cardiovascular system, such as ventricular remodeling and arrhythmogenesis.

Pathologic Consequences of Adrenergic Activation

Myocardial Stunning with Sudden Sympathoadrenergic Stimulation. The pathologic consequences of acute adrenergic activation are manifested in the profound, reversible left ventricular dysfunction precipitated by sudden emotional stress, a syndrome known as "stress cardiomyopathy" (17). Such acute, stress-induced myocardial dysfunction has been referred to as "takotsubo cardiomyopathy" (18–20) and "transient left ventricular apical ballooning" (21,22). Although the exact mechanism remains unknown, supraphysiologic levels of plasma catecholamines and stress-related neuropeptides in patients with stress cardiomyopathy suggest an association between sympathoadrenergic stimulation and myocardial stunning (23). It has been surmised that the high catecholamine state causes microvascular (24,25) and epicardial coronary arterial vasospasm (26,27) as well as direct myocyte injury (28–34).

Decreased β-Adrenergic Responsiveness. Prolonged adrenergic stimulation affects the functional state of adrenoceptors as well as their density on the cell surface (35). The net result is an impaired ability of the heart to respond to further adrenergic stimulation, which translates into a reduced capacity to mount a stress response. The cellular mechanisms responsible include receptor desensitization (36–39), internalization (40), lysosomal degradation (41), and down-regulation (42–45). Desensitization of the β receptor occurs as sustained stimulation induces β agonist receptor kinase (βARK) activity, which recruits arrestins to the adrenoceptor G protein subunit and causes conformational changes in the receptor (46–49). This conformational change uncouples β receptor from G protein activity. Yet another uncoupling mechanism involves cAMP-triggered phosphorylation of the β-receptor, preventing interaction of G_s with the receptor. Receptor desensitization occurs rapidly and is a short-term change. More relevant to chronic adrenergic activation, as is seen in chronic heart failure, is the long-term inhibitory mechanism of receptor sequestration and down-regulation.

Sequestration is a rapid and reversible process by which receptors are actively removed from the plasma membrane and internalized into an endosomal sorting system. Sequestration and internalization also decouples the β-adrenoceptor from agonists and G protein, further limiting the positive inotropic and chronotropic effects of sympathoadrenergic stimulation. The process of receptor down-regulation is not as well delineated but likely involves a combination of accelerated receptor removal from the plasma membrane and decreased rate of receptor synthesis. A slower process than sequestration, down-regulation ultimately results in the destruction of adrenoceptors.

In congestive heart failure, there is a selective down-regulation of β_1-receptors but not β_2-receptors (50–56). The density of the β_1-receptor may be decreased by as much as 50% to 70% (57), resulting in a relative up-regulation of cardiac β_2-receptors.

Remodeling—Fibrosis, Apoptosis, Hypertrophy. The above mechanisms of desensitization, sequestration, and down-regulation effectively diminish any beneficial compensatory results of chronic adrenergic activation. Yet chronic adrenergic activation has deleterious effects on the cardiovascular system beyond those mediated by negative feedback mechanisms. On the physiologic level, sympathoadrenergically-triggered peripheral vasoconstriction increases both preload and afterload, placing additional mechanical stress on the failing myocardium. The long-term mechanical stress contributes to ventricular remodeling, leading to a dilated, less contractile ventricle.

Chronic adrenergic activation also produces cellular and molecular abnormalities that contribute to the progressive decline of myocardial function. Although inaccessible to either agonists or G proteins, sequestered adrenoceptors continue to participate in growth-stimulating signal transduction pathways via arrestin and MAP kinase, which results in the promotion of cardiac cell growth and hypertrophy (58). Norepinephrine itself has toxic cardiac effects, causing cell death by both necrosis and apoptosis. The cardiotoxicity of catecholamines has been recognized since at least 1907, when catecholamine-induced cardiac necrosis was first reported (59). The primary mechanism of norepinephrine-induced toxicity has since been determined to be cAMP-mediated calcium overload, the results of which are diminished cardiomyocyte viability and decreased protein synthesis in remaining viable cardiomyocytes (60). Apoptosis has been implicated as one of the molecular mechanisms leading to end stage heart disease, regardless of etiology of cardiomyopathy (61–66). Studies in adult rat ventricular myocytes and transgenic mice have demonstrated promotion of cardiomyocyte apoptosis by β_1 adrenergic receptor stimulation and a downstream cAMP-dependent mechanism (likely involving the mitogen-activated protein kinase superfamily), as well as variable inhibition of

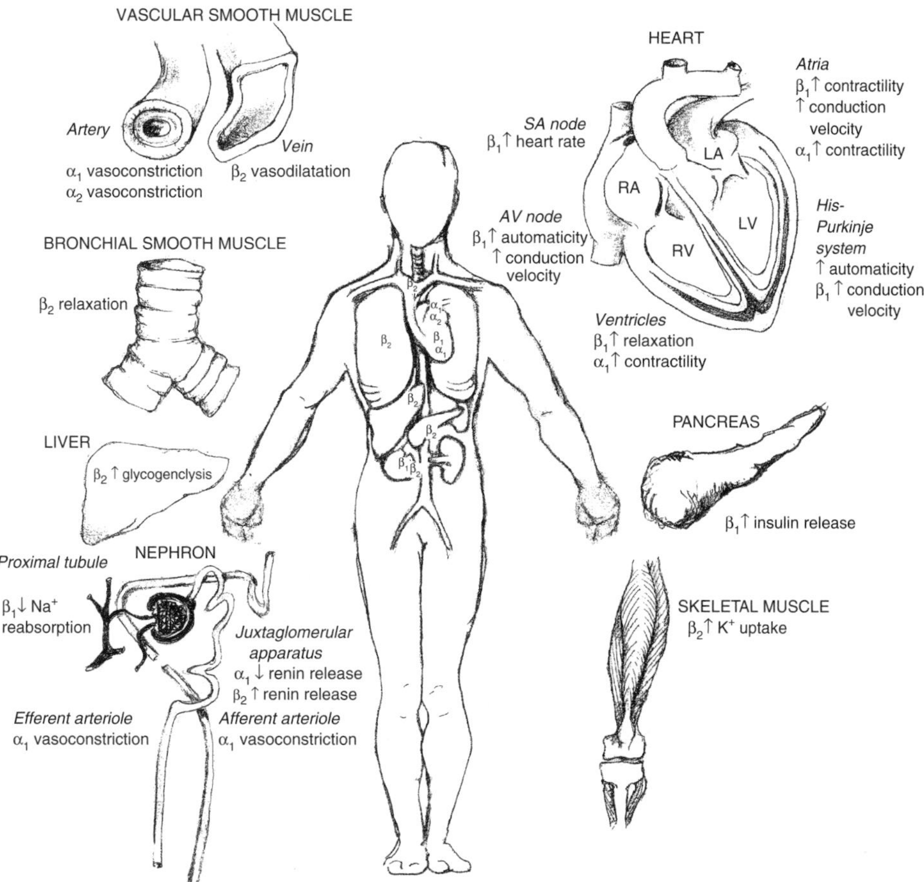

Figure 1 Distribution and function of adrenoceptors.

cardiomyocyte apoptosis by β_2 adrenergic receptor stimulation and its coupled effector pathways (65,67–73).

Arrhythmogenicity. In chronic heart failure, death ensues from either progressive heart failure or sudden death, which may have cardiac or non-cardiac causes (5,6,74). Data suggest that a significant proportion of sudden deaths are due to ventricular fibrillation (74). A high catecholamine state has been associated with increased arrhythmogenicity via decreased threshold for ventricular fibrillation (75–78). Furthermore, β-blockers have demonstrated a protective effect on sudden death in conditions of hypertension (79), post-myocardial infarction (80), and chronic heart failure (5,6), lending additional proof that adrenergic activation promotes arrhythmogenesis.

Mortality. Prolonged activation of the adrenergic system is not only maladaptive, causing progressive deterioration of cardiac function, but also predictive of poor prognosis. Plasma norepinephrine levels have long been known to proportionately correlate with heart failure severity and mortality (2,3,81–84). Early in congestive heart failure, cardiac output and plasma catecholamines are normal at rest. However, with exercise, cardiac output is limited and plasma catecholamines increase to abnormally high levels (1). As the disease progresses, plasma norepinephrine levels become elevated even at rest, with the degree of elevation directly reflecting the severity of cardiac dysfunction (2,84). The V-HeFT II trial established a direct relation between plasma norepinephrine and mortality, as those with lowest plasma norepinephrine levels had the lowest cumulative mortality rates.

EVIDENCE FOR THE ROLE OF BETA-BLOCKADE

As our understanding of the role of the adrenergic signaling pathway in the pathophysiology of heart failure has grown, so has the therapeutic potential of β-adrenoceptor antagonists. The first report of β-blocker use in congestive heart failure came from an observational study by Waagstein et al. in 1975 (85) in which seven patients with advanced cardiomyopathy showed echocardiographic and symptomatic improvement of ventricular function with β-blockade. Multiple studies have shown that treatment with β-blockers is associated with significant physiologic and hemodynamic improvements, including increases in left ventricular ejection fraction (EF) and cardiac index and a decrease in LV end diastolic pressure (86–96). Furthermore, β-blockers also decrease cardiac arrhythmias and sudden cardiac death (74,75,79,80,97–99).

In this section we will review the major clinical trials of β-blockers in the management of chronic heart failure, starting with those that demonstrated physiologic benefit with β-blocker use, then those that demonstrated symptomatic, morbidity, and, finally, mortality benefit (Table 3).

Physiologic/Functional Benefit

Australia, New Zealand (ANZ) Heart Failure Research

This randomized controlled trial of carvedilol in 415 patients with New York Heart Association (NYHA) Class II–IV heart failure was conducted in six hospitals in New Zealand and 14 hospitals in Australia over 19 months. The rationale behind the study was that beta-blockers, by improving left ventricular function, could improve exercise and functional ability in patients with heart failure due to ischemic disease. The target carvedilol dose was 25 mg BID. Although beneficial effects on left ventricular function and size were maintained for at least one year after treatment, carvedilol had no clear effect on exercise performance, symptoms, or episodes of worsening heart failure. There was an overall 21% reduction in combined endpoint of death and hospital admission. However, when only death was examined, there was no significant difference between the two groups. There were also no significant differences in treadmill exercise time, distance walked in 6 minutes, or NYHA functional class (100,101).

Multi-center Oral Carvedilol Heart Failure Assessment (MOCHA)

This multi-center, placebo-controlled trial aimed to establish the efficacy and safety of carvedilol in improving exercise tolerance in 345 subjects with mild to moderate, stable chronic heart failure. Three different doses of carvedilol were studied: low (6.25 mg), medium (12.5 mg), and high (25 mg), each given twice daily. Following an up-titration period of 2–4 weeks, patients were treated for an average of 6 months. Baseline heart failure management at time of study entry included angiotensin converting enzyme inhibitors (ACE-I), digitalis, and loop-diuretics in more than 90% of the patients.

Approximately 30% of patients in each group were also treated with vasodilators. Submaximal exercise tolerance was measured by the 6-minutes walk test and 9-minutes self-powered treadmill test. Carvedilol had no effect on either measure of exercise tolerance but was associated with dose-related improvements in LV function as reflected by EF. Furthermore, the all-cause actuarial mortality risk and hospitalization rate in carvedilol-treated patients were significantly lower (102). Since this study was not designed to evaluate the effect of carvedilol therapy on mortality, the mortality rates were assessed primarily as a safety end point.

Symptomatic Improvement

Prospective Randomized Evaluation of Carvedilol on Symptoms and Exercise (PRECISE)

The effect of carvedilol on symptomatic status, with exercise tolerance as the primary end-point, was studied in this multi-centered, double-blind, randomized controlled trial of 278 patients with moderate to severe heart failure (NYHA Class III–IV). An open-label run-in period of two weeks ensured that only those who tolerated carvedilol at a dose of 6.25 mg bid were randomized into the study. Patients remained on a background therapy of ACE-I, digoxin, and diuretics as they were treated with either placebo or carvedilol (target dose of 25 mg to 50 mg twice daily). Carvedilol treatment led to not only improved ejection fraction and reduced combined morbidity and mortality risk but also to symptomatic improvement and lower risk of clinical deterioration, as measured by NYHA functional class and the patient's or physician's global assessment. Of note, there was no significant, consistent improvement in the carvedilol group with respect to the primary end-point of exercise tolerance as measured by the 6-minute walk test and 9-minute treadmill test (103). Mortality rates were determined as part of the safety assessment.

U.S. Carvedilol Heart Failure Study—Mild CHF

In the same issue of *Circulation* in which the MOCHA and PRECISE trials were published, Colucci et al. reported the effects of carvedilol on the clinical progression of heart failure in patients with mild heart failure due to left ventricular systolic dysfunction. Almost all the patients in this study were NYHA functional class II. Although clinical severity of heart failure in these randomized patients was mild, left ventricular ejection fraction was markedly reduced, averaging 23%. Nearly all patients received triple therapy of ACE-I, digoxin, and diuretics at baseline. Open-label run-in and up-titration periods were also incorporated into the study design. The primary end-point was clinical progression of heart failure, defined as death due to heart failure, hospitalization for heart failure, or the need for sustained increases in heart failure medications. Secondary end-points included changes in left ventricular ejection fraction, NYHA functional class, heart failure symptom score, global patient assessment, and quality of life. Carvedilol reduced clinical progression of heart failure by 48% over the 12-month follow-up period. Significant improvements were also seen in several secondary end-points. Despite a reduction in all-cause mortality with carvedilol treatment, quality of life (as assessed by the Minnesota Living with Heart Failure scale) and exercise tolerance (as measured by the 9-minute treadmill test) were not affected by carvedilol (104).

Table 2 Summary of Large Randomized Clinical Trials of β-Blocker in Chronic Heart Failure

Trial (β-blocker)	Design	n	NYHA	LVEF	Follow-up (months)	Dose(mg/d)		Primary endpoint	Study result
						Target	Mean		
MDC (Metoprolol)	Placebo-controlled	383	II–III	<40%	12	100–150	108	Combined mortality and need for transplant	No benefit but benefit on 2° endpoints
CIBIS-I (Bisoprolol)	Placebo-controlled	641	III–IV	<40%	22.8	5	3.8	Mortality	No benefit but morbidity benefit seen
USCP (Carvedilol)	Placebo-controlled	1094	II–IV	≤35%	6–12	50–100	45	All-cause mortality hospitalization for cardiac cause	Significant benefit
CHF		366	II		12	50–100	n/a	Clinical progression combined end point of death, hospitalization, or medication change due to CHF	Significant benefit
MOCHA	Dose comparison	345	II–III		6	12.5 25 50	12.5 24.6 47.4	Efficacy: Submax exercise tolerance	No effect but dose-related improvement on LV function and survival

PRECISE		278	III–IV		6	50–100	n/a	Symptoms and exercise capacity	Benefit on symptoms, combined morbidity and mortality, and risk of progression
Severe CHF		131	III–IV		6	50	n/a	Quality of life	No benefit but improvement of LVEF
ANZ (Carvedilol)	Placebo-controlled	415	II–III		19	50	41	LVEF ETT and exercise tolerance	Benefit on LVEF but not exercise tolerance
CIBIS-II (Bisoprolol)	Placebo-controlled	2647	III–IV	≤35%	16.8	10	7.7	All-cause mortality	Significant benefit
MERIT-HF (Metoprolol XL)	Placebo-controlled	3991	II–IV	≤40%	12	200	159	All-cause mortality combined all-cause mortality and all-cause hospitalization	Significant benefit
BEST (Bucindolol)	Placebo-controlled	2708	III–IV	≤35%	24	100–200	152	All-cause mortality	Significant reduction in cardiac-related deaths but not in all-cause mortality
COPERNICUS (Carvedilol)	Placebo-controlled	2289	IV	<25%	10.4	50	35.6	All-cause mortality combined mortality and hospitalization	35% reduction in all-cause mortality with carvedilol
COMET (Carvedilol/metoprolol)	Comparison	3029	II–IV	≤35%	58	50 (c) 100 (m)	41.8 85	All-cause mortality combined mortality and hospitalization	Extended survival with carvedilol

Abbreviations: CHF, chronic heart failure; LVEF, left ventricular ejection fraction; LV, left ventricular.

Morbidity Benefit

The Metoprolol in Dilated Cardiomyopathy Trial (MDC)

One of the earliest large, multi-centered, randomized controlled trials of beta-blockade in heart failure, MDC studied the effect of metoprolol in 383 patients with NYHA class II–III heart failure. The primary combined end-point in this trial was mortality and morbidity, with morbidity captured as the need for cardiac transplant. The study employed a run-in period and then a subsequent up-titration period to a study target daily dose of 100–150 mg. Metoprolol conferred no statistically significant benefit on the primary end-point but did significantly retard clinical deterioration via a reduced need for cardiac transplant (4). Metoprolol also improved ejection fraction, quality of life, and exercise capacity compared to placebo. There was no difference in hospitalization.

The Cardiac Insufficiency Bisoprolol Study—I (CIBIS-I)

Although it failed to demonstrate a survival benefit, CIBIS-I established significant morbidity benefit with bisoprolol treatment in patients with moderate to severe heart failure. In this study of 641 patients with NYHA class III–IV heart failure of various etiologies, bisoprolol was associated with improved NYHA functional status and decreased hospitalizations due to cardiac decompensation over the follow-up period (mean 1.9 years) (105). All patients received background diuretic and vasodilator therapy during the study.

Mortality Benefit

The Beta-Blocker Evaluation of Survival Trial (BEST)

The effect of bucindolol on patients with more advanced heart failure was later revisited in BEST, a double-blind randomized controlled trial of 2708 patients with NYHA Class III–IV heart failure. No difference in the primary end-point of all-cause mortality was seen between the bucindolol and placebo groups. However, the trial was terminated early (average follow up of 2 years) at the recommendation of the data and safety monitoring board because risk of the secondary end-point, death from cardiovascular causes, was indeed lower in the bucindolol group. Risk of heart transplantation or death, as well as hospitalization for heart failure, was also lower with bucindolol treatment (12).

U.S. Carvedilol Heart Failure Study

This stratified, multi-center, randomized controlled trial pooled together the data from MOCHA, PRECISE, and two other trials to assess the effect of carvedilol on the occurrence of death or hospitalization for cardiovascular reasons. The 1094 patients with chronic heart failure enrolled in the study were assigned to one of four protocols based upon their exercise capacity. Patients were randomized to either placebo or carvedilol only after successful completion of an open-label run-in period. A titration period was incorporated into the design study, with a target dose of 25 mg–50 mg twice daily based on patient weight. Background therapy with an ACE-I, digoxin, and diuretics was continued during the study. A 65% reduction in overall mortality risk was attributed to carvedilol treatment, thereby leading to early termination of the study. Furthermore, carvedilol therapy was associated with a 27% reduction in the risk of hospitalization for cardiovascular causes and a 38% reduction in the combined risk of hospitalization or death (105,106).

The Metoprolol CR/XL Randomized Intervention Trial in Congestive Heart Failure (MERIT-HF)

Extended-release metoprolol was tested for treating NYHA Class II–IV heart failure in 3991 patients. Randomization to placebo or metoprolol CR/XL was preceded by a single-blind placebo run-in period. Titration toward a target dose of 200 mg daily occurred over an 8-week period. The two primary end points were all-cause mortality and all-cause mortality in combination with all-cause hospitalization. As with BEST and the US Carvedilol Heart Failure Study, MERIT-HF was also terminated early on the recommendation of an independent safety monitoring board. All-cause mortality was 34% lower in metoprolol treated patients than placebo patients. Metoprolol reduced the combined end-point of mortality and all-cause hospitalization by 19%. There were 31% fewer deaths from all causes and hospitalizations for heart failure in the metoprolol group. All-cause hospitalization alone was lowered by 13%, hospitalization for all heart-related causes by 20%, and hospitalization for worsening heart failure by 32%. (6,105,106)

The Cardiac Insufficiency Bisoprolol Study II (CIBIS-II)

Whereas CIBIS-I demonstrated only morbidity benefit with bisoprolol treatment, CIBIS-II demonstrated a 33% reduction in all-cause mortality with bisoprolol treatment. The study enrolled 2647 patients with NYHA Class III–IV heart failure and ejection fractions $\leq$35%, with an average EF of 27%. All patients received standard therapy with ACE inhibitors and diuretics, and were randomized to either placebo or bisoprolol, titrated to a target dose of 10 mg daily and followed over a mean of 1.3 years. The study was stopped early because bisoprolol showed a significant benefit on the primary end-point of overall, all-cause survival. Bisoprolol reduced the risk of death by 33% and the risk of cardiac-related death by 44%. Bisoprolol patients also had fewer overall hospitalizations, as well as fewer combined cardiovascular deaths and cardiovascular hospitalizations. The benefits of bisoprolol were independent of either severity or etiology of heart failure (5).

The Carvedilol Prospective Randomized Cumulative Survival Trial (COPERNICUS)

Although CIBIS-I and II, MERIT-HF, BEST, and the US Carvedilol Heart Failure Study all included patients with more advanced heart failure, NYHA Class IV heart failure patients comprised a small portion (3–16%) of the study population in those trials. COPERNICUS is particularly significant since its patients had the most advanced heart failure of any large-scale clinical trial of beta-blockade to date. All 2289 patients had NYHA Class III–IV heart failure of various etiologies and left ventricular ejection fractions $<$25%. Ischemic cardiomyopathy was twice as common as non–ischemic cardiomyopathy. Patients were symptomatic at rest or with minimal activity, despite treatment with an ACE-I and diuretics. While the mean EF was $<$20%, patients did not have any evidence of volume overload upon study entry. Randomization to either placebo or carvedilol was followed by titration over several weeks from an initiation dose of 3.125 mg twice a day to a target dose of 25 mg twice a day. The primary end-point was all-cause mortality; secondary end-points included the combined risk of death and hospitalization as well as patient self-assessment of clinical status. The trial was terminated early when the data and safety monitoring board noted a highly significant effect on mortality in the patients treated with carvedilol. The all-cause mortality rate was 35% lower in the carvedilol group than in the placebo group; the survival benefit was notable as early as 4 months and the difference in survival widened over the next 2 years.

Table 3 β-Blockers Used in Mortality Clinical Trials of Chronic Heart Failure Patients

Drug (trade name)	Adrenergic selectivity	Ancillary properties
Bisoprolol (Zebeta®)	β_1	None
Bucindolol (Bextra®)	β_1, β_2	Vasodilatory
Carvedilol (Coreg®)	α_1,β_1, β_2	Vasodilatory, antioxidant
Metoprolol tartrate (Lopressor®)	β_1	None
Metoprolol succinate (Toprol XL®)	β_1	None

Source: Adapted from Ref. 108.

The survival benefit attributable to carvedilol was independent of patient gender, age, ejection fraction, etiology of cardiomyopathy, or hospitalization within the previous year. With respect to secondary end-points, carvedilol reduced the risk of death or any hospitalization by 24%, the risk of death or any cardiac hospitalization by 27%, and the risk of death or any heart failure hospitalization by 31%. COPERNICUS demonstrated that even the highest risk heart failure patients not only tolerated beta-blockade with carvedilol with fewer serious adverse effects but also benefited significantly with respect to mortality and morbidity (8–10,107).

The Carvedilol or Metoprolol European Trial (COMET)

As β-blockers differ in their pharmacologic profiles (i.e., adrenergic receptor selectivity and ancillary properties) (Table 3), the COMET study set out to compare the effects of carvedilol and short-acting metoprolol (tartrate) on mortality and morbidity in patients with mild to severe chronic heart failure. Three thousand and twenty-nine patients with NYHA Class II–IV heart failure were randomized to either carvedilol or metoprolol in a parallel-group study design. Patients were titrated to a target dose of 25 mg twice a day for carvedilol and 50 mg twice a day for metoprolol. All-cause mortality was 34% for carvedilol and 40% for metoprolol, reflecting a 17% reduction in mortality with carvedilol over metoprolol. There was no significant difference between the two treatment groups in the composite end-point of mortality and hospitalization. The study suggested that carvedilol extends survival in heart failure patients compared to metoprolol (11).

However, the pharmacodynamic considerations and hemodynamic data of the COMET trial suggest disparate degrees of β_1-blockade attained with carvedilol and metoprolol tartrate (immediate-release). Without equivalent β_1-blockade in the two treatment groups, no potential incremental benefits of selective- versus nonselective-adrenergic blockade can be concluded. Furthermore, metoprolol tartrate was found by the MDC trial to have no significant benefit on the combined end point of mortality and need for cardiac transplantation (109). It was the long-acting formulation of metoprolol, metoprolol succinate, that demonstrated a survival benefit in heart failure (6).

Summary: Collectively, these randomized controlled clinical trials have assessed the safety and efficacy of β-blockers in tens of thousands of patients with stable, chronic heart failure of wide-ranging severity. The benefits of β-blockers on cardiac physiology, heart failure symptoms, functional status, morbidity, and mortality have been demonstrated across gender, age, and race, regardless of the etiology of heart failure and despite optimized medical management with ACEI, diurectics, and, in some, digitalis. Yet the efficacy of β-blockers cannot be considered a class effect, as xamoterol, bucindolol, and short-acting metoprolol (tartrate) do not confer an overall mortality benefit in heart failure patients (12,109,110). As such, the ACC/AHA guidelines for the evaluation and management of chronic heart failure in adults recommend the inclusion of any one of the proven β-blockers—bisoprolol, long-acting metoprolol (succinate), or carvedilol—in the management of post–myocardial infarction stage B heart failure, stage B heart failure with reduced LVEF, and stable stage C heart failure.

CLINICAL GUIDELINES

Based on the evidence presented in the previous sections, β-blockade has become a front-line therapy for the treatment of heart failure. However, the application of β-blockade to individual patients continues to evolve in the context of new device and pharmacologic therapies, new clinical research data, and accumulating clinical experience. Here we offer guidelines for using β-blockers that are based in part on American Heart Association and American College of Cardiology consensus statements (111), with the caveat that these recommendations will continue to evolve.

Choice of Beta-Blocker

While bisoprolol, metoprolol succinate, and carvedilol have all demonstrated therapeutic benefits in chronic heart failure, their relative efficacies have not been directly compared. Given the variation in adrenoceptor selectivity and ancillary properties amongst the three β-blockers, disparities in survival benefit might be expected. In fact, the COMET trial suggested additional survival benefit with carvedilol over metoprolol tartrate. However, metoprolol succinate, not metoprolol tartrate, was shown to reduce all-cause mortality in the MERIT-HF trial. Metoprolol tartrate failed to show any benefit on the combined primary end-point of mortality or need for cardiac transplant in the MDC trial. How carvedilol compares to an equivalent target dose of metoprolol succinate remains unanswered. In the absence of any evidence identifying one particular β-blocker as the most effective medication, any one of the three β-blockers with proven mortality benefit may be used in the management of chronic heart failure.

Relationship to Other Heart Failure Medications

β-blockers should be initiated in all patients with stable heart failure as soon as left ventricular dysfunction is diagnosed, even if patients are asymptomatic. Sufficient disease stability, however, is required. That is, patients should be relatively euvolemic, should not be hospitalized in an intensive care unit, and should not have had any recent treatment with an intravenous positive inotropic agent. If a patient does not satisfy these conditions of clinical stability, management should be optimized first with other heart failure medications (i.e., diuretics). Once disease stability is attained, the patient can then be re-assessed for β-blockade.

Even if clinically stable, patients with the slightest evidence or recent history of fluid retention should be prescribed diuretics while on β-blockers. The initiation of β-blockers can at times be accompanied by an exacerbation of fluid retention (112–114), making diuretics necessary for maintaining sodium and fluid balance.

Assuming patient clinical stability, β-blockade should be initiated regardless of a patient's regimen with other heart failure medications. The benefits of β-blockade, as evidenced in the numerous randomized controlled trials, are additive even in patients receiving treatment with ACE-I and diuretics (5,6,9,11,106). Furthermore, most patients in the large randomized controlled β-blocker trials were not on high doses of ACE-I. In view of that, ACE-I need not be up-titrated to target doses attained in clinical trials of ACE-I before β-blockers are incorporated into heart failure management. The addition of a β-blocker to low-dose ACE-I improves heart failure symptoms and reduces the risk of disease progression or death more so than even increasing the dose of ACE-I (115,116).

In fact, β-blockade can be started in combination with or prior to ACE-I therapy without fear of increased adverse side effects. Under-utilization and delayed initiation of β-blockers are in large part due to the common perception that β-blockers are not as well tolerated as ACE-I in heart failure, and to the concern that concomitant ACE-I-mediated after-load reduction is crucial to off-load the failing heart prior to initiating β-blockade. However, a double-blind, randomized, parallel-group study of carvedilol and enalapril in patients with mild chronic heart failure found no significant differences in adverse events or withdrawals between those patients treated with carvedilol alone, enalapril alone, or the combination of carvedilol and enalapril. Although the study compared safety and tolerability of treatment and was not designed or powered for assessing morbidity and mortality outcomes, combination therapy with carvedilol and enalapril resulted in trends toward fewer cardiovascular and heart failure events than monotherapy (117).

Titration Strategies: Target Dose, Titration Interval

β-blockers should be started at very low doses and up-titrated over several weeks. In clinical trials, the starting dose of bisoprolol was 1.25 mg daily (5); metoprolol succinate, 12.5 mg or 25 mg daily, depending on NYHA functional status (6); and carvedilol, 3.125 mg twice daily (9,11,106). Bisoprolol was titrated in dosing increments of 1.25 mg to 2.5 mg over titration intervals of one to four weeks for a target dose of 10 mg daily. Up-titrations of carvedilol and metoprolol were performed as dose doublings every two weeks to target doses of 25–50 mg twice daily and 200 mg once daily, respectively. Lower doses were prescribed only if patients could not tolerate higher doses. Physicians should aim for the target doses used in clinical trials as the effectiveness of low dose β-blockers has never been evaluated.

Patients, particularly those with more severe heart failure, should be closely monitored throughout the titration period for evidence of symptomatic bradycardia and fluid retention. Weight gain reflective of fluid retention should be immediately managed with higher doses of concomitant diuretics, and incremental up-titration of β-blockers should be withheld until side effects subside. Various clinical studies on β-blocker titration failure and tolerability, however, have found that titration failure is independent of severity of heart failure and that even patients with more advanced heart failure tolerate β-blockade without increased risk of clinical deterioration (118–121).

Continuation During Decompensation and Inotrope Use

Despite the significant beneficial effects of β-blockers and other heart failure medications, congestive heart failure remains a progressive disease in which patients are susceptible to episodic decompensation. Sudden withdrawal of chronic β-blockade can lead to further clinical deterioration and worsening heart failure (122, 123), arguing for continued β-blocker treatment during heart failure exacerbations. Yet, should β-blockade be continued in patients with decompensated heart failure requiring intravenous inotropic support? Does the choice of intravenous inotropic agent affect hemodynamic and clinical outcomes? Does the choice of β-blocker influence efficacy of inotropic agent?

The most commonly used inotropic drugs used to treat patients with decompensated heart failure are the β-adrenergic receptor agonist dobutamine and the type III phosphodiesterase inhibitors (PDE) milrinone and enoximone. A partial β_1-adrenoceptor agonist with post–synaptic β_2-vasodilatory and α_1-vasoconstrictive activity, dobutamine improves cardiac output without significant change in systemic vascular resistance. Milrinone and enoximone inhibit type III PDE, raising cAMP levels in the myocardium and vascular smooth muscle, which then trigger a signaling cascade involving protein kinase A, phospholamban, and L-type calcium channel phosphorylation. Type III PDE inhibition ultimately produces positive lusitropic and inotropic effects, leading to greater cardiac output. One distinguishing difference between these two classes of inotropic drugs is that type III PDE inhibitors act distally to the β-adrenergic receptor. Thus, while the inotropic effects of dobutamine depend upon the availability of β-adrenoceptors and on the β-adrenergic pathway, the lusitropic and inotropic effects of type III PDE inhibitors do not.

The safety of concurrent β-blockade in heart failure patients receiving inotropic therapy has been addressed in retrospective observational analyses only. A small study found that carvedilol titration could be achieved in NYHA Class IIIb–IV heart failure patients who required intermittent intravenous milrinone therapy, with similar success rates as in patients with NYHA Class II–IIIa, after reaching a stable clinical state with milrinone and triple oral therapy of ACE-I, diuretics, and digoxin. Most patients showed improvement in functional class with combination intermittent milrinone infusion and carvedilol titration and, furthermore, were successfully weaned off intravenous inotropic support (121).

The Outcomes of a Prospective Trial of Intravenous Milrinone for Exacerbations of Chronic Heart Failure (OPTIME-CHF) was a multi-center, randomized, double-blind placebo-controlled trial of milrinone in patients hospitalized for heart failure exacerbation. An observational analysis by Gattis et al. compared the clinical outcomes between patients treated with β-blockers versus those not on β-blockers at time of admission. The data revealed no difference in clinical events between the two patient groups, suggesting that continuation of chronic β-blocker therapy in patients admitted for heart failure exacerbation does not increase the risk of adverse clinical events, even when patients require milrinone infusion therapy. Furthermore, β-blockers did not appear to diminish the effect of therapies used for worsening heart failure, including intravenous inotropic support, or prolong length of hospital stay (124).

Studies of dobutamine response in the presence of β-blockade, however, have yielded different results (125–127). β-blockade with carvedilol does blunt the hemodynamic response to dobutamine. Relatively high doses of dobutamine are required to produce improvements in cardiac output. Although dobutamine increases cardiac output, it also increases systemic and pulmonary pressures, thereby increasing left ventricular stroke work index more so than milrinone at comparable doses (126).

The differential hemodynamic responses to PDE inhibitors and dobutamine in patients on chronic β-blockers are attributable to more than just the β-adrenoceptor-independent mechanism of PDE inhibitors. In the failing human heart, high catecholamine levels desensitize the β-adrenergic signaling pathway by down-regulating β_1-adrenoceptors (128–130) and up-regulating inhibitory G-protein (131–134). Chronic β-blockade may enhance the hemodynamic responses to PDE inhibitors via normalization of up-regulated inhibitory G-proteins levels (135). Additionally, PDE inhibitors improve diastolic function through their lusitropic effects, and improve cardiac index without increasing myocardial oxygen consumption.

Metra et al. further demonstrated that the hemodynamic response is influenced not only by the inotropic agent but also the β-blocker used. The favorable effects of dobutamine—dose-dependent increase in cardiac index, heart rate, and stroke volume index, and dose-dependent decrease in ventricular filling pressures—were diminished only slightly by metoprolol but were nearly extinguished by carvedilol (127). The contrasting effects of the β-blockers may be explained by the selectivity of the β-adrenoceptor antagonists as well as the responses to chronic β-blockade. A non–selective β-blocker, carvedilol also blocks β_2-adrenoceptors and does not up-regulate β_1-adrenergic receptor density (136). These two properties may inhibit the effects of dobutamine, which acts upon both β_1- and β_2-adrenoceptors to a greater degree than selective β_1-blockade by metoprolol. In contrast with dobutamine, the hemodynamic responses to enoximone were maintained or enhanced during concomitant β-blockade with either metoprolol or carvedilol (127). This finding is consistent with the mechanism of action of type III PDE inhibitors, which is distal to and independent of β-adrenergic receptors.

These studies favor the use of milrinone or enoximone over dobutamine to provide inotropic support in severely decompensated heart failure patients on chronic β-blockade, particularly carvedilol.

Consideration for Pacer Placement

β-blocker therapy, despite its proven mortality and morbidity benefits, remains under-prescribed in chronic heart failure. Fewer than a third of heart failure patients in recent large randomized clinical trials were on baseline β-blocker therapy (137,138). The ADHERE registry (Acute Decompensated Heart Failure National Registry) revealed that of 105,388 eligible heart failure patients admitted to community hospitals for heart failure exacerbations, fewer than a half were receiving β-blocker therapy prior to admission (139). Only about 70% of heart failure patients receiving care at specialized heart failure outpatient clinics were treated with chronic β-blocker therapy (140). Physician hesitancy in either initiating or up-titrating β-blocker therapy may be attributed to concerns over worsening heart failure, hypotension, and bradycardia, all of which could be potentially stabilized by cardiac resynchronization therapy (CRT). Aranda et al. addressed this question of implementing CRT for the purpose of initiating and optimizing b-blocker therapy (141). In this retrospective analysis, CRT was found to permit not only up-titration of β-blockers in heart failure patients but also reintroduction of β-blocker therapy in patients who had been previously intolerant of β-blockade.

Adverse Effects and Drug Interactions

β-blocker therapy can cause various adverse effects, such as fluid retention with worsening heart failure (112–114), fatigue, bradycardia, and hypotension. Patients therefore must be monitored for these adverse reactions when initiated and titrated on β-blockers.

Although the fluid retention associated with β-blockade is initially asymptomatic, it can ultimately worsen heart failure symptoms. Fluid retention is best reflected by increases in body weight. As such, physicians should closely monitor patients' weight and adjust concomitant diuretics accordingly. β-blocker-associated fatigue generally resolves spontaneously within several weeks, but the sense of malaise and weakness can be severe enough to limit β-blocker therapy. Fatigue can typically be managed by dose reductions of the β-blocker. However, if the fatigue is ever accompanied by peripheral hypoperfusion, β-blockade should be ceased and reinitiated at a later time. The bradycardia and hypotension associated with β-blockade are generally asymptomatic and require no treatment. However, if symptomatic bradycardia (i.e., light-headedness or dizziness) or second- or third-degree heart block occurs, the β-blocker dose should be reduced. If hypotension is accompanied by light-headedness, dizziness, or blurred vision, other anti-hypertensive medications (i.e., ACE-I) should be reduced in dose. Also, medication regimens should be re-assessed for possible drug interactions that may potentiate the effects of β-blockers on cardiac conduction or blood pressure, and, where appropriate, substitutions should be made. CRT has been shown to have a potential role in managing symptomatic bradycardia, hypotension, and heart block during β-blockade therapy (141), but the evidence for cardiac pacing with or without CRT in β-blockade optimization is limited.

FUTURE DIRECTIONS

Even with the morbidity and mortality benefits of β-blockers now firmly established, the challenge remains in improving their rate of utilization in the management of chronic heart failure. One area of investigation that may enhance the application of β-blockade therapy is that of β-adrenergic receptor polymorphisms and their associations with clinical progression of heart failure and responsiveness to β-blocker treatment (142–144). Whether the non–selective β-blocker carvedilol is indeed superior to the selective metoprolol or whether a patient tolerates β-blockade initiation and titration may well depend upon polymorphisms in the β-adrenergic receptor genes, as suggested by some studies (145–148). Large, prospective, multi-center trials, however, are needed to validate such theories before pharmacogenomic approaches can be incorporated into practice guidelines and used to individualize the treatment of patients with heart failure. Until then, it is the physician's prerogative to include any of the clinical trial-proven β-blockers in the standard therapy of chronic heart failure.

ACKNOWLEDGMENT

We thank Dr. Mariell Jessup for her critical review of this chapter.

REFERENCES

1. Chidsey CA, Braunwald E, Morrow AG, Mason DT. Myocardial norepinephrine concentration in man. Effects of reserpine and of congestive heart failure. N Engl J Med 1963; 269:653–658.
2. Thomas JA, Marks BH. Plasma norepinephrine in congestive heart failure. Am J Cardiol 1978; 41:233–243.
3. Cohn JN, Levine TB, Olivari MT, et al. Plasma norepinephrine as a guide to prognosis in patients with chronic congestive heart failure. N Engl J Med 1984; 311:819–823.
4. Waagstein F, Bristow MR, Swedberg K, et al. Beneficial effects of metoprolol in idiopathic dilated cardiomyopathy. Metoprolol in dilated cardiomyopathy (MDC) trial study group. Lancet 1993; 342:1441–1446.
5. The Cardiac Insufficiency Bisoprolol Study II (CIBIS-II): a randomised trial. Lancet 1999; 353:9–13.
6. Effect of metoprolol CR/XL in chronic heart failure: Metoprolol CR/XL Randomised Intervention Trial in Congestive Heart Failure (MERIT-HF). Lancet 1999; 353:2001–2007.
7. Hjalmarson A, Goldstein S, Fagerberg B, et al. Effects of controlled-release metoprolol on total mortality, hospitalizations, and well-being in patients with heart failure: the metoprolol CR/XL randomized intervention trial in congestive heart failure (MERIT-HF). MERIT-HF study Group. JAMA 2000; 283:1295–1302.

8. Packer M, Coats AJ, Fowler MB, et al. Effect of carvedilol on survival in severe chronic heart failure. N Engl J Med 2001; 344:1651–1658.
9. Packer M, Fowler MB, Roecker EB, et al. Effect of carvedilol on the morbidity of patients with severe chronic heart failure: results of the carvedilol prospective randomized cumulative survival (COPERNICUS) study. Circulation 2002; 106:2194–2199.
10. Krum H, Roecker EB, Mohacsi P, et al. Effects of initiating carvedilol in patients with severe chronic heart failure: results from the COPERNICUS Study. JAMA 2003; 289:712–718.
11. Poole-Wilson PA, Swedberg K, Cleland JG, et al. Comparison of carvedilol and metoprolol on clinical outcomes in patients with chronic heart failure in the carvedilol or metoprolol european trial (COMET): randomised controlled trial. Lancet 2003; 362:7–13.
12. A trial of the beta-blocker bucindolol in patients with advanced chronic heart failure. N Engl J Med 2001;344:1659–1667.
13. Katzung BF, ed. Basic and Clinical Pharmacology. New York: McGraw-Hill Medical, 2004.
14. Dorn GW, Brown JH. Gq signaling in cardiac adaptation and maladaptation. Trends Cardiovasc Med 1999; 9:26–34.
15. Bristow MR, Ginsburg R, Umans V, et al. Beta 1- and beta 2-adrenergic-receptor subpopulations in nonfailing and failing human ventricular myocardium: coupling of both receptor subtypes to muscle contraction and selective beta 1-receptor down-regulation in heart failure. Circ Res 1986; 59:297–309.
16. Brodde OE, Schuler S, Kretsch R, et al. Regional distribution of beta-adrenoceptors in the human heart: coexistence of functional beta 1- and beta 2-adrenoceptors in both atria and ventricles in severe congestive cardiomyopathy. J Cardiovasc Pharmacol 1986; 8:1235–1242.
17. Wittstein IS, Thiemann DR, Lima JA, et al. Neurohumoral features of myocardial stunning due to sudden emotional stress. N Engl J Med 2005; 352:539–548.
18. Kurisu S, Sato H, Kawagoe T, et al. Tako-tsubo-like left ventricular dysfunction with ST-segment elevation: a novel cardiac syndrome mimicking acute myocardial infarction. Am Heart J 2002; 143:448–455.
19. Kurisu S. Transient left ventricular hypocontraction induced by emotional stress with immobilization: an animal model of tako-tsubo cardiomyopathy in humans? Circ J 2002; 66:985–986.
20. Ueyama T, Kasamatsu K, Hano T, Yamamoto K, Tsuruo Y, Nishio I. Emotional stress induces transient left ventricular hypocontraction in the rat via activation of cardiac adrenoceptors: a possible animal model of 'tako–tsubo' cardiomyopathy. Circ J 2002; 66:712–713.
21. Tsuchihashi K, Ueshima K, Uchida T, et al. Transient left ventricular apical ballooning without coronary artery stenosis: a novel heart syndrome mimicking acute myocardial infarction. angina pectoris-myocardial infarction investigations in Japan. J Am Coll Cardiol 2001; 38:11–18.
22. Desmet WJ, Adriaenssens BF, Dens JA. Apical ballooning of the left ventricle: first series in white patients. Heart 2003; 89:1027–1031.
23. Wittstein IS, Thiemann DR, Lima JA, et al. Neurohumoral features of myocardial stunning due to sudden emotional stress. N Engl J Med 2005; 352:539–548.
24. Sadamatsu K, Tashiro H, Maehira N, Yamamoto K. Coronary microvascular abnormality in the reversible systolic dysfunction observed after noncardiac disease. Jpn Circ J 2000; 64:789–792.
25. Bybee KA, Prasad A, Barsness GW, et al. Clinical characteristics and thrombolysis in myocardial infarction frame counts in women with transient left ventricular apical ballooning syndrome. Am J Cardiol 2004; 94:343–346.
26. Kurisu S. Transient left ventricular hypocontraction induced by emotional stress with immobilization: an animal model of tako-tsubo cardiomyopathy in humans? Circ J 2002; 66:985–986.
27. Lacy CR, Contrada RJ, Robbins ML, et al. Coronary vasoconstriction induced by mental stress (simulated public speaking). Am J Cardiol 1995; 75:503–505.

28. Bolli R, Marban E. Molecular and cellular mechanisms of myocardial stunning. Physiol Rev 1999; 79:609–634.
29. Cebelin MS, Hirsch CS. Human stress cardiomyopathy. Myocardial lesions in victims of homicidal assaults without internal injuries. Hum Pathol 1980; 11(2):123–132.
30. Drislane FW, Samuels MA, Kozakewich H, Schoen FJ, Strunk RC. Myocardial contraction band lesions in patients with fatal asthma: possible neurocardiologic mechanisms. Am Rev Respir Dis 1987; 135:498–501.
31. Mann DL, Kent RL, Parsons B, Cooper G. Adrenergic effects on the biology of the adult mammalian cardiocyte. Circulation 1992; 85:790–804.
32. Neil-Dwyer G, Walter P, Cruickshank JM, Doshi B, O'Gorman P. Effect of propranolol and phentolamine on myocardial necrosis after subarachnoid haemorrhage. Br Med J 1978; 2:990–992.
33. Singal PK, Kapur N, Dhillon KS, Beamish RE, Dhalla NS. Role of free radicals in catecholamine-induced cardiomyopathy. Can J Physiol Pharmacol 1982; 60:1390–1397.
34. Wilkenfeld C, Cohen M, Lansman SL, et al. Heart transplantation for end-stage cardiomyopathy caused by an occult pheochromocytoma. J Heart Lung Transplant 1992; 60:363–366.
35. Hein L, Kobilka BK. Adrenergic receptor signal transduction and regulation. Neuropharmacology 1995; 34:357–366.
36. Dorn GW, Brown JH. Gq signaling in cardiac adaptation and maladaptation. Trends Cardiovasc Med 1999; 9:26–34.
37. Collins S, Bouvier M, Lohse MJ, Benovic JL, Caron MG, Lefkowitz RJ. Mechanisms involved in adrenergic receptor desensitization. Biochem Soc Trans 1990; 18:541–544.
38. Lohse MJ. Molecular mechanisms of membrane receptor desensitization. Biochim Biophys Acta 1993; 1179:171–188.
39. Pippig S, Andexinger S, Daniel K, et al. Overexpression of beta-arrestin and beta-adrenergic receptor kinase augment desensitization of beta 2-adrenergic receptors. J Biol Chem 1993; 268:3201–3208.
40. Ungerer M, Bohm M, Elce JS, Erdmann E, Lohse MJ. Altered expression of beta-adrenergic receptor kinase and beta 1-adrenergic receptors in the failing human heart. Circulation 1993; 87:454–463.
41. Muntz KH, Zhao M, Miller JC. Downregulation of myocardial beta-adrenergic receptors. Receptor subtype selectivity. Circ Res 1994; 74:369–375.
42. Bouvier M, Collins S, O'Dowd BF, et al. Two distinct pathways for cAMP-mediated downregulation of the beta 2-adrenergic receptor. Phosphorylation of the receptor and regulation of its mRNA level. J Biol Chem 1989; 264:16786–16792.
43. Fowler MB, Laser JA, Hopkins GL, Minobe W, Bristow MR. Assessment of the beta-adrenergic receptor pathway in the intact failing human heart: progressive receptor downregulation and subsensitivity to agonist response. Circulation 1986; 74:1290–1302.
44. Muntz KH, Zhao M, Miller JC. Downregulation of myocardial beta-adrenergic receptors. Receptor subtype selectivity. Circ Res 1994; 74:369–375.
45. Nozawa T, Igawa A, Yoshida N, et al. Dual-tracer assessment of coupling between cardiac sympathetic neuronal function and downregulation of beta-receptors during development of hypertensive heart failure of rats. Circulation 1998; 97:2359–2367.
46. Luttrell LM, Ferguson SS, Daaka Y, et al. Beta-arrestin-dependent formation of beta2 adrenergic receptor-Src protein kinase complexes. Science 1999; 283:655–661.
47. Iaccarino G, Tomhave ED, Lefkowitz RJ, Koch WJ. Reciprocal in vivo regulation of myocardial G protein-coupled receptor kinase expression by beta-adrenergic receptor stimulation and blockade. Circulation 1998; 98:1783–1789.
48. Lohse MJ, Benovic JL, Codina J, Caron MG, Lefkowitz RJ. beta-Arrestin: a protein that regulates beta-adrenergic receptor function. Science 1990; 248:1547–1550.
49. Pippig S, Andexinger S, Daniel K, et al. Overexpression of beta-arrestin and beta-adrenergic receptor kinase augment desensitization of beta 2-adrenergic receptors. J Biol Chem 1993; 268:3201–3208.

50. Altschuld RA, Starling RC, Hamlin RL, et al. Response of failing canine and human heart cells to beta 2-adrenergic stimulation. Circulation 1995; 92:1612–1618.
51. Bristow MR, Ginsburg R, Umans V, et al. Beta 1- and beta 2-adrenergic-receptor subpopulations in nonfailing and failing human ventricular myocardium: coupling of both receptor subtypes to muscle contraction and selective beta 1-receptor down-regulation in heart failure. Circ Res 1986; 59:297–309.
52. Brodde OE, Schuler S, Kretsch R, et al. Regional distribution of beta-adrenoceptors in the human heart: coexistence of functional beta 1- and beta 2-adrenoceptors in both atria and ventricles in severe congestive cardiomyopathy. J Cardiovasc Pharmacol 1986; 8:1235–1242.
53. Fowler MB, Laser JA, Hopkins GL, Minobe W, Bristow MR. Assessment of the beta-adrenergic receptor pathway in the intact failing human heart: progressive receptor down-regulation and subsensitivity to agonist response. Circulation 1986; 74:1290–1302.
54. Maurice JP, Shah AS, Kypson AP, et al. Molecular beta-adrenergic signaling abnormalities in failing rabbit hearts after infarction. Am J Physiol 1999; 276:H1853–H1860.
55. Muntz KH, Zhao M, Miller JC. Downregulation of myocardial beta-adrenergic receptors. Receptor subtype selectivity. Circ Res 1994; 74:369–375.
56. Ungerer M, Bohm M, Elce JS, Erdmann E, Lohse MJ. Altered expression of beta-adrenergic receptor kinase and beta 1-adrenergic receptors in the failing human heart. Circulation 1993; 87:454–463.
57. Maurice JP, Shah AS, Kypson AP, et al. Molecular beta-adrenergic signaling abnormalities in failing rabbit hearts after infarction. Am J Physiol 1999; 276:H1853–H1860.
58. Engelhardt S, Hein L, Wiesmann F, Lohse MJ. Progressive hypertrophy and heart failure in beta1-adrenergic receptor transgenic mice. Proc Natl Acad Sci USA 1999; 96:7059–7064.
59. Josue O. Hypertrophie cardiaque causee par l'adrenaline et la toxine typhique. C R Soc Biol (Paris) 1907; 63:285–286.
60. Mann DL, Kent RL, Parsons B, Cooper G. Adrenergic effects on the biology of the adult mammalian cardiocyte. Circulation 1992; 85:790–804.
61. Bing OHL. Hypothesis: apoptosis may be a mechanism for the transition to heart failure with chronic pressure overload. J Mol Cell Cardiol 1994; 26:943–948.
62. Gottlieb RA, Burleson KO, Kloner RA, Babior BM, Engler RL. Reperfusion injury induces apoptosis in rabbit cardiomyocytes. J Clin Invest 1994; 94:1621–1628.
63. Itoh G, Tamura J, Suzuki M. DNA framentation of human infarcted myocardial cells demonstrated by the nick end labeling method and DNA agarose gel electrophoresis. Am J Pathol 1995; 146:1325–1331.
64. Narula J, Haider N, Virmani R, et al. Apoptosis in myocytes in end-stage heart failure. N Engl J Med 1996; 335:1182–1189.
65. Reed JC, Paternostro G. Postmitochondrial regulation of apoptosis during heart failure. Proc Natl Acad Sci USA 1999; 96:7614–7616.
66. Tanaka M, Ito H, Adachi S. Hypoxia induces apoptosis with enhanced expression of Fas antigen messenger RNA in cultured neonatal rat cardiomyocytes. Circ Res 1994; 75:426–433.
67. Colucci WS, Sawyer DB, Singh K, Communal C. Adrenergic overload and apoptosis in heart failure: implications for therapy. J Card Fail 2000; 1:1–7.
68. Colucci WS. Apoptosis in the heart. N Engl J Med 1996; 335:1224–1226.
69. Communal C, Singh K, Pimentel DR, Colucci WS. Norepinephrine stimulates apoptosis in adult rat ventricular myocytes by activation of the beta-adrenergic pathway. Circulation 1998; 98:1329–1334.
70. Communal C, Singh K, Sawyer DB, Colucci WS. Opposing effects of beta(1)- and beta(2)-adrenergic receptors on cardiac myocyte apoptosis: role of a pertussis toxin-sensitive G protein. Circulation 1999; 100:2210–2212.
71. Port JD, Bristow MR. Altered beta-adrenergic receptor gene regulation and signaling in chronic heart failure. J Mol Cell Cardiol 2001; 33:887–905.
72. Singh K, Communal C, Sawyer DB, Colucci WS. Adrenergic regulation of myocardial apoptosis. Cardiovasc Res 2000; 45:713–719.

73. Singh K, Xiao L, Remondino A, Sawyer DB, Colucci WS. Adrenergic regulation of cardiac myocyte apoptosis. J Cell Physiol 2001; 189:257–265.
74. Rankin AC, Cobbe SM. Arrhythmias and sudden death in heart failure: can we prevent them?. In: McMurray JJV, Cleland JGF, eds. Heart Failure in Clinical Practice. London: Martin Dunitz Ltd, 1996:189–205.
75. Packer M. Pathophysiological mechanisms underlying the effects of beta-adrenergic agonists and antagonists on functional capacity and survival in chronic heart failure. Circulation 1990; 82:I77–I88.
76. Zipes DP. Sympathetic stimulation and arrhythmias. N Engl J Med 1991; 325:656–657.
77. Meredith IT, Broughton A, Jennings GL, Esler MD. Evidence of a selective increase in cardiac sympathetic activity in patients with sustained ventricular arrhythmias. N Engl J Med 1991; 325:618–624.
78. Raeder EA, Verrier RL, Lown B. Intrinsic sympathomimetic activity and the effects of beta-adrenergic blocking drugs on vulnerability to ventricular fibrillation. J Am Coll Cardiol 1983; 1:1442–1446.
79. Olsson G, Tuomilehto J, Berglund G, et al. Primary prevention of sudden cardiovascular death in hypertensive patients: mortality results from the MAPHY study. Am J Hypertens 1991; 4:151–158.
80. Olsson G, Wikstrand J, Warnold I, et al. Metoprolol-induced reduction in postinfarction mortality: pooled results from five double-blind randomized trials. Eur Heart J 1992; 13:28–32.
81. Cohn JN, Johnson GR, Shabetai R, et al. Ejection fraction, peak exercise oxygen consumption, cardiothoracic ratio, ventricular arrhythmias, and plasma norepinephrine as determinants of prognosis in heart failure. The V-HeFT VA cooperative studies group. Circulation 1993; 87:V15–V16.
82. Francis GS, Cohn JN, Johnson G, Rector TS, Goldman S, Simon A. Plasma norepinephrine, plasma renin activity, and congestive heart failure. Relations to survival and the effects of therapy in V-HeFT II. The V-HeFT VA cooperative studies group. Circulation 1993; 87:VI40–VI48.
83. Richards AM, Doughty R, Nicholls MG, et al. Neurohumoral prediction of benefit from carvedilol in ischemic left ventricular dysfunction. Australia–New Zealand heart failure group. Circulation 1999; 99:786–792.
84. Francis GS, Goldsmith SR, Cohn JN. Relationship of exercise capacity to resting left ventricular performance and basal plasma norepinephrine levels in patients with congestive heart failure. Am Heart J 1982; 104:725–731.
85. Waagstein F, Hjalmarson A, Varnauskas E, Wallentin I. Effect of chronic beta-adrenergic receptor blockade in congestive cardiomyopathy. Br Heart J 1975; 37:1022–1036.
86. Barone FC, Campbell WG, Jr, Nelson AH, Feuerstein GZ. Carvedilol prevents severe hypertensive cardiomyopathy and remodeling. J Hypertens 1998; 16:871–884.
87. Patten RD, Udelson JE, Konstam MA. Ventricular remodeling and its prevention in the treatment of heart failure. Curr Opin Cardiol 1998; 13:162–167.
88. Basu S, Senior R, Raval U, van der DR, Bruckner T, Lahiri A. Beneficial effects of intravenous and oral carvedilol treatment in acute myocardial infarction. A placebo-controlled, randomized trial. Circulation 1997; 96:183–191.
89. Feldman RL, Prida XE, Hill JA. Systemic and coronary hemodynamic effects of combined oral alpha- and beta-adrenergic blockade (labetalol) in normotensive patients with stable angina pectoris and positive exercise stress tests. Clin Cardiol 1988; 11:383–388.
90. Gilbert EM, Abraham WT, Olsen S, et al. Comparative hemodynamic, left ventricular functional, and antiadrenergic effects of chronic treatment with metoprolol versus carvedilol in the failing heart. Circulation 1996; 94:2817–2825.
91. Metra M, Nardi M, Giubbini R, Dei CL. Effects of short- and long-term carvedilol administration on rest and exercise hemodynamic variables, exercise capacity and clinical conditions in patients with idiopathic dilated cardiomyopathy. J Am Coll Cardiol 1994; 24:1678–1687.

92. Bellenger NG, Rajappan K, Rahman SL, et al. Effects of carvedilol on left ventricular remodelling in chronic stable heart failure: a cardiovascular magnetic resonance study. Heart 2004; 90:760–764.
93. Doughty RN, Whalley GA, Walsh HA, Gamble GD, Lopez-Sendon J, Sharpe N. Effects of carvedilol on left ventricular remodeling after acute myocardial infarction: the CAPRICORN echo substudy. Circulation 2004; 109:201–206.
94. Dubach P, Myers J, Bonetti P, et al. Effects of bisoprolol fumarate on left ventricular size, function, and exercise capacity in patients with heart failure: analysis with magnetic resonance myocardial tagging. Am Heart J 2002; 143:676–683.
95. Yaoita H, Sakabe A, Maehara K, Maruyama Y. Different effects of carvedilol, metoprolol, and propranolol on left ventricular remodeling after coronary stenosis or after permanent coronary occlusion in rats. Circulation 2002; 105:975–980.
96. Khattar RS, Senior R, Soman P, van der DR, Lahiri A. Regression of left ventricular remodeling in chronic heart failure: comparative and combined effects of captopril and carvedilol. Am Heart J 2001; 142:704–713.
97. Furberg CD, Hawkins CM, Lichstein E. Effect of propranolol in postinfarction patients with mechanical or electrical complications. Circulation 1984; 69:761–765.
98. Goldstein S. Clinical studies on beta blockers and heart failure preceding the MERIT-HF trial. Metoprolol CR/XL randomized intervention trial in heart Failure. Am J Cardiol 1997; 80:50J–53J.
99. Takusagawa M, Komori S, Matsumura K, et al. The inhibitory effects of carvedilol against arrhythmias induced by coronary reperfusion in anesthetized rats. J Cardiovasc Pharmacol Ther 2000; 5:105–112.
100. Australia–New Zealand Heart Failure Research Collaborative Group. Effects of carvedilol, a vasodilator-beta-blocker, in patients with congestive heart failure due to ischemic heart disease. Circulation 1995; 92:212–218.
101. Australia/New Zealand Heart Failure Research Collaborative Group. Randomised, placebo-controlled trial of carvedilol in patients with congestive heart failure due to ischaemic heart disease. Lancet 1997; 349:375–380.
102. Bristow MR, Gilbert EM, Abraham WT, et al. Carvedilol produces dose-related improvements in left ventricular function and survival in subjects with chronic heart failure. MOCHA investigators. Circulation 1996; 94:2807–2816.
103. Packer M, Colucci WS, Sackner-Bernstein JD, et al. Double-blind, placebo-controlled study of the effects of carvedilol in patients with moderate to severe heart failure. The PRECISE trial. Prospective randomized evaluation of carvedilol on symptoms and exercise. Circulation 1996; 94:2793–2799.
104. Colucci WS, Packer M, Bristow MR, et al. Carvedilol inhibits clinical progression in patients with mild symptoms of heart failure. US carvedilol heart failure study group. Circulation 1996; 94:2800–2806.
105. CIBIS Investigators and Committees. A randomized trial of beta-blockade in heart failure. The cardiac insufficiency bisoprolol study (CIBIS). Circulation 1994; 90:1765–1773.
106. Packer M, Bristow MR, Cohn JN, et al. The effect of carvedilol on morbidity and mortality in patients with chronic heart failure. U.S. carvedilol heart failure study group. N Engl J Med 1996; 334:1349–1355.
107. Fowler MB. Carvedilol prospective randomized cumulative survival (COPERNICUS) trial: carvedilol in severe heart failure. Am J Cardiol 2004; 93:35B–39B.
108. Foody JM, Farrell MH, Krumholz HM. beta-Blocker therapy in heart failure: scientific review. JAMA 2002; 287:883–889.
109. The Metoprolol in Dilated Cardiomyopathy (MDC) Trial Study Group. Three-year follow-up of patients randomised in the metoprolol in dilated cardiomyopathy trial. Lancet 1998; 351:1180–1181.
110. The Xamoterol in Severe Heart Failure Study Group. Xamoterol in severe heart failure. Lancet 1990; 336:1–6.

111. Hurh SA, Abraham W, Chin MH, et al. ACC/AHA, 2005 guideline update for the diagnosis and management of chronic heart failure in the adult: a report of the American College of cardiology/American Heart Association Task Force on Practice Guidelines (Writing Committee to Uptate the 2001 Guideline for the Evaluation and Management of Heart Failure). American College: Cardiology Web Site. Available at: http://www.acc.org/clinical/guidelines/failure/index.pdf.
112. Epstein SE, Braunwald E. The effect of beta adrenergic blockade on patterns of urinary sodium excretion. Studies in normal subjects and in patients with heart disease. Ann Intern Med 1966; 65:20–27.
113. Weil JV, Chidsey CA. Plasma volume expansion resulting from interference with adrenergic function in normal man. Circulation 1968; 37:54–61.
114. Gaffney TE, Braunwald E. Importance of the adrenergic nervous system in the support of circulatory function in patients with congestive heart failure. Am J Med 1963; 34:320–324.
115. Packer M, Poole-Wilson PA, Armstrong PW, et al. Comparative effects of low and high doses of the angiotensin-converting enzyme inhibitor, lisinopril, on morbidity and mortality in chronic heart failure. ATLAS study group. Circulation 1999; 100:2312–2318.
116. The NETWORK Investigators. Clinical outcome with enalapril in symptomatic chronic heart failure; a dose comparison. Eur Heart J 1998; 19:481–489.
117. Komajda M, Lutiger B, Madeira H, et al. Tolerability of carvedilol and ACE-inhibition in mild heart failure. Results of CARMEN (Carvedilol ACE-inhibitor remodelling mild CHF evaluatioN). Eur J Heart Fail 2004; 6:467–475.
118. Anthonio RL, van Veldhuisen DJ, Breekland A, Crijns HJ, van Gilst WH. Beta-blocker titration failure is independent of severity of heart failure. Am J Cardiol 2000; 85:509–512 see also A11.
119. Gottlieb SS, Fisher ML, Kjekshus J, et al. Tolerability of beta-blocker initiation and titration in the metoprolol CR/XL randomized intervention trial in congestive heart failure (MERIT-HF). Circulation 2002; 105:1182–1188.
120. Krum H. Tolerability of carvedilol in heart failure: clinical trials experience. Am J Cardiol 2004; 93:58B–63B.
121. Kumar A, Choudhary G, Antonio C, et al. Carvedilol titration in patients with congestive heart failure receiving inotropic therapy. Am Heart J 2001; 142:512–515.
122. Swedberg K, Hjalmarson A, Waagstein F, Wallentin I. Adverse effects of beta-blockade withdrawal in patients with congestive cardiomyopathy. Br Heart J 1980; 44:134–142.
123. Waagstein F, Caidahl K, Wallentin I, Bergh CH, Hjalmarson A. Long-term beta-blockade in dilated cardiomyopathy. Effects of short- and long-term metoprolol treatment followed by withdrawal and readministration of metoprolol. Circulation 1989; 80:551–563.
124. Gattis WA, O'Connor CM, Leimberger JD, Felker GM, Adams KF, Gheorghiade M. Clinical outcomes in patients on beta-blocker therapy admitted with worsening chronic heart failure. Am J Cardiol 2003; 91:169–174.
125. Bollano E, Tang MS, Hjalmarson A, Waagstein F, Andersson B. Different responses to dobutamine in the presence of carvedilol or metoprolol in patients with chronic heart failure. Heart 2003; 89:621–624.
126. Lowes BD, Tsvetkova T, Eichhorn EJ, Gilbert EM, Bristow MR. Milrinone versus dobutamine in heart failure subjects treated chronically with carvedilol. Int J Cardiol 2001; 81:141–149.
127. Metra M, Nodari S, D'Aloia A, et al. Beta-blocker therapy influences the hemodynamic response to inotropic agents in patients with heart failure: a randomized comparison of dobutamine and enoximone before and after chronic treatment with metoprolol or carvedilol. J Am Coll Cardiol 2002; 40:1248–1258.
128. Bohm M. Alterations of beta-adrenoceptor-G-protein-regulated adenylyl cyclase in heart failure. Mol Cell Biochem 1995; 147:147–160.
129. Bristow MR, Anderson FL, Port JD, et al. Differences in beta-adrenergic neuroeffector mechanisms in ischemic versus idiopathic dilated cardiomyopathy. Circulation 1991; 84:1024–1039.

130. Brodde OE. Beta 1- and beta 2-adrenoceptors in the human heart: properties, function, and alterations in chronic heart failure. Pharmacol Rev 1991; 43:203–242.
131. Bohm M, Gierschik P, Jakobs KH, et al. Increase of Gi alpha in human hearts with dilated but not ischemic cardiomyopathy. Circulation 1990; 82:1249–1265.
132. Bohm M, Gierschik P, Jakobs KH, et al. Increase of Gi alpha in human hearts with dilated but not ischemic cardiomyopathy. Circulation 1990; 82:1249–1265.
133. Feldman AM, Cates AE, Veazey WB, et al. Increase of the 40,000-mol wt pertussis toxin substrate (G protein) in the failing human heart. J Clin Invest 1988; 82:189–197.
134. Neumann J, Schmitz W, Scholz H, von Meyerinck L, Doring V, Kalmar P. Increase in myocardial Gi-proteins in heart failure. Lancet 1988; 2:936–937.
135. Bohm M, Deutsch HJ, Hartmann D, Rosee KL, Stablein A. Improvement of postreceptor events by metoprolol treatment in patients with chronic heart failure. J Am Coll Cardiol 1997; 30:992–996.
136. Bristow MR. Beta-adrenergic receptor blockade in chronic heart failure. Circulation 2000; 101:558–569.
137. Intravenous nesiritide versus nitroglycerin for treatment of decompensated congestive heart failure: a randomized controlled trial. JAMA 2002; 287:1531–1540.
138. Cuffe MS, Califf RM, Adams KF, Jr, et al. Short-term intravenous milrinone for acute exacerbation of chronic heart failure: a randomized controlled trial. JAMA 2002; 287:1541–1547.
139. Adams KF, Jr, Fonarow GC, Emerman CL, et al. Characteristics and outcomes of patients hospitalized for heart failure in the United States: rationale, design, and preliminary observations from the first 100,000 cases in the acute decompensated heart failure national registry (ADHERE). Am Heart J 2005; 149:209–216.
140. Gupta R, Tang WH, Young JB. Patterns of beta-blocker utilization in patients with chronic heart failure: experience from a specialized outpatient heart failure clinic. Am Heart J 2004; 147:79–83.
141. Aranda JM, Jr, Woo GW, Conti JB, Schofield RS, Conti CR, Hill JA. Use of cardiac resynchronization therapy to optimize beta-blocker therapy in patients with heart failure and prolonged QRS duration. Am J Cardiol 2005; 95:889–891.
142. Forleo C, Resta N, Sorrentino S, et al. Association of beta-adrenergic receptor polymorphisms and progression to heart failure in patients with idiopathic dilated cardiomyopathy. Am J Med 2004; 117:451–458.
143. Small KM, McGraw DW, Liggett SB. Pharmacology and physiology of human adrenergic receptor polymorphisms. Annu Rev Pharmacol Toxicol 2003; 43:381–411.
144. Liggett SB, Wagoner LE, Craft LL, et al. The Ile164 beta2-adrenergic receptor polymorphism adversely affects the outcome of congestive heart failure. J Clin Invest 1998; 102:1534–1539.
145. Johnson JA, Zineh I, Puckett BJ, McGorray SP, Yarandi HN, Pauly DF. Beta 1-adrenergic receptor polymorphisms and antihypertensive response to metoprolol. Clin Pharmacol Ther 2003; 74:44–52.
146. Kaye DM, Smirk B, Williams C, Jennings G, Esler M, Holst D. Beta-adrenoceptor genotype influences the response to carvedilol in patients with congestive heart failure. Pharmacogenetics 2003; 13:379–382.
147. Mialet PJ, Rathz DA, Petrashevskaya NN, et al. Beta 1-adrenergic receptor polymorphisms confer differential function and predisposition to heart failure. Nat Med 2003; 9:1300–1305.
148. Terra SG, Pauly DF, Lee CR, et al. beta-Adrenergic receptor polymorphisms and responses during titration of metoprolol controlled release/extended release in heart failure. Clin Pharmacol Ther 2005; 77:127–137.

8

Inotropic Therapy in Heart Failure Management

Lisa M. Mielniczuk
Division of Cardiology, Department of Medicine, Brigham and Women's Hospital, Boston, Massachusetts, U.S.A.

Anju Nohria
Advanced Heart Disease Section, Division of Cardiovascular Medicine, Department of Medicine, Brigham and Women's Hospital, Harvard Medical School, Boston, Massachusetts, U.S.A.

INTRODUCTION

Chronic heart failure (HF) affects nearly five million individuals and causes more than 200,000 deaths each year (1). Decompensated HF is a rapidly growing problem and accounts for nearly one million admissions annually in the United States. Despite optimal medical management, readmission rates remain as high as 30%–60% in the first six months after an admission for decompensated HF (2). The goals of HF management are to alleviate symptoms, improve quality of life, and prolong survival. Inotropic therapy remains one of the most controversial treatment modalities in HF. Despite this, inotropes are often employed in the acute management of decompensation as bridging strategies to definitive treatment, and for palliation of symptoms at the end of life (Fig. 1). This chapter reviews the currently available inotropic agents, their mechanisms of action, trial data regarding their use in patients with HF, and clinical scenarios where their use might be indicated.

THE CARDIAC CONTRACTILE APPARATUS

The sarcomere represents the basic contractile unit of the myocyte. The sarcomere is composed of thick and thin filaments that interact to cause sarcomere shortening and myocyte contraction. The thick filaments consist of myosin and the thin filaments are composed of the three proteins: actin, tropomyosin, and troponin. Each myosin molecule contains two heads that interact with actin, and are the sites of myosin ATPase, an enzyme that hydrolyzes ATP, which is required for myosin-actin cross-bridge formation. Each molecule of tropomyosin binds to about 6–7 molecules of actin and each tropomyosin molecule is in turn attached to the troponin complex. The troponin complex is made up of three subunits: troponin-T, which attaches to tropomyosin; troponin-C, which serves as

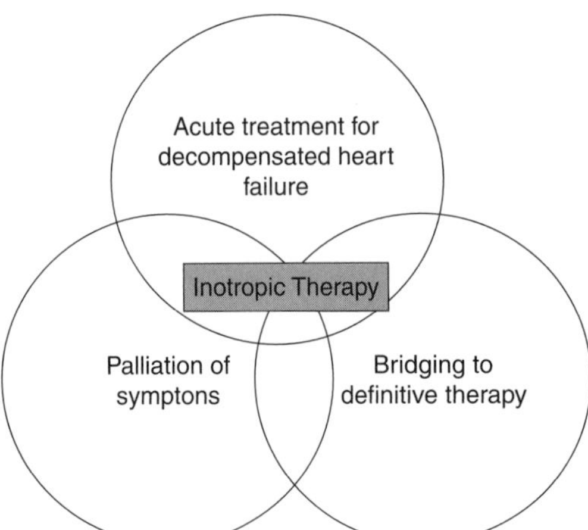

Figure 1 The role of inotropic therapy in advanced heart failure management. The management of advanced heart failure patients may involve the use of inotropic therapy in each of these patient realms. Although similarities exist, the goals of therapy can often be quite diverse.

a binding site for calcium (Ca^{++}) during excitation-contraction coupling; and troponin-I, which inhibits the myosin binding site on actin (Fig. 2).

When a myocyte is depolarized by an action potential, Ca^{++} enters the cell through L-type channels located on the sarcolemma. This in turn triggers the release of Ca^{++} from the sarcoplasmic reticulum (SR) through ryanodine receptors. This increases the intracellular Ca^{++} concentration and free Ca^{++} binds to troponin-C, inducing a conformational change in the troponin complex such that troponin-I exposes a site on the

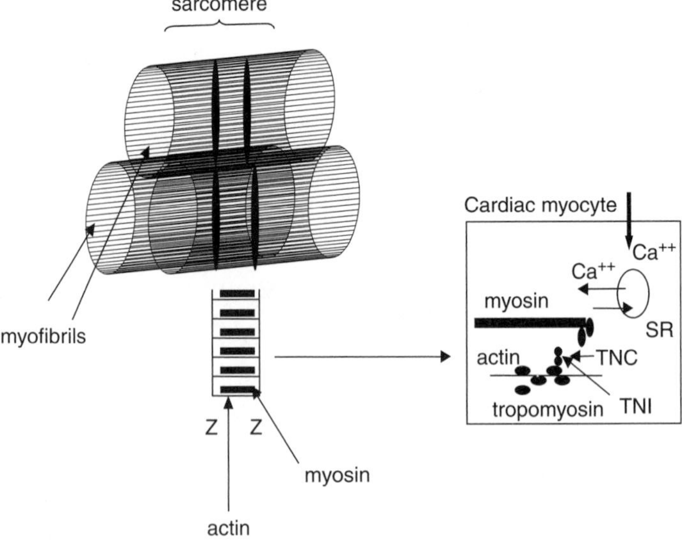

Figure 2 Myocyte contractile apparatus. The cardiac myocyte is composed of myofibrils, each of which contains a myofilament. The sarcomere lies between two Z-lines. The thick filament (myosin) contains two heads having ATPase activity. The thin filament is made up of actin, tropomyosin, and troponin (TN). TN-C brings calcium released by the sarcoplasmic reticulum (SR). TN-I inhibits actin-myosin binding until calcium binds to TN-C.

actin molecule that binds to the myosin head. Binding of actin and myosin results in ATP hydrolysis and ratcheting of the actin-myosin filaments to result in sarcomere shortening and myocyte contraction. At the end of phase 2 of the action potential, intracellular Ca^{++} concentrations are decreased by sequestration into the SR via an ATP-dependent Ca^{++} pump (SERCA) and by removal from the cell by the sodium- Ca^{++} exchange pump. This lowering of cytosolic Ca^{++} removes Ca^{++} from troponin-C and induces a conformational change that inhibits myosin-actin binding and restores sarcomere length (3).

MECHANISM OF ACTION OF INOTROPIC THERAPY

The traditional hemodynamic model suggests that HF is primarily a defect in cardiac contractility, and that drugs that increase cardiac contractility (positive inotropes) may have a positive effect. Mechanisms that increase the concentration of intracellular Ca^{++} increase the amount of ATP hydrolyzed and the force generated by actin-myosin interaction, as well as the velocity of shortening. Physiologically, cytosolic Ca^{++} concentrations are influenced primarily by beta-adrenergic stimulation that results in an increase in intracellular levels of cyclic adenosine monophosphate (cAMP). Increased cAMP activates protein kinase C that results in increased Ca^{++} entry into the cell through the L type Ca^{++} channels. Other mechanisms for increasing intracellular Ca^{++} concentrations include activation of the inositol 3 phosphate (IP_3) pathway, which increases Ca^{++} release from the SR, and inhibition of phospholamban phosphorylation, which leads to decreased Ca^{++} uptake by the SR. Another mechanism includes enhancement of the sensitivity or affinity of troponin-C for Ca^{++}. The various calcium regulatory pathways and potential therapeutic modalities are depicted in Figure 3.

Currently, there are three major classes of inotropic agents that are used clinically in patients with left ventricular dysfunction: (1) agents that increase intracellular levels of cAMP by direct stimulation of the beta-adrenergic receptor or by inhibiting phosphodiesterase; (2) drugs that inhibit the sodium-potassium ATPase pump, which thereby increasing intracellular sodium and thus cytosolic Ca^{++} levels; and (3) the new class of calcium sensitizing agents. The most commonly used intravenous agents are the beta-adrenergic receptor agonists (dopamine and dobutamine) and the phosphodiesterase inhibitor, milrinone (4).

Beta Adrenergic Agonists

Dopamine

The catecholamine, dopamine, is a sympathomimetic with both direct and indirect effects. It is formed in the body by the decarboxylation of levodopa, and is both a neurotransmitter in its own right (in the brain) and a precursor of epinephrine and norepinephrine. Dopamine stimulates α, β, and dopaminergic receptors and has both cardiac and vascular effects. It differs from epinephrine and norepinephrine in that it dilates renal and mesenteric blood vessels and increases urine output, apparently by a specific dopaminergic mechanism. This effect is predominant at low infusion rates ≤ 2 micrograms/kg per minute. At slightly higher infusion rates (2 to 10 micrograms/kg per minute), the β-receptor mediated increase in cAMP becomes more apparent, and at 10 to 20 micrograms/kg per minute, the α-mediated vasoconstrictive effects predominate. The major toxicities accompanying dopamine use include increased incidence of arrhythmias and complications related to excessive vasoconstriction, such as ischemia.

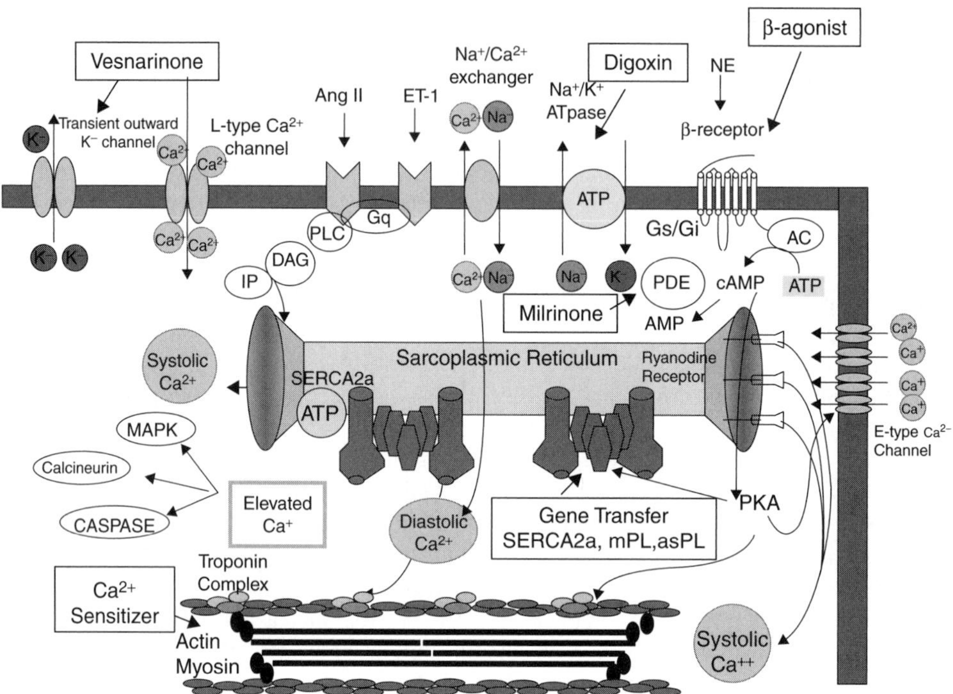

Figure 3 Effects of inotropic therapy on intracellular calcium handling in cardiac myocytes. Depolarization of membrane by action potential leads to opening of voltage-gated L-type calcium (Ca^{2+}) channels, which allows entry of small amount of Ca^{2+} into cell. Through coupling mechanism between L-type Ca^{2+} channel and sarcoplasmic reticulum (SR) release channels (ryanodine receptors), larger amount of Ca^{2+} is released, which activates myofilaments, leading to contraction. During relaxation, Ca^{2+} is accumulated back into SR by SR Ca^{2+} ATPase pump (SERCA2a) and extruded extracellularly by sarcolemmal Na^+/Ca^{2+} exchanger. Digoxin inhibits Na^+/K^+ ATPase pump, which increases intracellular Na^+. This results in increase in intracellular Ca^{2+} via Na^+/Ca^{2+} exchanger, which leads to enhanced Ca^{2+} loading of SR and increase in Ca^{2+} release. Phosphodiesterase inhibitors (PDEI) block breakdown of cAMP, which increases its intracellular level and activates PKA. Calcium sensitizers increase sensitivity of myofilaments to Ca^{2+}, enhancing myofilament activation for any concentration of Ca^{2+}. Vesnarinone prolongs action potential duration through modulation of K^+ channels, thereby prolonging opening of L-type calcium channels and increasing Ca^{2+} entry. Through gene transfer of SERCA2a (5), modified phospholamban (mPL) (6), or antisense phospholamban (asPL) (7), SRATPase activity can be increased, which enhances SR Ca^{2+} content, inotropic and lusitropic state. At level of cardiomyocyte, several stimuli, including endothelin-1 (ET-1), phenylephrine, and angiotensin, are involved in development of hypertrophy through Gq-coupled receptors. They induce activation of phospholipase C (PLC) and diacylglycerol (DAG), which increases levels of inositol triphosphate (IP3). IP3 induces release of calcium from SR. Increased cytosolic calcium induces mitogen-activated protein kinases (MAPKs) and activates calcineurin and caspases that contribute to apoptosis. *Abbreviations*: Ang II, angiotensin II; NE, norepinephrine; PDE, phosphodiesterase; PKA, protein kinase A; PKC, protein kinase C. *Source*: From Ref. 8.

The interest in "renal dose dopamine" has developed from the effect on dopaminergic receptors in animal models. Whether low dose ($\leq$2 micrograms/kg per minute) dopamine enhances renal function in patients with renal dysfunction in the setting of a normal circulation is controversial (9). In HF patients, the anecdotal natriuretic and diuretic effects seen with low dose dopamine are likely due to enhanced cardiac output and decreased systemic vascular resistance (SVR); however, there is no concrete data supporting its use to prevent renal dysfunction in this patient population. Fenoldopam, a benzazapine derivative, is a selective dopamine 1 receptor antagonist that acts as a vasodilator in the peripheral arteries and as a diuretic in the kidneys. Although, fenoldopam has been shown to improve hemodynamics and renal blood flow in HF patients, there are no trials addressing renal outcomes with this agent in HF patients (10).

Dobutamine

Dobutamine is one of the most commonly used inotropes in HF management. Dobutamine is a synthetic catecholamine that stimulates β1-receptors in the heart with positive inotropic and chronotropic effects. There is a modest decrease in left ventricular filling pressures and SVR due to a combination of direct vascular effects (activation of β2-receptors) and withdrawal of sympathetic tone (11). Unlike dopamine, dobutamine does not affect dopaminergic receptors and has little effect on α-receptors. Heart rate, atrial, and ventricular arrhythmias, and symptoms of ischemia are all increased with the use of dobutamine. Therefore, when dobutamine therapy is considered, it should be used at the lowest effective dose. Diuresis and renal function may improve at doses of 1–2 micrograms/kg per minute, however, more severe hypoperfusion may require higher doses. There is likely little additional benefit in doses above 10–15 micrograms/kg per minute and other agents should be considered. Dobutamine use for extended periods has been associated with a hypersensitivity reaction resulting in peripheral eosinophilia and occasional eosinophilic myocarditis. Therefore, patients on chronic dobutamine infusions should be monitored for this complication at regular intervals.

Phosphodiesterase Inhibitors

Milrinone

Milrinone belongs to a class of inotropes that selectively inhibit phosphodiesterase (PDE) III, the enzyme that catalyzes the breakdown of cAMP. In the myocardium, milrinone can exert both positive inotropic and lusitropic effects, and in the systemic and pulmonary vasculature, milrinone is a potent vasodilator. Cardiac output is increased due to an increase in stroke volume, and arterial and venous vasodilation result in a decrease of cardiac filling pressures, pulmonary pressures, and often mean arterial pressure. The degree to which cardiac output increases and SVR decreases can vary, and excessive vasodilation can lead to hypotension. This is rarely seen with dobutamine or dopamine. Milrinone is associated with less elevation in heart rate than dopamine or dobutamine (12); however, atrial and ventricular arrhythmias can still occur. Another unique feature of this drug is the prolonged half-life. The pharmacological half-life of dopamine and dobutamine can be measured in minutes, while the elimination half-life of milrinone is 2.5 hr. The physiologic effects of milrinone can last up to 6 hr and may be even more prolonged in patients with renal dysfunction. Thus the dose of milrinone has to be appropriately adjusted in patients with renal dysfunction. (See Table 1 for the hemodynamic and pharmacologic differences between commonly used inotropes.) Milrinone may be a more attractive choice in patients who are on chronic beta antagonist therapy as it works via a beta-adrenergic independent mechanism.

Table 1 Hemodynamic Effect of Positive Inotropic Agents

	Dobutamine	Dopamine (low dose)	Dopamine (high dose)	Milrinone
CO	↑	↑↔	↑↔↓	↑
PCWP	↓	↔	↑	↓↓
SVR	↓	↓	↑↑	↓↓
HR	↑	↔↑	↑	↔
T ½ (min)	2.4	2	2	150
Arrhythmia risk	↑↑	↑	↑↑	↑

Abbreviations: CO, cardiac output; PCWP, pulmonary capillary wedge pressure; SVR, systemic vascular resistance.
Source: Adapted from Ref. 13.

Inhibitors of the Sodium–Potassium ATPase Pump

Digoxin

Digoxin is the only oral inotrope approved for use in the management of chronic HF. The myocardial cellular effect of digoxin results from inhibition of the sodium–potassium ATPase pump. As the sodium–potassium ATPase pump is inhibited, there is a transient increase in intracellular sodium close to the sarcolemma, which in turn promotes calcium influx by the sodium–calcium exchange mechanism. The acute hemodynamic effects of digoxin include increase in cardiac output and a fall in venous pressure. The action of digoxin on slowing atrioventricular (AV) conduction and prolonging the refractory period, is primarily dependent on increased vagal tone and only to a minor extent on the direct effect of digoxin (13). Although early clinical studies suggested increased risk by the acute withdrawal of digoxin in HF patients (14,15), a prospective trial of digoxin use in 6800 patients failed to show a mortality benefit for digoxin in HF (16). However, there was a trend towards decreased risk of death due to worsening HF with digoxin (risk ratio, 0.88; 95% confidence interval, 0.77 to 1.01; $p=0.06$) and fewer patients were hospitalized for worsening HF (26.8% vs. 34.7%; $p<0.001$). A posthoc analysis of the DIG trial suggested that serum digoxin levels >0.8 ng/mL were associated with increased mortality (17). Furthermore, digoxin use was associated with a significantly higher risk of death among women (adjusted hazard ratio for the comparison with placebo, 1.23; 95% confidence interval, 1.02 to 1.47), but it had no significant effect among men (adjusted hazard ratio, 0.93; 95% confidence interval, 0.85 to 1.02; $P=0.014$ for the interaction). This may be attributed to the increased toxicity seen with higher serum digoxin levels in patients with lower body mass (18). Digoxin use requires frequent monitoring of potassium levels, especially in patients with renal dysfunction, and the concomitant doses of other medications (such as amiodarone and coumadin) may need to be adjusted in patients taking digoxin.

Calcium Sensitizers

Levosimendan

This class of inotropic agents represents a novel therapeutic approach. The most studied is levosimendan, which is not yet approved for use in the United States. Levosimendan enhances myocardial contractility by binding to the amino terminal of cardiac troponin C and increasing the calcium sensitivity of the cardiac contractile proteins in a calcium dependent manner. It does not alter intracellular free calcium or cyclic AMP levels. It also leads to vasodilation by the opening of ATP sensitive potassium channels. Clinically it has been associated with increased cardiac output, and reduction in both pulmonary capillary wedge pressure and SVR (19). Because these drugs delay the dissociation of calcium from the contractile apparatus, there was concern that calcium sensitizers may adversely affect diastolic function. This has not been demonstrated in animal studies. It is believed that the binding to troponin C is less avid when cytosolic calcium levels decrease during diastole (20). Levosimendan has two active metabolites, OR 1855 and OR 1896. While the drug itself has a half-life of approximately 1 hr, the serum metabolite levels peak 48 hr after drug discontinuation and have a half-life of 70–80 hr.

MECHANISMS OF HARM

Despite their beneficial effects on hemodynamics, inotropic therapy is acutely associated with increased morbidity and may increase mortality through a number of mechanisms. Acutely inotropic agents may exacerbate underlying ischemia or ventricular arrhythmias (4). The increase in cardiac contractility may come at the expense of increased myocardial oxygen demand, especially when high doses of agents are used. The stimulation of contractility in hibernating myocardium without restoration of blood flow may increase short-term myocardial contractility at the expense of accelerating apoptosis and further degeneration of myocardial function (21,22). As mentioned above, drug specific adverse effects include increased filling pressures and digital ischemia with high doses of dopamine, the development of eosinophilic myocarditis with chronic dobutamine use, and hypotension with milrinone.

Clinical trials of inotropic therapy have demonstrated increased morbidity and mortality (23). Despite the increased risk, there are certain clinical scenarios where the benefits may outweigh the risks associated with inotrope use. The decision to use inotropic therapy in a patient with advanced HF must be made with a clear understanding of the specific treatment goals and knowledge of the inherent risks. In most cases, the lowest effective dose for the shortest duration is the preferable strategy when inotropic therapy is deemed necessary.

INOTROPE THERAPY IN ACUTE DECOMPENSATED HF

Acute decompensation of chronic HF is one of the most common reasons for admission to hospital. In the United States, almost 75% of all costs related to HF are those that are related to admission and inpatient care (24). Patients with acute decompensation should be evaluated for the presence of congestion and adequacy of perfusion. Those patients, who have evidence of high filling pressures with sub-optimal perfusion, the "wet and cold" profile, are at the highest risk for mortality (25). Current consensus is that such patients may require vasoactive therapy in addition to diuretics to restore compensation (26). Among these patients, those who have a marginal or low SVR may benefit from short-term inotropic therapy to improve symptoms and end-organ perfusion.

The usefulness and safety of routine intravenous inotropic therapy for the treatment of acute decompensated HF was evaluated in the Outcomes of a Prospective Trial of Intravenous Milrinone for Exacerbations of Chronic Heart Failure (OPTIME CHF) study (12). Patients admitted with decompensated systolic HF and not felt to require inotropic therapy were randomized to receive either 48 to 72 hr of milrinone or placebo in addition to standard therapy. There was no difference in the end-points of days hospitalized for cardiovascular causes ($p=0.71$) or mortality ($p=0.41$) within 60 days of randomization between the two groups. Treatment failure was more common in the milrinone group and this was largely attributed to increased incidence of sustained hypotension (10% vs. 3% in the placebo arm, $p<0.001$), more atrial arrhythmias (4.6% vs. 1.5%, $p=0.004$), and a trend towards more ventricular arrhythmias. The results of this trial suggest that the routine administration of milrinone is not warranted in all patients admitted with decompensated HF. However, this trial did not address outcomes with inotrope use in the group of patients who have evidence of severe hypoperfusion manifested by cardiogenic shock or persistent hypotension with end-organ dysfunction. These patients may clearly need a short course of inotropes to establish hemodynamic stability. The Levosimendan compared with Dobutamine in severe Low-Output HF (LIDO) study randomized patients who were admitted to the hospital and felt to require inotropes to either 24 hr of intravenous levosimendan or dobutamine. All patients were required to have an ejection fraction <35% and a cardiac index <2.5 L/min with a PCWP >15 mmHg. The investigators demonstrated that the primary endpoint of hemodynamic response at 24 hr (greater than 30% increase in cardiac output and 25% decrease in PCWP) was greater in the levosimendan group (28% vs. 15%, $p=0.022$), without any difference in the symptoms of HF. Furthermore, there was a trend towards reduced mortality in the levosimendan group compared to the placebo group at 1 mo ($p=0.049$). Dobutamine use was associated with more arrhythmias (mostly atrial) and ischemic symptoms while patients in the levosimendan group were more likely to experience headaches or hypotension (27). These data suggest that levosimendan may prove more efficacious and safe than dobutamine in patients admitted with severe low-output failure. A randomized trial comparing the efficacy of short-term levosimendan to placebo in patients with decompensated HF has been completed but the results have not yet been published.

Inotropes vs. Vasodilators in Acute Decompensated HF

Patients with advanced decompensated HF can have low cardiac output with markedly elevated SVR in addition to high intracardiac filling pressures. When vasoconstriction is present, hemodynamics may be improved by either intravenous vasodilators or inotropic infusions (28). The advantages of intravenous vasodilation need to be balanced against the risk of hypotension, a complication that is more prevalent in patients whose SVR is not markedly elevated prior to therapy.

In general, there are few data to guide the choice of vasodilators versus inotropes in the population in whom additional therapy is needed. Low and high dose intravenous nesiritide has been compared to dobutamine infusions in patients admitted with advanced decompensated HF (29). While both nesiritide and dobutamine were equally effective at improving signs and symptoms of HF, dobutamine use was associated with an increased incidence of premature ventricular beats and ventricular tachycardia compared to nesiritide. A retrospective analysis of an open-label study evaluating the efficacy of nesiritide in patients with decompensated HF, compared the outcomes in patients receiving nesiritide to those treated with dobutamine. In this study nesiritide use was associated with a decreased rate of re-admission and reduced 6-mo mortality compared to dobutamine (30). Analysis of the Evaluation Study of Congestive Heart Failure and Plumonary Catheterization Effectiveness (ESCAPE) trial, which evaluated the use of pulmonary artery catheters on outcomes of death and rehospitalization at 6 mo also suggested that inotrope use increased the risk of death and rehospitalization while vasodilators did not (31). Similar results have been found in the Acute Decompensated Heart Failure National Registry (ADHERE®) Acute Decompensated Heart Failure National Registry (32).

The routine addition of intravenous inotropic therapy to all patients with acute decompensated HF is not warranted and could increase morbidity and mortality. Patients who have evidence of low cardiac output complicated by end organ dysfunction and hypotension may benefit from short courses of intravenous inotropic therapy. The choice of inotrope, and the decision between inotrope and vasodilator, will depend on the individual patient hemodynamic profile. In general, the lowest effective inotropic dose should be used, and the duration of therapy should be minimized as much as possible, with early transition to appropriate oral therapy.

INOTROPE USE IN CHRONIC HF

As HF progresses, there are patients in whom it becomes very difficult to wean intravenous inotropic therapy without further compromise. These patients are felt to be "inotrope dependent," and although many of these patients can still be successfully weaned onto oral vasodilator therapy in centers with dedicated HF programs, there remain a few patients who would not survive hospital discharge without ongoing inotropic support (33). Inotrope dependence is often manifested as sustained symptomatic hypotension, recurrent congestive symptoms, or worsening renal function without inotropic therapy. It is felt that dependence should be defined by functional limitation and not measured by hemodynamic parameters (8). In addition multiple attempts should be made to wean inotropes, often with hemodynamic monitoring, which may lead to better adjustment of vasodilator therapy. This may take a significant time period; one study reported the mean inpatient stay of 21 days prior to defining inotrope dependence (34). Patients who are felt to be inotrope-dependent have the worst prognosis. The continued use of inotropes can be viewed as a bridge to a transplant or left ventricular assist device (LVAD) placement in eligible patients, or as a palliative method of controlling symptoms in end of life care.

Risk and Mortality of Chronic Inotrope Use

Without cardiac transplantation, survival is clearly limited in patients who are inotrope-dependent. In one study, the mortality of 36 inotrope-dependent patients was 94% at one year (34). Based on collected experiences, the anticipated mortality rate at six months is more than 50% and few survivors will remain at 2 years (8). Long term inotrope use often requires an indwelling line increasing the risk of line related infection and sepsis. Other complications associated with this therapy include arrhythmias and sudden cardiac death, the development of tolerance and persistent decline in organ function and nutritional status.

Bridging to Transplant

In patients who are waiting for cardiac transplantation, inotropic therapy may provide the bridge needed before an organ becomes available. There are little data to guide the clinician about the choice and safety of this strategy. One randomized trial of 36 hospitalized patients awaiting transplant suggested that both milrinone and dobutamine produced a similar hemodynamic and risk profile, with much less expense incurred with dobutamine (35). Whether these patients can be safely discharged home to await transplant is also not known, however, concomitant implantable cardioverter defibrillator therapy would be warranted at a minimum. The best way to bridge these patients to a transplant is not known; no study has compared LVAD placement to inotropic infusions. The

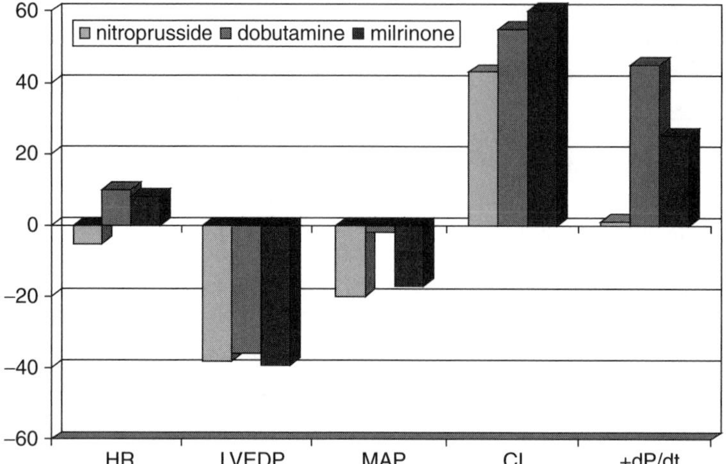

Figure 4 Relative hemodynamic effects of nitroprusside, dobutamine and milrinone. Data shown as percentage change from baseline. *Abbreviations*: HR, heart rate; LVEDP, left ventricular end diastolic pressure; MAP, mean arterial pressure; CI, cardiac index; +dP/dt, maximum development of pressure over time. *Source*: Modified from Ref. 28.

choice of bridging therapy will likely depend on the patient's risk of LVAD surgery, infection, and arrhythmia, as well as on the experience with LVAD management in the referring center (Fig. 4).

Inotropes as Destination Therapy

Many patients who are inotrope dependent are not candidates for cardiac transplantation. In these patients, chronic inotropic therapy is occasionally considered as a method of controlling refractory decompensated symptoms. In a recent analysis from the Randomized Evaluation of Mechanical Assistance for the Treatment of Congestive

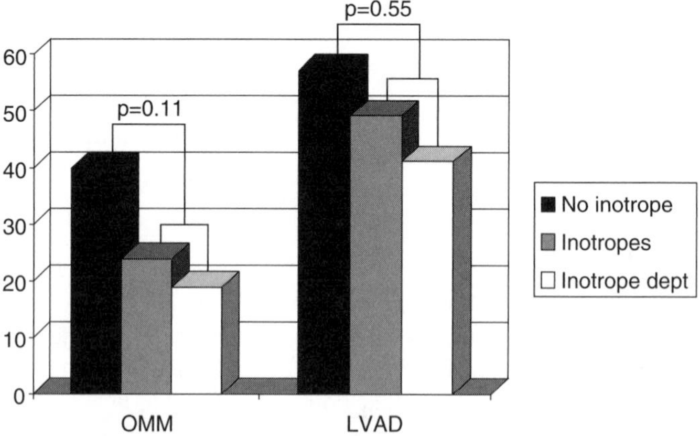

Figure 5 One-year survival (%) according to inotrope use in REMATCH patients. Numbers on Y axis represent percentage of survival at one year. The p values represent the difference between the three groups in each category. *Abbreviations*: OMM, optimal medical therapy; LVAD, left ventricular assist device. *Source*: Adapted from Ref. 36.

Heart Failure (REMATCH) trial, patients who were felt to be inotrope dependent tended to have a worse mortality than patients who were not on inotropes at the start of the trial. However, inotrope-dependent patients who were randomized to a LVAD had a greater one-year survival than patients who maintained optimal medical therapy (including inotropes) (Fig. 5) (8). Although destination LVAD is an option in very select patients, many patients who are inotrope dependent without options for cardiac transplant, also have comorbidites that would preclude a destination LVAD strategy. The use of continuous outpatient inotropic infusions at the end of life is increasing. In a recent survey of 71 US HF programs, more than 95% of responding physicians indicated willingness to use outpatient inotropic infusions; although 80% had seen worsening HF, 69% had seen infectious complications, and 50% had seen sudden death during such infusions (8). In these patients, palliation of symptoms, rather than prolongation of life, is the goal of therapy. When this strategy was evaluated in a small number of inotrope dependent patients, 64% of the 36 patients followed had one or less re-admission to hospital after discharge on home inotropic infusion. The six-month survival in these patients was only 26% with a one-year survival of 6%. The authors identified that continuous inotropic infusion allowed the majority of these advanced HF patients to be discharged home with only one or less re-admission at the end of life. This may be an important goal of therapy for some patients (34).

Methods of Chronic Inotropic Support

When chronic inotropic therapy is considered, multiple strategies have been considered, including oral therapy as well as either intermittent or continuous intravenous infusions. Unfortunately, the success has been extremely limited, with consistent increased risk of morbidity and mortality associated with chronic inotrope use.

Chronic Intravenous Inotropic Support

Continuous intravenous infusions of inotropes are an option in patients with refractory advanced HF. When evaluated in a clinical trial, they have been found to be an independent predictor of mortality (37). The limited data available also does not support the use of intermittent intravenous infusions. There are no large scale, double-blind, placebo-controlled trials to evaluate the use of intermittent intravenous inotropic therapy. Small studies have produced variable results, ranging from mild improvements in hemodynamics (38) and non-significant trends toward less hospitalization at the cost of increased mortality (23,39). Given the lack of convincing evidence of benefit, and the demonstration of increased mortality, neither intermittent nor continuous intravenous inotropic infusions can be recommended as a routine management strategy in advanced HF. In patients with end-stage disease and refractory symptoms, this therapy may have a role in the palliation of symptoms. But the goal of symptom control and comfort at the potential cost of increased mortality needs to be understood by both patient and physician. Patients with NYHA class IV HF have described a willingness to accept therapies that carry increased risk if symptoms might be improved (40).

Chronic Oral Inotropic Support

Ideally, chronic oral inotropic therapy would eliminate the line-related complications associated with chronic intravenous infusions. Thus, if proven safe and effective, oral inotropic therapy could be a preferred strategy in these patients. Unfortunately, the results of many long-term trials of oral inotropic therapy have been disappointing (Table 2).

Table 2 Mortality in Randomized Controlled Trials of Oral Inotropic Therapy

Trial	Inotrope	Number	Mortality
PROMISE (41)	Milrinone	1088	28% increase in risk of death (p=0.04)
VEST (42)	Vesnarinone	3833	11% increase in risk of death[a] (p=0.02)
PRIME II (43)	Ibopamine	1906	Hazard ratio for death 1.26 (p=0.02)
PICO (44)	Pimodendan	317	Hazard ratio for death 1.8 (p>0.05)
EMOTE (50)	Enoximone	202	Hazard ratio 1.2 (p=0.32)

[a]Mortality increase refers to the 60 mg dose compared to placebo.

Small studies have suggested a short-term benefit on hemodynamics; however, larger, sufficiently powered studies have demonstrated increased mortality.

Vesnarinone is an oral inotropic agent that decreases the delayed outward and inward rectifying potassium currents; increases intracellular sodium by the prolonged opening of sodium channels; and increases the inward calcium current via mild inhibition of PDE (45). During an initial dose finding study, the low dose of vesnarinone (60 mg) was associated with a 62% decrease in the relative risk of death in comparison to placebo (46). However, the larger Vesnarinone trial (VEST) did not substantiate the positive results of early clinical studies and demonstrated an increased mortality at both the 30 mg and 60 mg doses when compared to placebo. This increased mortality was largely attributed to arrhythmic death (42).

Selective PDE inhibitors, such as milrinone, are available in oral formulations and have demonstrated benefits on hemodynamics and exercise tolerance in small studies (47). The Prospective Randomized Milrinone Survival Evaluation (PROMISE) study was designed to evaluate the potential impact of oral milrinone on mortality in 1088 patients with advanced HF. The trial was stopped prematurely after a significant 28% increase in all-cause mortality in patients receiving oral milrinone was found (41). Another oral PDE inhibitor, enoximone, has been shown to increase mortality compared to placebo when used in high doses (4–6 mg/kg per day) in patients with moderate to moderately severe HF (48). However, lower doses ($\leq$3 mg/kg per day) have been shown to improve short-term symptoms and exercise capacity without an increase in adverse events (49). Large-scale trials evaluating the long-term outcomes of low dose enoximone in patients with functional NYHA class III to IV HF are currently underway (ESSENTIAL I and II). The recently completed Enoximone in Intravenous Inotrope-Dependent Subjects Study (EMOTE) evaluated the utility of oral enoximone as a means to wean patients off intravenous inotropic therapy. The primary outcome was the number of days patients were alive and free of intravenous inotropic therapy in the first 30 days following the initial wean of intravenous inotropic support. There were 202 patients randomized to either placebo or enoximone (25–50 mg tid) therapy. Although there was no statistical difference in the primary endpoint at 30 days, there was a trend for more patients to be intravenous inotrope–free in the enoximone group throughout the 180 days of follow-up, with a significant difference at 90 days. In patients who did require reintroduction of intravenous support, the mean time to intravenous therapy (32% risk reduction, p=0.04), and the mean number of rehospitalization days (43% risk reduction, p=0.49) was less in the enoximone group. Importantly there was no increase in arrhythmic events or significant increase in mortality over 26 weeks (50). This is the first oral inotropic therapy to be tested in a randomized trial that suggests some clinical benefit without significantly increased risk. Future confirmatory studies are needed before this therapy can be advocated in the advanced HF population.

FUTURE DIRECTIONS OF INOTROPIC THERAPY

With advancements in medical and device therapy, more patients with chronic HF are surviving much longer than previously experienced. It is estimated that more than 100,000 patients with poor systolic function and ventricular dilatation have advanced HF, or symptoms at rest or with minimal exertion, despite optimized medical therapy (51). Despite the history of disappointing results with inotropic therapy, the challenge still exists to develop a successful inotropic strategy. This may involve combined therapeutic interventions with preexisting agents or the development of novel inotropic drugs.

Adjusting Current Therapeutic Strategies

As with the small Phase II trials of enoximone, it is possible that currently available inotropic therapies would be less toxic if used in lower doses (49,52). Whether lower doses would have the same hemodynamic benefits with reduced risk is not known.

The safety and efficacy of inotropic therapy, specifically PDE inhibitors may be enhanced by concurrent treatment with beta-blockade. The underlying premise is that beta-blockers could attenuate the potential arrhythmic risks with PDE inhibitors while still providing a mechanism for the physiologic inotropic effects to occur. Preliminary data has suggested that the beneficial effects of milrinone are enhanced in the presence of beta-blocker therapy (53). Larger studies (Milrinone in the PROBE trial and Enoximone in the EMPOWER trial) evaluating the combined strategy of PDE inhibition with beta-blockers are currently in progress.

Novel Pharmacological Agents

The currently available intravenous inotropes stimulate cAMP and increase intracellular Ca^{++} either through β-adrenergic receptor stimulation or PDE inhibition. It is believed that the increased cytosolic Ca^{++}contributes to the risk of arrhythmias seen. Ca^{++}-sensitizing agents act by increasing the sensitivity of the myofilaments to Ca^{++} without increasing the absolute amount of cytosolic Ca^{++}. Levosimendan, an intravenous PDE inhibitor with Ca^{++}-sensitizing properties, continues to show promise in improving hemodynamics and symptoms, with less risk than traditional inotropic therapy (27). Larger randomized trials sufficiently powered to detect mortality need to be completed before this agent can be advocated as an alternative to our current therapies. Other agents with novel mechanisms of action are also being developed. This includes drugs that modulate sodium channels or the $Na+/K+$adenosine triphosphate pump (54). Biologic-based therapies to increase myocardial efficiency are also being developed. Xanthine oxidase inhibition has been shown to reduce myocardial oxygen consumption without a decrease in contractility (55). Other potential biologic therapies to improve myocardial efficiency include thyroid and growth hormone analogs and agents to improve myocardial metabolism, such as glucagon-like peptide 1 and ranolazine, a partial fatty acid oxidase inhibitor.

Targeted Gene Expression

Another method to improve Ca^{++} handling in the cell is through the development of gene transfer techniques. These techniques have been utilized to demonstrate improved contractility and survival after viral transfection of the SR calcium ATPase (SERCA-2) into small animals and pigs (5). Similar findings have been obtained with an adenovirus that encodes antisense RNA of phosphlamban (6). Future investigation will help to define the role of these novel approaches in improving contractile performance of the heart in humans.

CONCLUSIONS AND RECOMMENDATIONS

The number of patients with advanced cardiac disease continues to increase. Because cardiac transplantation is performed in less than 2400 patients annually in the United States, many of the 100,000 HF patients with symptoms at rest or with minimal exertion will not have this therapeutic option (36). This imbalance between organ supply and demand continues to increase, and alternative therapeutic strategies are required to minimize the morbidity of patients with advanced cardiac disease.

The medical management of HF patients continues to evolve. There has been a gradual shift towards medical therapy and neurohormonal strategies that were initially contraindicated in chronic HF (beta-blockers), and away from agents that act purely as positive inotropic support. However, the increasing numbers of patients with advanced HF challenges us to develop alternative inotropic strategies that have the same hemodynamic and symptomatic benefits without the risks of increased morbidity and mortality. It is

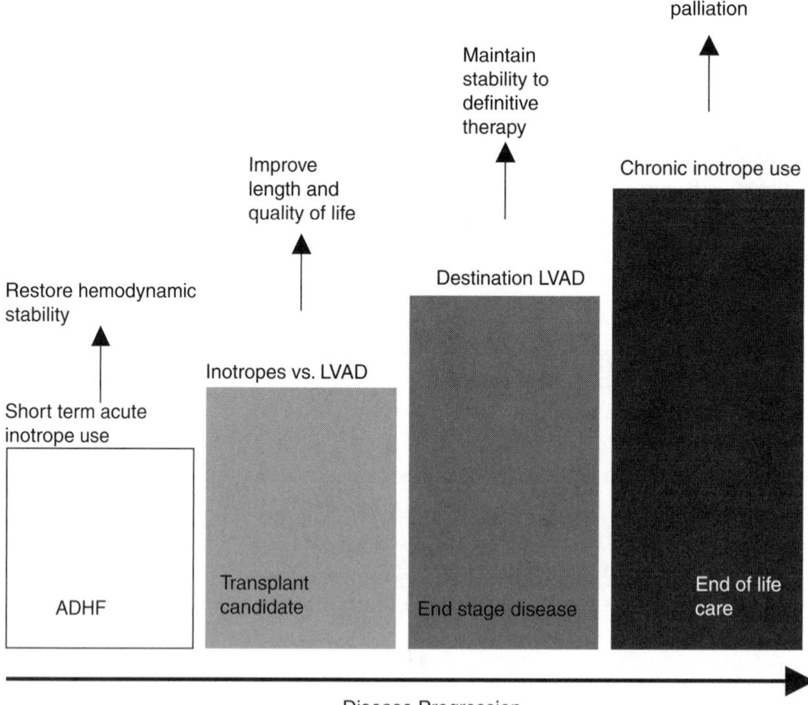

Figure 6 The therapeutic options and treatment goals involving inotropic therapy in advanced heart failure care. As heart failure disease progresses, the therapeutic options and treatment goals involving the use of inotropic therapy may change. *Abbreviations*: ADHF, advanced decompensated heart failure; LVAD, left ventricular assist device; QOL, quality of life.

possible that newer inotropic agents, lower doses, or combined therapy might represent safer alternatives; however, this needs to be confirmed in larger, randomized studies. In the interim, there remains a population of patients in which inotropic therapy seems warranted. It is important to recognize that the objectives and goals of therapy will be mandated by the individual situation (Fig. 6).

1. The acute management of decompensated HF: Patients with acute decompensated HF with evidence of poor end-organ perfusion may benefit from a short course of intravenous inotropic therapy. This strategy should be reserved for patients failing standard therapy, including vasodilators. Inotropic support should be started at the lowest possible dose and titrated to clinical effect. The duration of inotropic support should be minimized, with early attempts to wean to oral/standard therapy once stabilized. All patients on inotropes should have continuous telemetry monitoring, and avoidance of any elements that can exacerbate arrhythmic or ischemic complications (hypokalemia or hypomagnesemia).
2. Bridge to definitive therapy: There are patients with chronic HF who may require additional support in order to survive to definitive therapy, including transplantation. Currently there are two strategies with which to bridge these patients, chronic inotropic support and ventricular assist device therapy. There is no data to guide the clinician in this decision; however, it requires a careful assessment of risks, benefits, and program experience. In those patients in whom chronic inotropic support is deemed necessary, multiple attempts should be made to wean the inotropic therapy. Patients should only be considered inotrope dependent after they have repeatedly demonstrated a failure to wean because of worsening clinical status. All patients in whom home inotropic therapy is considered as a bridge to transplantation should have an implantable cardioverter defibrillator placed prior to discharge.
3. Palliation of symptoms: There are patients with very advanced cardiac disease who are not candidates for cardiac transplantation. When these patients are deemed inotrope dependent, the focus of continued therapy shifts from survival to symptom alleviation. Some patients, such as those in REMATCH, may be eligible for ventricular assist device therapy as destination care. However, for the majority of patients with end-stage cardiac disease, mechanical assist devices are not an option, often because of comorbities that might affect survival or increase the risk of the surgery. There may be a role for inotropic support in these patients; however, the goals of therapy may be to improve symptoms, or allow patients to be discharged with the dignity of dying at home. It is clear that inotropic support may increase the risk of mortality, at the benefit of improving comfort and quality of life. Consideration should be given to terminating defibrillator therapy in patients receiving inotropes as palliative care.

REFERENCES

1. Hunt SA, Baker DW, Chin MH, et al. ACC/AHA guidelines for the evaluation and management of chronic HF in the adult: executive summary. A report of the American college of Cardiology/American Heart Association Task Force on Practice Guidelines (Committee to revise the 1995 Guidelines for the Evaluation and Management of Heart Failure). J Am Coll Cardiol 2001; 38:2101–2113.

2. Krumholz HM, Chen YT, Wang Y, Vaccarino V, Radford MJ, Horwitz RI. Predictors of readmission among elderly survivors of admission with heart failure. Am Heart J 2000; 139:72–77.
3. Katz A. Molecular and cellular basis of contraction. In: Colucci WS, ed. Atlas of Heart Failure. Boston: Current Medicine, 2002:2–17.
4. Felker GM, O'Connor CM. Inotropic therapy for heart failure: an evidence-based approach. Am Heart J 2001; 142:393–401.
5. del Monte F, Hajjar RJ. Targeting calcium cycling proteins in heart failure through gene transfer. J Physiol 2003; 546:49–61.
6. Hoshijima M, Ikeda Y, Iwanaga Y, et al. Chronic suppression of heart-failure progression by a pseudophosphorylated mutant of phospholamban via in vivo cardiac rAAV gene delivery. Nat Med 2002; 8:864–871.
7. del Monte F, Harding SE, Dec GW, et al. Targeting phospholamban by gene transfer in human heart failure. Circulation 2002; 105:904–907.
8. Stevenson LW. Clinical use of inotropic therapy for heart failure: looking backward or forward? Part II: chronic inotropic therapy. Circulation 2003; 108:492–497.
9. Friedrich JO, Adhikari N, Herridge MS, Beyene J. Meta-analysis: low-dose dopamine increases urine output but does not prevent renal dysfunction or death. Ann Intern Med 2005; 142:510–524.
10. Francis GS, Wilson BC, Rector TS. Hemodynamic, renal, and neurohumoral effects of a selective oral DA1 receptor agonist (fenoldopam) in patients with congestive heart failure. Am Heart J 1988; 116:473–479.
11. Stevenson LW. Management of Acute Decompensation. Houston: Saunders, 2004 pp. 579–601.
12. Cuffe MS, Califf RM, Adams KF, Jr., et al. Short-term intravenous milrinone for acute exacerbation of chronic heart failure: a randomized controlled trial. JAMA 2002; 287:1541–1547.
13. Opie L, Gersh B. Digitalis, acute inotropes and inotropic dilators. In: Opie LGB, ed. Drugs for the Heart. Philadelphia: WB Saunders, 2001:154–186.
14. Packer M, Gheorghiade M, Young JB, et al. Withdrawal of digoxin from patients with chronic heart failure treated with angiotensin-converting-enzyme inhibitors. RADIANCE Study. N Engl J Med 1993; 329:1–7.
15. Uretsky BF, Young JB, Shahidi FE, Yellen LG, Harrison MC, Jolly MK. Randomized study assessing the effect of digoxin withdrawal in patients with mild to moderate chronic congestive heart failure: results of the PROVED trial. PROVED Investigative Group. J Am Coll Cardiol 1993; 22:955–962.
16. The Digitalis Investigation Group. The effect of digoxin on mortality and morbidity in patients with heart failure. N Engl J Med 1997; 336:525–533.
17. Rathore SS, Curtis JP, Wang Y, Bristow MR, Krumholz HM. Association of serum digoxin concentration and outcomes in patients with heart failure. JAMA 2003; 289:871–878.
18. Rathore SS, Wang Y, Krumholz HM. Sex-based differences in the effect of digoxin for the treatment of heart failure. N Engl J Med 2002; 347:1403–1411.
19. Slawsky MT, Colucci WS, Gottlieb SS, et al. Acute hemodynamic and clinical effects of levosimendan in patients with severe heart failure. Study Investigators. Circulation 2000; 102:2222–2227.
20. Haikala H, Linden IB. Mechanisms of action of calcium-sensitizing drugs. J Cardiovasc Pharmacol 1995; 26:S10–S19.
21. Singh K, Communal C, Sawyer DB, Colucci WS. Adrenergic regulation of myocardial apoptosis. Cardiovasc Res 2000; 45:713–719.
22. Elsasser A, Schlepper M, Klovekorn WP, et al. Hibernating myocardium: an incomplete adaptation to ischemia. Circulation 1997; 96:2920–2931.
23. Oliva F, Latini R, Politi A, et al. Intermittent 6-month low-dose dobutamine infusion in severe heart failure: DICE multicenter trial. Am Heart J 1999; 138:247–253.

24. Polanczyk CA, Rohde LE, Dec GW, DiSalvo T. Ten-year trends in hospital care for congestive heart failure: improved outcomes and increased use of resources. Arch Intern Med 2000; 160:325–332.
25. Nohria A, Tsang SW, Fang JC, et al. Clinical assessment identifies hemodynamic profiles that predict outcomes in patients admitted with heart failure. J Am Coll Cardiol 2003; 41:1797–1804.
26. Nohria A, Lewis E, Stevenson LW. Medical management of advanced heart failure. JAMA 2002; 287:628–640.
27. Follath F, Cleland JG, Just H, et al. Efficacy and safety of intravenous levosimendan compared with dobutamine in severe low-output heart failure (the LIDO study): a randomised double-blind trial. Lancet 2002; 360:196–202.
28. Colucci WS, Wright RF, Jaski BE, Fifer MA, Braunwald E. Milrinone and dobutamine in severe heart failure: differing hemodynamic effects and individual patient responsiveness. Circulation 1986; 73:III175–III183.
29. Burger AJ, Horton DP, LeJemtel T, et al. Effect of nesiritide (B-type natriuretic peptide) and dobutamine on ventricular arrhythmias in the treatment of patients with acutely decompensated congestive heart failure: the PRECEDENT study. Am Heart J 2002; 144:1102–1108.
30. Silver MA, Horton DP, Ghali JK, Elkayam U. Effect of nesiritide versus dobutamine on short-term outcomes in the treatment of patients with acutely decompensated heart failure. J Am Coll Cardiol 2002; 39:798–803.
31. Elakayam U, Tasissa G, Binanay C, et al. Use and impact of inotropes and vasodilator therapy during heart failure hosptialization in the ESCAPE trial. Circulation 2004; 110:111–515.
32. Yancey C, Fonarow G, Abraham W, et al. Clinical differences between high and low mortality risk stratified patients hospitalized with acutely decompensated heart failure: ADHERE Registry data. J Card Fail 2004; 10:S128.
33. Stevenson LW. The cul-de-sac at the end of the road. J Card Fail 2003; 9:188–191.
34. Hershberger RE, Nauman D, Walker TL, Dutton D, Burgess D. Care processes and clinical outcomes of continuous outpatient support with inotropes (COSI) in patients with refractory endstage heart failure. J Card Fail 2003; 9:180–187.
35. Aranda JM, Jr., Schofield RS, Pauly DF, et al. Comparison of dobutamine versus milrinone therapy in hospitalized patients awaiting cardiac transplantation: a prospective, randomized trial. Am Heart J 2003; 145:324–329.
36. Stevenson LW, Miller LW, Desvigne-Nickens P, et al. Left ventricular assist device as destination for patients undergoing intravenous inotropic therapy: a subset analysis from REMATCH (Randomized Evaluation of Mechanical Assistance in Treatment of Chronic Heart Failure). Circulation 2004; 110:975–981.
37. O'Connor CM, Gattis WA, Ryan TJ. The role of clinical nonfatal end points in cardiovascular phase II/III clinical trials. Am Heart J 2000; 139:S143–S154.
38. Hatzizacharias A, Makris T, Krespi P, et al. Intermittent milrinone effect on long-term hemodynamic profile in patients with severe congestive heart failure. Am Heart J 1999; 138:241–246.
39. Dies F, Krell MJ, Whitlow P, et al. Intermittent dobutamine in ambulatory outpatients with chronic heart failure. Circulation 1986; 74:II38.
40. Lewis EF, Johnson PA, Johnson W, Collins C, Griffin L, Stevenson LW. Preferences for quality of life or survival expressed by patients with heart failure. J Heart Lung Transplant 2001; 20:1016–1024.
41. Packer M, Carver JR, Rodeheffer RJ, et al. Effect of oral milrinone on mortality in severe chronic heart failure. The PROMISE Study Research Group. N Engl J Med 1991; 325:1468–1475.
42. Cohn JN, Goldstein SO, Greenberg BH, et al. A dose-dependent increase in mortality with vesnarinone among patients with severe heart failure. Vesnarinone Trial Investigators. N Engl J Med 1998; 339:1810–1816.

43. Hampton JR, van Veldhuisen DJ, Kleber FX, et al. Randomized study of the effect of ibopamine on survival in patients with advanced severe heart failure. Second Prospective Randomized study of Ibopamine on Mortaility and Efficacy (PRIME II) Investigators. Lancct 1997; 349:971–977.
44. Lubsen J, Just H, Hjalmarsson AC, et al. Effect of pimobendan on exercise capacity in patients with heart fialure: main results from the Pimobendan in Congestive Heart Failure (PICO) trial. Heart 1996; 76:223–231.
45. Focaccio A, Peeters G, Movsesian M, et al. Mechanism of action of OPC-8490 in human ventricular myocardium. Circulation 1996; 93:817–825.
46. Feldman AM, Bristow MR, Parmley WW, et al. Effects of vesnarinone on morbidity and mortality in patients with heart failure. Vesnarinone Study Group. N Engl J Med 1993; 329:149–155.
47. Shipley JB, Tolman D, Hastillo A, et al. Milrinone: basic and clinical pharmacology and acute and chronic management. Am J Med Sci 1996; 1996:201–206.
48. Uretsky BF, Jessup M, Konstam MA, et al. Multicenter trial of oral enoximone in patients with moderate to moderately severe congestive heart failure. Lack of benefit compared with placebo. Enoximone Multicenter Trial Group. Circulation 1990; 82:774–780.
49. Lowes BD, Higginbotham M, Petrovich L, et al. Low-dose enoximone improves exercise capacity in chronic heart failure. Enoximone Study Group. J Am Coll Cardiol 2000; 36:501–508.
50. Bristow MR. Oral enoximone in intravenous dependent subjects (EMOTE) Heart Failure Society of America 8th Annual Scientific Meeting. Toronto, Canada, 2004.
51. William V. Expert panel review of NHLBI total artificial heart program:1999.
52. Narahara KA. Oral enoximone therapy in chronic heart failure: a placebo-controlled randomized trial. The Western Enoximone Study Group. Am Heart J 1991; 121:1471–1479.
53. Bohm M, Deutsch HJ, Hartmann D, Rosee KL, Stablein A. Improvement of postreceptor events by metoprolol treatment in patients with chronic heart failure. J Am Coll Cardiol 1997; 30:992–996.
54. DeLuca L, Proietti P, Palombaro G, et al. New positive inotropic agents in the treatment of left ventricular dysfunction. Ital Heart J 2004; 5:635–675.
55. Cappola TP, Kass DA, Nelson GS, et al. Allopurinol improves myocardial efficiency in patients with idiopathic dilated cardiomyopathy. Circulation 2001; 104:2407–2411.

9
Statins, Inflammation, and Cardiomyopathy: Old Pathways, New Targets

Charles J. Lowenstein and Munekazu Yamakuchi
Department of Medicine, Johns Hopkins University School of Medicine, Baltimore, Maryland, U.S.A.

INTRODUCTION

Clinical trials of 3-hydroxy-3-methyl-glutaryl-CoA (HMG-CoA) reductase inhibitors (statins) have presented clinicians with a puzzle. Statins not only improve survival of patients at high risk for coronary heart disease with elevated low density lipoprotein (LDL) cholesterol, but also benefit patients with moderate risk and average LDL levels. Even more puzzling, statins may also benefit patients with dilated cardiomyopathy by decreasing symptoms and increasing the ejection fraction. Most puzzling of all, recent studies have found that statins improve outcomes in diseases as diverse as cancer, osteoporosis, and Alzheimer's Disease—all diseases in which LDL is not thought to play a significant role. These novel benefits of statins have raised the question: Do statins benefit patients by decreasing lipids, modulating inflammation, or through other pathways?

THE DISCOVERY OF STATINS: FROM MICROBES TO LIPIDS

The Japanese microbiologist Akira Endo discovered statins while screening fungi for novel antibiotics at the Sankyo Drug company. In 1973, he isolated a compound from a *Penicillium* mold that inhibited HMG-CoA reductase; Dr. Endo named this compound compactin (1). Although he soon found that compactin lacked antimicrobial activity, Dr. Endo realized that it might lower lipids in patients with elevated cholesterol. He showed that compactin lowered plasma cholesterol in mice, chickens, dogs, and monkeys (2). In 1976, Dr. Endo and colleagues administered compactin to a Japanese girl with homozygous Familial Hypercholesterolemia: mevastatin lowered her plasma cholesterol from approximately 400 to 320 mg/dl (3). Spurred on by Dr. Endo's research, scientists at Merck Research Laboratories in 1978 discovered another HMG-CoA reductase inhibitor from *Aspergillus*, and named it lovastatin (4). However, Merck suspended work on lovastatin because of reports of animal toxicity of compactin (5). After additional animal studies and pilot human studies of toxicity, Merck decided to restart clinical trials of lovastatin in patients with hypercholesterolemia.

ANTI-CHOLESTEROL EFFECTS OF STATINS: THE MOST DECORATED MOLECULE IN BIOLOGY

Cholesterol is a lipid found in cell membranes that is also necessary for the synthesis of steroid hormones and bile acid. Biosynthesis of cholesterol involves over 30 enzymes. Since thirteen Nobel prizes have been awarded to scientists who studied the synthesis and transport of cholesterol, Brown and Goldstein in their Nobel Prize lecture in 1985 called cholesterol "the most highly decorated small molecule in biology"(6). The rate limiting step in the biosynthesis of cholesterol is the conversion of mevalonate to HMG-CoA to mevalonate by HMG-CoA reductase (Fig. 1). Statins inhibit HMG-CoA reductase, thereby decreasing production not only of cholesterol, but also of cholesterol precursors such as geranyl pyrophosphate and farnesyl pyrophosphate.

Most cholesterol in the plasma is transported as cholesteryl esters in the hydrophobic core of lipoprotein particles, including LDL. Statins decrease plasma LDL through a complex regulatory mechanism. By inhibition of HMG-CoA reductase, statins decrease cholesterol levels inside hepatocytes, leading to an increase in LDL receptor synthesis, thereby increasing clearance of plasma LDL. Thus statins both decrease hepatic production of LDL and increase LDL clearance from the plasma. Since patients with Familial Hypercholesterolemia had elevated LDL cholesterol and premature coronary artery disease, and since subjects with elevated LDL cholesterol had an increased risk

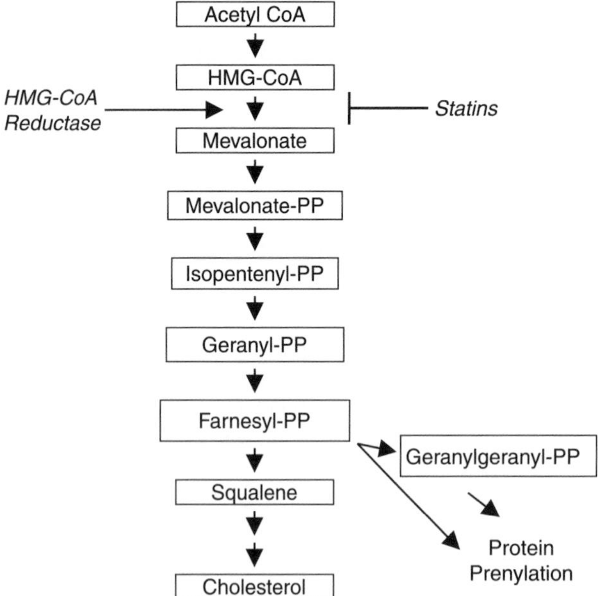

Figure 1 The cholesterol biosynthetic pathway. Statins inhibit 3-hydroxy-3-methyl-glutaryl-CoA (HMG-CoA) reductase, the enzyme that converts HMG-CoA into mevalonate. One of the metabolites of mevalonate is farnesyl pyrophosphate (farnesyl-PP), which is not only a precursor of cholesterol, but can also be attached to proteins, serving as a membrane anchor.

of coronary artery disease, pharmaceutical companies started clinical trials to see if statins could lower LDL and decrease coronary heart disease.

CLINICAL TRIALS OF STATINS AND LDL CHOLESTEROL: THE LOWER THE BETTER

Early human trials showed that statins improved outcome in a wide variety of patients. Statin treatment of patients with a prior myocardial infarction and elevated lipids (such as the Scandinavian Simvastatin Survival Study, and the Long Term Intervention with Pravastatin in Ischemic Disease trial) showed that statins could reduce LDL by 35% and decrease mortality as much as 30% (7,8). Statins appeared to help patients with higher levels of LDL, reinforcing the concept that statins improve survival by decreasing LDL. Statin treatment also improved outcomes in patients without a myocardial infarction but with high LDL levels (including the West of Scotland Coronary Prevention Study) (9). Intensive lipid lowering even reduced cardiovascular events (but not mortality) in patients with coronary heart disease but LDL levels less than 130 mg/dl (Treating to New Targets trial) (10). In all of these studies, statins were of most benefit to subjects with higher LDL levels.

Although the clinical benefit of statins is greater in patients with higher LDL cholesterol levels, statins still improve cardiovascular outcomes in patients with moderate LDL levels. Statins benefited patients with moderate LDL and prior myocardial infarction (in the Cholesterol and Recurrent Events trial), high risk of disease (in the Heart Protection Study, and the Anglo-Scandinavian Cardiac Outcomes Trial), and even those without heart disease (Air Force/Texas Coronary Atherosclerosis Prevention Study) (11–14).

Clinical trials of statins have not been designed specifically to identify the optimal LDL level—a threshold below which LDL lowering has no clinical impact. Perhaps average levels of cholesterol in adults in the industrialized Western world are higher than the ideal level, a much lower level is found in adults in developing countries (15). Thus one possible explanation for the benefit of statins in patients with moderate cholesterol is that even these moderate levels of cholesterol are too high: the lower LDL cholesterol is, the better the outcome. However, another possible explanation is that statins have other clinical effects in addition to their impact upon LDL.

CLINICAL STUDIES OF STATINS AND INFLAMMATION: LOWERING LDL, INFLAMMATION, OR BOTH?

Inflammation plays a pivotal role in all phases of atherogenesis, from fatty streak development to formation of fibrous plaques to plaque rupture (16–18). Injury to the arterial wall activates endothelial cells which trigger macrophage infiltration into the vessel wall. Macrophages ingest lipids, form foam cells which coalesce into fatty streaks, and then release inflammatory cytokines. Smooth muscle cells become activated by these inflammatory signals, proliferating and migrating into a fibrous cap, and secreting enzymes that destabilize the plaque. Plaque rupture causes thrombosis and myocardial infarction. Inflammatory markers are elevated in patients with atherosclerosis, in particular, components of the Acute Phase Response such as interleukin-6, serum amyloid A, secretory phospholipase A2, and C-reactive protein (CRP) (16–18). Inflammatory markers predict the risk of cardiovascular events such as myocardial infarction, not only in patients with atherosclerosis, but also in apparently healthy men and women (19,20). Of these inflammatory markers, CRP levels have the largest magnitude of predictive value (21).

Statins decrease inflammatory markers in patients with a broad spectrum of cardiovascular disease. Statins decrease CRP levels in patients with acute coronary syndrome and myocardial infarction (22–25). Statins even decrease CRP levels in patients without known atherosclerosis (24,26,27). For example, lovastatin reduced the CRP level by 15% in 6000 men and women with average LDL cholesterol levels enrolled in the AF/TexCAPS trial (23). Smaller clinical trials have shown that statin therapy of patients with elevated LDL decreases additional inflammatory markers, such as tumor necrosis factor-α, soluble P-selectin, von Willebrand Factor, ICAM-1, interleukin-2, and interleukin-6 (28–31). Thus statins decrease inflammation in a variety of patients.

The clinical benefit of statins is associated with decreasing inflammation. For example, patients with acute coronary syndrome have better outcomes when treated with statins, and the patients with the lowest levels of inflammatory markers have the fewest cardiovascular events (23). In patients without prior coronary artery disease, the benefit from statins is correlated with the decrease in CRP (21). These data suggest that statins improve outcomes in part by decreasing inflammation.

However, it is difficult to separate the anti-inflammatory properties of statins from their lipid lowering effects. The ability of statins to decrease inflammation may simply be the result of lowering LDL cholesterol. After all, LDL cholesterol, in particular, oxidized LDL, damages endothelial cell function, stimulates smooth muscle cell migration and proliferation, triggers macrophage expression of inflammatory genes, and activates smooth muscle proliferation—all critical steps in atherogenesis (16–18,32). Since LDL has pro-inflammatory effects, lowering LDL would also be expected to suppress inflammation. The only way to prove rigorously that the anti-inflammatory and anti-lipid effects of statins are independent would be to administer placebo or statin to patients, while clamping LDL cholesterol at a constant level by simultaneously infusing LDL particle. Such a trial would be clinically challenging, ethically dubious, and unlikely to be performed!

Clinical trials show that statins decrease inflammatory markers, and that the benefit of statins is associated with the decrease in inflammation. Perhaps this is due to the pro-inflammatory effect of LDL. But cellular and animal studies have identified novel anti-inflammatory targets of statins that are independent of cholesterol.

STATINS BLOCK INTEGRINS AND LEUKOCYTE TRAFFICKING

Statins directly block vascular inflammation—a critical step in atherogenesis. Leukocyte trafficking from the blood into the vessel wall depends upon a series of steps: leukocyte rolling along the vessel wall, leukocyte activation, leukocyte adherence to the vessel wall, diapedesis between endothelial cells into the vessel wall, and migration into the atheromatous plaque. The central stage of leukocyte trafficking, leukocyte adherence to the endothelial cell, is mediated by the interaction of adhesion molecules: $\alpha_1\beta_2$ integrin on the leukocyte surface binds to intercellular adhesion molecule-1 (ICAM-1) displayed on the endothelial surface (33).

Statins block leukocyte binding to endothelial cells by disrupting the interaction between $\alpha_1\beta_2$ integrin and ICAM-1 (34–36). Lovastatin and simvastatin bind directly to $\alpha_1\beta_2$ integrin, causing an allosteric shift in the integrin's adhesion binding site, inhibiting the ability of integrin to interact with ICAM-1, and thus blocking leukocyte attachment to the endothelium. This effect does not depend upon statin inhibition of HMG-CoA reductase, since a compound structurally related to statins that cannot inhibit HMG-CoA reductase also binds to $\alpha_1\beta_2$ integrin and blocks integrin-ICAM interactions (35). This leukocyte integrin is the only statin target that has been identified, other than HMG-CoA reductase.

STATINS DECREASE ISOPRENYLATION OF SIGNALING PROTEINS: RHO

By inhibiting HMG-CoA reductase, statins block the synthesis of cholesterol precursors that also serve as important subunits for post-translational modification of cellular proteins. Statins block the synthesis of farnesyl pyrophosphate (farnesyl-PP) and geranylgeranyl pyrophosphate (geranylgeranyl-PP) (Fig. 1). When these isoprenoid intermediates are attached to proteins, they serve as membrane anchors, localizing the modified protein to the cellular membrane. Over 100 proteins can be prenylated, including small guanosine triphosphate binding proteins (G-proteins) within the Rho, Rab, and Rac family (37). Since membrane targeting of these proteins is critical to their function, statin inhibition of prenylation impairs the function of these G-proteins.

Which G-proteins are targets of statins? Rho regulates cell shape, migration, and gene transcription; and prenylation is necessary for Rho functions. Statin therapy decreases prenylation of Rho, and consequently blocks Rho translocation to the inner surface of the cellular membrane (38,39). Statins block the ability of Rho to stimulate the pro-inflammatory transcription nuclear factor kappaB in endothelial cells, and to activate endothelial production of pro-coagulant microparticles (40–42). Statins also inhibit prenylation and activation of the G-protein Ras, thereby limiting smooth muscle cell proliferation (43). Thus, statins have wide-ranging effects upon activation of vascular cells through statin control of signals that localize proteins.

STATINS IMPROVE ENDOTHELIAL FUNCTION: NITRIC OXIDE

Statins also inhibit inflammation by modulating nitric oxide (NO) production (Fig. 2). Endothelial cells produce NO from endothelial NO synthase (eNOS), which converts arginine and molecular oxygen into citrulline and NO (44–46). Triggered by agonists such as bradykinin or acetylcholine, endothelial cells activate eNOS, leading to the synthesis of NO. NO plays an important role in protecting the vasculature from atherosclerosis, blocking leukocyte trafficking, platelet adhesion, and smooth muscle cell proliferation. Endothelial dysfunction is one of the earliest manifestations of atherogenesis, and is characterized in part by the inability of endothelial cells to produce NO (47–49).

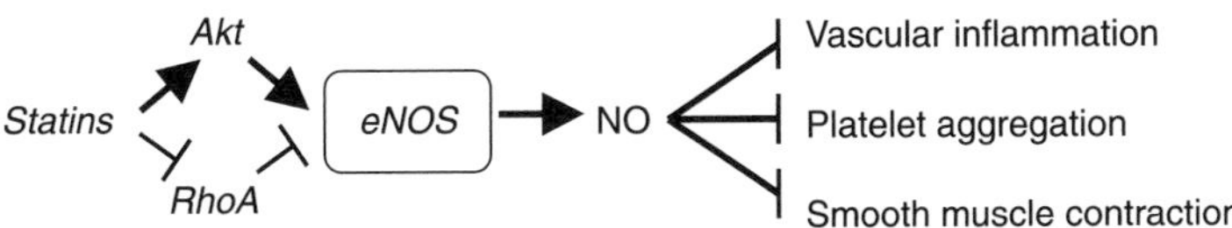

Figure 2 Statins increase nitric oxide synthesis. Statins increase endothelial NO synthase (eNOS) expression by inhibiting the G-protein RhoA and eNOS activation by stimulating the kinase Akt.

Statin therapy improves endothelial function in patients, increasing vasomotor responses to endothelial agonists (47–49). Statins can increase NO production by several mechanisms. First, statins can decrease LDL and oxidized LDL cholesterol levels, which normally inhibit eNOS expression and activity (50,51). Next, statins increase expression of eNOS protein through inhibition of Rho, which normally destabilizes eNOS mRNA transcripts (38). In addition, statins increase the bioavailability of NO by decreasing reactive oxygen species that would otherwise convert NO into the pro-inflammatory peroxynitrite (49). Finally, statins activate Akt, a protein kinase that phosphorylates eNOS and boosts NO synthesis (52). By activating Akt, statins also promote the survival of endothelial cells. Thus statins promote endothelial function through a variety of pathways that converge upon NO.

STATINS DECREASE VASCULAR INFLAMMATION: BLOCKADE OF EXOCYTOSIS

Statins also decrease vascular inflammation by blocking the first step in leukocyte trafficking into the vessel wall (Fig. 3). Inflammation of the vessel wall—triggered by cholesterol, hypoxia, or cytokines—activates rapid release of endothelial granules called Weibel-Palade bodies (53). These granules store P-selectin inside endothelial cells (54). Exocytosis of Weibel-Palade bodies causes P-selectin translocation from the interior to the exterior of the endothelial cell, where it interacts with the selectin receptors P-Selectin Glycoprotein Ligand-1 (PSGL-1) on leukocytes. This interaction between P-selectin on endothelial cells and PSGL-1 leukocytes mediates leukocyte rolling along the vascular wall, the first step in vascular inflammation.

Statins decrease vascular inflammation in part through a novel mechanism: blockade of endothelial exocytosis. Statins activate eNOS; the NO produced by eNOS then inhibits the exocytic machinery within endothelial cells by chemically modifying N-ethylmaleimide sensitive factor (NSF), the molecular motor of exocytosis (55). NO inhibition of NSF blocks exocytosis and externalization of P-selectin, thereby decreasing leukocyte rolling (55). By inhibiting exocytosis, statins decrease inflammation and necrosis in mice after myocardial infarction (56). However, statins have no effect upon exocytosis and myocardial infarction in mice lacking eNOS. Thus the ability of statins to inhibit

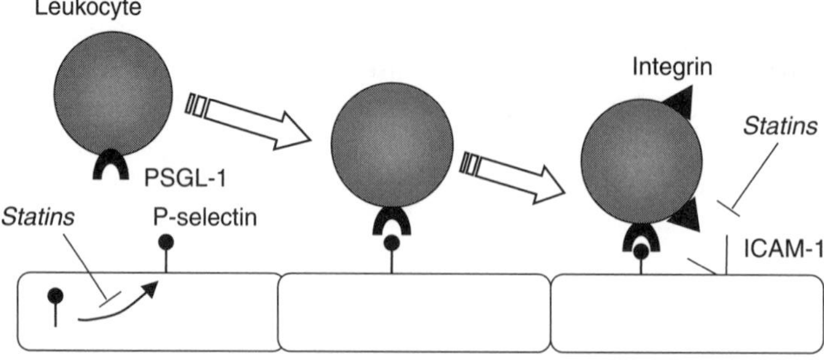

Figure 3 Statins decrease vascular inflammation. Statins block leukocyte interactions with endothelial cells by inhibiting endothelial release of P-selectin and by interrupting intercellular adhesion molecule (ICAM) binding to integrins.

exocytosis depends upon NO. Taken together, these observations suggest a novel mechanism by which statins decrease vascular inflammation.

STATINS AND CARDIOMYOPATHY

A few tantalizing clinical trials suggest that statins also benefit patients with idiopathic dilated cardiomyopathy—a disease not usually linked to LDL cholesterol. In one study, 60 patients with non-ischemic dilated cardiomyopathy NYHA class II were treated with placebo or simvastatin for 14 weeks. Statin treatment slightly improved symptoms of heart failure, and increased the ejection fraction from 34% to 41% (57). A smaller study showed that 20 weeks of cerivastatin treatment improved symptoms but not ejection fraction in 8 patients, compared to 7 patients receiving placebo (58). These trials are small but encourage further large-scale trials of statins for cardiomyopathy patients that include survival as a primary end-point.

Small clinical trials suggest that statins may benefit patients with dilated cardiomyopathy. How? Several mechanisms may explain the potential benefits of statins (Fig. 4). Statins decrease systemic inflammation. Tumor necrosis factor-α, interleukin-1β, and interleukin-6 are increased in patients with heart failure (59–61). Cytokines may contribute to cardiomyopathy directly by damaging cardiac myocytes or indirectly by attracting leukocytes which release mediators toxic to cardiac myocytes (62). As discussed above, statins can decrease inflammation by cholesterol dependent and independent pathways. Statins lowered tumor necrosis factor and interleukin-6 levels in patients with dilated cardiomyopathy, compared to placebo (57,58).

Statins may also benefit patients with cardiomyopathy by reversing endothelial dysfunction. In patients with dilated cardiomyopathy, vasodilation is impaired, in part due to decreased NO synthesis. Vasoconstriction is further heightened by increased levels of endothelin. Statins improve vasomotor function by increasing expression of eNOS, inhibiting superoxide production, and decreasing expression of endothelin (63,64). Increased NO, in turn, leads to decreased oxygen consumption (65,66). Statins may also improve microvascular function by mobilizing endothelial progenitor cells from the bone marrow (67,68). Supporting this idea, statin therapy accelerates the re-endothelialization of blood vessels and improves neovascularization of the myocardium (69,70). The mechanism by which statins mobilize endothelial stem cells is unclear, but it may include

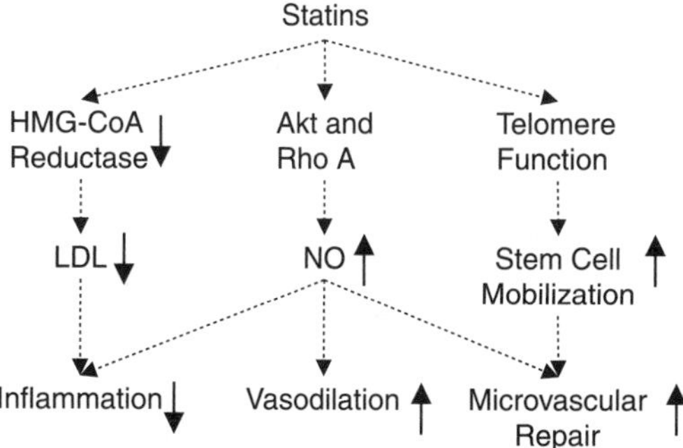

Figure 4 Potential benefits of statins for patients with cardiomyopathy. In addition to lowering low density lipoprotein (LDL) cholesterol, statins also decrease inflammation, improve vasodilation, and accelerate microvascular repair.

activation of eNOS or modulation of telomere function during endothelial stem cell proliferation (70,71). Thus, statins may improve endothelial function by multiple mechanisms in patients with cardiomyopathy.

CONCLUSIONS: THE TRUE SIGNIFICANCE OF STATIN ANTI-INFLAMMATORY EFFECTS

The major clinical benefit of statins is probably derived from lowering LDL. However, in the 30 yr since the discovery of statins, research has uncovered important anti-inflammatory effects of statins which may also benefit patients to a lesser degree. Some of the anti-inflammatory effects of statins are due to a decrease in LDL cholesterol, which itself is pro-inflammatory. But statins also decrease inflammation by cholesterol independent mechanisms. Statins block two distinct steps of leukocyte entry into the vessel wall. In addition, statins block post-translational modification of small G-proteins that would otherwise transduce inflammatory responses within the vessel wall. Finally, statins improve endothelial function by stimulating synthesis of NO, which itself has anti-inflammatory properties, and which can mobilize endothelial stem cells which repair damaged vessels.

Although the anti-inflammatory effects of statins may have less clinical benefit than the LDL lowering properties, research into statins have revealed new inflammatory pathways that modulate atherosclerosis and cardiomyopathy. The true significance of the discovery of these pleitropic effects of statins may be the identification of novel targets, which, in turn, will lead to the development of new anti-inflammatory therapies for patients with heart disease.

REFERENCES

1. Endo A, Kuroda M, Tsujita Y. ML-236A, ML-236B, and ML-236C, new inhibitors of cholesterogenesis produced by Penicillium citrinium. J Antibiot (Tokyo) 1976; 29:1346–1348.
2. Endo A. The discovery and development of HMG-CoA reductase inhibitors. J Lipid Res 1992; 33:1569–1582.
3. Yamamoto A, Sudo H, Endo A. Therapeutic effects of ML-236B in primary hypercholesterolemia. Atherosclerosis 1980; 35:259–266.
4. Alberts AW, Chen J, Kuron G, et al. Mevinolin: a highly potent competitive inhibitor of hydroxymethylglutaryl-coenzyme A reductase and a cholesterol-lowering agent. Proc Natl Acad Sci USA 1980; 77:3957–3961.
5. Tobert JA. Lovastatin and beyond: the history of the HMG-CoA reductase inhibitors. Nat Rev Drug Discov 2003; 2:517–526.
6. Brown MS, Goldstein JL. 1985 Nobel laureates in medicine. J Investig Med 1996; 44:14–23.
7. Randomized trial of cholesterol lowering in 4444 patients with coronary heart disease: the Scandinavian Simvastatin Survival Study (4S). Lancet 1994; 344:1383–1389.
8. White HD, Simes RJ, Anderson NE, et al. Pravastatin therapy and the risk of stroke. N Engl J Med 2000; 343:317–326.
9. Shepherd J, Cobbe SM, Ford I, et al. Prevention of coronary heart disease with pravastatin in men with hypercholesterolemia. West of Scotland Coronary Prevention Study Group. N Engl J Med 1995; 333:1301–1307.
10. LaRosa JC, Grundy SM, Waters DD, et al. Intensive lipid lowering with atorvastatin in patients with stable coronary disease. N Engl J Med 2005; 352:1425–1435.

11. Sacks FM, Pfeffer MA, Moye LA, et al. The effect of pravastatin on coronary events after myocardial infarction in patients with average cholesterol levels. Cholesterol and Recurrent Events Trial investigators. N Engl J Med 1996; 335:1001–1009.
12. MRC/BHF Heart Protection Study of cholesterol lowering with simvastatin in 20,536 high-risk individuals: a randomised placebo-controlled trial. Lancet 2002; 360:7–22.
13. Sever PS, Dahlof B, Poulter NR, et al. Prevention of coronary and stroke events with atorvastatin in hypertensive patients who have average or lower-than-average cholesterol concentrations, in the Anglo-Scandinavian Cardiac Outcomes Trial–Lipid Lowering Arm (ASCOT-LLA): a multicentre randomised controlled trial. Lancet 2003; 361:1149–1158.
14. Downs JR, Clearfield M, Weis S, et al. Primary prevention of acute coronary events with lovastatin in men and women with average cholesterol levels: results of AFCAPS/TexCAPS. Air Force/Texas Coronary Atherosclerosis Prevention Study. JAMA 1998; 279:1615–1622.
15. Verschuren WM, Jacobs DR, Bloemberg BP, et al. Serum total cholesterol and long-term coronary heart disease mortality in different cultures. Twenty-five-year follow-up of the seven countries study. JAMA 1995; 274:131–136.
16. Hansson GK. Inflammation, atherosclerosis, and coronary artery disease. N Engl J Med 2005; 352:1685–1695.
17. Libby P. Inflammation in atherosclerosis. Nature 2002; 420:868–874.
18. Ross R. Atherosclerosis—an inflammatory disease. N Engl J Med 1999; 340:115–126.
19. Ridker PM, Cushman M, Stampfer MJ, Tracy RP, Hennekens CH. Inflammation, aspirin, and the risk of cardiovascular disease in apparently healthy men. N Engl J Med 1997; 336:973–979.
20. Ridker PM, Hennekens CH, Buring JE, Rifai N. C-reactive protein and other markers of inflammation in the prediction of cardiovascular disease in women. N Engl J Med 2000; 342:836–843.
21. Ridker PM. Clinical application of C-reactive protein for cardiovascular disease detection and prevention. Circulation 2003; 107:363–369.
22. Kinlay S, Schwartz GG, Olsson AG, et al. High-dose atorvastatin enhances the decline in inflammatory markers in patients with acute coronary syndromes in the MIRACL study. Circulation 2003; 108:1560–1566.
23. Ridker PM, Cannon CP, Morrow D, et al. C-reactive protein levels and outcomes after statin therapy. N Engl J Med 2005; 352:20–28.
24. Albert MA, Danielson E, Rifai N, Ridker PM. Effect of statin therapy on C-reactive protein levels: the pravastatin inflammation/CRP evaluation (PRINCE): a randomized trial and cohort study. JAMA 2001; 286:64–70.
25. Ridker PM, Rifai N, Pfeffer MA, Sacks F, Braunwald E. Long-term effects of pravastatin on plasma concentration of C-reactive protein. The Cholesterol and Recurrent Events (CARE) Investigators. Circulation 1999; 100:230–235.
26. Musial J, Undas A, Gajewski P, Jankowski M, Sydor W, Szczeklik A. Anti-inflammatory effects of simvastatin in subjects with hypercholesterolemia. Int J Cardiol 2001; 77:247–253.
27. Ridker PM, Rifai N, Lowenthal SP. Rapid reduction in C-reactive protein with cerivastatin among 785 patients with primary hypercholesterolemia. Circulation 2001; 103:1191–1193.
28. Solheim S, Seljeflot I, Arnesen H, Eritsland J, Eikvar L. Reduced levels of TNF alpha in hypercholesterolemic individuals after treatment with pravastatin for 8 weeks. Atherosclerosis 2001; 157:411–415.
29. Romano M, Mezzetti A, Marulli C, et al. Fluvastatin reduces soluble P-selectin and ICAM-1 levels in hypercholesterolemic patients: role of nitric oxide. J Investig Med 2000; 48:183–189.
30. Bickel C, Rupprecht HJ, Blankenberg S, et al. Influence of HMG-CoA reductase inhibitors on markers of coagulation, systemic inflammation and soluble cell adhesion. Int J Cardiol 2002; 82:25–31.
31. Zubelewicz-Szkodzinska B, Szkodzinski J, Romanowski W, et al. Simvastatin decreases concentration of interleukin-2 in hypercholesterolemic patients after treatment for 12 weeks. J Biol Regul Homeost Agents 2004; 18:295–301.
32. Witztum JL, Steinberg D. Role of oxidized low density lipoprotein in atherogenesis. J Clin Invest 1991; 88:1785–1792.

33. Hynes RO. Integrins: a family of cell surface receptors. Cell 1987; 48:549–554.
34. Kallen J, Welzenbach K, Ramage P, et al. Structural basis for LFA-1 inhibition upon lovastatin binding to the CD11a I-domain. J Mol Biol 1999; 292:1–9.
35. Weitz-Schmidt G, Welzenbach K, Brinkmann V, et al. Statins selectively inhibit leukocyte function antigen-1 by binding to a novel regulatory integrin site. Nat Med 2001; 7:687–692.
36. Frenette PS. Locking a leukocyte integrin with statins. N Engl J Med 2001; 345:1419–1421.
37. Winter-Vann AM, Casey PJ. Post-prenylation-processing enzymes as new targets in oncogenesis. Nat Rev Cancer 2005; 5:405–412.
38. Laufs U, Liao JK. Post-transcriptional regulation of endothelial nitric oxide synthase mRNA stability by Rho GTPase. J Biol Chem 1998; 273:24266–24271.
39. Guijarro C, Blanco-Colio LM, Ortego M, et al. 3-Hydroxy-3-methylglutaryl coenzyme a reductase and isoprenylation inhibitors induce apoptosis of vascular smooth muscle cells in culture. Circ Res 1998; 83:490–500.
40. Perona R, Montaner S, Saniger L, Sanchez-Perez I, Bravo R, Lacal JC. Activation of the nuclear factor-kappaB by Rho, CDC42, and Rac-1 proteins. Genes Dev 1997; 11:463–475.
41. Martin G, Duez H, Blanquart C, et al. Statin-induced inhibition of the Rho-signaling pathway activates PPARalpha and induces HDL apoA-I. J Clin Invest 2001; 107:1423–1432.
42. Tramontano AF, O'Leary J, Black AD, Muniyappa R, Cutaia MV, El-Sherif N. Statin decreases endothelial microparticle release from human coronary artery endothelial cells: implication for the Rho-kinase pathway. Biochem Biophys Res Commun 2004; 320:34–38.
43. Campbell M, Allen WE, Sawyer C, Vanhaesebroeck B, Trimble ER. Glucose-potentiated chemotaxis in human vascular smooth muscle is dependent on cross-talk between the PI3K and MAPK signaling pathways. Circ Res 2004; 95:380–388.
44. Sessa WC. eNOS at a glance. J Cell Sci 2004; 117:2427–2429.
45. Michel T, Feron O. Nitric oxide synthases: which, where, how, and why? J Clin Invest 1997; 100:2146–2152.
46. Lloyd-Jones DM, Bloch KD. The vascular biology of nitric oxide and its role in atherogenesis. Annu Rev Med 1996; 47:365–375.
47. Davignon J, Ganz P. Role of endothelial dysfunction in atherosclerosis. Circulation 2004; 109:III27–III32.
48. Freedman JE, Loscalzo J. Endothelial dysfunction and atherothrombotic occlusive disease. Drugs 1997; 54:41–49 discussion 9-50.
49. Cai H, Harrison DG. Endothelial dysfunction in cardiovascular diseases: the role of oxidant stress. Circ Res 2000; 87:840–844.
50. Liao JK, Shin WS, Lee WY, Clark SL. Oxidized low-density lipoprotein decreases the expression of endothelial nitric oxide synthase. J Biol Chem 1995; 270:319–324.
51. Uittenbogaard A, Shaul PW, Yuhanna IS, Blair A, Smart EJ. High density lipoprotein prevents oxidized low density lipoprotein-induced inhibition of endothelial nitric-oxide synthase localization and activation in caveolae. J Biol Chem 2000; 275:11278–11283.
52. Kureishi Y, Luo Z, Shiojima I, et al. The HMG-CoA reductase inhibitor simvastatin activates the protein kinase Akt and promotes angiogenesis in normocholesterolemic animals. Nat Med 2000; 6:1004–1010.
53. Weibel ER, Palade GE. New Cytoplasmic Components In Arterial Endothelia. J Cell Biol 1964; 23:101–112.
54. Bonfanti R, Furie BC, Furie B, Wagner DD. PADGEM (GMP140) is a component of Weibel-Palade bodies of human endothelial cells. Blood 1989; 73:1109–1112.
55. Matsushita K, Morrell CN, Cambien B, et al. Nitric oxide regulates exocytosis by S-nitrosylation of N-ethylmaleimide-sensitive factor. Cell 2003; 115:139–150.
56. Yamakuchi M, Greer JJ, Cameron SJ, et al. HMG-CoA Reductase Inhibitors Inhibit Endothelial Exocytosis and Decrease Myocardial Infarct Size. Circ Res 2005.
57. Node K, Fujita M, Kitakaze M, Hori M, Liao JK. Short-term statin therapy improves cardiac function and symptoms in patients with idiopathic dilated cardiomyopathy. Circulation 2003; 108:839–843.

58. Laufs U, Wassmann S, Schackmann S, Heeschen C, Bohm M, Nickenig G. Beneficial effects of statins in patients with non-ischemic heart failure. Z Kardiol 2004; 93:103–108.
59. Levine B, Kalman J, Mayer L, Fillit HM, Packer M. Elevated circulating levels of tumor necrosis factor in severe chronic heart failure. N Engl J Med 1990; 323:236–241.
60. Torre-Amione G, Kapadia S, Benedict C, Oral H, Young JB, Mann DL. Proinflammatory cytokine levels in patients with depressed left ventricular ejection fraction: a report from the Studies of Left Ventricular Dysfunction (SOLVD). J Am Coll Cardiol 1996; 27:1201–1206.
61. Kubota T, McNamara DM, Wang JJ, et al. Effects of tumor necrosis factor gene polymorphisms on patients with congestive heart failure. VEST Investigators for TNF Genotype Analysis. Vesnarinone Survival Trial. Circulation 1998; 97:2499–2501.
62. Sekiguchi K, Li X, Coker M, et al. Cross-regulation between the renin–angiotensin system and inflammatory mediators in cardiac hypertrophy and failure. Cardiovasc Res 2004; 63:433–442.
63. Wassmann S, Laufs U, Baumer AT, et al. HMG-CoA reductase inhibitors improve endothelial dysfunction in normocholesterolemic hypertension via reduced production of reactive oxygen species. Hypertension 2001; 37:1450–1457.
64. Hernandez-Perera O, Perez-Sala D, Navarro-Antolin J, et al. Effects of the 3-hydroxy-3-methylglutaryl-CoA reductase inhibitors, atorvastatin and simvastatin, on the expression of endothelin-1 and endothelial nitric oxide synthase in vascular endothelial cells. J Clin Invest 1998; 101:2711–2719.
65. Loke KE, Messina EJ, Mital S, Hintze TH. Impaired nitric oxide modulation of myocardial oxygen consumption in genetically cardiomyopathic hamsters. J Mol Cell Cardiol 2000; 32:2299–2306.
66. Mital S, Magneson A, Loke KE, Liao J, Forfia PR, Hintze TH. Simvastatin acts synergistically with ACE inhibitors or amlodipine to decrease oxygen consumption in rat hearts. J Cardiovasc Pharmacol 2000; 36:248–254.
67. Vasa M, Fichtlscherer S, Adler K, et al. Increase in circulating endothelial progenitor cells by statin therapy in patients with stable coronary artery disease. Circulation 2001; 103:2885–2890.
68. Llevadot J, Murasawa S, Kureishi Y, et al. HMG-CoA reductase inhibitor mobilizes bone marrow—derived endothelial progenitor cells. J Clin Invest 2001; 108:399–405.
69. Abraham SS, Osorio JC, Homma S, et al. Simvastatin preserves cardiac function in genetically determined cardiomyopathy. J Cardiovasc Pharmacol 2004; 43:454–461.
70. Landmesser U, Engberding N, Bahlmann FH, et al. Statin-induced improvement of endothelial progenitor cell mobilization, myocardial neovascularization, left ventricular function, and survival after experimental myocardial infarction requires endothelial nitric oxide synthase. Circulation 2004; 110:1933–1939.
71. Spyridopoulos I, Haendeler J, Urbich C, et al. Statins enhance migratory capacity by upregulation of the telomere repeat-binding factor TRF2 in endothelial progenitor cells. Circulation 2004; 110:3136–3142.

10
Atrial Arrhythmia

Aamir Cheema and Hugh Calkins
Division of Cardiology, Department of Medicine, Johns Hopkins University School of Medicine, Baltimore, Maryland, U.S.A.

INTRODUCTION

Atrial arrhythmias are extremely common among patients with heart failure. The purpose of this chapter is to review the types and treatment of atrial arrhythmias which occur in the setting of heart failure. Particular attention is focused on atrial fibrillation and atrial flutter as these are by far the most common types of atrial arrhythmias which occur in this setting.

ATRIAL FIBRILLATION

Overview and Clinical Significance

Atrial fibrillation (AF) is the most common sustained tachyarrhythmia in humans, affecting more than two million people in the United States (1). The most common symptoms of AF are palpitations, dizziness, dyspnea, and fatigue. The presence of AF increases all-cause mortality and is associated with a five-fold increased risk of stroke (2). A large number of risk factors have been associated with the development of AF. These include age, structural heart disease, male gender, and obesity (3–6). Age is among the most important risk factors for the development of AF. The overall prevalence of AF in the United States is 2.3% in people older than 40 yr and 5.9% in those older than 65 yr. The number of patients with AF is likely to increase by 2.5 fold during the next 50 yr, reflecting the growing proportion of elderly individuals (7).

AF has been shown to cause structural and electrophysiologic remodeling of the atrium (8). These basic research findings can easily be translated to the clinical situation where it is well known that the duration of an AF episode is a profound determinant of whether sinus rhythm can be restored and maintained. The enlarged left atrial size commonly observed in patients with long standing AF can also be attributed to this atrial remodeling.

Relationship Between Atrial Fibrillation and Heart Failure

Eugene Braunwald recently declared that "AF and heart failure are the two new epidemics of cardiovascular disease" (9). Both result in economic cost, morbidity, and mortality. Both increase in the elderly (incidence doubles with each additional decade of life) and both have a propensity to coexist due to shared risk factors. The interaction of two conditions generates a vicious cycle, with AF enhancing the development of congestive heart failure and vice versa. In Framingham Heart Study (10), among 1470 subjects, 41% of congestive heart failure (CHF) patients developed AF and 42% of AF patients developed CHF. AF may be the underlying rhythm in up to 50% of the patients with severe heart failure (11). In AF subjects, the presence of development of CHF was associated with 2–3 fold increase in mortality.

There are three factors during AF, which can adversely affect impact hemodynamic function: loss of synchronous atrial mechanical activity, irregularity of ventricular response, and inappropriately rapid heart rate. This hemodynamic deterioration was seen in a prospective observational study (12). The development of new-onset chronic AF in heart failure patients was associated with a significant worsening of NYHA functional class (mean 2.4–2.9) and a significant reduction in cardiac index (mean 1.8–2.2). Heart failure by itself confers a risk of stroke and thromboembolism. The risk appears to be additive to that of AF (13–15). In SAVE trial (15), every 5% decrease in EF was associated with 18% increase of risk of stroke.

Management

In all heart failure patients with AF, there are four major issues that must be addressed: (1) prevention of systemic embolization, (2) reversion to sinus rhythm, (3) maintenance of sinus rhythm, and (4) control of the ventricular rate.

Prevention of Systemic Embolization in CHF Patients with Atrial Fibrillation and/or Atrial Flutter

Perhaps the single most important aspect of management of patients with CHF and AF is anticoagulation. Evidence from randomized controlled trials (16–20) indicates that in patients with AF, moderate to severe LV systolic dysfunction substantially increases the risk of cardioembolic events. According to ACC/AHA guidelines, warfarin, adjusted to achieve an INR of 2 to 3, should be administered in patients with heart failure and paroxysmal or chronic AF regardless of patient age (21–24).

Rate Versus Rhythm Control

Whether the "rate control" or "rhythm control" approach to AF is optimal in the setting of AF and HF remains a topic of debate. The rationale for restoring and maintaining sinus rhythm includes the potential reduction of symptoms, improved exercise tolerance, a lower risk of stroke, better quality of life, and the potential for better survival (25). Although this approach is inherently attractive, there have been no prospective randomized clinical trials which have demonstrated better outcomes among patients treated with a rate or rhythm control strategy. The AFFIRM study compared these two treatment strategies in more than 4000 patients with minimally symptomatic AF. No difference in outcomes was noted. It is important to note, however, that this does not disprove the hypothesis that if we were able to effectively and safely restore sinus rhythm that outcomes may have been improved. It is important to recognize that in the AFFIRM trial, as with all other rate versus rhythm control trials, many patients randomized to "rhythm control" were in AF, whereas a significant proportion of patients randomized to rate control were in sinus rhythm. In a recent report from the AFFIRM investigators, "on-treatment" analysis revealed that the presence of sinus rhythm was associated with 47% decrease in the risk of death (26). Several other observations support the concept that if sinus rhythm could be safely and effectively restored, this may be the optimal approach to management. In the CHF-STAT trial (27), heart failure patients on amiodarone who spontaneously converted to sinus rhythm and maintained it during the follow-up period had significantly lower mortality as compared to those who remained in AF ($p=0.04$). In the DIAMOND substudy (28), dofetilide had no effect on all-cause mortality but restoration and maintenance of sinus rhythm in patients with heart failure and AF/atrial flutter was associated with significant reduction in mortality ($P<0.0001$). Another important study which supports the value of rhythm control is a recent study by Hsu et al. (29). These investigators compared the outcomes of catheter ablation of AF among 58 patients with CHF and AF and a comparison group with AF but with normal ventricular function. (29). This study demonstrated that catheter ablation had similar efficacy in these two patient groups (78% in the patients with CHF vs. 84% in controls with the use of antiarrhythmic drugs, 69% and 71%, respectively without the use of antiarrhythmic drugs) and that restoration and maintenance of sinus rhythm by catheter ablation resulted in a significant improvement in ventricular function. This study was not powered adequately to assess the effect on mortality.

At the end of the day, it remains difficult to be certain whether rate or rhythm control is the optimal approach. There have been no prospective randomized clinical trials to address this issue. And to the extent that a safe and highly effective approach to restoration and maintenance of sinus rhythm in heart failure patients does not exist, it appears unlikely that these data will be forthcoming any time soon.

In our experience, every effort should be made to restore and maintain sinus rhythm in patients with heart failure, particularly among those in whom it is anticipated that the AF is truly symptomatic.

RHYTHM CONTROL

In this section of the chapter we discuss approaches that may be employed for rhythm control.

Reversion to Normal Sinus Rhythm

An important first step in restoring and maintaining sinus rhythm is electrical cardioversion. Although a number of pharmacologic approaches have been described, in our experience these are of little value, and electrical cardioversion should be relied on as the primary approach for restoration of sinus rhythm. When considering cardioversion it is important to pay careful attention to the issue of anticoagulation. Patients either should be systemically anticoagulated for 3 wk before and after cardioversion ($INR>2.0$) or a TEE should be performed prior to cardioversion to rule out a left atrial clot. If the TEE approach is used, it is important to be certain that systemic anticoagulation should be maintained for 4 wk after cardioversion. And unless this is a first episode of AF, current guidelines would suggest that all CHF patients with AF should be anticoagulated indefinitely (30).

Maintenance of Normal Sinus Rhythm

The long-term maintenance of sinus rhythm can be achieved by pharmacological or non-pharmacological methods.

Pharmacological Rhythm Control

According to the ACC/AHA/EHS guidelines, amiodarone and dofetilide should be the first-line agents to maintain sinus rhythm in heart failure patients because of proven safety and efficacy of these medications and increased pro-arrhythmic activity seen with Class IA/IC antiarrhythmic drugs and sotalol (31). Another concern with the use of Class I antiarrhythmic drugs in CHF patients is the associated negative inotropic effect (32–34).

Amiodarone. Amiodarone is a Class III antiarrhythmic drug. The safety and efficacy of low-dose amiodarone (<400 mg/day) has been validated (35,36). The major benefits of the use of low-dose amiodarone in heart failure are its neutral effect on survival (37), the lack of negative inotropic effect and absent or little pro-arrhythmic effect (35). In a meta-analysis of four randomized controlled trials (35) consisting of 738 patients, there were no cases of torsades de pointes. Interestingly, 3 cases of pro-arrhythmia occurred in the placebo group. In the CHF-STAT trial (38), patients with AF and CHF were randomized to either amiodarone or placebo and followed for four years. Amiodarone was associated with a greater likelihood of reverting to sinus rhythm (31% vs. 8%) and significantly lower mean (20%) and maximum (22%) ventricular rates as compared to placebo. Moreover, the patients initially in sinus rhythm had a lesser likelihood of developing AF (4.1% vs. 8.3%) if they were on amiodarone. In Canadian Trial of Atrial Fibrillation (CTAF), 430 patients were randomized (39) to either amiodarone or a second group (sotalol or propafenone in an open-label fashion). Over a mean follow-up of 458 days, 35% of patients on amiodarone had recurrence of AF compared with 63% of patients on propafenone or sotalol ($P<0.001$). The probability of remaining in SR over 1 yr with amiodarone was 69% versus 39% for propafenone or sotalol ($P<0.001$). The major early side effect of amiodarone (during loading) in patients with moderate or severe left ventricular systolic dysfunction was found to be bradyarrhythmia, requiring discontinuation of digoxin or permanent pacemaker placement in a significant proportion of patients (32% and 19%, respectively) in a retrospective study of 37 patients (40).

Although amiodarone is considered to be the most effective antiarrhythmic agent for treatment of AF, its use is limited by the development of side effects. The most common side effects associated with amiodarone include corneal microdeposits (>90%), photosensitivity (25–75%),increased liver transaminases (15–50%), cough with infiltrates on chest radiography and reduced DLCO (1–15%), hypo- and hyperthyroidism (2–24%) and gastrointestinal (30%) and neurological (3–30%) side effects (41–44). In an 11-year follow-up study of a subset of patients in CIDS study, 50% of the patients taking amiodarone eventually required discontinuation or dose reduction (45).

Dofetilide. Dofetilide is another antiarrhythmic agent which can be used for treatment of AF in heart failure patients. Dofetilide is a pure Class III antiarrhythmic agent that was recently approved for treatment of AF. It selectively inhibits K current. It has no negative inotropic actions and has no effect on sinus node function or cardiac conduction. In the DIAMOND CHF trial, it was shown to be effective and safe in preventing recurrent AF in CHF patients (46). It was shown to reduce the risk of all-cause or CHF-related hospitalizations (46). In a pooled subgroup analysis of DIAMOND studies (28), dofetilide had no effect on all-cause mortality but the restoration and maintenance of sinus rhythm was associated with a significant reduction in mortality (P<0.0001). In DIAMOND CHF trial (46), after cardioversion to sinus rhythm (either pharmacological or electrical), those treated with dofetilide were more likely to be in sinus rhythm (57% versus 28%). Among patients in sinus rhythm at baseline, those treated with dofetilide were less likely to develop AF (2% versus 6%). In the patients with normal QTc interval (<429 msec), dofetilide was associated with a significant reduction in mortality (risk ratio 0.4) while mortality was increased in those with QTc >479 msec (risk ratio 1.3). The most significant adverse effect associated with dofetilide was torsades de pointes, seen in 3.3% of patients (46).

Dofetilide can only be initiated on an in patient basis because of the risk of proarrhythmia. (47,48). The dose of dofetilide is based on patient weight and creatinine clearance. The most common adverse event is bradycardia followed by significant QT prolongation, ventricular arrhythmia, heart failure, rapid ventricular response, conduction abnormalities, hypotension, and stroke. The greatest risk is in the first 24 hr, in elderly patients and in patients with previous myocardial infarction (47).

Non-pharmacological Rhythm Control

If pharmacologic attempts at maintenance of sinus rhythm fail or are associated with significant side effects, nonpharmacologic approaches can be considered. Catheter ablation of AF is now performed in most major EP laboratories throughout the world. Catheter ablation of AF is performed in most centers using a circumferential approach with or without pulmonary vein isolation. These approaches involve the creation of continuous encircling lesions around the two left and two right pulmonary veins (49–51). A recent worldwide survey reported the outcomes of 8745 patients who underwent catheter ablation of AF at 90 distinct centers worldwide (50). The overall success rate (no AF, off drugs) was 52%. An additional 23.9% of patients were rendered AF free with antiarrhythmic therapy.

Less is known about the efficacy of catheter ablation in patients with AF and heart failure. The majority of pulmonary vein isolation procedures have been performed in patients with preserved left ventricular systolic function (52–56). However, a significant percentage of patients with AF have reduced systolic function (57). There have been two recent studies which have examined this question (29,58). In one study (29), 58 patients with CHF who underwent catheter ablation for AF, were compared to 58 patients without CHF who also underwent catheter ablation, matched according to age, sex and AF type. At 12 mo follow-up, 69% of patients with CHF and 71% of controls were in sinus rhythm without the administration of antiarrhythmic drugs (78% and 84% respectively, with antiarrhythmic drugs). The patients with CHF had significant improvement in LV function (mean increase in EF of 21% and fractional shortening of 11%, respectively $p<0.001$), LV dimensions (mean decreases in the diastolic and systolic diameters of 6 and 8 mm respectively, $p<0.001$). Among the subset of patients with presumed tachycardia-mediated cardiomyopathy (without structural heart disease and with inadequate prior rate control), 92% had a marked improvement in LVEF with ablation (an increase of $\geq 20\%$ or an increase to a final EF of $\geq 55\%$). The EF improved significantly not only in patients with concurrent structural heart disease and those with inadequate rate control before ablation, but also in those without coexisting heart disease and adequate rate control before ablation, supporting the recent finding that irregular rhythm decreases the cardiac output, independent of heart rate (59). In another study (60), after pulmonary vein isolation, there was a significant improvement in quality of life and about 75% of the patients with impaired EF remained AF free at the end of follow-up. There was a non-significant rise of 4.6% in EF.

Although both of the above-mentioned studies were nonrandomized, restoration and maintenance of sinus rhythm with catheter ablation in patients with AF and CHF without the use of antiarrhythmic drugs was shown to be a safe and effective option. Before recommending it as the first-line therapy for general population, randomized studies with more patients are needed. Catheter ablation for AF was recently developed and is still evolving. It is technically challenging and has a significant learning curve and potential risks. Further developments are needed to make it safer and easier. If rhythm control therapy is chosen, concurrent AV nodal blockade should be considered to prevent an exacerbation of CHF due to a rapid ventricular response in the case of recurrence of AF and to prevent a 1:1 response in the case of recurrence of atrial flutter.

RATE CONTROL

Rate control is an approach that can be used for treatment of AF patients either as primary therapy or if antiarrhythmic therapy or nonpharmacologic approaches are unsuccessful.

Pharmacological Rate Control

There are three classes of drugs which are widely used for rate control of AF: calcium channel blockers, beta-blockers, and digoxin. Although amiodarone is also effective for rate control, its side effect profile is such that it should not be relied on for rate control due to the high likelihood of developing side effects. A recent study reported the outcomes of a head-to-head comparison of several different rate control strategies. This crossover, open-label outpatient study was conducted comparing the effects of digoxin, diltiazem, and atenolol on the exercise-induced changes of ventricular rate in patients with chronic AF (61). The results of this study demonstrated that beta-blockers are most effective for rate control and that digoxin is least effective for rate control. Not surprisingly, combination therapy was more effective than monotherapy. Based on the results of this study, as well as the well-established benefits of beta-blockade and digoxin in the treatment of heart failure patients, we prefer to employ these two drugs for pharmacologic rate control in this setting.

Beta-Blockers

As noted above, beta-blockers are considered to be the most effective rate control medication in patients with AF. There are no data on the safety and efficacy of the use of beta-blockers in acute AF in patients with left ventricular dysfunction. Thus, their use in this setting has to be individualized. A few studies have investigated the role of beta-blockers in the long-term rate control of chronic AF in the setting of left ventricular dysfunction. In a recent retrospective analysis of the US Carvedilol Heart Failure Trials Program (62), carvedilol was associated with a significant improvement in left ventricular ejection fraction (from 23% to 33% with carvedilol and 24% to 27% with placebo, $P=0.001$) in patients with chronic AF and CHF. A trend toward a reduction in the combined end-point of death or CHF-related hospitalization was also observed ($p=0.055$). Other studies have also shown that beta-blockers control ventricular rate effectively, improve ventricular function, and are well tolerated when added to digoxin (63–65). However, great care should be used when initiating beta-blockers in patients with AF and CHF.

Digoxin

Despite its widespread use in heart failure patients who have AF, digoxin is only minimally effective in slowing the ventricular response to AF (66). Because of this, digoxin is commonly used in conjunction with beta-blockers or calcium channel blockers. A randomized, double-blind, placebo-controlled trial in patients with persistent AF and CHF demonstrated that the combination of digoxin and carvedilol was more effective in controlling ventricular rate as compared to digoxin or carvedilol alone (67).

Diltiazem

Limited experience (67–71) suggests that intravenous diltiazem is safe and more effective than digoxin for rate control in patients with heart failure and acute onset AF. The negative inotropic effect of diltiazem in the patients with acute AF and severe CHF is probably offset by a significant reduction in heart rate and peripheral vascular resistance. This explains the lack of significant reduction in ejection fraction and cardiac index despite significant reduction in mean arterial pressure and pulmonary capillary wedge pressure, observed in studies (72,73). Although the long-term use of ditiazem for rate control of AF in CHF patients has been shown to be beneficial in some series of CHF patients, other studies question its safety particularly in patients with severe heart failure. At this point we would suggest that diltiazem not be considered a first-line option for rate control in CHF patients. However, in selected situations, particularly when beta-blockers are contraindicated, diltiazem may be of value (74–76).

Non-pharmacological Rate Control

Catheter ablation of the AV junction and placement of a permanent pacemaker is a safe and highly effective approach to achieving rate control among patients with AF and CHF. A randomized controlled trial (77) has confirmed the effectiveness of this approach in controlling symptoms in patients with CHF, at 12-month follow-up. Ozcan et al. recently reported a study of 350 patients who underwent ablation of atrioventricular node and implantation of a permanent pacemaker (78). This study showed that in the absence of underlying heart disease, survival among patients with AF after ablation of AV node was similar to expected survival in the general population. However, a history of CHF was shown to be an independent predictor of death ($P=0.02$) after a mean follow-up of 36 mo, as compared to general population. In another study (79), the same authors studied the long-term survival in the patients with AF and CHF who underwent AV node ablation. This study included 58 patients with CHF who were followed up for a mean of 40 mo following AV node ablation. The results of this study demonstrated that after ablation, the LVEF nearly normalized ($\geq 45\%$) in 16 study patients (29%), in whom observed survival was comparable to that of normal subjects ($p=0.37$). Survival worsened in the patients with persistent LV dysfunction despite undergoing ablation (79), underscoring the impact of improvement in LV function after the procedure. It is particularly notable that a number of studies have reported that ventricular function may improve following ablation of the AV junction. This likely reflects the fact that in a subset of patients, AF with a rapid ventricular response can cause a reversible tachycardia-induced cardiomyopathy (80–84).

One potential down side of catheter ablation of the AV node and placement of a permanent pacemaker, is that this creates ventricular dyssynchrony as a result of stimulation of the right ventricular apex. In effect, this results in the same physiology as observed in patients with a LBBB. A recent study (PAVE trial) randomized patients undergoing AV node ablation to placement of a standard single chamber pacemaker or to placement of a biventricular pacemaker (85). One hundred eighty-four patients with chronic AF and CHF (NYHA class I–III) were randomly assigned to BiV pacing or standard RV pacing following AV junction ablation. At six months, BiV pacing was associated with significantly greater six-minute walking distance, peak oxygen consumption with exercise, and exercise duration. No significant change was seen in LVEF among patients with BiV pacing, while the LVEF fell from 45% to 41% in patients treated with RV pacing (85).

Isolated RV pacing has been shown to worsen heart failure and increase the frequency of AF (86,87). Upgrading to BiV pacing after chronic RV pacing in 20 patients with AF, CHF, and prior AV nodal ablation, was shown to improve the myocardial function (88).

ACE Inhibitors and Prevention of AF

A number of randomized studies have demonstrated that treatment with ACE inhibitors may also reduce AF. Trandolapril reduced the incidence of AF in a large cohort of post-MI patients with significant LV systolic dysfunction (89). Whether this effect was due to post-remodeling effect of ACE inhibitors post-MI or primary antiarrhythmic effect of ACE inhibitors on atrial myocardium preventing the onset of AF is not clear. In a recent meta-analysis of 7 randomized trials (90), there was a significant difference in the pooled development of AF in the people who were on ACE inhibitors or ARBs, as compared to controls ($P=0.003$). There is evidence for antiarrhythmic properties of ACE inhibitors, although the mechanism is unclear (91,92). Proposed mechanisms are reduction of atrial premature beats, reduction of atrial pressure (93), and increase in local bradykinin (94).

ATRIAL FLUTTER

Overview and Clinical Significance

Atrial flutter is also common in heart failure patients. Atrial flutter generally has a regular atrial rate varying from 250 to 350 bpm in the absence of antiarrhythmic therapy. There is generally 2:1 or 4:1 conduction to the ventricle resulting in a ventricular response of approximately 75 bpm. Like AF, atrial flutter is important because it can cause symptoms and also can increase stroke risk. The symptoms associated with atrial flutter result from the rapid rate, and loss of effective atrial contraction. Although the exact incidence of atrial flutter is unknown, it is estimated to be present in about 10% of the patients presenting with a supraventricular tachycardia (95). The overall incidence in general population increases markedly with age, ranging from 5 per 100,000 person-years under age 50 to 587 per 100,000 person-years over age 80 (96). The risk of developing atrial flutter increases 3.5 times in the patients with heart failure (96).

Atrial flutter is a macroreentrant arrhythmia that involves a single reentry circuit. The most common type of atrial flutter can be recognized by the presence of characteristic saw tooth flutter waves in the inferior leads and a positive flutter wave in V1. This type of atrial flutter results from a circuit which is confined to the right atrium and travels around the tricuspid annulus in a counterclockwise direction. The cavo-tricuspid isthmus is a critical component of the reentry circuit.

Relationship Between Atrial Flutter and Heart Failure

In a population-based study, among 118 new cases of atrial flutter, 16% were attributable to heart failure (96). Atrial flutter causes an increase in the mean right and left atrial pressure (97) and can cause tachycardia-induced cardiomyopathy or worsen pre-existing heart failure.

Management

Similar to AF, there are four goals of management: prevention of systemic embolization (discussed above in AF section), reversion to normal sinus rhythm, maintenance of normal sinus rhythm, and control of the ventricular rate.

Reversion to Normal Sinus Rhythm

Atrial flutter is generally an incessant arrhythmia that does not terminate spontaneously. There are three approaches that can be used to terminate atrial flutter. The most common approach is electrical cardioversion. The technique is identical to that used for AF, although lower energy settings are generally effective. The same guidelines for anticoagulation also apply. A second approach is to use overdrive pacing to terminate atrial flutter. This technique involves pacing the atrium 20 to 50 bpm faster than the atrial flutter rate. Although it is highly effective, this approach is impractical unless the patient is postoperative and external wires are on the atrium, or if the patient has a pacemaker capable of rapid atrial pacing for termination of atrial flutter. The third approach to termination of atrial flutter is catheter ablation. This will be described in more detail below.

Although pharmacologic cardioverion can be performed, it has only limited efficacy. Ibutilide is considered to be the most effective antiarrhythmic agent for acute termination of atrial flutter. Stambler et al. (98) recently reported that intravenous ibutilide had a higher efficacy in atrial flutter than fibrillation (63% versus 31%, P< .0001) but 8.3% patients developed polymorphic ventricular tachycardia. It is for this reason that we rarely, if ever, employ ibutilide for pharmacologic cardioversion of atrial flutter.

Maintenance of Normal Sinus Rhythm

Catheter ablation is considered to be first-line therapy for treatment of atrial flutter. Catheter ablation of atrial flutter involving the cavo-tricuspid isthmus is a very safe and highly effective procedure. Catheter ablation of atrial flutter is commonly performed on an outpatient basis. Two catheters are placed in the heart—a multipolar mapping catheter and the ablation catheter. RF energy is delivered between the tricuspid valve and in inferior vena cava. Most studies have reported an acute efficacy for this procedure greater than 90% with a less than 1% risk of complications (99–109). Although pharmacologic therapy can also be used for treatment of atrial flutter, a recent randomized trial reported that catheter ablation was superior to pharmacologic therapy with propafenone (80% vs. 36% respectively, P<0.01) (110).

Control of Ventricular Rate

The goals of controlling the ventricular response in a CHF patient are the same as in AF, i.e., to reduce symptoms, prevent hemodynamic instability and pulmonary edema and prevent tachycardia-induced cardiomyopathy. Intravenous diltiazem is the drug of choice for acute control of atrial flutter in patients with normal LV function. It should be used with caution in advanced heart failure, although limited evidence (68) suggests that it may be safe. There are no data on the safety and efficacy of intravenous beta-blockers in acute atrial flutter in the patients with CHF and their use should be individualized in this setting. Digoxin can be the first-line drug in acute atrial flutter in CHF (although efficacy is relatively low) and it can be given with beta-blockers or calcium channel blockers. It can also be used to achieve long-term control of ventricular rate in a patient with CHF. A larger dose of digoxin is needed to control the ventricular rate than used in AF because a greater AV nodal refractoriness must be produced (111). The higher doses of digoxin necessary to control the ventricular response to atrial flutter may result in serum levels associated with increased mortality. Therefore, digoxin should probably not be used alone to control rate in atrial flutter if the patient has CHF.

OTHER SUPRAVENTRICULAR TACHYCARDIAS

Overview, Clinical Significance, and Management

Although AF and atrial flutter are the most important supraventricular arrhythmias observed in patients with CHF, any type of supraventricular arrhythmias may be observed. Perhaps the most common type of SVT following AF and atrial flutter is paroxysmal supraventricular tachycardia resulting from AV node reentry or a concealed or manifest accessory pathway. Catheter ablation is considered first line in the management of these arrhythmias. Success rates in excess of 95% with complication rates of <3% are routinely achieved in virtually all EP laboratories. There is little role for antiarrhythmic therapy in the treatment of these types of supraventricular arrhythmias. A less common type of SVT is atrial tachycardia. Atrial tachycardia may either be focal or multifocal. Focal atrial tachycardias are also highly amenable to treatment with catheter ablation. Multifocal atrial tachycardia (MAT) is characterized by variability in P wave morphology. MAT can occur in the presence of any heart disease or acute critical illness like sepsis or recent surgery, particularly when associated with CHF or underlying lung disease. Treatment must be aimed at correcting any correctable underlying disorder which includes pulmonary and cardiac disease, hypokalemia, and hypomagnesemia. The use of antiarrhythmic drugs has generally been disappointing (112). Radiofrequency modification of AV junction has been shown to be effective in refractory MAT cases (113).

CONCLUSION

In conclusion, supraventricular arrhythmias are common among patients with heart failure. By far the most common types are AF and atrial flutter. For each of these arrhythmias systemic anticoagulation is essential. Although definitive data are still lacking, efforts to restore and maintain sinus rhythm are generally warranted. And if unsuccessful, rate control strategies can be employed. AF is generally treated initially with antiarrhythmic drugs. If these are ineffective or poorly tolerated, catheter ablation of AF has become a promising new option. Typical atrial flutter can be treated safely and effectively with catheter ablation (unless the patient has decompensated CHF), which is considered to be the first-line therapy. The approach to treatment of paroxymal supraventricular tachycardia and other types of atrial tachycardias is similar to the approach used in non-heart failure patients. It is especially important to be vigilant for the possibility that a patient's CHF may be due to a rate-related cardiomyopathy, which is reversible with effective rate control.

REFERENCES

1. Feinberg WM, Blackshear JL, Laupacis A, Kronmal R, Hart RG. Prevalence, age distribution, and gender of patients with atrial fibrillation, analysis and implications. Arch Intern Med. 155 1995.
2. Wolf PA, Kannel WB, McGee DL, Meeks SL, Bharucha NE, McNamara PM. Duration of atrial fibrillation and imminence of stroke: the Framingham study. Stroke 1983; 14:664–667.
3. Majeed A, Moser K, Carroll K. Trends in the prevalence and management of atrial fibrillation in general practice in England and Wales, 1994–1998: analysis of data from the general practice research database. Heart 2001; 86:284–288.
4. Feinberg WM, Blackshear JL, Laupacis A, Kronmal R, Hart RG. Prevalence, age distribution, and gender of patients with atrial fibrillation. Analysis and implications. Arch Intern Med 1995; 155:469–473.
5. Go AS, Hylek EM, Phillips KA, et al. Prevalence of diagnosed atrial fibrillation in adults: national implications for rhythm management and stroke prevention: the AnTicoagulation and Risk Factors in Atrial Fibrillation (ATRIA) Study. JAMA 2001; 285:2370–2375.
6. Wang TJ, Parise H, Levy D, et al. Obesity and the risk of new-onset atrial fibrillation. JAMA 2004; 282:2471–2477.
7. Go AS, Hylek EM, Phillips KA, et al. Prevalence of diagnosed atrial fibrillation in adults: national implications for rhythm management and stroke prevention: the Anticoagulation and Risk Factors in Atrial Fibrillation (ATRIA) Study. JAMA 2001; 285:2370–2375.
8. Wijffels MC, Kirchhof CJ, Dorland R, Allessie MA. Atrial fibrillation begets trial fibrillation. A study in awake chronically instrumented goats. Circulation 1995; 92:1954–1968.
9. Braunwald E. Shattuck lecture—cardiovascular medicine at the turn of the millennium: triumphs, concerns, and opportunities. N Engl J Med 1997; 337:1360–1369.
10. Wang TJ, Larson MG, Levy D, et al. Temporal relations of atrial fibrillation and congestive heart failure and their joint influence on mortality: the Framingham Heart Study. Circulation 2003; 107:2920–2925. Epub 2003 May 27.
11. Effects of enalapril on mortality in severe congestive heart failure. Results of the Cooperative North Scandinavian Enalapril Survival Study (CONSENSUS). The CONSENSUS Trial Study Group. N Engl J Med 1987; 316:1429–1435.
12. Pozzoli M, Cioffi G, Traversi E, et al. Predictors of primary atrial fibrillation and concomitant clinical and hemodynamic changes in patients with chronic heart failure: a prospective study in 344 patients with baseline sinus rhythm. J Am Coll Cardiol 1998; 32:197.
13. Lip GY. Intracardiac thrombus formation in cardiac impairment: the role of anticoagulant therapy. Postgrad Med J 1996; 72:731–738.
14. The Stroke Prevention in Atrial Fibrillation Investigators. Predictors of thromboembolism in atrial fibrillation: II. Echocardiographic features of patients at risk. Ann Intern Med 1992; 116:6–12.
15. Loh E, Sutton MS, Wun CC, et al. Ventricular dysfunction and the risk of stroke after myocardial infarction. N Engl J Med 1997; 336:251–257.
16. The effect of low-dose warfarin on the risk of stroke in patients with nonrheumatic atrial fibrillation. The Boston Area Anticoagulation Trial for Atrial Fibrillation Investigators. N Engl J Med 1990; 323:1505–1511.
17. Ezekowitz MD, Bridgers SL, James KE, et al. Warfarin in the prevention of stroke associated with nonrheumatic atrial fibrillation. Veterans affairs stroke prevention in nonrheumatic atrial fibrillation Investigators. N Engl J Med 1992; 327:1406–1412.
18. Petersen P, Boysen G, Godtfredsen J, Andersen ED, Andersen B. Placebo-controlled, randomised trial of warfarin and aspirin for prevention of thromboembolic complications in chronic atrial fibrillation. The copenhagen AFASAK study. Lancet 1989; 1:175–179.
19. Connolly SJ, Laupacis A, Gent M, Roberts RS, Cairns JA, Joyner C. Canadian Atrial Fibrillation Anticoagulation (CAFA) Study. J Am Coll Cardiol 1991; 18:349–355.
20. Stroke prevention in atrial fibrillation study. Final results. Circulation 1991; 84:527–539.

21. Laupacis A, Albers G, Dalen J, Dunn M, Feinberg W, Jacobson A. Antithrombotic therapy in atrial fibrillation. Chest 1995; 108:352S–359S.
22. Prystowsky EN, Benson DW, Jr, Fuster V, et al. Management of patients with atrial fibrillation. A Statement for Healthcare Professionals. From the Subcommittee on Electrocardiography and Electrophysiology, American Heart Association. Circulation 1996; 93:1262–1277.
23. Weigner MJ, Caulfield TA, Danias PG, Silverman DI, Manning WJ. Risk for clinical thromboembolism associated with conversion to sinus rhythm in patients with atrial fibrillation lasting less than 48 hours. Ann Intern Med 1997; 126:615–620.
24. Gallagher MM, Hennessy BJ, Edvardsson N, et al. Embolic complications of direct current cardioversion of atrial arrhythmias: association with low intensity of anticoagulation at the time of cardioversion. J Am Coll Cardiol 2002; 40:926–933.
25. Waldo AL. Management of atrial fibrillation: the need for affirmative action. Am J Cardiol 1999; 84:698–700.
26. The AFFIRM investigators. Relationships between sinus rhythm, treatment, and survival in the AFFIRM study. Circulation 2004; 109:1509–1513.
27. Deedwania PC, Singh BN, Ellenbogen K, Fisher S, Fletcher R, Singh SN. Spontaneous conversion and maintenance of sinus rhythm by amiodarone in patients with heart failure and atrial fibrillation: observations from the veterans affairs congestive heart failure survival trial of antiarrhythmic therapy (CHF-STAT). The Department of Veterans Affairs CHF-STAT Investigators. Circulation 1998; 98:2574–2579.
28. Pedersen OD, Bagger H, Keller N, Marchant B, Kober L, Torp-Pedersen C. Efficacy of dofetilide in the treatment of atrial fibrillation-flutter in patients with reduced left ventricular function: a Danish investigations of arrhythmia and mortality on dofetilide (diamond) substudy. Circulation 2001; 104:292–296.
29. Hsu LF, Jais P, Sanders P, et al. Catheter ablation for atrial fibrillation in congestive heart failure. N Engl J Med 2004; 351:2373–2383.
30. Fuster V, Ryden LE, Asinger RW, et al. ACC/AHA/ESC guidelines for the management of patients with atrial fibrillation: Executive summary. A report of the American College of Cardiology/American Heart Association Task Force on Practice Guidelines and the European Society of Cardiology Committee for Practice Guidelines and Policy Conferences (Committee to develop guidelines for the management of patients with atrial fibrillation). Developed in collaboration with the North American Society of Pacing and Electrophysiology. J Am Coll Cardiol 2001; 38:1231 no abstract available.
31. Lehmann MH, Hardy S, Archibald D, quart B, MacNeil DJ. Sex difference in risk of torsade de pointes with d,l-sotalol. Circulation 1996; 94:2535–2541.
32. Folk RH. Proarrhythmia in patients treated for atrial fibrillation or flutter. Ann Int Med 1992; 117:141–150.
33. Flaker GC, et al. Antiarrhythmic drug therapy and cardiac mortality in atrial fibrillation. J Am Coll Card 1992; 20:527–532.
34. Coplen SE, et al. Efficacy and safety of quinidine therapy for maintenance of sinus rhythm after cardioversion: a meta-analysis of randomized controlled trials. Circulation 1990; 82:1106–1116.
35. Vorperian VR, Havighurst TC, Miller S, January CT. Adverse effects of low dose amiodarone: a meta-analysis. J Am Coll Cardiol 1997; 30:791–798.
36. Deedwania PC, Singh BN, Ellenbogen K, Fisher S, Fletcher R, Singh SN. Spontaneous conversion and maintenance of sinus rhythm by amiodarone in patients with heart failure and atrial fibrillation: observations from the veterans affairs congestive heart failure survival trial of antiarrhythmic therapy (CHF-STAT). The Department of Veterans Affairs CHF-STAT Investigators. Circulation 1998; 98:2574–2579.
37. Effect of prophylactic amiodarone on mortality after acute myocardial infarction and in congestive heart failure: meta-analysis of individual data from 6500 patients in randomised trials. Amiodarone Trials Meta-Analysis Investigators. Lancet 1997; 350:1417–1424.

38. Deedwania PC, Singh BN, Ellenbogen K, Fisher S, Fletcher R, Singh SN. Spontaneous conversion and maintenance of sinus rhythm by amiodarone in patients with heart failure and atrial fibrillation: observations from the veterans affairs congestive heart failure survival trial of antiarrhythmic therapy (CHF-STAT). The Department of Veterans Affairs CHF-STAT Investigators. Circulation 1998; 98:2574–2579.
39. Roy D, Talajic M, Dorian P, et al. Amiodarone to prevent recurrence of atrial fibrillation. Canadian Trial of Atrial Fibrillation Investigators. N Engl J Med 2000; 342:913–920.
40. Weinfeld MS, Drazner MH, Stevenson WG, Stevenson LW. Early outcome of initiating amiodarone for atrial fibrillation in advanced heart failure. J Heart Lung Transplant 2000; 19:638–643.
41. Goldschlager N, Epstein AE, Naccarelli G, Olshansky B, Singh B. Practical guidelines for clinicians who treat patients with amiodarone. Practice guidelines subcommittee, North American society of pacing and electrophysiology. Arch Intern Med 2000; 160:1741–1748.
42. Vorperian VR, Havighurst TC, Miller S, January CT. Adverse effects of low dose amiodarone: a meta-analysis. J Am Coll Cardiol 1997; 30:791–798.
43. Harjai KJ, Licata AA. Effects of amiodarone on thyroid function. Ann Intern Med 1997; 126:63–73. Review.
44. Harjai KJ, Licata AA. Amiodarone induced hyperthyroidism: a case series and brief review of literature. Pacing Clin Electrophysiol 1996; 19:1548–1554. Review.
45. Bokhari F, Newman D, Greene M, et al. Long-term comparison of the implantable cardioverter defibrillator versus amiodarone: eleven-year follow-up of a subset of patients in the Canadian implantable defibrillator study (CIDS). Circulation 2004; 110:112–116.
46. Torp-Pedersen C, Moller M, Bloch-Thomsen PE, et al. Danish investigations of arrhythmia and mortality on dofetilide study group. Dofetilide in patients with congestive heart failure and left ventricular dysfunction. N Engl J Med 1999; 341:857–865.
47. Maisel WH, Kuntz KM, Reimold SC, et al. Risk of initiating antiarrhythmic drug therapy for atrial fibrillation in patients admitted to a university hospital. Ann Intern Med 1997; 127:281–284.
48. Hauser TH, Pinto DS, Josephson ME, Zimetbaum P. Safety and feasibility of a clinical pathway for the outpatient initiation of antiarrhythmic medications in patients with atrial fibrillation or atrial flutter. Am J Cardiol 2003; 91:1437–1441.
49. Vasamreddy CR, Dalal D, Eldadah Z, et al. Safety and efficacy of circumferential pulmonary vein catheter ablation of atrial fibrillation. Heart Rhythm 2005; 2:42–48.
50. Cappato R, Calkins H, Chen SA, Skanes A, et al. Worldwide survey on the methods, efficacy, and safety of catheter ablation for human atrial fibrillation. Circulation 2005; 111:1100–1105. Epub 2005 Feb 21.
51. Vasamreddy CR, Jayam V, Bluemke DA, Calkins H. Pulmonary vein occlusion: an unanticipated complication of catheter ablation of atrial fibrillation using the anatomic circumferential approach. Heart Rhythm 2004; 1:78–81.
52. Haissaguerre M, et al. Electrophysiological end point for catheter ablation of AF initiated from multiple pulmonary venous foci. Circulation 2000; 101:1409–1417.
53. Haissaguerre M, et al. Spontaneous initiation of AF by ectopic beats originating in the pulmonary veins. NEJM 1998; 339:659–666.
54. Pappone C, et al. Morbidity, mortality and quality of life after circumferential pulmonary vein ablation for AF. JACC 2003; 42:185–197.
55. Chen SA, et al. Initiation of AF by ectopic beats originating from the pulmonary veins: electrophysiologic characteristics, pharmacological responses, and effects of radiofrequency ablation. Circulation 1999; 100:1879–1886.
56. Pappone C, et al. Circumferential radiofrequency ablation of pulmonary vein ostia: a new anatomic approach for curing AF. Circulation 2000; 102:2619–2628.
57. Redfield MM, et al. Tachycardia-induced cardiomyopathy: a common cause of ventricular dysfunction in patients with AF referred for AV-nodal ablation. Mayo Clin Proc 2000; 75:790–795.

58. Pozzoli M, Cioffi G, Traversi E, Pinna GD, Cobelli F, Tavazzi L. Predictors of primary atrial fibrillation and concomitant clinical and hemodynamic changes in patients with chronic heart failure: a prospective study in 344 patients with baseline sinus rhythm. J Am Coll Cardiol 1998; 32:197–204.
59. Daoud EG, Weiss R, Bahu M, et al. Effect of an irregular ventricular rhythm on cardiac output. Am J Cardiol 1996; 78:1433–1436.
60. Michael S, Chen, et al. Pulmonary vein isolation for the treatment of AF in patients with impaired systolic function. J of Am Coll Cardiol 2004; 43:1004–1009.
61. Farshi R, Kistner D, Sarma JS, Longmate JA, Singh BN. Ventricular rate control in chronic atrial fibrillation during daily activity and programmed exercise: a crossover open-label study of five drug regimens. J Am Coll Cardiol 1999; 33:304–310.
62. Joglar JA, Acusta AP, Shusterman NH, et al. Effect of carvedilol on survival and hemodynamics in patients with atrial fibrillation and left ventricular dysfunction: retrospective analysis of the US Carvedilol Heart Failure Trials Program. Am Heart J 2001; 142:498–501.
63. Kudoh M. Clinical studies on long-term combined therapy of digitalis and xamoterol for patients with mild and moderate CHF accompanied by atrial fibrillation. Teikyo Med J 1988; 16:65–74.
64. Yahalom J. Beta-adrenergic blockade as adjunctive oral therapy in patients with chronic atrial fibrillation. Chest 1977; 71:592–596.
65. Cristodorescu R, et al. The heart rate slowing effect of pindolol in patients with digitalis resistant atrial fibrillation and heart failure. Rev Roum Med-Med Int 1986; 24:207–215.
66. Hou ZY, et al. Acute treatment of recent onset AF and flutter with a tailored dosing regimen of intravenous amiodarone. Eur Heart J 1995; 16:521–528.
67. Khand AU, Rankin AC, Martin W, et al. Carvedilol or digoxin for the treatment of atrial fibrillation in heart failure patients? (Abstract) Eur Heart J. 2000; 21:740.
68. Goldenberg IF, Lewis WR, Dias VC, Heywood JT, Pedersen WR. Intravenous diltiazem for the treatment of patients with atrial fibrillation or flutter and moderate to severe congestive heart failure. Am J Cardiol 1994; 74:884–889.
69. Heywood JT, Graham B, Marais GE, Jutzy KR. Effects of intravenous diltiazem on rapid atrial fibrillation accompanied by congestive heart failure. Am J Cardiol 1991; 67:1150–1152.
70. Packer M, et al. Comparative negative inotropic effects of nifedipine and diltiazem in patients wit severe left ventricular dysfunction. Am J Card 1984; 54:733–737.
71. Materne P, Legrand V, Vandormael M, Collignon P, Kulbertus HE. Hemodynamic effects of intravenous diltiazem with impaired left ventricular function. Am J Cardiol 1984; 54:733–737.
72. Walsh RW, Porter CB, Starling MR, O'Rourke RA. Beneficial hemodynamic effects of intravenous and oral diltiazem in severe congestive heart failure. J Am Coll Cardiol 1984; 3:1044–1050.
73. Kulick DL, McIntosh N, Campese VM, et al. Central and renal hemodynamic effects and hormonal response to diltiazem in severe congestive heart failure. Am J Cardiol 1987; 59:1138–1143.
74. Goldstein RE, et al. Diltiazem increases late-onset congestive heart failure in post-infarction patients with early reduction in ejection fraction. Circulation 1991; 83:52–60.
75. Liao YH. Interventional study of diltiazem in dilated cardiomyopathy: a report of multiple centre clinical trial in China. Chinese Cooperative Group of Diltiazem Intervention Trial in Dilated Cardiomyopathy. Int J Cardiol 1998; 64:25–30.
76. Figulla HR, Gietzen F, Zeymer U, et al. Diltiazem improves cardiac function and exercise capacity in patients with idiopathic dilated cardiomyopathy. Results of the Diltiazem in Dilated Cardiomyopathy Trial. Circulation 1996; 94:346–352.
77. Brignole M, Menozzi C, Gianfranchi L, et al. Assessment of atrioventricular junction ablation and VVIR pacemaker versus pharmacological treatment in patients with heart failure and chronic atrial fibrillation: a randomized, controlled study. brignoleomninet.it. Circulation 1998; 98:953–960.

78. Ozcan C, Jahangir A, Friedman PA, et al. Long-term survival after ablation of the atrioventricular node and implantation of a permanent pacemaker in patients with atrial fibrillation. N Engl J Med 2001; 344:1043–1051.
79. Ozcan C, Jahangir A, Friedman PA, et al. Significant effects of atrioventricular node ablation and pacemaker implantation on left ventricular function and long-term survival in patients with atrial fibrillation and left ventricular dysfunction. Am J Cardiol 2003; 92:33–37.
80. Twidale N, Sutton K, Bartlett L, et al. Effects on cardiac performance of atrioventricular node catheter ablation using radiofrequency current for drug-refractory atrial arrhythmias. Pacing Clin Electrophysiol 1993; 16:1275–1284.
81. Edner M, Caidahl K, Bergfeldt L, Darpo B, Edvardsson N, Rosenqvist M. Prospective study of left ventricular function after radiofrequency ablation of atrioventricular junction in patients with atrial fibrillation. Br Heart J 1995; 74:261–267.
82. Heinz G, Siostrzonek P, Kreiner G, Gossinger H. Improvement in left ventricular systolic function after successful radiofrequency His bundle ablation for drug refractory, chronic atrial fibrillation and recurrent atrial flutter. Am J Cardiol 1992; 69:489–492.
83. Twidale N, Manda V, Nave K, Seal A. Predictors of outcome after radiofrequency catheter ablation of the atrioventricular node for atrial fibrillation and congestive heart failure. Am Heart J 1998; 136:647–657.
84. Kay GN, Ellenbogen KA, Giudici M, et al. The Ablate and Pace Trial: a prospective study of catheter ablation of the AV conduction system and permanent pacemaker implantation for treatment of atrial fibrillation. APT Investigators. J Interv Card Electrophysiol 1998; 2:121–135.
85. Data presented at the 2004 Scientific Sessions of the American College of Cardiology.
86. Wilkoff BL, Cook JR, Epstein AE, et al. Dual-chamber pacing or ventricular backup pacing in patients with an implantable defibrillator: the Dual Chamber and VVI Implantable Defibrillator (DAVID) Trial. JAMA 2002; 288:3115–3123.
87. Sweeney MO, Hellkamp AS, Ellenbogen KA, et al. Adverse effect of ventricular pacing on heart failure and atrial fibrillation among patients with normal baseline QRS duration in a clinical trial of pacemaker therapy for sinus node dysfunction. Circlulation 2003; 107:2932–2937. Epub 2003 Jun 2.
88. Leon AR, Greenberg JM, Kanuru N, et al. Cardiac resynchronization in patients with congestive heart failure and chronic atrial fibrillation: effect of upgrading to biventricular pacing after chronic right ventricular pacing. J Am Coll Cardiol 2002; 39:1258–1263.
89. Pedersen OD, Bagger H, Kober L, Torp-Pedersen C. Trandolapril reduces the incidence of atrial fibrillation after acute myocardial infarction in patients with left ventricular dysfunction. Circulation 1999; 100:376–380.
90. Madrid AH, Peng J, Zamora J, et al. The role of angiotensin receptor blockers and/or angiotensin converting enzyme inhibitors in the prevention of atrial fibrillation in patients with cardiovascular diseases: meta-analysis of randomized controlled clinical trials. Pacing Clin Electrophysiol 2004; 27:1405–1410.
91. Budaj A, Cybulski J, Cedro K, et al. Effects of captopril on ventricular arrhythmias in the early and late phase of suspected acute myocardial infarction. Randomized, placebo-controlled substudy of ISIS-4. Eur Heart J 1996; 17:1506–1510.
92. Campbell RW. ACE inhibitors and arrhythmias. Heart 1996; 76:79–82.
93. Kontopoulos AG, Athyros VG, Papageorgiou AA, Boudoulas H. Effect of quinapril or metoprolol on circadian sympathetic and parasympathetic modulation after acute myocardial infarction. Am J Cardiol 1999; 84:1164–1169.
94. Cleland, et al. Bradykinin and ventricular function. Eur Heart J 2000; 2:H20–H29.
95. Bialy D, et al. Hospitalization for arrhythmias in the United States: importance of atrial fibrillation. J Am Coll Cardiol 1992; 19:716. Abstract.
96. Granada J, Uribe W, Chyou PH, et al. Incidence and predictors of atrial flutter in the general population. J Am Coll Cardiol 2000; 36:2242–2246.
97. Alboni P, Scarfo S, Fuca G, Paparella N, Mele D. Atrial and ventricular pressures in atrial flutter. Pacing Clin Electrophysiol 1999; 22:600–604.

98. Stambler BS, Wood MA, Ellenbogen KA, Perry KT, Wakefield LK, VanderLugt JT. Efficacy and safety of repeated intravenous doses of ibutilide for rapid conversion of atrial flutter or fibrillation. Ibutilide Repeat Dose Study Investigators. Circulation 1996; 94:1613–1621.
99. Poty H, Saoudi N, Abdel Aziz A, Nair M, Letac B. Radiofrequency catheter ablation of type 1 atrial flutter. Prediction of late success by electrophysiological criteria. Circulation 1995; 92:1389–1392.
100. Schumacher B, Pfeiffer D, Tebbenjohanns J, Lewalter T, Jung W, Luderitz B. Acute and long-term effects of consecutive radiofrequency applications on conduction properties of the subeustachian isthmus in type I atrial flutter. J Cardiovasc Electrophysiol 1998; 9:152–163.
101. Tai CT, Chen SA, Chiang CE, et al. Long-term outcome of radiofrequency catheter ablation for typical atrial flutter: risk prediction of recurrent arrhythmias. J Cardiovasc Electrophysiol 1998; 9:115–121.
102. Nabar A, Rodriguez LM, Timmermans C, Smeets JL, Wellens HJ. Isoproterenol to evaluate resumption of conduction after right atrial isthmus ablation in type I atrial flutter. Circulation 1999; 99:3286–3291.
103. Calkins H, Leon AR, Deam AG, Kalbfleisch SJ, Langberg JJ, Morady F. Catheter ablation of atrial flutter using radiofrequency energy. Am J Cardiol 1994; 73:353–356.
104. Calkins H, Canby R, Weiss R, et al. 100W Atakr II Investigator Group. Results of catheter ablation of typical atrial flutter. Am J Cardiol 2004; 94:437–442.
105. Atiga WL, Worley SJ, Hummel J, et al. Prospective randomized comparison of cooled radiofrequency versus standard radiofrequency energy for ablation of typical atrial flutter. Pacing Clin Electrophysiol 2002; 25:1172–1178.
106. Calkins H. Catheter ablation of atrial flutter: do outcomes of catheter ablation with "large-tip" versus "cooled-tip" catheters really differ? J Cardiovasc Electrophysiol 2004; 15:1131–1132.
107. Lickfett L, Calkins H. Catheter ablation for cardiac arrhythmias. Minerva Cardioangiol 2002; 50:189–207.
108. Wu RC, Berger R, Calkins H. Catheter ablation of atrial flutter and macroreentrant atrial tachycardia. Curr Opin Cardiol 2002; 17:58–64.
109. Calkins H. Catheter ablation for cardiac arrhythmias. Med Clin North Am 2001; 85:473–502 xii.
110. Natale A, Newby KH, Pisano E, et al. Prospective randomized comparison of antiarrhythmic therapy versus first-line radiofrequency ablation in patients with atrial flutter. J Am Coll Cardiol 2000; 35:1898–1904.
111. Smith TW. Digitalis. Mechanisms of action and clinical use. Engl l J Med 1988; 318:358–365.
112. Kastor JA. Multifocal atrial tachycardia. N Engl J Med 1990; 322:1713–1717.
113. Ueng KC, Lee SH, Wu DJ, Lin CS, Chang MS, Chen SA. Radiofrequency catheter modification of atrioventricular junction in patients with COPD and medically refractory multifocal atrial tachycardia. Chest 2000; 117:52–59.

11

Management of Ventricular Arrhythmias in Heart Failure

Usha B. Tedrow and William G. Stevenson
Cardiovascular Division, Brigham and Women's Hospital, Harvard Medical School, Boston, Massachusetts, U.S.A.

INTRODUCTION

Ventricular arrhythmias in patients with heart failure often contribute to clinical decompensation, and can cause sudden death. Because ventricular arrhythmias are nearly ubiquitous in heart failure, ambient arrhythmias represent only a portion of the many important considerations in assessing sudden death risk. Implantable cardiac defibrillators are considered for an increasing number of heart failure patients to prophylax against arrhythmic sudden death. Some patients require adjunctive antiarrhythmic drug therapy and occasionally catheter ablation to reduce the frequency of ventricular arrhythmias. The etiologic diversity of patients with heart failure impacts the incidence of arrhythmias and diagnostic as well as therapeutic strategies. Because of the complexities, potential risks and benefits of these therapeutic modalities, it is essential that management is integrated between patient, heart failure specialist, and electrophysiologist.

VENTRICULAR ARRHYTHMIAS AND SUDDEN CARDIAC DEATH

Sudden cardiac death accounts for 20% to 50% of the mortality in patients with heart failure. Ventricular arrhythmias are an important cause of these heart failure deaths, and implantable defibrillators (ICDs) are warranted for many high-risk patients. Other mechanisms of sudden death also occur, which ICDs do not prevent (1–4). Bradyarrhythmias caused 41% of in-hospital unexpected cardiac arrests in one series (4). Conduction disease associated with heart failure, myocardial ischemia, antiarrhythmic and beta-adrenergic blocking drugs, and hyperkalemia are important potential contributors. Bradyarrhythmias and pulseless electrical rhythm may be a more common presentation of cardiac arrest in nonischemic cardiomyopathies (NICM) as compared to ischemic cardiomyopathies (ICM). Compared to stable outpatients, patients hospitalized with advanced heart failure may have a higher incidence of electromechanical dissociation as a cause of sudden death (1,5). Unexpected and unrecognized acute myocardial infarction, pulmonary embolism, stroke, and ruptured aortic aneurysms also cause some of these deaths.

In chronic dilated cardiomyopathy, the incidence of sudden death increases with the severity of heart failure (6–15). In patients with minimal to modest symptoms of heart failure, the annual risk of sudden death ranges from 2%–6% per year. Those with more advanced symptoms, New York Heart Association functional class III to IV, have a risk of 5%–12% per year. As the severity of heart failure increases, deaths due to pump failure increase to a greater extent than sudden deaths (7). Thus the proportion of sudden deaths decreases from 50%–80% for mild to moderate heart failure, to 5%–30% for severe heart failure (2,16,17). ICDs provide effective therapy for most episodes of ventricular tachycardia (VT) or fibrillation, which has been shown to improve survival. In the Sudden Cardiac Death in Heart Failure Trial (SCD HeFT), ICD therapy in class II and III heart failure patients with EF $<35\%$ reduced mortality by 23% over 5 yr (absolute reduction of 7%) and was superior to therapy with amiodarone, which had no benefit (18). The major limitation of defibrillator therapy is that it does nothing for the substrate responsible for the arrhythmia. VT recurrences and ICD shocks can cause serious symptoms (19,20), and frequent episodes of symptomatic VT require antiarrhythmic drug therapy or catheter ablation.

Monomorphic Ventricular Tachycardia

Ischemic Heart Disease

Patients with ICM typically have large areas of infarction (Fig. 1A). Surviving myocyte bundles within areas of prior infarction can create channels of slow conduction of electrical impulses that can form the substrate for reentry circuits (21,22). The VT that results is typically monomorphic, with each QRS complex resembling the preceding and following QRS complex (Fig. 2). Because the arrhythmia substrate is relatively fixed and stable, VT is usually inducible in the electrophysiology laboratory with programmed stimulation. Induction of arrhythmia in these controlled circumstances is useful in several situations. When the diagnosis of a wide QRS tachycardia is uncertain, initiation of the arrhythmia allows confirmation of the diagnosis, distinguishing monomorphic VT from supraventricular tachycardia conducted with aberrancy. For patients with recurrent VT the location of the reentry circuit can potentially be identified and ablated. The ability to induce VT in the electrophysiology laboratory also predicts an increased risk of VT or cardiac arrest during follow-up, which usually warrants consideration of ICD implantation (23). However, it is important to recognize that in patients with poor ventricular function, absence of inducible VT does not necessarily convey a low sudden death risk and implantation of an ICD may still be associated with a survival benefit (23,24,64).

Nonischemic Dilated Cardiomyopathy

In patients with idiopathic nonischemic dilated cardiomyopathy (NICM), large areas of scar or infarction are usually absent (Fig. 1B) and programmed stimulation rarely induces sustained monomorphic VT if it has not occurred spontaneously (25,26). A negative electrophysiology study has little prognostic value (27–31). Interestingly, of the uncommon NICM patients who develop sustained monomorphic VT, most have evidence of large areas of ventricular scar associated with a reentry circuit (32). The scar may be a consequence of replacement fibrosis from the myopathic process itself or due to infarcts from embolism of left ventricular or atrial thrombus to a coronary artery. Scars causing VT

(A)

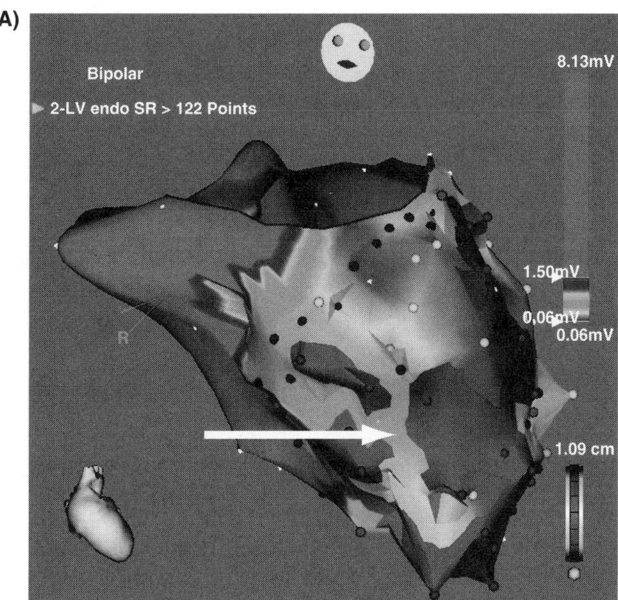

(B)

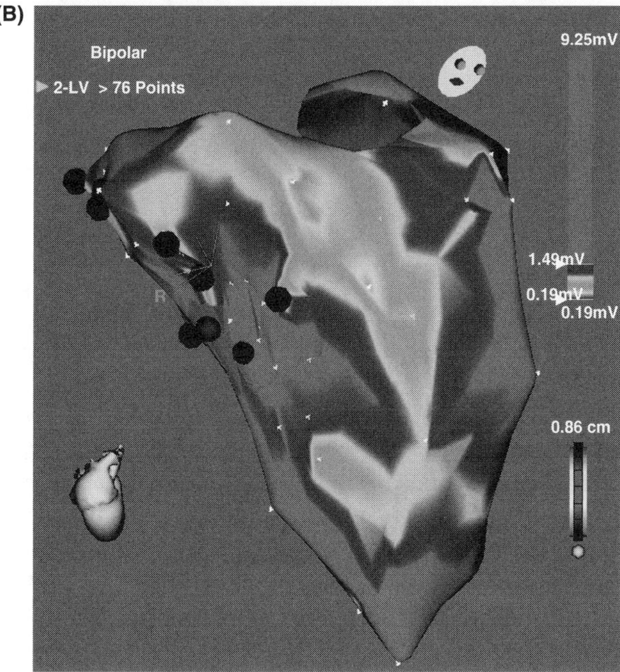

Figure 1 Left ventricular electroanatomic maps from two patients with ventricular tachycardia due to ischemic (**A**) and nonischemic (**B**) cardiomyopathy are shown. Maps were created during left ventricular mapping by moving a catheter from point to point on the ventricle. Points on the map are coded in grayscale for electrogram amplitude in millivolts (mV). Areas in medium gray represent normal myocardium, and lighter areas (<1.5 mV) are abnormal scars or infarcts. Areas of dark gray represent unexcitable scar. Notably the ischemic cardiomyopathy has a large area of low voltage anteroapical scar. Areas of surviving myocyte bundles within the scar are denoted by the arrow. The nonischemic cardiomyopathy has patchy low voltage disease without large areas of dense scar.

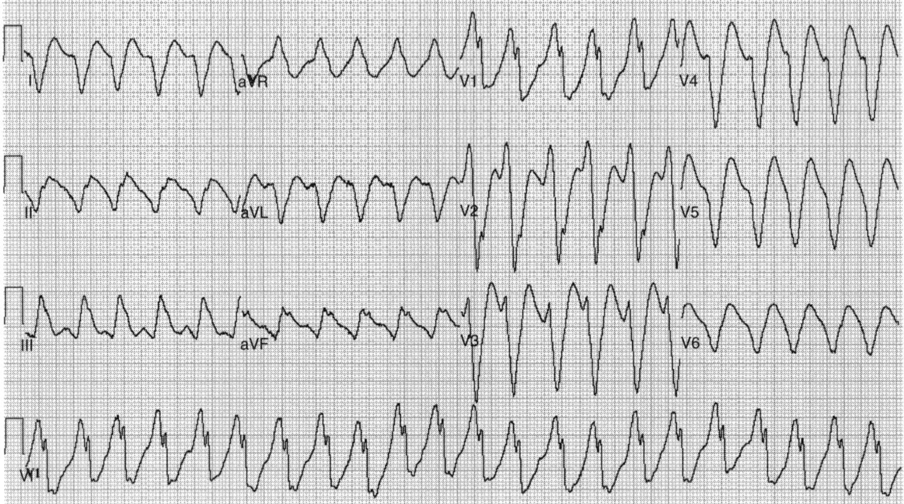

Figure 2 Shown is a 12 lead ECG of sustained monomorphic ventricular tachycardia in a patient with ischemic cardiomyopathy.

in the absence of coronary artery disease should prompt consideration of arrhythmogenic right ventricular dysplasia (ARVD), sarcoidosis, and Chagas' disease (33–40).

Arrhythmogenic Right Ventricular Dysplasia

ARVD or cardiomyopathy is a term that refers to a group of genetic disorders characterized by ventricular arrhythmias and preferential involvement of the right ventricle. The free wall of the right ventricle is most commonly affected in this disease characterized by myocyte replacement with fatty or fibrofatty tissue (Fig. 3) (41,42). Aneurysms can form in the typical "triangle of dysplasia," which includes the outflow tract of the right ventricle, the inflow area near the tricuspid valve, and the apex of the right ventricle (41). The left ventricle is involved in up to 76% of patients with advanced disease (35). Inheritance is typically autosomal dominant, though a recessive variant has been described. Several different genetic mutations have been described including genes coding for cell adhesion proteins (plakoglobin and plakophilin), and the ryanodine receptor (43,44). Over 75% of patients have T-wave inversions in the right precordium. Delayed activation of portions of the RV can produce notches at the end of the QRS, particularly in the anterior precordial leads, referred to as epsilon waves and contribute to abnormal signal averaged ECG (42,45). Ventricular arrhythmias are common, and may result both from the abnormal infiltrated tissue as well as from disrupted autonomic innervation of the ventricle (46). Monomorphic VT with a left bundle branch block configuration is the most common arrhythmia, although ventricular fibrillation is also a risk. Patients with sustained monomorphic VT should receive an ICD to prophylax against sudden death (47,48).

Sarcoidosis

Sarcoidosis is a systemic disease of cryptic origin marked by granuloma formation and immune response, most commonly in the pulmonary and lymphatic tissues. Clinically evident cardiac involvement is present in approximately 5% of cases (49,50). Isolated cardiac disease is uncommon. The most common manifestation of cardiac involvement is

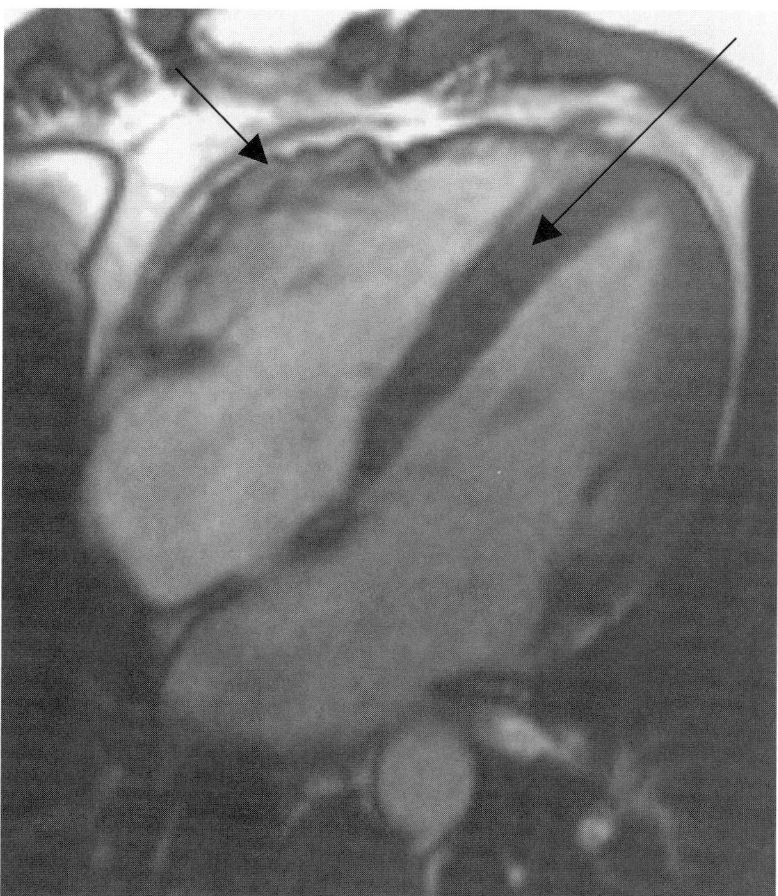

Figure 3 Shown is a fat suppressed MRI image from a patient with arrhythmogenic right ventricular dysplasia. The long arrow indicates the interventricular septum. The anterior wall of the right ventricular (*short arrow*) myocardium appears less dark than the septum in this fat-suppressed image. *Source*: Courtesy of Dr. Raymond Kwong, Brigham and Women's Hospital, Boston, Massachusetts, U.S.A.

AV block, as a consequence of granuloma formation in the basal interventricular septum (Fig. 4) (51). One-third of patients have complete heart block, and 60% have right bundle branch block (49). VT is the second most common cardiac manifestation affecting 20% of patients, and is typically the consequence of granuloma and scar formation in the ventricles. Predominantly right ventricular involvement can mimic right ventricular dysplasia. Atrial fibrillation and flutter can also occur but less commonly. Ablation and antiarrhythmic drugs may be required to control frequent episodes of VT. There is some evidence that early therapy with corticosteroids may be helpful in patients with refractory VT (52,53).

Chagas' Disease

Chagas' disease is associated with chronic infections by the parasite *Trypanosoma cruzi*. The parasite is endemic to Mexico and Central and South America. Approximately 16 to 18 million people in endemic areas are infected with *T. cruzi*, and 10% to 30% of those infected will develop symptomatic chronic Chagas' disease years or decades later (54).

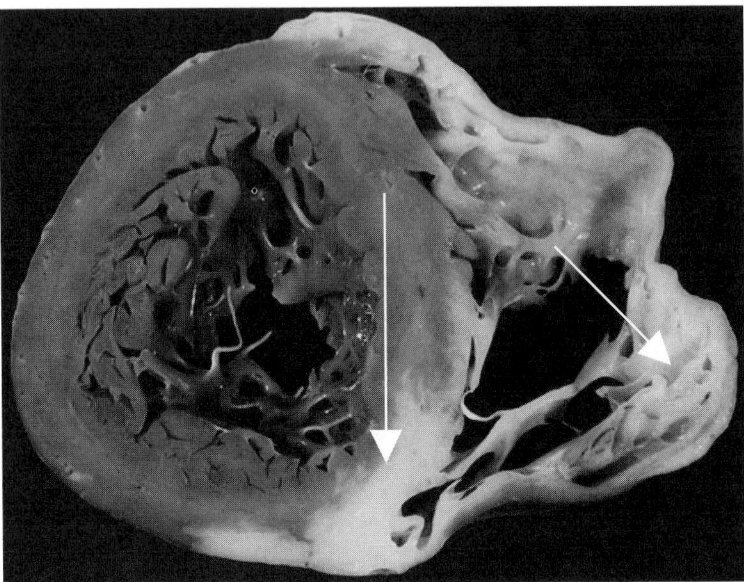

Figure 4 A gross pathology specimen from a patient with cardiac sarcoidosis is shown. The long arrow indicates an area of scarring within the interventricular septum. The right ventricle (*short arrow*) also exhibits extensive prominent scarring. This right ventricular involvement occasionally makes clinical differentiation between sarcoidosis and arrhythmogenic right ventricular dysplasia difficult.

The cardiac disease is characterized by biventricular enlargement, thinning of the ventricular walls, apical aneurysms, and mural thrombi. In the chronic form, lymphocytic infiltration, fibrosis, atrophy of myocardial cells, and absence of trypanosomes is typical. Atrioventricular conduction is often affected, resulting in right bundle-branch block, left anterior fascicular block, or complete atrioventricular block (55). VT is common and may dominate the clinical picture (56). The VT is inducible at electrophysiologic study and associated with large areas of ventricular scar. Catheter ablation often requires an epicardial approach and can help control recurrences when amiodarone therapy fails (57).

Bundle Branch Reentry VTs

Dilated heart failure is commonly associated with conduction system disease. Slowing of conduction in the specialized conduction system can lead to monomorphic VT due to a circulating reentry wavefront down the right bundle branch, through the interventricular septum and up the left bundle branch, referred to as bundle branch reentry. Tachycardia typically has a left bundle branch block type of QRS configuration. Less frequently the circuit revolves in the opposite direction giving rise to a right bundle branch block configuration. Bundle branch reentry is found in approximately 8% of patients with ventricular dysfunction and monomorphic VTs (58). This type of VT should be particularly suspected as the cause of VT in patients with nonischemic dilated cardiomyopathies, including those associated with valvular heart disease and muscular dystrophies, in whom it may account for over a third of sustained monomorphic VTs (32,59). Bundle branch reentry VT is inducible by programmed stimulation and is amenable to cure by catheter ablation of the right bundle branch. Other VTs may be present and AV conduction is often severely impaired warranting placement of an ICD with back up pacing in many patients.

Idiopathic VT Causing Tachycardia-Induced Cardiomyopathy

Incessant tachycardia from any cause can cause a tachycardia induced cardiomyopathy. Supraventricular arrhythmias are the most common cause but this can also occur with idiopathic VT (60). The most common idiopathic VT originates from the right ventricular outflow tract, giving rise to a left bundle branch block configuration QRS with an axis directed inferiorly. Arrhythmogenic RV dysplasia is an important consideration in the differential diagnosis. If recognized in time, elimination of tachycardia by catheter ablation or medications can be followed by marked improvement of ventricular function, in some cases to normal. Ongoing surveillance is warranted because rapid deterioration of ventricular function may occur if the arrhythmia recurs and sudden deaths have been reported (60).

Evaluation and Therapy for Sustained Monomorphic VT

Following restoration of sinus rhythm, potential precipitating and aggravating factors should be sought and corrected. The underlying heart disease should be defined. The major role of electrophysiologic testing after an episode of sustained monomorphic VT is to confirm the diagnosis when supraventricular tachycardia with aberrancy is a consideration, and to guide catheter ablation therapy of the VT, if needed. It should be recognized that sustained monomorphic VT is associated with an underlying structural abnormality in the vast majority of cases and that 20% to 40% of patients will have recurrences during the following two years regardless of correction of myocardial ischemia or other potential aggravating factors. Even when monomorphic VT occurs with elevated serum cardiac enzymes indicating infarction, the risk of recurrent VT remains high despite treatment for ischemia (61). Implantation of an ICD is recommended and is more effective in preventing sudden death than therapy with amiodarone (62). ICDs can often terminate the arrhythmia by painless, antitachycardia pacing. If recurrent episodes of VT causing symptomatic ICD therapies occur, antiarrhythmic drugs or catheter ablation can be considered at that time.

Patients with periods of high frequency of VT, typically more than 3 episodes of VT per 24 hr, are referred to as having VT storm. Intravenous amiodarone, and measures to reduce sympathetic tone, including sedation and assisted ventilation are often helpful adjuncts to antiarrhythmic drugs that act to decrease adrenergic tone in the setting of incessant VT (63). Episodes of VT are a marker for mortality, even when an ICD prevents arrhythmic death, and patients with VT storm or frequent VT have an increased incidence of death from pump failure during short term follow-up (19,64). If drug therapy is ineffective or the medication side effects are intolerable, catheter ablation should be pursued (65). When frequent or incessant arrhythmias cannot be controlled, placement of a ventricular assist device as destination therapy or as a bridge to cardiac transplantation is an option for some patients.

Sustained Polymorphic VT

Polymorphic VT has a continually changing QRS complex, and is often caused by potentially reversible conditions. Acute myocardial ischemia or infarction is a common etiology and warrants evaluation. Torsade de pointes associated with QT interval prolongation is the other major form of polymorphic VT. Less commonly, polymorphic VT is associated with cardiomyopathy or prior infarction without clear precipitating triggers.

Torsade de Pointes

Polymorphic VT associated with QT interval prolongation is referred to as torsade de pointes (66). Any cause of QT interval prolongation can cause torsade de pointes, and hypokalemia, bradycardia, drugs such as sotalol, dofetilide, ibutilide, quinidine, n-acetylprocainamide, haloperidol, and erythromycin are relatively common causes. A more extensive list is available at the www.QTdrugs.org web site maintained by the University of Arizona.

Chronic heart failure is accompanied by ventricular hypertrophy which is manifest not only as an increase in ventricular mass, but also as cellular hypertrophy, changes in ionic currents, and alterations in the ventricular interstitium. Repolarizing potassium currents are reduced, delaying repolarization and prolonging action potential duration. Impaired intracellular calcium handling promotes increased activity of the sodium–calcium exchanger which also contributes to action potential prolongation (67–73). Action potential prolongation is manifest on the surface ECG as QT interval prolongation.

These electrophysiologic changes may increase the susceptibility of patients with heart failure to the polymorphic VT and the increasing risk of drug induced proarrhythmia in heart failure (68,74). Potassium and magnesium depletion from chronic diuretic therapy also promote arrhythmias and torsade de pointes (15,75–77). In one series of patients with heart failure, torsade de pointes caused 13% of cardiac arrests (78,79). Administration of the potassium channel blocking antiarrhythmic drug dofetilide to patients with heart failure was associated with a 5% risk of torsade de pointes or marked QT prolongation even when precautions were taken to exclude susceptible patients (80). Patients who have had torsade de pointes to one agent remain at risk for recurrence when exposed to other agents that prolong the QT interval (74).

The potential susceptibility to torsade de pointes warrants several precautions in patients with heart failure. Patients treated with antiarrhythmic drugs that prolong the QT interval, (sotalol, dofetilide, quinidine, procainamide, ibutilide, or disopyramide) should have therapy initiated in-hospital with electrocardiographic monitoring and careful observation for the occurrence of marked QT prolongation and torsade de pointes. Amiodarone is an exception, which has a much lower risk of torsade de pointes, and can be safely initiated out of hospital for most patients. Even amiodarone should be avoided, however, in heart failure patients who have had torsade de pointes to another agent unless they have an implanted defibrillator (74).

Torsade de pointes is often "bradycardia-dependent" or "pause dependent," with a characteristic initiating sequence (Fig. 5). A sudden increase in R-R interval, as may occur following a premature beat, creates a pause. The QT interval of the beat terminating the pause is prolonged, and characteristically the first beat of the tachycardia interrupts the

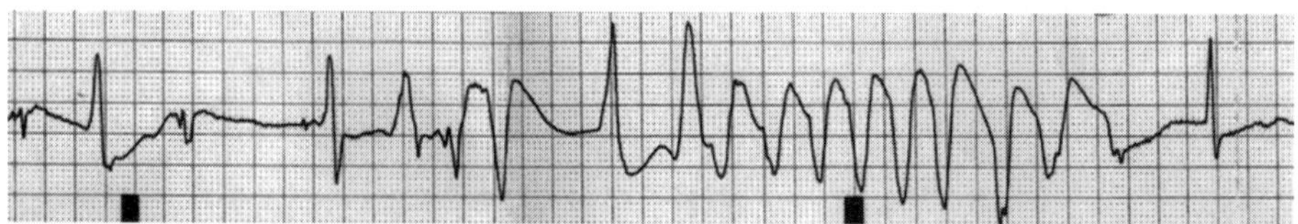

Figure 5 Shown is an episode of torsade de pointes initiated by a long-short R-R interval.

T-wave of that beat. Interventions that increase heart rate and shorten refractoriness are protective. Emergent treatment is intravenous administration of magnesium sulfate. If episodes continue, therapy directed at accelerating the heart rate with intravenous administration of isoproterenol and/or transvenous pacing is warranted.

Patients who have had torsade de pointes should avoid all drugs that prolong the QT interval. Although amiodarone prolongs the QT interval, torsade de pointes is uncommon, possibly because it also blocks ionic currents that also cause the arrhythmia. Patients with heart failure are particularly susceptible to torsade de pointes and therapy with amiodarone is not protective (68,74). Treatment with an ICD is reasonable. ICDs also provide pacing to prevent bradycardia and to suppress pauses following premature beats that may help prevent polymorphic VT (81).

Syncope

Although syncope can be due to orthostatic hypotension aggravated by diurectics and vasodilators, a careful evaluation and consideration for ICD placement is warranted. Among 491 consecutive patients with advanced heart failure, Middlekauff et al. found that 12% had a history of syncope (17). In 45% of these patients, syncope was attributed to a cardiac arrhythmia. Orthostatic hypotension or a non-cardiac cause was identified in 25%, and no clear cause was identified in 30% of patients. The rate of sudden death during the following year was 45%. The sudden death risk was similar for patients with identifiable cardiac causes and presumptively identified noncardiac causes of syncope, suggesting that even when an apparently benign explanation is found, patients with heart failure and syncope remain at high risk for sudden death.

In patients with NICM and syncope, a negative electrophysiologic study does not indicate a low risk. Knight and coworkers implanted ICDs in 14 patients with nonischemic cardiomyopathy, unexplained syncope, and a negative electrophysiology study. During an average follow-up of 2 yr, half of the patients received therapy from the ICD for VT or ventricular fibrillation (82). Of 639 consecutive patients with non-ischemic cardiomyopathy referred for heart transplantation reported by Fonarow and coworkers, 147 (23%) had a history of syncope (83). Twenty-five of these patients received an ICD; 40% received an appropriate shock for VT and none died suddenly during a mean follow-up of 22 mo. Of the 122 patients who had a history of syncope but did not receive an ICD, 15% died suddenly during follow-up. Actuarial survival at 2 yr was 84.9% with an ICD therapy and 66.9% with conventional therapy.

Based on the above data, implantation of an ICD is a reasonable consideration for most patients with heart failure and unexplained syncope (82,83).

Nonsustained VT and Ventricular Ectopic Activity

Ventricular ectopic activity and nonsustained VT of 3 or more consecutive beats are common in heart failure patients; 34% to 79% of patients have one or more runs of nonsustained VT on 24-hr ambulatory recordings (16,84,85). These are typically short; only 30% of patients have runs >5 beats in duration (16). Fast, long runs of nonsustained VT and polymorphic VT should prompt a careful search for possible myocardial ischemia and causes of torsade de pointes. Frequent ventricular ectopy and nonsustained VT are markers for increased mortality and sudden death, but appear to reflect the severity of underlying heart failure and ventricular dysfunction, rather than a specific arrhythmia risk (16,84,85). Furthermore, suppression of nonsustained VT with antiarrhythmic drug therapy does not improve survival (86). Occasionally ventricular ectopic activity is due to an aggravating factor that requires treatment, or is a marker for hemodynamic deterioration. Hyper- or hypokalemia, hypoxemia, apneic periods during sleep and myocardial ischemia are potential causes that deserve evaluation when a marked change in the frequency of ectopic activity occurs (87–90). Asymptomatic arrhythmias should, in general, not receive specific antiarrhythmic therapy unless there is concern that very frequent arrhythmias are having a negative impact on ventricular function.

Coronary Artery Disease with Depressed LV Function and Nonsustained VT

Nonsustained VT is clearly a risk factor for sustained VT and cardiac arrest in patients with depressed ventricular function due to coronary artery disease. In the Multicenter Unsustained Tachycardia Trial (MUSTT) 2202 patients with prior myocardial infarction, left ventricular ejection fraction less that 40%, and nonsustained VT (23) had electrophysiology testing. Inducible sustained VT was found in 35%. Inducible patients were randomized either to a control group who did not receive antiarrhythmic therapy or to a treatment group. The active treatment group received antiarrhythmic drug therapy guided by electrophysiologic testing. An ICD was used when arrhythmia could not be controlled by drugs. The five-year rate of sudden death or resuscitation from cardiac arrest was 32% for the patients who did not receive antiarrhythmic therapy as compared to 25% for those assigned to antiarrhythmic therapy. The benefit of treatment was due to ICDs, which were implanted in 46% of patients in the treatment group. Patients with an ICD had a 5-year rate of sudden death or cardiac arrest of 9% compared to 37% for patients treated with antiarrhythmic drugs. While symptomatic heart failure was not required for trial entry, New York Heart Association Class II or III symptoms were present in 63% of patients. These data support the use of an ICD in patients with ejection fractions between 30% and 40% with nonsustained ventricular arrhythmias and inducible VT at electrophysiology study, provided that the severity of heart failure and other comorbidities do not preclude an ICD.

ANTIARRHYTHMIC DRUGS

Antiarrhythmic drugs must be used cautiously with careful assessment of risk and benefit in patients with heart failure. The potential for drug toxicity is increased by diminished hepatic or renal excretion and drug interactions are common. In addition, depressed ventricular function is associated with a greater risk of drug-induced proarrhythmia, such as polymorphic VT (e.g., torsade de pointes). Many drugs have negative inotropic effects that can aggravate heart failure.

Antiarrhythmic Effects of Beta-Adrenergic Blockers

Beta-adrenergic blockers are a first-line therapy for many arrhythmias. These agents have antiarrhythmic effects and demonstrated efficacy for improving mortality and reducing sudden death in heart failure (91–93). In addition, beta-adrenergic blockers can help diminish symptoms of palpitations from premature ventricular contractions (94). Many ventricular arrhythmias are aggravated by sympathetic stimulation. Beta-adrenergic blockers are also effective in reducing the frequency of many ventricular arrhythmias and sudden death in patients with heart failure (95,96). In addition, sympathetic stimulation can blunt or reverse the electrophysiologic effects of amiodarone and other antiarrhythmic drugs. A combination of a beta-adrenergic blocker with another antiarrhythmic drug can be synergistic. Aggravation of bradyarrhythmias is the major arrhythmia-related adverse effect.

Class I Sodium Channel Blocking Antiarrhythmic Drugs

The class I antiarrhythmic drugs are largely reserved for control of frequent symptomatic arrhythmias in patients who have an implantable defibrillator when amiodarone, dofetilide, or sotalol are less attractive options. Class I sodium channel blocking drugs (mexiletine, tocainide, procainamide, quinidine, disopyramide, flecainide, and propafenone) have negative inotropic effects (with the possible exception of quinidine) (79,97). Blockade of sodium channels diminishes intracellular sodium and thereby may decrease intracellular calcium by its effect on the sodium–calcium exchanger (the opposite effect of digitalis). Quinidine may lack negative inotropic effects because vasodilation and QT interval prolongation, which allow additional time for calcium to enter during the plateau phase of the action potential, may offset the negative inotropic effects of the sodium channel blockade. In addition to a long-term risk of drug-induced systemic lupus erythematosis, procainamide is metabolized to N-acetylprocainamide (NAPA), which is a Class III antiarrhythmic drug that has QT prolonging effects of its own and accumulates in patients with renal insufficiency.

Class I antiarrhythmic drugs also have a potential for proarrhythmia that is likely aggravated by the electrophysiologic changes of heart failure and hypertrophy (98,99). These adverse effects of Class I antiarrhythmic drugs likely explain the increases in mortality observed when these agents were administered to patients with prior myocardial infarction, to patients with heart failure and atrial fibrillation, and to patients who had been resuscitated from a cardiac arrest (92,98,100).

Amiodarone

Amiodarone is the major option for chronic antiarrhythmic drug therapy in patients with heart failure, largely because it is relatively safe from a cardiac standpoint (101–103). Amiodarone blocks cardiac sodium, potassium, and calcium currents and has sympatholytic effects. It has activity against both ventricular and supraventricular arrhythmias. Individual trials have found either benefit or no effect on mortality (101,102). An early meta-analysis of randomized trials in patients with heart failure concluded that amiodarone reduced mortality by 17% and reduced sudden death by 23% (104). Amiodarone therapy was compared to ICD and no antiarrhythmic therapy in 2521 patients with Class II and III heart failure enrolled in the SCD HeFT. Five-year total mortality was similar in amiodarone and placebo treated groups and inferior to that of patients who received an ICD. Interestingly, in the relatively small group with the most severe heart failure, with Class III symptoms, amiodarone was associated with worse mortality than placebo (18). Use of amiodarone is therefore reserved for arrhythmias that are symptomatic or have an adverse effect on heart failure. In the Optimal Pharmacological Therapy in Implantable Cardioverter Defibrillator Patients (OPTIC) trial, amiodarone was more effective than sotalol or conventional beta blockade in reducing ICD shocks in a randomized 3 arm schema. Additionally, amiodarone was less often discontinued than sotalol in the 18-month study (105).

Ventricular proarrhythmia during initiation of amiodarone therapy is unusual and it has been initiated in the outpatient setting without an increase in mortality (101,102,104). Bradyarrhythmias due to potent effects on the sinus and AV nodes are the major cardiac risk, occurring in 1%–7% of patients in randomized trials, and in up to a third of patients in some case series (104,106).

In patients with compensated heart failure, oral amiodarone is well tolerated from a hemodynamic standpoint when administered at a loading dose of 600 to 800 mg daily for one to two weeks (101–103,106,107) In patients with advanced heart failure, administration of the loading dose and, in particular, large oral doses (e.g., >1200 mg daily) can exacerbate heart failure.

Noncardiac toxicities are a major problem. In randomized trials 41% of patients discontinue therapy by 2 yr due to real or perceived side effects. The true incidence of side effects is lower, as indicated by the observation that placebo was discontinued in 27% of patients in these trials (104). However, it is often difficult to distinguish an amiodarone-induced side effect from symptoms of heart failure. Amiodarone induced pulmonary toxicity occurs in approximately 1% of patients per year of therapy (108), and chronic therapy at doses exceeding 300 mg per day increases the risk. A chest radiograph should be obtained annually. Annual pulmonary function tests are recommended by some physicians, particularly for those patients taking a daily dose in excess of 300 mg. A decrease in diffusing capacity can indicate development of pulmonary toxicity (109). When pulmonary toxicity is suspected, a right heart catheterization to assess the possibility of pulmonary vascular congestion, and a high resolution chest computed tomography scan to assess interstitial fibrosis can be helpful in distinguishing pulmonary toxicity from heart failure (109,110).

Thyroid abnormalities occur in up to 18% of patients (111). Hypothyroidism is easily managed with thyroid replacement therapy and does not generally warrant discontinuation of amiodarone. Hyperthyroidism is a much more difficult problem, and can be refractory to management with antithyroid medications. Because the gland is saturated with iodine from the amiodarone, thyroid ablation with radioactive iodine is not possible. Discontinuation of the drug and medical therapy for hyperthyroidism in consultation with an endocrinologist is often required. Routine thyroid stimulating hormone (TSH) assay every 6 mo, as well as assessment of hepatic transaminases at those times for potential liver toxicity, are reasonable.

Additionally, long term use of amiodarone is associated with corneal and cutaneous deposits which are mainly cosmetic difficulties for the patient. In contrast, optic neuritis and peripheral neuropathy are also associated with use of amiodarone, and warrant discontinuation of the drug.

Dofetilide

Dofetilide is a Class III antiarrhythmic drug that is FDA approved for therapy of atrial fibrillation. It blocks the repolarizing potassium current I_{Kr}, increasing action potential duration and the QT interval. Its major toxicity is proarrhythmia from torsade de pointes, which occurs in more than 3% of patients (80). It is renally excreted with a plasma half-life of 9.5 hr. It requires initiation in-hospital with continuous electrocardiographic monitoring for a minimum of 72 hr to detect the development of QT prolongation and torsade de pointes. It should not be administered to patients with significant renal insufficiency (calculated creatinine clearance <20 ml/min). Taking these precautions and avoiding drug administration to patients with prolonged QT intervals, dofetilide can be administered safely to patients with heart failure. The Danish Investigations of Arrhythmia and Mortality on Dofetilide Study (DIAMOND) showed that, in patients with Class III of IV heart failure, during a median follow-up of 18 mo, there was no difference in mortality between dofetilide-treated and placebo groups (80). Dofetilide-treated patients were less likely to be re-hospitalized for exacerbation of heart failure (30% compared to 38%), possibly due to a reduction in atrial fibrillation. There is to date minimal data on the efficacy of dofetilide in controlling ventricular arrhythmias.

Sotalol

Sotalol is a mixture of two stereoisomers. The *d* isomer has Class III effects similar to dofetilide, from blockade of the potassium current I_{Kr}. The *l* isomer is a potent nonselective beta-adrenergic blocker. Sotalol has not been specifically evaluated in heart failure patients. In survivors of myocardial infarction who have depressed ventricular function, chronic therapy with the *d* isomer of sotalol increases mortality (112). Sotalol causes torsade de pointes with a similar incidence to that of dofetilide, and can aggravate bradyarrhythmias and heart failure through its beta-blocking effects. Therapy should be initiated in-hospital during continuous electrocardiographic monitoring. It also has a renal route of excretion and should be avoided in patients with renal insufficiency. Its antiarrhythmic efficacy for atrial fibrillation is less than that of amiodarone (113).

Antiarrhythmic Drug Interactions with ICDs

Many patients with ICDs require antiarrhythmic drug therapy to control supraventricular arrhythmias (most commonly atrial fibrillation and flutter) or reduce episodes of VT. In the presence of an ICD, the potential for fatal drug-induced proarrhythmia is low. The ICD will terminate torsade de pointes and provide pacing for bradyarrhythmias. Antiarrhythmic drugs can impede effective ICD termination of arrhythmias and should be used cautiously.

Some antiarrhythmic drugs can increase the energy required for defibrillation. At the time of ICD implantation, defibrillation testing is performed by inducing ventricular fibrillation and observing that an ICD shock will terminate fibrillation. Most ICDs are capable of providing a 31 to 42 J shock. A 10 J safety margin is recommended and confirmed by demonstrating that ventricular fibrillation is terminated by a shock 10 J below the maximum energy available from the ICD. Amiodarone and sodium channel blockers typically increase the energy required for defibrillation. If the defibrillation threshold is close to the maximal energy of the ICD, antiarrhythmic drug therapy may increase it such that maximal energy shocks from the ICD are no longer effective. Class III antiarrhythmic drugs that block potassium channels, such as sotalol and dofetilide, may decrease the defibrillation threshold. In general, repeat defibrillation testing is warranted when chronic therapy with an antiarrhythmic drug is administered, with the possible exceptions of beta-blockers, sotalol, and dofetilide.

SUMMARY AND CONCLUSIONS

Ventricular arrhythmias are common in patients with heart failure, either as a consequence of exacerbation of underlying disease or as the primary culprit leading to decompensation. Underlying etiologic factors influence prognosis as well as appropriate aggressiveness of therapy. A collaborative effort between patient, heart failure physician, and electrophysiologist is essential in managing the underlying disease, selecting antiarrhythmic medication, implanting defibrillators, and employing catheter ablation for optimal management of these tachycardias.

REFERENCES

1. Pratt CM, Greenway PS, Schoenfeld MH, et al. Exploration of the precision of classifying sudden cardiac death. Implications for the interpretation of clinical trials. Circulation 1996; 93:519–524.
2. Uretsky BF, Thygesen K, Armstrong PW, et al. Acute coronary findings at autopsy in heart failure patients with sudden death: results from the assessment of treatment with lisinopril and survival (ATLAS) trial. Circulation 2000; 102:611–616.
3. Stevenson WG, Sweeney MO. Arrhythmias and sudden death in heart failure. Jpn Circ J 1997; 61:727–740.
4. Faggiano P, d'Aloia A, Gualeni A, et al. Mechanisms and immediate outcome of in-hospital cardiac arrest in patients with advanced heart failure secondary to ischemic or idiopathic dilated cardiomyopathy. Am J Cardiol 2001; 87:655–657.
5. Grubman EM, Pavri BB, Shipman T, et al. Cardiac death and stored electrograms in patients with third-generation implantable cardioverter–defibrillators. J Am Coll Cardiol 1998; 32:1056–1062.
6. Anonymous. Effect of enalapril on survival in patients with reduced left ventricular ejection fractions and congestive heart failure. The SOLVD Investigators. N Engl J Med 1991; 325:293–302.
7. Anonymous. Effect of metoprolol CR/XL in chronic heart failure: metoprolol CR/XL randomised intervention trial in congestive heart failure (MERIT-HF). Lancet 1999; 353:2001–2007.
8. Cohn JN, Johnson GR, Shabetai R, et al. Ejection fraction, peak exercise oxygen consumption, cardiothoracic ratio, ventricular arrhythmias, and plasma norepinephrine as determinants of prognosis in heart failure. The V-HeFT VA Cooperative Studies Group. Circulation 1993; 87:V15–V16.
9. Anonymous. The cardiac insufficiency bisoprolol study II (CIBIS-II): a randomised trial. Lancet 1999; 353:9–13.
10. Anonymous. Effects of enalapril on mortality in severe congestive heart failure. Results of the Cooperative North Scandinavian Enalapril Survival Study (CONSENSUS). The CONSENSUS Trial Study Group. N Engl J Med 1987; 316:1429–1435.
11. Nagele H, Rodiger W. Sudden death and tailored medical therapy in elective candidates for heart transplantation. J Heart Lung Transplant 1999; 18:869–876.
12. Uretsky BF, Sheahan RG. Primary prevention of sudden cardiac death in heart failure: will the solution be shocking? J Am Coll Cardiol 1997; 30:1589–1597.
13. Cohn JN, Goldstein SO, Greenberg BH, et al. A dose-dependent increase in mortality with vesnarinone among patients with severe heart failure. Vesnarinone Trial Investigators. N Engl J Med 1998; 339:1810–1816.
14. Pitt B, Poole-Wilson PA, Segal R, et al. Effect of losartan compared with captopril on mortality in patients with symptomatic heart failure: randomised trial—the Losartan Heart Failure Survival Study ELITE II. Lancet 2000; 355:1582–1587.
15. Pitt B, Zannad F, Remme WJ, et al. The effect of spironolactone on morbidity and mortality in patients with severe heart failure. Randomized aldactone evaluation study investigators. N Engl J Med 1999; 341:709–717.
16. Teerlink JR, Jalaluddin M, Anderson S, et al. Ambulatory ventricular arrhythmias in patients with heart failure do not specifically predict an increased risk of sudden death. PROMISE (Prospective Randomized Milrinone Survival Evaluation) Investigators. Circulation 2000; 101:40–46.
17. Stevenson WG, Stevenson LW, Middlekauff HR, et al. Sudden death prevention in patients with advanced ventricular dysfunction. Circulation 1993; 88:2953–2961.
18. Bardy GH, Lee KL, Mark DB, et al. Amiodarone or an implantable cardioverter–defibrillator for congestive heart failure. N Engl J Med 2005; 352:225–237.

19. Exner DV, Pinski SL, Wyse DG, et al. Electrical storm presages nonsudden death: the antiarrhythmics versus implantable defibrillators (AVID) trial. Circulation 2001; 103:2066–2071.
20. Credner SC, Klingenheben T, Mauss O, et al. Electrical storm in patients with transvenous implantable cardioverter–defibrillators: incidence, management and prognostic implications. J Am Coll Cardiol 1998; 32:1909–1915.
21. de Bakker JM, van Capelle FJ, Janse MJ, et al. Slow conduction in the infarcted human heart. 'zigzag' course of activation. Circulation 1993; 88:915–926.
22. Stevenson WG, Friedman PL, Sager PT, et al. Exploring postinfarction reentrant ventricular tachycardia with entrainment mapping. J Am Coll Cardiol 1997; 29:1180–1189.
23. Buxton AE, Lee KL, Fisher JD, et al. A randomized study of the prevention of sudden death in patients with coronary artery disease. Multicenter Unsustained Tachycardia Trial Investigators. N Engl J Med 1999; 341:1882–1890 [erratum appears in N Engl J Med 2000 Apr 27;342:1300].
24. Moss AJ, Hall WJ, Cannom DS, et al. Improved survival with an implanted defibrillator in patients with coronary disease at high risk for ventricular arrhythmia. Multicenter Automatic Defibrillator Implantation Trial Investigators. N Engl J Med 1996; 335:1933–1940.
25. Stevenson WG, Stevenson LW, Weiss J, et al. Inducible ventricular arrhythmias and sudden death during vasodilator therapy of severe heart failure. Am Heart J 1988; 116:1447–1454.
26. Turitto G, Ahuja RK, Caref EB, et al. Risk stratification for arrhythmic events in patients with nonischemic dilated cardiomyopathy and nonsustained ventricular tachycardia: role of programmed ventricular stimulation and the signal-averaged electrocardiogram. J Am Coll Cardiol 1994; 24:1523–1528.
27. Hammill SC, Trusty JM, Wood DL, et al. Influence of ventricular function and presence or absence of coronary artery disease on results of electrophysiologic testing for asymptomatic nonsustained ventricular tachycardia. Am J Cardiol 1990; 65:722–728.
28. Lindsay BD, Osborn JL, Schechtman KB, et al. Prospective detection of vulnerability to sustained ventricular tachycardia in patients awaiting cardiac transplantation. Am J Cardiol 1992; 69:619–624.
29. Das SK, Morady F, DiCarlo L, Jr., et al. Prognostic usefulness of programmed ventricular stimulation in idiopathic dilated cardiomyopathy without symptomatic ventricular arrhythmias. Am J Cardiol 1986; 58:998–1000.
30. Meinertz T, Treese N, Kasper W, et al. Determinants of prognosis in idiopathic dilated cardiomyopathy as determined by programmed electrical stimulation. Am J Cardiol 1985; 56:337–341.
31. Poll DS, Marchlinski FE, Buxton AE, et al. Usefulness of programmed stimulation in idiopathic dilated cardiomyopathy. Am J Cardiol 1986; 58:992–997.
32. Delacretaz E, Stevenson WG, Ellison KE, et al. Mapping and radiofrequency catheter ablation of the three types of sustained monomorphic ventricular tachycardia in nonischemic heart disease. J Cardiovasc Electrophysiol 2000; 11:11–17.
33. Ellison KE, Friedman PL, Ganz LI, et al. Entrainment mapping and radiofrequency catheter ablation of ventricular tachycardia in right ventricular dysplasia. J Am Coll Cardiol 1998; 32:724–728.
34. Pinski SL. The right ventricular tachycardias. J Electrocardiol 2000; 33:103–114.
35. Corrado D, Basso C, Thiene G, et al. Spectrum of clinicopathologic manifestations of arrhythmogenic right ventricular cardiomyopathy/dysplasia: a multicenter study. J Am Coll Cardiol 1997; 30:1512–1520.
36. Anonymous. Case records of the Massachusetts General Hospital. Weekly clinicopathological exercises. Case 20-2000. A 61-year-old man with a wide-complex tachycardia. N Engl J Med 2000; 342:1979–1987.
37. Marcus FI, Fontaine G. Arrhythmogenic right ventricular dysplasia/cardiomyopathy: a review. Pacing Clin Electrophysiol 1995; 18:1298–1314.
38. Fontaine G, Fontaliran F, Hebert JL, et al. Arrhythmogenic right ventricular dysplasia. Annu Rev Med 1999; 50:17–35.

39. Inoue S, Shinohara F, Sakai T, et al. Myocarditis and arrhythmia: a clinico-pathological study of conduction system based on serial section in 65 cases. Jpn Circ J 1989; 53:49–57.
40. Delacretaz E, Stevenson WG, Winters GL, et al. Ablation of ventricular tachycardia with a saline-cooled radiofrequency catheter: anatomic and histologic characteristics of the lesions in humans. J Cardiovasc Electrophysiol 1999; 10:860–865.
41. Marcus F, Towbin JA, Zareba W, et al. Arrhythmogenic right ventricular dysplasia/cardiomyopathy (ARVD/C): a multidisciplinary study: design and protocol. Circulation 2003; 107:2975–2978.
42. Corrado D, Fontaine G, Marcus FI, et al. Arrhythmogenic right ventricular dysplasia/cardiomyopathy: need for an international registry. Study Group on Arrhythmogenic Right Ventricular Dysplasia/Cardiomyopathy of the Working Groups on Myocardial and Pericardial Disease and Arrhythmias of the European society of Cardiology and of the Scientific Council on Cardiomyopathies of the World Heart Federation. Circulation 2000; 101:E101–E106.
43. Basso C, Wichter T, Danieli GA, et al. Arrhythmogenic right ventricular cardiomyopathy: clinical registry and database, evaluation of therapies, pathology registry, DNA banking. Eur Heart J 2004; 25:531–534.
44. Sen-Chowdhry S, Lowe MD, Sporton SC, et al. Arrhythmogenic right ventricular cardiomyopathy: clinical presentation, diagnosis, and management. Am J Med 2004; 117:685–695.
45. Nasir K, Bomma C, Tandri H, et al. Electrocardiographic features of arrhythmogenic right ventricular dysplasia/cardiomyopathy according to disease severity: a need to broaden diagnostic criteria. Circulation 2004; 110:1527–1534.
46. Wichter T, Schafers M, Rhodes CG, et al. Abnormalities of cardiac sympathetic innervation in arrhythmogenic right ventricular cardiomyopathy: quantitative assessment of presynaptic norepinephrine reuptake and postsynaptic beta-adrenergic receptor density with positron emission tomography. Circulation 2000; 101:1552–1558.
47. Roguin A, Bomma CS, Nasir K, et al. Implantable cardioverter–defibrillators in patients with arrhythmogenic right ventricular dysplasia/cardiomyopathy. J Am Coll Cardiol 2004; 43:1843–1852.
48. Wichter T, Paul M, Wollmann C, et al. Implantable cardioverter/defibrillator therapy in arrhythmogenic right ventricular cardiomyopathy: single-center experience of long-term follow-up and complications in 60 patients. Circulation 2004; 109:1503–1508.
49. Bargout R, Kelly RF. Sarcoid heart disease: clinical course and treatment. Int J Cardiol 2004; 97:173–182.
50. Silverman KJ, Hutchins GM, Bulkley BH. Cardiac sarcoid: a clinicopathologic study of 84 unselected patients with systemic sarcoidosis. Circulation 1978; 58:1204–1211.
51. Abeler V. Sarcoidosis of the cardiac conducting system. Am Heart J 1979; 97:701–707.
52. Walsh MJ. Systemic sarcoidosis with refractory ventricular tachycardia and heart failure. Br Heart J 1978; 40:931–933.
53. Wilkins CE, Barron T, Lowrimore MG, et al. Cardiac sarcoidosis: two cases with ventricular tachycardia and review of cardiac involvement in sarcoid. Tex Heart Inst J 1985; 12:377–383.
54. Kirchhoff LV. Changing epidemiology and approaches to therapy for Chagas disease. Curr Infect Dis Rep 2003; 5:59–65.
55. Hagar JM, Rahimtoola SH. Chagas' heart disease. Curr Probl Cardiol 1995; 20:825–924.
56. d'Avila A, Splinter R, Svenson RH, et al. New perspectives on catheter-based ablation of ventricular tachycardia complicating Chagas' disease: experimental evidence of the efficacy of near infrared lasers for catheter ablation of Chagas' VT. J Interv Card Electrophysiol 2002; 7:23–38.
57. Sosa E, Scanavacca M, d'Avila A, et al. Nonsurgical transthoracic epicardial catheter ablation to treat recurrent ventricular tachycardia occurring late after myocardial infarction. J Am Coll Cardiol 2000; 35:1442–1449.
58. Lopera G, Stevenson WG, Soejima K, et al. Identification and ablation of three types of ventricular tachycardia involving the his-purkinje system in patients with heart disease. J Cardiovasc Electrophysiol 2004; 15:52–58.

59. de Bakker JM, van Capelle FJ, Janse MJ, et al. Fractionated electrograms in dilated cardiomyopathy: origin and relation to abnormal conduction. J Am Coll Cardiol 1996; 27:1071–1078.
60. Nerheim P, Birger-Botkin S, Piracha L, et al. Heart failure and sudden death in patients with tachycardia-induced cardiomyopathy and recurrent tachycardia. Circulation 2004; 110:247–252.
61. Woelfel A, Wohns DH, Foster JR. Implications of sustained monomorphic ventricular tachycardia associated with myocardial injury. Ann Intern Med 1990; 112:141–143.
62. The Antiarrhythmics Versus Implantable Defibrillators (AVID) Investigators. A comparison of antiarrhythmic-drug therapy with implantable defibrillators in patients resuscitated from near-fatal ventricular arrhythmias. N Engl J Med 1997; 337:1576–1583.
63. Nademanee K, Taylor R, Bailey WE, et al. Treating electrical storm: sympathetic blockade versus advanced cardiac life support-guided therapy. Circulation 2000; 102:742–747.
64. Moss AJ, Greenberg H, Case RB, et al. Long-term clinical course of patients after termination of ventricular tachyarrhythmia by an implanted defibrillator. Circulation 2004; 110:3760–3765.
65. Soejima K, Suzuki M, Maisel WH, et al. Catheter ablation in patients with multiple and unstable ventricular tachycardias after myocardial infarction: short ablation lines guided by reentry circuit isthmuses and sinus rhythm mapping. Circulation 2001; 104:664–669.
66. Passman R, Kadish A. Polymorphic ventricular tachycardia, long Q–T syndrome, and torsades de pointes. Med Clin N Am 2001; 85:321–341.
67. Tomaselli GF, Marban E. Electrophysiological remodeling in hypertrophy and heart failure. Cardiovasc Res 1999; 42:270–283.
68. Tomaselli GF, Rose J. Molecular aspects of arrhythmias associated with cardiomyopathies. Curr Opin Cardiol 2000; 15:202–208.
69. Nabauer M, Kaab S. Potassium channel down-regulation in heart failure. Cardiovasc Res 1998; 37:324–334.
70. Marban E. Heart failure: the electrophysiologic connection. J Cardiovasc Electrophysiol 1999; 10:1425–1428.
71. Jongsma HJ. Modulation of gap junction properties in failing hearts. J Cardiovasc Electrophysiol 1999; 10:1421–1424.
72. Priebe L, Beuckelmann DJ. Simulation study of cellular electric properties in heart failure. Circ Res 1998; 82:1206–1223.
73. Pogwizd SM, Qi M, Yuan W, et al. Upregulation of Na(+)/Ca(2+) exchanger expression and function in an arrhythmogenic rabbit model of heart failure. Circ Res 1999; 85:1009–1019.
74. Middlekauff HR, Stevenson WG, Saxon LA, et al. Amiodarone and torsades de pointes in patients with advanced heart failure. Am J Cardiol 1995; 76:499–502.
75. Cooper HA, Dries DL, Davis CE, et al. Diuretics and risk of arrhythmic death in patients with left ventricular dysfunction. Circulation 1999; 100:1311–1315.
76. Galinier M, Pathak A, Fourcade J, et al. Depressed low frequency power of heart rate variability as an independent predictor of sudden death in chronic heart failure. Eur Heart J 2000; 21:475–482.
77. Nolan J, Batin PD, Andrews R, et al. Prospective study of heart rate variability and mortality in chronic heart failure: results of the United Kingdom heart failure evaluation and assessment of risk trial (UK-heart). Circulation 1998; 98:1510–1516.
78. Middlekauff HR, Wiener I, Saxon LA, et al. Low-dose amiodarone for atrial fibrillation: time for a prospective study? Ann Intern Med 1992; 116:1017–1020.
79. Stevenson WG. Mechanisms and management of arrhythmias in heart failure. Curr Opin Cardiol 1995; 10:274–281.
80. Torp-Pedersen C, Moller M, Bloch-Thomsen PE, et al. Dofetilide in patients with congestive heart failure and left ventricular dysfunction. Danish Investigations of Arrhythmia and Mortality on Dofetilide Study Group. N Engl J Med 1999; 341:857–865.

81. Viskin S. Cardiac pacing in the long QT syndrome: review of available data and practical recommendations. J Cardiovasc Electrophysiol 2000; 11:593–600.
82. Knight BP, Goyal R, Pelosi F, et al. Outcome of patients with nonischemic dilated cardiomyopathy and unexplained syncope treated with an implantable defibrillator. J Am Coll Cardiol 1999; 33:1964–1970.
83. Fonarow GC, Feliciano Z, Boyle NG, et al. Improved survival in patients with nonischemic advanced heart failure and syncope treated with an implantable cardioverter–defibrillator. Am J Cardiol 2000; 85:981–985.
84. Singh SN, Fisher SG, Carson PE, et al. Prevalence and significance of nonsustained ventricular tachycardia in patients with premature ventricular contractions and heart failure treated with vasodilator therapy. Department of Veterans Affairs CHF STAT Investigators. J Am Coll Cardiol 1998; 32:942–947.
85. Doval HC, Nul DR, Grancelli HO, et al. Nonsustained ventricular tachycardia in severe heart failure. Independent marker of increased mortality due to sudden death. GESICA-GEMA Investigators. Circulation 1996; 94:3198–3203.
86. Bigger JT, Jr. Implications of the cardiac arrhythmia suppression trial for antiarrhythmic drug treatment. Am J Cardiol 1990; 65:3D–10D; discussion 68D–71D.
87. Davies SW, John LM, Wedzicha JA, et al. Overnight studies in severe chronic left heart failure: arrhythmias and oxygen desaturation. Br Heart J 1991; 65:77–83.
88. Javaheri S. Effects of continuous positive airway pressure on sleep apnea and ventricular irritability in patients with heart failure. Circulation 2000; 101:392–397.
89. Javaheri S, Corbett WS. Association of low PaCO2 with central sleep apnea and ventricular arrhythmias in ambulatory patients with stable heart failure. Ann Intern Med 1998; 128:204–207.
90. Javaheri S, Parker TJ, Liming JD, et al. Sleep apnea in 81 ambulatory male patients with stable heart failure. Types and their prevalences, consequences, and presentations. Circulation 1998; 97:2154–2159.
91. Exner DV, Dries DL, Waclawiw MA, et al. Beta-adrenergic blocking agent use and mortality in patients with asymptomatic and symptomatic left ventricular systolic dysfunction: a post hoc analysis of the studies of left ventricular dysfunction. J Am Coll Cardiol 1999; 33:916–923.
92. Kennedy HL, Brooks MM, Barker AH, et al. Beta-blocker therapy in the cardiac arrhythmia suppression trial. CAST Investigators. Am J Cardiol 1994; 74:674–680.
93. Exner DV, Reiffel JA, Epstein AE, et al. Beta-blocker use and survival in patients with ventricular fibrillation or symptomatic ventricular tachycardia: the antiarrhythmics versus implantable defibrillators (AVID) trial. J Am Coll Cardiol 1999; 34:325–333.
94. Khand AU, Rankin AC, Kaye GC, et al. Systematic review of the management of atrial fibrillation in patients with heart failure. Eur Heart J 2000; 21:614–632.
95. Naccarelli GV, Lukas MA. Carvedilol's antiarrhythmic properties: therapeutic implications in patients with left ventricular dysfunction. Clin Cardiol 2005; 28:165–173.
96. Deedwania PC, Gottieb S, Ghali JK, et al. Efficacy, safety and tolerability of beta-adrenergic blockade with metoprolol CR/XL in elderly patients with heart failure. Eur Heart J 2004; 25:1300–1309.
97. Ravid S, Podrid PJ, Lampert S, et al. Congestive heart failure induced by six of the newer antiarrhythmic drugs. J Am Coll Cardiol 1989; 14:1326–1330.
98. Flaker GC, Blackshear JL, McBride R, et al. Antiarrhythmic drug therapy and cardiac mortality in atrial fibrillation. The stroke prevention in atrial fibrillation investigators. J Am Coll Cardiol 1992; 20:527–532.
99. Stevenson WG, Stevenson LW, Middlekauff HR, et al. Improving survival for patients with atrial fibrillation and advanced heart failure. J Am Coll Cardiol 1996; 28:1458–1463 [erratum appears in J Am Coll Cardiol 1997 Dec;30:1902].
100. Kuck KH, Cappato R, Siebels J, et al. Randomized comparison of antiarrhythmic drug therapy with implantable defibrillators in patients resuscitated from cardiac arrest: the cardiac arrest study hamburg (CASH). Circulation 2000; 102:748–754.

101. Nul DR, Doval HC, Grancelli HO, et al. Heart rate is a marker of amiodarone mortality reduction in severe heart failure. The GESICA-GEMA Investigators. Grupo de Estudio de la Sobrevida en la Insuficiencia Cardiaca en Argentina-Grupo de Estudios Multicentricos en Argentina. J Am Coll Cardiol 1997; 29:1199–1205.
102. Singh SN, Fletcher RD, Fisher SG, et al. Amiodarone in patients with congestive heart failure and asymptomatic ventricular arrhythmia. Survival trial of antiarrhythmic therapy in congestive heart failure. N Engl J Med 1995; 333:77–82.
103. Massie BM, Shah NB, Pitt B, et al. Importance of assessing changes in ventricular response to atrial fibrillation during evaluation of new heart failure therapies: experience from trials of flosequinan. Am Heart J 1996; 132:130–136.
104. Anonymous. Effect of prophylactic amiodarone on mortality after acute myocardial infarction and in congestive heart failure: meta-analysis of individual data from 6500 patients in randomised trials. Amiodarone Trials Meta-Analysis Investigators. Lancet 1997; 350:1417–1424.
105. Connolly S. Optimal pharmacological therapy in implantable cardioverter defibrillator patients (OPTIC) trial. J Am Coll Cardiol 2005. Presented Abstract, March 2005.
106. Weinfeld MS, Drazner MH, Stevenson WG, et al. Early outcome of initiating amiodarone for atrial fibrillation in advanced heart failure. J Heart Lung Transplant 2000; 19:638–643.
107. Anonymous. A comparison of antiarrhythmic-drug therapy with implantable defibrillators in patients resuscitated from near-fatal ventricular arrhythmias. The antiarrhythmics versus implantable defibrillators (AVID) investigators. N Engl J Med 1997; 337:1576–1583.
108. Dusman RE, Staton MS, Miles WM, et al. Clinical features of amiodarone-induced pulmonary toxicity. Circulation 1990; 82:51–59.
109. Singh SN, Fisher SG, Deedwania PC, et al. Pulmonary effect of amiodarone in patients with heart failure. The Congestive Heart Failure-Survival Trial of Antiarrhythmic Therapy (CHF-STAT) Investigators (Veterans Affairs Cooperative Study no. 320). J Am Coll Cardiol 1997; 30:514–517.
110. Siniakowicz RM, Narula D, Suster B, et al. Diagnosis of amiodarone pulmonary toxicity with high-resolution computerized tomographic scan. J Cardiovasc Electrophysiol 2001; 12:431–436.
111. Loh KC. Amiodarone-induced thyroid disorders: a clinical review. Postgrad Med J 2000; 76:133–140.
112. Pratt CM, Camm AJ, Cooper W, et al. Mortality in the survival with ORal D-sotalol (SWORD) trial: why did patients die? Am J Cardiol 1998; 81:869–876.
113. Roy D, Talajic M, Dorian P, et al. Amiodarone to prevent recurrence of atrial fibrillation. Canadian Trial of Atrial Fibrillation Investigators. N Engl J Med 2000; 342:913–920.

12
Acute Heart Failure

Stuart D. Russell
Division of Cardiology, Department of Internal Medicine, The Johns Hopkins Hospital, Baltimore, Maryland, U.S.A.

INTRODUCTION

Acute heart failure can be defined as the sudden onset of heart failure in a patient that has never had a diagnosis of cardiac disease in the past or as an acute exacerbation of symptoms in someone who has chronic heart failure resulting in a hospitalization or a change in therapy. For the purposes of this chapter, "acute heart failure" will refer to exacerbations of heart failure in patients who already have chronic heart failure defined by symptomatic systolic dysfunction.

The incidence and prevalence of heart failure is increasing and subsequently there are more admissions for heart failure. From 1970 to 2002, the number of heart failure discharges has increased from less then 200,000 per year to almost 1,000,000 (1). This is in part related to the aging of the population, but also related to the improved survival after acute myocardial infarction. This increase in hospitalization rate has resulted in a huge increase in the cost of heart failure care in America. It is estimated that over 25.3 billion dollars will be spent on heart failure care in the United States in 2005 (1).

CLINICAL CONTEXT

There are three recently published studies that describe the current status of patients with acute heart failure (2–4). The Outcomes of a Prospective Trial of Intravenous Milrinone for Exacerbations of Chronic Heart Failure (OPTIME-CHF) trial randomized 951 patients admitted with an acute exacerbation of chronic heart failure to intravenous milrinone or placebo (2). As shown in Table 1, the mean age of these patients was 65 and their average ejection fraction was 23%. This is quite similar to the patients studied in the Vasodilation in the Management of Acute Chronic Heart Failure (VMAC) trial (3). This trial randomized 489 patients to nesiritide, nitroglycerin, or placebo. The mean age was 62 and the ejection fraction was 27%. In contrast, the Acute Decompensated Heart Failure National Registry (ADHERE) registry of patients admitted with heart failure but not enrolled in a clinic trial, reveals some interesting trends about the overall picture of patients being hospitalized with heart failure (4). Of 105,388 patients that had been enrolled in the registry since 2001,

Table 1 Comparison of Patients Admitted with Acute Heart Failure

	OPTIME[a]	VMAC[a]	ADHERE
Age (yrs)	66	62	72
Male sex (%)	68	60	48
Race			
White (%)	67	58	72
Black (%)	32	24	20
NYHA class			
II (%)	7	5	20
III (%)	45	42	44
IV (%)	48	45	32
Medical history			
Hypertension (%)	68	74	73
Myocardial infarction (%)	48	49	31
Atrial fibrillation (%)	30	34	31
Diabetes (%)	45	53	44
Physical findings			
SBP (mmHg)	120	121	144
Heart rate (bpm)	84	N/A	N/A
Baseline medications			
ACE inhibitor (%)	71	60	41
Angiotensin receptor blocker (%)	13	9	12
Beta blocker (%)	22	35	48
Diuretic (%)	90	87	70
Digoxin (%)	71	60	28

[a]Placebo arm for OPTIME and VMAC.

the mean age was 72.4 yr and 52% were women. This is a much older age group than has been studied in the clinical trials of angiotensin converting enzyme (ACE) inhibitors and beta-blockers where the average age was between 58 and 64 yr and the ejection fraction higher (34.4%) (5–11).

Despite differences in the age and ejection fraction of these patients (Table 1) the risk factors for heart failure are quite similar between the populations. Over half of the patients have a history of coronary artery disease and almost three quarters have a history of hypertension. Somewhat surprisingly, despite the proven benefits of ACE inhibitors and beta blockers on symptoms and survival, the use of these drugs was not optimal. In the OPTIME and VMAC trials, conducted at academic medical centers the use of ACE inhibitors and angiotensin receptor blockers (ARB) was 70%–80%. This contrasts to the ADHERE registry where just over half of the patients were on these medications. Similarly, the use of beta blockers was less than 50% in the ADHERE registry. Unfortunately, the use of these agents did not improve after being hospitalized. Only 66.1% of the patients felt eligible to receive an ACE inhibitor were discharged on one (4).

Being admitted to a hospital is a poor prognostic sign for patients with heart failure. The OPTIME-CHF trial demonstrated an incidence of death of 10% and death or readmission of 35% within 2 mo (2). Similarly, in the VMAC trial 20%–23% of the patients were readmitted within 30 days and the 6-month mortality was 20.8% for nitroglycerin and 25.1% for nesiritide (3). The current outcomes and prognosis for patients hospitalized with acute heart failure are quite poor and additional studies and novel therapies need to be studied. Additionally, the therapies that are beneficial need to be implemented in a standardized and routine fashion. This chapter will focus on the assessment and therapy for patients admitted to the hospital with an acute exacerbation of their chronic heart failure.

ASSESSMENT

Acute heart failure is a clinical syndrome involving multiple potential etiologies and clinical manifestations. Some patients may have an ischemic etiology and present with symptoms of dyspnea because of ongoing myocardial ischemia. Others may have eaten a high salt diet and have dyspnea due to fluid retention and volume overload. Finally, others may have progressively worsening cardiac function and present with dyspnea related to poor tissue perfusion from a low cardiac output. Prior to initiating therapy, it is important to differentiate between the many different potential etiologies resulting in admission and appropriately direct therapies based on these causes. Table 2 lists many of the potential exacerbating factors that contribute to an admission with acute heart failure (12).

Table 2 Cause and Precipitating Factors in Acute Heart Failure

Progression of pre-existing heart failure
Acute coronary syndromes
Myocardial infarction/unstable angina
Mechanical complication of acute myocardial infarction
Right ventricular infarction
Hypertensive crisis or urgency
Acute arrhythmia (ventricular tachycardia, atrial fibrillation or flutter, other supraventricular tachycardias)
Valvular regurgitation (acute or progression of chronic)
Severe aortic valve stenosis
Acute myocarditis
Cardiac tamponade
Aortic dissection
Noncardiovascular
Lack of compliance with diet or medical therapy
Volume overload
Infections
Severe brain insult
After major surgery
Reduction in renal function
Asthma
Drug abuse
Alcohol abuse
Pheochromocytoma
High output syndromes
Septicemia
Hyperthyroidism
Anemia
Shunt syndromes
Paget's disease

Source: From Ref. 12.

The treatment of someone with a hypertensive crisis will be much different than someone who presents with a low output syndrome.

In addition to thinking about the potential etiology, one must direct therapy based on the clinical manifestations that each patient presents. As first described by Forrester for patients with acute heart failure in the setting of acute myocardial infarction, dividing patients into four groups according to their tissue perfusion and volume status can be very helpful when deciding on therapy (13). Nohria et al. have further refined this system into four heart failure profiles (Fig. 1) (14). For a patient that presents with signs of congestion (history of orthopnea and/or paroxysmal nocturnal dyspnea, jugular venous distention, rales, hepatojugular reflux, ascites, peripheral edema), treatment with diuretics should be initiated. Conversely, signs of decreased perfusion (symptomatic hypotension, cold extremities, narrow pulse pressure, and worsening renal function) should be treated with vasodilators or inotropic agents.

Clinical Evaluation and Exam

Similar to other diseases, the evaluation begins with taking a complete history. This should be directed at determining potential exacerbating factors that have contributed to the acute decompensation (Table 2), the severity of the exacerbation, and the time course of the exacerbation (acute versus sub acute). Table 3 outlines parts of the history that should be focused on.

Some general questions can be quite helpful in determining the time course and potential etiologies of the exacerbation. Patients who have had a progressive decline over a few weeks to months will often have a slow progression of their heart failure and although need to be treated acutely, may also have a very different prognosis in the short and long term than the patient who had an episode of noncompliance and acute volume overload (see Section on Risk Stratifying). If the patient has gained weight, has that been a slow progression over two weeks or over two days? Similarly, the symptoms of increased weakness and fatigue can be quite informative. Daily activity is also a helpful marker of both the time course and the severity of the exacerbation. Has there been a marked reduction in activity for some time or was the patient active until a few days before admission? Finally, a history of dietary non-compliance, both for salt and volume intake should be obtained.

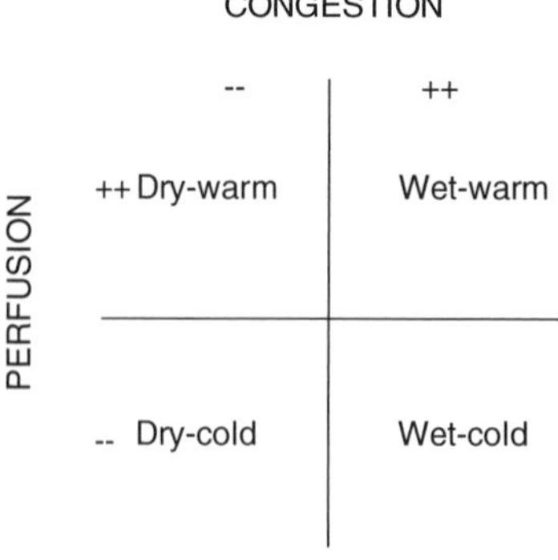

Figure 1 Diagram for assessing acute heart failure. Patients will usually present with evidence of poor (cold) or normal (warm) perfusion and evidence of volume overload (wet) or euvolemia (dry). *Source*: Adapted from Refs. 13 and 14.

Table 3 Clinical History in Acute Heart Failure

General
Weight change
Signs of infection (fever, chill, productive cough)
Weakness
Fatigue
Dietary non-compliance
Activity
Cardiac
Dyspnea
Orthopnea
Paroxysmal nocturnal dyspnea
Orthostatic symptoms
Chest pain
Palpitations
Pulmonary
Dyspnea
Cough
Hemoptysis
Gastrointestinal
Nausea
Vomiting
Abdominal pain
Anorexia
Renal
Nocturia
Oliguria
Periphery
Edema
Cool extremities
Neurologic
Mental status

The cardiac history is also quite helpful. Although dyspnea is one of the primary signs of heart failure, many patients with chronic heart failure will preferentially complain of fatigue. The severity of dyspnea, with and without exertion, can be helpful in following therapy outcomes. Orthopnea is a very helpful symptom for discerning heart failure exacerbations. Rarely do patients like to sleep on more than 2 pillows and the progression from their normal pillow count to sleeping on a wedge or sleeping in a recliner is quite instructive for the time course of the exacerbation. Similarly, when evaluating the patient in the hospital, the angle that they slept at the night before can be quite helpful in determining the adequacy of the diuresis. Once patients are sleeping flat or nearly flat in bed they are usually ready for discharge. Symptoms of coronary ischemia may be quite different and a broad range of questions to rule out ischemia as a potential exacerbating factor must be performed.

Cough is often associated with symptoms of volume overload and may be associated with pulmonary infections, which can cause heart failure exacerbations. Be careful to exclude infections before attributing all coughs and dyspnea to volume overload.

Gastrointestinal symptoms of heart failure are quite vague but can be telling. Patients with nausea and anorexia often have low output syndromes and are not perfusing their abdominal organs adequately. Conversely, acute volume overload can be associated with abdominal edema, like peripheral edema and can cause similar symptoms. Hepatic congestion may cause right upper quadrant pain and contribute to early satiety. Although never quantitated, in my experience gastrointestinal symptoms are more frequent in New York Heart Association (NYHA) functional class IV patients and appear to be a sign of worse disease.

Peripheral edema is one of the hallmarks of volume overload. In addition to the extremities, an increase in abdominal girth should also be evaluated.

The physical exam is the second important part of the assessment of patients with acute heart failure and helps to focus on potential therapies as well as the severity of the disease process. The exam should focus on the signs of volume overload, low cardiac output, and assess potential causes of deterioration (mitral regurgitation, thyroid disease, etc.). The reader is referred to textbooks on Physical Exam for the details on how to perform these maneuvers; this chapter will focus on the findings and how they relate to acute heart failure (15). As outlined in Table 4, although cardiac centered many other organ systems need to be closely evaluated during this exam. The vital signs should be used for the acute care of the patient, but one should also use them to evaluate the overall status of the patient. A low grade elevated temperature (<38°C) can occur in severe heart failure, but one must always search for other potential infections that may have caused the exacerbation. The blood pressure should be measured and if low, orthostatics should be performed. Many patients with heart failure will have systolic blood pressures below 100 mmHg, so determining the usual pressure is important before becoming concerned about hypotension. The pulse rate is probably the most important vital sign. Tachycardia can be secondary to thyroid abnormalities or anemia, but also is a sign of more severe heart failure. Arrhythmias, either atrial or ventricular, can be an exacerbating cause of heart failure. Finally, pulsus

Table 4 Physical Examination in Acute Heart Failure

Vital signs
Temperature
Blood pressure (orthostasis)
Heart rate (rate and pulse quality)
Respiratory rate (Cheyne-Stokes pattern)
Pulmonary
Rales
Wheezes
Dullness to percussion
Cardiac
Point of maximal impulse
Right ventricular heave
Jugular venous distention
S3 or S4
Loud P2
Murmurs
Abdominal
Hepatomegaly
Splenomegaly
Ascites
Periphery
Edema (including sacral)
Mental status

alternans, the alternating of strong and weak pulsations, is associated with severe heart failure (16,17). The respiratory rate helps to assess volume overload as tachypneic patients often have more fluid. Cheyne-Stokes respiration patterns are also associated with severe heart failure and may be evident even while awake. The presence of sleep apnea and a higher apnea/hypopnea index (the number of apneas and hypopneas per hour) have been associated with reduced maximal oxygen consumption and increased mortality (18,19). However, Cheyne-Stokes respirations have also been shown to increase in elderly patients and appear to be weakly associated with severity of illness in those over the age of 70 (20). Many times it can be helpful to ask the partner or hospital roommate about sleeping patterns since they are often awakened by the abnormal breathing pattern.

The pulmonary exam can be helpful to distinguish between a predominance of right-sided and left-sided heart failure. Auscultation of rales in the lungs is frequently heard in patients with acute heart failure. However, in patients with chronic heart failure who have developed compensatory mechanisms of pulmonary hypertension and improved lymphatic drainage, one many not hear rales even in the setting of high left sided filling pressures. Wheezes are often heard due to bronchial edema, usually in patients that are more acute and haven't had years to develop compensatory mechanisms. Pleural effusions can also occur in heart failure and percussion of the bases should always be performed.

There are many components to the cardiac exam which can be helpful. Palpation of the PMI provides an assessment of heart size and the chronicity of heart failure. Severe dilatation of the left ventricle does not happen acutely. If the patient has a normal size heart, one should think about different processes than in the massively dilated ventricle. A right ventricular heave is associated with increased pressure or volume overload and increased pulmonary pressures, which occur once the body has adapted to high filling pressures for some time. To judge the effects of therapy, the jugular venous pulsation is one of the most important physical exam findings. A normal jugular pulse should be less than 4 cm above the sternal angle. The jugular venous pulse has been shown to correlate with the pulmonary artery pressure by right heart catheterization and is a good surrogate for measuring left-sided filling pressures in most patients (21). Spending additional time and properly positioning the patient is important to determine the height of the venous pressure. Occasionally, the venous pulsation is high and even when the patient is sitting upright the peak cannot be found. With diuresis and time the pulse will then become visible. The presence of an S3 may be heard as part of the normal exam in children, but in adults is usually considered to be pathologic. When judging the effects of therapy, the intensity of S3 has been shown to correlate with the pulmonary capillary wedge pressure (22). This will not be helpful on the day of admission, but similar to the jugular venous pulse, can be used to follow the effectiveness of therapy as it may become softer with diuresis. The intensity of the pulmonic component of the second heart sound has been shown to correlate with the pulmonary systolic pressure (23). This is often heard over the left upper sternal border, but when the P2 is heard at the lower sternal border or the apex it is associated with elevated pressures, usually over 50 mmHg. Finally, one should listen carefully for murmurs. With heart failure and dilation of the left and right ventricles, tricuspid and mitral regurgitation can become quite prominent. With diuresis and reduction in ventricular size, these murmurs can diminish or disappear.

The abdominal exam is important to assess signs of volume overload. An enlarged liver or spleen is often associated with severe right-sided failure and can be used to assess the severity of heart failure. The presence of ascites secondary to elevated hepatic pressures yields similar information. Perhaps one of the most misunderstood parts of the abdominal exam is the hepatojugular reflex. A positive hepatojugular reflex is usually observed in states of low cardiac output. However, it can also be observed in constrictive pericarditis, pericardial tamponade, tricuspid insufficiency, and inferior vena caval obstruction (24,25).

Peripheral edema is quite common in heart failure and implies that there is some component of right-sided failure and volume overload. The extent of edema (thighs, genital, sacral) is important to evaluate when assessing adequacy of diuresis. One should be aware that patients may always have some peripheral edema due to venous insufficiency, but with the exception of other etiologies of total body edema (nephrotic syndrome, hypoalbuminemia, protein losing enteropathy, renal disease, venous obstruction, liver disease), edema in the thighs or over the sacrum would not result from venous disease alone.

STUDIES

A variety of laboratory studies and other testing should be performed in patients admitted with acute heart failure as outlined in Table 5 (26). These studies will aid in the diagnosis of potential exacerbating factors as well as in the therapy of the patient. Many of the laboratory tests are helpful for diagnosing factors that may have exacerbated the patient's chronic heart failure. Evidence of infection, anemia, renal dysfunction, hyperthyroidism, uncontrolled diabetes, and increased ischemia should all be ruled out. The severity of heart failure can be further elucidated by signs of volume overload [elevated liver function tests, low albumin, hyponatremia, brain natriuretic peptide (BNP)] (27–34). Finally, serum sodium and creatinine have both been shown to be independent prognostic risk factors for poor outcomes in patients with heart failure (27–29,35,36).

The laboratory studies are also important in the day-to-day care of the patients. Both potassium and magnesium are depleted with most diuretic therapies and need to be followed closely since low levels are associated with arrhythmias. Serum creatinine can sometimes by used to assess the adequacy of diuresis. Once the creatinine starts to rise, the patients are sufficiently diuresed and ready for discharge. One caveat to that general rule is

Table 5 Diagnostic Testing

Laboratory
Complete blood count[a]
Urinalysis[a]
Serum sodium, potassium, BUN, creatinine, glucose, magnesium, calcium, albumin, phosphorus[a]
Liver function tests
Prothrombin time
Consider
Brain natriuretic peptide or pro-brain natriuretic peptide
Thyroid-stimulating hormone (in patients with atrial fibrillation or unexplained heart failure)[a]
Creatinine kinase and troponin (if history of ischemia or chest pain)
EKG[a]
Chest X-ray[a]
Echocardiogram[a]
Consider
Right heart catheterization (to assess volume status and cardiac output)
Left heart catheterization (to assess for coronary artery disease if not performed previously)[a]

[a]These studies are recommended as Class I indications by the American College of Cardiology/American Heart Association Heart Failure Practice Guidelines (29).

in patients with baseline renal insufficiency or low cardiac output may have a quick rise in serum creatinine long before they are euvolemic.

The measurement of BNP levels is a recent advancement in the management of heart failure. In the Emergency Room, BNP levels have been used to evaluate the potential etiologies of dyspnea. In the Breathing Not Properly study, a cutoff of 100 pg/ml gave a diagnostic accuracy of 83% in distinguishing patients with heart failure from those with non-cardiac causes of dyspnea (37). For patients with a level above 500 pg/ml, heart failure is the most probable cause of their dyspnea. Despite the increases in BNP seen in patients with heart failure, the use of serial measurements of BNP in hospitalized patients to guide therapy has not been shown to be helpful. In fact, in a small study there was no correlation between a reduction in pulmonary capillary wedge pressure and BNP levels (38). One caveat to the use of BNP levels is that older age, female gender, and renal dysfunction can all be associated with increased levels (38–40). Conversely, obesity is associated with lower levels (41). At this time, BNP testing is emerging as a useful tool in the treatment of patients with heart failure, but more research needs to be performed to help ascertain the true value of this test. One should use a BNP level in conjunction with the overall clinical situation and not use an isolated level to guide therapy.

The electrocardiogram should be a normal part of the evaluation of every patient admitted with acute heart failure. It is essential for the assessment of acute coronary syndromes. Additionally, other potential causes of a heart failure exacerbation, including atrial and ventricular arrhythmias and myocarditis, can be detected. The electrocardiogram can also help to determine the severity of disease. Left and right atrial enlargement are signs of more chronic disease.

Echocardiography is almost mandatory in patients admitted with new onset heart failure. Determination of left and right ventricular function and size, wall motion abnormalities, valvular structure and function, as well as ventricular relaxation are all variables that should be obtained. Additionally, the estimate of pulmonary artery pressure from the tricuspid regurgitation jet provides a reliable estimate of left-sided filling pressures (42). In patients with chronic heart failure and a known reduction in ejection fraction that are admitted, obtaining an echocardiogram can still be quite helpful. Knowledge of ventricular size, further reductions in function, or worsening valvular abnormalities may alter therapy. The use of Doppler estimates of pulmonary pressure to follow the effectiveness of therapy has not been studied. Both the American College of Cardiology/American Heart Association and the European Society of Cardiology heart failure guidelines have a Class I recommendation for obtaining echocardiograms (12,26).

Coronary angiography is useful when clinically indicated for patients with acute coronary syndromes, but should not be routinely performed in patients admitted with heart failure. Conversely, right heart catheterization can be used to evaluate both the severity of the volume overload and the cardiac output when initiating therapy and when following the effects of therapy. The use of a right heart cath to guide therapy has proven to be useful in non-randomized studies. Fonarow et al. admitted 214 patients and used right heart catheter guided therapy to increase vasodilators and diuretics (43). They reduced hospital readmissions and improved functional status as measured by peak oxygen consumption. The percentage of patients on ACE inhibitors and other vasodilators at the time of discharge was also increased.

Support for the use of routine right heart catheterizations (RHC) was tempered by the SUPPORT study, which evaluated the use of a RHC for the routine care of patients who were critically ill (44). They found that patients who received RHC guided care had an increase in 30-day mortality. A subgroup analysis found that when used for patients with heart failure there was no change in mortality and therefore the National Institutes of Health sponsored another trial to evaluate the effectiveness of RHC guided therapy in patients admitted with acute heart failure. The results of this study have not yet been published but were presented at the American Heart Association 2004 Annual Scientific Session (45). The investigators found no difference in the primary end-point, days alive out of the hospital in 6 mo. Additionally, there was no difference in the secondary endpoints of survival or number of days hospitalized.

At this time, routine use of a right heart catheter to guide therapy in patients admitted with acutely decompensated heart failure is not indicated. At our institution, RHC are still performed but often the catheter is removed after the pressures and cardiac output have been measured instead of left in. This reduces the chance of infection or other catheter related complications yet still provides useful data. When done in patients who are close to discharge, we are often surprised to find that the pressures are still quite elevated even when the patients are symptomatically at baseline. Further diuresis is then performed in the hope that this will decrease hospital readmissions and improve quality of life. Additionally, RHC is still helpful for patients who are failing the usual medical therapy with hypotension and worsening renal function.

THERAPY

The goals of therapy during a hospitalization are to improve symptoms and stabilize the patient for long-term improvements in outcome. In patients with volume overload, this is often accomplished with aggressive diuresis. Other patients that present with low output symptoms may require changes in their vasodilators to improve their output. The long-term focus during a hospitalization should be on improving outcomes. This includes initiating therapies that have been shown to improve morbidity and mortality as well as using the opportunity to teach about diet and fluid management and improve compliance.

Since there are individual chapters devoted to the major groups of medicines used for the treatment of heart failure, this chapter will focus on the use of these agents in the acute, hospitalized setting.

Oxygen

Oxygen should be given to maintain an adequate oxygenation in order to prevent end organ dysfunction. A goal oxygen saturation of $>94\%$ is necessary to maintain tissue saturation. There are no data that the routine use of oxygen in patients that are not hypoxic is beneficial and therefore oxygen should not routinely be administered in all patients. One can also use oxygen and oxygen saturations to monitor the effectiveness of therapy. As fluid is removed from the lungs, oxygen saturations will improve and the oxygen can be weaned. Patients that continue to have an oxygen requirement and don't have other reasons for hypoxia probably need continued diuresis.

Angiotensin-Converting Enzyme Inhibitors

There is overwhelming evidence supporting the use of ACE inhibitors in patients with heart failure; however, these agents have never been studied in patients who are acutely decompensated (5–7,46). The mechanism of ACE inhibitors in theory should be quite beneficial to patients in acute heart failure. ACE inhibitors decrease renal vascular resistance and therefore improve renal blood flow and subsequent sodium and water excretion. Additionally, pulmonary and systemic vasodilation will reduce afterload and improve forward flow. In general, if the patient has already been on an ACE inhibitor when admitted to the hospital they can usually stay on it. There are some situations when the dose should be either reduced or the drug should be stopped, however, including patients who are hypotensive or have worsening renal function. Since ACE inhibitors preferentially dilate the efferent over the afferent glomerular arteriole, this can lead to a reduction in glomerular pressure and a reduction in glomerular filtration rate which may further exacerbate poor renal function.

Once the patient is stabilized, the ACE inhibitor should be restarted and up-titrated as tolerated by the blood pressure. When initiating an ACE inhibitor in a patient with marginal blood pressure or renal function, it is reasonable to start with a low dose of a short-acting agent such as captopril. If the patient tolerates this low dose, the dose can then be uptitrated and the agent can be switched to a longer acting, once-a-day agent for patient convenience. Studies have shown that aggressive vasodilation with ACE inhibitors prior to discharge in the setting of adequate diuresis leads to a significant reduction in rehospitalizations (43).

Beta-Blockers

Similar to ACE inhibitors, there are no data on the impact of beta blockers on patients admitted with an acute exacerbation of their chronic heart failure. Some advocate withdrawing the drug, others reduce the dose, and still others continue at the same dose if it appears that the patient has volume overload without evidence of poor perfusion. A retrospective analysis of the OPTIME-CHF trial looked at outcomes of patients who were on beta blockers at the time of admission compared to those not on a beta blocker. They further looked at the outcomes in patients who had their beta blocker withdrawn during the hospitalization (47). There was no difference in outcomes between the patients who were either on or not on a beta blocker at the time of admission. However, despite having very similar background characteristics, patients who had their beta blocker withdrawn during the hospitalization had a higher 60-day mortality rate, especially if they were treated with milrinone. While this is a retrospective analysis of a small population of patients, the routine practice of withdrawing beta blockers from patients at the time of admission does not seem warranted.

For patients not on beta blockers at the time of admission, the hospitalization should be utilized to initiate these agents prior to discharge. Despite the evidence that beta blockers have long term benefits, all of the large randomized clinical trials enrolled patients that were stable as outpatients (8–11). Based on these trials, the most recent guidelines of the Heart Failure Society of America state that in general beta blockers should not be routinely initiated during a hospitalization (48). Recently, the results of the Initiation Management Predischarge: Process for Assessment of Carvedilol Therapy in Heart Failure (IMPACT-HF) trial were presented (49). This was an open label randomized study of pre hospital discharge versus 2 wk post discharge initiation of the beta blocker carvedilol. The end-point was the number of patients treated with a beta blocker at 60 days. They found that 91.2% of the patients initiated pre discharge versus 73.4% of those initiated post-discharge were on a beta blocker at 60 days. Additionally, initiation prior to discharge was not associated with an increase in adverse events nor did it lengthen the hospital stay. Based on these data, once patients are euvolemic it is reasonable to initiate low-dose therapy with a beta blocker prior to discharge in patients that have not been on a beta blocker previously. For those patients that were on a beta blocker at the time of admission, unless the patient shows signs of poor end organ perfusion requiring inotropes the drug should be continued throughout the hospitalization.

Diuretics

Diuretic therapy is the mainstay of the therapy for acute heart failure secondary to volume overload. Within 15 min, furosemide administered intravenously causes venodilation and subsequent reduction in preload of both the left and right ventricles (50). Within 30 min, it acts on the kidney to inhibit sodium and water resorption resulting in diuresis. This quick acting agent provides symptomatic benefit for the patient with volume overload.

There are a few issues to consider when using diuretics. It is important to monitor for hypotension, electrolyte abnormalities, and renal function while administering diuretics. Hypotension may actually cause reduced flow to the kidney, worsening renal function and decreased diuresis. Diuretic induced hypokalemia and hypomagnesemia are both associated with ventricular arrhythmias. Finally, worsening renal function may be a sign of overdiuresis or poor cardiac output, necessititating the use of other agents to improve cardiac output. Additionally, worsening renal function has been shown to be an independent marker of a worse prognosis (35,36).

The use of diuretics induces activation of the neurohormonal system, especially the rennin-angiotensin and the sympathetic nervous system. Long-term activation of these systems has been shown to be detrimental. In both the Studies of Left Ventricular Dysfunction (SOLVD) and the Vasodilator-Heart Failure Trial II (V-HeFT II) trials, investigators have demonstrated that plasma levels of norepinephrine, renin, ANP, and AVP are elevated in patients with left ventricular dysfunction when compared with healthy control individuals (51,52). Furthermore, as NYHA functional class worsens, the levels of these neurohormones are increased. It is important to judiciously use diuretics to avoid this upregulation if possible.

No clinical trials have studied the efficacy of one diuretic versus another in patients with acute heart failure. In general, one must use a loop diuretic in a high enough dose of the diuretic to initiate and maintain a diuresis. In patients that are receiving high doses of a loop diuretic, the addition of a synergistic agent such as a thiazide that acts on the distal loop may be quite beneficial to assist with adequate diuresis (53–55). There is one study comparing intermittent bolus doses of intravenous furosemide with a continuous infusion (56). Patients receiving high doses of oral furosemide (>250 mg) were randomized to receive that dose by either continuous infusion or intravenous bolus. Patients receiving furosemide by continuous infusion had a greater urine output and a reduced incidence of adverse side effects.

Vasodilators

For patients that have congestion and adequate blood pressure, vasodilators can be quite helpful be reducing either preload or afterload in patients admitted with acute heart failure. Nitroglycerin improves the symptoms of heart failure by reducing pressures through direct pulmonary venodilation. Nitrates have been shown to reduce pulmonary capillary wedge pressure and systemic vascular resistance in patients admitted with acute heart failure (57). Additionally, patients receiving intravenous nitroglycerin reported an improvement in dyspnea and their overall sense of well being. One concern about the use of nitroglycerin is that patients develop tolerance to the drug over time and need to have the dose increased. For patients that are acutely diuresing and only require nitroglycerin for a couple of days, this may not be an issue. One study has examined the effects of high versus low doses of nitroglycerin. Cotter et al. randomized patients to either high nitroglycerin and low dose furosemide or low dose nitroglycerin and high dose furosemide (58). The group receiving high dose nitroglycerin had a decreased incidence of the end-point of mechanical ventilation arguing that increasing vasodilator doses may be more effective than increasing doses of diuretics for the treatment of refractory heart failure.

Nitroprusside is a mixed arterial and venodilator that reduces both preload and afterload. It can be useful for patients with hypertension and acute heart failure. Nitroprusside has not been studied in the treatment of patients with acute heart failure. In patients with acute myocardial infarction is has been shown to worsen mortality (59). Coronary blood flow may be shunted away from vessels with high-grade stenosis that cannot dilate and cause further ischemia in those territories (50). Although this is a different patient population, one should use caution with this agent in patients with a history of coronary artery disease. Nitroprusside should also be used cautiously due to the toxic effects of its metabolites, thiocyanide and cyanide, especially in patients with renal or hepatic insufficiency. In general, with the exception of patients with severe hypertension, other agents should be used for first-line vasodilator therapy.

The newest vasodilator is nesiritide, a recombinant human natriuretic peptide that activates guanylyl cyclase and increases intracellular cGMP levels. B-type natriuretic peptide (BNP) is the only neurohormone that is thought to be beneficial when upregulated in end stage heart failure. Endogenous BNP is stimulated to be released by stretching of the ventricles and acts as both an arterial and venodilator. This agent has been studied for use in acute heart failure. When initially compared to placebo, the use of nesiritide was associated with a 6 to 9.6 mmHg decrease in pulmonary capillary wedge pressure as well as improvements in clinical status, reduced dyspnea, and reduced fatigue (60). It was also compared to the usual intravenous agents used to treat acute heart failure including dobutamine (57% of patients), milrinone (19%), nitroglycerin (18%), dopamine (6%), and amrinone (1%). There were no significant differences in the clinical end-points of dyspnea or fatigue although the nesiritide group was associated with fewer intravenous diuretics being given (60).

The VMAC study compared nesiritide to nitroglycerin or placebo for three hours after which the placebo patients were randomized to nitroglycerin or nesiritide (57). There was a significant reduction in the pulmonary capillary wedge pressure in the nesiritide group compared to the nitroglycerin group at 3 hr, there was a significant reduction in the pulmonary capillary wedge pressure in the nesiritide group compared to the nitroglycerin group. Both were reduced compared to placebo. This reduction was sustained over 24 hr although the absolute difference between the two groups was only 1.9 mmHg. By 36 and 48 hr, there was no longer any statistical difference between the two groups. The investigators also assessed dyspnea and global clinical status of the patients. Despite demonstrating a reduction in pulmonary capillary wedge pressure, there were no significant differences in dyspnea or global clinical status at 24 hr when compared to nitroglycerin.

Nesiritide has also been compared to other vasoactive agents commonly used in patients admitted with acute, symptomatic, decompensated heart failure in an open label fashion (61). The predominant agent used in the control arm was dobutamine and all comparisons were made between the patients that received dobutamine and two doses of nesiritide. Dose changes, vasoactive agent changes, and the length of therapy were all left to the discretion of the investigator. The baseline characteristics of the patients were similar although the dobutamine group had more patients with an ischemic etiology and the high dose nesiritide patients had an increased prevalence of patients with a history of sudden death. The authors found that the median duration of drug infusion was less with nesiritide compared to dobutamine although this did not result in a difference in length of hospitalization. The readmission rate for heart failure trended towards a benefit with nesiritide although this did not reach statistical significance ($p=0.081$). However, compared with dobutamine the 6-mo mortality rate was reduced with the low dose (0.015 μg/kg/min) of nesiritide.

Based on the results of these two trials, nesiritide was approved for use in patients with acute, decompensated heart failure. Despite only being demonstrated to be a vasodilator in clinical trials, many now, perhaps incorrectly, use nesiritide as a first-line diuretic. Wang et al. recently demonstrated that this might not be the correct use for the drug (62). In a small trial of 15 patients hospitalized for heart failure with mild renal insufficiency (baseline creatinine of 1.8 mg/dL), a double-blind, placebo-controlled, crossover study randomized subjects to receive either placebo or nesiritide for 24 hr on consecutive days. There was no difference in glomerular filtration rate, renal plasma flow, urine output, or sodium excretion between the two agents. Sackner-Bernstein et al. have also recently published two manuscripts using data from the Food and Drug Administration website that suggest that nesiritide may be associated with a higher risk of death and worsening renal function compared to vasodilators and diuretics (63,64). This analysis was limited by lack of full access to data and no information on agents used after termination of the study drug. This assessment does give one caution when considering other agents such as vesnarinone and flosequinan that were initially promising and turned out to be detrimental (65–68). Further randomized studies comparing nesiritide to usual care should be performed to demonstrate its benefit as a diuretic and to assess its effect on morbidity and mortality (2). Until available, nesiritide use should be restricted to patients that have been studied, those admitted with acutely decompensated heart failure who would potentially benefit from a vasodilator therapy.

Inotropes

Improving contractility as a goal in the treatment of heart failure has been sought since 1785 when Withering published "An account of the foxglove and some of its medical uses, with practical remarks on dropsy and other diseases." Over 200 yr later, digoxin is still the most commonly used agent of this class of drugs. In addition to its reported clinical benefits, in the early 1920's Wiggers and Stimson showed that digitalis compounds increase ventricular pressure generation in the setting of a constant heart rate and afterload in both normal and failing hearts (69). Recently, based on the results of randomized trials digoxin has fallen out of favor as a therapy for patients with acute heart failure. The Randomized Assessment of Digoxin on Inhibitors of the Angiotensin-Converting Enzyme (RADIANCE) study and the PROVED study both helped to define digoxin's role in current practice. PROVED ($n=88$) and RADIANCE ($n=178$) were multi-center, double blind, randomized placebo-controlled trials with similar patient populations (70,71). In both trials, patients already on digoxin were randomized to continue digoxin therapy or placebo. The RADIANCE trial showed an increase in the relative risk ($RR=5.9$; 95% CI 2.1–17.2) of worsening heart failure in the group receiving placebo compared to those continuing digoxin (70). Placebo treated patients also had a deterioration in all measures of functional capacity (maximal exercise tolerance, submaximal exercise endurance, NYHA classification) and lower quality of life scores. PROVED demonstrated similar results (71). Patients receiving placebo had a higher percentage of treatment failures, decreased time to treatment failure, and significant worsening of maximal exercise performance. The combined results of these two trials demonstrate that withdrawal of digoxin in patients with stable heart failure results in deterioration of functional status, exercise capacity, and left ventricular ejection fraction. Although these studies provide valuable information, they were too short and too small to assess the impact of digoxin on mortality.

These studies were followed by the Digitalis Investigator Group (DIG) study, which evaluated the effect of digoxin on mortality and morbidity in patients with heart failure (72). The primary endpoint was mortality and secondary end-points included mortality from cardiovascular deaths, death from worsening heart failure, hospitalization for worsening heart failure, and hospitalization for other causes. This trial demonstrated a neutral effect on mortality, although a trend toward lower risk of mortality due to worsening heart failure was observed. However, there was a significant reduction in the number of hospitalizations due to worsening heart failure with 6% fewer hospitalizations overall in the digoxin group. When these end-points were combined, there was a significantly lower incidence of death due to worsening heart failure and hospitalization due to worsening heart failure in the digoxin group compared to placebo (Fig. 2).

If digoxin is used, appropriate dosing is important. There are no prospective randomized studies comparing outcomes associated with high ($\geq$1.2 ng/ml) and low ($\leq$1.2 ng/ml) digoxin concentrations; however, combined information from multiple retrospective studies supports a dosing strategy that targets serum digoxin concentrations of 0.5–1.0 ng/ml (73,74). These same studies have shown that the potential for toxicity without additional clinical benefit occurs at serum concentrations greater than 1.2 ng/ml. Additionally, it is important to recognize that multiple drug interactions occur. Table 6 shows some of the common interactions and appropriate dose changes.

While digoxin appears to have a beneficial effect in reducing heart failure hospitalizations, no studies have been performed in patients admitted with acute heart failure. It is reasonable to continue digoxin, but the initiation of digoxin has not been shown to improve the short-term outcomes of patients admitted with acute heart failure.

In contrast to digoxin, there have been studies of the inotropic agents milrinone and dobutamine in acute heart failure. The OPTIME-CHF investigators examined the use of

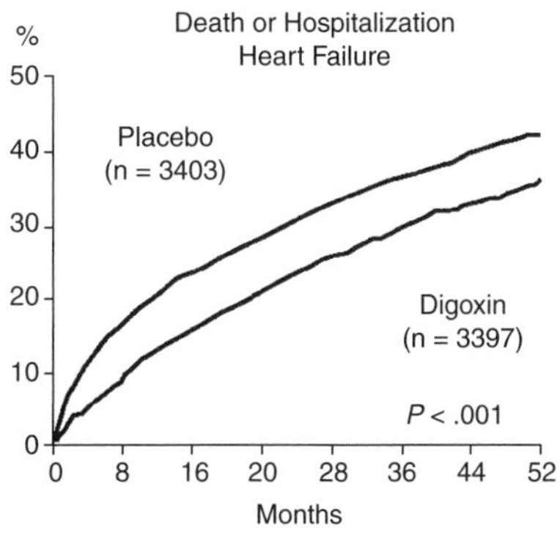

Figure 2 Results of Digitalis Investigator Group trial showing a reduction in the combined endpoint of death or heart failure hospitalization with digoxin when compared to placebo. *Source*: Adapted from Ref. 72.

Table 6 Drugs that Interact with Digoxin

Drug	Action	Rationale
Aluminum or magnesium containing antacids, bile acid binding resins, kaolin-pectin, psyllium, metoclopramide, sulfasalazine, neomycin	Avoid concomitant use or stagger administration time around digoxin (1 hr before, or 2–3 hr after)	Reduced absorption of digoxin; unpredictable absorption.
Erythromycin, clarithromycin, tetracycline	Possible reduction of digoxin dose up to 50% may be indicated in patients at risk of toxicity	Reduced activity of intestinal bacteria which metabolize ~20% of an oral digoxin dose, increasing the bioavailability of digoxin. Not significant with parenteral digoxin therapy
Quinidine, quinine, propafenone	Reduce digoxin dose by 50%	Reduced renal excretion, nonrenal clearance of digoxin, and tissue binding
Amiodarone	Reduce digoxin dose by 50%	Reduced renal and nonrenal clearance of digoxin may displace digoxin from tissue stores. Dose adjust digoxin for up to 6 mo after discontinuation of amiodarone
Verapamil, diltiazem (moderate)	Possible reduction of digoxin dose up to 50% with concomitant verapamil therapy may be indicated in patients at risk of toxicity	Reduction in non-renal clearance of digoxin
Itraconazole	Digoxin dose may require reduction by up to 50% if concomitant itraconazole therapy of $\geq$200 mg/day requiring a course of therapy of 10 or more days	Uncertain; possibly reduction in renal elimination and/or digoxin metabolism

the positive inotrope milrinone (2). Nine hundred and fifty-one patients admitted with an exacerbation of their chronic heart failure were randomized to either milrinone or placebo. The primary endpoint of cumulative days of cardiovascular hospitalization in the first 60 days after randomization was similar between the two groups. Similarly, there was no difference in 60-day mortality, in-hospital mortality, or the composite of death or readmission. The use of milrinone was associated with more hypotension and new atrial arrhythmias. One caveat to this study was that patients who were felt to require inotropes were not eligible for enrollment. Therefore, the sickest patients, who in theory might benefit most from the use of inotropes, were not enrolled. While that hypothesis has not been tested, it is clear that there is no benefit to routinely using milrinone in all patients admitted with heart failure.

Dobutamine compared to placebo has not been evaluated in acute heart failure, but outcomes of patients on dobutamine have been assessed in two different trials. The first was a trial with epoprostenol in patients with advanced heart failure (75). Of the 471 patients randomized, 80 were being treated with dobutamine at the time of randomization. In a retrospective analysis, the use of dobutamine was associated with a higher incidence of mortality (70.5% vs 37.1%). This was followed by a trial comparing dobutamine and nesiritide (61). Again, the use of dobutamine was associated with worse 6-mo mortality and more nonsustained ventricular tachycardia.

Currently, the use of either milrinone or dobutamine in patients admitted with acute heart failure should be reserved for those that exhibit manifestations of low perfusion and cannot be adequately diuresed. For patients on a beta blocker, the use of dobutamine should be considered carefully. Since dobutamine acts as a beta receptor agonist and since this same receptor is blocked by beta antagonists, high doses (>15 μg/kg/min) may be required to achieve a hemodynamic effect (76). In this situation, one should consider using milrinone, a phosphodiesterase inhibitor, or reducing the dose or discontinuing the beta blocker.

Future Therapy

There are many new agents that are being evaluated for use in patients with acute heart failure. These include vasopressin receptor antagonists, adenosine antagonists, and the calcium sensitizer levosimendan.

Through stimulation of V_2 receptors on the renal tubule collecting duct, vasopressin has been found to reduce the rate of free water secretion and concentrate the urine (77). This causes a decrease in urine production that has been found to be proportional to the concentration of plasma vasopressin. Recently, specific antagonists to vasopressin have been developed as potentially useful agents for patients with heart failure and hyponatremia. In patients with heart failure, although vasopressin levels are elevated their exact role is unclear. Vasopressin may cause edema and hyponatremia by activating the V_2 receptor and it may increase peripheral vascular resistance through the V_{1a} receptor located on vascular smooth muscle (78,79). Theoretically, antagonism of one or both of these receptors may be beneficial in patients with heart failure.

Studies with two of these agents have been published. Conivaptan, a dual receptor (V_{1A} and V_2) antagonist was evaluated in 142 patients randomized to either placebo or an intravenous dose of conivaptan at one of 3 different doses (80). These patients had NYHA II or III functional symptoms, but were stable outpatients that were admitted for placement of a right heart catheter and infusion of study drug. The investigators found a significant reduction in pulmonary capillary wedge and right atrial pressure. Additionally, urine output increased by 176 ± 18 mL/hr in the high dose conivaptan group.

Tolvaptan, a V_2 selective vasopressin receptor antagonist has also been studied in patients with heart failure. Gheorghiade et al. reported the results of 254 patients who were randomized to either placebo or 3 different doses of tolvaptan for 25 days (81). A decrease in body weight of about 1 kg was found after the first day that was maintained throughout the study. There was also an increase in urine volume and a normalization of serum sodium with tolvaptan.

A second dose-ranging study was performed with a primary end-point of change in body weight at 24 hr (82). Additionally, heart failure outcomes, including death, hospitalization, or unscheduled visits for heart failure at 60 days, were collected. Body weight at 24 hr after tolvaptan decreased compared to the placebo arm. This decrease occurred without a change in renal function or hypokalemia. There were no differences in the secondary outcome of worsening heart failure at 60 days. Additionally, there was an increase in serum sodium in the tolvaptan arms. If future studies confirm these positive results, these agents may become available for the treatment of acute heart failure, especially in patients with diuretic resistance and/or hyponatremia.

A second class of agents currently undergoing evaluation is the adenosine antagonists. Similar to vasopressin, adenosine levels are increased in patients with advanced heart failure and theoretically antagonism of the receptor will be beneficial (83). There are four different types of adenosine receptors that are present throughout the body (84). The A_1 receptor appears to have effects that could be detrimental to patients with heart failure. In the heart, intravenous boluses of adenosine are associated with profound bradycardia and negative inotropy. In the kidney, binding of adenosine to the A_1 receptor results in afferent arteriole vasoconstriction and a decrease in glomerular blood flow (85). Additionally, an acute increase in the sodium concentration in the proximal renal tubule leads to increased local adenosine production, which then causes further afferent arteriole vasoconstriction (86).

The effects of adenosine antagonism in patients with heart failure are currently under evaluation. The selective A_1 receptor antagonist BG9719 was studied in 12 patients with congestive heart failure (87). Patients were given placebo, BG9719, and furosemide on three different days and glomerular filtration rate, renal plasma flow, sodium excretion, and urine volume were measured. There was a significant decline in glomerular filtration rate, increased sodium excretion, and increased urine volume with furosemide compared to BG9719 or placebo.

A second study with BG9719 was performed in a group of 63 patients (88). Patients were given placebo or 1 of 3 doses of BG9719 on day 1 and then the same agent plus furosemide on a separate day in a double blind, crossover fashion. Infusion of BG9719 was associated with a urine output of over 700 ml in the subsequent 8 hr. Conversely, intravenous furosemide alone resulted in over 1500 ml of urine in 8 hr. The benefit of BG9719 appeared to be when used in combination with furosemide. The combination of the two agents resulted in a urine output of about 2200 ml of urine in 8 hr and there was no change in glomerular filtration rate from baseline. This compares to the furosemide alone group that experienced a decline in glomerular filtration rate of over 15%. Hence, the combination of an A_1 adenosine antagonist and furosemide might theoretically preserve renal function and promote natriuresis and diuresis in patients with acute heart failure.

The last agent currently undergoing evaluation is the calcium sensitizer levosimendan. This agent causes an inotropic response by increasing the sensitivity of troponin-C to intracellular levels of calcium (89). Additionally, it inhibits phosphodiesterase-III (similar to milrinone) and has a vasodilating effect. Levosimendan has been shown to improve stroke volume and decrease pulmonary capillary wedge pressure in patients admitted with decompensated heart failure (90). Further studies are needed to determine if this agent will be the first "safe" inotrope that can be used for the treatment of heart failure.

PRE-DISCHARGE GOALS

Teaching

One of the advantages of an acute heart failure admission is that other non medical issues can be dealt with during their stay. In contrast to an outpatient clinic visit where time is limited, detailed teaching can be done. This needs to be individualized for each patient. If a patient is admitted with decompensated heart failure for the first time, more time should be spent on general teaching about the disease and how it is treated. Conversely, for patients that demonstrate non-compliance to medications, fluid intake, or diet the teaching

Table 7 Optimal Therapy for Patients with Heart Failure

Prolong survival
ACE inhibitors
Angiotensin receptor blockers
Beta-blockers
Spironolactone (if NYHA functional class III or IV)
Statins (if ischemic)
ICD (if EF<35%)
Decrease symptoms
Digoxin
Biventricular pacemakers

should be focused on reinforcing appropriate behaviors. Post discharge care should also be focused on including abstinence from tobacco, measuring weight daily with instructions to self dose diuretics or call the care team, and further teaching about nutrition. Ideally, this should be a multidisciplinary approach that may include physicians, nurses, dieticians, pharmacists, and others involved in the care of heart failure patients. Detailed, written information should be provided as well to reinforce the teaching. This teaching should be provided for both the patient and their family members. Fonarrow et al. have shown that such an approach can result in a decrease in readmission rates and an improvement in functional status (43). By reducing readmission rates the cost savings was $9800 per patient. Similar cost savings has been shown by implementing this teaching in the outpatient setting (91). Whellan et al. reported on the development of an outpatient heart failure disease management program that reduced admissions for heart failure exacerbations saving the hospital $8571 per patient-year.

In addition to extensive teaching, the hospitalization should be used as an opportunity to ensure that patients are on the proper medical therapy for heart failure. Table 7 outlines medications and therapies that are indicated for patients with heart failure. If patients are admitted to the hospital with NYHA functional class III or IV heart failure, spironolactone should be added to their therapy as long as their renal function is normal and they do not have a history of hyperkalemia (92). Similarly, with the recent data showing a survival benefit with internal cardiac defibrillators, appropriate patients with an ejection fraction less than 35% should have one placed (93–95). Utilizing the time prior to hospital discharge when patients are almost euvolemic allows this procedure to be performed without a second hospitalization. Finally, it is important to arrange for appropriate outpatient follow-up soon after discharge. These patients should be followed frequently at first and only when stable can the time between outpatient visits lengthen.

Risk Stratifying

One question that often comes up when talking with the patient and their family is the future and their risk of death and rehospitalization. Although this can be difficult to estimate, it is an important issue to think about both for practical reasons for the family with planning and also for the physician. If a patient has a high risk of death or readmission, one should think about referral for cardiac transplantation (if eligible) or advanced alternative therapies like destination left ventricular assist device. Additionally, referral to intensive outpatient heart failure disease management programs may be helpful to improve outcomes. Although there has not been much research in this area, older age, NYHA functional class IV heart failure, lower systolic blood pressure and sodium, and higher blood urea nitrogen have all been shown to be associated with worsening outcomes (96).

SUMMARY

The incidence of heart failure is increasing and as the population ages more of these patients will be admitted with acute decompensations. There are three main issues when treating heart failure. Immediately try to improve symptoms by treating fluid overload and poor perfusion and by identifying and reversing the underlying cause of the exacerbation. Second, focus on optimizing the patient's fluid status and initiating appropriate therapy. Finally, try to alter the long term outcomes of the disease by establishing ideal therapies and educating those affected about the disease process and about how the patient and their family play an important role in their overall outcomes.

REFERENCES

1. American Heart Association. Heart Disease and Stroke Statistics-2005 Update. Dallas, Texas: American Heart Association; 2005.
2. Cuffe MS, Califf RM, Adams KF, et al. Short-term intravenous milrinone for acute exacerbation of chronic heart failure: a randomized controlled trial. JAMA 2002; 287:1541–1547.
3. Publication Commitee for the VMAC Investigators. Intravenous nesiritide vs. nitroglycerin for treatment of decompensated congestive heart failure: a randomized controlled trial. JAMA 2002; 287:1531–1540.
4. Adams KF, Fonarow GC, Emerman CL, et al. Characteristics and outcomes of patients hospitalized for heart failure in the United States: rationale, design, and preliminary observations from the first 100,000 cases in the Acute Decompensated Heart Failure National Registry (ADHERE). Am Heart J 2005; 149:209–216.
5. The SOLVD Investigators. Effect of enalapril on survival in patients with reduced left ventricular ejection fractions and congestive heart failure. N Engl J Med 1991; 325:293–302.
6. Cohn JN, Johnson G, Ziesche S, et al. A comparison of enalapril with hydralazine-isosorbide dinitrate in the treatment of chronic congestive heart failure. N Engl J Med 1991; 325:303–310.
7. The SOLVD Investigators. Effect of enalapril on mortality and the development of heart failure in asymptomatic patients with reduced left ventricular ejection fractions. N Engl J Med 1992; 327:685–691.
8. Packer M, Bristow MR, Cohn JN, et al. The effect of carvedilol on morbidity and mortality in patients with chronic heart failure. N Engl J Med 1996; 334:1349–1355.
9. Hjalmarson A, Goldstein S, Fagerberg B, et al. Effects of controlled-release metoprolol on total mortality, hospitalizations, and well being in patients with heart failure. JAMA 2000; 283:1295–1302.
10. Packer M, Coats AJS, Fowler MB, et al. Effect of carvedilol on survival in severe chronic heart failure. N Engl J Med 2001; 344:1651–1658.
11. Poole-Wilson PA, Swedberg K, Cleland JGF, et al. Comparison of carvedilol and metoprolol on clinical outcomes in patients with chronic heart failure n the Carvedilol Or Metoprolol European Trial (COMET): randomized controlled trial. Lancet 2003; 362:7–13.
12. Nieminen MS, Bohm M, Cowie MR, et al. Guidelines on the diagnosis and treatment of acute heart failure—full text. The Task Force on Acute Heart Failure of the European Society of Cardiology. Eur Heart J 2005; 26:1115–1140.
13. Forrester JS, Diamond GA, Swan HJ. Correlative classification of clinical and hemodynamic function after acute myocardial infarction. Am J Cardiol 1977; 39:137–145.

14. Nohria A, Tsang SW, Fang JC, et al. Clinical assessment identifies hemodynamic profiles that predict outcomes in patients admitted with heart failure. J Am Coll Cardiol 2003; 41:1797–1804.
15. Bickley LS. Bates' Guide to Physical Exam and History Taking. 8th ed.: Lippincott Williams and Wilkins, 2002.
16. White PD. Alternation of the pulse: a common clinical condition. Am J Med 1915; 150:82–97.
17. Edwards P, Cohen GI. Both diastolic and systolic function alternate in pulsus alternans: a case report and review. J Am Soc Echocardiogr 2003; 16:695–697.
18. Tremel F, Pepin JL, Veale D, et al. High prevalence and persistence of sleep apnoea in patients referred for acute left ventricular failure and medically treated over 2 months. Eur Heart J 1999; 20:1201–1209.
19. Lanfranchi PA, Braghiroli A, Bosimini E, et al. Prognostic value of nocturnal Cheyne-Stokes respiration in chronic heart failure. Circulation 1999; 99:1435–1440.
20. Mared L, Cline C, Erhardt L, Berg S, Midgren B. Cheyne-Stokes respiration in patients hospitalized for heart failure. Respir Res 2004; 5:14–20.
21. Drazner MH, Hamilton MA, Fonarow G, Creaser J, Flavell C, Stevenson LW. Relationship between right and left-sided filling pressures in 1000 patients with advanced heart failure. J Heart Lung Transplant 1999; 18:1126–1132.
22. Kono T, Rosman H, Alam M, Stein PD, Sabbah HN. Hemodynamic correlates of the third heart sound during the evolution of chronic heart failure. J Am Coll Cardiol 1993; 21:419–423.
23. Chen D, Pibarot P, Honos G, Durand LG. Estimation of pulmonary artery pressure by spectral analysis of the second heart sound. Am J Cardiol 1996; 78:785–789.
24. Ducas J, Magder S, McGregor M. Validity of hepatojugular reflux as a clinical test for congestive heart failure. Am J Cardiol 1983; 52:1299–1303.
25. Fowler NO. Examination of the heart: Part II—Inspection and palpation of venous and arterial pulses. Dallas: American Heart Association, 1967.
26. Williams JF, Bristow MR, Fowler MB, et al. Guidelines for the evaluation and management of heart failure. Report of the American College of Cardiology/American Heart Association Task Force on Practice Guidelines (Committee on Evaluation and Management of Heart Failure). J Am Coll Cardiol 1995; 26:1376–1398.
27. Packer M, Lee WH. Prognostic importance of serum sodium concentration and its modification by converting-enzyme inhibition in patients with severe chronic heart failure. Circulation 1986; 73:257–267.
28. Chin MH, Goldman L. Correlates of major complications or death in patients admitted to the hospital with congestive heart failure. Arch Int Med 1996; 156:1814–1820.
29. Oren RM. Hyponatremia in congestive heart failure. Am J Cardiol 2005; 95:2–7.
30. Koglin J, Pehlivanli S, Schwaiblmair M, Vogeser M, Cremer P, von Scheidt W. Role of brain natriuretic peptide in risk stratification of patients with congestive heart failure. J Am Coll Cardiol 2001; 38:1934–1941.
31. Gardner RS, Ozalp F, Murday AJ, Robb SD, McDonagh TA. N-terminal pro-brain natriuretic peptide. A new gold standard in predicting mortality in patients with advanced heart failure. Eur Heart J 2003; 24:1735–1743.
32. O'Neill JO, Bott-Silverman CE, McRae AT, et al. B-type natriuretic peptide levels are not a surrogate marker for invasive hemodynamics during management of patients with severe heart failure. Am Heart J 2005; 149:363–369.
33. Zaphirou A, Robb S, Murray-Thomas T, et al. The diagnostic accuracy of plasma BNP and NTproBNP in patients referred from primary care with suspected heart failure: results of the UK natriuretic peptide study. Eur J Heart Fail 2005; 7:537–541.
34. Verdiani V, Nozzoli C, Bacci F, et al. Pre-discharge B-type natriuretic peptide predicts early recurrence of decompensated heart failure in patients admitted to a general medical unit. Eur J Heart Fail 2005; 7:566–571.
35. Krumholz H, Chen Y, Vaccarino V, et al. Correlates and impact on outcomes of worsening renal function in patients >65 years of age with heart failure. Am J Cardiol 2000; 85:1110–1113.

36. Gottlieb SS, Abraham W, Butler J, et al. The prognostic importance of different definitions of worsening renal function in congestive heart failure. J Card Fail 2002; 8:136–141.
37. Maisel AS, Krishnaswamy P, Nowak RM, et al. Rapid measurement of B-type natriuretic peptide in the emergency diagnosis of heart failure. N Engl J Med 2002; 347:161–167.
38. Tang WHW, Girod JP, Lee MJ, et al. Plasma B-Type natriuretic peptide levels in ambulatory patients with established chronic symptomatic systolic heart failure. Circulation 2003; 108:2964–2966.
39. Redfield MM, Rodeheffer RJ, Jacobsen SJ, et al. Plasma brain natriuretic peptide concentration: impact of age and gender. J Am Coll Cardiol 2002; 40:976–982.
40. Wang TJ, Larson MG, Levy D, et al. Impact of age and sex on plasma natriuretic peptide levels in healthy adults. Am J Cardiol 2002; 90:254–258.
41. Wang TJ, Larson MG, Levy D, et al. Impact of obesity on plasma natriuretic peptide levels. Circulation 2004; 109:594–600.
42. Nagueh SF, Kopelen HA, Zoghbi WA. Feasibility and accuracy of doppler echocardiographic estimation of pulmonary artery occlusive pressure in the intensive care unit. Am J Cardiol 1995; 75:1256–1262.
43. Fonarow GC, Stevenson LW, Walden JA, et al. Impact of a comprehensive heart failure management program on hospital readmission and functional status of patients with advanced heart failure. J Am Coll Cardiol 1997; 30:725–732.
44. Connors AF, Speroff T, Dawson NV, et al. The effectiveness of right heart catheterization in the initial care of critically ill patients. JAMA 1996; 276:889–897.
45. Shah S, Patel M, Goyal A, et al. Highlights from the American heart association annual scientific sessions 2004: November 7–10, 2004. Am Heart J 2005; 149:240–253.
46. The CONSENSUS trial study group. Effects of enalapril on mortality in severe congestive heart failure: results of the Cooperative North Scandinavian Enalapril Survival Study (COPN-SENSUS). N Engl J Med 1987; 316:1429–1435.
47. Gattis WA, O'Connor CM, Leimberger JD, Felker GM, Adams KF, Gheorghiade M. Clinical outcomes in patients on beta-blocker therapy admitted with worsening chronic heart failure. Am J Cardiol 2003; 91:169–174.
48. Heart Failure Society of America Guideline Committee. HFSA guidelines for the management of patients with heart failure caused by left ventricular systolic dysfunction: pharmacologic approaches. J Card Fail 1999; 5:357–382.
49. Gattis WA, O'Connor CM, Gallup DS, Hasselblad V, Gheorghiade M, on behalf of the IMPACT-HF investigators and coordinators. Predischarge initiation of carvedilol in patients hospitalized for decompensated heart failure. J Am Coll Cardiol 2004; 43:1534–1541.
50. Jain P, Massie BM, Gattis WA, Klein L, Gheorghiade M. Current medical treatment for the exacerbation of chronic heart failure resulting in hospitalization. Am Heart J 2003; 145:S3–S17.
51. Francis GS, Benedict C, Johnstone DE, et al. Comparison of neuroendocrine activation in patients with left ventricular dysfunction with and without congestive heart failure. Circulation 1990; 82:1724–1729.
52. Francis GS, Cohn JN, Johnson G, Rector TS, Goldman S, Simon A, for the V-HeFT VA Cooperative Studies Group. Plasma norepinephrine, plasma renin activity, and congestive heart failure. Relations to survival and the effects of therapy in V-HeFT II. Circulation 1998; 87:VI-40–VI-48.
53. Dormans TP, Gerlag PG, Russel FG, Smits P. Combination diuretic therapy in severe congestive heart failure. Drugs 1998; 55:165–172.
54. Ellison DH. Diuretic therapy and resistance in congestive heart failure. Cardiology 2001; 96:132–143.
55. Kiyingi A, Field MJ, Pawsey CC, Yiannikas J, Lawrence JR, Arter WJ. Metolazone in treatment of severe refractory congestive cardiac failure. Lancet 1990; 335:29–31.
56. Dormans TP, van Meyel JJ, Gerlag PG, Tan Y, Russel FG, Smits P. Diuretic efficacy of high dose furosemide in severe heart failure: bolus injection high dose furosemide versus continuous infusion. J Am Coll Cardiol 1996; 28:376–382.

57. Publication Committee for the VMAC Investigators. Intravenous nesiritide vs nitroglycerin for treatment of decompensated congest heart failure. JAMA 2002; 287:1531–1540.
58. Cotter G, Metzkor E, Kaluski E, et al. Randomised trial of high-dose isosorbide dinitrate plus low-dose furosemide versus high-dose furosemide plus low-dose isosorbide dinitrate in severe pulmonary oedema. Lancet 1998; 351:389–393.
59. Cohn JN, Franciosa JA, Francis GS, et al. Effect of short-term infusion of sodium nitroprusside on mortality rate in acute myocardial infarction complicated by left ventricular failure: results of a veterans administration cooperative study. N Engl J Med 1982; 306:1129–1135.
60. Colucci WS, Elkayam U, Horton DP, et al. Intravenous nesiritide, a natriuretic peptide, in the treatment of decompensated congestive heart failure. N Engl J Med 2000; 343:246–253.
61. Silver MA, Horton DP, Ghali JK, Elkayam U. Effect of nesiritide versus dobutamine on short-term outcomes in the treatment of patients with acutely decompensated heart failure. J Am Coll Cardiol 2002; 39:798–803.
62. Wang DJ, Dowling TC, Meadows D, et al. Nesiritide does not improve renal function in patients with chronic heart failure and worsening serum creatinine. Circulation 2004; 110:1620–1625.
63. Sackner-Bernstein JD, Skopicki HA, Aaronson KD. Risk of worsening renal function with nesiritide in patients with acutely decompensated heart failure. Circulation 2005; 111:1487–1491.
64. Sackner-Bernstein JD, Kowalski M, Fox M, Aaronson K. Short-term risk of death after treatment with nesiritide for decompensated heart failure: a pooled analysis of randomized controlled trials. JAMA 2005; 293:1900–1905.
65. Packer M, Narahara KA, Elkayam U, et al. Double-blind, placebo-controlled study of the efficacy of flosequinan in patients with chronic heart failure. J Am Coll Cardiol 1993; 22:65–72.
66. Moe GW, Rouleau JL, Charbonneau L, et al. Neurohormonal activation in severe heart failure: relations to patient death and the effect of treatment with flosequinan. Am Heart J 2000; 139:587–595.
67. Feldman AM, Bristow MR, Parmley WW, et al. Effects of vesnarinone on morbidity and mortality in patients with heart failure. Vesnarinone study group. N Engl J Med 1993; 329:149–155.
68. Cohn JN, Goldstein SO, Greenberg BH. A dose-dependent increase in mortality with vesnarinone among patients with severe heart failure. Vesnarinone trial investigators. N Engl J Med 1998; 339:1810–1816.
69. Wiggers CJ, Stimson B. Studies on the cardiodynamic actions of drugs. III. The mechanism of cardiac stimulation by digitalis and g-strophanthin. J Pharmacol Exp Ther 1927; 30:251.
70. Packer M, Gheorghiade M, Young JB, et al. N Engl J Med 1993; 329:1–7.
71. Uretsky BF, Young JB, Shahidi FE, Yellen LG, Harrison MC, Jolly MK, on behalf of the PROVED investigative group. Randomized study assessing the effect of digoxin withdrawal in patients with mild to moderate chronic congestive heart failure: results of the PROVED trial. J Am Coll Cardiol 1993; 22:955–962.
72. The Digitalis Investigation Group. The effect of digoxin on mortality and morbidity in patients with heart failure. N Engl J Med 1997; 336:525–533.
73. Terra SG, Washam JB, Dunham GD, Gattis WA. Therapeutic range of digoxin's efficacy in heart failure: what is the evidence? Pharmacotherapy 1999; 19:1123–1126.
74. Rathore SS, Curtis JP, Wang Y, Bristow MR, Krumholz HM. Association of serum digoxin concentration and outcomes in patients with heart failure. JAMA 2003; 289:871–878.
75. O'Connor CM, Gattis WA, Uretsky BF, et al. Continuous intravenous dobutamine is associated with an increased risk of death in patients with advanced heart failure: insights from the Flolan International Randomized Survival Trial (FIRST). Am Heart J 1999; 138:78–86.
76. Lowes BD, Simon MA, Tsvetkova YO, Bristow MR. Inotropes in the beta blocker era. Clin Cardiol 2000; 23:11–16.

77. Russell SD, DeWald T. Vasopressin receptor antagonists: therapeutic potential in the management of acute and chronic heart failure. Am J Cardiovasc Drugs 2003; 3:13–20.
78. Goldsmith SR, Francis GS, Cowley AW, Levine TB, Cohn JN. Increased plasma arginine vasopressin levels in patients with congestive heart failure. J Am Coll Cardiol 1983; 1:1385–1390.
79. Goldsmith SR. Vasopressin: a therapeutic target in congestive heart failure? J Card Fail 1999; 5:347–356.
80. Udelson JE, Smith WB, Hendrix GH, et al. Acute hemodynamic effects of conivaptan, a dual V and V vasopressin receptor antagonist, in patients with advanced heart failure. Circulation 2001; 104:2417–2423.
81. Gheorghiade M, Niazi I, Ouyang J, et al. Vasopressin V_2—receptor blockade with tolvaptan in patients with chronic heart failure. Results from a double-blind, randomized trial. Circulation 2003; 107:2690–2696.
82. Gheorghiade M, Gattis WA, O'Connor CM, et al. JAMA 2004; 291:1963–1971.
83. Funaya J, Kitakaze M, Node K, Minamino T, Komamura K, Hori M. Plasma adenosine levels increase in patients with chronic heart failure. Circulation 1997; 95:1363–1365.
84. Fredholm BB, Ijzerman AP, Jacobson KA, Klotz KN, Linden J. International Union of Pharmacology. XXV. Nomenclature and classification of adenosine receptors. Pharmacol Rev 2001; 53:527–552.
85. Gottlieb SS. Renal effects of adenosine A_1—receptor antagonists in congestive heart failure. Drugs 2001; 61:1387–1393.
86. Schnermann J, Weihprecht H, Briggs JP. Inhibition of tubulo-glomerular feedback during adenosine 1 receptor blockade. Am J Physiol 1990; 258:F553–F561.
87. Gottlieb SS, Skettino SL, Wolff A, et al. Effects of BG9719 (CVT-124), an A_1—adenosine receptor antagonist, and furosemide on glomerular filtration rate and natriuresis in patients with congestive heart failure. J Am Coll Cardiol 2000; 35:56–59.
88. Gottlieb SS, Brater DC, Thomas I, et al. BG9719 (CVT-124), an A_1 adenosine receptor antagonist, protects against the decline in renal function observed with diuretic therapy. Circulation 2002; 105:1348–1353.
89. Hasenfuss G, Pieske B, Castell M, Kretschmann B, Maier LS, Just H. Influence of the novel inotropic agent levosimendan on isometric tension and calcium cycling in failing human myocardium. Circulation 1998; 98:2141–2147.
90. Slawsky MT, Colucci WS, Gottlieb SS, et al. Acute hemodynamic and clinical effects of levosimendan in patients with severe heart failure. Study investigators. Circulation 2000; 102:2222–2227.
91. Whellan DJ, Gaulden L, Gattis WA, et al. The benefit of implementing a heart failure disease management program. Arch Intern Med 2001; 161:2223–2228.
92. Pitt B, Zannad F, Remme WJ, et al. The effect of spironolactone on morbidity and mortality in patients with severe heart failure. Randomized aldactone evaluation study investigators. N Engl J Med 1999; 341:709–717.
93. Moss AJ, Zareba W, Hall WJ, et al. Prophylactic implantation of a defibrillator in patients with myocardial infarction and reduced ejection fraction. N Eng J Med 2002; 346:877–883.
94. Bristow MR, Saxon LA, Boehmer J, et al. Cardiac-resynchronization therapy with or without an implantable defibrillator in advanced chronic heart failure. N Eng J Med 2004; 350:2140–2150.
95. Bardy GH, Lee KL, Mark DB, et al. Amiodarone or an implantable cardioverter-defibrillator for congestive heart failure. N Eng J Med 2005; 352:225–237.
96. Felker GM, Adams KF, Konstam MA, O'Connor CM, Gheorghiade M. The problem of decompensated heart failure: nomenclature, classification, and risk stratification. Am Heart J 2003; 145:S18–S25.

13
Diastolic Heart Failure

Michael M. Givertz
Cardiovascular Division, Brigham and Women's Hospital, Harvard Medical School, Boston, Massachusetts, U.S.A.

James C. Fang
Advanced Heart Disease Section, Cardiovascular Division, Department of Medicine, Brigham and Women's Hospital, Harvard Medical School, Boston, Massachusetts, U.S.A.

DEFINITIONS AND CLASSIFICATION

Many patients with signs and symptoms of heart failure have normal or near normal left ventricular ejection fraction. In 1988, Kessler introduced the term "diastolic heart failure" to describe these patients (1). More recently, Aurigemma and Gaasch suggested a more comprehensive definition: "if effort intolerance and dyspnea develop in a patient with hypertensive left ventricular hypertrophy, normal ejection faction and abnormal left ventricular filling, especially in combination with venous congestion and pulmonary edema, it would be appropriate to use the term *diastolic heart failure* (2)." Alternatively, Grossman and others have proposed purely pathophysiologic definitions, such as filling of the left ventricle to a normal end-diastolic volume only at higher than normal pressure (3).

To avoid ambiguity in defining patient populations and promote standardization in practice, specific diagnostic criteria for diastolic heart failure have been developed. The European Study Group (4) proposed that three conditions must be simultaneously met to make a diagnosis of primary diastolic heart failure: (1) presence of signs or symptoms of heart failure; (2) presence of normal or only mildly abnormal left ventricular systolic function; and (3) evidence of abnormal left ventricular relaxation, filling, diastolic distensibility or diastolic stiffness (Table 1A). More recent criteria proposed by Vasan and Levy (5) considers both clinical presentation as well as documentation of systolic and diastolic function, and grades the likelihood of diastolic heart failure as possible, probable or definite (Table 1B).

Although classifying patients allows for standardization of practice, it is important to remember that systolic and diastolic heart failure are not mutually exclusive. While these terms underscore the predominant pathophysiologic mechanism operating in the individual patient, many patients with heart failure have abnormalities of both systole and diastole. In patients with ischemic cardiomyopathy, for example, systolic heart failure is caused by both the chronic loss of myocardium secondary to infarction and the acute loss

Table 1A Diagnostic Criteria for Diastolic Heart Failure: European Study Group

Criterion	Examples
Signs or symptoms of heart failure	Exertional dyspnea, orthopnea, gallop sounds, lung crepitations, pulmonary edema
Normal or mildly reduced left ventricular systolic function	LVEF $\geq$ 45% and LVEDIDI $<$ 3.2 cm/m^2; LVEDVI $<$ 102 ml/m^2
Abnormal left ventricular relaxation, filling, diastolic distensibility and diastolic stiffness	LV dP/dt$_{min}$ $<$ 1100 mmHg/sec; PFR $<$ 160 ml/sec/m^2; LVEDP $>$ 16 mmHg or mean PCWP $>$ 12 mmHg; b $>$ 0.27

Abbreviations: LVEF, left ventricular ejection fraction; LVEDIDI, left ventricular end-diastolic internal dimension index; LVEDVI, left ventricular end-diastolic volume index; LV dP/dt$_{min}$, peak negative left ventricular dP/dt; PFR, peak filling rate; LVEDP, left ventricular end-diastolic pressure; PCWP, pulmonary capillary wedge pressure; b, constant of LV chamber stiffness.
Source: Adapted from European Study Group on Diastolic Heart Failure: How to diagnose diastolic heart failure. Eur Heart J 1998; 19:990.

of contractility due to ischemia; diastolic heart failure is due to reduced compliance caused by chronic replacement fibrosis and the acute reduction in distensibility by ischemia.

Diastolic dysfunction should also be distinguished from diastolic heart failure. Some patients with diastolic dysfunction (e.g., abnormal left ventricular filling) do not have signs or symptoms of heart failure, while other patients with diastolic heart failure do not have demonstrable abnormalities of diastolic function. For these patients, heart failure with normal or preserved ejection fraction may be the more appropriate terminology. National guidelines recommend that every effort be made to exclude other possible explanations or disorders that may present in a similar manner (Table 2).

Table 1B Diagnostic Criteria for Diagnostic Heart Failure: Vasan and Levy

Criterion	Possible diastolic HF	Probable diastolic HF	Definite diastolic HF
Definitive evidence of HF	Signs and symptoms of HF, supporting lab tests[a], and response to diuretics	Signs and symptoms of HF, supporting lab tests[a], and response to diuretics	Signs and symptoms of HF, supporting lab tests[a], and response to diuretics
Objective evidence of normal LV systolic function	LVEF $\geq$ 50%, but not at the time of heart failure event	LVEF $\geq$ 50% within 72 hr of heart failure event	LVEF $\geq$ 50% within 72 hr of heart failure event
Objective evidence of LV diastolic dysfunction	No conclusive information	No conclusive information	Abnormal LV relaxation, filling and/or distensibility at cardiac catheterization

[a]Chest X-ray, B-type natriuretic peptide level.
Abbreviations: HF, heart failure; LV, left ventricular; LVEF, left ventricular ejection fraction.
Source: From Vasan RS, Levy D: Defining diastolic heart failure: a call for standardized diagnostic criteria. Circulation 2000; 101:2118.

Table 2 Differential Diagnosis in a Patient with Heart Failure and Preserved Ejection Fraction

Incorrect diagnosis of HF
Inaccurate measurement of LVEF
Primary valvular disease
Restrictive or infiltrative cardiomyopathy (e.g., amyloidosis, sarcoidosis)
Pericardial constriction
Episodic or reversible left ventricular systolic dysfunction
Severe hypertension and/or ischemia
High-output heart failure (e.g., due to thyrotoxicosis, anemia)
Chronic pulmonary disease with right heart failure
Pulmonary arterial hypertension

Abbreviations: HF, heart failure; LVEF, left ventricular ejection fraction.
Source: From Hunt SA, Abraham WT, Chin MH, et al: ACC/AHA 2005 guideline update for the diagnosis and management of chronic heart failure in the adult: a report of the American College of Cardiology/American Heart Association Task Force on Practice Guidelines (Writing Committee to Update the 2001 Guidelines for the Evaluation and Management of Heart Failure): developed in collaboration with the American College of Chest Physicians and the International Society for Heart and Lung Transplantation: endorsed by the Heart Rhythm Society. Circulation 2005; 112:e154–e235.

EPIDEMIOLOGY

Community-based, epidemiological studies have demonstrated that diastolic heart failure is common and is particularly prevalent in older patients, women, and those with a history of hypertension (Table 3) (6–8). Lindenfeld et al. (9) reviewed the medical records of 1,081 randomly selected Medicare patients hospitalized with heart failure and found that 25% of men and 45% of women had an ejection fraction greater than 40%. The prevalence of diastolic heart failure increased to 31% and 52%, respectively in patients greater than or equal to 85 yr of age (Fig. 1). The Acute Decompensated Heart Failure National Registry (ADHERE®) collected data on 105,388 patients hospitalized with a primary or secondary diagnosis of heart failure (10). Mean age was 72.4 yr, and 52% were women. Assessment of quantitative or qualitative left ventricular ejection fraction was obtained during or before hospitalization in 81%, and revealed that 46% had either normal or mild impairment of systolic function.

Follow-up data shows that patients hospitalized with heart failure and preserved ejection fraction have rates of functional decline and readmission that are similar to patients with systolic dysfunction (11). While some data suggests that long-term survival is similar among patients with systolic versus diastolic heart failure (7), most studies show that diastolic heart failure is associated with a lower risk of death (Table 4). Philbin et al. (12) assessed outcomes in 1,291 patients hospitalized for heart failure with left ventricular

Table 3 Epidemiology of Heart Failure by Ejection Fraction

Characteristics	Preserved EF (n=200)	Reduced EF (n=213)	P
Mean age, years	73	70	0.004
Female gender, %	63	35	0.001
HTN, %	80	65	0.001
CAD, %	24	76	0.0001
Diabetes, %	48	48	0.94

Abbreviations: EF, ejection fraction; HTN, hypertension; CAD, coronary artery disease.
Source: From Smith GL et al.: Outcomes in heart failure patients with preserved ejection fraction: mortality, readmission, and functional decline. J Am Coll Cardiol 2003; 42:1510.

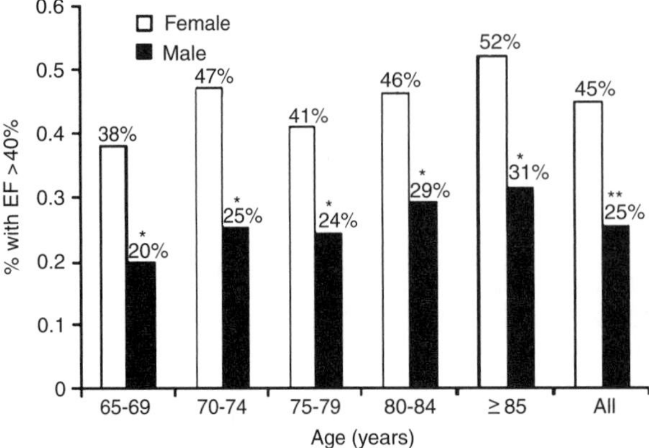

Figure 1 Percentage of Medicare patients with a principal discharge diagnosis of heart failure and ejection fraction <40% according to age and gender. *p<0.01 for individual age-group comparisons; **p<0.01, all women compared to all men. *Source*: From Ref. 9.

ejection fraction ≤0.39 (57%), 0.40 to 0.49 (18%) or ≥0.50 (24%) and found the lowest mortality in patients with preserved ejection fraction (Fig. 2). Interestingly, in this large cohort of patients with diastolic heart failure, angiotensin-converting enzyme (ACE) inhibitors were not associated with improved survival.

The incidence of diastolic heart failure is not well known. In one study of asymptomatic patients over the age of 65 with echocardiographic evidence of diastolic dysfunction, heart failure developed in up to 15% within five years (13). Restrictive left ventricular filling and left ventricular mass were strong independent predictors of incident heart failure.

Table 4 Mortality in Diastolic Versus Systolic Heart Failure

Study (Ref.)	Patients, n	Follow-up	Mortality with reduced EF	Mortality with preserved EF	RR of death with preserved EF
Cohn 1990 (82)	623	2.3 yr	19% per year	8% per year	0.42
Ghali 1992 (83)	78	2 yr	46%	26%	0.56
McDermott 1997 (84)	192	27 mo	35%	35%	0.97
Vasan 1999 (6)	73	5 yr	64%	32%	0.50
McAlister 1999 (85)	566	3 yr	38%	34%	NA
Philbin 2000 (12)	1291	6 mo	18%	15%	0.69
Masoudi 2003 (86)	413	6 mo	21%	13%	0.49

Abbreviations: EF, ejection fraction; RR, relative risk; NA, not available.

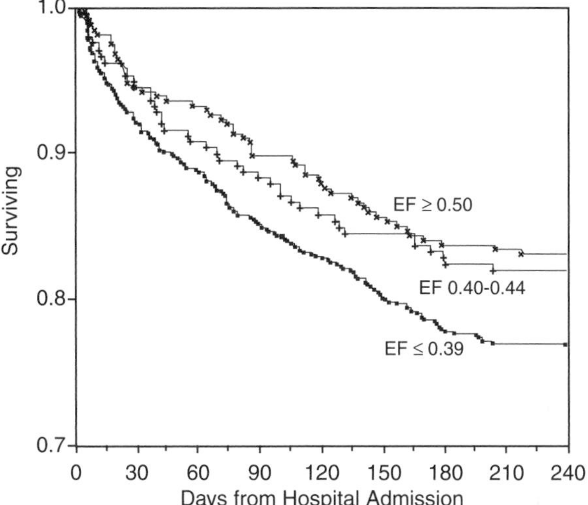

Figure 2 Kaplan–Meier curves showing proportion of patients with heart failure surviving after hospitalization stratified by ejection fraction. Crosses, ejection fraction (EF) greater than or equal to 0.50; plus signs, EF from 0.40 to 0.49; closed squares, EF less than or equal to 0.39. *Source*: From Ref. 12.

PATHOPHYSIOLOGY

Ventricular diastole is generally divided into four phases: isovolumic relaxation, rapid early filling, diastasis, and atrial systole. Although what constitutes an abnormality in each of these four phases, i.e., diastolic dysfunction, can generally be agreed upon, there is a lack of consensus as to the predominant pathophysiologic mechanism that underlies the clinical syndrome of diastolic heart failure. In large part, this lack of consensus results from the arbitrary nature of the clinical definition (4,5), the heterogeneity of the clinical syndrome (14), and the absence of well-characterized animal models (15). Furthermore, there is a paucity of simultaneous intracardiac pressure and volume data in the patient populations for which there is the greatest debate (16–18). Most importantly, it is difficult to completely separate concepts of diastolic function from considerations of ventricular systole since they are intimately linked (19,20). Despite these issues, recent work suggests that there are likely several mechanisms at work that help to define syndromes of diastolic heart failure.

If the clinical heterogeneity of diastolic heart failure is acknowledged, it is useful from a pathophysiologic perspective to consider two broad principal distinctions: "primary" forms of diastolic heart failure where intrinsic conditions of the myocardium directly result in diastolic dysfunction (e.g., restrictive cardiomyopathies) and "secondary" forms of diastolic heart failure where diastolic dysfunction is a consequence of the myocardial response to a given physiologic stimulus (e.g., hypertensive heart disease). Some investigators have suggested that the clinical presence of hypertension provides an easy and useful method of distinguishing these syndromes (16).

Primary diastolic heart failure syndromes are characterized by diastolic dysfunction in the absence of a physiologic loading condition that would lead to reactive ventricular hypertrophy and fibrosis, load-dependent changes in diastole or both. Acute ischemic heart disease, hypertrophic cardiomyopathy, and constrictive pericarditis fall into this category.

Other less common examples of primary diastolic heart failure include forms of restrictive cardiomyopathy (21) that are characterized by myocardial infiltration such as cardiac amyloidosis or hemochromatosis, endomyocardial fibrosis, and Fabry's disease. Hemodynamically, there is impedance to ventricular filling, impaired relaxation, relatively fixed small end-diastolic volumes, and biatrial enlargement. In these disorders, filling of the left ventricle to a normal end-diastolic volume occurs only at higher than normal end-diastolic pressures, i.e., a leftward and upward shift of the end-diastolic pressure-volume relationship, the traditional paradigm for diastolic dysfunction and heart failure (Fig. 3) (22,23).

The unifying characteristic of these conditions is abnormal active and/or passive relaxation (22,23). In this paradigm, abnormalities in active muscular relaxation, passive tissue chamber compliance, and/or extrinsic forces (such as pericardial constraint, vascular venous turgor, and right ventricular function) produce dysfunction in one of the four phases of diastole. For example, active muscular relaxation may be impaired when cytosolic calcium transients (e.g., acute ischemic heart disease) and/or contractile proteins (e.g., hypertrophic cardiomyopathy) are disturbed (24,25). Passive diastolic compliance may be influenced by both myocyte hypertrophy as well as changes in the extracellular matrix. Although this matrix is composed of several components including elastin, proteoglycans, and basement membrane proteins, fibrillar collagen has received the most attention as a pathologic offender (26,27). Fibrillar collagen is often abnormal in diseases associated with diastolic dysfunction and experimentally, when collagen metabolism is altered, diastolic function changes concomitantly (28,29). The cardiac endothelial and neurohormonal systems also contribute to ventricular relaxation and stiffness (30). Finally, salt and water avidity results from the neurohormonal activation that occurs as a result of the decreased distal delivery of sodium in the loop of Henle. In this setting, small chamber size leads to small stroke volumes and decreased cardiac output.

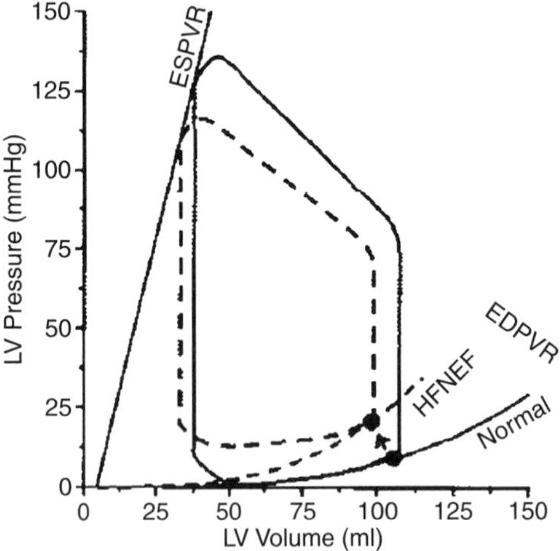

Figure 3 Traditional paradigm of diastolic heart failure. Note the displacement of the end-diastolic pressure volume relationship (EDPVR) up and to the left (*dotted lines*). Filling of the left ventricle to a normal end-diastolic volume only occurs at higher than normal end-diastolic pressures. Note that systolic pressure must fall in this paradigm if end-systolic pressure volume relationship (ESPVR) remains unchanged. *Abbreviation*: HFNEF, heart failure with normal ejection fraction. *Source*: From Ref. 32.

In secondary forms of diastolic heart failure, diastolic dysfunction may be the consequence of excessive preload (e.g., renal failure), afterload (e.g., hypertension) or both, with subsequent secondary changes in ventricular diastolic function. These types of diastolic heart failure are more common than the primary forms described previously. It was recently concluded that abnormalities in diastolic function alone are sufficient to explain the primary pathophysiologic process in such patients. Zile et al. (17) demonstrated a longer time constant of isovolumic relaxation and an upward and leftward shift of the end-diastolic pressure-volume relation in middle-aged men with a history of diastolic heart failure but without hypertrophy versus age-matched controls. However, epidemiologic studies consistently show that most patients with diastolic heart failure are predominantly elderly, female, hypertensive, and diabetic (31). These observations suggest that it is likely a subset of patients with diastolic heart failure that have a primary abnormality of LV filling and that these patients may be more accurately classified as having a type of restrictive cardiomyopathy or primary diastolic heart failure.

In the majority of patients with diastolic heart failure (i.e., elderly hypertensive women), it remains unclear whether diastolic dysfunction is primary and sufficient to explain the heart failure syndrome. Recent work has challenged the stiff heart paradigm (14,32). While available only in a small number of patients, invasively obtained pressure-volume data suggest that the end-diastolic pressure-volume relationship is variable (Fig. 4) (18,32). Abnormalities of diastolic function may reflect a reactive or secondary response of ventricular form and function to a more primary insult such as vascular stiffness (33). Since the rate and extent of myocardial relaxation is dependent upon ventricular load, timing of load in systole, and duration of systole, changes in vascular impedance would be expected to result in diastolic dysfunction (19). Furthermore, an increase in aortic stiffness leads to premature wave reflection and consequent increases in late systolic load and decreased diastolic coronary perfusion. Finally, abnormalities of systole often co-exist (34). Increases in ventricular systolic stiffness (i.e., end-systolic elastance) exacerbate the late systolic load of increased arterial elastance leading to premature cessation of systole, blood pressure lability, and exaggerated effects of vascular impedance on ventricular relaxation (14). Invasive pressure–volume data in small numbers of elderly women appear to confirm this hypothesis (Fig. 5) (18).

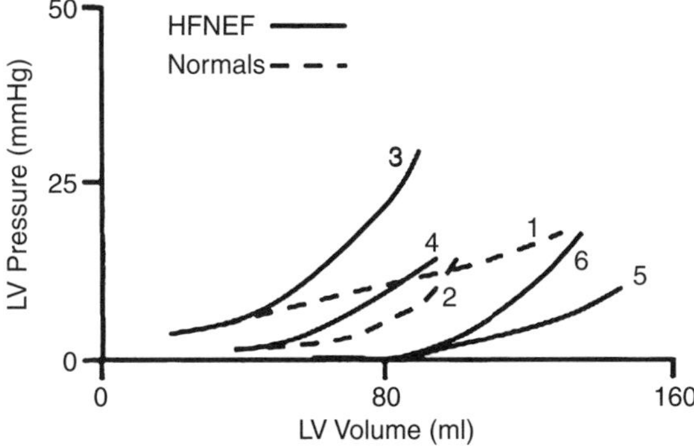

Figure 4 Invasively obtained end-diastolic volume relations (EDPVR) in patients with diastolic heart failure. In elderly subjects with diastolic heart failure, the EDPVR is quite variable and may be shifted to the left or right, or may not be significantly different from the normal relationship. *Source*: From Ref. 32.

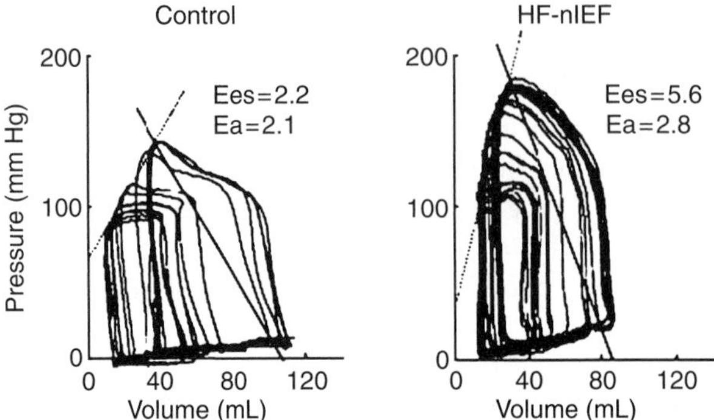

Figure 5 Ventricular–vascular coupling in diastolic heart failure. In an elderly patient with hypertension and heart failure with normal ejection fraction (HF-nlEF), pressure volume loops demonstrate an increase in both end systolic elastance (Ees) and arterial elastance (Ea), leading to premature cessation of systole, decreased stroke volume, and increased end-diastolic pressure. There is near matching of Ees and Ea in the control patient. *Source*: From Ref. 18.

Maladaptive volume regulation may also contribute to diastolic heart failure. Increasing evidence suggests that in elderly hypertensive patients with heart failure, volume expansion, renal dysfunction, and anemia (35) play important roles in disease progression. Maurer and colleagues (16) describe three pathophysiologic entities of diastolic heart failure, which can be characterized by specific pressure-volume relationships. Two of the three have been described above and are characterized by either a steep end-diastolic pressure-volume relation (i.e., primary diastolic heart failure, Fig. 3) or an increase in end-systolic elastance (i.e., vascular and ventricular stiffness, Fig. 5). The third mechanism suggests that patients are volume expanded and that the increase in end-diastolic pressure is due to movement up along a "normal" end-diastolic pressure-volume curve (Fig. 6A). Using control data derived from regression models incorporating age, gender and size, Maurer et al. (16) demonstrated higher than normal end-diastolic and end-systolic volumes in a group of predominately elderly female hypertensive subjects (Fig. 6B). Finally, the role of the kidney in these disorders remains unexplored. Although there appears to be neurohormonal activation (36), the direct stimuli for salt and water retention in the face of a normal cardiac output remain unknown. Concomitant anemia, obesity, baroreceptor dysfunction, and intrinsic kidney disease may play important roles in this paradigm.

CLINICAL ASSESSMENT

A number of clinical features and laboratory findings may be used to characterize patients with diastolic heart failure (Table 5). However, it is important to recognize that the clinical features of heart failure may be similar whether left ventricular ejection fraction is preserved or reduced, underscoring the need for evaluation of ventricular function in all patients with heart failure. Certain aspects of the history and physical examination may help to distinguish diastolic from systolic heart failure. For example, older patients with hypertensive heart disease and left ventricular hypertrophy often experience heart failure because of diastolic dysfunction, volume expansion or both.

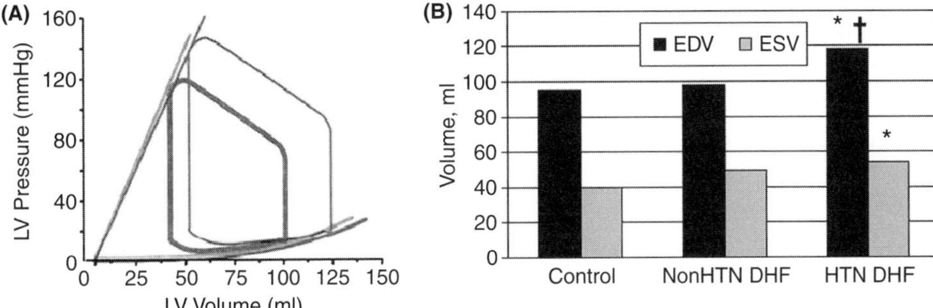

Figure 6 Volume overload in diastolic heart failure. (**A**) The end-diastolic pressure volume relationship (EDPVR) in a hypertensive patient with diastolic heart failure (*thin line*) compared to normal (*thick line*). The "volume overload" hypothesis suggests that the EDPVR is not shifted upward and to the left but rather that the end-diastolic volume is greater, and the end-diastolic pressure increases, due to movement up and out along a "normal" EDPVR curve (e.g., rightward shift). (**B**) Assessment of end-systolic (ESV) and end-diastolic volumes (EDV) using three-dimensional echocardiography. Non-hypertensive patients with diastolic heart failure (nonHTN DHF) have elevated end-diastolic pressures with relatively normal EDVs consistent with the traditional paradigm of diastolic heart failure. In contrast, patients with hypertension and diastolic heart failure (HTN DHF) have elevated end-diastolic pressures with increased EDVs and ESVs in support of the "volume overload" hypothesis. *$p<0.05$ versus control, †$p<0.05$ vs. non-HTN DHF. *Source*: From Ref. 16.

Noninvasive Imaging

Just as the physical examination lacks sensitivity and specificity for diastolic heart failure, the chest x-ray cannot reliably distinguish diastolic from systolic heart failure. However, findings such as pulmonary vascular redistribution, pulmonary edema and/or pleural effusions may be used to support a diagnosis of heart failure in patients with shortness of breath and preserved ejection fraction. The echocardiogram is an essential tool for management of patients with systolic or diastolic heart failure, and the baseline study should be used to quantify ejection fraction, and assess left ventricular chamber size and wall thickness. In addition, two–dimensional echocardiography can help to identify other causes of heart failure in patients with preserved ejection fraction, such as primary valvular disease (e.g., acute mitral regurgitation), isolated right heart failure, pulmonary arterial hypertension or infiltrative cardiomyopathy (e.g., cardiac amyloidosis). Doppler techniques, including assessment of mitral inflow velocity or pulmonary venous flow, can be used to assess left ventricular diastolic function; however, these velocities are generally load- and heart rate-dependent and lack appropriate specificity. Newer Doppler techniques, including tissue Doppler imaging, appear to be less sensitive to preload, but their clinical utility in the diagnosis and management of diastolic heart failure remains to be determined.

For patients in whom poor acoustic windows limit transthoracic techniques, a transesophageal echocardiogram may be performed to define cardiac structure and function. Alternatively, cardiac magnetic resonance (MRI) allows high-resolution imaging of the myocardium, cardiac chambers and valves and adjacent structures. For patients with heart failure and preserved ejection fraction, cardiac MRI may be used to rule out pericardial disease with high sensitivity or support a specific diagnosis such as hypertrophic cardiomyopathy (37), myocardial sarcoidosis (38) or cardiac hemochromatosis (39).

Table 5 Clinical Features of Systolic vs. Diastolic Heart Failure

Parameters	Systolic	Diastolic
History		
Coronary artery disease	+++	++
Hypertension	++	++++
Diabetes	++	++
Valvular heart disease	++++	+
Paroxysmal dyspnea	++	+++
Physical examination		
Cardiomegaly	+++	+
Soft heart sounds	++++	+
S_3 gallop	+++	+
S_4 gallop	+	+++
Hypertension	++	++++
Mitral regurgitation	+++	+
Rales	++	+
Edema	+++	+
Jugular venous distension	+++	+
Chest roentgenogram		
Cardiomegaly	+++	+
Pulmonary congestion	+++	+++
Electrocardiogram		
Left ventricular hypertrophy	++	++++
Q waves	++	+
Low voltage	+++	−
Echocardiogram		
Left ventricular hypertrophy	++	++++
Left ventricular dilation	++	−
Left atrial enlargement	++	++
Reduced ejection fraction	++++	−

Plus signs indicate "suggestive" (the number reflects relative weight). Minus signs indicate "not very suggestive."
Source: From Givertz MM, Colucci WS, Braunwald E: Clinical aspects of heart failure; pulmonary edema, high-output failure. In Zipes DP, Libby P, Bonow RO, Braunwald E (eds): Heart Disease: A Textbook of Cardiovascular Medicine, 7th ed. Philadelphia: Elsevier Saunders: 2005: 539–568.

Exercise Testing

Exercise testing may be used to determine the degree of exercise intolerance and assess for the presence of coronary artery disease in patients with diastolic heart failure. Kitzman et al. (40) measured resting and exercise hemodynamics in 7 patients with heart failure, normal ejection fraction and no significant ischemic or valvular heart disease. In patients with diastolic heart failure, pulmonary capillary wedge pressure increased markedly at peak exercise, and this increase in left ventricular filling pressure was not associated with an increase in cardiac output. Proposed mechanisms underlying this failure of the Frank Starling response include decreased distensibility (or compliance), loss of recoil, increased passive chamber stiffness and decreased coronary vasodilator reserve. Subcellular mechanisms of exercise intolerance have also been elucidated in animal models of heart failure, and include excess diastolic calcium and reduced adenosine triphosphate availability.

The abnormal cardiac output response to exercise contributes to leg fatigue, while an increase in pulmonary venous pressures causes a reduction in lung compliance resulting in dyspnea. Other factors contributing to impaired exercise tolerance in patients with diastolic heart failure include age, deconditioning, reduced aortic distensibility (41), skeletal muscle atrophy and endothelial dysfunction.

Invasive Testing

Cardiac catheterization remains the gold standard for assessment of hemodynamics and definition of coronary anatomy. Catheterization of the right side of the heart using a balloon-tipped catheter allows measurement of right and left-sided cardiac filling pressures, pulmonary artery pressures and cardiac output using either thermodilution or Fick techniques. Routine left heart catheterization allows measurement of left ventricular systolic and end-diastolic pressures. While hemodynamics are generally assessed at rest, measurements obtained during exercise may help to clarify the underlying pathophysiology and functional limitation in selected patients. However, due to the heterogeneous nature of the clinical syndrome, there is no single hemodynamic profile that defines a patient with diastolic heart failure. For example, a patient with primary diastolic heart failure (e.g., due to restrictive cardiomyopathy) may have elevated right and left-sided filling pressures, secondary pulmonary hypertension and low resting cardiac output, while a patient with diastolic heart failure secondary to hypertensive heart disease may have normal filling pressures at rest that increase inappropriately with exercise and are associated with an inadequate cardiac output response (40).

As proposed by Vasan and Levy, definite diastolic heart failure requires demonstration of abnormal LV relaxation, filling and/or distensibility at cardiac catheterization (Table 1B). Zile et al. (42) hypothesized that the vast majority of patients with heart failure and a normal ejection fraction exhibit abnormal LV diastolic function and therefore do not need invasive hemodynamic assessment. Of 63 patients with diastolic heart failure, 58 (92%) had a left ventricular end-diastolic pressure >16 mm Hg (mean 27 ± 7 mm Hg, range 7 to 48). In a subset of patients that underwent detailed assessment using a micromanometer-tipped catheter and Doppler echocardiography, the time constant of LV relaxation was abnormal in 79% (mean 59 ± 15 ms, range 32 to 110), and at least one index of diastolic function was abnormal in every patient. A follow-up hemodynamic study by the same investigators demonstrated normal LV systolic function, performance and contractility in patients with diastolic heart failure (43).

Biomarkers

B-type natriuretic peptide (BNP) is synthesized and secreted by the cardiac ventricles in response to an increase in wall stress or filling pressure. In patients with systolic heart failure, BNP levels are elevated in relation to disease severity and provide strong independent prognostic information. Recent data demonstrates that plasma BNP levels are also elevated in patients with diastolic heart failure and may predict survival. In animal models, myocardial BNP messenger RNA levels are increased during the transition from left ventricular hypertrophy to diastolic heart failure (44), and in patients who have received adriamycin, BNP levels are inversely correlated with measures of diastolic filling (45). In a cross-sectional echocardiographic study of patients with normal ejection fraction, elevated BNP levels were associated with diastolic dysfunction, with the highest levels seen in patients with a restrictive filling pattern (Fig. 7A) (46).

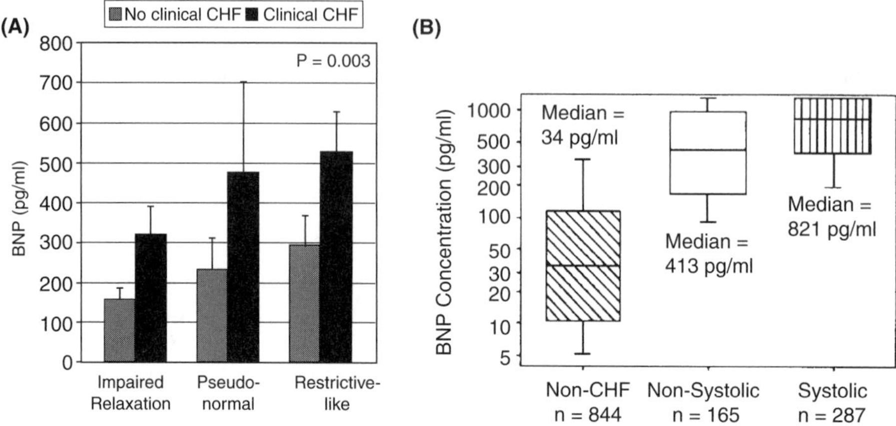

Figure 7 B-type natriuretic peptide (BNP) levels in diastolic heart failure. (**A**) Mean BNP levels in 119 patients referred for echocardiography and found to have normal systolic function and abnormal diastolic function. Comparison of three diastolic filling patterns (impaired relaxation, pseudonormal or restrictive-like) demonstrates that, as a group, patients with diastolic dysfunction and heart failure symptoms (clinical CHF) have higher BNP levels than patients with asymptomatic diastolic dysfunction (no clinical CHF). *Source*: From Ref. 46. (**B**) Box and whisker plots showing median BNP levels in patients presenting to the emergency department with dyspnea not due to heart failure (non-CHF) compared to patients with a final adjudicated diagnosis of diastolic (non-systolic) versus systolic heart failure. *Source*: From Ref. 47.

Maisel et al. (47) examined BNP levels in 452 patients with systolic versus diastolic heart failure who presented to the emergency room with shortness of breath. Patients with diastolic heart failure had lower BNP levels than those with systolic heart failure (Fig. 7B). However, BNP added only modest discriminatory value in differentiating these two groups of patients. Further studies show that BNP levels are elevated in diastolic heart failure independent of left ventricular hypertrophy (48). In a prospective echocardiographic study of patients with hypertension and diastolic heart failure, BNP levels were higher in patients with diastolic dysfunction and were independently related to blood pressure and age (49). However, nearly 80% of patients with diastolic dysfunction had levels less than 100 pg/mL. There is no randomized controlled data demonstrating a role for BNP-guided therapy of diastolic heart failure in the inpatient or outpatient setting.

TREATMENT

While large randomized trials have confirmed survival and other benefits of ACE inhibitors and beta-blockers in patients with systolic heart failure, there have been few trials of neurohormonal antagonists in patients with diastolic heart failure. As a result, therapy of diastolic heart failure is based on the results of clinical investigations in small groups of patients, and on pathophysiologic concepts (50). Principles of therapy as recommended by the American College of Cardiology/American Heart Association guidelines (51) include fluid and sodium restriction, heart rate and blood pressure control, prevention of myocardial ischemia, reduction in cardiac filling pressures and control of edema, and maintenance of sinus rhythm (Table 6). Neurohormonal antagonists to minimize symptoms and slow disease progression remain unproven. Additional non-pharmacologic strategies that have proven effective in systolic heart failure and should be

Table 6 ACC/AHA Recommendations for Management of Diastolic Heart Failure

Class	Recommendation	Level of evidence
I	Control systolic and diastolic hypertension	A
	Control ventricular rate in atrial fibrillation	C
	Diuretics to control pulmonary congestion and edema	C
IIa	Coronary revascularization if ischemia is having an adverse effect on diastolic function	C
IIb	Restoration of sinus rhythm if atrial fibrillation present	C
	Beta-blockers, ACE inhibitors, ARBs or calcium antagonists to minimize symptoms of HF	C
	Digoxin to minimize symptoms of HF	C

Abbreviations: ACE, angiotensin-converting enzyme; ARB, angiotensin receptor blocker; HF, heart failure. *Source*: From Hunt SA, Abraham WT, Chin MH, et al. ACC/AHA 2005 guideline update for the diagnosis and management of chronic heart failure in the adult: a report of the American College of Cardiology/American Heart Association Task Force on Practice Guidelines (Writing Committee to Update the 2001 Guidelines for the Evaluation and Management of Heart Failure): developed in collaboration with the American College of Chest Physicians and the International Society for Heart and Lung Transplantation: endorsed by the Heart Rhythm Society. Circulation 2005; 112:e154–e235.

generalized to patients with diastolic heart failure include weight loss, exercise and smoking cessation.

In general, positive inotropic agents should not be used in patients with diastolic heart failure as they may adversely affect myocardial energetics, induce ischemia and promote tachyarrhythmias. Results of the Digitalis Investigation Group trial, however, suggest that even patients with a normal ejection fraction may have fewer symptoms and reduced hospitalizations with digoxin. In 988 patients with heart failure and an ejection fraction greater than 45%, digoxin was associated with a non-significant reduction in the combined endpoint of death or heart failure hospitalization (52,53). The mechanism of benefit may not be related to digoxin's inotropic effect, but rather to improvements in parasympathetic tone and baroreceptor sensitivity (54).

Fluid and Sodium

Pulmonary venous congestion associated with diastolic dysfunction usually responds rapidly to preload reduction with diuretics, nitrates, or both. However, because of increased myocardial stiffness, a small decrease in LV volume can cause a marked decrease in LV filling pressure, stroke volume, and cardiac output, especially in primary forms of diastolic heart failure (see discussion in Pathophysiology). Therefore, it is important to avoid excessive preload reduction, which can cause symptomatic hypotension. Diuretic therapy should be initiated with a small dose of a loop diuretic (e.g., furosemide 20 mg). If effective diuresis is not achieved, the dose should be increased and/or a second diuretic agent (e.g., metolazone 2.5–5 mg) should be added. For patients presenting to the emergency room with acute pulmonary edema, oxygen, morphine and positive mask ventilation may be important adjunctive therapies to achieve clinical stabilization and avoid the need for intubation and mechanical ventilation. If acute pulmonary edema occurs in the setting of marked hypertension, intravenous nitroglycerin or nitroprusside can be used to rapidly lower blood pressure, with nitroglycerin being the preferred agent if an acute coronary syndrome is suspected based on associated symptoms (e.g., chest pain) or electrocardiographic changes (e.g., ST segment elevation or depression). Pulmonary edema associated with atrial fibrillation and a rapid ventricular response may respond to rate control with a beta-blocker or calcium channel blocker or in more urgent situations to electrical or chemical cardioversion.

Blood Pressure Control and LVH Regression

In diastolic heart failure due to hypertension, blood pressure control is important to prevent progression of left ventricular hypertrophy and possibly to promote its regression (55,56). In addition, effective antihypertensive therapy may improve diastolic filling properties, relieve the load on the left atrium, and help preserve sinus rhythm. Calcium channel blockers may reduce symptoms of diastolic heart failure not only by lowering blood pressure, but also by improving active, but not passive, ventricular relaxation (57). Antagonists of the renin angiotensin system (e.g., ACE inhibitors and angiotensin receptor blockers) may also improve ventricular relaxation, slow or reverse myocardial fibrosis and decrease left ventricular mass (56,58). Treatment of hypertension in the elderly with either diuretics or ACE inhibitors decreases the incidence of myocardial infarction, stroke and heart failure, with the greatest benefits seen in patients with ischemic heart disease (59).

While there is no evidence that ACE inhibitors improve survival in diastolic heart failure (12), the effect of an angiotensin receptor blockade on morbidity and mortality has been tested in a large randomized controlled trial. The Candesartan in Heart Failure-Assessment of Reduction in Mortality and Morbidity (CHARM)-Preserved Trial randomly assigned 3,023 patients with mild-moderate heart failure and an ejection fraction greater than 40% to receive candesartan (up to 32 mg daily) or placebo for a median of three years (60). Baseline medical therapy included ACE inhibitors in 19%, beta-blockers in 56%, and diuretics in 75%. Compared to placebo, candesartan reduced heart failure hospitalizations (230 vs. 279, $p=0.017$), but not cardiovascular deaths (170 vs. 170, $p=0.92$). A smaller study of patients with diastolic dysfunction and a hypertensive response to exercise demonstrated beneficial effects of losartan on exercise capacity and quality of life (61). Taken together, these studies suggest that activation of the renin-angiotensin system is an important target of therapy in diastolic heart failure. Data from the Heart Outcomes Protection Evaluation (HOPE) Study also supports the use of ACE inhibitors in high-risk patients with diabetes or evidence of vascular disease to prevent the development of diastolic heart failure (62).

Anti-ischemic Therapy

Patients with left ventricular hypertrophy are prone to subendocardial ischemia, even in the absence of coronary artery disease, due to supply–demand mismatch. Ischemia increases myocardial diastolic stiffness and exacerbates diastolic dysfunction. Since most coronary flow occurs in diastole, tachycardia with reduced diastolic filling time compromises subendocardial perfusion. Therefore, heart rate control is considered central to prevent or treat ischemia associated with diastolic heart failure. Beta-blockers and non-dihydropyridine calcium channel blockers are useful negative chronotropic agents in this setting. In patients with ischemic heart disease, percutaneous or surgical revascularization may be indicated to treat ischemia. However, acute pulmonary edema may recur in as many of 50% of patients despite successful revascularization (63).

Rate and Rhythm Control

Due to increased LV diastolic stiffness, patients with diastolic dysfunction have reduced passive LV filling in early and mid diastole and depend on an active atrial contribution to late ventricular filling. Maintenance of sinus rhythm is important for achieving adequate stroke volume and cardiac output. Electrical or chemical cardioversion should be considered for all patients with diastolic dysfunction and atrial fibrillation, although long-term survival may be similar whether a rate control or rhythm control strategy is used (64). While awaiting therapeutic anticoagulation, beta-blockers, calcium channel blockers, or digoxin may be used to control the ventricular response. Of these three, digoxin is the least likely to control ventricular response in patients with increased sympathetic activity and consideration should be given to combination therapy (e.g., digoxin and a beta-blocker). If cardioversion is not successful and drug therapy controls ventricular response at the expense of symptomatic bradycardia, pacing with or without ablation of the atrioventricular junction should be considered. However, caution needs to be exercised in primary forms of diastolic heart failure where stroke volumes are small and relatively fixed. In this setting, cardiac output may be dependent upon relative tachycardia to maintain blood pressure, and beta-blockers can lead to hemodynamic collapse. Furthermore, in patients with hypertensive and/or ischemic heart failure, dyssynchrony associated with chronic right ventricular pacing may contribute to disease progression and recurrence of atrial fibrillation (65). With regard to the long-term effects of anti-adrenergic therapy, there have been no large randomized controlled trials of beta-blockers in diastolic heart failure.

Exercise Training

The benefits of exercise training in patients with systolic heart failure are well documented (see Chapter 4), and include improvements in exercise tolerance, symptoms and quality of life as well as reverse ventricular remodeling (66). There are also data suggesting that exercise training reduces morbidity (e.g., hospitalizations) and possibly mortality in heart failure (67). Relevant pathophysiologic changes include an increase in the cardiac output response to exercise, improved endothelial function and skeletal muscle metabolism, reversal of ventilatory abnormalities and reduced sympathetic tone. There have been no randomized controlled trials with adequate patient numbers to prove the benefits of exercise training in patients with diastolic heart failure. However, exercise training favorably affects the consequences of aging, hypertrophy and ischemia, which may contribute to diastolic dysfunction (66). Furthermore, in patients with dilated cardiomyopathy, exercise training has been shown to improve diastolic function (68). Proposed mechanisms for reversal of diastolic dysfunction include reduced myocardial collagen content, improved calcium handling, and more efficient energy utilization.

Table 7 Therapy to Improve Exercise Tolerance in Diastolic Heart Failure

Etiology	Therapy
Hypertensive cardiomyopathy	Angiotensin receptor blockade
Hypertrophic cardiomyopathy	Nonsurgical septal reduction
Hemochromatosis	Phlebotomy
Acromegaly	Octreotide
Cardiac amyloidosis	Stem cell transplant

Beyond exercise training, therapies targeted to the underlying pathophysiology have also been shown to improve exercise tolerance in selected patients with primary forms of diastolic heart failure (Table 7).

NEW DIRECTIONS

Positive Lusitropes

In dogs with pacing-induced heart failure, intravenous infusion of BNP decreased LV end-diastolic pressure and accelerated Tau (69), while intracoronary infusion of a BNP receptor antagonist prolonged Tau (70). In an early clinical study, Clarkson et al. (71) evaluated the effects of intravenous BNP on resting and exercise hemodynamics in patients with diastolic heart failure. BNP did not affect resting hemodynamics, but attenuated the rise in pulmonary capillary wedge pressure and mean pulmonary artery pressure during exercise. Interestingly, endogenous BNP levels have been shown to increase with exercise in hypertensive patients with diastolic heart failure and may contribute to improved diastolic function (72). More recent studies with nesiritide (recombinant human BNP) demonstrate favorable effects on symptoms and hemodynamics in patients hospitalized with acute decompensated heart failure and either reduced or preserved ejection fraction. However, caution is advised regarding the use of nesiritide in normotensive patients as higher doses have been associated with symptomatic hypotension and worsening renal function (73). Other novel strategies to improve diastolic function in patients with heart failure and preserved ejection fraction include calcium sensitization (74) and gene therapy to increase calcium handling proteins (75).

Vascular Stiffness and Anti-fibrotic Therapy

Left ventricular fibrosis leading to impaired relaxation is postulated to be a key feature in diastolic heart failure. However, characteristic histopathologic changes have not been defined and recent attention has turned to increased ventricular systolic and vascular stiffness as a novel target of therapy (76). In large conduit arteries, degeneration of elastin and an increase in collagen content result in vascular stiffness and increased pulse wave velocity. In addition, advanced glycation end-products (AGE) contribute to cross-linking of collagen and reduced susceptibility to the activity of matrix metalloproteinases. In turn, AGE-related arterial stiffening may be accompanied by increases in ventricular systolic and diastolic stiffness. ALT-711 is a novel compound that breaks AGE-related collagen cross-links, and has been shown in animal models to decrease diastolic stiffness and aortic pulse wave velocity (77). In patients with hypertension, ALT-711 increased arterial compliance by 15% (78), while in patients with diastolic heart failure, ALT-711 improved symptoms and reduced LV mass but had no effect on exercise tolerance (79).

Aldosterone has also been implicated in the development of myocardial and vascular stiffness due to growth-promoting effects on vascular smooth muscle and increased collagen deposition (80). Eplerenone, a selective aldosterone receptor antagonist, has been shown to improve diastolic function in a rat model of heart failure (81). Mottram et al. (80) randomized 30 overweight patients with hypertension and diastolic heart failure to receive spironolactone 25 mg daily or placebo for 6 months. Spironolactone was associated with increases in strain rate and peak systolic strain and a decrease in posterior wall thickness. The effect of anti-fibrotic therapy with spironolactone on morbidity and mortality in patients with diastolic heart failure is currently being tested in a large National Institutes of Health sponsored study.

REFERENCES

1. Kessler KM. Heart failure with normal systolic function. Update of prevalence, differential diagnosis, prognosis, and therapy. Arch Intern Med 1988; 148:2109–2111.
2. Aurigemma GP, Gaasch WH. Clinical practice. Diastolic heart failure. N Engl J Med 2004; 351:1097–1105.
3. Grossman W. Diastolic dysfunction in congestive heart failure. N Engl J Med 1991; 325:1557–1564.
4. European Study Group on Diastolic Heart Failure. How to diagnose diastolic heart failure. Eur Heart J 1998; 19:990–1003.
5. Vasan RS, Levy D. Defining diastolic heart failure: a call for standardized diagnostic criteria. Circulation 2000; 101:2118–2121.
6. Vasan RS, Larson MG, Benjamin EJ, et al. Congestive heart failure in subjects with normal versus reduced left ventricular ejection fraction: prevalence and mortality in a population-based cohort. J Am Coll Cardiol 1999; 33:1948–1955.
7. Senni M, Redfield MM. Heart failure with preserved systolic function. A different natural history? J Am Coll Cardiol 2001; 38:1277–1282.
8. Masoudi FA, Havranek EP, Smith G, et al. Gender, age, and heart failure with preserved left ventricular systolic function. J Am Coll Cardiol 2003; 41:217–223.
9. Lindenfeld J, Fiske KS, Stevens BR, et al. Age, but not sex, influences the measurement of ejection fraction in elderly patients hospitalized for heart failure. J Card Fail 2003; 9:100–106.
10. Adams KF, Jr, Fonarow GC, Emerman CL, et al. Characteristics and outcomes of patients hospitalized for heart failure in the United States: rationale, design, and preliminary observations from the first 100,000 cases in the Acute Decompensated Heart Failure National Registry (ADHERE). Am Heart J 2005; 149:209–216.
11. Smith GL, Masoudi FA, Vaccarino V, et al. Outcomes in heart failure patients with preserved ejection fraction: mortality, readmission, and functional decline. J Am Coll Cardiol 2003; 41:1510–1518.
12. Philbin EF, Rocco TA, Jr, Lindenmuth NW, et al. Systolic versus diastolic heart failure in community practice: clinical features, outcomes, and the use of angiotensin-converting enzyme inhibitors. Am J Med 2000; 109:605–613.
13. Aurigemma GP, Gottdiener JS, Shemanski L, et al. Predictive value of systolic and diastolic function for incident congestive heart failure in the elderly: the cardiovascular health study. J Am Coll Cardiol 2001; 37:1042–1048.
14. Kass DA. Is heart failure with decent systole due to bad diastole? J Card Fail 2005; 11:188–190.
15. Munagala VK, Hart CY, Burnett JC, Jr., et al. Ventricular structure and function in aged dogs with renal hypertension: a model of experimental diastolic heart failure. Circulation 2005; 111:1128–1135.
16. Maurer MS, King DL, El Khoury RL, et al. Left heart failure with a normal ejection fraction: identification of different pathophysiologic mechanisms. J Card Fail 2005; 11:177–187.
17. Zile MR, Baicu CF, Gaasch WH. Diastolic heart failure—abnormalities in active relaxation and passive stiffness of the left ventricle. N Engl J Med 2004; 350:1953–1959.
18. Kawaguchi M, Hay I, Fetics B, et al. Combined ventricular systolic and arterial stiffening in patients with heart failure and preserved ejection fraction: implications for systolic and diastolic reserve limitations. Circulation 2003; 107:714–720.
19. Leite-Moreira AF, Correia-Pinto J, Gillebert TC. Afterload induced changes in myocardial relaxation: a mechanism for diastolic dysfunction. Cardiovasc Res 1999; 43:344–353.
20. Eichhorn EJ, Willard JE, Alvarez L, et al. Are contraction and relaxation coupled in patients with and without congestive heart failure? Circulation 1992; 85:2132–2139.
21. Kushwaha SS, Fallon JT, Fuster V. Restrictive cardiomyopathy. N Engl J Med 1997; 336:267–276.
22. Zile MR, Brutsaert DL. New concepts in diastolic dysfunction and diastolic heart failure: Part I: diagnosis, prognosis, and measurements of diastolic function. Circulation 2002; 105:1387–1393.

23. Zile MR, Brutsaert DL. New concepts in diastolic dysfunction and diastolic heart failure: Part II: causal mechanisms and treatment. Circulation 2002; 105:1503–1508.
24. Paulus WJ, Grossman W, Serizawa T, et al. Different effects of two types of ischemia on myocardial systolic and diastolic function. Am J Physiol 1985; 248:H719–H728.
25. Pak PH, Maughan L, Baughman KL, et al. Marked discordance between dynamic and passive diastolic pressure–volume relations in idiopathic hypertrophic cardiomyopathy. Circulation 1996; 94:52–60.
26. Weber KT. Extracellular matrix remodeling in heart failure. A role for de novo angiotensin II generation. Circulation 1997; 96:4065–4082.
27. Weber KT, Brilla CG. Pathological hypertrophy and cardiac interstitium. Fibrosis and renin-angiotensin-aldosterone system. Circulation 1991; 83:1849–1865.
28. Villari B, Campbell SE, Hess OM, et al. Influence of collagen network on left ventricular systolic and diastolic function in aortic valve disease. J Am Coll Cardiol 1993; 22:1477–1484.
29. Kato S, Spinale FG, Tanaka R, et al. Inhibition of collagen cross-linking: effects on fibrillar collagen and ventricular diastolic function. Am J Physiol 1995; 269:H863–H868.
30. Brutsaert DL, Fransen P, Andries LJ, et al. Cardiac endothelium and myocardial function. Cardiovasc Res 1998; 38:281–290.
31. Vasan RS, Benjamin EJ, Levy D. Prevalence, clinical features and prognosis of diastolic heart failure: an epidemiologic perspective. J Am Coll Cardiol 1995; 26:1565–1574.
32. Burkhoff D, Maurer MS, Packer M. Heart failure with a normal ejection fraction: is it really a disorder of diastolic function? Circulation 2003; 107:656–658.
33. Mitchell GF, Tardif JC, Arnold JM, et al. Pulsatile hemodynamics in congestive heart failure. Hypertension 2001; 38:1433–1439.
34. Yu CM, Lin H, Yang H, et al. Progression of systolic abnormalities in patients with "isolated" diastolic heart failure and diastolic dysfunction. Circulation 2002; 105:1195–1201.
35. Klapholz M, Maurer M, Lowe AM, et al. Hospitalization for heart failure in the presence of a normal left ventricular ejection fraction: results of the New York heart failure registry. J Am Coll Cardiol 2004; 43:1432–1438.
36. Kitzman DW, Little WC, Brubaker PH, et al. Pathophysiological characterization of isolated diastolic heart failure in comparison to systolic heart failure. JAMA 2002; 288:2144–2150.
37. Moon JC, McKenna WJ, McCrohon JA, et al. Toward clinical risk assessment in hypertrophic cardiomyopathy with gadolinium cardiovascular magnetic resonance. J Am Coll Cardiol 2003; 41:1561–1567.
38. Smedema JP, Snoep G, van Kroonenburgh MP, et al. Evaluation of the accuracy of gadolinium-enhanced cardiovascular magnetic resonance in the diagnosis of cardiac sarcoidosis. J Am Coll Cardiol 2005; 45:1683–1690.
39. Pomerantz S, Siegelman ES. MR imaging of iron depositional disease. Magn Reson Imaging Clin N Am 2002; 10:105–120.
40. Kitzman DW, Higginbotham MB, Cobb FR, et al. Exercise intolerance in patients with heart failure and preserved left ventricular systolic function: failure of the Frank-Starling mechanism. J Am Coll Cardiol 1991; 17:1065–1072.
41. Hundley WG, Kitzman DW, Morgan TM, et al. Cardiac cycle-dependent changes in aortic area and distensibility are reduced in older patients with isolated diastolic heart failure and correlate with exercise intolerance. J Am Coll Cardiol 2001; 38:796–802.
42. Zile MR, Gaasch WH, Carroll JD, et al. Heart failure with a normal ejection fraction: is measurement of diastolic function necessary to make the diagnosis of diastolic heart failure? Circulation 2001; 104:779–782.
43. Baicu CF, Zile MR, Aurigemma GP, et al. Left ventricular systolic performance, function, and contractility in patients with diastolic heart failure. Circulation 2005; 111:2306–2312.
44. Yamamoto K, Masuyama T, Sakata Y, et al. Local neurohumoral regulation in the transition to isolated diastolic heart failure in hypertensive heart disease: absence of AT1 receptor downregulation and "overdrive" of the endothelin system. Cardiovasc Res 2000; 46:421–432.
45. Nousiainen T, Vanninen E, Jantunen E, et al. Natriuretic peptides during the development of doxorubicin-induced left ventricular diastolic dysfunction. J Intern Med 2002; 251:228–234.

46. Lubien E, DeMaria A, Krishnaswamy P, et al. Utility of B-natriuretic peptide in detecting diastolic dysfunction: comparison with Doppler velocity recordings. Circulation. 2002; 105:595–601.
47. Maisel AS, McCord J, Nowak RM, et al. Bedside B-Type natriuretic peptide in the emergency diagnosis of heart failure with reduced or preserved ejection fraction. Results from the breathing not properly multinational study. J Am Coll Cardiol 2003; 41:2010–2017.
48. Yamaguchi H, Yoshida J, Yamamoto K, et al. Elevation of plasma brain natriuretic peptide is a hallmark of diastolic heart failure independent of ventricular hypertrophy. J Am Coll Cardiol 2004; 43:55–60.
49. Mottram PM, Leano R, Marwick TH. Usefulness of B-type natriuretic peptide in hypertensive patients with exertional dyspnea and normal left ventricular ejection fraction and correlation with new echocardiographic indexes of systolic and diastolic function. Am J Cardiol 2003; 92:1434–1438.
50. Bonow RO, Udelson JE. Left ventricular diastolic dysfunction as a cause of congestive heart failure. Mechanisms and management. Ann Intern Med 1992; 117:502–510.
51. Hunt SA, Abraham WT, Chin MH, et al. ACC/AHA 2005 guideline update for the diagnosis and management of chronic heart failure in the adult: a report of the American College of Cardiology/American Heart Association Task Force on Practice Guidelines (Writing Committee to Update the 2001 Guidelines for the Evaluation and Management of Heart Failure): developed in collaboration with the American College of Chest Physicians and the International Society for Heart and Lung Transplantation: endorsed by the Heart Rhythm Society. Circulation 2005; 112:e154–e235.
52. The Digitalis Investigation Group. The effect of digoxin on mortality and morbidity in patients with heart failure. N Engl J Med 1997; 336:525–533.
53. Gheorghiade M, Adams KF, Jr., Colucci WS. Digoxin in the management of cardiovascular disorders. Circulation 2004; 109:2959–2964.
54. Hauptman PJ, Kelly RA. Digitalis. Circulation 1999; 99:1265–1270.
55. Mathew J, Sleight P, Lonn E, et al. Reduction of cardiovascular risk by regression of electrocardiographic markers of left ventricular hypertrophy by the angiotensin-converting enzyme inhibitor ramipril. Circulation 2001; 104:1615–1621.
56. Gottdiener JS, Reda DJ, Massie BM, et al. Effect of single-drug therapy on reduction of left ventricular mass in mild to moderate hypertension: comparison of six antihypertensive agents. The Department of Veterans Affairs Cooperative Study Group on Antihypertensive Agents. Circulation 1997; 95:2007–2014.
57. Kass DA, Wolff MR, Ting CT, et al. Diastolic compliance of hypertrophied ventricle is not acutely altered by pharmacologic agents influencing active processes. Ann Intern Med 1993; 119:466–473.
58. Friedrich SP, Lorell BH, Rousseau MF, et al. Intracardiac angiotensin-converting enzyme inhibition improves diastolic function in patients with left ventricular hypertrophy due to aortic stenosis. Circulation 1994; 90:2761–2771.
59. Kostis JB, Davis BR, Cutler J, et al. Prevention of heart failure by antihypertensive drug treatment in older persons with isolated systolic hypertension. SHEP Cooperative Research Group. JAMA 1997; 278:212–216.
60. Yusuf S, Pfeffer MA, Swedberg K, et al. Effects of candesartan in patients with chronic heart failure and preserved left-ventricular ejection fraction: the CHARM-Preserved Trial. Lancet 2003; 362:777–781.
61. Warner JG, Jr, Metzger DC, Kitzman DW, et al. Losartan improves exercise tolerance in patients with diastolic dysfunction and a hypertensive response to exercise. J Am Coll Cardiol 1999; 33:1567–1572.
62. Yusuf S, Sleight P, Pogue J, et al. Effects of an angiotensin-converting-enzyme inhibitor, ramipril, on cardiovascular events in high-risk patients. The Heart Outcomes Prevention Evaluation Study Investigators. N Engl J Med 2000; 342:145–153.

63. Kramer K, Kirkman P, Kitzman D, et al. Flash pulmonary edema: association with hypertension and reoccurrence despite coronary revascularization. Am Heart J 2000; 140:451–455.
64. Wyse DG, Waldo AL, DiMarco JP, et al. A comparison of rate control and rhythm control in patients with atrial fibrillation. N Engl J Med 2002; 347:1825–1833.
65. Sweeney MO, Hellkamp AS, Ellenbogen KA, et al. Adverse effect of ventricular pacing on heart failure and atrial fibrillation among patients with normal baseline QRS duration in a clinical trial of pacemaker therapy for sinus node dysfunction. Circulation 2003; 107:2932–2937.
66. Pina IL, Apstein CS, Balady GJ, et al. Exercise and heart failure: a statement from the American heart association committee on exercise, rehabilitation, and prevention. Circulation 2003; 107:1210–1225.
67. Belardinelli R, Georgiou D, Cianci G, et al. Randomized, controlled trial of long-term moderate exercise training in chronic heart failure: effects on functional capacity, quality of life, and clinical outcome. Circulation 1999; 99:1173–1182.
68. Belardinelli R, Georgiou D, Cianci G, et al. Exercise training improves left ventricular diastolic filling in patients with dilated cardiomyopathy. Clinical and prognostic implications. Circulation 1995; 91:2775–2784.
69. Lainchbury JG, Burnett JC, Jr, Meyer D, et al. Effects of natriuretic peptides on load and myocardial function in normal and heart failure dogs. Am J Physiol Heart Circ Physiol 2000; 278:H33–H40.
70. Hart CY, Hahn EL, Meyer DM, et al. Differential effects of natriuretic peptides and NO on LV function in heart failure and normal dogs. Am J Physiol Heart Circ Physiol 2001; 281:H146–H154.
71. Clarkson PB, Wheeldon NM, MacFadyen RJ, et al. Effects of brain natriuretic peptide on exercise hemodynamics and neurohormones in isolated diastolic heart failure. Circulation 1996; 93:2037–2042.
72. Mottram PM, Haluska BA, Marwick TH. Response of B-type natriuretic peptide to exercise in hypertensive patients with suspected diastolic heart failure: correlation with cardiac function, hemodynamics, and workload. Am Heart J 2004; 148:365–370.
73. Sackner-Bernstein JD, Skopicki HA, Aaronson KD. Risk of worsening renal function with nesiritide in patients with acutely decompensated heart failure. Circulation 2005; 111:1487–1491.
74. Hasenfuss G, Pieske B, Castell M, et al. Influence of the novel inotropic agent levosimendan on isometric tension and calcium cycling in failing human myocardium. Circulation 1998; 98:2141–2147.
75. Miyamoto MI, del Monte F, Schmidt U, et al. Adenoviral gene transfer of SERCA2a improves left-ventricular function in aortic-banded rats in transition to heart failure. Proc Natl Acad Sci USA 2000; 97:793–798.
76. Redfield MM. Treating diastolic heart failure with AGE crosslink breakers: thinking outside the heart failure box. J Card Fail 2005; 11:196–199.
77. Vaitkevicius PV, Lane M, Spurgeon H, et al. A cross-link breaker has sustained effects on arterial and ventricular properties in older rhesus monkeys. Proc Natl Acad Sci USA 2001; 98:1171–1175.
78. Kass DA, Shapiro EP, Kawaguchi M, et al. Improved arterial compliance by a novel advanced glycation end-product crosslink breaker. Circulation 2001; 104:1464–1470.
79. Little WC, Zile MR, Kitzman DW, et al. The effect of alagebrium chloride (ALT-711), a novel glucose cross-link breaker, in the treatment of elderly patients with diastolic heart failure. J Card Fail 2005; 11:191–195.
80. Mottram PM, Haluska B, Leano R et al. Effect of aidosterone antagonism on myocardial dysfunction in hypertensive patients with diastolic heat failure. Circulation 2004; 110:558–565.
81. Masson S, Staszewsky L, Annoni G, et al. Eplerenone, a selective aldosterone blocker, improves diastolic function in aged rats with small-to-moderate myocardial infarction. J Card Fail 2004; 10:433–441.

14
Diagnosis and Management of Secondary Pulmonary Hypertension

Anna R. Hemnes and Hunter C. Champion
Divisions of Cardiology and Pulmonary and Critical Care Medicine, Department of Medicine, Johns Hopkins University School of Medicine, Baltimore, Maryland, U.S.A.

INTRODUCTION

Pulmonary hypertension (PH) is defined as a mean pulmonary arterial pressure of greater than 25 mmHg at rest or greater than 30 mmHg with exercise with a pulmonary vascular resistance greater than 3.0 mmHg/l/min. Recently, the World Health Organization convened a conference to re-classify PH based on underlying mechanisms of pathophysiology and pathobiology. Thus, the old terminology of primary and secondary PH has been replaced; the current classification subdivides PH into subgroups of pulmonary arterial hypertension, which includes idiopathic pulmonary arterial hypertension previously known as primary PH, or PH associated with connective tissue disease and chronic systemic-to-pulmonary shunt, left heart disease, pulmonary vascular disorders, hypoxemia or respiratory disorders, chronic thromboembolic disease, and other miscellaneous disorders. The focus of this chapter is PH in the setting of advanced heart failure, both from chronic systemic-to-pulmonary shunt and left heart disease.

PATHOPHYSIOLOGY

As prescribed by Ohm's law relating change in pressure to flow multiplied by resistance, pulmonary arterial pressure is comprised of three components —flow, pulmonary vascular resistance and pulmonary venous pressure in the following relationship: PA mean $= (Q \times PVR) + Ppv$, where Q is flow, PVR is pulmonary vascular resistance, and Ppv is pulmonary vascular pressure. Ppv is clinically measured as the pulmonary capillary wedge pressure. Thus, the pathophysiologic mechanisms driving PH development are: increased pulmonary blood flow, rise in pulmonary vascular resistance, or rise in pulmonary capillary wedge pressure. Heart failure can produce PH via several mechanisms, depending on the underlying cause of disease. Dilated cardiomyopathy associated with left ventricular dysfunction or mitral stenosis, for example, result in increased pulmonary venous pressure. Alternatively, congenital left to right intracardiac shunts produce increased flow through the pulmonary vasculature with resultant PH. Interestingly, previous research has shown that PH will not rise until pulmonary blood flow reaches 2.5 times normal (1).

PATHOLOGY AND BASIC SCIENCE

The earliest pulmonary pathologic finding in patients with elevated left heart filling pressures is an edematous alveolar-capillary wall (2). Over time, the increased intraluminal pressure alters the pathology of the pulmonary arteries with development of intimal fibrosis, medial hypertrophy of the muscular pulmonary arteries, and extension of the muscular layer into smaller branches of the arterial tree (3). The characteristic plexiform lesion of pulmonary arterial hypertension is generally not present in PH due to left heart disease, but is present in chronic systemic-to-pulmonary shunt (4). This dissimilarity underlies the different pathophysiologic mechanisms for the development of PH in these patient populations: the former with PH due to increased venous pressure and the latter primarily due to increased flow.

Basic science work has pointed to multiple possible mechanisms that drive increased pulmonary vascular resistance in patients with elevated left heart filling pressures. Nitric oxide (NO), synthesized by NO synthase, has been noted to be an important mediator of vascular tone in patients with PH. NO diffuses into adjacent smooth muscle cells where it activates soluble guanylyl cyclase and subsequently increases cyclic guanosine monophosphate (cGMP) levels. Elevated cGMP alters smooth muscle cell relaxation by inhibiting calcium release from the sarcoplastic reticulum and other downstream pathways (5). In human studies of normal controls and heart failure patients with normal PVR using N^g-monomethyl-L-arginine (L-NMMA), a NO synthase inhibitor, vasoconstriction was found after intrapulmonary infusion of the compound. Alternatively, when administered to patients with heart failure and PH, L-NMMA resulted in an augmented vasoconstrictor response (6). These and other data suggest that basal pulmonary arterial NO generation is deficient in patients with PH and heart failure and that PH development in this patient population may in part be due to loss of NO-dependent vasodilation (5,7,8). Our data demonstrate that in heart failure, PDE5, the enzyme that degrades cGMP in the vasculature, is markedly upregulated and limits NO/cGMP/PKG signaling. This observation provides new insights as to the pathophysiology of this disease process, suggesting that a loss of vascular reactivity in advanced heart failure may be due interruption of normal signaling via PDE5 upregulation.

As has been shown to be important in left heart failure (9), the neurohormonal axis plays a critical role in pulmonary vascular resistance in humans as well. Studies have shown that lisinopril attenuates hypoxic vasoconstriction in humans (10). This and additional data confirm the importance of the renin-angiotensin-aldosterone system to PH (11). A detailed discussion of the neurohormonal axis in heart failure can be found in the chapters of vasodilators, diuretics, and beta-blockers in this publication.

Additionally, research has suggested that angiotensin II, a potent pulmonary vasoconstrictor (12), promotes activated endothelin, which regulates vascular tone (13). The two sub-types, endothelin-1 (ET-1) and endothelin-2 (ET-2), exert their effects on the pulmonary vasculature via the endothelin A (ETA) and endothelin B (ETB) receptors. ETA receptors are located on vascular smooth muscle cells and mediate growth and vasoconstriction, whereas ETB receptors are found on vascular endothelial cells and promote vasodilation via release of NO and prostacyclin (5,7,14). ET-1 levels have been shown to be elevated in patients with PH due to congenital heart disease as well as idiopathic and secondary PH (15,16). In patients with severe heart failure, ET-1 levels have been shown to correlate with pulmonary vascular resistance and pulmonary arterial pressures, suggesting the clinical importance of this molecule in patients with left ventricular failure (17). Moreover, direct infusion of the ETA selective antagonist sitaxsentan into the pulmonary arteries of patients with chronic heart failure resulted in dose-dependent decrease in PVR, suggesting a causative role for endothelin in development of PH in patients with heart failure (18).

EPIDEMIOLOGY AND CLINICAL EVALUATION

The prevalence of PH in patients with congestive heart failure is 25%–50% (19–21). In one study evaluating patients with dilated cardiomyopathy by echocardiography, 26% had an estimated pulmonary arterial systolic pressure greater than 40 mmHg (19), while invasive hemodynamics in a similar patient population estimate a prevalence at 44% (22). PH in patients with congestive heart failure has been linked to prognosis. In the echocardiographic study by Abramson et al. 89% of affected patients either died or were hospitalized at 28 mo, compared with 2% of patients without PH (19). Cappola et al. found that mean systemic pressure and mean pulmonary arterial pressure were the most important hemodynamic predictors of mortality in a diverse group of patients with the new diagnosis of cardiomyopathy (23).

History

Symptoms due to PH may be difficult to differentiate from those attributable to underlying cardiac dysfunction. Classic symptoms of PH include fatigue, lethargy, dyspnea, and exertional syncope due to an inability to augment cardiac output during exercise. In addition, patients may also experience exertional angina from right ventricular hypertrophy with insufficient vascular supply. This pain is not easily distinguished from typical angina associated with coronary flow limitation from atherosclerotic coronary disease. Less frequent symptoms include cough, hemoptysis and hoarseness. Recurrent laryngeal nerve irritation from pulmonary artery enlargement can result in hoarse voice, known as Ortner's syndrome (24). When overt right heart failure is present, lower extremity edema and ascites are also prominent physical findings.

The nature of the cardiac derangement and its duration are central to understanding an individual patient's potential to be successfully treated. Barriers to alleviation of persistent elevation in left heart filling pressures should be identified during the history, with particular attention to determination of reversible ischemia and valvular heart disease.

While it is often evident clinically that PH is due to elevated left heart filling pressures or underlying congenital heart disease, consideration should be given to other conditions that may either be confused with PH associated with left heart disease or may be concomitantly present. Although right heart catheterization is essential to the evaluation of this disorder, history and physical examination frequently give clues to other underlying etiologies. A history of hypoxemic lung disease or sleep disordered breathing may point to PH associated with intrinsic lung disease, obesity or congestive heart failure. Similarly, in a patient with multiple risk factors or a suggestive history for pulmonary embolism, chronic thromboembolic disease should be investigated. Additional factors that may be associated with pulmonary arterial hypertension, including HIV, thyroid or liver disease, anorexogen use, or collagen vascular disease should be queried.

Physical Examination

Physical examination findings depend on the severity of the disorder in the pulmonary vasculature and the degree of right ventricular dysfunction (25). In all subtypes of PH a loud P2 is frequently heard, and as the right heart dilates a tricuspid regurgitation murmur is present. A right-sided third or fourth heart sound may be present depending on the severity of right heart decompensation. Additional findings may include a right ventricular heave, jugular venous pressure elevation and prominent "v" waves, ascites and peripheral edema (24). These physical findings are general to PH and their manifestation may be overshadowed in patients with other prominent findings such as valvular heart disease or left ventricular dysfunction.

Echocardiography

Essential to the evaluation of the patient with clinical left heart failure or congenital heart disease, echocardiography can also suggest the presence of PH. PH is often implied by an elevated tricuspid regurgitant jet velocity. The degree of left ventricular dysfunction by echocardiography has been shown not to correlate with the presence of PH in studies comparing echocardiographic data with right heart catheterization (20,22). In a study by Capomolla et al., in which patients with decompensated heart failure underwent echocardiography and right heart catheterization, the degree of catheter measured PH was found to correlate closely to the echocardiographic diastolic early and late atrial filling ratio (E/A ratio) (22).

Laboratory and Radiologic Evaluation

The goal of laboratory and radiologic studies is to confirm that PH is due to advanced left heart failure or systemic-to-pulmonary shunting. Thus testing should be judiciously applied as indicated by history and physical examination. In excluding alternative diagnoses to PH due to left heart disease, serologic studies should be ordered for patients with a suspicion of collagen vascular disease, HIV, or hepatitis. Chest computed tomogram to evaluate interstitial lung disease or emphysema may be warranted if symptoms or previous radiographs are suggestive. Lastly, ventilation perfusion scan and, if needed, pulmonary angiogram should be performed in those patients with a suggestive history of pulmonary embolism.

Differential Diagnosis

Certain processes can be challenging to differentiate from PH associated with left heart disease. Pulmonary veno-occlusive disease is a rare disorder characterized by extensive occlusion of pulmonary veins and venules by fibrous tissue. Classically chest computed tomography of this disorder shows ground glass opacities as well as pleural effusions that could be confused with pulmonary venous hypertension due to left heart disease (26). This diagnosis should be considered in patients with radiographs consistent with congestive heart failure with normal left ventricular function on examination and echocardiography. Pulmonary capillary hemagiomatosis, which may appear radiographically similar to pulmonary veno-occlusive disease, is characterized by capillary proliferation invading pulmonary interstitium and vessels with resultant vascular occlusion and PH (26). Patients generally present with recurrent hemoptysis in addition to the usual symptoms of PH. These diagnoses require surgical biopsy to confirm.

Right Heart Catheterization

The cornerstone of the evaluation of PH in left heart disease remains the right heart catheterization. PH is diagnosed when the mean pulmonary arterial pressure is greater than 25 mmHg at rest or 30 mmHg with exercise or when the PVR is >3.0 Wood units. An elevated pulmonary capillary wedge pressure confirms that the etiology is due to left heart disease. Frequently depressed cardiac index and low mixed venous saturation are found. The degree of the PH depends on the chronicity of the insult in the pulmonary vasculature. The normal adult right ventricle is capable of generating systolic pressures of 45 to 50 mm Hg in the setting of an acute increase in afterload, as in acute pulmonary embolism. Right ventricular failure ensues if afterload is further increased (21). In a hypertrophied right ventricle, systolic pressures of 80–100 mmHg are possible; however with an ischemic, infracted, or myopathic process, the right ventricle is not capable of producing such elevated pressures and failure occurs at lower mean pulmonary arterial pressures (21).

Equally important as confirming the presence of PH is the determination of reversibility, as this establishes a patient's eligibility for cardiac transplantation. While a number of agents have been used to determine reversibility, the most commonly administered in the evaluation of left heart failure are dopamine, dobutamine, and milrinone. All of these medications have direct vasodilatory effects on the pulmonary vasculature in addition to acting as positive inotropes with subsequent decrease in left atrial filling pressure. Milrinone is the most potent pulmonary vasodilator, followed by dobutamine and dopamine respectively. While oxygen, NO, and nitroprusside can result in pulmonary vasodilation, they are not as potent as the inotropes. Pulmonary vascular resistance has traditionally been used to determine appropriate candidates for transplantation, with a PVR of 3 Wood units or less at rest or with maximal vasodilation being optimal (27).

MANAGEMENT

Medical Management of Pulmonary Hypertension Associated with Left Heart Disease

Despite the prevalence of PH in patients with advanced cardiac failure, there is a paucity of clinical data directed specifically at its treatment. Generally accepted management strategies, published reports, as well as possible future therapies will be discussed below.

General Considerations

Recalling Ohm's law, PVR is closely linked to pulmonary vascular pressure, or left atrial filling pressure. As PH in patients with left heart failure is closely linked to pulmonary capillary wedge pressure, it stands to reason that the mainstay of management of PH in patients with left heart failure is normalization of the wedge pressure (20). A retrospective review of patients admitted to the hospital with heart failure exacerbations and secondary PH with pulmonary arterial catheters in place, showed improved hemodynamics including mean pulmonary arterial pressure, cardiac index, and improved symptoms in patients treated with nesiritide which lowered pulmonary capillary wedge pressure (28). Thus, close attention must be paid to optimization of fluid status and lowering filling pressures in those with PH due to left sided heart failure.

As hypoxia can contribute to vasoconstriction, it is recommended to normalize PaO2 in all patients with PH, such that the oxygenation saturation is 90% or greater or the PaO2 is >60 mmHg (29).

Calcium channel blockers, while helpful in the management of vaso-responsive pulmonary arterial hypertension (30), are not specifically used to treat PH due to left heart disease. As in general heart failure therapy, calcium blocking agents remain indicated only when systemic hypertension persists despite maximal neurohormonal blockade.

The Neurohormonal Axis

The neurohormonal axis should be treated, including spironolactone, afterload reduction with ACE-inhibitors or ARBs, and beta-blockers when tolerated. While there are no survival data to support their use in human PH associated with left heart dysfunction, ACE inhibitors have been shown in animal models of PH to attenuate pulmonary pressor response (10).

Inotropes

Inotropes are frequently used in the hemodynamic evaluation of PH to determine vasoreactivity. Chronic inotrope infusion, with a goal of increasing myocardial contractility, decreasing wedge pressure and subsequently decreasing pulmonary vascular resistance, has also been evaluated (31–34). Of the three most frequently used inotropes—dopamine, dobutamine and milrinone—milrinone appears to be the most potent pulmonary vasodilator (31,35). While long term oral milrinone has been associated with an increased mortality in patients with severe heart failure in the pre-AICD era, the use of milrinone infusion has been advocated as a treatment for elevated pulmonary vascular resistance in cardiac transplant candidates. Indeed, milrinone has been shown to decrease pulmonary artery pressure, pulmonary capillary wedge pressure and pulmonary vascular resistance in patients with chronic infusions from 24–63 days (33,34). Similar findings have been described with dobutamine in a head-to-head comparison with milrinone; dobutamine was less expensive and associated with similar outcomes (34). While not recommended as standard therapy for all patients, chronic inotrope therapy can be useful in a select group awaiting cardiac transplantation with rising or already elevated pulmonary vascular resistance, as a means of dropping pulmonary resistance and thereby improving transplant suitability. In patients who are not transplant candidates, chronic inotrope therapy can be useful for symptomatic relief as a palliative intervention.

Endothelin-Receptor Antagonists

Given the importance of endothelin in PH associated with left heart failure in both animal models and humans, the use of endothelin-receptor blockers has been investigated in patients with heart failure. Unfortunately the results have been less promising than animal data would suggest (36). The ENABLE (Endothelin Antagonist Bosentan for Lowering cardiac Events in heart failure) study was a phase 3 evaluation of low-dose bosentan, a non-selective ETA and ETB antagonist, in patients with chronic heart failure and an ejection fraction $<35\%$. In this study, 1613 patients were randomized to placebo or bosentan at 125 mg daily with a mean length of follow up of 18 mo. There was no difference in the primary endpoint of all-cause mortality or hospitalization between the two groups; however, there was an increase in early worsening of heart failure necessitating hospitalization in the bosentan treatment arm (37). Similar early worsening of heart failure was noted in the REACH-I (Research on Endothelin Antagonism in Chronic Heart failure) Study, which randomized patients with heart failure and an ejection fraction <35% to high dose (500 mg twice daily) bosentan or placebo. Additionally, this trial was stopped early due to worsening liver function abnormalities in the treatment arm. In those patients who completed the study protocol of 26 wk, there was a significant improvement in the NYHA class in the treatment group (38). However, none of these studies specifically targeted patients with PH or measured hemodynamics. Moreover, these trials involved the use of agents that were nonselective in their antagonism of the ET_A and ET_B receptors. It is possible that selective antagonism of the ET_A receptor will prove superior to non-selective antagonists with respect to PH. From our own experience, endothelin antagonists such as bosentan can be helpful in the treatment of patients with PH secondary to non-systolic heart failure with well-managed volume status.

Prostacyclin Analogs

Other therapies that have been proven successful in pulmonary arterial hypertension have been attempted in patients with PH due to left heart failure, including prostacyclin. The acute administration of epoprostanol, a prostacyclin analog, to patients with heart failure and secondary PH has been shown to improve hemodynamics (39–41). Unfortunately, the results of the FIRST (Flolan International Randomized Survival Trial) trial showed an increased mortality in patients with left heart failure treated long term with epoprostanol in the pre-AICD era. The positive inotropic action of prostacyclin at therapeutic doses is hypothesized to explain the increased mortality seen in patients with heart failure treated with this drug (40). In patients with heart failure and secondary PH, iloprost, an inhaled prostacyclin analog, has been shown to have beneficial effects on hemodynamics, including decrease in mean pulmonary artery pressure and increase in cardiac index; however, long term data are lacking currently in this patient population (42).

Future Directions

PDE5 inhibitors such as sildenafil, which increase intracellular cGMP and subsequently promote vascular relaxation, may be shown to be useful in the long-term therapy of PH associated with left heart failure. A hemodynamic study of 14 patients with heart failure who were administered 25 mg or 50 mg thrice daily sildenafil for 24 hr showed a marked drop in pulmonary vascular resistance and a decrease in pulmonary artery pressure, with a trend to greater improvement in the group with the higher dose. The drug was safe and well tolerated in this patient population (43). At our institution we have treated patients with severe left heart disease and associated PH with sildenafil and found success in dropping pulmonary vascular resistance as well as decreasing the need for inotrope therapy or ventricular assist device placement. Long-term trial data in large numbers of patients is lacking at this time, however this may prove to be an exciting venue for future therapeutic options.

Medical Management of PH Associated with Chronic Systemic-to-Pulmonary Shunt

There is significantly more data for the management of pulmonary arterial hypertension associated with chronic systemic-to-pulmonary shunt, as this disorder is associated with similar pathologic findings as the other causes of pulmonary arterial hypertension and has been included in trials of numerous medications for this disorder. While the numbers of included patients remain small, the results are promising.

General Considerations

In a patient with a chronic systemic-to-pulmonary shunt, consideration should be given to correction of the shunt, if possible, to diminish flow through the pulmonary vasculature. Often, at the time the patient presents, this is not technically possible or the procedure poses excessive risk to the patient. As above, correction of hypoxemia is indicated whenever possible. Additionally, limited data suggest benefit to anticoagulation in patients with pulmonary arterial hypertension whenever possible, with a goal international normalized ratio of 1.5–2.5 times normal (30,44–46). Similarly, as described above for patients with PH associated with left heart disease, optimization of fluid status is paramount to symptom relief as well as to improvement in hemodynamics.

Prostacyclin Analogs

The prostacyclin analog epoprostanol has been shown to improve mortality in patients with idiopathic pulmonary arterial hypertension (47). In chronic systemic-to-pulmonary shunt, mortality benefit has not been described with this drug. However, in a study of 20 patients with NYHA class II-IV congenital heart disease and PH treated with continuous infusion of epoprostanol for one year, mean pulmonary artery pressure fell by 21%, and cardiac index and pulmonary vascular resistance improved. Importantly, NYHA functional class and exercise capacity improved (48). Similar improvement in functional capacity has been noted in this patient population when treated with oral beraprost, which is not available in the United States at this time (49). Inhaled iloprost has not yet been evaluated in patients with congenital left-to-right shunt. In general, epoprostanol has been reserved for the sickest patients as it requires an in-dwelling catheter and has significant side effects. The risks associated with this therapy and the alteration in quality of life is only outweighed by the survival benefit in those patients with severe pulmonary arterial hypertension.

Endothelin-Receptor Antagonists

The non-selective ETA and ETB receptor antagonist bosentan has been shown to be effective in idiopathic pulmonary arterial hypertension and that associated with systemic sclerosis (50). Recent data now supports its use in PH associated with congenital heart disease and left-to-right shunt. In an open label noncontrolled trial, patients with congenital heart disease and systemic to pulmonary shunt with associated class II–IV PH received weight-based dosing of oral bosentan, ranging from 31.25 to 125 mg twice daily for 16 wk. An improvement was found in WHO class, exercise tolerance, and mean pulmonary artery pressure (51). A mortality benefit was not found in this short-term trial. Monthly transaminases should be measured in patients receiving this medication to monitor rare and generally reversible hepatotoxicity.

PDE5 Inhibition

Chronic PDE5 inhibition via sildenafil has been shown to be an effective short-term vasodilator in patients with pulmonary arterial hypertension (52). New data show the efficacy of this therapy chronically in patients with pulmonary arterial hypertension. In the

SUPER trial, placebo or sildenafil was administered at 20, 40, or 80 mg orally three times daily to patients with class I–IV pulmonary arterial hypertension, some of whom had underlying systemic-to-pulmonary shunt. After one year of therapy, there was an increase in 6 mo walk time and improvement in pulmonary vascular resistance in the treatment group (52a). Overall, bosentan and sildenafil are good choices for patients with less advanced symptoms, e.g. class II or III. Given their low risk profile and potential benefit, bosentan and sildenafil are recommended as first line therapy for patients with class II or III symptoms. In patients who fail with a single agent, the two drugs can be combined.

Surgical Management

Surgical Management of Advanced Left Heart Failure

While cardiac transplantation remains the definitive management for patients with refractory advanced left heart failure, new procedures may offer improved quality of life for patients with associated PH who may not yet qualify or are not candidates for transplantation. A recent case report by Healey et al. described a 63 yr old woman with a non-ischemic dilated cardiomyopathy, refractory heart failure and a widened QRS complex who had right heart catheterization before and five months after an atrio-biventricular pacemaker placement. Prior to the device placement she had no response to inhaled NO and a PVR of 10.1 Wood units; after 5 mo her PVR had dropped to 4.5 Wood Units. Wedge pressure was 26 mmHg and 15 mmHg respectively (53). This report suggests there may be a role for cardiac resynchronization therapy in management of PH associated with advanced left heart disease.

More invasive procedures, such as ventricular assist devices, have been evaluated for the management of advanced left heart failure with PH (54,55). A European trial of left ventricular assist devices as a bridge to transplantation followed six patients with mean pulmonary arterial pressure 25 mmHg or greater for six months after device placement. They were able to demonstrate decreased PVR and decreased systolic pulmonary pressures (54). Right ventricular assist devices, while commonly used post-operatively from cardiac surgery, have not been studied in the chronic setting for management of left heart disease with fixed PH (56). Cardiac support devices, which are surgically placed mesh sleeves that surround the heart and reduce stress-mediated myocardial stretch, have not yet been shown to improve pulmonary hemodynamics in patients with moderate congestive heart failure and cannot be advocated as management for PH associated with left heart disease at this time (57), but show promise and warrant further investigation.

The gold standard for management of refractory left heart failure is cardiac transplantation. Pre-operative PH is a predictor of mortality with cardiac transplantation (58–60), thus precluding many patients from undergoing this procedure. Currently, most clinicians consider a PVR of 6 Wood units or greater than 3 Wood units with maximal vasodilation to be a contraindication to transplantation (27). In a patient with unacceptably high PVR, therapies discussed in medical management, such as inotrope infusion or ventricular assist device, should be considered. Nonetheless, replacement of the failing left ventricle can markedly improve pulmonary hemodynamics. Previous authors have shown by echocardiography and invasive hemodynamic measurements that there is resolution of elevated PVR and right ventricular dysfunction after cardiac transplantation (61).

Surgical Management of Pulmonary Hypertension Associated with Systemic-to-Pulmonary Shunt

In patients with advanced heart failure due to systemic-to-pulmonary shunt, the gold standard of management is cardiac transplantation. In those patients who have associated PH, heart-lung transplantation is indicated, as without transplanted lungs the new heart would develop right ventricular failure when faced with the afterload of a remodeled pulmonary vasculature. Outcomes for this population of patients undergoing transplantation are unchanged from the general population (62). Patients with intermediate elevations of PVP may be considered for heterotopic heart transplantation (piggy back heart), allowing the new and old heart to eject into the pulmonary vascular bed.

REFERENCES

1. Paraskos J. Pulmonary heart disease including pulmonary embolism. In: Parmley WW, Chatterjee K, eds. Cardiology. Philadelphia: Lippincott, 1987.
2. Haworth SG, Hall SM, Panja M. Peripheral pulmonary vascular and airway abnormalities in adolescents with rheumatic mitral stenosis. Int J Cardiol 1988; 18:405–416.
3. Harris P. The Human Circulation. 3rd ed. New York: Churchill Livingstone, 1986.
4. Kidd L, et al. Second natural history study of congenital heart defects. Results of treatment of patients with ventricular septal defects. Circulation 1993; 87:138–151.
5. Moraes DL, Colucci WS, Givertz MM. Secondary pulmonary hypertension in chronic heart failure: the role of the endothelium in pathophysiology and management. Circulation 2000; 102:1718–1723.
6. Cooper CJ, et al. The influence of basal nitric oxide activity on pulmonary vascular resistance in patients with congestive heart failure. Am J Cardiol 1998; 82:609–614.
7. Porter TR, et al. Endothelium-dependent pulmonary artery responses in chronic heart failure: influence of pulmonary hypertension. J Am Coll Cardiol 1993; 22:1418–1424.
8. Celermajer DS, Cullen S, Deanfield JE. Impairment of endothelium-dependent pulmonary artery relaxation in children with congenital heart disease and abnormal pulmonary hemodynamics. Circulation 1993; 87:440–446.
9. Jessup M, Brozena S. Heart failure. N Engl J Med 2003; 348:2007–2018.
10. Cargill RI, Lipworth J. Lisinopril attenuates acute hypoxic pulmonary vasoconstriction in humans. Chest 1996; 109:424–429.
11. Anand IS, et al. Pathogenesis of congestive state in chronic obstructive pulmonary disease. Studies of body water and sodium, renal function, hemodynamics, and plasma hormones during edema and after recovery. Circulation 1992; 86:12–21.
12. Lipworth BJ, Dagg KD. Vasoconstrictor effects of angiotensin II on the pulmonary vascular bed. Chest 1994; 105:1360–1364.
13. Lerman A, Burnett JC, Jr., Intact and altered endothelium in regulation of vasomotion. Circulation 1992; 86:III12–III19.
14. Tuder RM, et al. The pathobiology of pulmonary hypertension. Endothelium. Clin Chest Med 2001; 22:405–418.
15. Stewart DJ, et al. Increased plasma endothelin-1 in pulmonary hypertension: marker or mediator of disease? Ann Intern Med 1991; 114:464–469.
16. Staniloae C, et al. Reduced pulmonary clearance of endothelin in congestive heart failure: a marker of secondary pulmonary hypertension. J Card Fail 2004; 10:427–432.
17. Cody RJ, et al. Plasma endothelin correlates with the extent of pulmonary hypertension in patients with chronic congestive heart failure. Circulation 1992; 85:504–509.
18. Ooi H, Colucci WS, Givertz MM. Endothelin mediates increased pulmonary vascular tone in patients with heart failure: demonstration by direct intrapulmonary infusion of sitaxsentan. Circulation 2002; 106:1618–1621.

19. Abramson SV, et al. Pulmonary hypertension predicts mortality and morbidity in patients with dilated cardiomyopathy. Ann Intern Med 1992; 116:888–895.
20. Enriquez-Sarano M, et al. Determinants of pulmonary hypertension in left ventricular dysfunction. J Am Coll Cardiol 1997; 29:153–159.
21. Rich S. Pulmonary hypertension. In: Braunweld E, Zipes DP, Libby P, Bonow RO, eds. A Textbook of Cardiovascular Medicine. Philadelphia: W.B. Saunders Company, 2001.
22. Capomolla S, et al. Invasive and non-invasive determinants of pulmonary hypertension in patients with chronic heart failure. J Heart Lung Transplant 2000; 19:426–438.
23. Cappola TP, et al. Pulmonary hypertension and risk of death in cardiomyopathy: patients with myocarditis are at higher risk. Circulation 2002; 105:1663–1668.
24. Gaine SP, Rubin LJ. Primary pulmonary hypertension. Lancet 1998; 352:719–725.
25. Rich S, et al. Primary pulmonary hypertension. A national prospective study. Ann Intern Med 1987; 107:216–223.
26. Pietra GG, et al. Pathologic assessment of vasculopathies in pulmonary hypertension. J Am Coll Cardiol 2004; 43:25S–32S.
27. Natale ME, Pina IL. Evaluation of pulmonary hypertension in heart transplant candidates. Curr Opin Cardiol 2003; 18:136–140.
28. O'Dell KM, et al. Nesiritide for secondary pulmonary hypertension in patients with end-stage heart failure. Am J Health Syst Pharm 2005; 62:606–609.
29. Rubin LJ, Rich S. Medical management. In: Rubin LJ, ed. Primary Pulmonary Hypertension. New York: Marcel Dekker, 1997:271–286.
30. Rich S, Kaufmann E, Levy PS. The effect of high doses of calcium-channel blockers on survival in primary pulmonary hypertension. N Engl J Med 1992; 327:76–81.
31. Young JB, Moen EK. Outpatient parenteral inotropic therapy for advanced heart failure. J Heart Lung Transplant 2000; 19:S49–S57.
32. Zewail AM, et al. Intravenous milrinone in treatment of advanced congestive heart failure. Tex Heart Inst J 2003; 30:109–113.
33. Mehra MR, et al. Safety and clinical utility of long-term intravenous milrinone in advanced heart failure. Am J Cardiol 1997; 80:61–64.
34. Aranda JM, Jr., et al. Comparison of dobutamine versus milrinone therapy in hospitalized patients awaiting cardiac transplantation: a prospective, randomized trial. Am Heart J 2003; 145:324–329.
35. Givertz MM, et al. Effect of bolus milrinone on hemodynamic variables and pulmonary vascular resistance in patients with severe left ventricular dysfunction: a rapid test for reversibility of pulmonary hypertension. J Am Coll Cardiol 1996; 28:1775–1780.
36. Mishima T, et al. Effects of long-term therapy with bosentan on the progression of left ventricular dysfunction and remodeling in dogs with heart failure. J Am Coll Cardiol 2000; 35:222–229.
37. Kalra PR, Moon JC, Coats AJ. Do results of the ENABLE (Endothelin Antagonist Bosentan for Lowering Cardiac Events in Heart Failure) study spell the end for non-selective endothelin antagonism in heart failure? Int J Cardiol 2002; 85:195–197.
38. Packer M, et al. Clinical effects of endothelin receptor antagonism with bosentan in patients with severe chronic heart failure: results of a pilot study. J Card Fail 2005; 11:12–20.
39. Sueta CA, et al. Safety and efficacy of epoprostenol in patients with severe congestive heart failure. Epoprostenol Multicenter Research Group. Am J Cardiol 1995; 75:34A–43A.
40. Montalescot G, et al. Effects of prostacyclin on the pulmonary vascular tone and cardiac contractility of patients with pulmonary hypertension secondary to end-stage heart failure. Am J Cardiol 1998; 82:749–755.
41. Yui Y, et al. Prostacyclin therapy in patients with congestive heart failure. Am J Cardiol 1982; 50:320–324.
42. Sablotzki A, et al. Iloprost improves hemodynamics in patients with severe chronic cardiac failure and secondary pulmonary hypertension. Can J Anaesth 2002; 49:1076–1080.
43. Alaeddini J, et al. Efficacy and safety of sildenafil in the evaluation of pulmonary hypertension in severe heart failure. Am J Cardiol 2004; 94:1475–1477.

44. Bjornsson J, Edwards WD. Primary pulmonary hypertension: a histopathologic study of 80 cases. Mayo Clin Proc 1985; 60:16–25.
45. Fuster V, et al. Primary pulmonary hypertension: natural history and the importance of thrombosis. Circulation 1984; 70:580–587.
46. Humbert M, Sitbon O, Simonneau G. Treatment of pulmonary arterial hypertension. N Engl J Med 2004; 351:1425–1436.
47. Barst RJ, et al. A comparison of continuous intravenous epoprostenol (prostacyclin) with conventional therapy for primary pulmonary hypertension. The Primary Pulmonary Hypertension Study Group. N Engl J Med 1996; 334:296–302.
48. Rosenzweig EB, Kerstein D, Barst RJ. Long-term prostacyclin for pulmonary hypertension with associated congenital heart defects. Circulation 1999; 99:1858–1865.
49. Galie N, et al. Effects of beraprost sodium, an oral prostacyclin analogue, in patients with pulmonary arterial hypertension: a randomized, double-blind, placebo-controlled trial. J Am Coll Cardiol 2002; 39:1496–1502.
50. Rubin LJ, et al. Bosentan therapy for pulmonary arterial hypertension. N Engl J Med 2002; 346:896–903.
51. Apostolopoulou SC, et al. Effect of the oral endothelin antagonist bosentan on theclinical, exercise, and haemodynamic status of patients with pulmonary arterial hypertension related to congenital heart disease. Heart 2005.
52. Michelakis E, et al. Oral sildenafil is an effective and specific pulmonary vasodilator in patients with pulmonary arterial hypertension: comparison with inhaled nitric oxide. Circulation 2002; 105:2398–2403.
52a. Galie N, Ghofrani HA, Torbicki A, et al. Sildenafil Use in Pulmonary Arterial Hypertension (SUPER) study group. N Engl J Med 2005; 353:2148–2157.
53. Healey JS, Davies RA, Tang AS. Improvement of apparently fixed pulmonary hypertension with cardiac resynchronization therapy. J Heart Lung Transplant 2004; 23:650–652.
54. Salzberg SP, et al. Normalization of high pulmonary vascular resistance with LVAD support in heart transplantation candidates. Eur J Cardiothorac Surg 2005; 27:222–225.
55. Al-Khaldi A, et al. Left ventricular unloading in a patient with end-stage cardiomyopathy and medically unresponsive pulmonary hypertension. Artif Organs 2004; 28:158–160.
56. Stobierska-Dzierzek B, Awad H, Michler RE. The evolving management of acute right-sided heart failure in cardiac transplant recipients. J Am Coll Cardiol 2001; 38:923–931.
57. Starling RC, Jessup M. Worldwide clinical experience with the CorCap Cardiac Support Device. J Card Fail 2004; 10:S225–S233.
58. Delgado JF, et al. Impact of mild pulmonary hypertension on mortality and pulmonary artery pressure profile after heart transplantation. J Heart Lung Transplant 2001; 20:942–948.
59. Kirsch M, et al. Pretransplantation risk factors for death after heart transplantation: the Henri Mondor experience. J Heart Lung Transplant 1998; 17:268–277.
60. Erickson KW, et al. Influence of preoperative transpulmonary gradient on late mortality after orthotopic heart transplantation. J Heart Transplant 1990; 9:526–537.
61. Bhatia SJ, et al. Time course of resolution of pulmonary hypertension and right ventricular remodeling after orthotopic cardiac transplantation. Circulation 1987; 76:819–826.
62. Jayakumar KA, Addonizio LJ, Kichuk-Chrisant MR, et al. Cardiac transplantation after the Fontan or Glenn procedure. J Am Coll Cardiol 2004; 44:2065–2072.

PART III: DEVICE THERAPY

15
Cardiac Resynchronization Therapy

Michael O. Sweeney
CRM Research and Cardiac Arrhythmia Service, Brigham and Women's Hospital, Harvard Medical School, Boston, Massachusetts, U.S.A.

A HEART FAILURE EPIDEMIC

There are 4–5 million people living with chronic heart failure and an additional 400,000 newly diagnosed yearly (1–3). The incidence of heart failure is 10 per 1000 for individuals that are over 65 yr of age. The increasing incidence of heart failure is due primarily to the advancing age of the population with coronary artery disease, which is now the principal cause of heart failure associated with reduced ventricular function (dilated cardiomyopathy, DCM) (4). Mortality due to progressive heart failure associated with DCM has declined. In the Framingham study total mortality was 24% and 55% within 4 yr of developing symptomatic heart failure for women and men, respectively (4). These statistics approximate well the natural history of heart failure as the subject population was untreated by contemporary standards. Recognition of the beneficial effects of ACE inhibitors, diuretics, digoxin and beta-blockade has yielded substantial reductions in mortality due to progressive pump failure. However, despite these improvements in medical therapy, symptomatic heart failure still confers a 20–25% risk of premature death in the first 2½ yr after diagnosis.

ABNORMAL ELECTRICAL TIMING IN HEART FAILURE ASSOCIATED WITH DCM

Disordered electrical timing frequently accompanies heart failure associated with DCM. Disordered electrical timing alters critical mechanical relationships that further impair left ventricular (LV) performance. It is now recognized that there are 4 levels of electromechanical abnormalities associated with heart failure due to DCM.

Prolonged Atrioventricular (AV) Delay

Optimal AV coupling is necessary for maximum ventricular pumping performance. The normal AV interval results in atrial contraction just before the pre-ejection (isovolumic) period of ventricular contraction that maximizes ventricular filling (LV end diastolic pressure, or pre-load) and cardiac output by the Starling mechanisms. This optimal timing relationship also results in filling throughout diastole, prevents diastolic mitral regurgitation (MR) and maintains mean left atrial pressure at low levels (Fig. 1).

Alterations in the AV coupling can be understood by analysis of Doppler mitral inflow patterns (Fig. 2). Prolonged AV conduction disrupts these relationships and may degrade ventricular performance. Significantly prolonged AV conduction results in displacement of atrial contraction earlier in diastole such that atrial contraction may occur immediately after, or even within, the preceding ventricular contraction. This may result in atrial contraction before venous return is completed and reduce the atrial contribution to

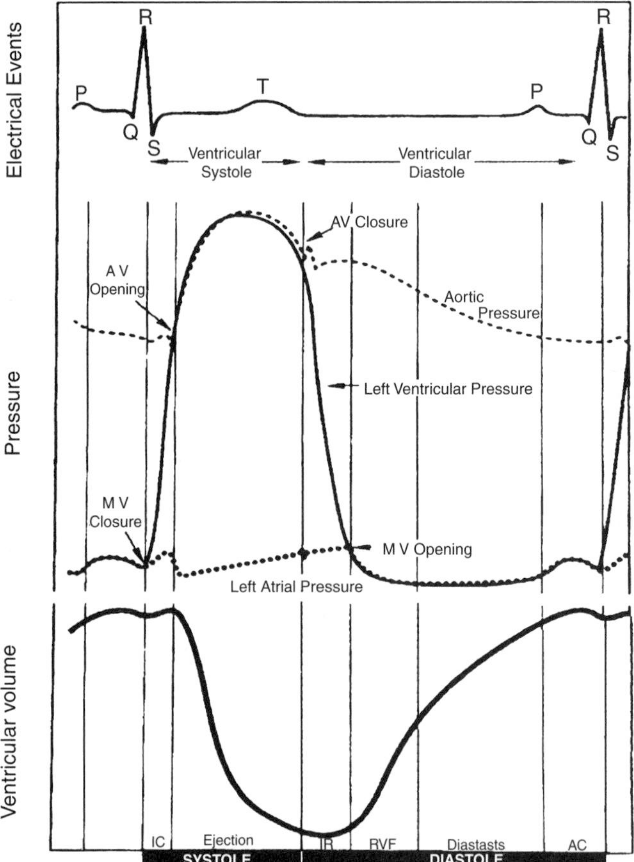

Figure 1 Events of the cardiac electrical cycle. Atrial contraction followed by relaxation produces a negative pressure gradient, causing a surge of blood in the LV at end diastole. Reversal of the AV pressure gradient initiates MV closure because of a rapid decrease in pressure between the MV cusps pulling them into apposition. A brief period of isovolumetric contraction exists after MV closure and before AV opening during which the max rate of pressure change (peak + dP/dt) occurs. Rapid ejection occurs during ventricular systole and is terminated when ventricular pressure falls below aortic pressure, closing the AV. A brief period of isovolumic relaxation follows during which the max rate of pressure decline (peak-dP/dt) occurs. As the LV pressure continues to decline and fall below atrial pressure, the MV opens and diastolic ventricular filling begins. Normal diastolic filling is characterized by an initial rapid increase in ventricular filling during early diastole followed by a slow phase of filling during mid-diastole. A second rapid increase in ventricular filling occurs in late diastole as a result of atrial contraction.

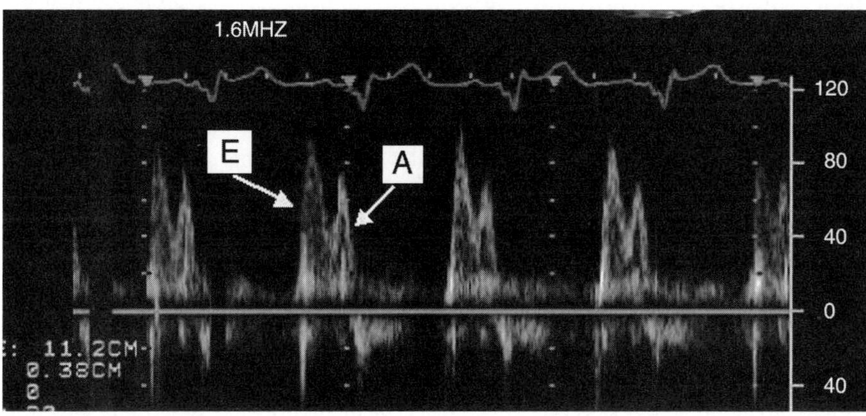

Figure 2 Doppler mitral inflow patterns. This figure shows LV filling velocities from a patient with dilated cardiomyopathy, LBBB and first degree AVB, recorded at the level of the mitral leaflet tips (apical window) with pulsed-wave Doppler. The mitral flow velocity curve is composed of the peak initial velocity (E wave) and the velocity at atrial contraction (A wave). This comprises the diastolic filling period, which is the interval from the onset of the E velocity to the cessation of the A velocity. Note characteristic EA fusion due to the combined effects of delayed LV activation (LBBB) and delayed AV conduction (first degree AVB).

pre-load, thereby diminishing ventricular volume and contractile force. Early atrial contraction may also initiate early mitral valve closure, limiting diastolic filling time. Diastolic MR may also occur with prolonged AV conduction because of premature and incomplete mitral valve closure (Fig. 3).

Interventricular and Intraventricular Delay

Normal ventricular electrical activation is rapid and homogeneous with minimal temporal dispersion throughout the wall. This elicits a synchronous mechanical activation and ventricular contraction. Exploration of the link between the sequence of cardiac electrical activation and mechanical function is one of the most exciting contemporary areas of research in heart failure. But recognition of the importance of normal ventricular activation patterns for optimal pumping function dates back 75 years. Wiggers observed that asynchronous delayed activation of the ventricular musculature induced by electrical

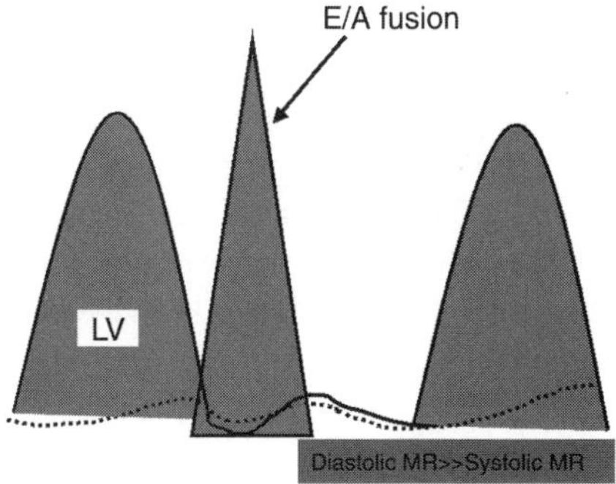

Figure 3 Schematic representation of hemodynamic effects of prolonged native atrioventricular conduction on left ventricular performance.

stimulation had adverse hemodynamic consequences in mammals and proposed that the more muscle activated before excitation of the Purkinje system, the greater the asynchrony and the weaker the resulting contraction (5). Forty years later RC Schlant reached similar conclusions and stated that asynchronous ventricular activation imposed by significant interventricular conduction delay left bundle branch block (LBBB) was hemodynamically disadvantageous due to loss of the "idioventricular kick" (6). This is a term applied to improved systolic function attributed to the greater stretch and increased contractility of later contracting areas imparted by earlier contraction of other areas of the ventricle.

Chronic DCM is often accompanied by delayed ventricular electrical activation manifested as prolonged QRS duration (QRSd), most commonly in the form of LBBB. The prevalence of prolonged QRSd in heart failure associated with DCM varies but appears to be in the range of 25–50%. Prolonged QRSd is a potent predictor of mortality in heart failure associated with DCM. In the VEST study, which assessed the efficacy of vesnarinone in patients with DCM and Class II–IV heart failure, age, creatinine, ejection fraction, heart rate, and QRSd were found to be independent predictors of mortality. Cumulative survival from all-cause mortality decreased proportionally with QRSd. The relative risk of the widest QRSd group was 5 times greater than the narrowest (7). The association between LBBB in DCM and increased risk of sudden death and total mortality in DCM has subsequently been demonstrated in large population studies (8).

Optimal inter- and intra-ventricular coupling is more important than AV coupling for maximum ventricular pumping function. Interventricular coupling refers to coordinated contraction of the right ventricle (RV) and the left ventricle (LV). *Interventricular delay* refers to a relative delay in mechanical activation of each ventricle, most commonly LBBB where the RV begins its contraction before the LV. The delay in onset of LV activation results in reversal of the normal sequence between RV and LV mechanical events that persists throughout the cardiac cycle (9). Asynchronous ventricular contraction and relaxation results in dynamic changes in ventricular pressures and volumes throughout the cardiac cycle. This results in abnormal septal deflections that alter the regional contribution to global ejection fraction. Earliest ventricular depolarization is recorded over the anterior surface of the RV and latest at the basal-lateral LV. In canine models with induced LBBB, increasing the delay between RV and LV contraction increases the delay between the upslope of LV and RV systolic pressure. The increase in interventricular delay was associated with decreased LV +dP/dt and decreased stroke work, presumptively the result of ventricular interdependence and impairment of the septal contribution to LV ejection due to displacement after onset of RV ejection (10).

Pacing models can be used to induce asynchronous ventricular activation, with early activation occurring at the pacing site (11,12). Regions of late activation are subject to greater wall stress and develop local myocyte hypertrophy accompanied by reductions in sarcoplasmic reticulum calcium-ATPase and phospholamban (13). Chronic asynchronous ventricular activation redistributes the mechanical load within the ventricular wall and leads to reduction of blood flow and myocardial wall thickness over the site of early activation (12,14). This ventricular remodeling may contribute to progression of heart failure. In addition to these effects, delayed, sequential activation of papillary muscles may aggravate MR (15).

Intraventricular Delay

The third level of synchrony exists within each ventricle. Rapid spread of contraction from the LV septum endocardially to the base of the heart creates coordinated, efficient contraction. With LBBB, and delayed propagation of the electrical impulse across the LV, the septum begins contraction substantially earlier than the lateral wall. When one segment of the ventricle, such as the septum, contracts earlier than another segment, such as the lateral wall, the lateral wall stretches, absorbing some of the initial force, then begins its late contraction, stretching the septum. Shortening of earlier activated regions is wasted work because pressure is low and no ejection is occurring. Delayed shortening of late activated regions occurs at higher wall stress because the early regions have already developed tension, yet it is also characterized by wasted work because the early regions may now undergo paradoxical stretch. The resulting contraction is mechanically inefficient, with diminished ejection at an increased metabolic cost. This is accompanied by increased end systolic volume and wall stress and reduced LV +dP/dt and diastolic filling time. The net result is an acute decline in systolic function of about 20%.

Intramural Delay

Studies of activation maps have shown different activation timing and sequence between endocardial and transmural activation. This suggests the possibility of intramural activation delay between the endocardial and myocardial layer (16). The negative effects, if any, of intramural delay on ventricular pumping function, are uncertain.

CARDIAC RESYNCHRONIZATION THERAPY (CRT)

Recognition of the contribution of disordered electrical timing to reduced venticular performance suggested the possibility that pacing techniques could favorably modulate contractile dyssynchrony and delayed AV timing. The fundamental premise of this therapeutic strategy is that LV pre-excitation may correct inter- and intra-ventricular conduction delays and permit optimization of left-sided AV delay, thereby improving ventricular pumping function.

The first report of the potential hemodynamic benefit of left univentricular pacing used epicardial leads placed on the high right atrium and lateral LV free wall during surgery for aortic valve replacement in patients with LBBB (17). De Teresa et al. (17) noted that LV ejection fraction was maximal when septal motion was simultaneous with free wall contraction and diminished when septal and free wall motion were dyssynchronous, such as during spontaneous activation with LBBB or during right ventricular (RV) apical pacing. The term "cardiac resynchronization" was first used 10 years later when Cazeau et al. (18) used epicardial leads on all 4 cardiac chambers to modify the ventricular activation sequence and improve hemodynamic performance in heart failure due to DCM accompanied by LBBB.

Mechanisms of CRT

Improved Pumping Function: AV Optimization and Ventricular Resynchronization

Correction of physiologically disadvantageous prolonged AV conduction (*AV optimization*) can be achieved with LV pre-excitation. Optimization of the AV interval during CRT can be demonstrated by examining mitral flow velocity curves using 2-D echocardiography.

When LV pre-excitation is inadequate, the result is similar to a prolonged AV interval as shown in Fig. 3. Note atrial contraction occurs too early and does not contribute to increased LVEDP (absence of A wave on mitral inflow velocity). Atrial contraction occurs before venous return is completed causing reduced ventricular volume and

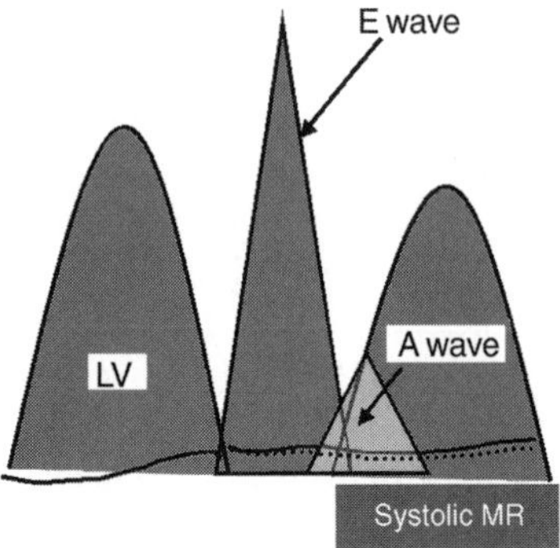

Figure 4 Schematic representation of hemodynamic effects of too short an atrioventricular interval on left ventricular performance.

contractile force. It may also initiate early mitral valve closure, thereby limiting diastolic filling time. Diastolic MR may also occur because once closed, the mitral valve may drift open again before ventricular contraction.

When the programmed AV interval is too short, LV pre-excitation occurs too early relative to atrial systole (Fig. 4). Note that filling occurs throughout all of diastole. With a long AV delay, atrial contraction now occurs simultaneously with LV contraction resulting in increased left atrial pressure and loss of atrial contribution to ventricular systole, reducing cardiac output. A shorter AV interval lengthens the diastolic filling period by abolishing premature mitral valve closure due to the LV-left atrial pressure gradient seen with long AV delays. This also eliminates diastolic MR. However, the diastolic filling period should not be used as the only guideline to optimize the AV interval. Despite optimization of the diastolic filling period, hemodynamic deterioration will occur at too short an AV interval if atrial contraction occurs against a closed mitral valve. This could result in a decrease in cardiac output and increase in mean left atrial pressure despite optimization of the diastolic filling period.

LV pre-excitation at the optimal AV interval is shown in Figure 5. The relation of atrial contraction to the onset of ventricular contraction is now optimal, resulting in diastolic filling throughout the entire diastolic filling period. An appropriate relation now exists between mechanical left atrial and LV contraction so that mean left atrial pressure is maintained at a low level with left atrial contraction occurring just before LV contraction.

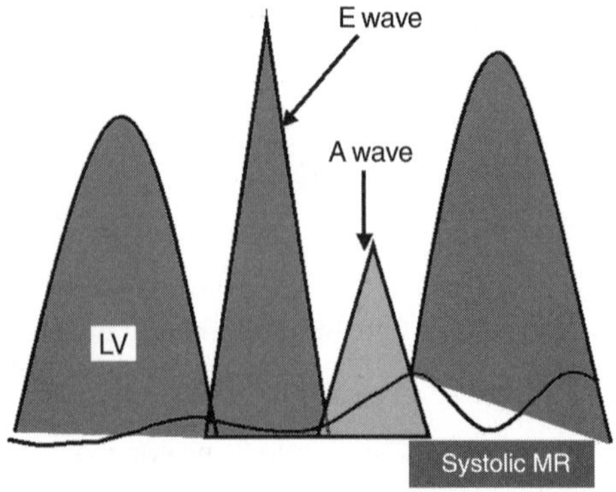

Figure 5 Schematic representation of hemodynamic effects of optimal atrioventricular interval on left ventricular performance.

This causes an increase in LVEDP (preload) and cardiac output. Note diastolic MR is eliminated and systolic MR is reduced.

Acute hemodynamic studies have shown that AV delay is a significant determinant of changes in all LV systolic parameters (+dP/dt, aortic systolic pressure, aortic pulse pressure) (19). For CRT "responders" (see below) LV+dP/dt and aortic pulse pressure AV delay functions are positive and unimodal, with a peak effect at approximately 50% of the native PR interval. The optimal AV delays for the same pacing chamber and parameter vary widely among patients and often differed for pulse pressure and LV+dP/dt within an individual (19). The acute increase in LV +dP/dt with optimal AV delay may be in the range of 15–45% (19,20).

The hemodynamic benefit of LV pre-excitation is primarily due to *ventricular resynchronization* rather than AV optimization. The decreased LV+dP/dt and decreased stroke work associated with interventricular delay can be eliminated by CRT (10) and improvements in RV to LV delay correlate with improvements in EF (21). Furthermore, CRT improves pumping function while decreasing myocardial energy consumption (22).

Reverse Left Ventricular Remodeling

In addition to improvement in acute hemodynamic performance, it has now been clearly demonstrated that CRT improves chronic LV pumping function. This improvement is accompanied by Doppler echocardiographic (conventional two-dimensional and tissue imaging) evidence of reverse LV remodeling (23–25). These remodeling effects include reduction in LV volume, redistribution of cardiac mass, reduced mitral orifice size and reduced MR.

Other Effects of CRT: Reduction in Functional Mitral Regurgitation

Functional MR frequently accompanies DCM and results from an imbalance between the closing and tethering forces that act on the mitral leaflets as elegantly described by Breithardt et al. (15). This is strongly dependent on alterations in ventricular shape as the tethering forces that act on the mitral leaflets are greater in dilated, more spherical ventricles. These geometric changes alter the balance between tethering and closing forces and impede effective mitral closure. Ventricular dilatation and increased chamber sphericity increase the distance between the papillary muscles to the enlarged mitral annulus as well as to each other, restricting leaflet motion and increasing the force needed for effective mitral valve closure. This mitral valve closing force is determined by the systolic LV pressure-left atrial pressure difference, which is called the transmitral pressure gradient. Under these conditions, the mitral regurgitant orifice area will be largely determined by the phasic changes in transmitral pressure. Increasing the transmitral pressure can reduce the effective regurgitant orifice area. CRT acutely reduces the severity of functional MR and this reduction is quantitatively related to an increase in LV+dp/dt max and transmitral pressure (15). This is distinct from the reduction in MR due to reduced LV dimensions from remodeling associated with chronic CRT.

Functional MR may also occur due to delayed sequential activation of the papillary muscles due to intraventricular delay (15). This accounts for the acute hemodynamic deterioration reported in some patients after ablation of the AV junction and institution of RV apical pacing, which mimics LBBB (26,27). This can be ameliorated by CRT (28).

IMPLEMENTATION OF CRT

There are currently three approaches to achieving LV pacing. The transvenous approach utilizes specially designed delivery sheaths and tools for cannulating the coronary sinus in order to permit delivery of pacing leads into the epicardial venous circulation serving the LV free wall. LV pacing lead placement can also be achieved under direct visualization using a cardiac surgical approach. Finally, transvenous LV endocardial pacing via transseptal puncture has been described in the rare circumstance where neither the transvenous epicardial nor surgical options are viable (29,30).

Approach to Transvenous Left Ventricular Lead Placement

Early attempts at epicardial LV pacing via the coronary veins utilized standard endocardial pacing leads designed for RV pacing or coronary sinus leads designed for left atrial pacing (31). This approach was met with predictable difficulties, including lead dislodgement, high pacing thresholds and inability to reach the target coronary venous branch. Currently available tools and techniques achieve a >90% transvenous LV lead placement success rate.

Typically, the coronary sinus is cannulated with a specially designed sheath that serves as a workstation for LV lead placement. Such sheaths are available in a variety of diameters and shapes intended to overcome unpredictable anatomic variation in right heart anatomy. Though directional sheaths permit unassisted cannulation of the coronary sinus ostium in some cases, most implanters cannulate the coronary sinus with a deflectable electrophysiology catheter or a coronary angiography catheter. The sheath is then advanced into the coronary sinus body using the catheter as a railing system (Fig. 6).

Once the coronary sinus is successfully cannulated, retrograde venography is performed to delineate the coronary venous anatomy (Fig. 7). This is done with a standard balloon occlusion catheter and hand injections of contrast. Care must be taken to achieve a good seal within the main body of the coronary sinus in order to obtain maximal opacification of the distal vasculature. Underfilling the coronary venous system is a common mistake that may result in failure to identify potentially suitable targets for LV

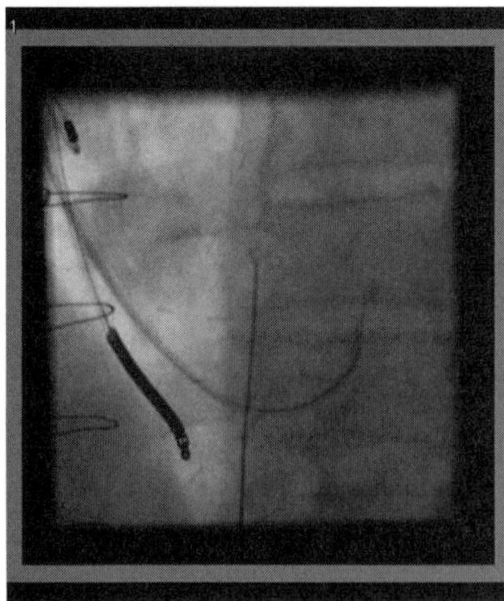

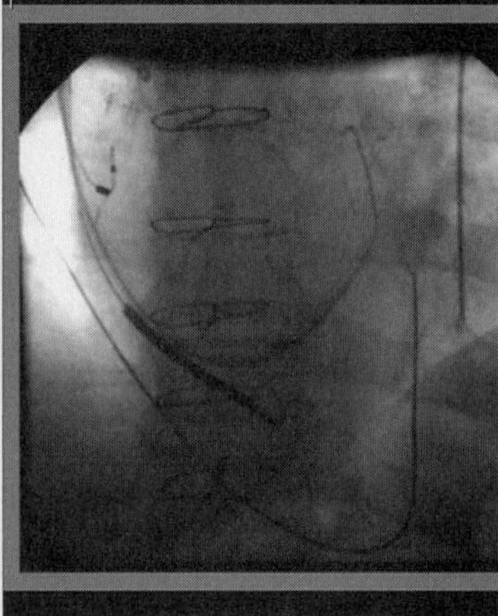

Figure 6 Cannulation of the coronary sinus using a coronary guide catheter and an over-the-wire technique. Note LV lead delivery sheath within main body of coronary sinus.

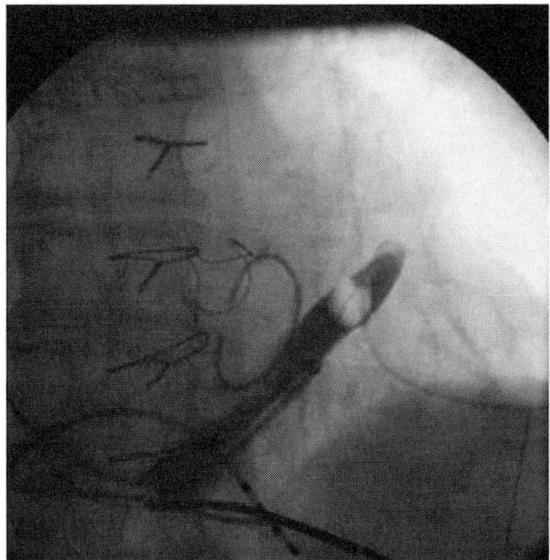
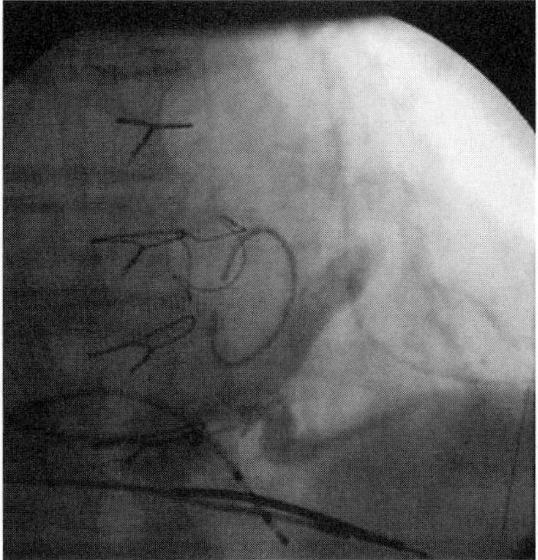

Figure 7 Retrograde coronary venogram via femoral approach. (*Left*) Note large lateral veins. (*Right*) Note two large lateral veins revealed by a more proximal injection in the CS. The ostium of this vein was occluded by the balloon during the first injection.

pacing lead placement. Occasionally, the inflated balloon will occlude the ostium of a suitable branch vessel for LV lead placement, therefore occlusive venography at multiple levels within the main CS is advisable (Fig. 7).

Currently available transvenous LV pacing leads may be either stylet driven or use over-the-wire delivery similar to percutaneous coronary intervention. Fixation relies primarily on "wedging" the lead tip into a distal site within the target vein such that the outer diameter of the lead closely approximates the inner luminal diameter of the vein. Some current LV lead designs incorporate one or more tines, which may assist with fixation by catching on a coronary venous valve or promoting thrombosis, but are probably otherwise irrelevant. Active fixation technologies are in development and will likely incorporate various self-retaining bends or cants that compress the distal segment of the lead against the outer wall of the vein and the epicardial surface of the heart.

Factors Limiting Successful Transvenous LV Lead Placement

Complex and unpredictable anatomic and technical considerations may preclude successful delivery of the LV lead to an optimal pacing site.

Inability to Cannulate the Coronary Sinus

It is difficult to estimate the true percentage of cases in which the coronary sinus cannot be cannulated because this is clearly influenced by operator experience. It is probably in the range of 1–5%. When the coronary sinus cannot be located by the superior approach, an adaptation of the inferior approach described for complex electrophysiology procedures is often successful in localizing the CS ostium (Fig. 7).

Coronary Venous Anatomy: Absent or Inaccessible Target Veins

The coronary venous circulation demonstrates considerably more variability than the parallel arterial circulation (Fig. 8). Careful studies of retrograde coronary venography have revealed that the anterior interventricular vein is present in 99% of patients and the middle cardiac vein is present in 100%. These veins are generally undesirable for LV pre-excitation

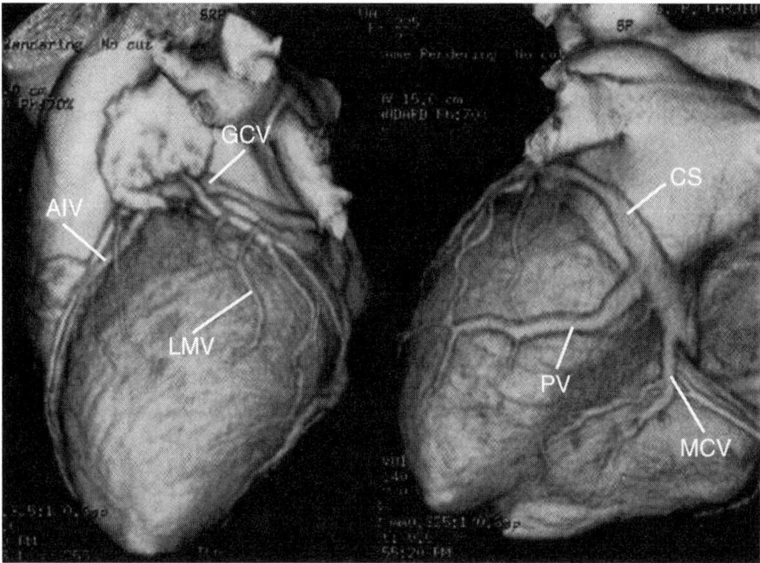

Figure 8 Three-dimensional reconstruction of epicardial coronary venous anatomy using computed tomography. *Source*: From Tada H, et al. How to discriminate pulmonary vein potentials from atrial potentials. J Cardiovasc Electrophysiol 2003; 14:1385.

because they do not reach the late activated portion of the LV free wall. Unfortunately, approximately 50% patients have only a single vein serving the LV free wall. Anatomically, this is a lateral marginal vein in slightly more than 75% and a true posterior vein that ascends the free wall in approximately 50% of patients (32). Thus, as many as 20% of patients may not have a vein that reaches the optimal LV free wall site for delivery of CRT. In some instances target veins are present but too small for cannulation with existing lead systems, or paradoxically too large to achieve mechanical fixation (Figs. 9 and 10).

Coronary Venous Tortuosity

Another commonly encountered difficulty in transvenous LV lead placement is tortuosity of the target vessel take-off or main segment. These anatomic constraints can be extremely difficult to overcome and often require the use of multiple LV lead design and delivery systems (Fig. 11).

High LV Stimulation Thresholds and Phrenic Nerve Stimulation

The principal limitation of the transvenous approach is that the selection of sites for pacing is entirely dictated by navigable coronary venous anatomy. A commonly encountered problem is that an apparently suitable target vein delivers the lead to a site where ventricular capture can be achieved at only very high output voltages or not at all. This presumably relates to the presence of scar on the epicardial surface of the heart underlying the target vein and cannot be anticipated by fluoroscopic examination *a priori* (Fig. 12). If this is not successful, surgical placement of LV leads permits more detailed mapping of viable sites in the anatomic region of interest (Fig. 12).

A second common problem is that the target vein delivers the lead to a site that results in phrenic nerve stimulation and diaphragmatic pacing. This can be difficult to demonstrate during implantation when the patient is supine and sedated but may be immediately evident when the patient is active and changes body positions, even in the

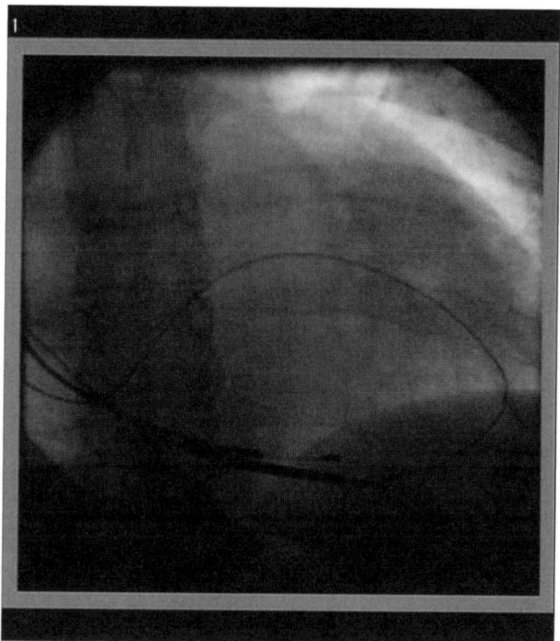

Figure 9 Retrograde coronary venogram demonstrated a very large lateral marginal vein descending to the LV apex. The LV lead descended to terminus of lateral marginal vein and into middle cardiac vein, circumnavigating the LV. Despite attempts with multiple leads, mechanical stability could not be achieved more proximally within the vein.

absence of lead dislodgement. Occasionally, if there is a significant differential in the capture thresholds for phrenic nerve stimulation versus LV capture, this can be overcome by manipulation of LV voltage output. However, many experienced implanters recognize that once phrenic nerve stimulation is observed acutely (during implantation), it is almost invariably encountered during follow-up despite manipulation of output voltages and, therefore, alternative site LV pacing is sought (Fig. 13). As with high LV capture thresholds, occasionally phrenic nerve stimulation can be overcome by repositioning the LV lead more proximally within the target vein (Fig. 14).

Approach to Surgical Left Ventricular Lead Placement

The first clinical trial of CRT utilized a hybrid epicardial LV, endocardial RV pacing lead configuration for multisite ventricular stimulation simply because the technique for transvenous epicardial LV pacing had not been developed (33).

There are several current approaches to surgical placement of LV pacing leads. Many surgeons still use a full left lateral thoracotomy, which permits full visualization of the LV free wall, but results in significant postoperative pain and an extended recovery period. More recently, a minimally invasive approach has been developed. In this approach, the patient is prepped lying on their right side with left arm suspended over their head. Two or three "porthole" incisions are made in the left axillary space for access to the LV free wall (Fig. 15). Two epicardial LV leads are typically placed using the obtuse marginal branches of the circumflex coronary artery as regional landmarks, approximately 1 cm apical to the mitral annulus. After the leads are placed, the capped terminal pins are tunneled to a provisional pocket on the chest wall. The patient is then re-prepped and

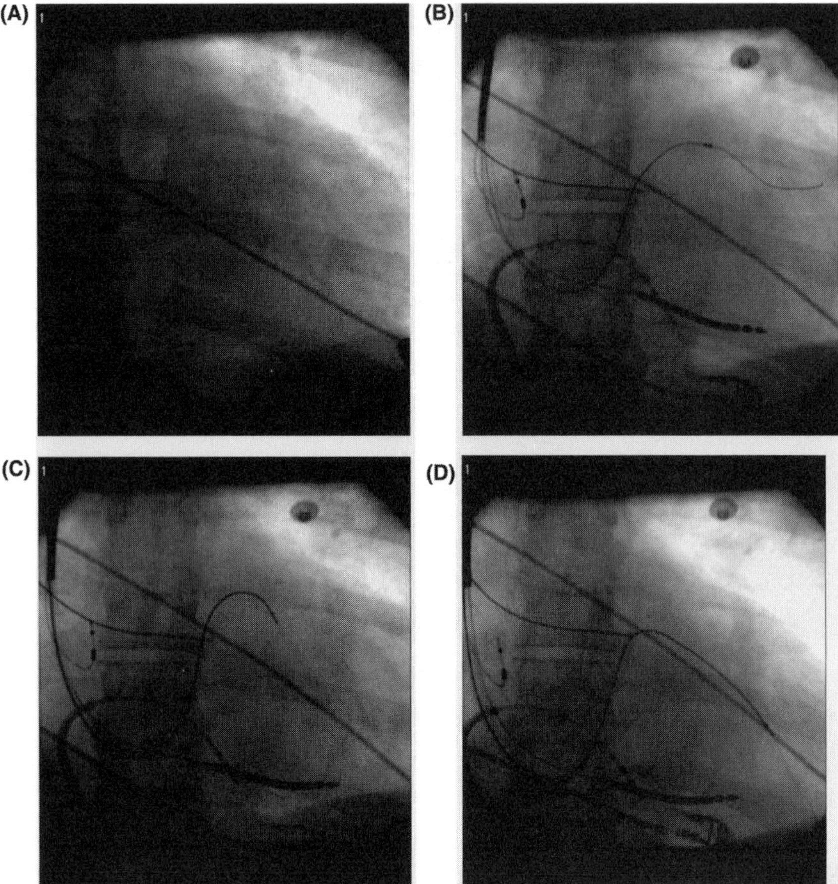

Figure 10 (**A**). "Shepherd's Crook" take-off of lateral marginal vein, with kink just beyond second bend. (**B**). 4-French over-the-wire LV lead cannot navigate venous kinking. (**C**), (**D**). Alternate 4-French over-the-wire lead successfully navigated kinked portion of vein.

draped on their back; the provisional pocket is opened and terminal pins are tunneled to the pectoral pocket. One critical difference in patient preparation for surgical versus transvenous LV lead placement is that it is better to have the patient a little "dry" (well diuresed) in the former and a little "wet" (diuretics withheld) in the latter. In the case of the transvenous approach, adequate hydration may minimize the risk of contrast-induced renal failure. In contrast, during the surgical approach volume overload may increase lung volume. This increases the hemodynamic consequences of single lung ventilation, particularly on right heart function and may limit LV visualization if complete left lung deflation cannot be achieved.

Optimal LV Lead Placement

The optimal site for LV pacing is an unsettled and complex consideration. It is probably true that the optimal site varies between patients and is likely to be modified by venous anatomy, regional and global LV mechanical function, myocardial substrate, characterization of electrical delay and other factors. The success of resynchronization is dependent on pacing from a site that causes a change in the sequence of ventricular

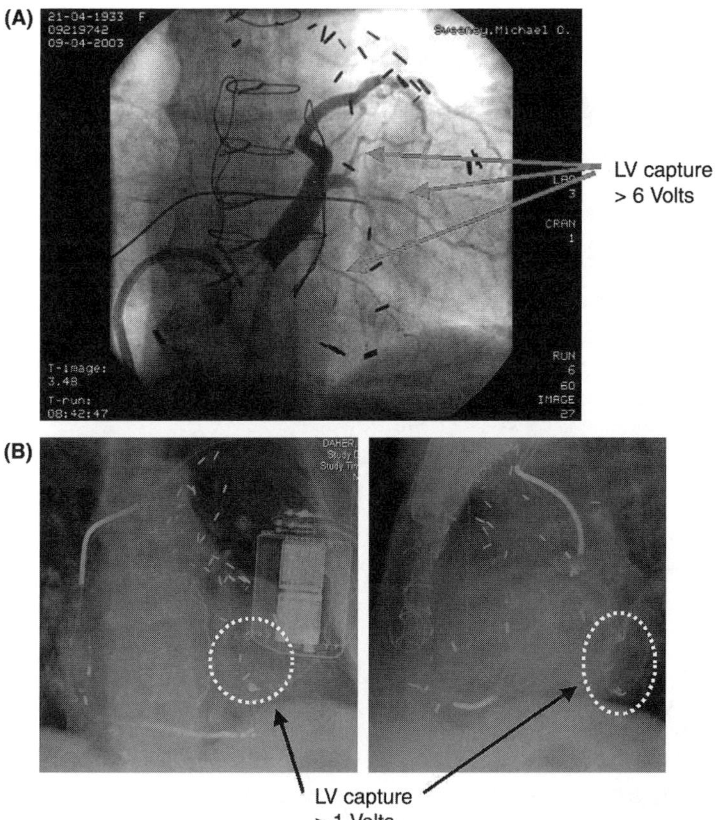

Figure 11 (**A**) Multiple diminutive lateral marginal veins. LV pacing threshold exceeded 6 volts in all locations due to epicardial scar due to prior infarct (note surgical clips associated with prior coronary revascularization). (**B**) Chest radiographs of surgically placed epicardial LV pacing leads in same patient. Note LV free wall position of leads approximates obtuse marginal artery location in circumflex territory, where epicardial mapping identified viable sites for LV pacing.

activation that translates to an improvement in cardiac performance. Such systolic improvement and mechanical resynchronization does not require electrical synchrony and explains the lack of correlation between change in QRSd and clinical response to CRT. Ideally the pacing site or sites that produce the greatest hemodynamic effect would be selected.

However, current clinical evidence permits some generalizations regarding LV pacing site selection for optimal acute hemodynamic response. At least 3 different independent investigations comparing the acute effects of different pacing sites in similar DCM populations have reported parallel evidence that stimulation site is a primary determinant of CRT hemodynamic benefit.

Auricchio et al (33,34) showed a positive correlation between the magnitude of pulse pressure and LV+dP/dT increases and LV pacing site. The percent increases in pulse pressure and LV+dP/dT averaged over all AV delays were significantly larger at mid-lateral free wall LV epicardial pacing sites compared to any other sample LV region. Furthermore, increases at the mid-anterior sites were smaller than all other sites.

These observations were extended in an analysis of 30 patients enrolled in the PATCH-CHF II trial (Fig. 16) (35). LV stimulation was delivered at the lateral free wall or

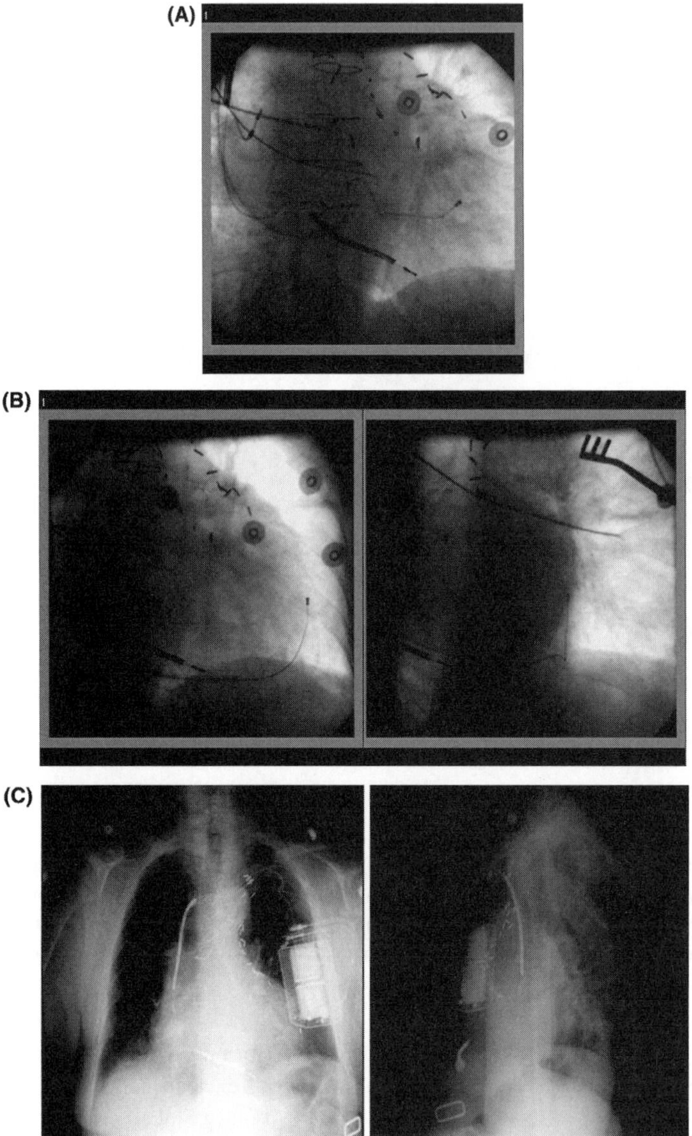

Figure 12 (**A**) LV lead is positioned in a lateral marginal vein but this site was rejected due to insuperable phrenic nerve stimulation. (**B**) Repositioning of the LV lead in a large posterior vein, which ascended the LV free wall, and eliminated phrenic nerve stimulation. (**C**) Chest radiographs of LV lead in posterior vein.

mid-anterior wall. Free wall sites yielded significantly larger improvements in LV + dP/dT and pulse pressure than anterior sites. Furthermore, in one third of patients stimulation at anterior sites worsened acute LV hemodynamic performance, whereas free wall stimulation improved it, and the opposite pattern was never observed. This difference in acute hemodynamic response correlated with intrinsic conduction delays (Fig. 17). This may be interpreted as evidence that stimulating a later activated LV region produces a larger response because it more effectively restores regional activation synchrony. Thus, the negative effect of anterior wall stimulation at all AV delays in some patients may

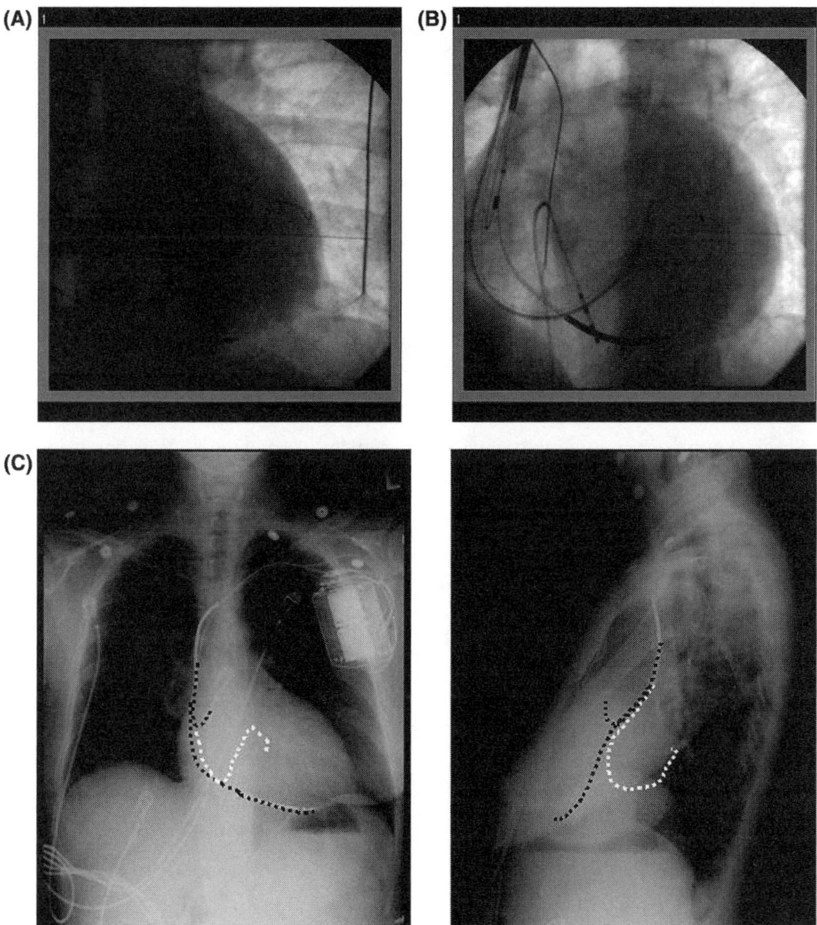

Figure 13 (**A**) LV lead positioned in lateral marginal vein. This site was rejected due to insuperable phrenic nerve stimulation. (**B**) Repositioning of a larger diameter LV lead more proximally in the same vein eliminated phrenic nerve stimulation. (**C**) Chest radiograph of LV lead in proximal segment of lateral marginal vein.

be due to pre-excitation of an already relatively early activated site thereby exaggerating intraventricular dyssynchrony (36)

Interestingly, in PATH-CHF a small number of patients with heart failure and LBBB achieved optimal hemodynamic improvement with RV versus LV or biventricular pacing (37). Electroanatomic mapping has demonstrated that the RV apex is frequently delayed in LBBB and in select patients, LV pre-excitation can be achieved by RV apical pacing due to early breakthrough into the left ventricle at this site (Angelo Auricchio, MD, Personal Communication).

Methods for identifying the best site during implantation are not yet of proven clinical benefit. Furthermore, even if optimal LV pacing sites could be identified *a priori*, access to such sites is potentially constrained by variations in coronary venous anatomy. Despite rapid evolution of implantation techniques, including guiding sheaths and catheters and over-the-wire delivery systems, a suitable pacing site on the LV free wall cannot be achieved in 5–10% of patients. Even when the coronary venous anatomy is suitable and navigable, some free wall sites are rejected due to unacceptably high pacing

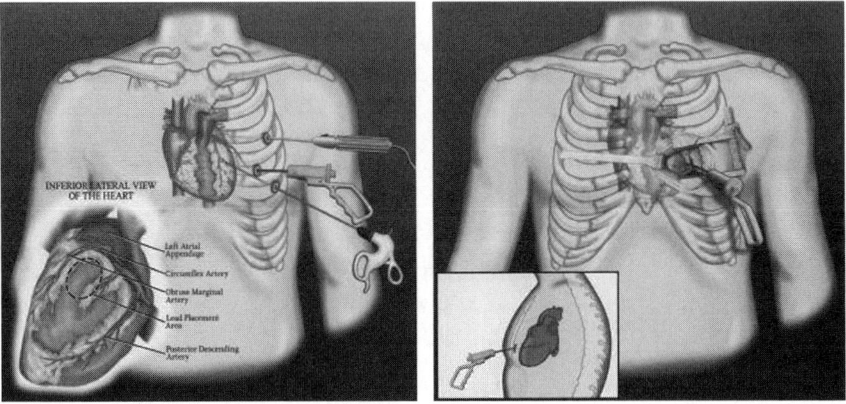

Figure 14 Surgical approach to minimally invasive placement of epicardial LV pacing leads via "port hole" approach (*left*) or limited left lateral thoracotomy (*right*).

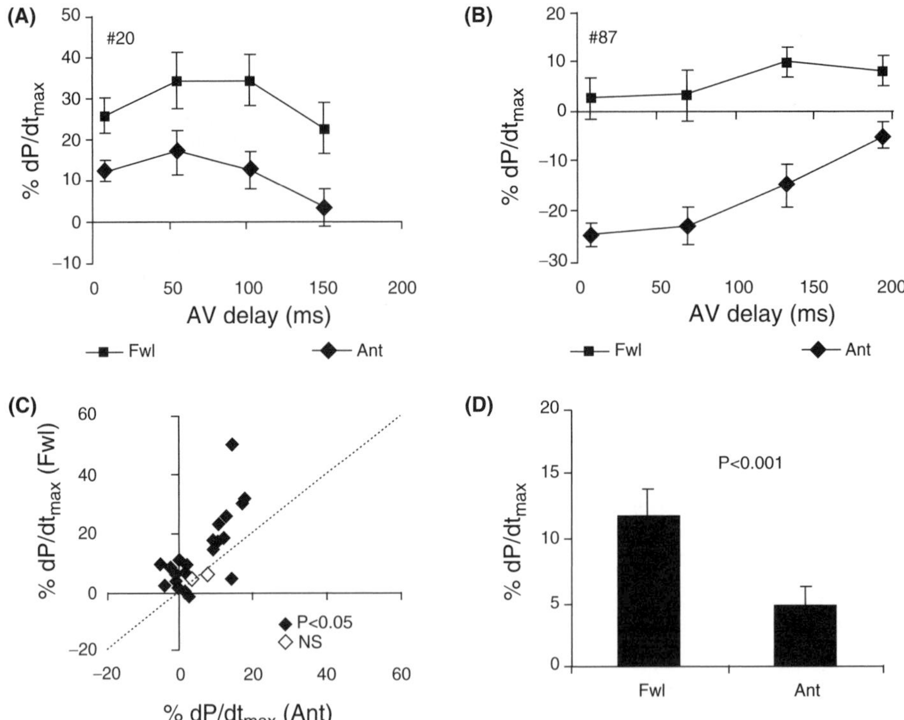

Figure 15 Effect of CRT stimulation site on acute hemodynamic response. (**A**) CRT responder at all AV delays. (**B**) CRT non-responder at all AV delays. (**C**) LV stimulation was delivered at free wall (FWL) or anterior wall (ANT) sites. Points above line of equality indicate patients with significantly larger LV + dP/dT and pulse pressure at FWL versus ANT sites. (**D**) Larger LV + dP/dT at FWL versus ANT sites. In one third of patients stimulation at ANT sites worsened hemodynamic function, whereas FWL stimulation improved it. The opposite pattern was never observed. See text for details.

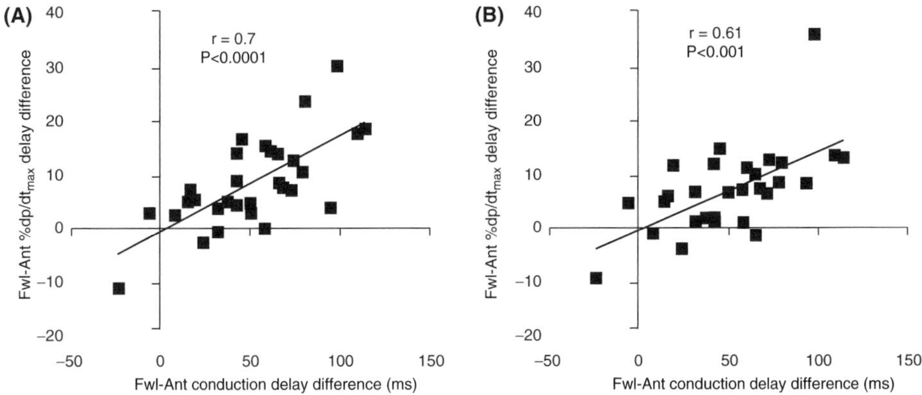

Figure 16 Correlation between free wall (FWL) and anterior wall (ANT) intrinsic conduction delay differences and the LV + dP/dt_{max} response differences during FWL and ANT stimulation for LV CRT (**A**) and BV CRT (**B**). Positive conduction delay differences correspond to more delayed FWL activation. Positive LV + dP/dt_{max} differences correspond to a larger FWL stimulation response (percentage change from baseline).

thresholds related to epicardial scar or unavoidable phrenic nerve stimulation. Surgical placement of epicardial LV pacing leads or endocardial LV stimulation (29) are options when the coronary venous approach fails.

CRT PACING SYSTEMS

Leads and Electrodes

Non-independently Programmable Ventricular Polarity Configurations

Transvenous and epicardial LV pacing leads may be either unipolar or bipolar, though the former dominates current applications. Multiple ventricular pacing polarity configurations

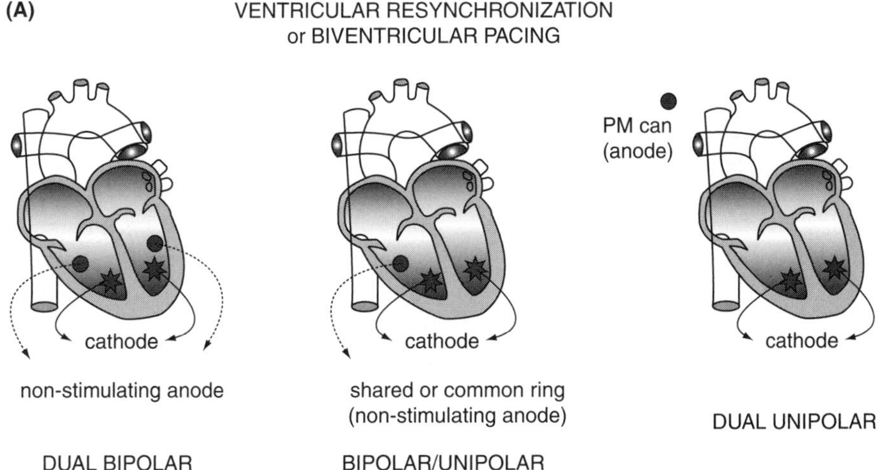

Figure 17 (**A**) Various combinations of lead polarities for biventricular pacing. (**B**) Lead polarities and configurations for transvenous and epicardial biventricular pacing. (*Continued*)

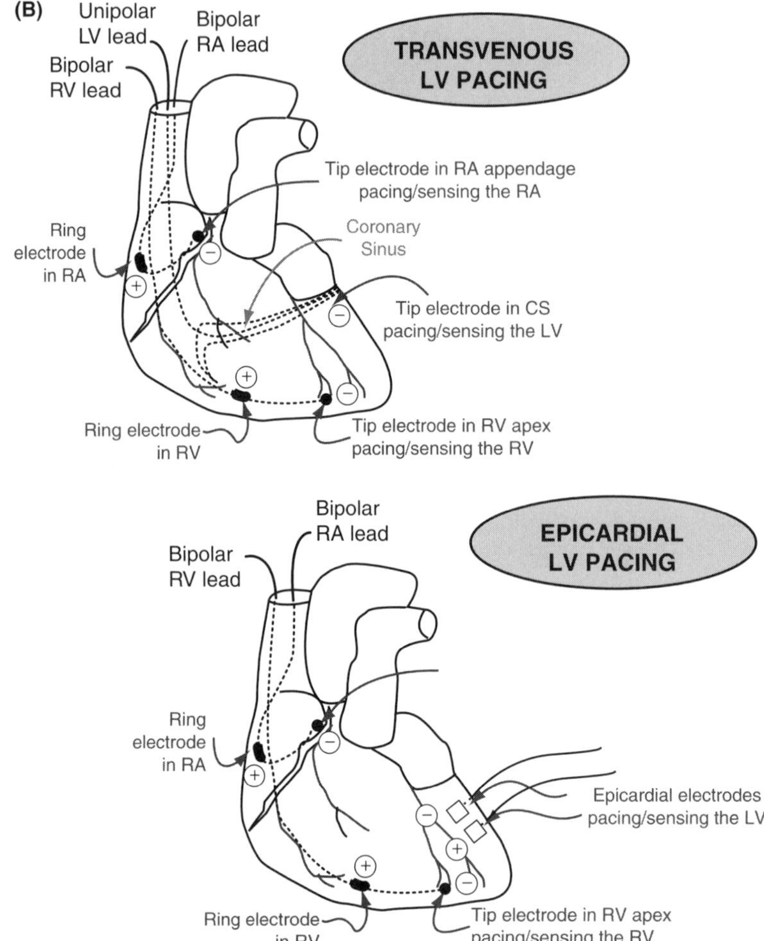

Figure 17 (*Continued from previous page*)

are therefore possible. Since programmed polarity settings are common to both ventricular leads and since the type (bipolar or unipolar) of these leads may not be the same, the following considerations apply.

In a dual bipolar polarity configuration, both lead tips are the active electrodes (cathodes) and the ring(s) are the common (non-stimulating) anode. However, the type of ventricular leads implanted define the pacing/sensing vector (Fig. 18). With 2 unipolar leads, the bipolar setting results in no pacing or sensing. If both leads are bipolar, both rings act as the common electrode. If one lead is bipolar (RV) and the other lead is unipolar (typically LV), the ring on the bipolar lead acts as the common electrode (non-stimulating anode). This configuration results in "shared-ring" bipolar pacing and sensing. This hybrid bipolar/unipolar stimulation configuration is employed in most contemporary CRT pacing systems.

In a dual unipolar polarity configuration, the lead tips are the active electrodes; the noninsulated device case is the common electrode (Fig. 18). This configuration is uncommonly used in CRT pacing systems and is not feasible in CRTD systems due to the concerns regarding ventricular oversensing.

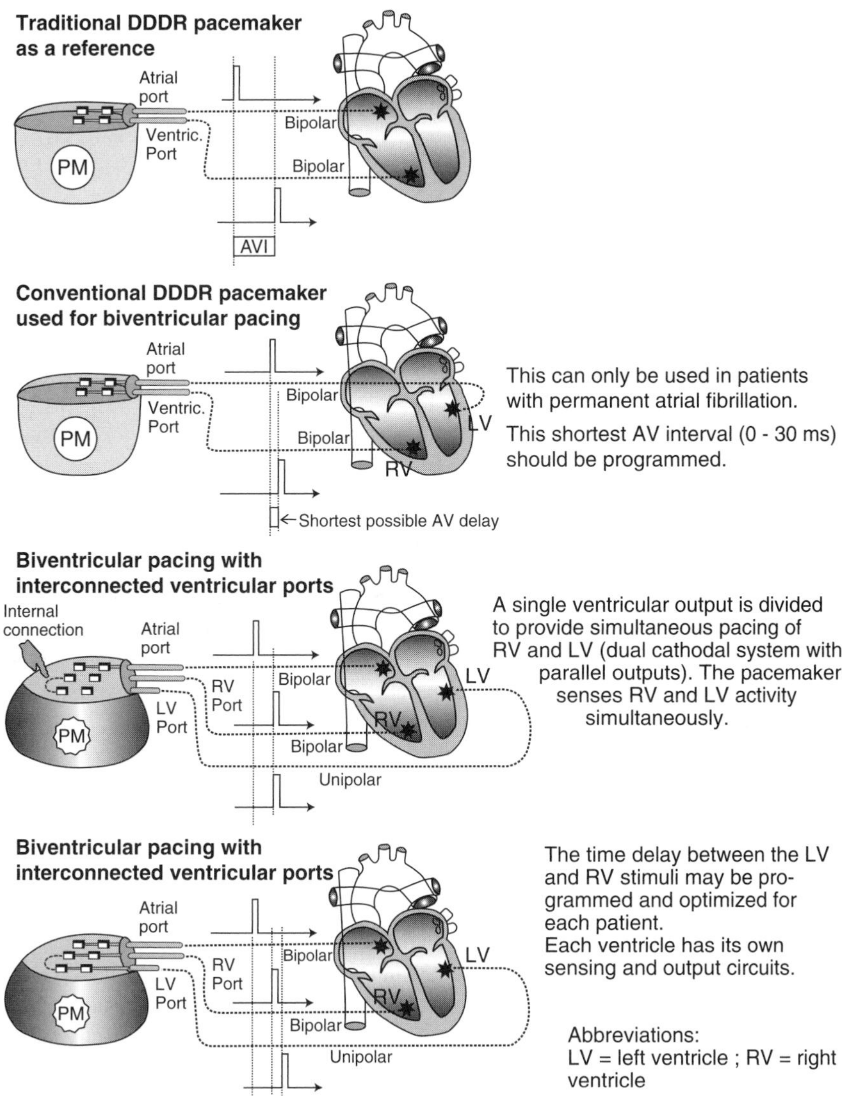

Figure 18 Various pulse generator configurations for biventricular pacing

Pulse Generators

Conventional dual chamber pulse generators or specially designed multisite pacing pulse generators may be used for CRT applications. A conventional dual chamber pulse generator is well-suited for CRT in patients with permanent AF. In this situation, the ventricular port is used for the RV lead and the atrial port is used for the LV lead. This permits programming of independent outputs and ventricular–ventricular timing by manipulation of the AV delay. The programming mode can be either DDD/R or DVI/R (see below). A conventional dual chamber pulse generator can also be used for atrial-synchronous biventricular pacing. The single ventricular output must be divided to provide simultaneous stimulation of the RV and LV (dual cathodal system with parallel outputs). This is achieved with a Y-adaptor and results in simultaneous RV and LV sensing, which may result in ventricular double-counting and loss of CRT (see later) or

- Sensed Signal May Have 2 Distinct Depolarizations.
- Special Consideration Required For Selecting
  - Refractory Periods
  - Sensitivity

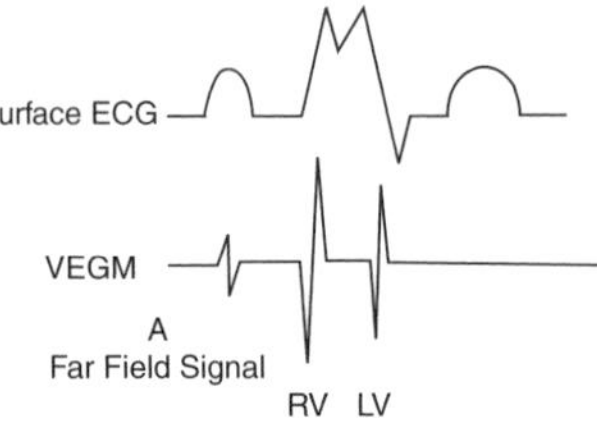

Figure 19 Origin of temporally dispersed RV and LV electrograms during biventricular sensing.

pacemaker inhibition in the case of LV lead dislodgement into the coronary sinus with sensing of atrial activity (Fig. 19).

First generation multisite pacing pulse generators similarly provide a single ventricular output for simultaneous RV and LV stimulation, however, two separate ventricular channels internally connect in parallel. This connection is made for both the lead tip and ring connections and eliminates the need for a Y-adaptor. However, this configuration still provides simultaneous RV and LV sensing with associated limitations.

Second generation multisite pacing pulse generators have independent ventricular ports. Each ventricular lead therefore has separate sensing and output circuits. This arrangement permits optimal programming of outputs and time delay between RV and LV stimulation for each patient. It also eliminates the potential complications of biventricular sensing.

Biventricular or Univentricular Stimulation for CRT

It is important to note that uncertainty about the requirement of RV stimulation during CRT, uneasiness about long term LV lead performance, and unavailability of pacing systems with separately programmable ventricular outputs influenced the use of biventricular pacing, as opposed to left univentricular pacing, in large scale randomized clinical trials. A particular concern is LV lead dislodgement with risk for potentially lethal bradycardia and has a reported incidence of 5 to 10% in larger studies. However, there is some scientific evidence that RV stimulation might not be necessary for optimal CRT response. Left univentricular pacing alone has acute hemodynamic effects that are similar or superior to those achieved with biventricular pacing in some patients (24,38–40). Blanc and coworkers recently extended these observations (41). Functional capacity (6 min walk and maximal O2 uptake), ventricular size and function, and blood norepinephrine levels prior to and after 12 mo of left univentricular pacing were evaluated in 22 patients with DCM, LBBB, and NYHA Class III or IV heart failure. The LV lead was placed in a lateral coronary vein when possible and all patients had sinus rhythm to allow atrial synchronous left univentricular pacing with an AV delay initially programmed to 100 ms. Significant improvements in functional capacity, echocardiographic MR, and LV end diastolic diameter were observed with a favorable trend towards improvement in LVEF. Thus these results are encouraging and support persistent benefit (at least to one year) of left univentricular pacing in some patients.

At present it is not possible to identify patients who will respond better to LV alone compared to biventricular pacing, or neither; and it is not clear how to identify the optimal pacing site. Other factors will warrant RV lead placement in many patients.

Patients with reduced LV ejection fraction and at least moderately symptomatic heart failure are at risk for sudden cardiac death due to ventricular arrhythmias. This risk can be reduced by ICD therapy. Current ICD systems require a RV lead for tachyarrhythmia sensing and high voltage therapies and have a long record of safety and reliability. Further data on the safety and reliability of LV leads for tachyarrhythmia sensing and possibly defibrillation (42) are essential before RV leads are abandoned in CRT pacing and CRT defibrillation systems. It is likely that systems incorporating an RV lead will continue to predominate. If LV pacing systems can become as reliable as RV pacing systems, the paradigm could shift.

PROGRAMMING CONSIDERATIONS IN CRT

Pacing Modes

Pacemaker modes are classified by up to 5 designations which indicate in order of listing the (1) chamber(s) paced and (2) sensed (active, ventricular or dual = A,V,D), (3) response to sensing (triggered, embedded or dual T,I,D), (4) rate modulation [rate modulated or none (R or O) or (5) site of pacing (atrium, ventricle, dual—A, V, D)].

It is axiomatic that for maximal delivery of CRT ventricular pacing must be continuous. DDD mode guarantees AV synchrony and ventricular pacing with all atrial events in the physiologic heart rate range. However, DDD mode increases the probability of atrial pacing (depending upon programmed lower rate limit) that may alter the left sided AV timing relationship due to interatrial conduction time and atrial pacing latency.

VDD mode guarantees the absence of atrial pacing and synchronizes all atrial events to ventricular pacing at the programmed AV delay. However, if the sinus rate is below the lower programmed rate limit, AV synchrony is lost because the VDD mode is operationally VVI.

Although conventional dual chamber pacemakers are not designed for biventricular pacing and generally do not allow programming of an AV delay of zero, or near zero, they are being increasingly used with their shortest AV delay (0–30 ms) for CRT in patients with permanent AF. The advantages include programming flexibility, elimination of the Y adaptor (required for conventional VVIR devices), protection against far-field sensing of atrial activity (an inherent risk of dual cathodal devices with simultaneous sensing from both ventricles) and cost. When a conventional dual chamber PM is used for CRT, the LV lead is usually connected to the atrial port and the RV lead to the ventricular port. This provides for (1) LV stimulation before RV activation (LV preexcitation), (2) protection against ventricular asystole related to oversensing of far-field atrial activity when the LV lead is dislodged towards the AV groove. The DVIR mode is ideally suited for this application. The DVIR mode behaves like the VVIR mode except that there are always two closely coupled independent ventricular stimuli thereby facilitating comprehensive evaluation of RV and LV pacing and sensing performance. The DVIR mode also provides absolute protection against far-field sensing of atrial activity in case of LV lead dislodgement since no sensing occurs on the "atrial" (LV) lead in the DVIR mode.

Ventricular Double-Counting Causing Loss of CRT and Spurious Ventricular Therapies

In first generation CRT and CRTD systems, pacing and sensing occurs from RV and LV simultaneously. Double counting involves the spontaneous wide QRS complex of LBBB (Fig. 20). This produces temporal separation of RV and LV electrograms (EGM). The

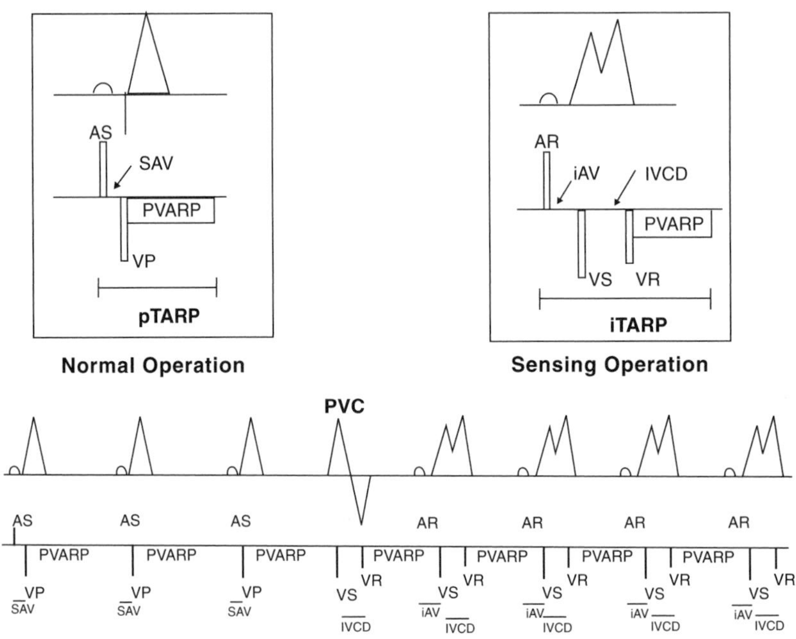

Figure 20 Onset of ventricular double-counting and failure to deliver CRT due to loss of atrial tracking during CRT. See text for details.

degree of separation depends on the severity of the interventricular conduction delay and the location of the electrodes. The LV EGM may be sensed sometime after detection of the RV EGM if the LV signal extends beyond the relatively short ventricular blanking period initiated by RV sensing. This is more likely to occur when a long post-ventricular atrial refractory period (PVARP) is programmed. During sinus tachycardia and first degree AV block the P wave may be displaced into the PVARP where it cannot be tracked. This results in loss of ventricular pacing and CRT. This situation is commonly triggered by PVARP extensions after a premature ventricular contraction (PVC). Spontaneous AV conduction occurs in the form of a preempted upper rate Wenckebach response with loss of ventricular pacing and CRT (Fig. 21). In CRTD systems, this may result in ventricular double counting and misclassification of sinus tachycardia or rapidly conducted AF as ventricular tachycardia (VT) resulting in spurious therapies. During true ventricular episodes, such as VT, the LV EGM may precede the RV EGM and may result in spurious shocks because the rate is misclassified as VF.

Failure to deliver CRT at high sinus rates can be minimized by shortening the PVARP, increasing the upper tracking limit and deactivating the PVC response in the DDD/R mode. Additionally, AF should be aggressively treated to prevent rapid ventricular response and emergence of spontaneous QRS complexes. New CRT systems prevent ventricular double-counting by employing an IVRP (intreventricular ventricular refractory period). Ventricular sensed events (i.e., LV sensing) during the IVRP do not restart PVARP (Fig. 22).

AV Optimization

AV optimization is important for maximal hemodynamic response to CRT but not essential, since ventricular pumping function can be improved by CRT even in the

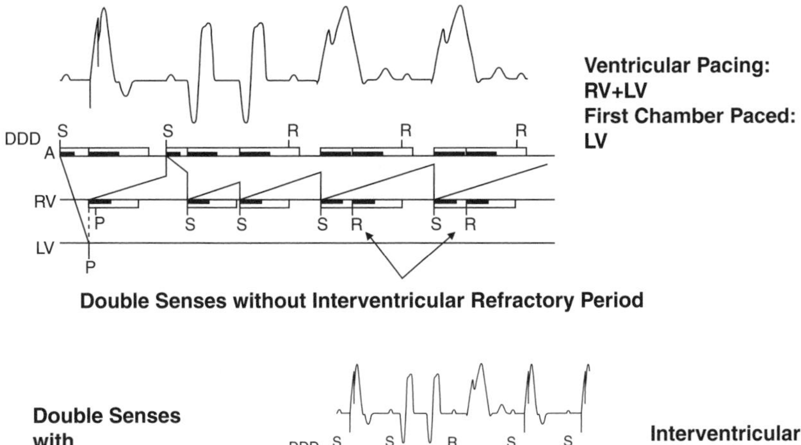

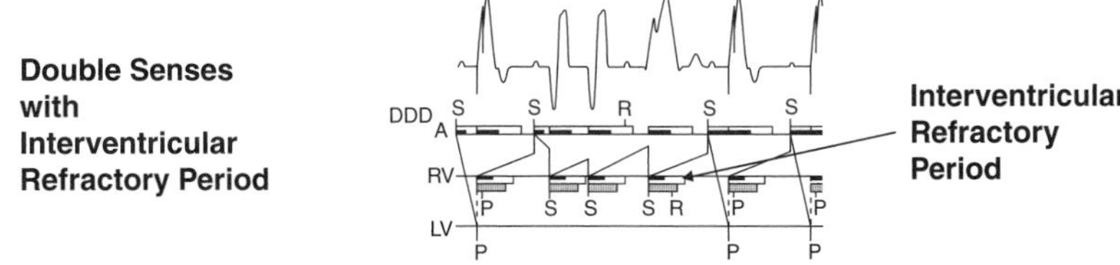

Figure 21 Prevention of ventricular double-counting with an inter-ventricular refractory period. See text for details.

presence of permanent AF. Nonetheless, acute hemodynamic studies have consistently demonstrated that AV optimization "re-times" the left atrial-left ventricular relationship and can result in 15–40% improvement in indices of LV systolic performance acutely. Furthermore, small changes in AV delay may nullify hemodynamic benefit of CRT.

Presently, two methods of AV optimization are commonly applied. One method uses an echo-guided Doppler analysis of transmitral blood flow velocities to approximate an optimal timing relationship between atrial systole and ventricular filling. This is a rather tedious process and may be physiologically unsound since the basis for the technique was derived from studies of patients with permanent AV block and conventional dual chamber pacing with RV apical stimulation. Nonetheless, this was the technique for AV optimization used in the MIRACLE study (43). Empiric observation suggested that most optimized AV delays derived using this technique were in the range of 80–100 ms

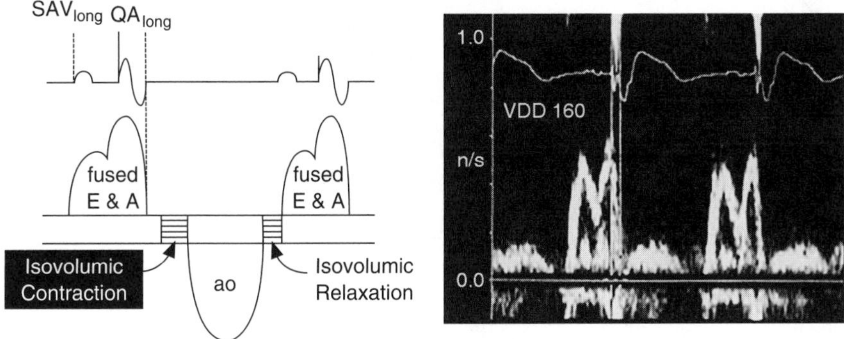

Figure 22 Doppler echo of transmitral blood flow with long AV delay. When the AV delay is too long, mitral valve closure may be not be complete, since atrial contraction is not followed by a properly timed ventricular systole. LV pressure increases above the LA pressure at the end of the diastolic filling period and results in diastolic or "pre-systolic" MR.

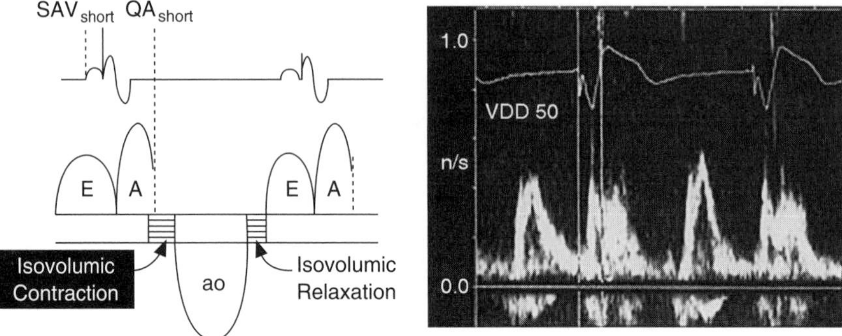

Figure 23 Doppler echo of transmitral blood flow with short AV delay. Note truncation of diastolic filling period due to premature closure of mitral valve (atrial and ventricular contraction occur simultaneously).

regardless of other considerations. The process of AV optimization using this technique is shown in Figures 23–25.

A second approach to AV optimization for maximal positive change in LV + dP/dt is derived from the intrinsic AV interval measured from the local right atrial and RV endocardial EGMs using 2 linear equations (44). If the native QRSd is >150 ms, then estimated optimal AV delay (EOAVD) = AxiAVI + B (ms) and EOAVD = CxiAVI + D (ms), where iAVI = intrinsic AV interval, A = 0.7, B = −55 ms, and D = 0 ms. These regression formulas can be very closely approximated by the following simple rules: the estimated optimal programmed AV delay for patients with QRSd > 150 msec is 50% of the intrinsic AV interval and 75% for QRSd of 120 to 150 msec. This strategy was used in the study design of the Comparison of Medical Therapy, Pacing, and Defibrillation in Heart Failure (COMPANION) trial (45) that showed significant reductions in mortality and heart failure hospitalizations with CRT at 1 year.

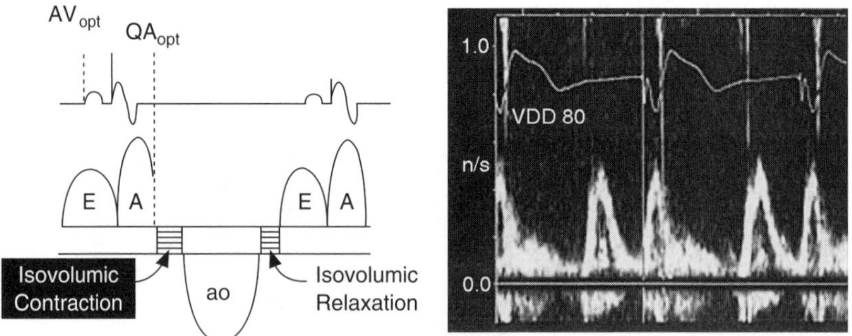

Figure 24 Doppler echo of transmitral blood flow at optimal AV delay. The relation of atrial contraction to the onset of ventricular contraction is now optimal, resulting in diastolic filling throughout the entire diastolic filling period. An appropriate relation now exists between mechanical left atrial and left ventricular contraction so that mean left atrial pressure is maintained at a low level with left atrial contraction occurring just before left ventricular contraction. AV optimization is noted by return of the normal E-A separation. Transmitral flow and LV diastolic filling time are increased, which improves to increased CO. If a large amount of diastolic MR can be abolished, a beneficial effect is obtained because of lower left atrial and higher left ventricular preload at the onset of ventricular contraction.

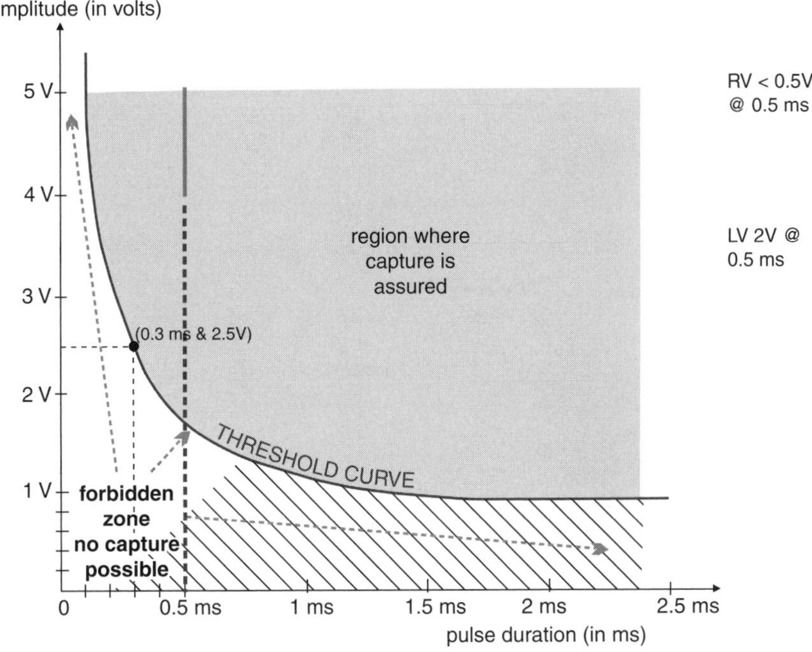

Figure 25 Strength-duration curve considerations for biventricular pacing. The ventricular output must exceed the capture threshold for the chamber with the highest threshold, typically the LV, in common cathodal systems.

It is almost certainly true that the optimal AV delay will likely differ as heart rate and cardiac loading conditions change, such that the optimal AV delay at one point in time may not predict optimal AV timing under other conditions. Furthermore, the importance of AV delay optimization at rest for chronic clinical and hemodynamic effect remains to be shown.

Pacing Outputs

It is critically important that voltage output be adjusted to exceed ventricular capture threshold for LV and RV in common cathodal devices. Since there are commonly differences in capture thresholds between ventricular chambers, this means that the voltage output must exceed capture threshold in the chamber with highest threshold (usually the LV) (Fig. 26). Newer pulse generators that permit independent programming of ventricular output provide greater flexibility in this regard. Similarly, RV and LV voltage output may be separately programmable in the situation where a standard DDD device is used to provide RV and LV stimulation in the DVI mode for CRT in permanent AF (see above).

Inter-ventricular Timing

Implantation of a biventricular pacing system with separately programmable LV and RV stimulation outputs and timing delay would allow adjustments to be made during follow-up. It is presently unclear what benefit, if any, manipulation of inter-ventricular timing would provide during biventricular pacing (24). This is highlighted by the emerging evidence (above) that univentricular LV pacing is probably either equivalent or superior to biventricular pacing acutely and chronically.

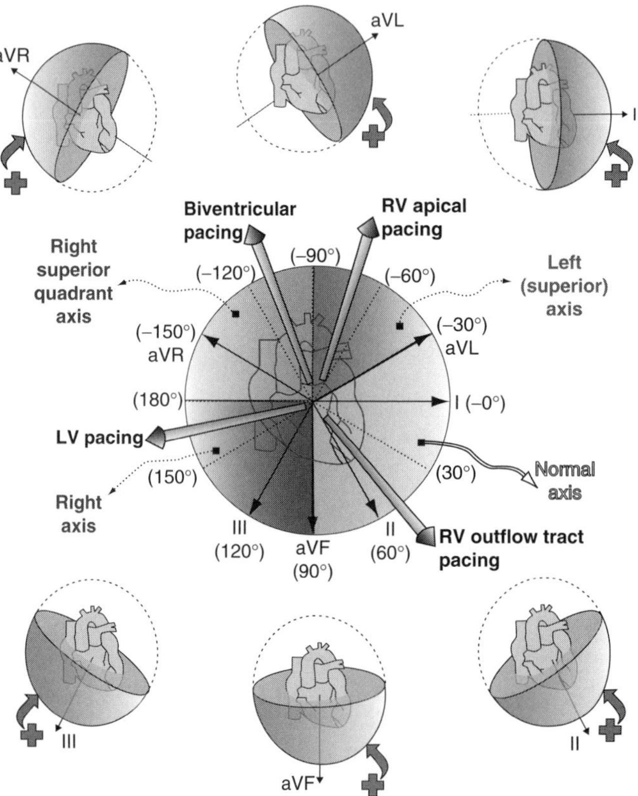

Figure 26 Mean QRS axis in the frontal plane during ventricular pacing.

CRT PACEMAKER ELECTROCARDIOGRAPHY/DETERMINING LV AND RV CAPTURE

The 12-lead EKG is essential to ascertain RV and LV capture during followup of CRT systems without separately programmable ventricular outputs. It is recognized that 5 distinct 12-lead ventricular activation patterns may be seen during threshold determination. These are (1) intrinsic rhythm during loss of RV and LV capture or pacing inhibition (native QRS), (2) isolated RV stimulation, (3) isolated LV stimulation, (4) biventricular stimulation, and (5) biventricular stimulation with anodal capture (Figs. 27–32).

Ventricular pacing thresholds should ideally be performed independently and in the VVI mode at a rate superceding the prevailing ventricular rate so as to obtain continuous ventricular capture without fusion. Alternately, thresholds can be performed in the VDD or DDD mode at very short AV delays to ensure full ventricular capture without fusion. In general it is advisable to initiate threshold determinations at maximum output (voltage and pulse duration) since there is often a significant differential in capture thresholds between RV and LV.

In devices without separately programmable ventricular outputs RV and LV capture can only be determined by EKG analysis during common ventricular voltage decrement.

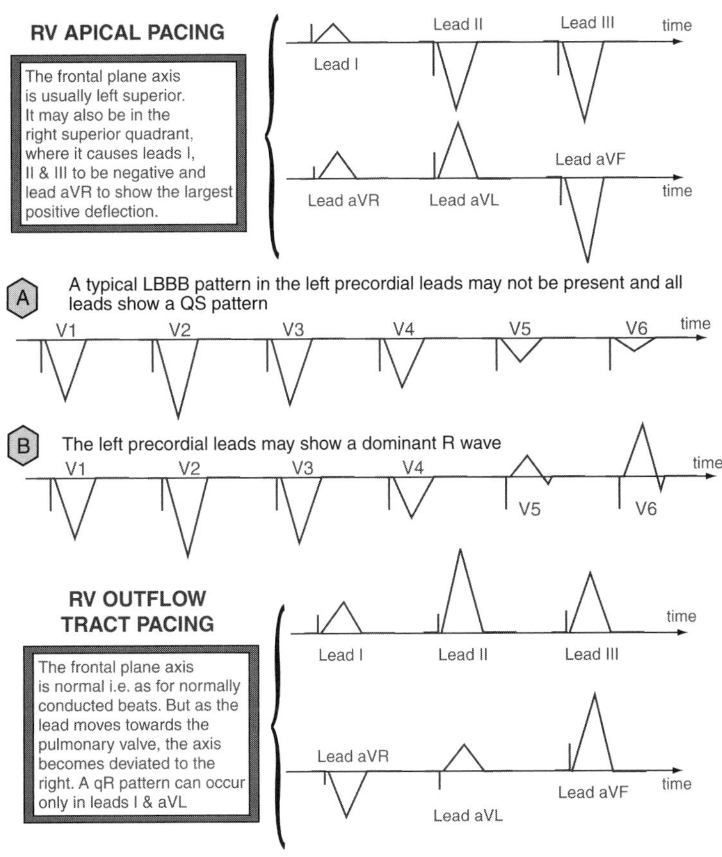

Figure 27 EKG QRS patterns during RV pacing from different sites.

This requires inspection of a 12-lead EKG to demonstrate a change in electrical axis that confirms independent LV and RV capture.

Pacing from the RV apex produces a negative paced QRS complex in the inferior leads simply because the activation starts in the inferior part of the heart and travels superiorly away from the inferior leads. The mean QRS frontal plan axis is superior either in the left or right superior quadrant. Pacing from the RVOT produces a frontal plane axis that is "normal", meaning, inferiorly directed (positive QRS in inferior leads). Isolated LV pacing produces a rightward axis, similar to maximal ventricular pre-excitation over a left-sided accessory pathway. Biventricular pacing (RV + LV) produces a right superior axis as a result of fusion of RV and LV electrical axes. A qR or Qr complex in lead I is rare in uncomplicated RV apical pacing. It is present in 90% of cases of biventricular pacing. In biventricular pacing, loss of the q or Q wave in lead I is 100% predictive of loss of LV capture.

CRT Responders and Nonresponders

Despite the technical limitations for achieving reliable, long-term transvenous LV stimulation, the majority of appropriately selected patients respond to CRT. Nonetheless, approximately 18–30% of patients fail to respond clinically to CRT. In some cases failure

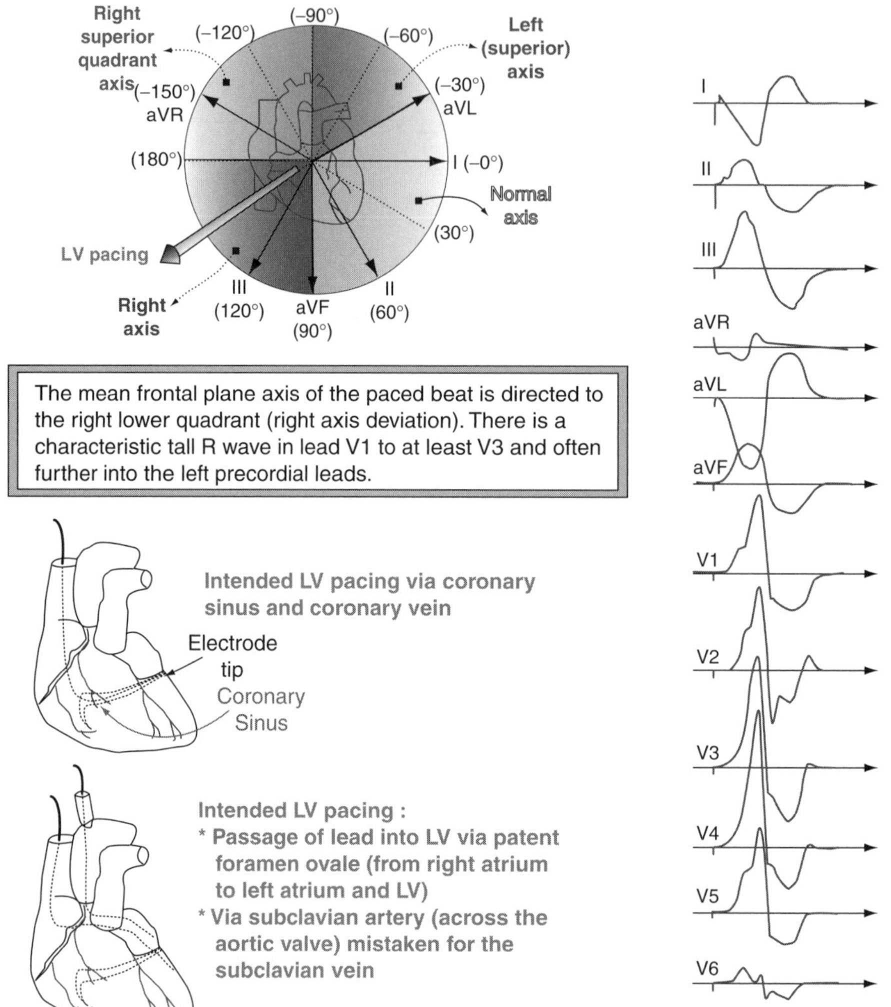

Figure 28 EKG QRS patterns during LV free wall pacing.

to respond may simply indicate that despite delayed ventricular activation, mechanical activation is not dyssynchronous. It is likely, however, that technical limitations are a major factor. In the MIRACLE study a lateral marginal vein site serving the LV free wall was obtained in only 43% of patients. This number is probably an overestimate since the larger diameter stylet driven leads used during MIRACLE typically traverse the "Shepherd's Crook" curve of the anterior interventricular vein before they descend the LV. Many of the "lateral" sites were probably really anterolateral rather than true lateral marginal vein sites. Thus, at least 57% patients in MIRACLE may have had suboptimal LV lead positions. It is conceivable that some of these patients were actually made worse by CRT due to LV pacing at suboptimal sites, particularly among the patients with relatively narrow QRSd (less than 150 ms) (35). As reviewed previously, CRT with stimulation at a LV free wall site consistently improves short-term systolic function more than stimulation at an anterior site does (Figs. 33 and 34). These differences may account for the varied results and large individual difference observed among clinical studies.

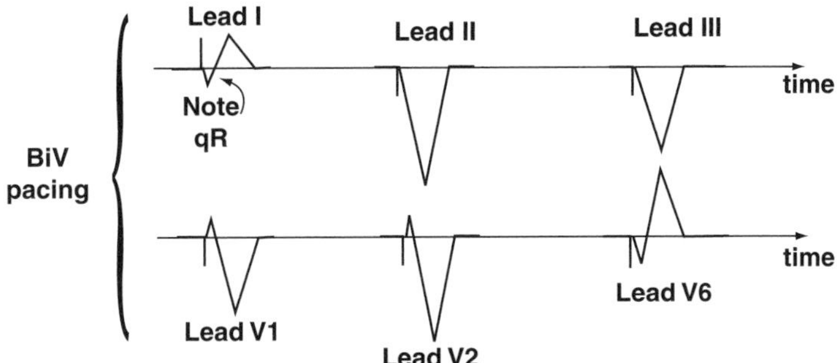

To show ventricular capture in pacemakers with a common output, lower the voltage and/or the pulse width. The left ventricle (LV) will lose capture first in almost all cases because pacing threshold is higher than that of the right ventricle (RV).
Loss of capture in one ventricle will cause a change in the morphology of the beats in the 12-lead ECG. Examination of a single lead may be misleading.

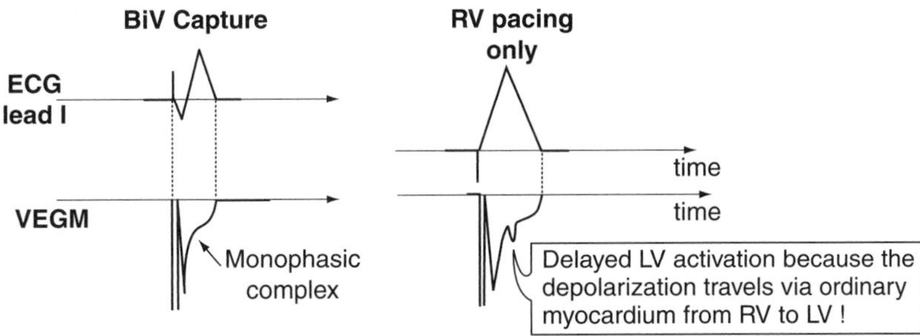

* A change in frontal plane axis may corroborate loss of capture in one ventricle
* Simultaneous recording of ECG, markers and ventricular electrogram (VEGM) is very helpful
* Beware of ventricular fusion beats with the conducted spontaneous QRS complex. The absence of fusion is verified by shortening the AV delay whereupon no change in QRS morphology should take place

Figure 29 Analysis of EKG QRS patterns to ascertain RV and LV capture in CRT systems without separately programmable ventricular outputs.

PATIENT SELECTION FOR CRT

Ventricular dyssynchrony is the pathophysiologic target of CRT. Techniques for selecting patients with significant ventricular dyssynchrony likely to benefit from CRT are rapidly evolving. The optimal criteria would identify all patients with a high probability of response and reject all patients with a low probability of response. To date, QRSd determined from the surface EKG has been most extensively evaluated as a selection criteria for CRT on the premise that electrical delay is a reliable marker for spatially dispersed mechanical activation. Numerous studies have reproducibly demonstrated that baseline QRSd is an important predictive indicator of acute hemodynamic improvement with CRT. Auricchio et al. (19) showed that there was a positive correlation between

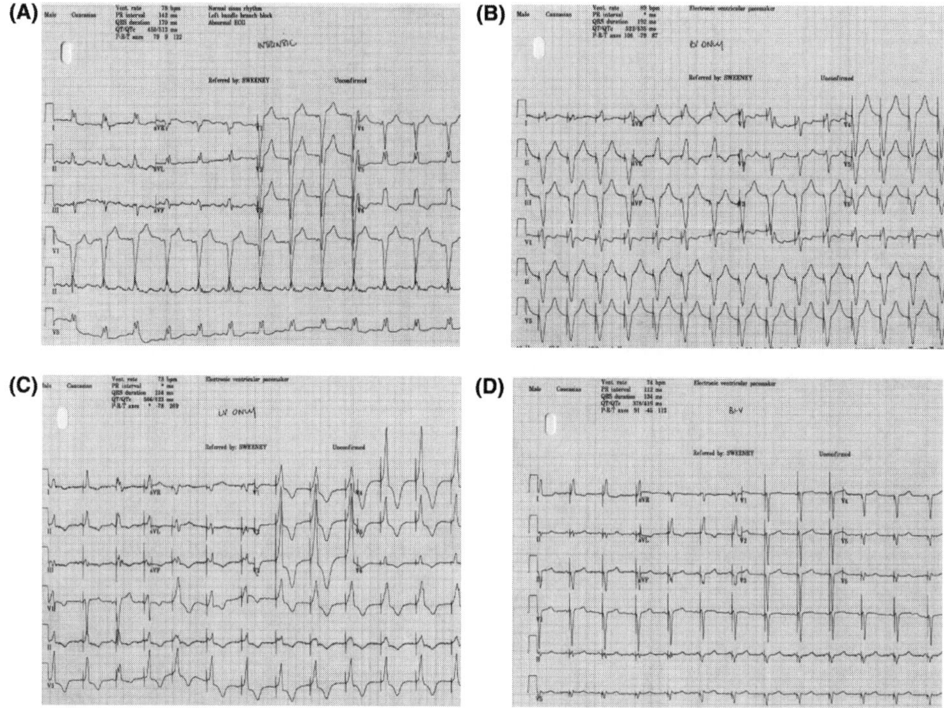

Figure 30 (**A**) Intrinsic ventricular activation (LBBB). (**B**) RV only pacing. (**C**) LV only pacing. (**D**) Biventricular pacing.

the surface QRSd and the percentage of change in LV + dP/dt and pulse pressure during CRT. This observation was corroborated by Nelson et al. (Table 1) (20). Baseline QRSd modestly predicted systolic response, as assessed by maximal rate of pressure defined as % change in LV + $dP/dt_{max} = 0.61 \times QRS_d - 70.2$. Combining baseline QRSd and LV + dP/dt_{max} improved the predictive accuracy for identifying CRT clinical responders. Patients with baseline QRSd $\geq$ 155 ms and baseline LV + $dP/dt_{max} \leq 700$ mmHg/s consistently yielded the greatest acute hemodynamic response to CRT (% change LV + $dP/dt_{max} \geq 25\%$).

Prediction curves for contractile function response using baseline QRSd derived from the PATH-CHF and PATH-CHF II studies are shown in Figure 35 (46). The specificity curve indicates that 80% of CRT nonresponders had a QRSd < 150 ms. The sensitivity curve indicates that 80% of CRT responders had a QRSd > 150 ms. The overlap between these QRSd ranges was populated with CRT responders and nonresponders. The predictive accurary of QRSd to separate responders from nonresponders is fairly constant around 80% with a threshold cut-off between 120 and 150 ms. If the QRSd is > 150 ms, the likelihood of CRT response is greater. An important qualification is that this analysis is based on acute hemodynamic response to CRT. It is possible that acute hemodynamic response does not correlate precisely with chronic clinical improvement. However, these observations appear to be corroborated by the COMPANION Trial, where little or no benefit of CRT or CRTD on death or heart failure hospitalization was observed among patients with baseline QRSd < 150 ms (45).

QRSd may not reliably predict CRT response for several reasons. It is important to remember that QRSd reflects both RV and LV activation. In many patients with LBBB, the delay in ventricular activation resides entirely within the left ventricle, as anticipated.

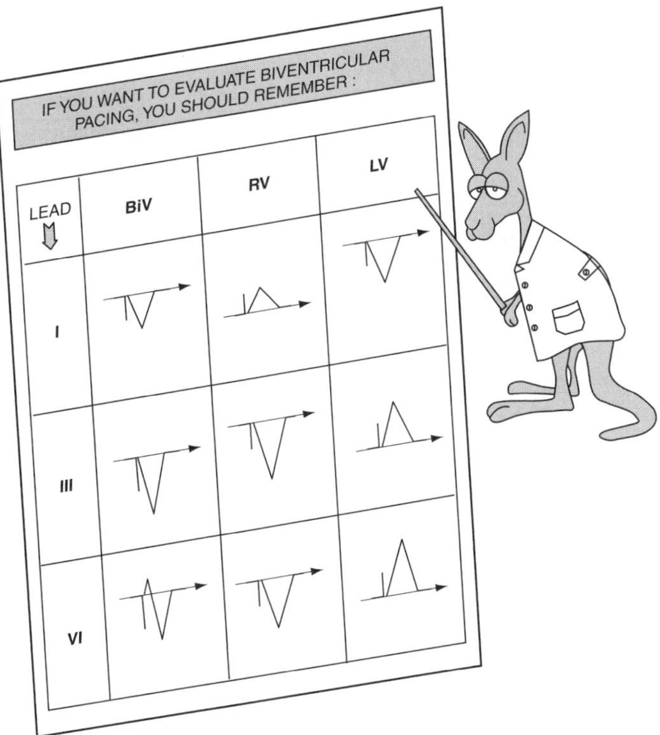

Figure 31 EKG clues for assessing LV capture.

However, in some patients with LBBB, delayed RV activation accounts for a significant proportion of electrical delay manifest on the surface EKG (Fig. 36). Another reason is the intriguing observation that a prolonged QRSd may not be accompanied by dyssynchronous mechanical activation (47). In this situation, despite electrically delayed ventricular activation CRT would not be anticipated to modify mechanical performance.

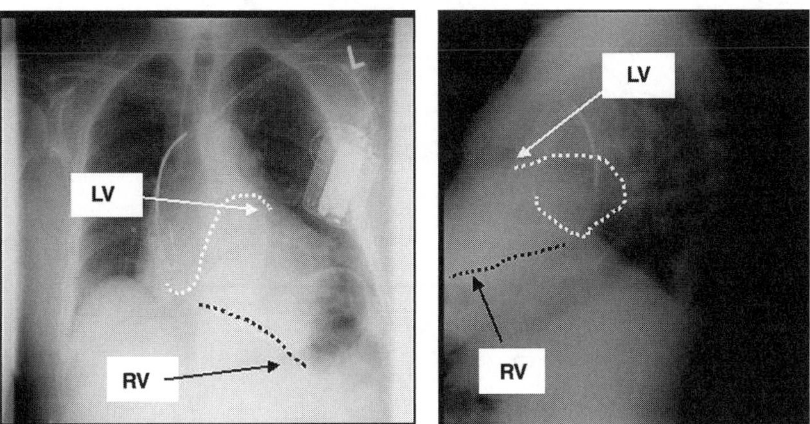

Figure 32 CRT nonresponder. Note position of LV lead in anterior interventricular vein and lack of spatial separation of RV and LV leads in lateral view. This patient required a left ventricular assist device within days of CRT implantation, followed by cardiac transplantation.

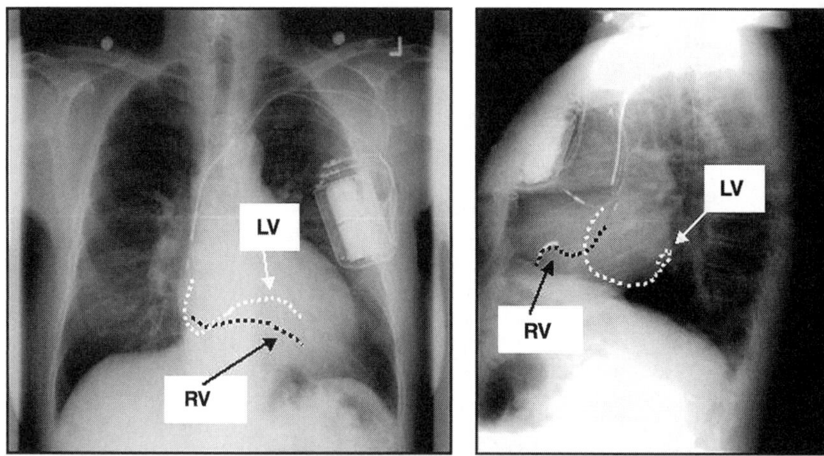

Figure 33 CRT responder. Note position of LV lead in lateral marginal vein on LV free wall. Note spatial separation of RV and LV leads in lateral view. This patient had a two step improvement in NYHA Class (IV to II), reduction in MR from severe to trace, and improvement in LVEF from 20% to 35%.

Recognition of the potential limitations of QRSd for predicting CRT response has stimulated interest in techniques for directly measuring baseline ventricular dyssynchrony. Intraventricular synchrony can be assessed echocardiographically from the delay between the maximal posterior displacement of the septum and the maximal displacement of the LV posterior wall measured from an M-mode short axis view of the LV. Pitzalis et al. (48) found that the delay between septal and posterior wall LV motion improved from a mean of 192 msec to a mean of 14 msec after 1 month of CRT, and was the only

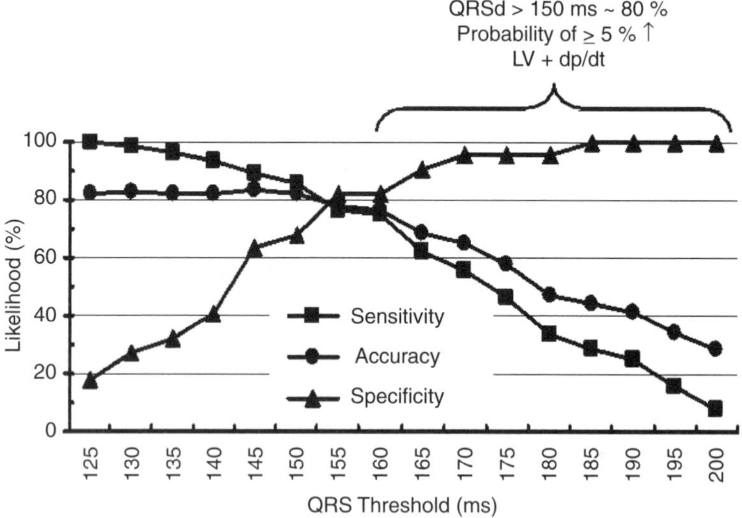

Figure 34 Sensitivity, specificity, and accuracy likelihoods are plotted for different QRS thresholds between 120 and 200 ms using acute hemodynamic data from PATH CHF and PATH-CHF II. Specificity curve indicates that 80% of nonresponders have QRSd <150 ms. Sensitivity curve indicates that 80% of responders have QRSd >150 ms. CRT response is defined as >5% acute increase in LV+dP/dt.

Table 1 ACC/AHA/NASPE Guidelines for CRT in Patients with Congestive Heart Failure and Dilated Cardiomyopathy

Advanced symptomatic heart failure (NYHA III–IV) refractory to optimal medical therapy
LVEF $\leq$35%
QRS duration > 130 ms

Abbreviations: CRT, cardiac resynchronization therapy; NYHA, New York Heart Association; LVEF, left ventricular ejection fraction.

echocardiographic marker (including interventricular delay, ejection fraction, mitral regurgitant duration and mitral regurgitant area) associated with a favorable response to CRT, defined as a greater than 15% improvement in LV systolic volume index.

Another promising echocardiographic technique to identify dyssynchrony and target patients for CRT is Doppler strain rate imaging. This utilizes tissue Doppler signals to quantify the rate of regional myocardial deformation, providing a sensitive estimate of regional myocardial shortening and lengthening that correlates with LV + dP/dt and systolic function in healthy and diseased hearts (49). In LBBB Doppler strain imaging demonstrates maximal septal contraction occurring before aortic valve opening and accompanied by lateral wall lengthening, consistent with studies in animal models (11). The septum then lengthens after aortic valve opening and does not contribute to ejection. Peak lateral wall contraction is observed very late in systole and persists into the postsystolic period. During CRT, systolic contraction can be demonstrated to occur simultaneously in both septal and lateral walls, contributing equally to ejection (50). The utility of this technique in patient selection for CRT remains to be defined in clinical trials but preliminary results appear encouraging. Ventricular dyssynchrony detected by tissue Doppler imaging has been shown to predict acute and chronic response (including remodeling) to CRT in several studies (51,52).

Numerous clinical variables have also been evaluated for predicting likelihood of CRT responsiveness. Baseline contractile function indexed by LV + dP/dt_{max} has been shown to inversely correlate with its subsequent change during LV pacing. Heart failure functional class is positively correlated with CRT response. In several studies, equivalent benefit was observed with CRT in NYHA Class III–IV patients but no significant benefit in Class II (43,53). Ejection fraction has not been shown to correlate with likelihood of CRT

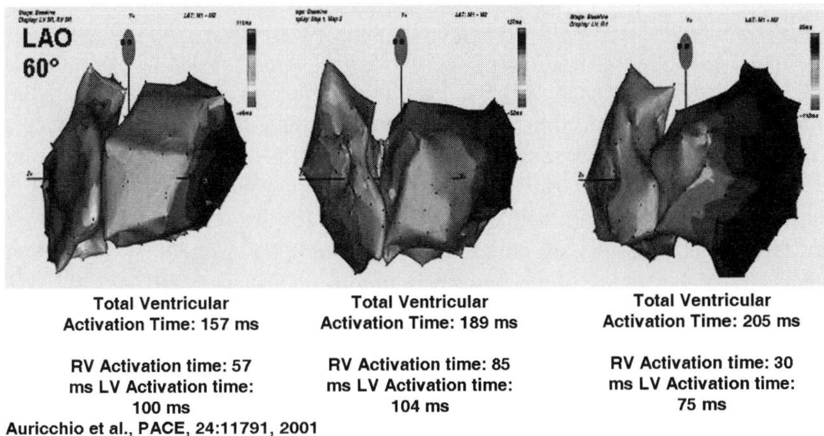

Figure 35 Electroanatomic endocardial activation maps showing heterogeneity of electrical delay in LBBB. See text for details.

response in any study. Some studies have suggested that ischemic CMP is less likely to respond to CRT than NDCMP, but not others. Sinus rhythm does not appear to be necessary for CRT response. Patients in permanent AF had a similar acute hemodynamic response as sinus rhythm in PATH-CHF and similar long-term function improvements in other trials (43,54–56). There are very limited data on CRT in RBBB that suggests the possibility of similar intermediate term response as LBBB in one trial (57) but not another (45).

Further complicating the matter of patient selection for CRT is the fascinating observation that some patients with DCM and significant mechanical dyssynchrony have a normal or near-normal QRSd (58–61).

In summary, 80% of patients with QRSd > 150 ms will have a hemodynamic improvement with CRT and the probability of response is positively correlated with QRSd. Patients with QRSd < 150 ms are less likely to respond to CRT though this is not uniformly true. Improvements in asynchrony seem to be the determinant of the improvements obtained with CRT, and this may be independent of QRSd. Patients with more advanced heart failure symptoms are more likely to respond to CRT than patients with less severe symptoms. There is limited data suggesting that patients with NDCMP respond more consistently than ischemic CMP and LBBB more consistently than RBBB. Permanent atrial fibrillation does not preclude CRT response.

Finally, RV apical pacing may cause prolonged QRSd and ventricular desynchronization. Ventricular desynchronization imposed by ventricular pacing even when AV synchrony is preserved causes increased left atrial diameters and reduced LV fractional shortening (62) and is associated with increased risks of atrial fibrillation, heart failure and death among patients with normal baseline QRSd (63,64). Therefore, it is logical to speculate that multisite (RV+LV) or alternate single site (LV) pacing may be more physiologic among patients in whom ventricular dyssynchrony is due to unavoidable ventricular pacing (i.e., persistent heart block). Intriguing studies suggest that pacing at the LV septum or apex maintains ventricular pumping function at sinus rhythm levels despite pacing-induced QRSd prolongation, possibly because of early engagement of the specialized conduction system resulting in a more physiologic propagation of electrical conduction (65).

CLINICAL TRIALS OF CRT

CRT is an effective adjunctive treatment for moderately to severely symptomatic heart failure associated with depressed LV function and ventricular dyssynchrony (Table 2) (43,54,66). The aggregate experience with CRT in clinical trials involving more than 3500 patients demonstrates a consistent clinical benefit. The magnitude of the benefits is modest and concordant. These include about a 1-step improvement in NYHA class, a 10-point improvement in quality of life measures, a 1–2 ml/kg/min improvement in peak VO2, a 50–70 meter improvement in 6-min hall walk, and a trend towards reduced heart failure hospitalizations. A meta-analysis of randomized trials of CRT using first generation pacing systems in 1634 patients found that heart failure deaths were reduced by 51% (from 3.5% to 1.7%) and heart failure hospitalizations were reduced by 29% (67).

CLINICAL TRIALS OF CRT/DEFIBRILLATION (CRTD)

Sudden cardiac death is the leading cause of mortality in the United States (Table 3). It is estimated that 200,000–400,000 sudden deaths occur annually (68). The vast majority of

Table 2 Randomized Trials of CRT: Enrollment Criteria and Results

Study	Design	N	NYHA	QRSd	LVEF	LVEDD
PATH-CHF	Randomized, single blind, controlled	42	II–IV	>120	<35	NA
VIGOR-CHF	Randomized, controlled	53	II–IV	>120	<30	NA
PATH-CHF II	Acute hemodynamic	43	II–IV	>120	<30	NA
InSync OUS	Uncontrolled	81	III–IV	>150	<35	>60
MUSTIC	Uncontrolled	67	III–IV	>150	<35	>60
MIRACLE	Randomized, double-blind, controlled	266	III–IV	>130	<35	<55

Study	Baseline NYHA	3 mo NYHA	Baseline QRSd	3 mo QRSd	Baseline LVEF	3 mo LVEF
PATH-CHF	3.0±0.3	2.0±0.7	NA	NA	NA	NA
InSync OUS	3.37	2.15	179	143	20.9	23.9
MUSTIC	NA	NA	176±19	NA	23.0±7	NA
MIRACLE	3.0±0.3	2.0±0.3[a]	160	150	23.3	26.5

Study	Baseline peak VO2	3 mo peak VO2	Baseline QOL	3 mo QOL	Baseline 6 min walk	3 mo 6 min walk
PATH-CHF	13.9±0.8	17.0±1.1	49.0±4	21.0±4	362±18	443±13
InSync OUS	NA	NA	55	34	299	418
MUSTIC	13.7±3.9	16.2±4.7	51.0±20	29.0±21	320±97	399.2±100
MIRACLE	13.9	15.1	59.2±19	39.6±24[a]	314±84	339±127[a]

[a]6 mo comparison.

Abbreviations: CRT, cardiac resynchronization therapy; LVEF, left ventricular ejection fraction; LVEDD, left ventricular end diastolic dimension; NYHA, New York Heart Association; QOL, Minnesota Living with Heart Failure Quality of Life; VO_2, oxygen uptake determination.

these deaths occur among patients with symptomatic heart failure associated with reduced LV function. In the Framingham study, the sudden death rate for patients with heart failure was 9 times the general age-adjusted population rate (4). The annual incidence of sudden death is expected to increase coincident with the increasing incidence of heart failure. There are 4–5 million people living with chronic heart failure and an additional 400,000 newly diagnosed yearly (3). The increasing incidence of heart failure is due primarily to the advancing age of the population with coronary artery disease, which is now the principal cause of heart failure associated with reduced ventricular function (4).

Advances in medical therapy have reduced mortality and transformed heart failure into a chronic illness. In the Framingham study, population total mortality was 24% and 55% within 4 yr of developing symptomatic heart failure for women and men, respectively (4). These statistics approximate the natural history of heart failure as the subject population was untreated by contemporary standards. Recognition of the beneficial effects of ACE inhibitors, ARBs, diuretics and beta-blockade has yielded substantial reductions in mortality due to progressive pump failure. However, despite these

Table 3 Randomized Trials of CRTD for Primary and Secondary Prevention of Sudden Death and Treatment of Congestive Heart Failure

	MIRACLE ICD	CONTAK CD	COMPANION
Target population	CHF+QRSd prolongation + ICD	CHF + QRSd prolongation + ICD	CHF + QRSd prolongation + ICD
Treatment	ICD vs. CRTD	ICD vs. CRTD	CRT vs. CRTD vs. medical management
Patients enrolled	364	581	1602
Arrhythmia qualifier	ICD indication	ICD indication	ICD indication
LVEF (%) qualifier	≤ 35	<35	$\leq 35+$ LVEDD≥ 60 mm[a]
CHF qualifier (NYHA Class)	II–IV	II–IV	III–IV
QRS duration qualifier (ms)	>120	>130	>120
Improvement in NYHA class	65% decreased 1 class vs. 50% control	23% decreased 1 class, 11.6% decreased 2 classes vs. control	Not reported
Improvement in 6 min hall walk (m)	No difference	35 overall; 47 Class IV	Not reported
Improvement in QOL	7.2 ± 2.0	6	Not reported
Improvement in VO_2 (ml/kg/min)	1.1	0.9 overall; 1.8 Class IV	Not reported
Death or CHF hospitalization	Not reported	Not reported	40% ↓ CRTD, 35% ↓ CRT
Death	Not reported	Not reported	36% ↓ CRTD, 24% ↓ CRT
Comments	Single blind	Double blind	PR >150 ms; Single blind; mortality reduction with CRT not stat. significant

Not reported, indicates data has not been published.
Abbreviations: CRTD, cardiac resynchronization therapy+defibrillation; LVEF, left ventricular ejection fraction; LVEDD, left ventricular end-diastolic dimension; NYHA, New York Heart Association; QOL, Minnesota Living with Heart Failure Quality of Life; VO_2, oxygen uptake determination.

improvements in medical therapy, symptomatic heart failure still confers a 20–25% risk of premature death in the first two and a half years after diagnosis. Approximately 50% of these premature deaths are sudden and attributable to VT or ventricular fibrillation (VF). This proportionate contribution of sudden death to total mortality in heart failure associated with reduced LV function has not changed substantially between the Framingham data and the modern era.

Survival from out-of-hospital cardiac arrest remains abysmal; it is estimated that less than 20% of victims will leave the hospital alive (69). The principal reason for this dismal statistic is unavailability, or delayed time to, successful defibrillation. Prevention, or at least effective treatment, of the first episode of cardiac arrest is thus critically important.

These realities have focused attention on identification and treatment of patients at risk for sudden death due to ventricular arrhythmias.

The results of large scale randomized treatment trials in patients with reduced LV function and VF or hemodynamically unstable sustained uniform VT that occurs spontaneously or can be induced, consistently demonstrate a survival advantage associated with ICD therapy compared to antiarrhythmic drugs (70–74). Accordingly, ICD therapy can be recommended as first-line treatment for primary and secondary prevention of sudden cardiac death in these settings.

A similar mortality benefit for ICD therapy was subsequently demonstrated in MADIT II among patients with ischemic cardiomyopathy and LV ejection fraction < 30% without prior electrophysiology study (75). These findings were extended in SCD-HeFT which demonstrated a 23% mortality reduction among patients with ischemic or NDCMP, NYHA Class II–III heart failure and LV ejection fraction ≤ 35% (76). The mortality reduction among patients with ischemic cardiomyopathy approximated that observed in MADIT II and validates the findings of that study. More importantly, the equivalent mortality reduction among patients with NDCMP definitively demonstrates that the primary prevention mortality benefits of ICD therapy seen in ischemic CMP are transferable to NDCMP. Accordingly, ICD therapy can be recommended as first-line treatment for primary prevention of sudden cardiac death in either of these settings.

The incidence of ventricular dysynchrony (usually LBBB or other interventricular conduction delay) as designated by prolonged QRSd > 120 ms among patients with chronic congestive heart failure and reduced systolic function is in the range of 35–40% (77,78). It is not surprising, therefore, that intense interest has focused on CRT combined with ICD therapy for prevention of sudden death and treatment of congestive heart failure. Despite impressive technical hurdles, CRT has been successfully hybridized with conventional ICD therapy delivery systems and implanted successfully in humans.

CONTAK CD, MIRACLE ICD, AND COMPANION

Three studies of CRTD involving > 2500 patients have been reported. The study populations were similar to trials of CRT (without defibrillation capability) except there was a conventional indication for ICD therapy. CONTAK CD showed a significant improvement in NYHA Class, 6-min hall walk, peak V02 and standardized quality of life (79). Post-hoc analysis showed that the greatest benefit was observed in the patients with the most advanced heart failure. However, the primary goal of a 25% reduction in heart failure, as measured by a composite outcome of death, heart failure hospitalization, worsening heart failure requiring other interventions, and ventricular arrhythmis, was not met. Patients receiving CRTD had a 21% reduction in this composite endpoint ($p = 0.17$). However, the study was probably underpowered to detect significant differences in this composite endpoint, particularly because 80% of the patients were NYHA I or II after 6 mo of CRTD. MIRACLE ICD showed a reduction in NYHA Class and improvement in quality of life but not 6-min hall walk (53). Importantly, neither of these studies provided data on the effect of CRTD on mortality and limited data on whether the clinical benefits of CRT or CRTD are sustainable for more than 12 months.

The COMPANION trial compared CRT, CRTD and optimal medical therapy among 1602 patients with DCM (ischemic and nonischemic), LV ejection fraction < 35%, QRSd > 120 ms and PR interval > 150 ms. Mortality was reduced by CRTD (36%) and CRT (24%), although only the reduction associated with CRTD was statistically significant (45).

Retrospective analysis of these and other ICD trials clearly demonstrates that the mortality benefit of ICD therapy is almost entirely confined to older patients with the most severely depressed LV systolic function and more advanced symptomatic heart failure. However, it is crucial to recognize that none of the ICD trials cited above specified heart failure as a requisite for entry, and even though the majority of patients had mild to moderate heart failure symptoms (NYHA Class II or III) many were not receiving optimal medical therapy. Though post-hoc analysis has consistently demonstrated a mortality benefit among the "sickest" patients *in ICD trials* (80), none of these trials prior to SCD-HeFT and COMPANION specifically enrolled heart failure patients. Patients with severely reduced LVEF and highly symptomatic heart failure may pose unique problems for mortality reduction using ICD therapy. These patients are at equivalently high risk for lethal ventricular arrhythmias and death due to progressive heart failure. Mortality generally increases with increasing NYHA functional class however the proportion of sudden deaths declines from 50–80% among patients with Class II symptoms to 5–30% among patients with Class IV symptoms (81,82). Furthermore, sudden bradyarrhythmic death in advanced heart failure (83) may occur spontaneously or after successful termination of VT/VF storms" in ICD patients ("cardiac annihilation") (84) and further diminish the mortality benefit of ICD therapy.

REFERENCES

1. Schocken DD, Arrieta MI, leaverton PE, Ross EA. Prevalence and mortality of congestive heart failure in the United States. J Am Coll Cardiol 1992; 20:301–306.
2. Ho KKL, Anderson KM, Kannel WB, et al. Survival after the onset of congestive heart failure in the Framingham Heart Study subjects. Circulation 1993; 88:107–115.
3. Massie BM, Shah NB. Evolving trends in the epidemiologic factors of heart failure. Am Heart J 1997; 133:703–712.
4. Kannel WB, Plehn JF, Cupples A. Cardiac failure and sudden death in the Framingham Study. Am Heart J 1988; 115:869–875.
5. Wiggers C. The muscular reactions of the mammalian ventricles to artificial surface stimuli. Am J Physiol 1925; 73:346–378.
6. Schlant RC. Idioventricular kick. Circulation 1966; 33:III-209.
7. Gottipaty VK, Krelis SP, Lu F, for the VEST Investigators, et al. The resting electrocardiogram provides a sensitive and inexpensive marker of prognosis in patients with chronic congestive heart failure. J Am Coll Cardiol 1999; 33:145A. Abstract.
8. Baldasseroni S, Opasich C, Gorini M, Italian Network on Congestive Heart Failure Investigators, et al. Left bundle branch block is associated with increased 1-yr sudden and total mortality rate in 5517 outpatients with congestive heart failure: a report from the Italian network on congestive heart failure. Am Heart J 2002; 143:398–405.
9. Grines CL, Boshore TW, Boudoulas H, Olson S, Shafer P, Wooley CF. Functional abnormalities in isolated left bundle branch block: the effect of interventricular asynchrony. Circulation 1989; 79:845–853.
10. Verbeek XA, Vernooy K, Peschar M. Intra-ventricular resynchronization for optimal left ventricular function during pacing in experimental left bundle branch block. J Am Coll Cardiol 2003; 42:558–567.
11. Prinzen FW, Hunter WC, Wyman BT, et al. Mapping of regional myocardial strain and work during ventricular pacing: experimental study using magnetic resonance imaging tagging. J Am Coll Cardiol 1999; 33:1735–1742.
12. Prinzen FW, Augustijn CH, Arts T, Allessi MA, Reneman RS. Redistribution of myocardial fiber strain and blood flow by asynchronous activation. Am J Physiol 1990; 259:H300–H308.

13. Spragg DD, Leclercq C, Loghmani M, et al. Regional alterations in protein expression in the dyssynchronous failing heart. Circulation 2003; 108:929–932.
14. Prinzen FW, Cheriex EC, Delhaas T, et al. Asymmetric thickness of the left ventricular wall resulting from asynchronous electric activation: a study in dogs with ventricular pacing and in patients with left bundle branch block. Am Heart J 1995; 130:1045–1053.
15. Breithardt OA, Sinha AM, Schwammenthal E, et al. Acute effects of cardiac resynchronization therapy on functional mitral regurgitation in advanced systolic heart failure. J Am Coll Cardiol 2003; 203:765–770.
16. Auricchio A, Fantoni C, Regoli F, et al. Characterization of left ventricular activation in patients with heart failure and left bundle branch block. Circulation 2004; 109:1133–1139.
17. de Teresa E, Chamorro JL, Pulpon LA, et al. An even more physiologic pacing. Changing the sequence of activation. In: Steinbech KGD, Laskovics A et al, eds. Cardiac pacing. Proceedings of the VIIth world symposium on cardiac Pacing. Darmstadt, Germany: Steinkoopff Verlag, 1984:395–400.
18. Cazeau S, Ritter P, Bakdach S, et al. Four chamber pacing in dilated cardiomyopathy. Pacing Clin Electrophysiol 1994; 17:1974–1979.
19. Auricchio A, Stellbrink C, Block M, et al. Effect of pacing chamber and atrioventricular delay on acute systolic function of paced patients with congestive heart failure. The Pacing Therapies for Congestive Heart Failure Study Group. The Guidant Congestive Heart Failure Research Group. Circulation 1999; 99:2993–3001.
20. Nelson GS, Curry CW, Wyman BT, et al. Predictors of systolic augmentation from left ventricular preexcitation in patients with dilated cardiomyopathy and intraventricular conduction delay. Circulation 2000; 101:2703–2709.
21. Kerwin WF, Botvinick EH, O'Connell JW, et al. Ventricular contraction abnormalities in dilated cardiomyopathy: effect of biventricular pacing to correct interventricular dyssynchrony. J Am Coll Cardiol 2000; 35:1221–1227.
22. Nelson GS, Berger RD, Fetics BJ, et al. Left ventricular or biventricular pacing improves cardiac function at diminished energy cost in patients with dilated cardiomyopathy and left bundle branch block. Circulation 2000; 105:3053–3059.
23. St John Sutton MG, Plappert T, Abraham WT, for the MIRACLE Study Group, et al. Effect of cardiac resynchronization therapy on left ventricular size and function in chronic heart failure. Circulation 2003; 105:1985–1990.
24. Sogaard P, Egeblad H, Pedersen AK, et al. Sequential versus simultaneous biventricular resynchronization for severe heart failure: evaluation by tissue Doppler imaging. Circulation 2002; 106:2078–2084.
25. Lau CP, Yu CM, Chau E, et al. Reversal of left ventricular remodeling by synchronous biventricular pacing in heart failure. Pacing Clin Electrophysiol 2000; 23:1722–1725.
26. Van Oosterhout MFM, Prinzen FW, Arts T, et al. Asynchronous electrical activation induces asymmetrical hypertrophy of the left ventricular wall. Circulation 1998; 98:588–595.
27. Cannan CR, Higano ST, Holmes DR. Pacemaker induced mitral regurgitation: an alternative form of pacemaker syndrome. Pacing Clin Electrophysiol 1997; 20:735–738.
28. Nunez A, Alberga MT, Cosio FG, et al. Severe mitral regurgitation with right ventricular pacing successfully treated with left ventricular pacing. Pacing Clin Electrophysiol 2002; 25:226–230.
29. Garrigue S, Jais P, Espil G. Comparison of chronic biventricular pacing between epicardial and endocardial left ventricular stimulation using doppler tissue imaging in patients with heart failure. Am J Cardiol 2001; 88:858–862.
30. Jais P, Douard H, Shah DC, Barold S, Barat JL, Clementy J. Endocardial biventricular pacing [see comments]. Pacing Clin Electrophysiol 1998; 21:2128–2131.
31. Daubert CJ, Ritter P, LeBreton H, et al. Permanent left ventricular pacing with transvenous leads inserted into the coronary veins. Pacing Clin Electrophysiol 1998; 21:239–345.

32. Meisel E, Pfeiffer D, Engelmann L, et al. Investigation of coronary venous anatomy by retrograde venography in patients with malignant ventricular tachycardia. Circulation 2001; 104:442–447.
33. Auricchio A, Stellbrink C, Sack S, et al. The pacing therapies for congestive heart failure (PATH-CHF) study: rationale, design, and endpoints of a prospective randomized multicenter study. Am J Cardiol 1999; 83:130D–135D.
34. Auricchio A, Klein H, Tockman B, et al. Transvenous biventricular pacing for heart failure: can the obstacles be overcome? Am J Cardiol 1999; 83:136D–142D.
35. Butter C, Auricchio A, Stellbrink C, et al, for the Pacing Therapy for Chronic Heart Failure II Study Group. Effect of resynchronization therapy stimulation site on the systolic function of heart failure patients. Circulation 2001; 104:3026–3029.
36. Fauchier L, Marie O, Casset-Senon D, Babuty D, Cosnay P, Fauchier JP. Interventricular and intraventricular dyssynchrony in idiopathic dilated cardiomyopathy: a prognostic study with fourier phase analysis of radionuclide angioscintigraphy. J Am Coll Cardiol 2002; 40:2031–2033.
37. Auricchio A, Stellbrink C, Sack S, Group PTiCHFP-CS, et al. Long-term clinical effect of hemodynamically optimized cardiac resynchronization therapy in patients with heart failure and ventricular conduction delay. J Am Coll Cardiol 2002; 39:2026–2033.
38. Blanc JJ, Etienne Y, Gilard M, et al. Evaluation of different ventricular pacing sites in patients with severe heart failure: results of an acute hemodynamic study. Circulation 1997; 96:3273–3277.
39. Kass DA, Chen CH, Curry C, et al. Improved left ventricular mechanics from acute VDD pacing in patients with dilated cardiomyopathy and ventricular conduction delay. Circulation 1999; 99:1567–1573.
40. Touiza A, Etienne Y, Gilard M, et al. Long-term left ventricular pacing: assessment and comparison with biventricular pacing in patients with severe congestive heart failure. J Am Coll Cardiol 2001; 38:1966–1970.
41. Blanc JJ, Bertault-Valls V, Fatemi M, et al. Long-term benefits of left univentricular pacing in patients with congestive heart failure. Circulation 2004; 109(14):1741–1744.
42. Butter C, Meisel E, Engelmann L, et al. Human experience with transvenous biventricular defibrillation using an electrode in a left ventricular vein. Pacing Clin Electrophysiol 2002; 25:324–331.
43. Abraham WT, Fisher WG, Smith AL, for the MIRACLE Study Group, et al. Cardiac resynchronization in chronic heart failure. N Eng J Med 2002; 346:1845–1853.
44. Auricchio A, Kramer A, Spinelli J, et al. Can the optimum dosage of resynchronization therapy be derived from the intracardiac electrogram? J Am Coll Cardiol 2002; 39:124. Abstract.
45. Bristow MR, Saxon LA, Boehmer J, the Comparison of Medical Therapy P, and Defibrillation in Heart Failure (COMPANION) Investigators, et al. Cardiac-resynchronization therapy with or without an implantable defibrillator in advanced chronic heart failure. N Engl J Med 2004; 350:2140–2150.
46. Kadhiresan V, Vogt J, Auricchio A, et al. Sensitivity and specificity of QRS duration to predict acute benefit in heart failure patients with cardiac resynchronization. Pacing Clin Electrophysiol 2000; 23:555. Abstract.
47. Bax JJ, Mohoek SG, Marwick TJ, et al. Left ventricular dyssynchrony predicts benefit of cardiac resynchronization therapy in patients with end-stage heart failure before pacemaker implantation. Am J Cardiol 2003; 92:1238–1240.
48. Pitzalis MD, Iacoviello M, Romito R, et al. Cardiac resynchronization therapy tailored by echocardiographic evaluation of ventricular asynchrony. J Am Coll Cardiol 2002; 40:1615–1622.
49. D'Hooge J, Heimdal A, Jamal F, et al. Regional strain and strain rate measurements by cardiac ultrasound: principles, implementation and limitations. Eur J Echocardiography 2000; 1:154–170.
50. Breithardt OA, Stellbrink C, Herbots L, et al. Cardiac resynchronization therapy can reverse abnormal myocardial strain distribution in patients with heart failure and left bundle branch block. J Am Coll Cardiol 2003; 42:486–494.

51. Baxx JJ, Yu C-M, Lin H, et al. Comparison of acute changes in left ventricular volume, systolic and diastolic functions, and intraventricular synchronicity after biventricular pacing and right ventricular pacing for congestive heart failure. Am Heart J 2003; 145:G1–G7.
52. Yu CM, Chau E, Sanderson EJ, et al. Tissue doppler echocardiographic evidence of reverse remodeling and improved synchronicity by simultaneous delaying regional contraction after biventricular pacing therapy in heart failure. Circulation 2002; 105:438–445.
53. Young JB, Abraham WT, Smith AL, Multicenter InSync ICD Randomized Clinical Evaluation (MIRACLE ICD) Trial Investigators, et al. Combined cardiac resynchronization and implantable cardioversion defibrillation in advanced chronic heart failure: the MIRACLE ICD Trial. JAMA 2003; 289:2394–2685.
54. Auricchio A, Stellbrink C, Sack S, et al. Long-term benefit as a result of pacing resynchronization in congestive heart failure: results of the PATH-CHF Trial. Circulation 2000; 102:II-693A.
55. Linde C, Leclerc C, Rex S, et al. Long-term benefits of biventricular pacing in congestive heart failure: Results from the Multisite Stimulation in Cardiomyopathy (MUSTIC) Study. J Am Coll Cardiol 2002; 40:111–118.
56. Linde C, Braunschweig F, Gadler F, Bailleul C, Daubert JC. Long-term improvement in quality of life by biventricular pacing in patients with chronic heart failure: Results from the MUSTIC Study. Am J Cardiol 2003; 91:1090–1095.
57. Aranda JM, Curtis AB, Conti JB, Stejskal-Peterson S. Do heart failure patients with right bundle branch block benefit from cardiac resynchronization therapy? Analysis of the MIRACLE Study J Am Coll Cardiol 2002; 39:96A. Abstract.
58. Yu C-M, Yang H, Lau C-P, et al. Regional left ventricular mechanical asynchrony in patients with heart disease and normal QRS duration. Pacing Clin Electrophysiol 2003; 26:562–570.
59. Achilli A, Sassara M, Ficili S, et al. Long term effectiveness of cardiac resynchronization therapy in patients with refractory heart failure and "narrow" QRS duration. J Am Coll Cardiol 2003; 42:2117–2124.
60. Kass DM. Predicting cardiac resynchronization response by QRS duration. J Am Coll Cardiol 2003; 42:2125–2127.
61. Gaspirini M, Mantica M, Galimberti P, et al. Beneficial effects of biventricular pacing in patients with a "narrow" QRS duration. Pacing Clin Electrophysiol 2003; 26:169–174.
62. Nielsen JC, Kristensen L, Andersen HR, Mortensen PT, Pedersen O, Pedersen AK. A randomized comparison of atrial and dual-chamber pacing in 177 consecutive patients with sick sinus syndrome: echocardiographic and clinical outcome. J Am Coll Cardiol 2003; 42:614–623.
63. Sweeney MO, Hellkamp AS, Ellenbogen KA, et al. Adverse effect of ventricular pacing on heart failure and atrial fibrillation among patients with normal baseline QRS duration in a clinical trial of pacemaker therapy for sinus node dysfunction. Circulation 2003; 23:2932–2937.
64. The DAVID Trial Investigators. Dual-chamber pacing or ventricular backup pacing in patients with an implantable defibrillator: the Dual Chamber and VVI Implantable Defibrillator (DAVID) Trial. JAMA 2002; 288:3115–3123.
65. Peschar M, de Swart H, Michels KJ, Reneman RS, Prinzen FW. Left ventricular septal and apex pacing for optimal pump function in canine hearts. J Am Coll Cardiol 2003; 41:1218–1226.
66. Cazeau S, Leclerlq C, Lavergne T, et al. Effects of multisite biventricular pacing in patients with heart failure and intraventricular conduction delay. N Engl J Med 2001; 344:873–880.
67. Bradley DJ, Bradley EA, Baughman KL, et al. Cardiac resynchronization and death from progressive heart failure: a meta-analysis of randomized controlled trials. JAMA 2003; 289:730–740.
68. Gillum RF. Sudden coronary death in the United States. Circulation 1989; 79:756–765.
69. Moss AJ. Sudden cardiac death and national health. Pacing Clin Electrophysiol 1993; 16:2190–2191.

70. The Antiarrhythmics versus Implantable Defibrillator (AVID) Investigators. A comparison of antiarrhythmic-drug therapy with implantable defibrillators in patients resuscitated from near-fatal ventricular arrhythmias. N Engl J Med 1997; 337:1576–1583.
71. Kuck KH, Cappato R, Siebels J, Ruppel F, for the CASH Investigators. Randomized comparison of antiarrhythmia drug therapy with implantable defibrillators in patients resuscitated from cardiac arrest: the Cardiac Arrest Study Hamburg (CASH). Circulation 2000; 102:748–754.
72. Connolly SJ, Gent M, Roberts RS, et al. for the CIDS Investigators. Canadian implantable defibrillator study (CIDS): a randomized trial of the implantable cardioverter defibrillator against amiodarone. Circulation 2000; 101:1297–1302.
73. Moss AJ, Hall WJ, Cannom DS, et al. for the Multicenter Automatic Defibrillator Implantation Trial Investigators. Improved survival with an implanted defibrillator in patients with coronary disease at high risk for ventricular arrhythmia. N Engl J Med 1996; 335:1940–1993.
74. Buxton AE, Lee KL, Fisher JD, Josephson ME, Prystowsky EN, Hafley G. for the Multicenter Unsustained Tachycardia Trial Investigators. A randomized study of the prevention of sudden death among patients with coronary artery disease. N Engl J Med 1999; 341:1882–1890.
75. Moss AJ, Zareba W, Hall WJ, et al. for the Multicenter Automatic Defibrillator Implantation Trial II Investigators. Prophylactic implantation of a defibrillator in patients with myocardial infarction and reduced ejection fraction. N Engl J Med 2002; 346:877–883.
76. Bardy GH, Lee KL, Mark DB, et al. for the Sudden Cardiac Death in Heart Failure Trial (SCD-HeFT) Investigators. Amiodarone or an implantable cardioverter-defibrillator for congestive heart failure. N Engl J Med 2005; 352:225–237.
77. Shamim W, Francis DP, Yousufuddin M, et al. Intra-ventricular conduction delay: a prognostic marker in congestive heart failure. Int J Cardiol 1999; 70:171–178.
78. Gerber TC, Nishimura R, Holmes DR, et al. Left ventricular and biventricular pacing in congestive heart failure. Mayo Clin Proc 2001; 706:803–812.
79. Higgins SL, Hummel JD, Niazi IK, et al. Cardiac resynchronization therapy for the treatment of heart failure and intraventricular conduction delay and malignant ventricular tachyarrhythmia. J Am Coll Cardiol 2003; 42:1454–1459.
80. Moss AJ. Implantable cardioverter defibrillator therapy: the sickest patients benefit the most. Circulation 2000; 101:1638–1640.
81. MERIT-HF Study Group. Effect of metoprolol CR/XL in chronic heart failure: metoprolol CR/XL randomized intervention trial in congestive heart failure (MERIT-HF). Lancet 1999; 353:2001–2007.
82. Uretsky B, Sheahan G. Primary prevention of sudden cardiac death in heart failure: will the result be shocking? J Am Coll Cardiol 1997; 30:1589–1597.
83. Luu M, Stevenson WG, Saxon LA, Stevenson LW. Diverse mechanisms of unexpected cardiac arrest in heart failure. Circulation 1989; 80:1675–1680.
84. Mitchell LB, Pineda EA, Titus JL, Bartosch PM, Benditt DG. Sudden death in patients with implantable cardioverter defibrillators: importance of post-shock electromechanical dissociation. J Am Coll Cardiol 2002; 39:1323–1328.

16

Device Therapy for Advanced Heart Disease: The Role of Implantable Defibrillators

Akshay S. Desai

Advanced Heart Disease Section, Division of Cardiovascular Medicine, Department of Medicine, Brigham and Women's Hospital, Harvard Medical School, Boston, Massachusetts, U.S.A.

Bruce A. Koplan

Cardiovascular Division, Brigham and Women's Hospital, Harvard Medical School, Boston, Massachusetts, U.S.A.

BACKGROUND: SUDDEN CARDIAC DEATH

Sudden death, often as a consequence of lethal ventricular arrhythmias, is an important cause of cardiovascular mortality, accounting for 300,000–400,000 deaths annually in the United States (1). Nearly 80% of individuals who die suddenly from cardiac causes have evidence of underlying coronary artery disease or prior myocardial infarction (2,3). The risk of sudden death increases with worsening left ventricular function and heart failure symptoms (4,5). As a consequence, patients with advanced heart failure are at particularly high risk for sudden cardiac death (SCD). In the Framingham Heart Study, the age-adjusted sudden death rate for patients with heart failure was nine times that of the general population (6). Despite marked advances in medical therapy, it is estimated that roughly one-half of patients with depressed left ventricular ejection fraction (LVEF) and congestive heart failure (CHF) will die suddenly or require resuscitation from a cardiac arrest (7).

Sudden cardiac death results from a complex interaction between a suitable anatomic or functional substrate and an inciting trigger (8). Patients with heart failure due to coronary artery disease and prior myocardial infarction, dilated (nonischemic) cardiomyopathy, hypertrophic cardiomyopathy, or right ventricular dysplasia are especially vulnerable to arrhythmia due to the enhanced susceptibility of the scarred or myopathic ventricle to the effects of transient initiating events. While arrhythmic death is usually related to ventricular tachyarrhythmias, cardiac arrest from bradyarrhythmias or electromechanical dissociation, perhaps due to pulmonary emboli, electrolyte abnormalities (e.g. hyperkalemia), drugs (e.g. digitalis toxicity), or hypoxia, also occurs, particularly in patients with nonischemic cardiomyopathy (NICM) (9). The diversity of mechanisms of unexpected cardiac arrest in heart failure make prevention of sudden death particularly challenging in this population, with no single therapy likely to provide universal protection. Aside from beta-blocker therapy, antiarrhythmic drugs have been ineffective or even harmful when utilized for sudden death prevention (10). Device therapy, by contrast, has proven to be more beneficial.

From the time of its clinical introduction in 1980, the implantable cardioverter-defibrillator (ICD) has been shown to provide reliable and rapid detection and termination of ventricular tachyarrhythmias (11–13). The backup pacing available in all modern devices provides additional protection against bradyarrhythmias. In the modern era, adequate defibrillation thresholds can be achieved in over 98% of patients with transvenous lead systems, avoiding the need for thoracotomy (14). These devices have therefore become the cornerstone of therapy for prevention of sudden cardiac death in selected high-risk populations with advanced heart disease. This chapter will focus on the role of ICDs in the management of advanced heart disease and the identification of patients who are most likely to benefit from this therapy.

PREDICTING SUDDEN DEATH IN PATIENTS WITH HEART FAILURE

While both the severity of ventricular dysfunction and the magnitude of heart failure symptoms are important determinants of the risk of sudden death from arrhythmia (15) patients may be further categorized based on prior history of arrhythmia and the nature of their underlying heart disease. Patients with prior unexplained syncope or with resuscitated cardiac arrest are at substantial risk for sudden cardiac death (16,17,18). *Secondary* prevention of sudden death should therefore be distinguished from *primary* prevention of a first arrhythmic event. The etiology of heart failure may also be relevant. Patients with intramyocardial scarring due to coronary artery disease and prior myocardial infarction (*ischemic* cardiomyopathy) are at risk for ventricular tachycardia due to re-entry at the site of a healed infarct scar or primary ventricular fibrillation as a consequence of ongoing myocardial ischemia. Such mechanisms are less common in patients with *nonischemic* causes of heart failure (e.g. valvular heart disease, idiopathic or familial cardiomyopathy) despite the presence of potentially similar electrical substrate (19). Finally, while the severity of electrophysiologic abnormalities tracks in general with the severity of heart failure, the proportion of deaths due to cardiac arrhythmias decreases with worsening functional impairment. As a result, the specificity of clinical or noninvasive risk prediction criteria for sudden death is limited in patients with the most advanced disease, in whom death from progressive heart failure may play a larger proportionate role in mortality.

Several clinical criteria have been utilized to stratify the risk of sudden death in patients with advanced heart disease (Table 1). The most frequently utilized non-invasive risk stratification measurement is the left ventricular ejection fraction (LVEF). In nearly every study, the degree of left ventricular dysfunction is a major independent predictor of total and sudden cardiac mortality (20,21). The annualized risk of sudden death in medically managed patients with prior myocardial infarction and LVEF$\leq$0.30 is approximately 11% per year, while in similar patients with nonischemic cardiomyopathy, the estimated risk is slightly lower at 5–7% (20,22). Beyond EF, the presence of ambient, nonsustained ventricular arrhythmia, LV cavity enlargement, neurohormonal markers, or QRS widening may enhance overall mortality prediction, but these features do not specifically predict the vulnerability to fatal arrhythmias (23,24,25). Other non-invasive

Table 1 Indicators of an Increased Risk of Sudden Death from Arrhythmia

Variable	Measure	Predictive power
Conventional coronary risk factors High cholesterol High blood pressure Smoking Diabetes	Risk of underlying disease	Low power to discriminate the individual person at risk for sudden death from arrhythmia
Clinical markers NYHA functional class Ejection fraction	Extent of structural disease	High power to predict death from cardiac causes; relatively low specificity as predictors of death from arrhythmia
Ambient ventricular arrhythmia	Presence of transient triggers	
Frequency of premature ventricular depolarizations		Low overall power if not combined with other variables
Nonsustained ventricular tachycardia Sustained ventricular tachycardia		Higher predictive power, with low ejection fraction
Electrocardiographic variables	Presence of electrical abnormalities	
Standard ECG Left ventricular hypertrophy		Low power to predict death from arrhythmia
Width of QRS complex QT dispersion Specific abnormalities [e.g., prolonged QT interval, right bundle-branch block plus ST-segment elevation in lead V_1 (Brugada syndrome), ST-segment and T-wave abnormalities in leads V_1, and V_2 (right ventricular dysplasia), delta waves (Wolf–Parkinson–White syndrome)] High-resolution ECG		High degree of accuracy in identifying specific electrical abnormalities
Late potentials on signal-averaged electrocardiography		High negative predictive value but low positive predictive value
T-wave-alternans		Primary predictive value unknown
Markers of autonomic nervous function Heart-rate variability Baroreflex sensitivity	Presence of conditioning factors	Exact predictive value unknown
Electrophysiologic testing	Presence of permanent substrate for ventricular arrhythmias	High degree of accuracy in specific high-risk subgroups
Inducibility of sustained tachyarrhythmia by programmed electrical stimulation		

Abbreviations: ECG, electrocardiogram; NYHA, New York Heart Association.

measurements such as QT dispersion, T wave alternans, signal-averaged electrocardiogram, and heart rate variability have been associated with an increased risk of sudden death, but their clinical utility has been limited by either difficulties in measurement, poor reproducibility, or questionable positive predictive value in unselected patients with heart failure (3,20). To date, none of these adjunctive tests have been proven to discriminate benefit from ICD therapy in large clinical trials.

Given the limitations of noninvasive testing, invasive electrophysiologic study with programmed ventricular stimulation has been explored as a means of stratifying risk for sudden death. In the Multicenter Unsustained Tachycardia Trial (MUSTT) of patients with prior myocardial infarction and LVEF$\leq$0.40, inducibility of monomorphic ventricular tachycardia during programmed ventricular stimulation predicted a 6–9% per year risk of spontaneous sustained ventricular tachycardia or sudden death and identified patients that derived a survival benefit from ICD therapy (26). However, among patients with severely reduced ejection fraction, even those without inducible arrhythmias carry a measurably increased risk of sudden death compared to the general population (27). In contrast to ischemic cardiomyopathy, programmed ventricular stimulation is of limited utility in the population of patients with nonischemic cardiomyopathy (28). As ejection fraction alone may be an adequate discriminator of ICD benefit in many patients (see the results from the MADIT-II and SCD-HeFT trials below), programmed stimulation is frequently offered for risk stratification and selection for an ICD in patients in with LVEF 35–40% and ischemic heart disease.

SELECTION OF HEART FAILURE PATIENTS FOR DEFIBRILLATOR THERAPY

Implantable Defibrillators for Secondary Prevention of Sudden Cardiac Death

Patients who survive cardiac arrest or symptomatic, sustained ventricular tachycardia, merit some form of medical or device therapy due to the risk of recurrent events. The comparative benefits of antiarrhythmic drugs and implantable defibrillators for secondary prevention of sudden death in patients with underlying coronary artery disease has been the subject of four prospective, randomized clinical trials: the Antiarrhythmics Versus Implantable Defibrillators (AVID) (1) trial, the Cardiac Arrest Study Hamburg (CASH) (3), the Canadian Implantable Defibrillator Study (CIDS) (2) and a small Dutch study by Wever, et al. (29). Key characteristics for each of these trials are summarized in Table 2. In aggregate, the secondary prevention trials have randomized predominantly men over the age of 55 years with ischemic cardiomyopathy, LVEF$<$35%, and mild-moderate heart failure symptoms to therapy with ICD or antiarrhythmic drugs (predominantly amiodarone).

The largest of these trials, the AVID study, randomized 1016 patients with prior resuscitated VF arrest, sustained VT with syncope, or symptomatic VT and EF$\leq$40% to therapy with ICD or Class III antiarrhythmic drugs (96% amiodarone). Patients with a transient or correctable cause of VT/VF (e.g. ischemia, hypokalemia, or drug toxicity) were excluded. The majority of the patients enrolled had coronary artery disease (81%) and LV dysfunction, with a mean ejection fraction of 31%. While most patients had mild-moderate (NYHA II–III) symptoms of heart failure, nearly half denied functional limitation (NYHA class I). Despite nearly 20% crossover from drug therapy to ICD, the trial was terminated early due to evidence of reduced total mortality in the ICD arm. At two-years, 82% of those randomized to defibrillator were alive, compared to 75% of

Table 2 Randomized Trials of Implantable Defibrillators for the Secondary Prevention of Sudden Death

Characteristic	AVID	CASH	CIDS	Wever et al.
Design	ICD vs. AAD (96% amiodarone, 3% sotalol)	ICD vs. AAD (amiodarone/ metoprolol/ propafenone[a])	ICD vs. amiodarone	Early ICD vs. AAD (EP-study guided, 50% crossover to ICD)
Years of recruitment	1993–1997	1986–1997	1990–1997	1989–1993
# Pts. randomized	1016	288	659	60
# NICMP (%)	193 (19.0%)	36 (12.5%)	63 (9.6%)	0 (0%)
Inclusion criteria	VF, VT + syncope, or symptomatic VT + EF ≤ 40%	VF, VT + syncope, VT > 150 beats/ min + EF ≤ 35%, or syncope + inducible VT at EPS	VF	Previous MI + previous VT/VF arrest
Mean duration of follow up (mo)	18.2 ± 12.2	57 ± 34	36	27
Patients				
Age, mean (yr)	65	58	58	58
% Male	79%	80%	84.5%	90
NYHA III/IV	9.5%	18%	10.8%	2%
LVEF (%)	0.32 ± 0.13	0.46 ± 0.18	0.34 ± 0.14	0.30 ± 0.12
Meds (baseline)				
Beta-blocker	29.4%	1/3 Randomized to metoprolol	27.5%	25%
ACE/ARB	69.5%	42%	Not reported	47%
ICD type				(no details reported)
% Transvenous	93%	44%	84%	Minority
% Epicardial	5%	54%	10%	Majority
Endpoints (ICD vs. control)				
Total mortality	18% vs. 25% at 2 yrs	17% vs. 25% at 2 yrs	15% vs. 21% at 2 yrs	14% vs. 35% (crude)
RRR	32%, $p < 0.02$	32%, $p = \text{NS}$	30%, $p = \text{NS}$	–
Arrhythmic mortality	3.0% vs. 7.4% (crude)	1.5% vs. 5.1% (crude)	3.0%/yr vs. 4.5%/yr ($p = 0.09$)	3.4% vs. 12.9% (crude) Very few events[a]

[a]Propafenone arm in CASH terminated early due to excess mortality (all sudden deaths); data presented for ICD versus amio/metoprolol.

Abbreviations: ICD, implantable cardioverter-defibrillator; AAD, antiarrhythmic drug; AVID, Amiodarone Versus Implantable Defibrillator Trial; CASH, Cardiac Arrest Study Hamburg; CIDS, Canadian Implantable Defibrillator Study; NICMP, nonischemic cardiomyopathy; VF, ventricular fibrillation; VT, ventricular tachycardia; LVEF, left ventricular ejection fraction; NYHA, New York Heart Association functional class; CHF, congestive heart failure; ACE, angiotensin converting enzyme inhibitor; ARB, angiotensin receptor-blocker; RRR, relative risk reduction.

those randomized to drug therapy (RR 0.73, 95% CI 0.52–0.94, $p<0.02$) (Fig. 1); this benefit was entirely due to reduction in sudden deaths from ICD therapy relative to antiarrhythmic drugs (30).

Overall, the results of all four large randomized trials of antiarrhythmic drugs versus ICD therapy in the secondary prevention setting consistently suggest a survival benefit to ICD therapy. A meta-analysis of pooled data from AVID, CASH, and CIDS indicates a 28% relative reduction in the risk of overall mortality and a 50% reduction in the risk of arrhythmic death for ICD versus amiodarone (Fig. 2) (31). Ejection fraction, in particular, is an important discriminator of ICD benefit, with less difference seen in outcomes between ICD- and amiodarone-treated patients with LVEF$>$35% (Fig. 3) (32).

ICD therapy should therefore be considered as first-line treatment for patients with ischemic heart disease and LVEF$\leq$40% who present with VF, unexplained syncope, or symptomatic, sustained ventricular tachycardia. Device therapy should be considered only after potential triggers of ventricular arrhythmia (such as ischemia, electrolyte disturbances, or drug toxicity) have been investigated and addressed. However, since even patients with a "corrected" cause for VT or VF may remain at high risk for sudden death, the decision regarding device implantation must be individualized (33).

ICD Therapy for Secondary Prevention in Patients with Nonischemic Cardiomyopathy

The majority of cardiac arrest survivors studied in large clinical trials have had evidence of prior myocardial infarction or underlying coronary artery disease. Across all the four largest trials enrolling a total of 2023 patients, only 291 patients (14.4%) could be classified as having NICM. Pooled analysis of NICM patients in AVID and

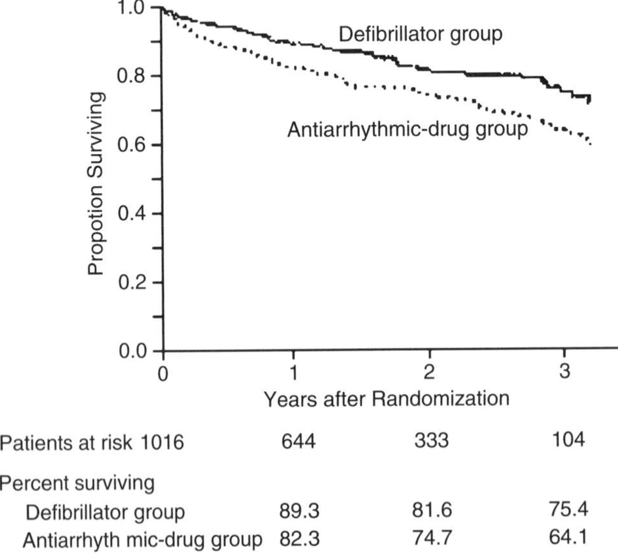

Patients at risk 1016	644	333	104
Percent surviving			
Defibrillator group	89.3	81.6	75.4
Antiarrhyth mic-drug group	82.3	74.7	64.1

Figure 1 Kaplan–Meier estimates of the probability of survival in the AVID trial, showing a significant survival benefit to implantable cardioverter-defibrillator therapy over therapy with antiarrhythmic drugs ($p<0.02$ by log-rank test).

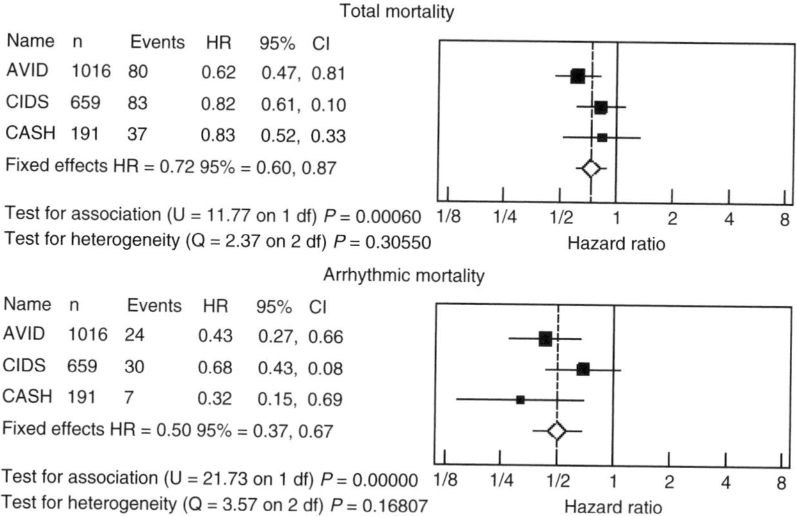

Figure 2 Total and arrhythmic mortality from the pooled analysis of trials of implantable cardioverter-defibrillator (ICD) in secondary prevention. Overall, there is a marked reduction in total mortality associated with ICD therapy that is attributable primarily to a statistically significant reduction in the risk of arrhythmic death. See text for explanation.

CIDS suggests a 31% reduction in mortality that remained statistically nonsignificant, but is comparable to the estimated risk reduction in patients with ischemic cardiomyopathy (21). Despite the lack of prospective, randomized studies, however, there is ample data supporting the benefit to ICDs in secondary prevention among patients with NICM. Observational epidemiologic studies suggest that up to 30% of deaths in patients with NICM may be sudden (34). Mortality in medically treated patients with NICM and a prior history of syncope may exceed 30% (35) at two years,

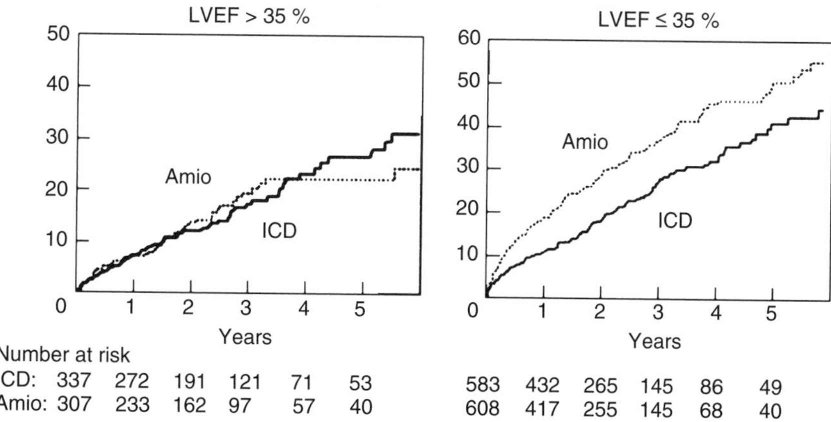

Figure 3 Cumulative risk of overall mortality, pooled from the secondary prevention trials (AVID, CASH, and CIDS) and stratified by ejection fraction. Ejection fraction is an important discriminatory of benefit, with nearly all of the benefit of implantable cardioverter-defibrillator therapy relative to amiodarone accruing to patients with EF≤35%.

while patients with NICM and prior unexplained syncope treated with a defibrillator experience a high frequency of appropriate device therapies (36–38). ICD therapy is indicated in patients NICM with resuscitated cardiac arrest requiring defibrillation, or symptomatic, sustained VT. Furthermore, ICD therapy can be considered in patients with NICM and prior syncope where either invasive or noninvasive evaluation has failed to identify a cause.

Implantable Defibrillators for Primary Prevention of Sudden Cardiac Death

Only a small fraction of sudden cardiac deaths occur in patients with a previous episode of cardiac arrest and survival from out-of-hospital cardiac arrest remains poor, largely due to a delay in the time to defibrillation (39). These observations have fueled increasing interest in primary prevention of sudden death, both by expanding public access to external defibrillators and by identifying populations of patients at high risk for sudden death who might benefit from prophylactic defibrillator implantation. In the absence of critical coronary artery disease or an underlying arrhythmic predisposition (such as long-QT syndrome, arrhythmogenic right ventricular dysplasia, or the Brugada syndrome) patients with preserved left ventricular function are at relatively low risk for fatal ventricular arrhythmias. Clinical trials of ICDs in primary prevention have therefore focused instead on patients felt to be at highest risk for sudden cardiac death—those with left ventricular dysfunction and symptomatic heart failure, the vast majority of whom have underlying coronary artery disease.

ICD Therapy for Primary Prevention in Patients with Ischemic Cardiomyopathy

As noted in the previous chapter, the persistence of viable myocardium within islands of infarct scar provides the electrical substrate for re-entrant ventricular arrhythmias. The comparative benefits of ICD therapy versus conventional medical therapy for sudden death prophylaxis in patients with ischemic cardiomyopathy have been the subject of five large, randomized clinical trials over the last decade: the Multicenter Automated Defibrillator Implantation Trials (MADIT (40) and MADIT II (41)), the Coronary Artery Bypass Graft-Patch Trial (CABG-Patch (42)), the Multicenter Unsustained Tachycardia Trial (MUSTT (43)), and the Defibrillator In Acute Myocardial Infarction Trial (DINAMIT (44)). Important characteristics and results of each of these trials are summarized in Table 3. Two additional trials enrolling patients with both ischemic cardiomyopathy and nonischemic cardiomyopathy have also been performed: the Sudden Cardiac Death Heart Failure Trial (SCD-HeFT) and the Comparison of Medical Therapy, Pacing, and Defibrillation in Heart Failure (COMPANION) Trial.

MADIT

The MADIT trial randomized 196 patients with coronary artery disease, LVEF $\leq$35%, and spontaneous nonsustained VT who had inducible, nonsuppressible monomorphic VT with programmed ventricular stimulation at electrophysiologic study to therapy with an implantable defibrillator or conventional medical therapy. Of those randomized to medical therapy, 80% received amiodarone, while 11% received Class IA antiarrhythmic drugs and 9% received no specific antiarrhythmic therapy. Patients with NYHA Class IV heart failure were excluded. A significant reduction in mortality was seen in ICD-treated

Table 3 Randomized Trials of Implantable Defibrillators for the Primary Prevention of Sudden Death in Patients with Coronary Artery Disease

Characteristic	MADIT	CABG-patch	MUSTT	MADIT-II	DINAMIT
Design	ICD vs. AAD (80% amiodarone, 11% Class IA AAD)	ICD vs. usual care (no protocol driven AAD)	EPS-guided rx (ICD or AAD) vs. no AAD (26% Class IA, 10% amiodarone, 9% sotalol)	ICD vs. conventional therapy	ICD vs. conventional therapy
Years of recruitment	1990–1996	1990–1997	1990–1996	1997–2001	1998–2003
# Pts. randomized	196	900	704	1232	674
Inclusion criteria	CAD+ EF≤35%+ NSVT +inducible, nonsuppressible sustained monomorphic VT	CAD undergoing CABG+ EF≤35%+ abnormal SAECG	CAD+ EF≤40%+ NSVT +inducible VT at EPS	CAD +EF≤30%	Recent MI+ EF≤35%+ abnormal autonomic function
Mean duration of follow up (mo)	27	32±16	39	20	30±13
Patients					
Age, mean (yr)	63	63	67	65	62
% Male	92%	84%	90%	85%	76%
NYHA II/III	65%	73%	63%	60%	87%
LVEF (%)	0.26±0.07	0.27±0.06	0.30	0.23±0.05	0.28±0.05
Meds (baseline, ICD vs. AAD)					
Beta-blocker	27% vs. 15%	17.9% vs. 24.0%	29% vs. 51%[a]	70%	87%
ACE/ARB	60% vs. 55%	54.7% vs. 53.8%	72% vs. 77%[a]	70%	95%
ICD type					
% Transvenous	53%	0%	Not reported	97.2%	94%
% Epicardial	47%	97.3%	Not reported	0%	0%
Endpoints (ICD vs. control)					
Total mortality	16% vs. 34% at 1 yr	27% vs. 24% at 4 yrs	24% vs. 55% at 5 yrs[b]	14% vs. 19.8% at 1.8 yr	7.5% vs. 6.9% per yr
Hazard ratio for mortality	0.46, $p<0.009$	1.07, $p=0.64$ (NS)	0.40, $p<0.001$	0.69, $p=0.016$	1.08, $p=0.66$ (NS)

(Continued)

Table 3 Randomized Trials of Implantable Defibrillators for the Primary Prevention of Sudden Death in Patients with Coronary Artery Disease (*Continued*)

Characteristic	MADIT	CABG-patch	MUSTT	MADIT-II	DINAMIT
Arrhythmic mortality	3.2% vs. 13.0% (crude)	3.4% vs. 6.2% (crude)	9% vs. 37%[b]	Not reported	1.5% vs. 3.5% per yr 0.42, $p=0.009$

[a]Reported rates are for EPS-guided therapy versus control.
[b]Reported rates are for ICD versus non-ICD among patients randomized to EPS-guided therapy.
Abbreviations: ICD, implantable cardioverter-defibrillator; AAD, antiarrhythmic drug; MADIT, Multicenter Automated Defibrillator Implantation Trial; CABG, coronary artery bypass grafting; MUSTT, Multicenter Unsustained Tachycardia Trial; VF, ventricular fibrillation; VT, ventricular tachycardia; LVEF, left ventricular ejection fraction; NYHA, New York Heart Association functional class; CHF, congestive heart failure; ACE, angiotensin converting enzyme inhibitor; ARB, angiotensin receptor-blocker.

patients. The mortality at one year was 16% in the ICD group and 34% in the conventional therapy group. Most of the benefit to ICD therapy was due to a reduction in arrhythmic mortality (3.2% vs. 13%). Despite some study limitations, MADIT was a landmark trial, documenting potential benefit to prophylactic ICD implantation in selected, high risk patients with ischemic cardiomyopathy, paving the way for a series of confirmatory trials and expanding indications for ICD therapy.

CABG-Patch

The CABG-Patch trial examined the potential benefit to ICD therapy in a different subset of patients with coronary artery disease and LV dysfunction. In this study, 900 patients with LVEF $\leq$35%, an abnormal signal-averaged electrocardiogram, and coronary artery disease slated for bypass surgery were randomized to implantation of an epicardial ICD system at the time of surgery or usual perioperative care. The trial results were dramatically different than in the MADIT trial, with termination for futility at a mean follow-up duration of 32 months. Mortality in the ICD-treated patients was 27%, versus 24% in the conventional therapy arm at four years, generating a hazard ratio of 1.07 for all-cause mortality ($p=0.64$, NS).

The differential benefit of ICD therapy in MADIT and CABG-Patch may have more than one explanation. Mortality in CABG-Patch likely included a larger proportion of perioperative, non-arrhythmic deaths that would be uninfluenced by ICD therapy. All patients received epicardial ICD systems, while nearly half received transvenous systems in MADIT. Patients enrolled in MADIT had inducible VT at EP study, while those in CABG-Patch qualified on the basis of an abnormal signal-averaged ECG; this may have led to inclusion of a population at lower-risk of arrhythmic death. Patients in CABG-Patch underwent surgical revascularization, which may have had independent antiarrhythmic benefits in this population, reducing the margin for benefit of ICD therapy. Finally, the CABG-Patch trial did not take into account the possibility for improvement of ventricular function after revascularization, while the subjects in the MADIT trial had to have reduced ejection fraction documented at least three months after any bypass surgery.

MUSTT

The MUSTT trial randomized patients with coronary artery disease, LVEF$\leq$40%, and asymptomatic unsustained ventricular tachycardia to a strategy of antiarrhythmic therapy (including drugs and defibrillators) guided by electrophysiologic (EP) study or no antiarrhythmic therapy. The primary endpoint, a composite of cardiac arrest or arrhythmic death, was significantly lower in the group randomized to EP testing, with the reduction in mortality and morbidity mainly due to a reduction in arrhythmic death in the patients receiving an implantable defibrillator because of inducible ventricular tachycardia during programmed stimulation. Sudden death rates at five years were 9% in the ICD arm, 32% in those receiving antiarrhythmic drugs, and 37% for those receiving no antiarrhythmic therapy (RR for ICD vs. non-ICD patients$=$0.24, $p<0.001$); antiarrhythmic drug therapy in this population, predominantly with class IA antiarrhythmic drugs, was associated with no mortality benefit relative to control. The MUSTT study thus demonstrated that electrophysiologic study can be utilized effectively to risk stratify patients with ischemic cardiomyopathy and guide ICD therapy for primary prevention of sudden death. It also reinforced the concept that even if they are effective in acute suppression arrhythmias, antiarrhythmic drugs are less effective than defibrillators with regard to sudden death prevention.

MADIT II

The MADIT II trial randomized patients with prior myocardial infarction ($>$1 month prior to entry) and LVEF$\leq$30% to ICD or conventional medical therapy. During an average follow-up of 20 months, mortality was significantly lower in the ICD group (14.2%) compared to conventional medical therapy (19.8%) (Fig. 4). This trial demonstrated that a LVEF$<$30% in patients with ischemic cardiomyopathy was sufficient alone to discriminate patients who would derive a mortality benefit from ICD therapy. Based upon the results of MUSTT and MADIT-II, a reasonable strategy for primary prevention of sudden death in patients with ischemic heart disease is to offer ICD therapy in patients with LVEF$\leq$30%, and programmed ventricular stimulation in patients with LVEF between 30% and 40% with ICD therapy when ventricular tachycardia is inducible (45).

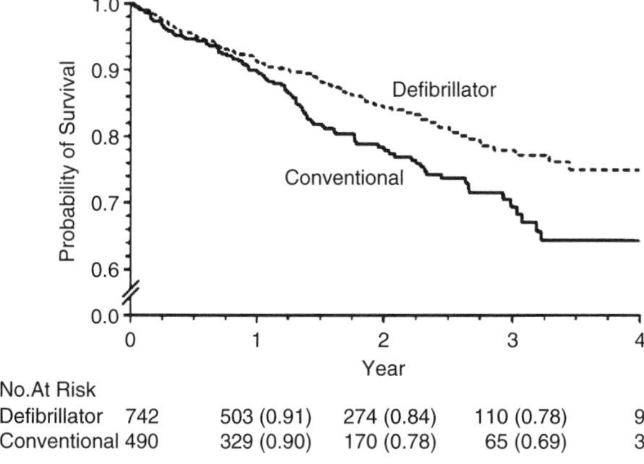

Figure 4 Kaplan–Meier estimates of the probability of survival in the two arms of the MADIT II trial. The difference in survival between the two groups was significant (nominal $p=0.007$, by the log-rank test).

Enthusiasm for broad application of prophylactic ICD therapy has been tempered only slightly by the trend of increased heart failure hospitalizations in ICD-treated patients in MADIT II, perhaps as a consequence of unnecessary and deleterious right ventricular apical pacing.

DINAMIT

The DINAMIT trial was designed to extend the MADIT II observations to a population with recent myocardial infarction, based on the recognition that the risk of arrhythmia is greatest in the days immediately following myocardial infarction. The trial randomized patients who had a myocardial infarction within 6–40 days of enrollment, an ejection fraction $\leq$35%, and evidence of impaired autonomic function (manifest as depressed heart rate variability or elevated average HR on 24-hour Holter monitoring) to ICD or conventional therapy. Nearly all patients had symptomatic heart failure and were optimally treated with ace-inhibitors, beta-blockers, and diuretics. In contrast to prior trials of device therapy, no difference in overall mortality was observed in the two treatment groups over 30 months of follow-up. While ICD therapy was associated with a statistically significant reduction in arrhythmic death, this benefit was offset by an increase in death from non-arrhythmic (though largely cardiovascular) causes.

The lack of clear benefit to ICD therapy in DINAMIT has been challenging to explain. The close proximity of ICD implantation to myocardial infarction may be a relevant factor. Though peri-infarct ventricular arrhythmias are common, the incidence of sudden death is markedly reduced by modern medical therapy (particularly coronary revascularization and beta-blockade) and falls off rapidly within the first 30 days after infarction, coincident with healing of the acute injury. Subsequently, the mortality rate in stable infarct survivors increases steadily as a function of time, with the greatest risk of death seen in those most remote from infarction. ICD benefit in MADIT II, therefore, was greatest in those most temporally removed from their infarct (46). Based upon the results of DINAMIT, there is no evidence to support ICD therapy for primary prevention of sudden death in the early post-infarction setting with newly documented reduced ejection fraction.

ICD Therapy for Primary Prevention in Patients with Nonischemic Cardiomyopathy

Patients with NICM comprise a heterogeneous group of patients in whom identification of those at high risk for sudden death is complicated by the inadequate predictive accuracy of both electrophysiologic study and available noninvasive tests for arrhythmia risk prediction (47,48). Recognition that deteriorating left ventricular function, independent of etiology, is associated with an increased risk of sudden cardiac death (49) has prompted efforts to explore the benefit of prophylactic ICD therapy in the population of patients with NICM (Table 4).

The largest trial to date of ICD therapy for primary prevention of sudden death that included a significant proportion of patients with NICM is the SCD-HeFT trial (50). This study randomized patients with congestive heart failure and left ventricular ejection fraction $\leq$35% to therapy with ICD, amiodarone, or placebo. Heart failure symptoms (70% NYHA Class II, 30% Class III) were a precondition for enrollment. Nearly half of the 2521 patients enrolled had nonischemic cardiomyopathy. ICD therapy was associated with a statistically significant reduction in overall mortality (22%) relative to placebo (29%) at five years follow-up while amiodarone failed to confer the same mortality benefit (Fig. 5). Importantly, there was a non-significant trend to benefit in the subgroup of NICM patients, a result replicated in the Defibrillators in Non-Ischemic Cardiomyopathy

Table 4 Randomized Trials of Implantable Defibrillators for the Primary Prevention of Sudden Death Enrolling Patients with Nonischemic Cardiomyopathy (NICM)

Characteristic	Cat	Amiovirt	Definite	SCD-HeFT	Companion
Design	ICD vs. medical therapy	ICD vs. amiodarone	ICD vs. medical therapy	ICD vs. amiodarone vs. placebo	CRT-D vs. CRT vs. medical rx (2:2:1)
Years of recruitment	1991–1997	1996–2000	1998–2002	1997–2001	2000–2002
# Pts. randomized	104	103	458	2521	(CRT-D vs. med only) 903
# NICM	104 (100%)	103 (100%)	458 (100%)	1211 (48%)	394 (43.6%)
Inclusion criteria	NICM (<9 mos duration) +EF≤30%	NICM (mean 3.2 yrs duration) +EF≤35% +NSVT	NICM (mean 2.8 yrs duration) +EF≤35% +NSVT or frequent PVC's	CHF (Class II/III) +EF≤30%	CHF (Class III/IV) +EF≤35% +QRS≥120 ms+ PR≥150 ms
Mean duration of follow up (mo)	66±26.4	24±14.4	29±14.4	45.5	15
Patients					
Age, mean (yr)	52	59	58	60	67
% Male	80%	70%	71%	76%	67%
NYHA II/III	34.6%	20%	21%	100%	87%
LVEF (%)	0.24±0.07	0.23±0.09	0.21±0.14	0.25±0.05	0.22
Meds (base line, ICD vs. cntrl)					
Beta-blocker	3.8%	51.5%	84.9%	69% (all groups)	69% vs. 66%
ACE/ARB	96.2%	85%	96.7%	96% (all groups)	90% vs. 89%
ICD type					
% Transvenous	~100%	~100%	99.1%	98%	91%
% Epicardial	0%	0%	0%	0%	0%
Endpoints (ICD vs. control)					
Total mortality	8% vs. 9% at 2 yrs	13% vs. 12% at 3 yrs	7.9% vs. 14.1% at 2 yrs	22% vs. 29% at 5 yrs	16% vs. 25%
Hazard ratio for mortality	0.89, p=NS	1.08, p=0.8 (NS)	0.65, p=0.08 (NS)	0.77, p=0.007	0.64, p=0.003
Arrhythmic mortality	Not reported	No significant difference	1.3% vs. 6.1% (p=0.006)	Not reported	Not reported

Abbreviations: NICM, nonischemic cardiomyopathy; ICD, implantable cardioverter-defibrillator; CRT-D, cardiac resynchronization therapy+defibrillator; NSVT, non-sustained ventricular tachycardia; PVC, premature ventricular contraction; LVEF, left ventricular ejection fraction; NYHA, New York Heart Association functional class; CHF, congestive heart failure; ACE, angiotensin-converting enzyme inhibitor; ARB, angiotensin receptor=blocker; NS, not significant.

Treatment Evaluation (DEFINITE) trial enrolling exclusively patients with NICM (51). While earlier trials (CAT (52), AMIOVIRT (53)) failed to demonstrate a benefit of ICD therapy in this population, the small numbers of patients enrolled may account for the different results. One further study, the Comparison of Medical Therapy, Pacing, and Defibrillation in Heart Failure (COMPANION) Trial (54), randomized patients with heart failure, ICM or NICM, and QRS duration >120 ms in a 1:2:2 ratio to receive optimal pharmacologic therapy alone (OPT) or in combination with cardiac resynchronization therapy with either a pacemaker (CRT) or pacemaker-defibrillator (CRT-D). CRT-D reduced all-cause mortality relative to OPT (HR0.64, $p=0.003$), and this result remained significant in the subgroup with NICM. Since cardiac resynchronization therapy may in itself reduce mortality in appropriately selected heart failure patients (55), the incremental benefit of ICD therapy is difficult to discern. Taken together, however, the randomized controlled trials of ICD therapy suggest a benefit of prophylactic defibrillator implantation in the broader population of patients with symptomatic heart failure and LV dysfunction, independent of etiology.

Integrating the Trial Data: ICD in Primary Prevention of Sudden Death

Overall, the data supporting the use of defibrillators in patients with advanced heart disease are most reproducible in the population of patients with ischemic cardiomyopathy. Though the initial trials of ICD therapy in this population utilized an arrhythmia qualifier for inclusion (nonsustained VT, late potentials on signal-averaged ECG, inducibility at electrophysiologic study), the results of the MADIT II trial suggest that prior myocardial infarction and LVEF$\leq$30% alone identify a population of patients likely to experience a reduction in all-cause mortality with ICD therapy.

The benefits of ICD therapy in primary prevention of sudden cardiac death, however, are not likely to be equal in all patients with coronary artery disease and LV

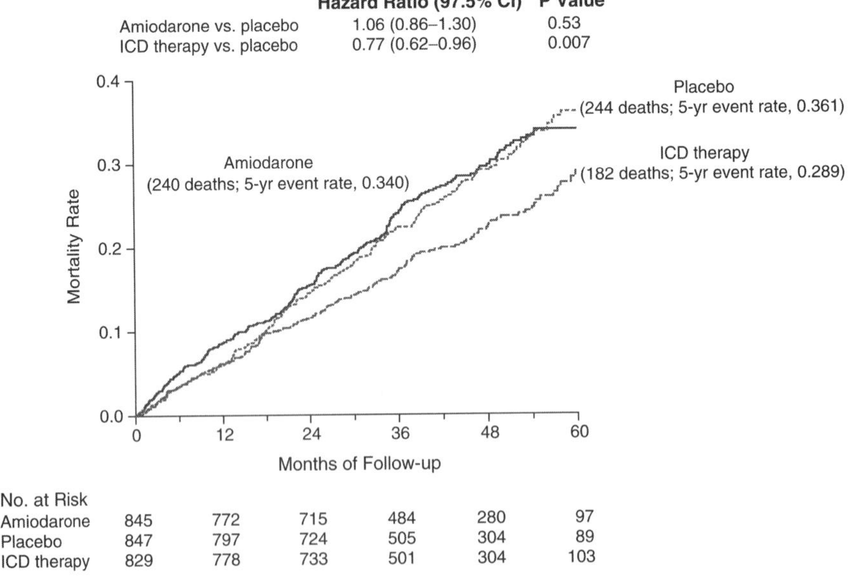

Figure 5 Kaplan–Meier estimates of the probability of survival in the SCD-HeFT trial. Implantable cardioverter-defibrillator therapy was associated with a statistically significant reduction in overall mortality relative to placebo, while amiodarone was not.

dysfunction. The DINAMIT trial results suggest that implantation of ICD in the peri-infarct setting may not be beneficial. Subgroup analyses of the CIDS and MADIT trials suggest that the greatest benefits of ICD therapy are seen in the patients with advanced heart failure who are at highest risk of arrhythmic death; in the MADIT population, LVEF ≤ 26%, QRS duration ≥ 120 ms, and history of treatment for symptomatic heart failure together identified a subset receiving a nearly 80% reduction in the hazard for all-cause mortality with ICD treatment (56). It should be emphasized, however, that patients with the most advanced heart failure symptoms (NYHA Class IV) have been systematically excluded from the defibrillator trials; since advancing heart failure is associated with an increased risk for both sudden and non-sudden (pump-failure-related) death, there may be diminishing returns to ICD therapy in the population with very late-stage disease. As with other conditions that might increase the short-term risk of death from non-arrhythmic causes, the clinical course of end-stage heart failure is unlikely to be altered by ICD implantation.

While no single trial of ICD in primary prevention has demonstrated a statistically significant reduction in mortality amongst patients with non-ischemic cardiomyopathy, the data in aggregate suggest that the relative benefit for this population is comparable to those with ischemic heart disease. A recent meta-analysis of 1854 patients with NICM enrolled in five separate trials of prophylactic ICD therapy suggested a composite 31% risk reduction in all-cause mortality relative to best medical therapy for heart failure that was robust in sensitivity analyses (Fig. 6) (57). Importantly, the relatively low annual mortality amongst medically treated patients in the primary prevention setting necessarily implies a small absolute mortality benefit to ICD therapy in NICM. Assuming a mortality of ~7% per year (as in the DEFINITE trial) and a 31% relative risk reduction, one could expect ICD therapy to result in an absolute reduction of ~2% per year in all-cause mortality. Though this benefit may be less than in secondary prevention, and slightly less than in those with concomitant coronary artery disease, however, it is now clear that prophylactic ICD therapy is efficacious in preventing sudden death in selected patients with

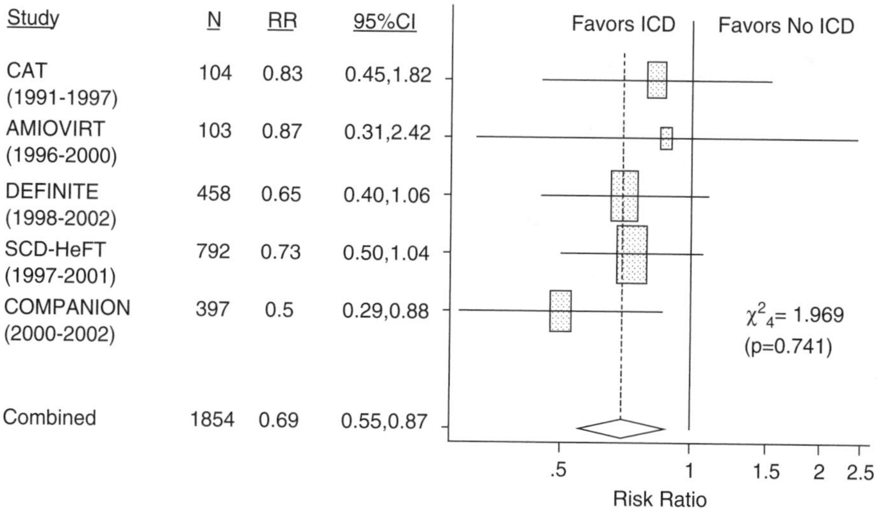

Figure 6 Fixed effects meta-analysis of prophylactic implantable cardioverter-defibrillator (ICD) therapy in nonischemic cardiomyopathy, demonstrating a statistically significant 31% overall reduction in mortality with ICD.

cardiomyopathy who meet the inclusion criteria for the trials discussed above (LVEF ≤ 30%, symptomatic heart failure [NYHA Class II–III]).

Device Selection and Implantation

The vast majority of modern ICD systems consist of two basic components: a pulse generator, which contains a battery, a capacitor, memory, and integrated circuitry necessary for coordinated device operation, and a lead system, which contains both shocking coils and electrodes for pacing and sensing. The pulse generator is typically implanted in a subcutaneous pocket in the left pectoral region in order to achieve an optimal vector for defibrillation of the heart between a shocking coil in the right ventricle, and the generator. An additional shocking coil is typically present on the right ventricular lead in the region of the superior vena cava-right atrial junction (Fig. 7). Virtually all systems are implanted transvenously, and may be configured for atrial, ventricular, or coronary sinus pacing for bradycardia or cardiac resynchronization in addition to tachycardia recognition and termination. The ICD functions by continuously monitoring the ventricular rate, and triggering sequential therapies (such as burst antitachycardia

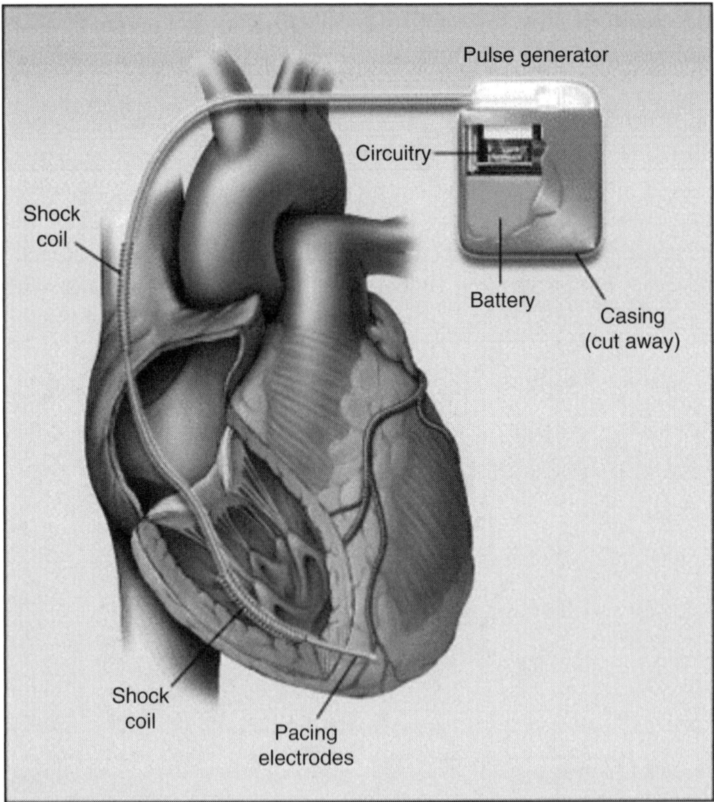

Figure 7 Diagram of a single-chamber implantable cardioverter-defibrillator system. The system consists of a pulse generator, usually implanted in a subcutaneous pocket in the pectoral region of the left chest, and a transvenous lead, with shock coils and pacing electrodes. Additional leads may be inserted into the generator header to permit atrial pacing and/or left ventricular pacing for cardiac resynchronization.

pacing or shocks of varying voltage) based on operator-programmed heart rate thresholds. Additional features include programs for discrimination between supraventricular and ventricular arrhythmias, and minimization of unnecessary ventricular pacing. Despite programs to attempt to discriminate supraventricular tachycardia from ventricular tachycardia, inappropriate therapies for atrial arrhythmias still occur.

Device Selection

The decision regarding what type of device to implant turns on two issues: first, the need for physiologic pacing support independent of defibrillation, which conditions the choice of single- or dual-chamber device; and second, the need for cardiac resynchronization, which usually requires implantation of leads for atrial and biventricular pacing as well as a pulse generator capable of supporting both resynchronization and defibrillation.

Ventricular pacing support is a critical feature of all ICDs, as there is a need to deliver antitachycardia pacing and to prevent potentially lethal bradycardia on either a continuing basis or after defibrillation. While a single-chamber device is adequate for many patients, dual-chamber devices may be necessary for those with indications for physiologic pacing support (e.g. sinus node dysfunction). In addition, dual-chamber devices offer the possible advantages of atrial electrogram storage, enhanced arrhythmia discrimination algorithms, and the potential to treat atrial arrhythmia by pacing or defibrillation.

The choice of a single-chamber ICD programmed for VVI pacing versus a dual chamber ICD programmed for DDD pacing in patients *without* a clear bradycardia pacing indication has been the subject of investigation. In the Dual Chamber and VVI Implantable Defibrillator (DAVID) trial (58), 506 patients with a left ventricular ejection fraction $\leq$40%, an indication for ICD, no atrial arrhythmias, and no indication for pacing underwent implantation of a dual chamber defibrillator and were then randomized to one of two programming modes: VVI pacing at 40 beats/min versus DDDR pacing at 70 beats/min. All patients received aggressive medical therapy for heart failure, and the primary endpoint was a composite of death or hospitalization for heart failure. At one year, 26.7% of the patients assigned to DDD pacing versus 16.1% of those assigned to VVI pacing achieved the composite endpoint of death or hospitalization for heart failure ($p < 0.05$), suggesting a potential increase in the rate of death or hospitalization in patients receiving dual-chamber pacing.

The apparent survival advantage to VVI-assigned patients, however, was confounded by a high frequency of obligate ventricular pacing in the DDD-assigned patients as a consequence of the high set rate (70 beats/min) and inadequate programmed AV delay. In patients with a narrow QRS complex at baseline, pacing from the RV apex mimics a myocardial activation pattern of left bundle branch block, desynchronizes left ventricular contraction and may lead to congestive heart failure (59). The frequency of ventricular pacing, rather than the pacing mode or choice of device, may be the critical factor governing outcomes in patients with heart failure and normal interventricular conduction. Indeed, this is a potential explanation for the slight increase in heart failure hospitalizations noted in ICD-treated patients in the MADIT II trial, and the association between cumulative ventricular pacing and risk of both heart failure and atrial fibrillation in patients with normal baseline QRS duration in the Mode Selection Trial of DDDR vs. VVIR pacing for sinus node dysfunction (60). Programming of single- or dual-chamber ICDs in patients with heart failure and intact ventricular synchrony should take into account the potentially deleterious effects of RV pacing and seek to maximize native ventricular activation.

Risks of Implantation

The evolution of the implantable defibrillator from a large abdominal device requiring thoracotomy for epicardial lead placement to a smaller, transvenous system has markedly reduced the incidence of procedural complications (Table 5). Mortality associated with defibrillator implant is less than 1% when a nonthoracotomy approach is utilized (61). Risks of implant also include a 1–2% risk of bleeding or infection, and risk of pneumothorax/hemothorax as a consequence of axilllary or subclavian venous puncture. Cardiac perforation during lead placement is uncommon but can lead to tamponade. Device testing is usually performed at insertion by induction of ventricular fibrillation to identify the threshold energy necessary for successful defibrillation; the device is typically programmed to deliver the first shock at 10 J greater than this threshold to ensure an adequate safety margin for effective device operation. Since active myocardial ischemia or decompensated heart failure can increase the risk of device implantation and testing, such problems must be addressed ahead of time. After successful insertion, generator life is variable and largely a function of current drain related to the frequency of pacing and device discharges (usually 5–6 yr).

Modern-generation defibrillators have a very high sensitivity for detection of lethal ventricular arrhythmias. This occurs at the expense of a rate of inappropriate delivery of therapy in the range of 15% or more per year despite technology to avoid inappropriate sensing and algorithms designed to differentiate supraventricular and ventricular arrhythmias (62). Fractures in a lead or failure in the insulation can cause false signals, which, when detected, prompt delivery of inappropriate shocks. Strong electromagnetic fields may interfere with the function of a defibrillator, and inappropriate therapy can result from noise due to devices that generate electrical current or magnetic fields (e.g., cautery and magnetic resonance imaging) or by the use of motors, appliances, cellular phones, and security and anti-theft devices.

Repeated shocks may also have important psychological effect, with many patients reporting significant anxiety with lasting impact on their physical functioning and mental well being (63). Interest in reducing the frequency of painful shocks has fueled an increasing preference for programming aggressive antitachycardia pacing to treat fast ventricular tachycardia and reserving high-energy shocks as a therapy of last resort (64).

CONCLUSIONS

A significant percentage of sudden deaths in patients with advanced heart disease can be treated effectively by ICDs. However, since sudden death due to stroke, pulmonary

Table 5 Implantable Defibrillator Therapy: Complications

Implant-related complications
Infection
Pneumothorax
Cardiac perforation/tamponade
Hematoma
Complications from ventricular fibrillation induction testing
Death
Device-related complications
Inappropriate shocks
Worsening heart failure from right ventricular pacing

Table 6 ACC/AHA/NASPE Guidelines for ICD Implantation, Adapted Based on January 2005 Centers for Medicare and Medicaid Services Decision

Class I	Class II	Class III
1. Cardiac arrest due to ventricular fibrillation (VF) or VT not due to a transient or reversible cause	Class IIa: Patients with LV ejection fraction of less than or equal to 35% and NYHA Class II or III heart failure who are at least one month post myocardial infarction and three months post coronary artery revascularization surgery. Patients with nonischemic dilated cardiomyopathy (NIDCM) > 9 months, NYHA Class II and III heart failure, and measured LVEF < 35%.	1. Syncope of undetermined cause in a patient without inducible ventricular tachyarrhythmias and without structural heart disease.
2. Spontaneous sustained VT in association with structural heart disease	Class IIb:	2. Incessant VT or VF.
3. Syncope of undetermined origin with clinically relevant, hemodynamically significant sustained VT or VF induced at electrophysiological study when drug therapy is ineffective, not tolerated, or not preferred	1. Cardiac arrest presumed to be due to VF when EP testing is precluded by other medical conditions.	3. VF or VT resulting from arrhythmias amenable to surgical or catheter ablation; for example, atrial arrhythmias associated with the Wolff-Parkinson-White syndrome, right ventricular outflow tract VT, idiopathic left ventricular tachycardia, or fascicular VT.
4. Nonsustained VT in patients with coronary disease, prior myocardial infarction (MI), LV dysfunction, and inducible VF or sustained VT at EP study that is not suppressible by a Class I antiarrhythmic drug	2. Severe symptoms (eg, syncope) attributable to ventricular tachyarrhythmias in patients awaiting cardiac transplantation.	4. Ventricular tachyarrhythmias due to a transient or reversible disorder (eg, AMI, electrolyte imbalance, drugs, or trauma) when correction of the disorder is considered feasible and likely to substantially reduce the risk of recurrent arrhythmia.
	3. Familial or inherited conditions with a high risk for life-threatening ventricular tachyarrhythmias such as long-QT syndrome or hypertrophic cardiomyopathy.	5. Significant psychiatric illnesses that may be aggravated by device implantation or may preclude systematic follow-up.
	4. Nonsustained VT with coronary artery disease, prior MI, LV dysfunction, and inducible sustained VT or VF at EP study.	

(Continued)

Table 6 ACC/AHA/NASPE Guidelines for ICD Implantation, Adapted Based on January 2005 Centers for Medicare and Medicaid Services Decision (*Continued*)

Class I	Class II	Class III
5. Spontaneous sustained VT in patients who do not have structural heart disease that is not amenable to other treatments	5. Recurrent syncope of undetermined etiology in the presence of ventricular dysfunction and inducible ventricular arrhythmias at EP study when other causes of syncope have been excluded.	6. Terminal illnesses with projected life expectancy less than six months.
	6. Syncope of unexplained etiology orfamily history of unexplained sudden cardiac death in association with typical or atypical right bundle-branch block and ST-segment elevations (Brugada syndrome).	7. Patients with coronary artery disease with LV dysfunction and prolonged QRS duration in the absence of spontaneous or inducible sustained or nonsustained VT who are undergoing coronary bypass surgery.
	7. Syncope in patients with advanced structural heart disease in which thorough invasive and noninvasive investigation has failed to define a cause.	8. NYHA Class IV drug-refractory congestive heart failure in patients who are not candidates for cardiac transplantation.

Class I: Conditions for which there is evidence and/or general agreement that a given procedure or treatment is useful and effective. *Class II*: Conditions for which there is conflicting evidence and/or a divergence of opinion about the usefulness/efficacy of a procedure or treatment. *IIa*: Weight of evidence/opinion is in favor of usefulness/efficacy. *IIb*: Usefulness/efficacy is less well established by evidence/opinion. *Class III*: Conditions for which there is evidence and/or general agreement that the procedure/treatment is not useful/effective and in some cases may be harmful.

Source: Gregoratos G, Abrams J, Epstein AE, et al. ACC/AHA/NASPE 2002 Guidelines update for implantation of cardiac pacemakers and antiarrhythmic devices–summary article: a report of the American College of Cardiology/American Heart Association Task Force on Practice Guidelines (ACC/AHA/NASPE Committee to Update the 1998 Pacemaker Guidelines). J Am Coll Cardiol 2002; 40:1703–1719.

emboli, hyperkalemia, myocardial infarction, and progressive pump failure may also occur, the relative benefit of a defibrillator in any given patient is determined by a balanced clinical assessment of the likelihood of death from primary arrhythmia and the likelihood of death from other causes. In the secondary prevention setting, where the risk of recurrent arrhythmia may exceed 30%, the benefits to ICD implantation are quite clear. In the primary prevention setting, where the absolute mortality risk is smaller, there is still a consistent and reproducible mortality reduction with ICD therapy in carefully selected patients with LV dysfunction and symptomatic heart failure, independent of etiology. A summary of currently accepted indications for ICD implantation is outlined in Table 6. Not all patients with reduced ejection fractions are appropriate for an ICD. A defibrillator in patients with end-stage heart disease or other conditions associated with limited survival may actually impair quality of life by delivering repeated shocks without meaningful prolongation of survival. Careful consideration should be given to patient preferences and overall prognosis in selection of candidates for device implantation. Despite the growing body of evidence supporting the use of defibrillators, the decision to implant an ICD must always be individualized.

REFERENCES

1. Zipes DP, Wellens HJJ. Sudden cardiac death. Circulation 1998; 98:2334–2351.
2. Myerburg RJ, Kessler KM, Castellanos A. Sudden cardiac death: epidemiology, transient risk, and intervention assessment. Ann Intern Med 1993; 119:1187–1197.
3. Huikuri HV, Castellanos A, Myerburg RJ. Sudden death due to cardiac arrhythmias. New Engl J Med 2001; 345:1473–1482.
4. Bigger JT. Relation between left ventricular dysfunction and ventricular arrhythmias after myocardial infarction. Am J Cardiol 1996; 57:8B–14B.
5. Bigger JT, Fleiss JL, Kleiger R, et al. The relationships among ventricular arrhythmias, left ventricular dysfunction, and mortality in the two years after myocardial infarction. Circulation 1984; 69:250–258.
6. Kannel WB, Plehn JF, Cupples A. Cardiac failure and sudden death in the Framingham study. Am Heart J 1988; 115:869–875.
7. Myerburg RJ, Castellanos A. In: Braunwald E, ed. Cardiac Arrest and Sudden Death. 6th ed. In: Heart Disease: A Textbook of Cardiovascular Medicine, 6th ed. Philadelphia, PA: WB Saunders, 2001:890–905.
8. Zipes DL, Wellens HJJ. Sudden cardiac death. Circulation 1998; 98:2334–2351.
9. Stevenson WG, Stevenson LW, Middlekauff HR, Saxon LA. Sudden death prevention in patients with advanced ventricular dysfunction. Circulation 1993; 88:2953–2961.
10. Epstein AE, Hallstrom, et al. Mortality following ventricular arrhythmia suppression by encainide, flecainide, and moricizine after myocardial infarction. The original design concept of the Cardiac Arrhythmia Suppression Trial (CAST). JAMA 1993; 270:2451–2455.
11. Mirowski M, Reid PR, Winkle RA, et al. Mortality in patients with implantable automatic defibrillators. Ann Intern Med 1983; 98:585–588.
12. Tchou PJ, Kadri N, Anderson J, Cacered JA, Jazayeri M, Akhtar M. Automatic implantable cardioverter defibrillators and survival of patients with left ventricular dysfunction and malignant arrhythmia. Ann Intern Med 1988; 109:529–534.
13. Zipes DP, Roberts D. For the Pacemaker-Cardioverter-Defibrillator Investigators. Results of the international study of the implantable pacemaker cardioverter-defibrillator: a comparison of epicardial and endocardial lead systems. Circulation 1995; 92:59–65.
14. Stevenson WG, Sweeney MO. Arrhythmias and sudden death in heart failure. Jpn Circ J 1997; 61:727–740.

15. Bigger JT, Jr, Fleiss JL, Kleiger R, et al. The relationships among ventricular arrhythmias, left ventricular dysfunction, and mortality in the two years after myocardial infarction. Circulation 1984; 69:250–258.
16. Knight BP, Goyal R, Pelosi F, et al. Outcome of patients with nonischemic dilated cardiomyopathy and unexplained syncope treated with an implantable defibrillator. J Am Coll Cardiol 1999; 33:1964–1970.
17. Steinberg JS, Beckman K, Greene HL, et al. Follow-up of patients with unexplained syncope and inducible ventricular tachyarrhythmias: Analysis of the AVID registry and an AVID substudy. J Cardiovasc Electrophysiol 2001; 12:996–1001.
18. Levine JH, Waller T, Hoch D, et al. Implantable cardioverter defibrillator: Use in patients with no symptoms and at high risk. Am Heart J 1996; 131:59–65.
19. Stevenson WG, Epstein LM. Predicting sudden death risk for heart failure patietns in the implantable cardioverter-defibrillator age. Circulation 2003; 107:514–516.
20. Moss AJ, Zareba W, Hall WJ, et al. Prophylactic implantation of a defibrillator in patients with myocardial infarction and reduced ejection fraction. N Engl J Med 2002; 346:877–883.
21. Grimm W, Christ M, Bach J. Noninvasive arrhythmia risk stratification in idiopathic dilated cardiomyopathy: Results of the marburg cardiomyopathy study. Circulation 2003; 108:2883–2891.
22. Desai AS, Fang JC, Maisel WH, Baughman KL. Implantable defibrillators for the prevention of mortality in patients with nonischemic cardiomyopathy: a meta-analysis of randomized, controlled trials. JAMA 2004; 292:2874–2879.
23. Goldman S, Johnson G, Cohn JN. Mechanism of death in heart failure: the vasodilator-heart failure trials. The V-HeFT VA cooperative studies group. Circulation 1993; 87:VI24–VI31.
24. Bode-Schnurbus L, Bocker D, Block M, et al. QRS duration: a simple marker for predicting cardiac mortality in ICD patients with heart failure. Heart 2003; 89:1157–1162.
25. Lee TH, Hamilton MA, Stevenson LW, et al. Impact of left ventricular cavity size on survival in advanced heart failure. Am J Cardiol 1993; 72:672–676.
26. Buxton AE, Lee KL, Fisher JD, et al. A randomized study of the prevention of sudden death in patients with coronary artery disease. Multicenter unsustained tachycardia investigators. N Engl J Med 1999; 341:1882–1890.
27. Buxton AE, Lee KL, DiCarlo L, et al. Electrophysiologic testing to identify patients with coronary artery disease who are at risk for sudden death. N Engl J Med 2000; 342:1937–1945.
28. Grimm W, Christ M, Bach J. Noninvasive arrhythmia risk stratification in idiopathic dilated cardiomyopathy: Results of the marburg cardiomyopathy study. Circulation 2003; 108:2883–2891.
29. Wever EF, Hauer RN, van Capelle FL, et al. Randomized study of implantable defibrillator as first-choice therapy versus conventional strategy in postinfarct sudden death survivors. Circulation 1995; 91:2195–2203.
30. The AVID Investigators. Causes of death in the antiarrhythmics versus implantable defibrillators (AVID) trial. J Am Coll Cardiol 1999; 34:1552–1559.
31. Connolly SJ, Hallstrom AP, Cappato R, et al. Meta-analysis of the implantable defibrillator secondary prevention trials. Eur Heart J 2000; 21:2071–2078.
32. Sheldon R, Connolly S, Krahn A, et al. Identification of patients most likely to benefit from implantable cardioverter-defibrillator therapy: the canadian implantable defibrillator study. Circulation 2000; 101:1660–1664.
33. Wyse DG, Friedman PL, Brodsky MA, et al. Life-threatening ventricular arrhythmias due to transient or correctable causes: high risk for death in follow-up. J Am Coll Cardiol 2001; 38:1718–1724.
34. Tamburro P, Wilber D. Sudden death in idiopathic dilated cardiomyopathy. Am Heart J 1992; 124:1035–1045.
35. Fonarow GC, Feliciano Z, Boyle NG, et al. Improved survival in patients with nonischemic advanced heart failure and syncope treated with an implantable cardioverter-defibrillator. Am J Cardiol 2000; 85:981–985.

36. Knight BP, Goyal R, Pelosi F, et al. Outcome of patients with nonischemic dilated cardiomyopathy and unexplained syncope treated with an implantable defibrillator. J Am Coll Cardiol 1999; 33:1964–1970.
37. Rankovic V, Karha J, Passman R, et al. Predictors of appropriate implantable cardioverter-defibrillator therapy in patients with dilated cardiomyopathy. Am J Cardiol 2002; 89:1072–1076.
38. Levine JH, Waller T, Hoch D, et al. Implantable cardioverter defibrillator: Use in patients with no symptoms and at high risk. Am Heart J 1996; 131:59–65.
39. Sweeney MO. Implantable cardioverter-defibrillators and cardiac resynchronization therapy. In: Manson JE, et al., eds, Clinical Trials in Heart Disease: A Companion to Braunwald's Heart Disease. Philadelphia, PA: WB Saunders, 2004
40. Moss AJ, Hall WJ, Cannom DS, et al. Improved survival with an implanted defibrillator in patients with coronary artery disease at high risk for ventricular arrhythmia. N Engl J Med 1996; 335:1940–1993.
41. Moss AJ, Zareba W, Hall WJ, et al. Prophylactic implantation of a defibrillator in patients with myocardial infarction and reduced ejection fraction. N Engl J Med 2002; 346:877–883.
42. Bigger JT, et al. Prophylactic use of implanted cardiac defibrillators in patients at high risk for ventricular arrhythmias after coronary artery bypass surgery. N Engl J Med 1997; 337:1569–1575.
43. Buxton AE, Lee KL, Fisher JD, et al. A randomized study of the prevention of sudden death among patients with coronary artery disease. N Engl J Med 1999; 341:1882–1890.
44. Hohnloser SH, Kuck KH, Dorian P, et al. Prophylactic use of an implantable defibrillator after acute myocardial infarction. NEJM 2004; 351:2481–2488.
45. Gregoratos G, Abrams J, Epstein AE, et al. ACC/AHA/NASPE Guidelines update for implantation of cardiac pacemakers and antiarrhythmic devices—summary article: a report of the American College of Cardiology/American Heart Association Task Force on Practice Guidelines (ACC/AHA/NASPE Committee to Update the 1998 Pacemaker Guidelines). J Am Coll Cardiol 2002; 40:1703–1719.
46. Wilber DJ, Zareba W, Hall WJ, et al. Time dependence of mortality risk and defibrillator benefit after myocardial infarction. Circulation 2004; 109:1082–1084.
47. Grimm W, Hoffmann J, Menz V, et al. Programmed ventricular stimulation for arrhythmia risk prediction in patients with idiopathic dilated cardiomyopathy and nonsustained ventricular tachycardia. J Am Coll Cardiol 1998; 32:739–745.
48. Grimm W, Christ M, Bach J. Noninvasive arrhythmia risk stratification in idiopathic dilated cardiomyopathy: Results of the Marburg Cardiomyopathy Study. Circulation 2003; 108:2883–2891.
49. Stevenson WG, Stevenson LW, Middlekauf HR, Saxon LA. Sudden death prevention in patients with advanced left ventricular dysfunction. Circulation 1993; 88:2953–2961.
50. Bardy GH, Lee KL, Mark DB, et al. Amiodarone or an implantable defibrillator for congestive heart failure. N Engl J Med 2005; 352:225–237.
51. Kadish A, Dyer A, Daubert JP, et al. Prophylactic defibrillator implantation in nonischemic dilated cardiomyopathy. N Engl J Med 2004; 350:2151–2158.
52. Bansch D, Antz M, Boczor S, et al. Primary prevention of sudden cardiac death in idiopathic dilated cardiomyopathy: The cardiomyopathy trial (CAT). Circulation 2002; 105:1453–1458.
53. Strickberger SA, Hummel JD, Bartlett TG, et al. Amiodarone versus implantable cardioverter-defibrillator: Randomized trial in patients with nonischemic dilated cardiomyopathy and asymptomatic nonsustained ventricular tachycardia—AMIOVIRT. J Am Coll Cardiol 2003; 41:1707–1712.
54. Bristow MR, Saxon LA, Boehmer J, et al. Cardiac-resynchronization therapy with or without an implantable defibrillator in advanced chronic heart failure. N Engl J Med 2004; 350:2140–2150.
55. Cleland JGF, Daubert J-C, Erdmann E, et al. The effect of cardiac resynchronization on morbidity and mortality in heart failure. N Engl J Med 2005; 352:1539–1549.

56. Moss AJ, Fadl Y, Zareba W, et al. Survival benefit with an implanted defibrillator in relation to mortality risk in chronic coronary heart disease. Am J Cardiol. 2001; 88:516–520.
57. Desai AS, Fang JC, Maisel WH, Baughman KL. Implantable defibrillators for the prevention of mortality in nonischemic cardiomyopathy: A meta-analysis of randomized controlled trials. JAMA 2004; 292:2874–2879.
58. Wilkoff BL, Cook JR, Epstein AE, et al. Dual-chamber pacing or ventricular backup pacing in patients with an implantable defibrillator: the dual chamber and VVI implantable defibrillator trial. JAMA 2002; 288:3115–3123.
59. Barold SS, Herweg B, Sweeney MO. Minimizing right ventricular pacing. Am J Cardiol 2005; 95:966–968.
60. Sweeney MO, Hellkamp AS, Ellenbogen KA, et al. Adverse effects of ventricular pacing on heart failure and atrial fibrillation among patients with normal baseline QRS duration in a clinical trial of pacemaker therapy for sinus node dysfunction. Circulation 2003; 107:2932–2937.
61. Zipes DP, Roberts D. Results of the international study of the implantable pacemaker cardioverter-defibrillator. A comparison of epicardial and endocardial lead systems. The pacemaker-cardioverter-defibrillator investigators. Circulation 1995; 92:59–65.
62. Gradaus R, Block M, Brachmann J, et al. Mortality, morbidity, and complications in 3344 patients with implantable cardioverter defibrillators: results fron the German ICD Registry EURID. Pacing Clin Electrophysiol 2003; 26:1511–1518.
63. Schron EB, Exner DV, Yao Q, et al. Quality of life in the antiarrhythmics versus implantable defibrillators trial: impact of therapy and influence of adverse symptoms and defibrillator shocks. Circulation 2002; 105:589–594.
64. Wathen MS, DeGroot PJ, Sweeney MO, et al. Prospective randomized multicenter trial of empirical antitachycardia pacing versus shocks for spontaneous rapid ventricular tachycardia in patients with implantable cardioverter-defibrillators: Pacing fast ventricular tachycardia reduces shock therapies (PainFREE Rx II) trial results. Circulation 2004; 110:2591–2596.

17
Device Therapy for Heart Failure

James C. Fang
Advanced Heart Disease Section, Cardiovascular Division, Department of Medicine, Brigham and Women's Hospital, Harvard Medical School, Boston, Massachusetts, U.S.A.

INTRA-AORTIC BALLOON COUNTERPULSATION (IABP)

In 1953, Kantrowitz and Kantrowitz conceived of a novel approach to improving coronary blood flow to the ischemic myocardium by delaying the arterial pulse into the diastolic period (1). They extended this principle of diastolic augmentation by stimulating a hemidiaphragm wrapped around the distal thoracic aorta in diastole, thereby providing the first description of an auxiliary ventricle (2). Simultaneously, Harken, working in the Harvard Surgical Research Laboratory, hypothesized that the rapid removal of blood from the arterial circulation during systole (and returned during diastole) could decrease the pressure work of the heart (3). Such a device, the "arterial counterpulsator" was built by Birtwell and saw brief clinical use but was limited by an inability to move the blood back and forth rapidly enough without excessive hemolysis (4). Clauss (5) and Moulopoulos (6), working independently, developed the use of an inflatable chamber within the aorta as an arterial counterpulsator. In 1968, Kantrowitz reported the successful resuscitation of a patient with medically refractory cardiogenic shock following a myocardial infarction using helium to rapidly inflate and deflate an intra-aortic balloon placed via the femoral artery (without the need for thoracic surgery) (7). The Datascope Corporation developed a percutaneously insertable device in 1979, introducing the modern era of emergent arterial counterpulsation (8). IABP has now become standard equipment in all institutions that offer advanced cardiovascular care due to its ease of placement, cost, availability, simplicity, and clinical track record. Its effectiveness has been well-documented and counterpulsation is now considered a Class I indication by the American College of Cardiology and the American Heart Association for the management of pharmacologically resistant cardiogenic shock (9). IABP is the most commonly used circulatory assist device in the world. The clinical use of IABP has also evolved rapidly and its contemporary use includes the support of the circulation during percutaneous coronary intervention, cardiac surgical procedures, and bridging of patients with both acute and chronic heart failure to more definitive therapies. Recent and future developments in counterpulsation technology are now testing the effectiveness and feasibility of using noninvasive counterpulsation, EECP, as well as surgically implanted permanent devices for the chronic management of heart failure.

The basic principle of counterpulsation is relatively simple: to augment diastolic coronary blood flow through inflation of an intravascular balloon during diastole and to decrease the pulsatile resistance to ventricular ejection through the rapid deflation of the intravascular balloon during systole. These actions improve myocardial oxygen supply and demand mismatch, increase the cardiac output, and improve end organ perfusion pressure. When instituted early in cardiogenic shock, counterpulsation increases human coronary blood flow by 34% with a concomitant change in myocardial metabolism from lactate production to lactate extraction and a decrease in myocardial oxygen consumption from 79% to 61% (10,11). However, without a more definitive therapy of shock, these improvements may wane quickly (12).

When deflation of the intra-aortic balloon is properly timed, ventricular afterload decreases due to the decrease in impedance to ventricular ejection as the aortic volume is suddenly diminished. Consequently, stroke volume increases by as much as 34% with the largest increases in those with the worst LV function (Fig. 1) (13). Myocardial wall stress also falls as left ventricular end-diastolic pressure decreases by as much as 40% and the

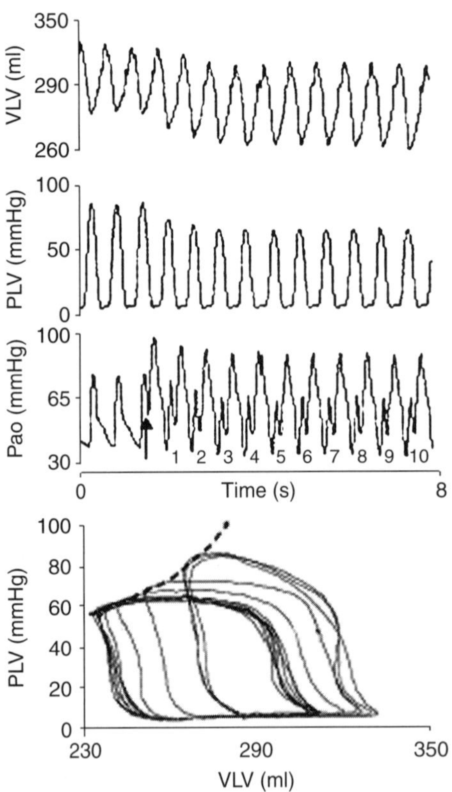

Figure 1 PV loop demonstrating effects of IABP. Patient has ejection fraction of 14% and NYHA III symptoms. Arrow signifies onset of counterpulsation. Beats 1–10 demonstrate decrease in systolic pressure and lowering of end-diastolic pressure with counterpulsation. PV loops demonstrate progressive increases in stroke volume (*right to left loops*) by decreasing both end-systolic and end-diastolic volume. Note nonlinear endsystolic elastance consistent with changes in contractility. *Abbreviations:* IABP, intra-aortic ballon counterpulsation; NYHA, New York Heart Association. *Source*: From Ref. 13.

peak LV systolic pressure falls by as much as 20% (14). Changes in systemic vascular resistance (SVR) are more difficult to quantify since mean arterial blood pressure, which is directly proportional to vascular resistance, can rise with IABP support, leading to the potential to overestimate the true vascular resistance using the calculated SVR. However, pulsatile resistance, or impedence, and ventricular vascular coupling improve measurably (15). Most importantly, contractile performance, as assessed by ejection fraction, dP/dT, and the endsystolic elastance also improves, presumably due the improved coronary blood flow, decreased aortic impedance (15), and improvements in ventricular mechanical synchrony, a powerful determinant of LV performance (Fig. 1) (14).

The hemodynamic effectiveness of IABP is dependent upon several factors including the position of the balloon within the descending thoracic aorta, the balloon displacement volume, the relationship of balloon to aortic diameter, the type of inflating gas, inflation/deflation timing, and hemodynamic variables such as circulating blood volume, blood pressure, and vascular resistance (16). The ideal position of the IABP is within 1 cm of the left subclavian artery origin. The blood displacement volume should be less than the ventricular stroke volume in order to prevent retrograde flow in the coronary arteries and aortic branches. The current standard volume is 40 cc for the average adult and approximates the lower limit of stroke volume in the failing heart. The balloon diameter should not be occlusive and is in general 75%–90% of the aortic diameter. Most commercially available devices range from 16–18 mm since the human mid-thoracic aorta is generally greater than 19 mm. Helium is the ideal gas since it is far less dense than carbon dioxide, which facilitates its rapid shuttling in and out of the intra-aortic balloon. Inflation and deflation timing is critical and typically gated to either the EKG or the intraaortic waveform. Early inflation and late deflation will lead to obstruction of ventricular ejection in late and early systole respectively, leading to increased myocardial afterload, myocardial oxygen consumption, increased ventricular preload, and decreased stroke volumes (13).

There is extensive published clinical experience with the short-term use (i.e., less than 5 days) of IABP for the management of acute ischemic heart disease and cardiogenic shock, and as adjunctive therapy for high-risk cardiac surgery and percutaneous coronary intervention. A discussion of IABP use for cardiac surgery and PCI can be found elsewhere (16,17). Indications, contraindications, and complications of IABP are listed in Tables 1–3. However, despite its AHA/ACC Class I indication and its effectiveness in published experiences, the use of counterpulsation in shock accompanying acute myocardial infarction varies widely. For example, in the GUSTO experience, only one

Table 1 Indications for Intra-aortic Balloon Counterpulsation

Cardiogenic shock
Acute mitral regurgitation
Acute ventricular septal defect
Myocardial infarction
Post cardiotomy syndrome
Aortic stenosis (uncommon)
Medically refractory unstable angina
Medically refractory severe heart failure
Unstable incessant ventricular arrhythmias
Support of high-risk percutaneous interventions
Support of high-risk cardiac surgical procedures
Bridging to heart transplantation

Table 2 Contraindications to Intra-aortic Balloon Counterpulsation

Significant aortic insufficiency
Aortic dissection
Obstructive iliofemoral arterial disease
Uncontrolled sepsis
Abdominal aortic aneurysm
Aortic prosthetic graft (relative contraindication)

third of U.S. centers employed counterpulsation for cardiogenic shock despite trends toward improved 30 day and one year mortality (18).

Although IABP is effective in reversing the hemodynamic picture of shock, survival may still be poor due to the level of illness. In early series of IABP for shock from acute myocardial infarction, survival was a sobering 16%–24% (19,20). Advances in cardiac surgery, interventional cardiology, and medical therapy for acute myocardial infarction and better patient selection have increased survival and more contemporary series of patients with myocardial infarction and shock demonstrate improved but still high mortality rates. In the largest published series of IABP use (4756 cases) from the Massachusetts General Hospital (MGH), which has used IABP since the late 1960's, mortality has decreased from 41% to 20% despite an increasing mean age (54 to 66 yr) (21). In part, this improvement in mortality reflects a change in the type of patient who receives IABP support at the MGH. Since 1968, the use of IABP for ischemic heart disease (with a mortality of 11.9%) has increased from 28.4% to 65.4% of all pumps used. In their series, mortality when IABP support is used for hemodynamic reasons (heart failure, hypotension, shock) was much higher at 38.2% but represented fewer proportional cases of their total recent experience. In this series, independent predictors of death included insertion in the operating room or intensive care unit, transthoracic insertion, age, procedure other than coronary angioplasty or coronary bypass surgery, or placement for cardiogenic shock.

In cardiogenic shock unrelated to coronary artery disease, IABP can be particularly useful since support may only need to be temporary, as in the case of fulminant myocarditis which typically presents with rapid catastrophic cardiovascular collapse but often abates within days (22,23). If spontaneous recovery does not occur, IABP allows the patient to be bridged to either mechanical assist devices and/or cardiac transplantation. In one series, only 3 to 4 days of counterpulsation was enough to allow for recovery of ventricular function when patients presented in this manner (23).

The prolonged use (greater than 5 days) of IABP, especially in severe refractory heart failure without shock, is less well documented. In such cases, prolonged support is often necessary before weaning of the device or more definitive therapy such as transplantation or high-risk cardiac surgery is entertained. Mechanical support with IABP may allow for the improvement in renal function, neurohormonal activation, and

Table 3 Complications of Intra-aortic Balloon Counterpulsation

Vascular obstruction (risk factors: PVD, female, percutaneous insertion)
Aortic trauma
Thrombocytopenia
Bleeding
Infection
Balloon rupture
Atheroembolic syndrome

nutritional status in such chronically ill patients. In an early series from 1977, Hagemeijer, et al. reported that 14 of 25 patients with NYHA III/IV heart failure following myocardial infarction survived for more than 3 mo after discontinuation of IABP support (duration up to 24 days) and 12 were considered to be NYHA II (24). In 1988, Freed and coworkers described 27 out of 733 cases that were supported for more than 20 days (range 20 to 71), 12 of whom had a history of heart failure (25). Not surprisingly, there were more complications (vascular, infectious, bleeding) when compared to those patients with less than 20 days of support but survival was comparable (63% for >20 days versus 57% for <20 days). Although all with a history of heart failure eventually died within six months of discharge, 7 of these patients were discharged to home following IABP removal without cardiac surgery. However, in the contemporary era of mechanical assist devices, most cases of refractory heart failure are only supported with IABP long enough to optimally time ventricular assist device insertion as a bridge to transplantation (26–29). The duration of support is extremely variable in such situations depending upon institutional practices and transplant waiting times but generally averages less than two weeks, although one notable report describes 327 days of IABP support until transplantation (30).

The effectiveness of IABP has led to numerous strategies to use arterial counterpulsation as a permanent strategy for chronic heart failure and permanently implanted aortic balloons are now being considered. Providing counterpulsation from outside the aorta has also been attempted with both skeletal muscle and balloons wrapped around the aorta that in essence squeeze the aorta to provide augmented diastolic pressure and counterpulsation. In fact, this method of arterial counterpulsation was the original strategy as first proposed by Kantrowicz in 1958 when he suggested wrapping the aorta in skeletal muscle from the diaphragm (2). The primary barrier of skeletal muscle fatigue has been overcome by the work of Acker and others by using low frequency electrical stimulation to transform skeletal muscle into fatigue resistant fibers in their work with cardiomyoplasty (31). The modern operation, dynamic aortomyoplasty, has been reported by several centers with modest success. In a report from Paris and Buenos Aires in 2002 (32), 15 patients underwent this procedure with the latissimus dorsi wrapped around the ascending aorta and conditioned with an electrical stimulator. Twelve patients survived to an average follow up of 18 mo and all were NYHA I–II. Cardiac index improved from 2.0 ± 0.3 to 2.6 ± 0.4, the end diastolic dimension decreased from 76.5 ± 9.9 to 71.8 ± 9.3, and oxygen consumption improved from 12.5 ± 3.2 to 14.7 ± 4.3. Australian investigators have used a balloon cuff wrapped around the ascending aorta, the C-Pulse™, to provide similar arterial counterpulsation (33). Although limited to patients without aortic root disease, it has the advantage of implantation without cardiopulmonary bypass, lack of contact with the circulation and blood elements, and the ability to be turned on and off for power source reasons without cardiovascular collapse.

Conventional percutaneous IABP has a firm role in the contemporary management of acute cardiovascular disease due to the efforts of many investigators over the years. Its role in the future for chronic heart failure remains to be determined but technologic developments could pave the way for automated permanently implanted IABP support. How such systems will compete with the ever more sophisticated mechanical ventricular assist device technology remains to be seen.

ENHANCED EXTERNAL COUNTERPULSATION (EECP)

Almost simultaneous to the development of intra-aortic counterpulsation was the development of an external noninvasive means of providing diastolic augmentation to

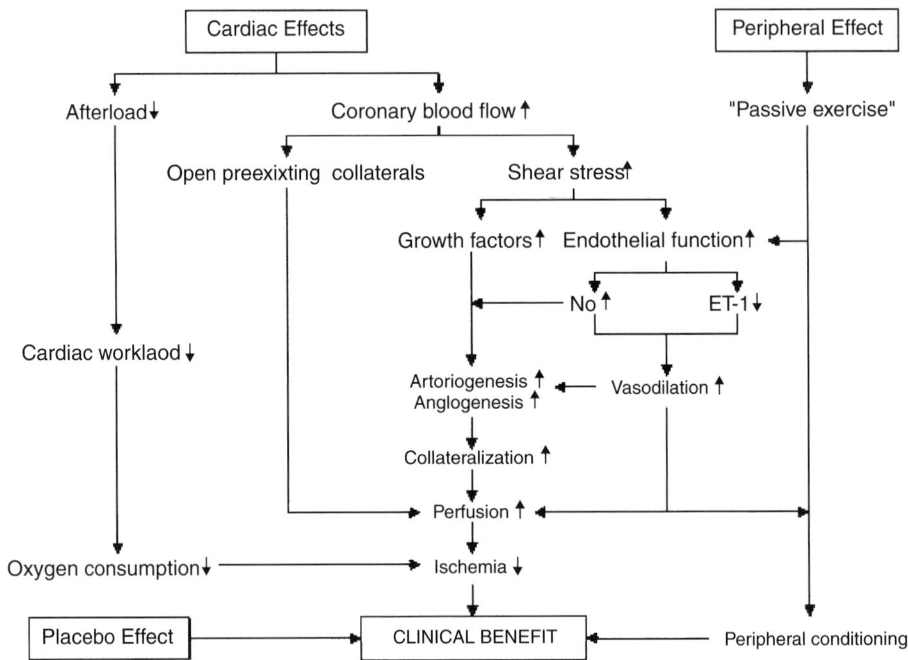

Figure 2 Potential mechanisms of benefit of EECP. The benefits of EECP include effects of decreased afterload from arterial counterpulsation, improved diastolic coronary blood flow, augmentation of venous return, and improvements in vascular function. However, a placebo effect or a training effect cannot be discounted. *Abbreviations:* EECP, enhanced external counterpulsation. *Source*: From Ref. 44.

coronary blood flow and afterload reduction for the left ventricle (34–37). However, in contrast to IABP, EECP also provides an increase in venous return since the lower extremity venous system is also "milked" during the external counterpulsation (Fig. 2). This additional action of EECP provides further improvements in cardiac output by Starling's law (38,39) and supplements the increase in stroke volume created by the improved diastolic coronary blood flow and reduction in vascular impedance (38,40). Soroff and Birtwell reported increases in diastolic blood pressure by 40%–50% and lowering of systolic blood pressure by as much as 30% with pulsed external positive pressure (41,42) with early prototypes of EECP. Intracoronary Doppler flow wire studies have confirmed the significant increase in coronary flow velocity by as much as 100% and an increase in coronary blood flow by 28% assessed by the TIMI frame count with angiography (Fig. 3) (43). Other mechanisms of action may also play a role in the effectiveness of EECP to treat angina from ischemic heart disease. Endothelial function appears to improve with EECP which predicts a clinical response to EECP for the relief of angina (44,45). This change may result from increased nitric oxide release as well as decreases in endothelin-1 (46). Stimulation of collateral blood flow through angiogenesis may also occur since release of several growth factors (human growth factor, beta fibroblast growth factor, vascular endothelial growth factor, monocyte chemoattractant protein-1) occurs with EECP (47). Others have suggested that EECP provides a physical training effect similar to exercise through decreases in peripheral resistance and heart responses to exercise (47,48). Finally, a placebo effect cannot be discounted due to the lack of appropriate controls in most clinical studies (Table 4).

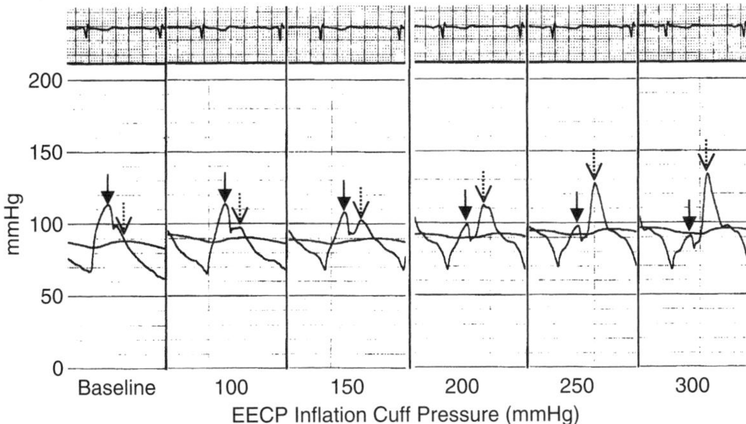

Figure 3 Effect of EECP on coronary pressure. With increasing EECP pressure, the diastolic coronary pressure increases (*dotted arrows*) and systolic pressure decreases (*solid arrows*). *Abbreviation:* EECP, enhanced external counterpulsation. *Source*: From Ref. 43.

Currently available technology uses three sets of lower extremities cuffs that are sequentially inflated from calf to upper thigh and buttocks in a pulsatile manner, beginning early in diastole and delivering up to 300 mmHg of external pressure (Fig. 4). Therapy can be titrated to provide the greatest diastolic augmentation ratio (area under systole / area under diastole in the arterial waveform) obtained from finger plethysmography (49). Patients typically undergo 35 one-hour daily treatments over the course of 5 to 7 wk. Contraindications to EECP include recent cardiac catheterization, severe peripheral vascular disease, decompensated heart failure, lower extremity deep venous thrombosis, severe hypertension, aortic insufficiency, arrhythmias that prevent EKG gating, and coumadin therapy (due to concerns for deep tissue bleeding). An important aspect of EECP is that there is generally little morbidity associated with this treatment if contraindications are honored. In the MUST-EECP study, the most common adverse events were non-device related and the only device related adverse event more common in the active treatment arm was skin abrasion, bruise, blister and pain of the legs and back (50). On the basis of clinical trial evidence, the FDA approved the device for the management of chronic angina in 1995.

Most of the clinical investigations for EECP have concentrated on the role of this therapy in ischemic heart disease. Since the early 1980s, numerous unblinded, uncontrolled studies and registries have suggested clinical benefits of EECP with improvements in quality of life, time to exercise-induced ST depression, exercise tolerance, and scintigraphic myocardial perfusion abnormalities (Table 4). However, in the only placebo controlled randomized prospective trial of EECP, the Multicenter Study of Enhanced External Counterpulsation (MUST-EECP), EECP was only modestly effective (50). In this study of 139 patients with positive exercise tests and angina, sham counterpulsation was provided by using only 75 mmHg of pressure which provided the appearance and feel of active EECP (which used 300 mmHg) but was insufficient to produce a change in blood pressure. Although there was a statistically significant difference in the time to ST segment depression (42 sec vs. 4 sec, $p=0.01$) and number of anginal episodes ($p<0.05$) between the two treatment groups, both groups experienced comparable increases in exercise duration and no significant differences in nitroglycerin use (50). These findings are in contrast to the observations from the more than 5000 patients in the International EECP Registry. In a study from the registry that examined

Table 4 Trials of EECP in Patients with Angina

Study	Year	N	Treatment duration (h)	Angina(% ≥1 CCS class)[a]	Nitrate use	Exercise tolerance (%)[a]	Time to ST depression	Carbine perfusion (%)[a]
Zheng et al.	1983	200	12	↓ (97)	N/A	N/A	N/A	N/A
Lawson et al.	1992	18	36	↓ (100)	↓	↑ (67)	N/A	↑ (78)
Lawson et al.	1996	27	35	N/A	N/A	↑ (81)	N/A	↑ (78)
Lawson et al.	1996	50	35	↓ (100)	↓	N/A	N/A	↑ (80)
Lawson et al.	1998	60	35	↓	N/A	↑	N/A	↑ (75)
Arem et al.	1999	139	35	↓	↓	↑	↑	N/A
Lawson et al.	2000	33	35–36	↓ (100)	↓	N/A	N/A	↑ (79)
Lawson et al.	2000	2,289	35	↓ (74)	N/A	N/A	N/A	N/A
Urns et al.	2001	12	35	N/A	N/A	↑	↑	↑
Masds et al.	2001	11	35	N/A	N/A	↑	↑	↑
Stys et al.	2001	395	35	↓ (88)	N/A	N/A	N/A	N/A
Barsness et al.	2001	978	35	↓ (81)	↓	N/A	N/A	N/A
Syes et al.	2002	175	35	↓ (83)	N/A	↑	N/A	↑ (83)

[a]When reported in the original article, the percentages of patients for whom the criteria applies are found in parenthesis.

Abbreviations: CCS, Canadian Cardiovascular Society; N/A, not assessed; EECP, enhanced external counterpulsation.

Source: From Ref. 44, 45.

1097 patients with primarily NYHA III–IV angina (87.5% with previous PCI or CABG and an average of 10.7 ± 13.2 anginal episodes/week), 74.9% had an improved NYHA functional class that was sustained at 2 yr following therapy and 50% had sustained improvement in their quality of life (51).

The use of EECP for hemodynamic reasons actually dates to the earliest clinical studies of this technology. In 1974, Soroff reported the first clinical use of such a device for the management of cardiogenic shock following a myocardial infarction (41). In an early randomized nonblinded experience in 258 patients with acute Killip II myocardial infarction, EECP improved short-term survival when used within the first 24 hr of symptoms (6.5% vs. 14.7%, $p < 0.05$) (52). Several lines of evidence suggest that EECP may be beneficial for chronic heart failure as well. As described previously, cardiac output can increase by as much as 25% (53,54). Improvements in arterial compliance also predict clinical benefit, which may favor ventricular vascular coupling and consequently ventricular performance (55). In an uncontrolled study of 11 patients with angina, atrial and brain natriuretic peptide levels also fell (56). Urano and colleagues reported improved

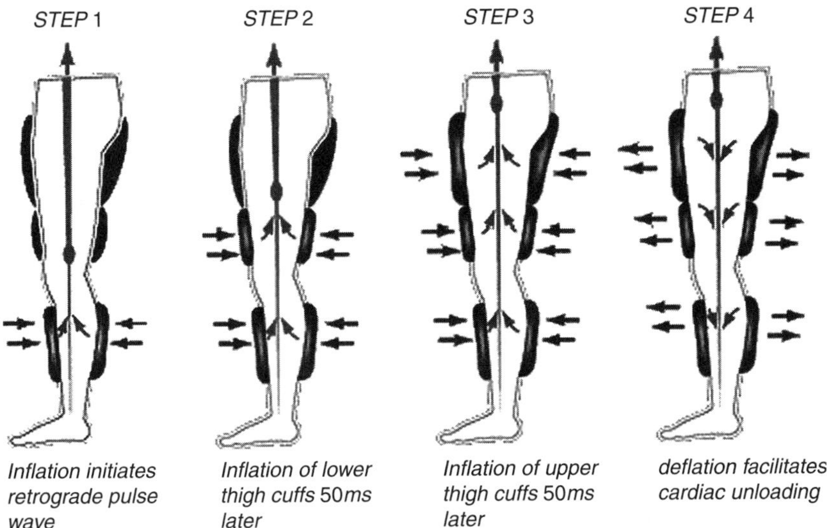

Figure 4 Sequential cuff inflation in EECP. Three sets of lower extremities cuffs are sequentially inflated from calf to upper thigh and buttocks in a pulsatile manner, beginning early in diastole and delivering up to 300 mmHg of external pressure. Therapy can be titrated to provide the greatest diastolic augmentation ratio (area under systole/area under diastole in the arterial waveform) obtained from finger plethysmography. *Abbreviation:* EECP, enhanced external counterpulsation. *Source*: From Ref. 115.

diastolic function in 12 patients with angina and normal LV systolic function with a fall in the end diastolic pressure, a rise in the peak LV filling rate, and a drop in the time to peak LV filling rate that correlated with a fall in BNP (57). Ejection fraction has also been reported to improve in a modest fashion (58). Despite concerns that increases in venous return may not be tolerated in patients with a history of heart failure, data from 746 patients in the International EECP Registry with heart failure found similar benefits in angina relief whether the EF was greater than or less than 35% and no difference in exacerbations of heart failure (5.4% in EF $<35\%$ vs. 3.1% in EF $>35\%$, $p=0.12$) (59). Finally, in an open pilot study of EECP in heart failure, 26 patients with an average EF of 23% experienced improved exercise tolerance and quality of life without serious adverse events (60). This preliminary evidence has formed the basis of the Prospective Evaluation of EECP in Heart Failure (PEECH) trial, a controlled randomized single blind study of 187 patients with NYHA II–III heart failure and an ejection fraction of $<35\%$ (61). Endpoints will include peak oxygen uptake, exercise duration time, quality of life, NYHA status, and neurohormonal markers. The trial will not provide a sham counterpulsation arm due to concerns that low levels of external pressure (i.e., 75 mmHg as used in the MUST-EECP study) may produce increases in venous return that would not be tolerated if concomitant afterload reduction were not provided (as is the case with conventional EECP using 300 mmHg). Blinding will be accomplished by separating the study investigators, who will blindly assess study endpoints, from the clinical team caring for the patient.

In summary, EECP offers a noninvasive method of arterial counterpulsation that may have a role in chronic heart failure. It is FDA approved for chronic angina and appears to benefit those with normal and impaired ventricular function and the effects appear to be sustained in a significant portion of patients for months to years. For those patients with persistent symptoms of heart failure despite optimal medical management, EECP can be offered but definitive support for its use in heart failure will need to await the results of trials such as PEECH.

CONTINUOUS POSITIVE AIRWAY PRESSURE (CPAP)

The use of supplemental oxygen for heart failure dates back to 1907 when Pembrey demonstrated that nasal oxygen therapy improves Cheyne-Stokes respirations (CSR) in heart failure (62). Since then, there has been an increasing recognition that such forms of therapy may be treating a common condition that often accompanies heart failure, sleep apnea. Since sleep is a time for cardiovascular rest, its disruption not surprisingly stresses cardiovascular health (63,64). It is now evident that sleep apnea is not only common but may also play a role in the progression of heart failure. Because obstructive sleep apnea (OSA) has a well-accepted and effective therapy, CPAP, there is increasing interest in targeting this aspect of heart failure.

There are two forms of sleep apnea, obstructive and central sleep apnea [CSA] (also known as CSR). OSA is defined as reductions or cessations in airflow during sleep in association with ongoing respiratory effort (65). OSA results from an instability of ventilatory control during sleep as well as anatomic narrowing of the upper airway and a loss of pharyngeal muscle tone, which may be exacerbated by soft tissue edema common in heart failure (66). In contrast, CSR is defined as cyclic reductions or cessations in airflow but without respiratory effort (Fig. 5) (67). Although rarely appreciated, CSR may occur while awake although classically occurring during sleep. The pathogenesis behind CSR is less clear but also appears in part to be due to an instability of ventilatory control that is initiated and sustained by chronic hypocapnia and a hypersensitivity of the respiratory control center to $PaCO_2$ (68), both common to heart failure (63). In heart failure patients with CSR, the awake and sleep $PaCO_2$ (33 mmHg) is below normal due to chronic hyperventilation (presumably due to stimulation of pulmonary vagal irritant receptors from pulmonary congestion) and lower than those heart failure patients without CSA despite similar ejection fractions and awake or sleep PaO_2 (69,70). In fact, raising the nocturnal $PaCO_2$ with inhaled CO_2 (69,71,72), or oxygen (73) can markedly attenuate CSR. When sleep ensues, an oscillation in ventilation occurs as the respiratory center tries to normalize the PaCO2 but under/overshoots the targeted $PaCO_2$ because of hypersensitivity of the control center to CO_2 and a time delay between the central ventilatory sensors and the peripheral ventilatory action of the lungs. This under/overshooting oscillation is then manifest clinically as alternating apneas and hyperpneas (Fig. 6).

Both OSA and CSR likely contribute to the progression of heart failure through chronic adrenergic stimulation from the intermittent nocturnal arousals that stem from intermittent hypoxias and hypercapnias. In a large community based cross sectional sleep survey of men and women, OSA conferred an independent relative risk of heart failure of 2.38 (74). Such chronic neurohormonal activation is central to the progression of heart failure. It also likely plays a role in hypertension (75) and unrecognized OSA is not uncommon in refractory hypertension. There may also be a hemodynamic consequence of sleep apnea through large swings in transmural wall stress and afterload during ventilation while asleep (76). In the context of chronic heart failure, when there is either poor lung compliance (from "wet" congested lungs) and/or obstruction of the upper airway (as a consequence of OSA), the inspiratory fall in pleural pressure required to ventilate the lungs can be substantial (77) and lead to major increases in left ventricular transmural pressure (or afterload) (78). In the morbidly obese patient, this phenomenon may be dramatic and even explain the cardiomyopathy of obesity (79). In addition, OSA appears

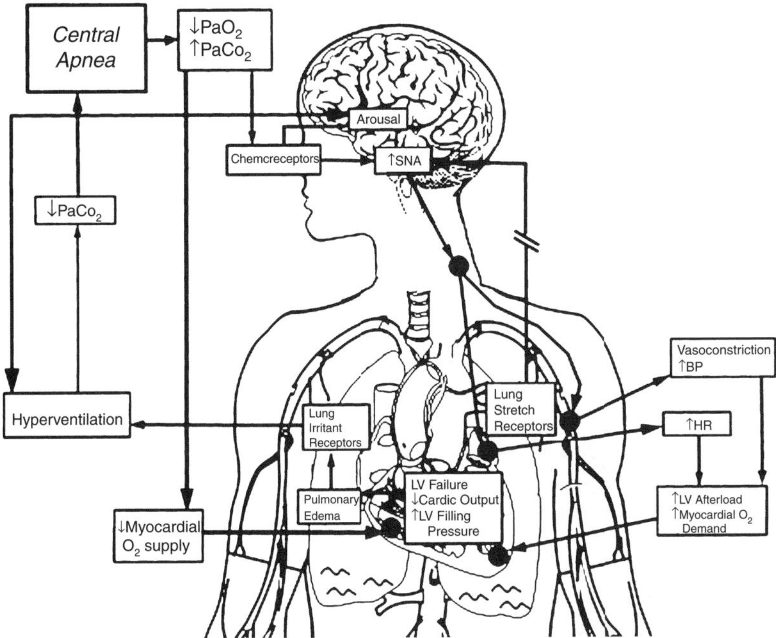

Figure 5 Pathogenesis of central sleep apnea. See text for explanation. *Source*: From Ref. 63.

to have an independent role in exacerbating pulmonary hypertension (80–82). Finally, CSR appears to be prevalent in patients with diastolic heart failure (83).

Sleep apnea is common in heart failure although studies vary in their definition of sleep apnea, the population study, and the background heart failure medical therapy (Table 5). Most patients with heart failure and sleep apnea will have both obstructive and central events. In the largest study of sleep apnea in heart failure patients, 70% of 450 New York Heart Association (NYHA) II–IV patients had sleep apnea (defined by an apnea-hyponea index [AHI] >10 episodes per hour): 33% with CSR and 37% with OSA (84). Although CSR is thought to be an affliction of patients with advanced stages of heart failure (85), it appears to affect both asymptomatic patients with left ventricular dysfunction (86) and heart failure patients with preserved left ventricular function, ie. diastolic heart failure (87). Symptoms of sleep apnea such as insomnia, snoring, and daytime somnolence may be present, but such symptoms are generally insensitive to the presence of either OSA or CSR. Some have suggested screening all heart failure patients due to the high prevalence of sleep-disordered breathing. In many cases, only the spouse may be aware of such symptoms. Risk factors for CSR are male gender, atrial fibrillation, age, and daytime hypocapnia; for OSA, age (women only) and obesity (men only) (84). Sleep apnea is also important to consider when there is frequent ventricular or atrial arrhythmias (84,88). Recent evidence suggests that CSR is an independent predictor of prognosis as well. In a report of 62 NYHA II–III heart failure patients, the cardiovascular mortality was significantly higher in those patients with an AHI >30 (50% vs. 26%) after a mean follow-up of 28 mo (89). In fact, the AHI was the best predictor of mortality in the multivariate analysis that considered demographic variables, Holter monitoring, exercise studies, echocardiography, and autonomic testing.

Definitive diagnosis of sleep apnea is made by in-laboratory overnight polysomnography, which involves the assessment of sleep with electroencephalogram (EEG), submental electromyogram (EMG), electrooculogram (EOG), thermistors, nasal pressure, electrocardiogram (EKG), anterior tibialis EMG, and pulse oximetry. The

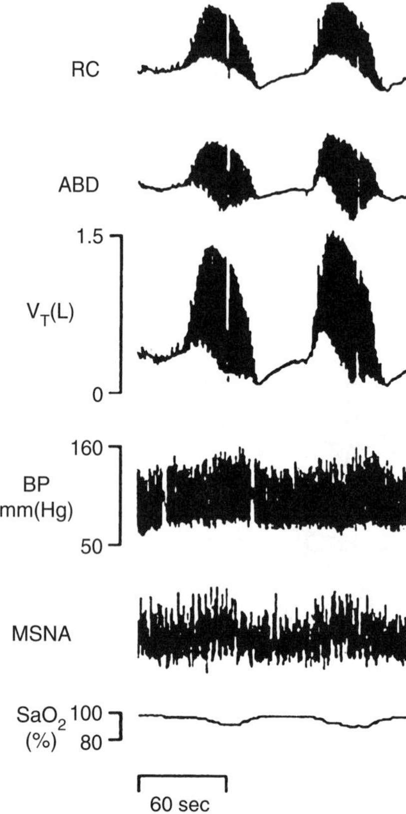

Figure 6 Cheyne–Stokes respirations in a patient with heart failure and atrial fibrillation. Central nature of apnea is indicated by absence of ribcage (RB) and abdominal (ABD) movement. Tidal volume [Vt (L)] waxes and wanes with dips in oxygen saturation (SaO2). Hemodynamic effects reflected in surges in blood pressure (BP) and muscle sympathetic nerve activity (MSNA). *Source*: From Ref. 63.

severity of sleep apnea is generally quantified by the apnea-hypopnea index (AHI), defined as the number of cessations or reductions in breathing per hour of sleep. Most investigators consider an AHI of greater than 10 to be clinically relevant but substantial variability exists in the literature (90).

Table 5 Prevalence of Sleep Disordered Breathing in Heart Failure

Study, year	No. of patients	Obstructive sleep apnea	Central sleep apnea
Lofaso, 1994	29	1 (5%)	8 (40%)
Chan, 1997	20	7 (35%)	4 (20%)
Javaheri, 1998	81	9 (11%)	32 (40%)
Staniforth	104	0	23 (22%)
Tremel, 1999	34	7 (20%)	21 (62%)
Sin, 1999	450	168 (37%)	148 (33%)
Lanfranchi, 2003	47	5 (11%)	17 (36%)
Villa, 2003	14	0	3 (21%)
Total	779	197 (25%)	256 (33%)

OSA has a well-established therapy, CPAP, that works by splinting open the collapsed pharyngeal airway and increasing functional residual capacity of the lung (65). In heart failure, the elimination of OSA appears to decrease transmural wall stress by preventing the dramatic negative intrapleural pressures that are consequence of pharyngeal obstruction and provides a nonpharmacologic form of afterload reduction (Fig. 7) (91). Furthermore, by preventing the hypoxias and hypercapnias, adrenergic stimulation can be prevented (92,93). There is also evidence that CPAP for OSA may also improve heart rate variability (94), reduce oxidative stress (95), and improve endothelial function (96). Some have likened the effects of CPAP in heart failure to nonpharmacologic beta blockade (64).

However, there are very few published randomized controlled studies that have examined the effects of CPAP for OSA in human heart failure. In one small study of 24 patients with NYHA II–III heart failure and OSA, CPAP for one month titrated to an average of 8.9 ± 0.7 cm H_20 for 6.2 ± 0.5 hr per night decreased systolic blood pressure, heart rate, and end systolic dimension as well as increased the ejection fraction by 9% (25.0 ± 2.8 to $33.8 \pm 2.4\%$) (97). In the only other randomized study, 54 patients were treated with CPAP for three months (98). Forty of the 54 completed the study and the mean EF was 35.5% with an average AHI of 28 (mild to moderate sleep apnea). Again, ejection fraction increased ($1.5 \pm 1.4\%$ vs. $5.0 \pm 1.0\%$, $p = 0.04$) with concomitant decreases in urinary norepinephrine excretion and improvements in quality of life. Interestingly, the improvements in quality of life did not include improvements in dyspnea or exercise capacity. Unfortunately, it is not likely that long-term effectiveness (ie. >3 mo) will be confirmed in future randomized data since there are strong ethical

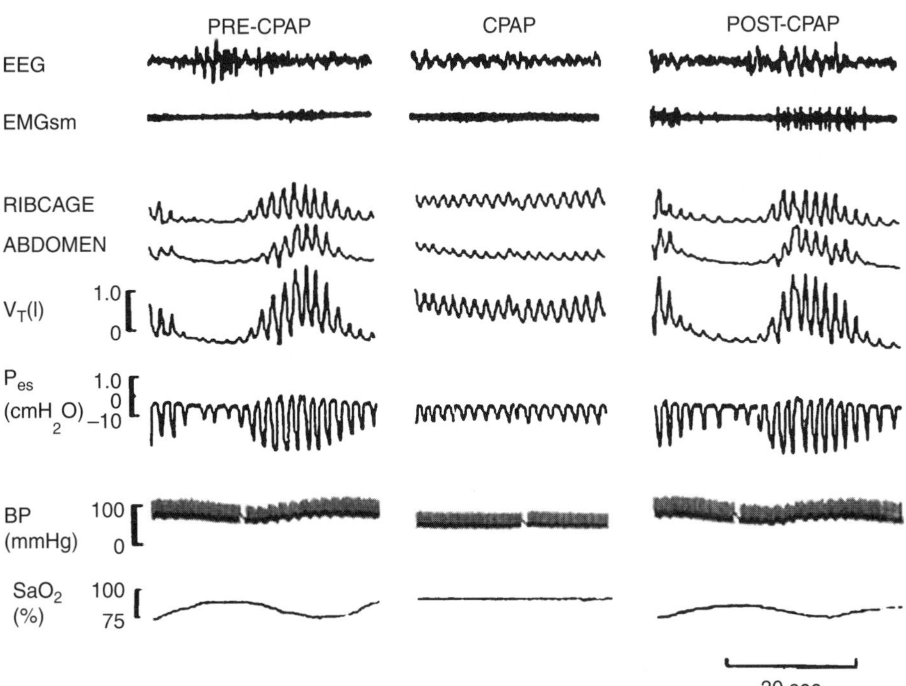

Figure 7 Effects of continuous positive airway pressure (CPAP) on obstructive sleep apnea in heart failure. CPAP prevents dips in oxygen saturation (SaO2), swings in intrapleural pressures (Pes), and lowers blood pressure (BP) while eliminating apneas (Vt) (*middle panel*). *Source*: From Ref. 64.

concerns to withholding CPAP for extended periods of time for the purposes of providing a control, "placebo" arm when CPAP is clinically indicated for the treatment of OSA in the absence of heart failure. However, some investigators point out that it is not clear CPAP has benefits in patients with OSA (without heart failure) in the absence of symptoms such as daytime somnolence (99).

CSR has no universally accepted form of therapy and there is still debate as to whether it needs treatment as all (63). The first strategy, however, is the optimization of medical management for heart failure, which should include establishment of euvolemia (100), RAS antagonists (101), and beta-blockers. In one small study, the ACE inhibitor, captopril, decreased apneic and desaturation episodes by 50% (101). However, care should be taken to avoid overdiuresis and contraction metabolic alkalosis that may exacerbate CSR (102). Maximal medical therapy should also include biventricular pacing in the appropriate patients since ventricular resynchronization alone may improve sleep disordered breathing (103). In a study of 24 patients with heart failure and left bundle branch block, cardiac resynchronization therapy decreased the AHI from19.2 $\pm$ 10.3 to 4.6 $\pm$ 4.4 ($p < 0.001$) and improved sleepiness in those with CSR. Theophylline (104) and nasal oxygen have also been tried with modest success in small studies. Oxygen, in particular, may improve CSR by increasing the difference between the baseline pCO2 and the pCO2 at the apneic threshold, decreasing the sympathetic stimulation of hypoxemias, and improving total body oxygen content (105). Limited studies have demonstrated that supplemental nasal oxygen in patients with heart failure improves sleep architecture, decreases CSR, decreases sympathetic activity, and improves exercise capacity (105). Again, longterm studies are lacking.

Similar to OSA, there are few randomized trials of CPAP for the treatment of CSR but there are plausible reasons to expect that CPAP would provide benefit. In an analogous manner to OSA, CPAP lowers transmural wall stress (91), decreases hypoxias and adrenergic stimulation (106), improves cardiac output (107), prevents venous return (108), and reduces arrhythmias (109). In 66 patients with heart failure (EF 20.2%, NHYA III/IV 38%), CPAP improved ejection fraction and decreased the risk of death and/or need for cardiac transplantation in those with CSR (110). In a larger recent randomized trial of CPAP for CSR in heart failure, the Canadian Continuous Positive Airway Pressure (CPAP) Trial for Congestive Heart Failure patients with CSA [CANPAP] (111), CSR was decreased (AHI decreased by 50%) and ejection fraction (LVEF 2.5%) and exercise capacity (six-minute walk, 20 meters) were improved. However, the trial, which studied NYHA II–IV heart failure patients with an EF $< 40\%$, was stopped due to the low event rate for the primary endpoint of all cause mortality and cardiac transplantation (112). Other substudy endpoints, such as effects of CPAP on cardiac arrhythmias, natriuretic peptides, and catecholamines, have yet to be reported. Final publication of this important trial is still pending but other studies are underway to test the hypothesis that CPAP can improve outcomes in heart failure.

It is important to note that many patients are unable to tolerate CPAP despite focused efforts to improve comfort and compliance. Many such patients therefore go untreated and consequently may suffer the sequelae of OSA. CPAP habituation clinics, knowledgeable respiratory therapists, patient education (113), and improved technologies to deliver CPAP (114) may all help to improve long-term compliance. Other strategies to treat OSA have included mandibular advancement devices, uvulopalatopharyngoplasty, and gastric reduction surgery but they have not been tested in heart failure populations.

Until more randomized clinical trial data is available, it is reasonable to screen for OSA when symptoms of sleep apnea (daytime somnolence, snoring, early morning headaches, late day fatigue) are present since treatment has proven effective in randomized studies of patients without heart failure. In heart failure patients without symptoms directly referable to sleep apnea syndromes, sleep studies and treatment could be considered when symptoms of heart failure persist despite optimal medical management. Special consideration to sleep apnea should also be entertained when difficult to control angina, arrhythmias, and hypertension complicate heart failure.

REFERENCES

1. Kantrowitz A. Experimental augmentation of coronary flow by retardation of the arterial pressure pulse. Surgery 1953; 34:678–687.
2. Kantrowitz A, Mc KW. The experimental use of the diaphragm as an auxiliary myocardium. Surg Forum 1958; 9:266–268.
3. Harken D. Counterpulsation: foundation and future, with a tribute to William Clifford Birtwell (1916–1978). In: Unger F, ed. Assisted Circulation. New York: Springer-Verlag, 1978:20–23.
4. Soroff HS, Giron F, Ruiz U, Birtwell WC, Hirsch LJ, Deterling RA, Jr. Physiologic support of heart action. N Engl J Med 1969; 280:693–704.
5. Clauss RH, Birtwell WC, Albertal G, et al. Assisted circulation I. The arterial counterpulsator. J Thorac Cardiovasc Surg 1961; 41:447–458.
6. Moulopoulos SD, Topaz SR, Kolff WJ. Extracorporeal assistance to the circulation and intraaortic balloon pumping. Trans Am Soc Artif Intern Organs 1962; 8:85–89.
7. Kantrowitz A, Tjonneland S, Freed PS, Phillips SJ, Butner AN, Sherman JL, Jr. Initial clinical experience with intraaortic balloon pumping in cardiogenic shock. JAMA 1968; 203:113–118.
8. Wolvek S. The evolution of the intra-aortic balloon: the datascope contribution. J Biomater Appl 1989; 3:527–543.
9. Antman EM, Anbe DT, Armstrong PW, et al. ACC/AHA guidelines for the management of patients with ST-elevation myocardial infarction: a report of the American College of Cardiology/American Heart Association Task Force on Practice Guidelines (Committee to Revise the 1999 Guidelines for the Management of Patients with Acute Myocardial Infarction). Circulation 2004; 110:588–636.
10. Mueller H, Ayres SM, Conklin EF, et al. The effects of intra-aortic counterpulsation on cardiac performance and metabolism in shock associated with acute myocardial infarction. J Clin Invest 1971; 50:1885–1900.
11. Kern MJ, Aguirre FV, Tatineni S, et al. Enhanced coronary blood flow velocity during intraaortic balloon counterpulsation in critically ill patients. J Am Coll Cardiol 1993; 21:359–368.
12. Leinbach RC, Buckley MJ, Austen WG, Petschek HE, Kantrowitz AR, Sanders CA. Effects of intra-aortic balloon pumping on coronary flow and metabolism in man. Circulation 1971; 43:I77–I81.
13. Schreuder JJ, Maisano F, Donelli A, et al. Beat-to-beat effects of intraaortic balloon pump timing on left ventricular performance in patients with low ejection fraction. Ann Thorac Surg 2005; 79:872–880.
14. Cheung AT, Savino JS, Weiss SJ. Beat-to-beat augmentation of left ventricular function by intraaortic counterpulsation. Anesthesiology 1996; 84:545–554.
15. Sakamoto T, Suzuki A, Kazama S, Komatsu S, Sasaki S, Shoji Y. Effects of timing on ventriculoarterial coupling and mechanical efficiency during intraaortic balloon pumping. Asaio J 1995; 41:M580–M583.
16. Kantrowitz A. Intraaortic balloon pumping in congestive heart failure. In: Hosenpud JaG BH, ed. Congestive Heart Failure. New York: Springer-Verlag, 1994:522–547.

17. Aroesty J. Intraaortic balloon counterpulsation and other circulatory assist devices. In: Baim DaG W, ed. Grossman's Cardiac Catheterization, Angiography, and Intervention. 6th ed. Philadelphia: Lippincott, Williams, and Wilkins, 2000:463–488.
18. Anderson RD, Ohman EM, Holmes DR, Jr, et al. Use of intraaortic balloon counterpulsation in patients presenting with cardiogenic shock: observations from the GUSTO-I Study. Global Utilization of Streptokinase and TPA for Occluded Coronary Arteries. J Am Coll Cardiol 1997; 30:708–715.
19. Scheidt S, Wilner G, Mueller H, et al. Intra-aortic balloon counterpulsation in cardiogenic shock. Report of a co-operative clinical trial. N Engl J Med 1973; 288:979–984.
20. Dunkman WB, Leinbach RC, Buckley MJ, et al. Clinical and hemodynamic results of intraaortic balloon pumping and surgery for cardiogenic shock. Circulation 1972; 46:465–477.
21. Torchiana DF, Hirsch G, Buckley MJ, et al. Intraaortic balloon pumping for cardiac support: trends in practice and outcome, 1968 to 1995. J Thorac Cardiovasc Surg 1997; 113:758–764; discussion 764–9.
22. Lieberman EB, Hutchins GM, Herskowitz A, Rose NR, Baughman KL. Clinicopathologic description of myocarditis. J Am Coll Cardiol 1991; 18:1617–1626.
23. Dembitsky WP, Moore CH, Holman WL, et al. Successful mechanical circulatory support for noncoronary shock. J Heart Lung Transplant 1992; 11:129–135.
24. Hagemeijer F, Laird JD, Haalebos MM, Hugenholtz PG. Effectiveness of intraaortic balloon pumping without cardiac surgery for patients with severe heart failure secondary to a recent myocardial infarction. Am J Cardiol 1977; 40:951–956.
25. Freed PS, Wasfie T, Zado B, Kantrowitz A. Intraaortic balloon pumping for prolonged circulatory support. Am J Cardiol 1988; 61:554–557.
26. O'Connell JB, Renlund DG, Robinson JA, et al. Effect of preoperative hemodynamic support on survival after cardiac transplantation. Circulation 1988; 78:III78–III82.
27. Oaks TE, Wisman CB, Pae WE, Pennock JL, Burg J, Pierce WS. Results of mechanical circulatory assistance before heart transplantation. J Heart Transplant 1989; 8:113–115.
28. Lazar JM, Ziady GM, Dummer SJ, Thompson M, Ruffner RJ. Outcome and complications of prolonged intraaortic balloon counterpulsation in cardiac patients. Am J Cardiol 1992; 69:955–958.
29. Birovljev S, Radovancevic B, Burnett CM, et al. Heart transplantation after mechanical circulatory support: four years' experience. J Heart Lung Transplant 1992; 11:240–245.
30. Ashar B, Turcotte LR. Analyses of longest IAB implant in human patient (327 days). Trans Am Soc Artif Intern Organs 1981; 27:372–379.
31. Acker M. Dynamic cardiomyoplasty and new prosthetic LV girdling devices. In: Fang JaC GS, ed. Surgical Management of Congestive Heart Failure. Totowa, NJ: Humana Press, 2005:225–238.
32. Trainini J, Cabrera Fischer EI, Barisani J, et al. Dynamic aortomyoplasty in treating end-stage heart failure. J Heart Lung Transplant 2002; 21:1068–1073.
33. Milson P. First Successful Implant of the Sunshine Heart Failure Device. Press Release May 9, 2005. From www.sunshineheart.com/news.
34. Soroff HS, Birtwell WC, Giron F, Collins JA, Deterling RA, Jr. Support of the systemic circulation and left ventricular assist by synchronous pulsation of extramural pressure. Surg Forum 1965; 16:148–150.
35. Giron F, Birtwell WC, Thrower WB, Soroff HS, Ruiz U, Deterling RA, Jr. A prosthetic left ventricle energized by an external replaceable actuator, and capable of intermittent or continuous pressure assist for the left ventricle. Surg Forum 1965; 16:146–148.
36. Ruiz U, Soroff HS, Birtwell WC, Deterling RA, Jr. External synchronous assisted circulation: experimental and clinical evaluation. Surg Forum 1968; 19:127–128.
37. Giron F, Birtwell WC, Soroff HS, Ruiz U, Collins JA, Deterling RA, Jr. Assisted circulation by synchronous pulsation of extramural pressure. Surgery 1966; 60:894–901.
38. Suresh K, Simandl S, Lawson WE, et al. Maximizing the hemodynamic benefit of enhanced external counterpulsation. Clin Cardiol 1998; 21:649–653.

39. Taguchi I, Ogawa K, Oida A, Abe S, Kaneko N, Sakio H. Comparison of hemodynamic effects of enhanced external counterpulsation and intra-aortic balloon pumping in patients with acute myocardial infarction. Am J Cardiol 2000; 86:1139–1141. A9.
40. Werner D, Schneider M, Weise M, Nonnast-Daniel B, Daniel WG. Pneumatic external counterpulsation: a new noninvasive method to improve organ perfusion. Am J Cardiol 1999; 84:950–952. A7–8.
41. Soroff HS, Cloutier CT, Birtwell WC, Begley LA, Messer JV. External counterpulsation. Management of cardiogenic shock after myocardial infarction. JAMA 1974; 229:1441–1450.
42. Soroff HS, Birtwell WC. Clinical evaluation in synchronous external counterpulsation in cardiogenic shock. J Cardiovasc Surg (Torino) 1973;752–756. Spec No.
43. Michaels AD, Accad M, Ports TA, Grossman W. Left ventricular systolic unloading and augmentation of intracoronary pressure and Doppler flow during enhanced external counterpulsation. Circulation 2002; 106:1237–1242.
44. Bonetti PO, Holmes DR, Jr, Lerman A, Barsness GW. Enhanced external counterpulsation for ischemic heart disease: what's behind the curtain? J Am Coll Cardiol 2003; 41:1918–1925.
45. Bonetti PO, Barsness GW, Keelan PC, et al. Enhanced external counterpulsation improves endothelial function in patients with symptomatic coronary artery disease. J Am Coll Cardiol 2003; 41:1761–1768.
46. Barsness GW. Enhanced external counterpulsation in unrevascularizable patients. Curr Interv Cardiol Rep 2001; 3:37–43.
47. Masuda D, Nohara K, Kataoka K, Hosokawa R, Kanbara N, Fujita M. Enhanced external counterpulsation promotes angiogenesis factors in patients with chronic stable angina (abstr). Circulation 2001; 104:II-445.
48. Lawson WE, Hui JC, Zheng ZS, et al. Improved exercise tolerance following enhanced external counterpulsation: cardiac or peripheral effect? Cardiology 1996; 87:271–275.
49. Michaels AD, Kennard ED, Kelsey SE, et al. Does higher diastolic augmentation predict clinical benefit from enhanced external counterpulsation?: Data from the International EECP Patient Registry (IEPR) Clin Cardiol 2001; 24:453–458.
50. Arora RR, Chou TM, Jain D, et al. The multicenter study of enhanced external counterpulsation (MUST-EECP): effect of EECP on exercise-induced myocardial ischemia and anginal episodes. J Am Coll Cardiol 1999; 33:1833–1840.
51. Michaels AD, Linnemeier G, Soran O, Kelsey SF, Kennard ED. Two-year outcomes after enhanced external counterpulsation for stable angina pectoris (from the International EECP Patient Registry [IEPR]). Am J Cardiol 2004; 93:461–464.
52. Amsterdam EA, Banas J, Criley JM, et al. Clinical assessment of external pressure circulatory assistance in acute myocardial infarction. Report of a cooperative clinical trial. Am J Cardiol 1980; 45:349–356.
53. Cohen LS, Mullins CB, Mitchell JH. Sequenced external counterpulsation and intraaortic balloon pumping in cardiogenic shock. Am J Cardiol 1973; 32:656–661.
54. Singh M, Holmes DR, Jr, Tajik AJ, Barsness GW. Noninvasive revascularization by enhanced external counterpulsation: a case study and literature review. Mayo Clin Proc 2000; 75:961–965.
55. Lakshmi MV, Kennard ED, Kelsey SF, Holubkov R, Michaels AD. Relation of the pattern of diastolic augmentation during a course of enhanced external counterpulsation (EECP) to clinical benefit (from the International EECP Patient Registry [IEPR]). Am J Cardiol 2002; 89:1303–1305.
56. Masuda D, Nohara R, Hirai T, et al. Enhanced external counterpulsation improved myocardial perfusion and coronary flow reserve in patients with chronic stable angina; evaluation by(13)N-ammonia positron emission tomography. Eur Heart J 2001; 22:1451–1458.
57. Urano H, Ikeda H, Ueno T, Matsumoto T, Murohara T, Imaizumi T. Enhanced external counterpulsation improves exercise tolerance, reduces exercise-induced myocardial ischemia and improves left ventricular diastolic filling in patients with coronary artery disease. J Am Coll Cardiol 2001; 37:93–99.

58. Gorscan J, Crawford L, Soran O. Improvement in left ventricular performance by enhanced external counterpulsation in patients with heart failure (abstr). J Am Coll Cardiol 2000; 35:230A.
59. Lawson WE, Silver MA, Hui JC, Kennard ED, Kelsey SF. Angina patients with diastolic versus systolic heart failure demonstrate comparable immediate and one-year benefit from enhanced external counterpulsation. J Card Fail 2005; 11:61–66.
60. Soran O, Fleishman B, Demarco T, et al. Enhanced external counterpulsation in patients with heart failure: a multicenter feasibility study. Congest Heart Fail 2002; 8:204–208 see also p. 227.
61. Feldman AM, Silver MA, Francis GS, De Lame PA, Parmley WW. Treating heart failure with enhanced external counterpulsation (EECP): design of the Prospective Evaluation of EECP in Heart Failure (PEECH) trial. J Card Fail 2005; 11:240–245.
62. Pembrey M. Observations on Cheyne-Stokes respiration. J Pathol Bacteriol 1908; 12:259–266.
63. Bradley TD, Floras JS. Sleep apnea and heart failure: part II: central sleep apnea. Circulation 2003; 107:1822–1826.
64. Bradley TD, Floras JS. Sleep apnea and heart failure: part I: obstructive sleep apnea. Circulation 2003; 107:1671–1678.
65. Malhotra A, White DP. Obstructive sleep apnoea. Lancet 2002; 360:237–245.
66. Shepard JW, Jr, Pevernagie DA, Stanson AW, Daniels BK, Sheedy PF. Effects of changes in central venous pressure on upper airway size in patients with obstructive sleep apnea. Am J Respir Crit Care Med 1996; 153:250–254.
67. Leung RS, Bradley TD. Sleep apnea and cardiovascular disease. Am J Respir Crit Care Med 2001; 164:2147–2165.
68. Narkiewicz K, Pesek CA, van de Borne PJ, Kato M, Somers VK. Enhanced sympathetic and ventilatory responses to central chemoreflex activation in heart failure. Circulation 1999; 100:262–267.
69. Naughton M, Benard D, Tam A, Rutherford R, Bradley TD. Role of hyperventilation in the pathogenesis of central sleep apneas in patients with congestive heart failure. Am Rev Respir Dis 1993; 148:330–338.
70. Hanly P, Zuberi N, Gray R. Pathogenesis of Cheyne-Stokes respiration in patients with congestive heart failure. Relationship to arterial PCO2. Chest 1993; 104:1079–1084.
71. Steens RD, Millar TW, Su X, et al. Effect of inhaled 3% CO2 on Cheyne-Stokes respiration in congestive heart failure. Sleep 1994; 17:61–68.
72. Naughton MT, Benard DC, Rutherford R, Bradley TD. Effect of continuous positive airway pressure on central sleep apnea and nocturnal PCO2 in heart failure. Am J Respir Crit Care Med 1994; 150:1598–1604.
73. Hanly PJ, Millar TW, Steljes DG, Baert R, Frais MA, Kryger MH. The effect of oxygen on respiration and sleep in patients with congestive heart failure. Ann Intern Med 1989; 111:777–782.
74. Shahar E, Whitney CW, Redline S, et al. Sleep-disordered breathing and cardiovascular disease: cross-sectional results of the Sleep Heart Health Study. Am J Respir Crit Care Med 2001; 163:19–25.
75. Portaluppi F, Provini F, Cortelli P, et al. Undiagnosed sleep-disordered breathing among male nondippers with essential hypertension. J Hypertens 1997; 15:1227–1233.
76. Sin DD, Fitzgerald F, Parker JD, et al. Relationship of systolic BP to obstructive sleep apnea in patients with heart failure. Chest 2003; 123:1536–1543.
77. Malone S, Liu PP, Holloway R, Rutherford R, Xie A, Bradley TD. Obstructive sleep apnoea in patients with dilated cardiomyopathy: effects of continuous positive airway pressure. Lancet 1991; 338:1480–1484.
78. Bradley TD, Hall MJ, Ando S, Floras JS. Hemodynamic effects of simulated obstructive apneas in humans with and without heart failure. Chest 2001; 119:1827–1835.
79. Kasper EK, Hruban RH, Baughman KL. Cardiomyopathy of obesity: a clinicopathologic evaluation of 43 obese patients with heart failure. Am J Cardiol 1992; 70:921–924.

80. Sforza E, Krieger J, Weitzenblum E, Apprill M, Lampert E, Ratamaharo J. Long-term effects of treatment with nasal continuous positive airway pressure on daytime lung function and pulmonary hemodynamics in patients with obstructive sleep apnea. Am Rev Respir Dis 1990; 141:866–870.
81. Weitzenblum E, Krieger J, Apprill M, et al. Daytime pulmonary hypertension in patients with obstructive sleep apnea syndrome. Am Rev Respir Dis 1988; 138:345–349.
82. Weitzenblum E. The effects of controlled oxygen therapy on ventricular function in patients with stable and decompensated cor pulmonale. Am Rev Respir Dis 1989; 139:285–286.
83. Fung JW, Li TS, Choy DK, et al. Severe obstructive sleep apnea is associated with left ventricular diastolic dysfunction. Chest 2002; 121:422–429.
84. Sin DD, Fitzgerald F, Parker JD, Newton G, Floras JS, Bradley TD. Risk factors for central and obstructive sleep apnea in 450 men and women with congestive heart failure. Am J Respir Crit Care Med 1999; 160:1101–1106.
85. Mansfield D, Kaye DM, Brunner La Rocca H, Solin P, Esler MD, Naughton MT. Raised sympathetic nerve activity in heart failure and central sleep apnea is due to heart failure severity. Circulation 2003; 107:1396–1400.
86. Lanfranchi PA, Somers VK, Braghiroli A, Corra U, Eleuteri E, Giannuzzi P. Central sleep apnea in left ventricular dysfunction: prevalence and implications for arrhythmic risk. Circulation 2003; 107:727–732.
87. Chan J, Sanderson J, Chan W, et al. Prevalence of sleep-disordered breathing in diastolic heart failure. Chest 1997; 111:1488–1493.
88. Javaheri S, Parker TJ, Liming JD, et al. Sleep apnea in 81 ambulatory male patients with stable heart failure. Types and their prevalences, consequences, and presentations. Circulation 1998; 97:2154–2159.
89. Lanfranchi PA, Braghiroli A, Bosimini E, et al. Prognostic value of nocturnal Cheyne-Stokes respiration in chronic heart failure. Circulation 1999; 99:1435–1440.
90. Sleep-related breathing disorders in adults: recommendations for syndrome definition and measurement techniques in clinical research. The Report of an American Academy of Sleep Medicine Task Force. Sleep 1999;22:667–689.
91. Naughton MT, Rahman MA, Hara K, Floras JS, Bradley TD. Effect of continuous positive airway pressure on intrathoracic and left ventricular transmural pressures in patients with congestive heart failure. Circulation 1995; 91:1725–1731.
92. Somers VK, Dyken ME, Clary MP, Abboud FM. Sympathetic neural mechanisms in obstructive sleep apnea. J Clin Invest 1995; 96:1897–1904.
93. Narkiewicz K, Kato M, Phillips BG, Pesek CA, Davison DE, Somers VK. Nocturnal continuous positive airway pressure decreases daytime sympathetic traffic in obstructive sleep apnea. Circulation 1999; 100:2332–2335.
94. Narkiewicz K, Montano N, Cogliati C, van de Borne PJ, Dyken ME, Somers VK. Altered cardiovascular variability in obstructive sleep apnea. Circulation 1998; 98:1071–1077.
95. Schulz R, Mahmoudi S, Hattar K, et al. Enhanced release of superoxide from polymorphonuclear neutrophils in obstructive sleep apnea. Impact of continuous positive airway pressure therapy. Am J Respir Crit Care Med 2000; 162:566–570.
96. Ip MS, Lam B, Chan LY, et al. Circulating nitric oxide is suppressed in obstructive sleep apnea and is reversed by nasal continuous positive airway pressure. Am J Respir Crit Care Med 2000; 162:2166–2171.
97. Kaneko Y, Floras JS, Usui K, et al. Cardiovascular effects of continuous positive airway pressure in patients with heart failure and obstructive sleep apnea. N Engl J Med 2003; 348:1233–1241.
98. Mansfield DR, Gollogly NC, Kaye DM, Richardson M, Bergin P, Naughton MT. Controlled trial of continuous positive airway pressure in obstructive sleep apnea and heart failure. Am J Respir Crit Care Med 2004; 169:361–366.
99. Barbe F, Mayoralas LR, Duran J, et al. Treatment with continuous positive airway pressure is not effective in patients with sleep apnea but no daytime sleepiness. a randomized, controlled trial. Ann Intern Med 2001; 134:1015–1023.

100. Solin P, Bergin P, Richardson M, Kaye DM, Walters EH, Naughton MT. Influence of pulmonary capillary wedge pressure on central apnea in heart failure. Circulation 1999; 99:1574–1579.
101. Walsh JT, Andrews R, Starling R, Cowley AJ, Johnston ID, Kinnear WJ. Effects of captopril and oxygen on sleep apnoea in patients with mild to moderate congestive cardiac failure. Br Heart J 1995; 73:237–241.
102. Bradley TD. Crossing the threshold: implications for central sleep apnea. Am J Respir Crit Care Med 2002; 165:1203–1204.
103. Sinha AM, Skobel EC, Breithardt OA, et al. Cardiac resynchronization therapy improves central sleep apnea and Cheyne-Stokes respiration in patients with chronic heart failure. J Am Coll Cardiol 2004; 44:68–71.
104. Sin DD, Bradley TD. Theophylline therapy for near-fatal Cheyne-Stokes respiration. Ann Intern Med 1999; 131:713–714 author reply.
105. Javaheri S. Pembrey's dream: the time has come for a long-term trial of nocturnal supplemental nasal oxygen to treat central sleep apnea in congestive heart failure. Chest 2003; 123:322–325.
106. Kaye DM, Mansfield D, Aggarwal A, Naughton MT, Esler MD. Acute effects of continuous positive airway pressure on cardiac sympathetic tone in congestive heart failure. Circulation 2001; 103:2336–2338.
107. Bradley TD, Holloway RM, McLaughlin PR, Ross BL, Walters J, Liu PP. Cardiac output response to continuous positive airway pressure in congestive heart failure. Am Rev Respir Dis 1992; 145:377–382.
108. Mehta S, Liu PP, Fitzgerald FS, Allidina YK, Douglas Bradley T. Effects of continuous positive airway pressure on cardiac volumes in patients with ischemic and dilated cardiomyopathy. Am J Respir Crit Care Med 2000; 161:128–134.
109. Javaheri S. Effects of continuous positive airway pressure on sleep apnea and ventricular irritability in patients with heart failure. Circulation 2000; 101:392–397.
110. Sin DD, Logan AG, Fitzgerald FS, Liu PP, Bradley TD. Effects of continuous positive airway pressure on cardiovascular outcomes in heart failure patients with and without Cheyne-Stokes respiration. Circulation 2000; 102:61–66.
111. Bradley TD, Logan AG, Floras JS. Rationale and design of the Canadian Continuous Positive Airway Pressure Trial for Congestive Heart Failure patients with Central Sleep Apnea—CANPAP. Can J Cardiol 2001; 17:677–684.
112. Bradley TD. CANPAP preliminary results. American College of Cardiology 2005. Orlando, FL.
113. Hoy CJ, Vennelle M, Kingshott RN, Engleman HM, Douglas NJ. Can intensive support improve continuous positive airway pressure use in patients with the sleep apnea/hypopnea syndrome? Am J Respir Crit Care Med 1999; 159:1096–1100.
114. Teschler H, Dohring J, Wang YM, Berthon-Jones M. Adaptive pressure support servo-ventilation: a novel treatment for Cheyne-Stokes respiration in heart failure. Am J Respir Crit Care Med 2001; 164:614–619.
115. www.vasomedical.com.

18
Revascularization

Prem S. Shekar and Gregory S. Couper
Division of Cardiac Surgery, Brigham and Women's Hospital, Harvard Medical School, Boston, Massachusetts, U.S.A.

INTRODUCTION AND EPIDEMIOLOGY OF ADVANCED ISCHEMIC HEART DISEASE

Congestive heart failure afflicts 2.3% of the U.S. population: 4.9 million people have the condition and 550,000 new cases are added every year. Its estimated cost for 2005 is 27.9 billion US dollars (1). Congestive heart failure has multiple etiologies but ischemic cardiomyopathy from coronary artery disease accounts for 75% of the patients. Twenty to twenty-five percent of heart failure patients have Class III or IV symptoms and 5%–10% have refractory symptoms. While over 80,000 patients have end stage heart disease, only 2000 transplants were performed in 1999 (2). Patients with advanced ischemic heart disease and heart failure may not be ideal candidates for heart transplantation since they are usually over 65 yr of age and have multiple co-morbidities that may exclude them. It becomes essential therefore to find other treatment modalities for advanced ischemic heart disease. Surgical revascularization is one of various options available to patients with advanced coronary artery disease. Surgical revascularization is a well-studied and recommended option for coronary disease but its role in patients with advanced heart disease is less well defined.

THE CONCEPTS OF NORMAL MYOCARDIUM, STUNNED HIBERNATING MYOCARDIUM, AND SCAR

Normal myocardium is cardiac muscle that is well perfused both at rest and exercise with normal metabolism and capable of generating the required contractile force. Myocardial stunning is defined as persistent cardiac dysfunction despite restoration of normal blood flow following a short period of ischemia (3). It is often seen in patients with acute coronary syndromes after reperfusion with thrombolysis or percutaneous coronary intervention (PCI). Normal contractile function returns in weeks to months. The contractile function of stunned myocardium can be restored by inotropes or an increase in extracellular sodium suggesting that the abnormality is unrelated to contractile proteins. Hibernating myocardium, on the other hand, describes a state of persistently impaired myocardial and left ventricular (LV) function at rest, due to chronically reduced coronary blood flow that can be partially or completely restored to normal if the myocardial oxygen supply demand relationship is favorably altered by improving blood flow or reducing oxygen demand (4). It is exquisitely regulated tissue successfully adapting its activity to the prevailing circumstances in a process of controlled active down-regulation (5). If the supply demand ratio is once again altered unfavorably, then infarction and necrosis occurs in this tissue. In contrast to myocardial stunning, hibernating myocardium is initially functional before proceeding to the structural phase that can be associated with a myriad of microscopic alterations in the contractile proteins, including loss of myofibrils, disorganization of the cytoskeleton and degeneration of the sarcoplasmic reticulum (6). This is probably related to changes in coronary microcirculation that could slowly improve, months after successful revascularization. Improvement is likely to be maximal and faster if intervention occurs before advanced structural changes have set in. Acute coronary occlusion without reperfusion or revascularization results in irreversible cell necrosis and myocardial infarction that eventually leads to a non-contractile fibrous scar in the ventricle.

CORONARY DISEASE, LEFT VENTRICULAR DYSFUNCTION, AND SURVIVAL

As described above, coronary artery disease can cause abnormalities in the contractile function of the heart related to different pathophysiological mechanisms. Stunning, hibernation and scar all produce impaired contraction of the cardiac muscle fibers that will result in impaired ventricular function and eventually the clinical syndrome of heart failure. There remains a complex interplay between these various components of myocardial dysfunction in patients with advanced ischemic heart disease. When the dyskinetic portion is more than 10% of the myocardial mass, ventricular remodeling begins and symptomatic heart failure will set in. It has been shown that when a myocardial infarction involves greater than 23% of the (LV) circumference, the ejection fraction (EF) drops below 45% resulting in a 3-yr mortality of 40%. Less extensive myocardial damage results in a 3-yr mortality of about 5% (7). This however did not depict the true risk in patients with hibernating myocardium. The 3-year mortality for patients with an EF $<43\%$ and no viable myocardium was 63%. That contrasts to a 13% mortality for similar patients with viable myocardium. This underlines the importance of ascertaining viability and early intervention in these patients to prevent irreversible changes and improve survival.

INVESTIGATIONAL MODALITIES

Electrocardiography (EKG)

While EKG remains a key test in the diagnosis of acute and chronic coronary syndromes, the findings may be variable and may not accurately identify the magnitude of the problem, and indeed, occasionally in a subset of patients with chronic coronary artery disease, it may even be normal. The EKG abnormalities can vary according to the duration, extent and location of the disease in addition to being affected by a multitude of other underlying abnormalities.

Exercise Stress Testing

This diagnostic modality is especially useful in patients with chest pain syndromes who have a moderate probability of coronary disease and a normal resting EKG. It has the greatest predictive value (90%) if typical chest discomfort occurs during exercise along with horizontal or downward sloping ST segment depression of 1 mm or more.

TESTS TO DETERMINE MYOCARDIAL VIABILITY

Myocardial viability means recoverable (with improvement of blood flow) myocardial tissue. This is of paramount significance to the current topic of discussion as it can affect outcomes. Nuclear cardiology techniques, stress echocardiography and cardiac magnetic resonance imaging (MRI) are some tests that can be used for this purpose.

Positron Emission Tomography (PET)

This may be the gold standard for determination of myocardial viability but availability of this technique has limited its use. The two components to this study involve determination of blood flow and viability of the muscle. The hypoperfused myocytes are metabolically more active and rely preferentially on glucose metabolism for energy. Hence the uptake of ^{18}F-deoxy glucose (FDG) by myocytes will mean viability (8). Normal myocardium has normal perfusion and metabolism while scar has decreased perfusion and metabolism. Hibernating myocardium will have decreased perfusion but normal metabolism. Studies have shown PET to be a good predictor for improvement in wall motion after revascularization (9).

Technetium Scintigraphy

This utilizes the technetium-based tracers ^{99m}Tc-sestamibi or ^{99m}Tc-tetrofosmin to assess myocardial viability. The distribution of these tracers is determined by perfusion and viability. Their widespread availability have made this a popular test for assessment of myocardial viability although its sensitivity and specificity are slightly lower than that of the PET scan at 81% and 60% respectively compared to the 90% and 70% of the FDG-PET (10).

Thallium Scintigraphy

This utilizes Thallium-201 as a tracer. Its patterns of distribution and redistribution help identify myocardial viability. Viable myocardium is an area of reduced uptake of the tracer at rest that fills in on the redistribution scan. Various inadequacies in this technique related to the redistribution phase, its inability to always differentiate between scar and hibernating myocardium and the need for reinjection and occasionally exercise make this a less desirable study especially when compared to the FDG-PET. It has been reported to have a sensitivity of 85% and specificity of 47% (8).

Dobutamine Stress Echocardiography

This test is based on the concept that stunned and hibernating myocardium are able to demonstrate an augmented contractile response when exposed to beta-adrenergic inotropes stimulation while scar tissue does not. This study involves the use of low dose dobutamine (<5 mcg/kg/min) and hypocontractile but viable myocardium is stimulated to contract but not at an inappropriately high level of oxygen demand. The sensitivity and specificity for this test are about 70% and 90% respectively indicating that it is less sensitive but more specific than the tests discussed above (11). The attractiveness of this investigation is its low cost and widespread availability. The issues revolving around poor acoustic windows due to obesity and lung disease could be resolved with the development of transesophageal dobutamine stress echocardiography.

Cardiac MRI

Cardiac MRI is a rapidly emerging non-invasive tool especially in the diagnosis and surgical management of heart disease. Myocardial blood flow is measured by quantifying the gadolinium-based contrast. Delayed hyperenhancement with gadolinium identifies areas of myocardial scar. The more transmural the hyperenhancement, the less likely it is to recover with revascularization. Areas of transmural hyperenhancement could be identified as potential areas of resection for surgical restoration of a remodeled ventricle (12). One study showed that 78% of non-hyperenhancing dysfunctional segments improved after revascularization (13). Cardiac MRI is gradually becoming a good tool to assess myocardial viability but constraints remain. Most important of these are the high cost, the problem of patients with pacemakers and defibrillators, and those who develop claustrophobic symptoms.

Cardiac Catheterization, Coronary Angiography, and Intravascular Ultrasound

All patients with coronary artery disease will need coronary angiography to determine the exact location of the coronary occlusions. Among patients with chronic stable angina who undergo angiography, 75% will have some from of critical one, two or three vessel coronary artery disease, while 5%–10% will have left main disease and 15% will have non-critical disease. The coronary angiogram serves as a tool that not only identifies lesions but also identifies potential locations for bypass grafting on the distal vessel. There are particular details that portend a hazard for the surgeon attempting to revascularize a patient. Diffusely calcified coronary ateries disease with multiple blocks along the entire length of the vessel could make bypass potentially difficult and suggest the need for an endarterectomy. The revascularization of such a vessel can be deemed as less than adequate and it is known that endarterectomized vessels do not have as good a long-term patency as conventional bypass (14). When diffusely calcified, coronary arteries may truly be unsuitable for bypass grafting. Calcification of the ascending aorta may be present in these cases that could dictate the conduct of the operation. Chronic total occlusions with no collateral refill of the distal vessel may suggest complete fibrotic occlusion of the vessel and therefore its unsuitability for bypass. Sometimes these patients would have had multiple angiograms in the past with or without percutaneous interventions and these may reveal the vessel that is now not seen. If the myocardium in this region is viable, experience suggests that a patent vessel may be found at surgery. Newer diagnostic modalities like the multidetector helical CT scans could help ascertain whether these totally occluded vessels are distally patent. Indeed, these advanced computed tomograms may eventually replace the invasive coronary arteriography completely.

Cardiac catheterization, although not always performed with coronary arteriography, is an important adjunct, especially in patients with advanced heart disease.

Important information gleaned from this test are the degree and chronicity of LV dysfunction as evidenced by the development of pulmonary hypertension and right ventricular failure. An assessment of the reversibility of the pulmonary hypertension could also be made. Patients with severe fixed pulmonary hypertension may fare poorly after surgical revascularization (15). Various valve gradients and valve orifice areas could be measured as these are often underestimated with non-invasive testing in patients with severe ventricular dysfunction.

Intravascular ultrasound is an infrequently used but valuable tool during coronary arteriography that can be used to assess cross-sectional dimensions and coronary artery structure and pathology especially when angiography provides equivocal findings like occult left main disease or ostial coronary lesion.

SELECTION OF PATIENTS FOR SURGICAL REVASCULARIZATION

Only 10% of patients on the waiting list will be transplanted. Recent studies indicate that 50% of patients with advanced ischemic heart disease and (LV) dysfunction will have hibernating myocardium (16). High-risk coronary artery bypass surgery (CABG) should be considered in all patients who have severe coronary artery disease and viable myocardium. All patients with known coronary artery disease and LV dysfunction should have tests for myocardial viability performed even if their predominant symptom is shortness of breath and they have mild or no angina. Segmental and global ventricular function is likely to improve after revascularization if viability studies demonstrate significant viable myocardium. In ischemic patients with heart failure and little or no angina, the presence of >25% viability and good target vessels indicated potential benefit from surgical revascularization (17).

Despite their potential candidacy for CABG from the standpoint of target vessels and a viable myocardium, a thorough assessment of the patient as a whole must be performed in order to ascertain operability. Patients with such severe coronary disease and LV dysfunction usually have other co-morbid conditions as well. They could have sequelae of severe peripheral vascular disease with carotid, mesenteric and other axial arterial involvement, sequelae of diabetes with renal impairment, sequelae of long-term smoking with severe chronic obstructive airway disease, previous cerebrovascular accidents and hepatic dysfunction. All these conditions in various combinations could make the overall mortality risk higher and in some cases prohibitive. Although, no recommendation is made to avoid surgery in these patients, only accurate analysis will allow better informed consent for an already high-risk operation. In addition, evaluation of the cardiorespiratory system for other sequelae of LV dysfunction such as pulmonary hypertension and right ventricular failure could determine the overall ability of the heart to tolerate this extensive procedure. Most of these patients usually need multiple additional procedures as well, the commonest being mitral valve reconstruction and/or LV restoration.

PRINCIPLES OF SURGICAL REVASCULARIZATION

It must be realized that the outcome of surgical revascularization in patients with advanced ischemic heart disease and heart failure is not determined by the number of bypass grafts performed but by targeted perfusion of hibernating but viable myocardium. It is not useful in revascularising vessels that supply non-viable myocardium. Although Westaby summarized the ethos for surgery in this high-risk population as simplicity, safety and speed (2), this should not be interpreted as minimalistic approach. One should perform all components to the operation identified as necessary during the preoperative evaluation. The patient that obviously needs an anterior wall reconstruction for a dyskinetic scar and mitral valve reconstruction is not going to get significant benefit from CABG alone in the effort to keep the operation simple. On the other hand, preoperative evaluation in these difficult patients should be complete and all interventions required should be identified and completed at surgery. This is the essence of a simple, safe and effective operation. A surgical procedure in these patients should never be a "fishing expedition" where new things are discovered and managed as the operation goes along. This is usually associated with poor outcomes.

TECHNICAL CONSIDERATIONS

Conduits for Surgical Revascularization, Grafting Techniques and Endarterectomy

A variety of conduits are available for CABG and they all have their potential advantages and disadvantages. Broadly, they can be divided into:

1. Venous conduits
2. Arterial conduits
3. Prosthetic conduits

Venous conduits have been used for CABG for many years. The commonly used venous conduit is the greater saphenous vein that was historically harvested through a linear incision along the medial side of the thigh but lately the development of endoscopic vein harvest techniques have helped minimize the potential leg complications of the open harvest techniques (18). The other venous conduits available are lesser saphenous, cephalic or basilic veins. Cryopreserved homograft veins may also be used as a last resort. Of the various venous conduits, the greater saphenous vein remains the conduit of choice with patency rates the best among the venous conduits. However concern still remains, as it is well known that 50% of vein grafts are occluded at 10 yr and 20%–40% have substantial stenosis in them (19). The patency rates of the other venous conduits are even lower with the worst patency rates of the cryopreserved homograft veins.

The left internal mammary arterial (LIMA) conduit had a significant impact on CABG surgery. Although it was the first conduit used for revascularization of the ventricular myocardium by Vineberg and later by Kolessov, its wide spread use occurred much later. The LIMA graft is usually placed on the left anterior descending artery (LAD) and it seems to have excellent long-term patency rates approaching 83% at 10 years. It also appears to be immune to the development of neointimal hyperplasia and has preserved endothelial function (20,21). The radial artery used as a free graft and the right internal mammary artery used as a free or in-situ graft come in as the second choice arterial conduits. The radial artery initially fell out of favor due to reports of spasm and high early occlusion rates. However, recent data suggest that it may have better long-term patency rates when compared to the venous grafts with minimal handling and judicious use of calcium-channel blockade (22). The radial artery is harvested through a linear incision in the non-dominant forearm with a balanced circulation in the hand demonstrated by a preoperative and/or intraoperative Allen's test. Endoscopic radial arterial harvest is now possible. The right internal mammary arterial graft when used as a free or in-situ (23) graft has lower patency rates than the LIMA graft but higher than venous conduits. Their widespread use has been restricted due to the higher incidence of postoperative wound and respiratory complications with bilateral mammary arterial harvest and increased operative times and dissection involved. Other infrequently used conduits are the gastroepiploic, inferior epigastric and inferior mesenteric arteries.

The other prosthetic conduits available for last resort use are the bovine IMA, Dacron and PTFE grafts that have poor intermediate term patency rates (19).

The various options for grafting include direct end (of conduit) to side (of coronary artery) technique or sequential bypass technique where multiple side to side bypasses are performed using a single conduit. The direct bypass technique is the time-honored method but each conduit will have to be separately anastomosed to the aorta or other vessel (innominate, subclavian or mammary arteries) for inflow. This may be a limiting factor in patients with short or diseased aortas and in reoperations. The sequential anastomosis is a solution to this issue where a single inflow could serve multiple distal anastomoses. The proponents of the sequential technique claim that this involves less manipulation of the ascending aorta with consequently lesser incidence of embolic events and increased graft patency rates related to increased velocity of blood flow from the supply of a larger vascular bed (24). The detractors question the wisdom of supplying a large portion of the myocardium from a single inflow.

Endarterectomy of the coronary arteries is now becoming reasonably commonplace in modern day CABG with diffuse coronary artery disease. This involves the coring out of the subintimal lipid deposit along the entire length of the involved coronary artery followed by bypass grafting. This exposes the media and consequently an increased risk of early graft closure. Endarterectomies are associated with increased complication rates like myocardial infarction and cardiac dysfunction. The key principles of endarterectomy are entire removal of the atheromatous plaque from the vessel especially in the distal segment, washout of debris from the coronary circuit with retrograde cardioplegia and aggressive long-term multi-drug anti-platelet therapy (25).

On-Pump, Off-Pump, and Other Options

Various options exist for CABG. These include the traditional on-pump CABG, the newer off-pump CABG and the most recent minimally invasive direct coronary artery bypass (MIDCAB) or the port access CABG or the totally endoscopic CABG (TECAB) among others. For purposes of this discussion, we will focus on the first two most commonly used techniques.

On-Pump CABG: The Management of Cardiopulmonary Bypass (CPB) and Myocardial Protection

The performance of coronary bypass grafting on an arrested heart with the use of CPB is the oldest and time-honored technique. The use of CPB involves the placement of cannulae in the ascending aorta and the right atrium. The oxygenation is achieved with the use of a membrane oxygenator and the blood is then pumped back using roller head pumps providing a continuous flow. This interface of blood with artificial surfaces and the change of pulsatile to continuous flow cause a systemic inflammatory response. The placement of a cannula in the ascending aorta and the performance of proximal anastomoses have been documented to increase cerebral atheroembolic events (26). However, with recent advances in imaging techniques with the epiaortic ultrasound and the development of the single clamp technique as well as proximal anastomotic devices, the incidence of atheroembolic complications have been markedly reduced (27–29). Recent studies indicate that on-pump techniques for CABG may provide a higher three-year survival and higher freedom from death or revascularization (30). While historically cardiac surgery on bypass was performed with moderate to deep hypothermia, currents trends are the use of mild hypothermia or tepid CPB with little or no adverse effects (31).

Although the safe institution of CPB is one aspect of on-pump CABG, the other more important aspect is one of myocardial protection. In order to perform the bypass in a still and bloodless field, the heart needs to be arrested and flaccid. This involves the placement of a clamp on the ascending aorta between the coronaries and the systemic circulation (proximal to the innominate artery) and selective perfusion of the coronary arteries with cardioplegia. Although numerous cardioplegia solutions have been developed, the corner stone remains the delivery of high dose potassium to the heart to achieve diastolic arrest. Crystalloid cardioplegia was in vogue during the early days of development of cardiac surgery but it has now been completely replaced by blood cardioplegia as blood is a more physiologic carrier medium with excellent buffering properties (32). Although the oxygen demand of the flaccid myocardium is extremely small, it is still quite important as these are metabolically active cells that need to be replenished from time to time. Cardioplegia has traditionally been delivered antegrade through the aortic root into the coronary arteries. In patients with coronary occlusions, this could lead to malperfusion of myocardium that is perfused by a coronary artery with high-grade stenosis. Retrograde cardioplegia was developed to overcome this disadvantage. A flexible catheter is inserted into the coronary sinus and blood cardioplegia is delivered at lower pressure into the coronary venous system. This venous system being valve-free will allow retrograde perfusion of the capillary bed and more uniform distribution of the cardioplegia. However, concern still exists about the protection of the right ventricle afforded by the retrograde cardioplegia (33). The current practice seems to favor the delivery of both antegrade and retrograde cardioplegia in all patients with dysfunctional ventricles. Although cold blood cardioplegia is still the norm, various surgeons have moved to warm blood cardioplegia. While the dose and frequency still remains a matter of personal choice, one could safely say that in an average adult person, the delivery of 1000cc of cold blood cardioplegia initially followed by 500cc through either route every 20–30 min affords adequate myocardial protection. Warm blood cardioplegia may require more frequent delivery (every 10 min) or continuous infusion (34). Various other combinations like terminal warm blood cardioplegia ("hot-shot") and substrate-enriched cardioplegia have been tried with benefit but have not achieved wide application due to the potential complexities. Topical cooling with cold saline or slush, once used quite frequently, has less application due to improved cardioplegia techniques as well as possible complications like phrenic nerve palsy (35).

Various studies have documented good results with on-pump CABG performed on patients with LV dysfunction with the operative mortality rates around 3–4% and a >80% 3-year survival rate (36–38).

Off-Pump CABG

This concept was developed to avoid the potential disadvantages of the systemic inflammatory response syndrome generated by the use of CPB and the atheroembolic complications of aortic cross clamping. Furthermore, creation of more global ischemia could potentially worsen the already poorly functioning ventricle.

This procedure has technical considerations of its own like the necessity to elevate, tilt, retract and compress the heart to facilitate coronary anastomosis. There is also the need to temporarily occlude the vessel to perform the bypass itself. Although various exposure and stabilizing devices have been developed to ensure minimal hemodynamic instability during these maneuvers, the dysfunctional ventricle does not always tolerate this well. It is still uncertain whether the group of patients with ischemic cardiomyopathy are better served by on or off pump CABG. While off-pump CABG is feasible, studies have not consistently demonstrated any statistically significant lower mortality rates (39–41). Off-pump CABG has been shown to have reduced transfusion requirements and lower cardiac enzyme leak but they may be associated with less complete revascularization than the on-pump group (42).

In summary, it would be prudent to say that the recommended operation for patients with advanced ischemic heart disease and LV dysfunction is an on-pump CABG with LIMA to the LAD and saphenous vein graft to the other coronaries. Individual practices and unique patient situations can always dictate alternate courses of action.

Reoperations

It is not uncommon to find patients with ischemic cardiomyopathy who have had previous cardiac surgery. More often than not, they have had previous CABG. This could be due to progression of disease in the native circulation and/or development of graft disease. A thorough preoperative evaluation is paramount. It is important to identify areas of viable myocardium and the ability to revascularize these areas. Identification of patent, patent but diseased and occluded grafts along with diseased or occluded native coronaries with or without collaterals will help guide the course of the reoperations. While the presence of graftable vessels in the areas of viable myocardium would suggest good response from CABG, areas of viable myocardium without bypassable arteries would be suitable for other revascularization strategies like transmyocardial laser. The reooperative approach to CABG in ischemic cardiomyopathy is similar to the first time approach. The recommended choice would still be on-pump CABG with LIMA and saphenous vein grafting. Issues with conduit availability due to previous usage or other disease states could lead to alternate conduit use and the presence of mediastinal adhesions or graft/cardiac chamber proximity to the posterior sternal table may dictate alternate CPB strategies. The technical complexities of reoperation CABG, in addition to the above, revolve around dissection of diseased grafts, prevention of coronary atheroembolic with consequent myocardial damage and location of the coronaries identified for bypass. Reoperative CABG remains a high-risk operation.

CABG, PCI, OR MEDICAL MANAGEMENT IN ISCHEMIC CARDIOMYOPATHY

The AWESOME trial indicated that the inpatient mortality was higher at 4% for CABG compared to 1% for PCI. However the gap starts to narrow with 30 day mortality being 5% and 3% respectively and the 3 yr survival being 79% and 80% respectively. However, the PCI group had less freedom from angina in this study (43).

A study by Toda et al. (44) showed that CABG achieved more complete revascularization, had improved cardiac event free survival at 3 yr (52% vs. 25%) and improvement in EF. There was no survival advantage noticed at 3 yr.

Caines et al. (45), in their analysis, concluded that there is a survival advantage with CABG over PCI or medical management. CABG offers more complete revascularization, freedom from angina at the cost of increased periprocedural morbidity and mortality. PCI is associated with increased rates of target vessel revascularization and is more cost-effective in the short-term but not in the long-term due to the need for multiple re-interventions.

The CASS study (46) clearly demonstrated a survival advantage for all patients especially those with ventricular dysfunction and severe three-vessel disease with CABG when compared to medial therapy (79% vs. 61% at 10 yr).

THE BENEFITS OF CABG IN LV DYSFUNCTION—WHO AND WHEN

Clearly the patients that will derive the greatest benefit from surgical revascularization are those that have discrete lesions in relatively good caliber coronary arteries and a large amount of dysfunctional yet viable hibernating myocardium. The benefits are certain irrespective of the methods and conduits used. Issues such as diffuse or calcific coronary disease will influence outcomes despite the presence of viable myocardium due to the need for more complex surgical interventions as will reoperations and major co-morbid states. Patients with large amounts of scar and little or no viable myocardium will gain little or no benefit from CABG. These patients will be better served by assist devices and/or transplantation.

While some patients may see benefit from revascularization within days of the procedure, most patients will take weeks or months to receive obvious benefit. This is the time taken by the hibernating myocardium to recover and redevelop cellular integrity with restored perfusion. Debates continue about the best procedure available—PCI with drug eluting stents or CABG. It is clear that medical therapy has little or no role. Most studies to date have favored CABG over PCI.

REFERENCES

1. http://www.americanheart.org/downloadable/heart/1105390918119HDSStats2005Update.pdf. Accessed 06/14/2005.
2. Westaby S. Coronary revascularization in ischemic cardiomyopathy. Surg Clin N Am 2004; 84:179–199.
3. Bonow RO. The hibernating myocardium: implications for management of congestive heart failure. Am J Cardiol 1995; 75:17A–25A.
4. Rahimtoola SH. The hibernating myocardium. Am Heart J 1989; 117:211–221.
5. Hearse DJ, Bolli R. Reperfusion induced injury: manifestations, mechanisms, and clinical relevance. Cardiovasc Res 1992; 26:101–108.
6. Schwarz ER, Schaper J, vom Dahl J, et al. Myocyte degeneration and cell death in hibernating human myocardium. J Am Coll Cardiol 1996; 27:1577–1585.
7. Yoshida K, Gould KL. Quantitative relation of myocardial infarct size and myocardial viability by positron emission tomography to left ventricular ejection fraction and 3-year mortality with and without revascularization. J Am Coll Cardiol 1993; 22:984–997.
8. Bax JJ, Wijns W, Cornel JH, Visser FC, Boersma E, Fioretti PM. Accuracy of currently available techniques for prediction of functional recovery after revascularization in patients with left ventricular dysfunction due to chronic coronary artery disease: comparison of pooled data. J Am Coll Cardiol 1997; 30:1451–1460.
9. Di Carli MF, Hachamovitch R, Berman DS. The art and science of predicting post revascularization improvement in left ventricular (LV) function in patients with severely depressed LV function. J Am Coll Cardiol 2002; 40:1744–1747.

10. Khabbaz KR, DeNofrio D, Kazimi M, Carpino PA. Revascularization options for ischemic cardiomyopathy: on-pump and off-pump coronary artery bypass surgery. Cardiology 2004; 101:29–36.
11. Cheitlin MD, Armstrong WF, Aurigemma GP, et al. ACC; AHA; ASE. ACC/AHA/ASE 2003 Guideline update for the clinical application of echocardiography: summary article. A report of the American college of cardiology/American heart association task force on practice guidelines (ACC/AHA/ASE committee to update the 1997 guidelines for the clinical application of echocardiography). J Am Soc Echocardiogr 2003; 16:1091–1110.
12. Dor V, Sabatier M, Montiglio F, Civaia F, Donato MD. Endoventricular patch reconstruction of ischemic failing ventricle. A single center with 20 years experience. Advantages of magnetic resonance imaging assessment. Heart Fail Rev 2005; 9:269–286.
13. Kim RJ, Wu E, Rafael A, et al. The use of contrast-enhanced magnetic resonance imaging to identify reversible myocardial dysfunction. N Engl J Med 2000; 343:1445–1453.
14. Abrahamov D, Tamaris M, Guru V, et al. Clinical results of endarterectomy of the right and left anterior descending coronary arteries. J Card Surg 1999; 14:16–25.
15. Mitropoulos FA, Elefteriades JA. Myocardial revascularization as a therapeutic strategy in the patient with advanced ventricular dysfunction. Heart Fail Rev 2001; 6:163–175.
16. Tjan TD, Kondruweit M, Scheld HH, et al. The bad ventricle—revascularization versus transplantation. Thorac Cardiovasc Surg 2000; 48:9–14.
17. Mickleborough LL, Maruyama H, Takagi Y, Mohamed S, Sun Z, Ebisuzaki L. Results of revascularization in patients with severe left ventricular dysfunction. Circulation 1995; 92:II73–II79.
18. Kiaii B, Moon BC, Massel D, et al. A prospective randomized trial of endoscopic versus conventional harvesting of the saphenous vein in coronary artery bypass surgery. J Thorac Cardiovasc Surg 2002; 123:204–212.
19. Eagle KA, Guyton RA, Davidoff R, et al. ACC/AHA Guidelines for coronary artery bypass graft surgery: a report of the American College of Cardiology/American Heart Association Task Force on Practice Guidelines (Committee to revise the 1991 Guidelines for coronary artery bypass graft surgery). American College of Cardiology/American Heart Association. J Am Coll Cardiol 1999; 34:1262–1347.
20. Loop FD. Internal-thoracic-artery grafts. Biologically better coronary arteries. N Engl J Med 1996; 334:263–265.
21. Amoroso G, Tio RA, Mariani MA, et al. Functional integrity and aging of the left internal thoracic artery after coronary artery bypass surgery. J Thorac Cardiovasc Surg 2000; 120:313–318.
22. Tatoulis J, Royse AG, Buxton BF, et al. The radial artery in coronary surgery: a 5-year experience—clinical and angiographic results. Ann Thorac Surg 2002; 73:143–148.
23. Shah PJ, Bui K, Blackmore S, et al. Has the in situ right internal thoracic artery been overlooked? An angiographic study of the radial artery, internal thoracic arteries and saphenous vein graft patencies in symptomatic patients Eur J Cardiothorac Surg 2005; 27:870–875.
24. Christenson JT, Simonet F, Schmuziger M. Sequential vein bypass grafting: tactics and long-term results. Cardiovasc Surg 1998; 6:389–397.
25. Byrne JG, Karavas AN, Gudbjartson T, et al. Left anterior descending coronary endarterectomy: early and late results in 196 consecutive patients. Ann Thorac Surg 2004; 78:867–873 discussion 873–4.
26. Kapetanakis EI, Stamou SC, Dullum MK, et al. The impact of aortic manipulation on neurologic outcomes after coronary artery bypass surgery: a risk-adjusted study. Ann Thorac Surg 2004; 78:1564–1571.
27. Hogue CW, Jr, Sundt TM, 3rd, Goldberg M, Barner H, Davila-Roman VG. Neurological complications of cardiac surgery: the need for new paradigms in prevention and treatment. Semin Thorac Cardiovasc Surg 1999; 11:105–115.
28. Aranki SF, Sullivan TE, Cohn LH. The effect of the single aortic cross-clamp technique on cardiac and cerebral complications during coronary bypass surgery. J Card Surg 1995; 10:498–502.

29. Akpinar B, Guden M, Sagbas E, Sanisoglu I, Ergenoglu MU, Turkoglu C. Clinical experience with the Novare Enclose II manual proximal anastomotic device during off-pump coronary artery surgery. Eur J Cardiothorac Surg 2005; 27:1070–1073.
30. Racz MJ, Hannan EL, Isom OW, et al. A comparison of short- and long-term outcomes after off-pump and on-pump coronary artery bypass graft surgery with sternotomy. J Am Coll Cardiol. 2004 February 18;43:557–564.
31. Ohata T, Sawa Y, Kadoba K, Masai T, Ichikawa H, Matsuda H. Effect of cardiopulmonary bypass under tepid temperature on inflammatory reactions. Ann Thorac Surg 1997; 64:124–128.
32. Cohen G, Borger MA, Weisel RD, Rao V. Intraoperative myocardial protection: current trends and future perspectives. Ann Thorac Surg 1999; 68:1995–2001.
33. Allen BS, Winkelmann JW, Hanafy H, et al. Retrograde cardioplegia does not adequately perfuse the right ventricle. J Thorac Cardiovasc Surg 1995; 109:1116–1126.
34. Isomura T, Hisatomi K, Sato T, Hayashida N, Ohishi K. Interrupted warm blood cardioplegia for coronary artery bypass grafting. Eur J Cardiothorac Surg 1995; 9:133–138.
35. Canbaz S, Turgut N, Halici U, Balci K, Ege T, Duran E. Electrophysiological evaluation of phrenic nerve injury during cardiac surgery—a prospective, controlled, clinical study. BMC Surg 2004; 4:2.
36. Elefteriades JA, Morales DL, Gradel C, Tollis G, Jr., Levi E, Zaret BL. Results of coronary artery bypass grafting by a single surgeon in patients with left ventricular ejection fractions < or =30%. Am J Cardiol 1997; 79:1573–1578.
37. Kron IL, Flanagan TL, Blackbourne LH, Schroeder RA, Nolan SP. Coronary revascularization rather than cardiac transplantation for chronic ischemic cardiomyopathy. Ann Surg 1989; 210:348–352.
38. Mickleborough LL, Carson S, Tamariz M, Ivanov J. Results of revascularization in patients with severe left ventricular dysfunction. J Thorac Cardiovasc Surg 2000; 119:550–557.
39. Arom KV, Flavin TF, Emery RW, Kshettry VR, Petersen RJ, Janey PA. Is low ejection fraction safe for off-pump coronary bypass operation? Ann Thorac Surg 2000; 70:1021–1025.
40. Meharwal ZS, Trehan N. Off-pump coronary artery bypass grafting in patients with left ventricular dysfunction. Heart Surg Forum 2002; 5:41–45.
41. Shennib H, Endo M, Benhamed O, Morin JF. Surgical revascularization in patients with poor left ventricular function: on- or off-pump? Ann Thorac Surg 2002; 74:S1344–S1347.
42. Kleisli T, Cheng W, Jacobs MJ, et al. In the current era, complete revascularization improves survival after coronary artery bypass surgery. J Thorac Cardiovasc Surg 2005; 129:1283–1291.
43. Morrison DA, Sethi G, Sacks J, et al. Angina With Extremely Serious Operative Mortality Evaluation (AWESOME). Percutaneous coronary intervention versus coronary artery bypass graft surgery for patients with medically refractory myocardial ischemia and risk factors for adverse outcomes with bypass: a multicenter, randomized trial. Investigators of the department of veterans affairs cooperative study #385, the Angina With Extremely Serious Operative Mortality Evaluation (AWESOME). J Am Coll Cardiol 2001; 38:143–149.
44. Toda K, Mackenzie K, Mehra MR, et al. Revascularization in severe ventricular dysfunction (15%<OR=LVEF<OR=30%): a comparison of bypass grafting and percutaneous intervention. Ann Thorac Surg 2002; 74:2082–2087.
45. Caines AE, Massad MG, Kpodonu J, Rebeiz AG, Evans A, Geha AS. Outcomes of coronary artery bypass grafting versus percutaneous coronary intervention and medical therapy for multivessel disease with and without left ventricular dysfunction. Cardiology 2004; 101:21–28.
46. Alderman EL, Bourassa MG, Cohen LS, et al. Ten-year follow-up of survival and myocardial infarction in the randomized Coronary Artery Surgery Study. Circulation 1990; 82:1629–1646.

19
Valvular Surgery in Cardiomyopathy

Frederick Y. Chen and Lawrence H. Cohn
Division of Cardiac Surgery, Brigham and Women's Hospital, Harvard Medical School, Boston, Massachusetts, U.S.A.

INTRODUCTION

Heart failure is a health care problem of enormous importance in the United States. As the leading cause of elderly hospitalizations, congestive heart failure (CHF) claims over 40,000 deaths per year and contributes to an additional 250,000. More than five million Americans are affected. An estimated half a million more individuals will be diagnosed with CHF every year (1). Currently, the only definitive treatment modality for CHF is cardiac transplantation. Though an effective option, the ~2000 heart transplants performed annually have essentially no significant epidemiological impact (2). With better treatment strategies continually evolving for coronary, valvular, and congenital heart disease, improved patient survival ultimately will translate into a gradual progression over time to cardiac failure in several of these patients. Myocardial function is at first compromised but compensated. Once hearts can no longer compensate, however, patients develop CHF. In pure economic terms, CHF costs the nation an estimated $10 to $50 billion annually. Clearly, more therapeutic options are needed.

In the context of this background, the concept of valvular disease in cardiomyopathy has recently received additional attention. Valvular surgery in the setting of low ejection fraction is rapidly becoming increasingly performed as one treatment methodology for this patient population. The possibility of serving as an intermediate step toward transplantation or as a final pathway in itself is attractive given the inadequacy of acceptable heart donors. By treating valvular pathology, these procedures serve to ameliorate or eliminate many of the symptoms.

The pathophysiology of cardiomyopathy progression is well described. Excluding the primary cardiomyopathies, secondary and extramyocardial cardiomyopathies produce remodeling that can be classified simplistically into two mechanistic pathways—pressure and volume overload. Overload results in some degree of cellular hypertrophy (3). Once in failure, the myocardium, without treatment intervention, ultimately spirals in an exorable downward pathway. Each version of overload has its own characteristic pathophysiology. With volume overload, there is abnormally increased filling of the ventricle during diastole. This results in an adaptative dilatation by the ventricle to accommodate the increased volume load imposed on it. With increase in left ventricular size, the volume overload increases.

With pressure overload, the ventricle is forced to pump blood against an abnormally high impedance, resulting in a compensatory hypertrophy and thickening of the myocardial wall. Such wall thickening can lead to subendocardial ischemia as well as diastolic dysfunction. This increases wall stress contributing to a vicious cycle, resulting in worse heart failure.

Valvular disease in the context of heart failure is a clear illustration of these concepts. In mitral regurgitation (MR), for example, volume overload of the heart causes ventricular dilatation. Dilatation results in annular dilatation and greater separation of the mitral valve leaflets, resulting in increased MR, which then has the corresponding effect on ventricular dilatation (4). Another example might be the presence of an atrial septal defect (ASD). Over time, right ventricular volume overload can occasionally occur. The compliance of the left heart tends to decrease as the ventricles thicken, leading to increased left to right shunting and further volume overload. Aortic stenosis represents the classic example of pressure overload. The ventricle is forced to work against increasing afterload, leading to compensatory hypertrophy, causing fibroblast proliferation, myocardial apoptosis, and subendocardial ischemia resulting in angina, syncope, or CHF.

In this chapter, we review the current concepts, controversies, and indications for valvular surgery in cardiomyopathy. Specifically, the aortic valve and mitral valve are addressed.

VALVULAR REPAIR OR REPLACEMENT IN CARDIOMYOPATHY

In the past, valvular replacement or repair in the context of cardiomyopathy was thought to be contraindicated. With significant comorbidities, often including age, COPD, and renal dysfunction, patients with this diagnosis were considered to be of high operative risk. Traditional valvular series from 10 to 20 years ago in the context of cardiomyopathy often reported operative mortality rates in the 10% to 20% range. Medical treatment was considered the best option.

This traditional paradigm of treatment has undergone significant change in the past 10 to 20 years. Although several reasons account for this shift in cardiac surgery, the evolution of cardiac surgery and anesthesiology form the basis of this change. Surgical techniques have been refined, including better myocardial protection and more homeopathic cardiopulmonary bypass (CPB). Blood cardioplegia, given at regular, routine intervals in an antegrade as well as retrograde fashion, is the accepted standard for myocardial preservation. Vacuum-assisted drainage and heparin-coated circuits are adjuncts contributing to improved CPB. Vacuum-assisted drainage allows for smaller cannulas to be used, enabling peripheral cannulation and minimally invasive approaches to valvular surgery. These advances have resulted in an overall decrease in cardiac surgery operative morbidity and mortality for all patients. This has led to broadened indications for surgery, including those patients previously perceived as too high risk. At Brigham and Women's Hospital, for instance, overall operative mortality for all patients over the age of 80 in the early 1990s was approximately 10%. By 2004, that operative mortality had fallen to 1%–2%.

The timing of operative intervention for valvular heart disease is critical for the management of these patients. With the trend of increasingly better operative outcomes in valve surgery, there has been a parallel trend to treat valvular disease earlier before the left ventricle sustains irreversible changes.

MITRAL VALVE SURGERY IN CARDIOMYOPATHY: A PROBLEM OF REGURGITATION

This new approach to treatment of patients with valvular disease is perhaps best exemplified in the context of mitral valve surgery. In the cardiomyopathic ventricle, the pathophysiology associated with the mitral valve is usually mitral reguvgitation (MR). Though mitral stenosis can occur in the setting of cardiomyopathy, the pathological process is usually rheumatic fever (RF), and the cardiomyopathy associated with RF occurs by a completely different mechanism. This condition is relatively rare, as mitral stenosis typically does not produce left ventricular dysfunction.

A significant percentage of the five million people with CHF have associated MR. The estimated incidence of significant MR in patients with dilated cardiomyopathy is approximately 60% (5). The etiology of MR in these patients is an abnormal geometry that results in poor coaptation of the valve leaflets. Two mechanisms are primarily responsible. Ventricular dilatation itself can cause mitral valve leaflets to not coapt as the annulus-ventricle complex enlarges (Fig. 1). In ischemic cardiomyopathy, inferior ischemia may cause selective posteromedial papillary muscle dysfunction with subsequent adverse effects on leaflet coaptation (P3 is the most commonly affected region of the posterior leaflet).

Regardless of the precise mechanism, the prognosis for patients with severe MR and compromised ventricular function is particularly poor, with a one-year actuarial survival of approximately 50% (6). In a study from Brigham and Women's, patients undergoing combined coronary bypass grafting and ring annuloplasty had decreased survival if there was residual MR (7).

As stated earlier, surgical correction of MR in patients with cardiomyopathy was considered to be associated with high risk (8). The thinking during this time was that with left ventricular dysfunction and MR, repairing or replacing the valve might significantly increase the afterload of the heart resulting in an even higher mortality. This was determined by the fact that up to 25% of the cardiac output was being injected back into the left atrium.

During this period, approximately 20 years ago, there was significant mortality associated with combined coronary artery bypass surgery and mitral valve replacement, reported to be between 10% and 20% (9).

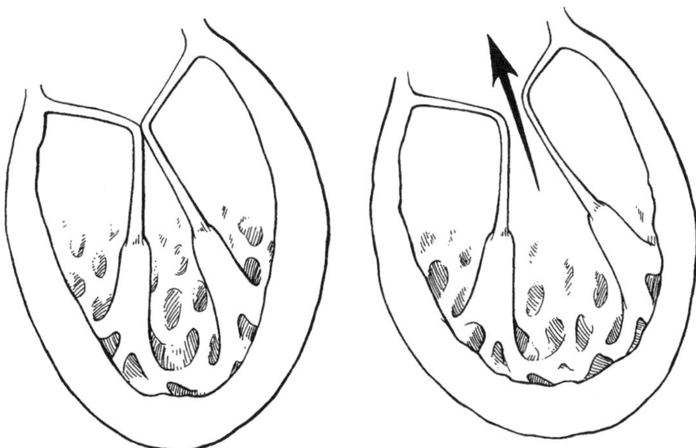

Figure 1 Mitral regurgitation occurs through leaflets that fail to coapt when the ventricle becomes dilated. *Source*: From Cohn LH. Cardiac Surgery in the Adult. New York: McGraw Hill, 2003.

Dr. Carpentier's original work with mitral valve repair was extended to patients with diminished ventricular function where he demonstrated that this concept was not valid (10). Subsequently Drs. Cohn and Cosgrove brought the concept of mitral valve repair to this United States (11,12). The benefits of mitral valve repair include maintaining the mitral annulus-chordae-papillary geometry is associated with preservation of ventricular function (13). This has lead to the general philosophy that mitral valve repair should be attempted in the majority of patients with MR. If a replacement is necessary, it is suggested that as much of the annulus-chordae-papillary geometry be maintained to again preserve as much ventricular systolic function as possible.

The application of mitral valve repair to patients with idiopathic cardiomyopathy was performed first by Dr. Bolling and associates (14) who performed mitral valve repair on a selected number of heart transplant patients. This resulted in increased postoperative ejection fraction, improvement in New york Heart Association (NYHA) functional class and a one-year actuarial survival of 75%. Patients with end-stage heart failure and associated MR have a two-year mortality as high as 80% without heart transplantation (15).

Similar outcomes of mitral valve repair in patients with diminished ventricular function were subsequently reported, including work at the Brigham and Women's Hospital (4). Survival of this group of patients at one year was 73% (Fig. 2). Similar results were obtained in other studies in which procedures were done with low surgical mortality and outcomes were associated with symptomatic relief and functional improvement (16,17).

Dr. Bolling and his group reported a 10-year follow-up of over 200 patients with cardiomyopathy and significant MR who underwent mitral valve repair (18). NYHA functional classification improved from a mean of 3.2 to 1.8 and ejection fraction increased from a mean of 16% to a mean of 26%. One, two, and five-year actuarial survival was 82%, 71%, and 52%, respectively.

A follow-up study from the same institution by Wu et al. (19) compared 126 patients who underwent mitral repair with 293 patients who did not undergo operation. This study showed no clear survival benefit associated with mitral valve repair in patients with significant MR and severe left ventricular dysfunction. The authors suggested that a randomized prospective control trial be carried out to further assess potential survival benefits with mitral valve repair in this group of severely ill patients.

Postoperative follow-up of these patients who underwent mitral valve repair from a variety of centers demonstrate good durability. Recurrence of MR has a number of etiologies including anterior leaflet repair as well as ventricular remodeling that occur

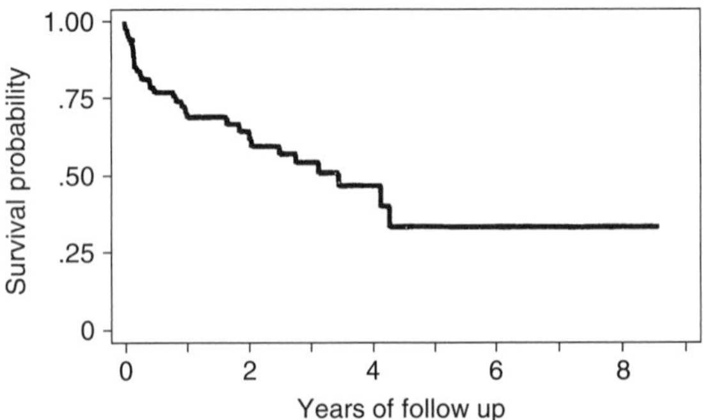

Figure 2 Survival of patients undergoing mitral valve repair with ejection fraction <0.30. One year survival is 73%. *Source*: From Ref. 4.

subsequent to the operative procedure. A variety of devices are being developed to decrease ventricular dilatation and allow corrective remodeling to occur. The ACORN cardiac support device, a polyester mesh design to be wrapped around the ventricles, is one of the first to be tested in a clinical trial (Fig. 3). Further investigation in this complex area of MR associated with cardiomyopathy needs to be performed. This hypothesis is one that could be addressed by a randomized clinical trial (20).

A reasonable set of guidelines for mitral valve surgery and cardiomypathy is the following:

1. The mitral valve should be repaired, and not replaced, if at all possible.
2. Surgery should be undertaken if:
    a. The patient is symptomatic, regardless of the degree of MR, and if the symptoms can be attributed to MR,
    b. Objective serial studies demonstrate evidence of continuing myocardial deterioration in mild to moderate MR,
    c. Asymptomatic severe MR exists with progressive left ventricular dilatation.

AORTIC VALVE SURGERY IN CARDIOMYOPATHY: AORTIC STENOSIS AND AORTIC REGURGITATION

Aortic Stenosis

The pathophysiology of critical aortic stenosis is well described. Pressure overload results in compensatory myocardial hypertrophy in an attempt to normalize the

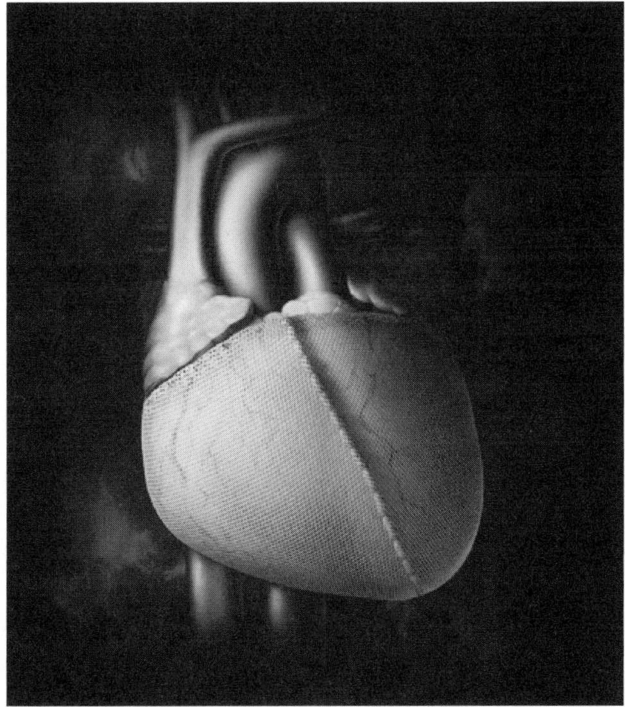

Figure 3 The ACORN cardiac support device. A polyester mesh is wrapped around the heart to prevent further ventricular remodeling and dilatation.

increased wall stress. Increasing levels of diastolic dysfunction subsequently occur as the ventricle thickens and stiffens. Fibroblasts and collagen proliferate in response to the pressure overload and contribute to this hypertrophy response. Increased subendocardial ischemia results as the myocardial wall further thickens. Such ischemia worsens any diastolic dysfunction. If left unchecked, irreversible cardiac dysfunction occurs and ultimately CHF.

Aortic valve replacement (AVR) is indicated whenever a patient becomes symptomatic or if the ventricle demonstrates any objective signs of dysfunction. Unlike mitral valve surgery, surgery for critical aortic stenosis and poor ventricular function has been an operation performed for a number of years. This philosophy has gained more enthusiasm over the last 20 years. Early results demonstrated that operative mortality ranged from 10%–20% (21–22), including one at our institution (23).

Improved surgical results in patients with critical aortic stenosis and left ventricular dysfunction are related to a variety of changes that have occurred in cardiac surgery and anesthesiology over these past two decades. Pereira et al. (24) reported on patients undergoing AVR for severe aortic stenosis and associated severe left ventricular dysfunction and a low transvalvular gradient. These patients were compared to a closely matched non-surgical group. Results indicated that AVR was associated with significantly better hospital mortality, 8% compared to the non-surgical group (14%). Patients undergoing AVR had reasonable long-term survival with 78% of patients living four years versus only 15% of patients who did not undergo operation. These long-term improved survival outcomes have been reported in other series (25,26). We offer surgery to patients with critical aortic stenosis and left ventricular dysfunction who have demonstrated reasonable functionality at home and before the onset of ventricular decompensation.

Severe AS, LV Dysfunction, and a Low Transvalvular Gradient: Special Considerations

A patient with aortic stenosis and poor ventricular function will receive significant benefit from AVR if the ventricle exhibits "contractile reserve." If there is a question of the degree of left ventricular dysfunction reversibility, contractile reserve is best assessed by Dobutamine stress echocardiography. It is defined as an increase in stroke volume $\geq$20% with low dose Dobutamine (27). There is also a school of thought that if the ventricular dysfunction is caused by severely increased afterload and not intrinsic myocardial dysfunction, AVR is indicated with the thought that left ventricular dysfunction is secondary to "afterload mismatch" (28).

The particular patient who has presumed significant aortic stenosis, left ventricular function, and a low transvalular gradient is somewhat more difficult to assess. There is some thought that with Dobutamine infusion there is an increase in stroke volume which results in opening a mildly diseased valve leading to a calculated area that is larger than expected. This concept is known as "pseudostenosis" by Carabello and associates (28). Another interpretation of a patient with presumed aortic stenosis, left ventricular dysfunction, and a low transvalvular gradient is that the ventricle is unable to generate enough cardiac output to produce a significant gradient.

A more accurate way to define the intrinsic property of the myocardium independent of preload and afterload would provide the best assessment of operative risks. Currently, however, our strategy is to offer AVR to any patient with critical aortic stenosis and left ventricular dysfunction who has demonstrated reasonable functionality at home and has a valve area of 0.8 cm^2 or less. Calcification of the aortic valve is another important finding in determining the timing for operation. Severe calcification, even in the presence of a questionable gradient but with symptoms, would prompt operative intervention. Our current technique is to perform the majority of AVRs though a mini-sternotomy.

Aortic Regurgitation

Unlike aortic stenosis, there is a significant component of both volume and pressure overload in aortic insufficiency (AI). AI results in eccentric hypertrophy and myocardial fibrosis. Increased diastolic wall stress occurs as the ventricle receives excess volume and pressure loading during diastole. Fibrosis of the myocardium develops. The thickened ventricle, in combination with decreased diastolic coronary perfusion, renders the patient vulnerable to angina. Permanent LV dysfunction is the end result.

Traditionally, AVR for AI has been recommended in patients that are symptomatic or whose ventricular function exhibits any objective signs of decompensation. With preserved ventricular function, AVR is well tolerated with low operative morbidity and mortality (29). If ventricular dysfunction is present (as assessed by preoperative ejection fraction), the indications for AVR are less clear. There are very few modern reports in the literature on AVR in the setting of cardiomyopathy, as the vast majority of patients undergo correction before cardiomyopathy develops. In general, the reported operative mortality for AVR in this condition ranges between 8%–15%. This operative mortality compares favorably with a five-year survival of between 20% and 66% in patients medically treated for severe AI and left ventricular dysfunction (30). Chaliki and associates reported on 450 patients with this condition, finding that preoperative ejection fraction was related to operative mortality (31), a similar finding in other studies. In patients with a preoperative ejection fraction of 35% or less, the operative mortality was 14% compared to an operative mortality of 3.7% in patients with an ejection fraction of 50% or greater. Our strategy is to offer AVR to the majority of patients with cardiomyopathy and severe AI.

CONCLUSIONS

The past 20 years have seen a dramatic improvement in cardiac surgery and anesthesiology in regards to technology, technique, support, valve technology, and perioperative care. With the current limited number of potential donor hearts, valve repair and/or replacement in these patients with severe left ventricular dysfunction is a reasonable option.

REFERENCES

1. American Heart Association. 2001 Heart and Stroke Statistical Update. Dallas, TX: American Heart Association, 2000.
2. United Network for Organ Sharing (UNOS): Annual report of the US scientific registry fro organ transplantation and the organ procurement and transplantation network. US Department of Health and Human Services, 1999.
3. Grossman W, Carabello BA, Gunther S, et al. Ventricular wall stress and the development of cardiac hypertrophy and failure. In: Alpert NR, ed. In: Perspectives in Cardiovascular Research. Myocardial Hypertrophy and Failure, Vol. 7. New York: Raven Press, 1993:1–15.
4. Chen FY, Adams DH, Aranki SF, et al. Mitral valve repair in cardiomyopathy. Circulation 1998; 98:II-124–II-127.

5. Junker A, Thayssen P, Nielsen B, et al. The hemodynamic and prognostic significance of echo-Doppler-proven mitral regurgitation in patients with dilated cardiomyopathy. Cardiology 1993; 83:14–20.
6. Stevenson LW, Fowler MB, Schroeder JS, et al. Poor survival of patients with idiopathic cardiomyopathy considered too well for transplantation. Am J Med 1987; 83:871–876.
7. Soltesz E. Personal Communication, 2005.
8. Rothlin ME. Severe mitral regurgitation with ejection fraction below 40%: pharmacological therapy is the treatment of choice. Schweiz Med Wochenschr 1997; 127:2035–2039.
9. DiSesa VJ, Cohn LH, Collins JJ, Jr., et al. Determinants of operative survival following combined mitral valve replacement and coronary revascularization. Ann Thorac Surg 1982; 34:482.
10. Carpentier A. Cardiac valve surgery: the "French correction". J Thorac Cardiovasc Surg 1983; 86:323–337.
11. Cohn LH, Couper GS, Kinchla NM, et al. Decreased operative risk of surgical treatment of mitral regurgitation with or without coronary artery disease. Journal of the American College of Cardiology 1990; 16:1575–1578.
12. Gillinov AM, Cosgrove DM, Blackstone EH, et al. Durability of mitral valve repair for degernerative disease. J Thorac Cardiovasc Surg 1998; 116:734.
13. Goldman ME, Mora F, Guarno T, et al. Mitral valvuloplasty is superior to valve replacement for preservation of left ventricular function: an intraoperative two-dimensional echocardiographic study. J Am Coll Cardiol 1987; 10:568–575.
14. Bolling SF, Deeb GM, Brunsting LA, et al. Early outcome of mitral valve reconstruction in patients with end-stage cardiomyopathy. J Thorac Cardiovasc Surg 1995; 109:676–683.
15. Blondheim DS, Jacobs LE, Kotler MN, et al. Dilated cardiomyopathy with mitral regurgitation: decreased survival despite a low frequency of left ventricular thrombus. Am Heart J 1991; 122:763–771.
16. Bishay ES, McCarthy PM, Cosgrove DM, et al. Mitral valve surgery in patients with severe left ventricular dysfunction. Eur J Card Thorac Surg 2000; 17:213–221.
17. Rothenburger M, Rukosujew A, Hammel D, et al. Mitral valve surgery in patients with poor left ventricular function. Thorac Cardiovasc Surg 2002; 50:351–354.
18. Romano MA, Bolling SF. Update on mitral repair in dilated cardiomyopathy. J Card Surg 2004; 19:396–400.
19. Wu AH, Aaronson KD, Bolling SF, et al. Impact of mitral valve annuloplasty on mortality risk in patients with mitral regurgitation and left ventricular systolic dysfunction. J Am Coll Cardiol 2005; 45:381–387.
20. Mehra MR, Griffith BP. Is mitral regurgitation a viable treatment target in heart failure? J Am Coll Cardiol 2005; 45:388–390.
21. Smith N, McAnulty JH, Rahimtoola SH, et al. Severe aortic stenosis with impaired left ventricular function and clinical heart failure: results of valve replacement. Circulation 1978; 58:255–264.
22. Henry WL, Bonow RO, Borer JS, et al. Observations on the optimum time for operative intervention for aortic valve replacement for aortic regurgitation from 1976–1983: impact of preoperative left ventricular function. Circulation 1985; 72:1244–1256.
23. Carabello BA, Green LH, Grossman W, et al. Hemodynamic determinants of prognosis of aortic valve replacement in critical aortic stenosis and advanced congestive heart failure. Circulation 1980; 62:42–48.
24. Pereira JJ, Lauer MS, Bashir M, et al. Survival after aortic valve replacement for severe aortic stenosis with low transvalvular gradients and severe left ventricular dysfunction. J Am Coll Cardiol 2002; 39:1356–1363.
25. Connolly HM, Oh JK, Orszulak TA, et al. Aortic valve replacement for aortic stenosis with severe left ventricular dysfunction. Prognostic indicators. Circulation 1997; 95:2395–2400.
26. Paul S, Mihaljevic T, Rawn JD, et al. Aortic valve replacement in patients with severely reduced left ventricular function. Cardiology 2004; 101:7–14.

27. Monin JL, Monchi M, Gest V, et al. Aortic stenosis with severe left ventricular dysfunction and low transvalvular pressure gradients. J Am Coll Cardiol 2001; 37:2101–2107.
28. Carabello BA. Ventricular function in aortic stenosis: how low can you go? J Am Coll Cardiol 2002; 39:1364–1365.
29. Bonow RO, Carabello B, de Leon AC, Jr., et al. Guidelines for the management of patients with valvular heart disease: executive summary. A report of the American College of Cardiology/American Heart Association Task Force on Practice Guidelines (Committee on Management of Patients with Valvular Heart Disease). Circulation 1998; 98:1949–1985.
30. Aronow WS, Ahn C, Kronzon I, et al. Prognosis of patients with heart failure and unoperated severe aortic valvular regurgitation and relation to ejection fraction. Am J Cardiol. 1994; 74(3): 286–288.
31. Chaliki HP, Mohty D, Avierinos JT, et al. Outcomes after aortic valve replacement in patients with severe aortic regurgitation and markedly reduced left ventricular function. Circulation 2002; 106:2687–2693.

20
Surgical Ventricular Remodeling

John V. Conte
Division of Cardiac Surgery, The Johns Hopkins Hospital, Baltimore, Maryland, U.S.A.

INTRODUCTION

Congestive heart failure (CHF) is a major health care problem facing western society. It is the leading cause of death in the United States and is expected to grow significantly in the years ahead. The health care costs are staggering and the costs are estimated at $100 billion today and $1 trillion by 2020 (1). Medical therapy is the mainstay of treatment for CHF of all etiologies and a detailed overview of the medical treatment of CHF is presented in this issue. Ischemic cardiomyopathy is the leading cause of CHF in western society. There are however, many patients for whom medical therapy is not effective and for whom surgical therapy is appropriate (2,3).

Coronary artery occlusion, if left untreated, will result in a transmural full thickness myocardial infarction. Following infarction, the left ventricle undergoes a well-described process of ventricular remodeling. Following an infarction of more than 30% of the left ventricular circumference, the remodeling causes a progressive dilation of the ventricle converting the normal elliptical left ventricle to a sphere (4). Early reperfusion via thrombolysis or angioplasty techniques may alter the normal of progression of the infarction from the endocardium to the epicardium resulting in a relative sparing of the epicardium. This partial thickness infarction may result in a normal appearing epicardium with less thinning of the ventricle as is seen in a full thickness infarction. This leads to the development of an akinetic segment as opposed to the dyskinetic segments commonly seen with full thickness infarctions. However, this thin layer of normal appearing myocardium does not change the negative remodeling process or the ultimate clinical outcomes. The GUSTO trial demonstrated that dilation does occur following thrombolysis for acute infarctions and the dilation seen early after infarction is a predictor of early and late mortality (5).

This remodeling process can result in a progressive dilation of the ventricle resulting in an increase in the end diastolic diameter and volume, an increase in left ventricular wall stress and oxygen demand, a loss of the natural elliptical shape with the development of a more rounded LV, the development of mitral insufficiency and ultimately a worsening of the global systolic function (6). The development of mitral regurgitation is due to factors specific to ventricular remodeling as well as unrelated leaflet issues. The first factor related to the remodeling process is the annular dilation due to the global ventricular enlargement. The second is restricted leaflet motion and reduced coaptation due to the global LV dilation or involvement of the papillary muscles with the infarction itself. These factors combine to prevent leaflet coaption or limit it in the proper plane resulting in central regurgitation. Superimposed leaflet pathology can worsen the functional regurgitation.

The prognosis of patients with ischemic cardiomyopathy is related to the left ventricular size and the impact that remodeling has had on the function of the remote non infracted zones (7). Progressive thinning and dilation of the remote areas leads to the development of a spherical rather than the normal elliptical shape of the heart. Clinically, the ongoing remodeling generates a progressive reduction in contractile force, worsening CHF and ultimately death (4–8).

Another aspect of the dysfunction that develops following infarction is the electrical and mechanical dyssynchrony that develops following infarction. Electrical dyssynchrony will be delt with in detail in other sections of this book but the concept is simply that abnormalities in the conduction system result in differential timing of left and right ventricular contraction resulting in overall diminished left ventricular function. This is treated in appropriate circumstances with biventricular pacing. Mechanical dyssynchrony is a phenomenon of impaired left ventricular function caused by nonuniform contraction, relaxation and filling of the ventricle due to juxtaposed areas of akinesis, dyskinesis and hypokinesis alongside normal areas. This has been associated with reduced survival (9).

Surgical techniques have been developed to arrest the progression and reverse the pathologic changes induced by the process of negative post infarction ventricular remodeling. This chapter will review these techniques and discuss the clinical outcomes that have been achieved.

HISTORY

The genesis of procedures whose goal is to remodel the ventricle following myocardial infarction is found in the history of left ventricular aneurysm surgery. Any discussion of the history of the development of surgery to remodel the left ventricle following myocardial infarction begins with Dr. Denton Cooley in 1958 when he performed the first linear left ventricular aneurysmectomy on cardiopulmonary bypass (CPB) to treat a true calcified ventricular aneurysm (10). Many other techniques and approaches were developed over the years to treat post-infarction ventricular aneurysms (11). Jatene used a technique of septoplasty and modified linear closure in the early 1980s (12). At the same time Dor and colleagues introduced the technique of endoventricular circular patch plasty which later came to bear his name in 1985 (13). His approach was unique in that it approached akinetic areas and dyskinetic aneurysms equally and later began to apply this technique to treat CHF. Cooley and colleagues later utilized a similar technique aneurysm resection by patching the anterior wall from within the ventricle but without the encircling purse string suture to reduce the volume of the anterior wall of the left ventricle (14,15). The concept of reconstructing the ventricle to a prescribed size based on the patient's size was introduced by Dor and popularized by Menicanti. This has led to the development of several commercial products to size the ventricle (16). Additional technical approaches include a linear closure and septoplasty approach described by Mickleborough and a concentric pursestring or "cerclage" technique followed by linear closure utilized by

McCarthy (17,18). The end result of two decades of surgical innovation is four techniques used for ventricular remodeling procedures today.

INDICATIONS FOR SURGERY

Classically, patients are candidates for SVR (Surgical Ventricular Remodeling) if they have had an anterior myocardial infarction, have a large area of akinesis or dyskinesis and have clinical evidence of CHF. Specific characteristics of patients who have successfully undergone SVR are shown in Table 1. Ideal candidates have a large area of akinesis/dyskinesis in the anteroseptal area, have retained function of the basilar and lateral portions of the heart, and have good right ventricular function. In addition, they should be candidates for revascularization and mitral valve repair if needed. Included in many clinical series of SVR are patients who have had anterior infarctions with areas of akinesis or dyskinesis who do not have heart failure. The indication for surgery in such patients is angina and the need for coronary artery revascularization. In such patients, the goal of therapy is to prevent the dilation and the clinical development of CHF which is an inevitable part of post-infarction remodeling. Relative contraindications are shown in Table 2. Many patients have additional cardiac conditions which will necessitate repair or replacement, and they should be candidates for surgical repair of any lesion that exists.

SURGICAL APPROACHES

The surgical goals in surgical ventricular remodeling are seen in Table 1. They include complete revascularization of all territories. Exclusion of the akinetic and dyskinetic segments with a concomitant reduction in the size of the nonfunctioning anteroseptal portion of the heart, recreation of the elliptical shape of the heart and a repair of any valvular incompetence by valve repair or replacement.

The techniques required to achieve these goals are varied but all procedures share in common standard surgical principles. The surgical procedure begins with standard arterial and venous cannulation for CPB. Since concomitant coronary artery bypass grafting is usually performed, the standard approach for CABG at that institution is utilized, including myocardial protection. If mitral valve repair or replacement is a strong possibility, cannulation of both inferior and superior cava is recommended. The left ventricle can be vented directly, through the right superior pulmonary vein, or through the

Table 1 Indications for Surgical Ventricular Restoration

Anteroseptal myocardial infarction
NYHA Class 3 or 4 CHF
Depressed ejection fraction %
Large area of akinesis/dyskinesis
Asynergy of >35% of LV
End diastolic volume index >150 cc/m2
End systolic volume index >60 cc/m2
Candidate for revascularization
Retained basilar heart function
Good right ventricular function

Table 2 Relative Contraindications to Surgical Ventricular Restoration

Multiple areas of infarction
Loss of basilar myocardial function
Pulmonary hypertension and right ventricular dysfunction
Unreconstructable coronary artery disease

aortic root. Prior to systemic heparinization, femoral arterial access is obtained to make the later placement of an intra-aortic balloon pump easier if necessary.

Once the patient is on CPB the sequence of procedures performed is dependent upon personal preference. Most commonly, CABG is performed first. Once this is accomplished, the SVR or the MVR can be performed next. The author performs the MVR to avoid potential disruption of the ventricular reconstruction with retraction to expose the mitral valve.

With the heart vented the left ventricle will often collapse demonstrating the area of thinned out scar (Fig. 1). This does not always happen and the absence of collapse does not contraindicate SVR. An incision is made into the anterior wall of the left through the area of scar. In a typical anterior infarction, this is extended to the apex and proximally parallel to the course of the left anterior descending coronary artery. Retention sutures are placed to aid in achieving and maintaining exposure.

The ventricle is inspected and any thrombus is removed. If there is suspicion that there is a large thrombus burden in the left ventricle preoperatively, it may be beneficial to perform a left atriotomy, as if approaching the mitral valve, and placing a sponge into the left atrium prior to opening the ventricle. This will prevent any particulate matter from falling through the mitral valve into an unretrievable location in the pulmonary veins. The sponge is later removed through the mitral valve and out the left ventricle after the ventriculotomy is performed, the thrombus is removed and the ventricle irrigated.

During inspection of the ventricle the extent as well as the transmurality of the scar is noted. A palpable transition zone between infarcted and noninfarcted muscle is often palpable. This is particularly so with full thickness infarctions but is notably absent in

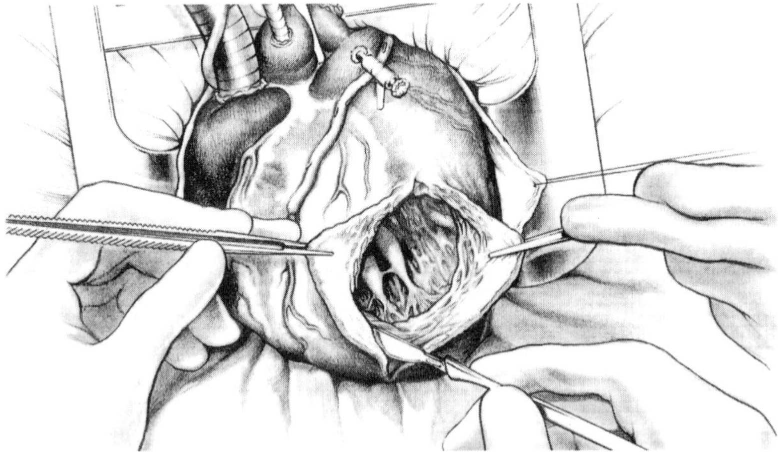

Figure 1 The anterior ventriculotomy is made lateral to and parallel to the left anterior descending coronary artery. This is extended to the apex and proximally to allow adequate exposure of the endocardium. *Source*: From Dor V. Surgical management of left ventricular aneurysms by the endoventricular circular patch plasty technique. Tech Card Thor Surg 1997; 2:139–50.

some patients who have received thrombolytics or percutaneous revascularization prior to widespread cell death. These patients demonstrate a mosaic pattern of ventricular scarring. Such ventricles often demonstrate akinesis rather than dyskinesis.The presence or absence of a transition zone is not known to be of clinical significant. The differences in the various operations are apparent from this point forward in the operations.

DOR PROCEDURE (ENDOVENTRICULAR CIRCULAR PATCH PLASTY)

At this point in the procedure an encircling purse string of 2-0 polypropylene suture is placed roughly at the "transition zone" between normal and infarcted myocardium (Fig. 2). This stitch actually defines the limits of the new anterior wall. This is commonly referred to as the "Fontan" stitch. The stitch is begun at the point selected to be the new apex and is run cephalad across the septum along the transition zone. It is recommended to include no more than one half of the septum regardless of the amount of scar left behind. The suture is carried across the anterior wall and down the anterolateral wall to the new apex. Deep, partial thickness bites into tough scar is recommended. If a second or more purse strings are used, they should be placed equidistant from the previous purse string. This is not a necessary step. The purse string is tied defining the outline of the new distal anterior wall. The purse string should not be tied in an attempt to close the ventriculotomy except in the rare instances of very small reconstructions. Doing so may cause the suture to pull through the endocardium, especially in patients without well formed scar tissue. If this was done it could result in a left ventricle which is more rounded than optimal. If a sizing device is utilized, it is left inflated while the purse string is tied.

Placement of the purse string is one of the key steps in the operation. It chooses the new apex of the heart and defines the outline of the new anterior wall. Selecting the location of the purse strings is usually done by personal preference. It can be done in a

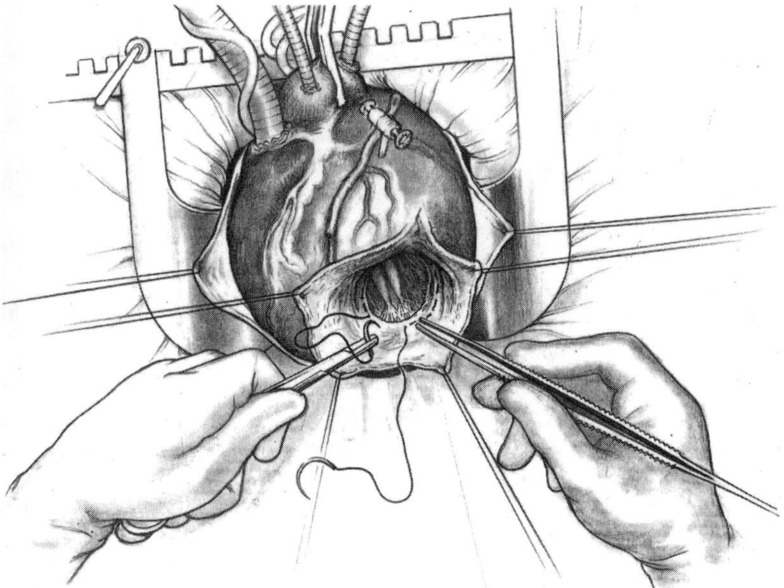

Figure 2 An encircling purse string suture is placed in the endocardium to outline the margins of the "new" anterior wall. *Source*: From Dor V. Surgical management of left ventricular aneurysms by the endoventricular circular patch plasty technique. Tech Card Thor Surg 1997; 2:139–50.

measured fashion using one of several commercially available sizing devices, by selecting a site based on experience or proximity to a landmark such as the papillary muscles, or at the border of infarcted and non infarcted tissue. Use of the so called "border zone" was most commonly recommended before the development of commercially available devices. If a sizing device is used a variety of methods of determining the size of the device to use have been recommended. Our method is to pick a device with a volume determined roughly by 50-60 cc/m2 body surface area. Obese patients will have the volume titrated down to 50 cc/m2 and cachetic patients will have the volume titrated up to 70 cc/m2.

The anterior wall is reconstructed utilizing a variety of techniques. A patch of Dacron is used if the remaining defect is greater than 2–3 cm long (Fig. 3). An oval shaped patch is cut to the appropriate size and is sutured in place closing the defect. Care is made to place the patch sutures around the anterior purse string. The patch may be sutured using a continuous or interrupted technique (Fig. 4). The sizing device is often left in place while half of the patch is sewn into place and is deflated and removed after this. Prior to completing the patch the left ventricular vent is shut off allowing the ventricle to fill with blood, forcing air to escape the ventricle through the partially completed closure. After the patch is sutured into place, or in the event of a small residual defect, a linear closure is performed superficial to the patch or purse string (Fig. 5). Horizontal mattress sutures, buttressed with bovine pericardium, is used as a first layer of closure. The second layer is a continuous running stitch of 2-0 polypropylene. If the defect is moderate in size, but not large enough for patching, a series of anterior purse string sutures can be placed to narrow the ventricular defect prior to placing the mattress sutures.

The mitral repair, if necessary, can be done at any time utilizing any technique preferred. An intra-ventricular repair as described by Menicanti is done through the ventriculotomy prior to performing the SVR (8). Our standard approach is to perform a

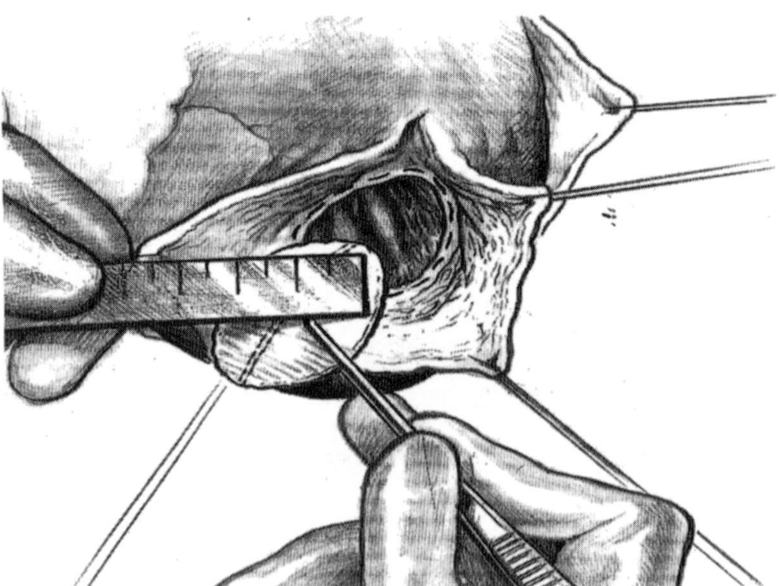

Figure 3 The anterior wall is reconstructed with a patch or by primary closure. Patching is optimally used for defects larger than 3 cm. *Source*: From Dor V. Surgical management of left ventricular aneurysms by the endoventricular circular patch plasty technique. Tech Card Thor Surg 1997; 2:139–50.

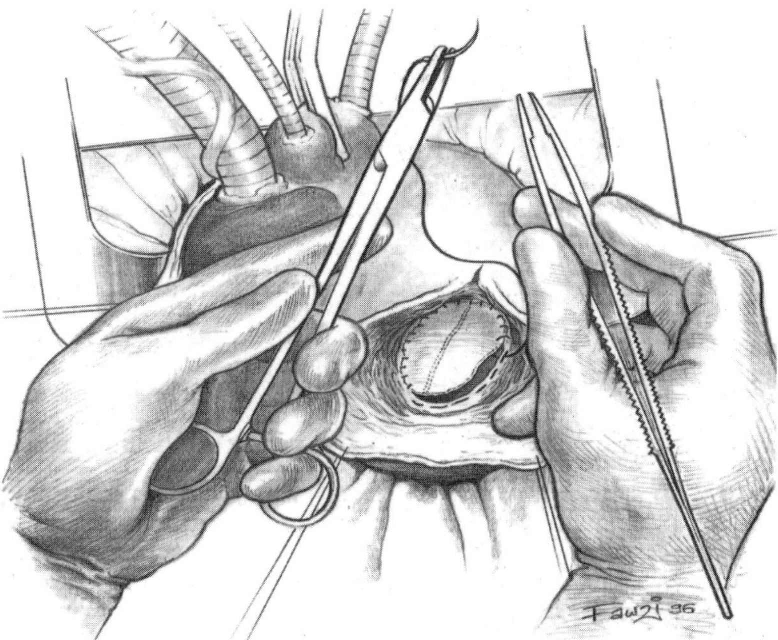

Figure 4 Patch sutures should be passed around the encircling anterior wall purse string for added strength. A variety of different materials may be used to patch the ventriculotomy. *Source*: From Dor V. Surgical management of left ventricular aneurysms by the endoventricular circular patch plasty technique. Tech Card Thor Surg 1997; 2:139–50.

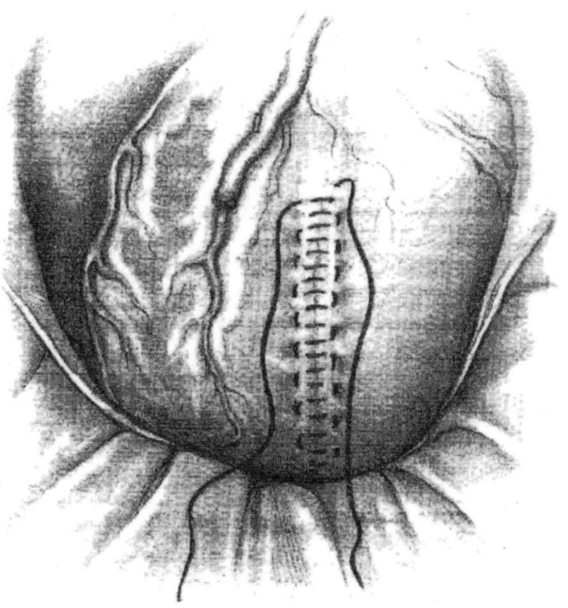

Figure 5 The remaining tissue of the anterior wall is reapproximated over the patch. *Source*: From Dor V. Surgical management of left ventricular aneurysms by the endoventricular circular patch plasty technique. Tech Card Thor Surg 1997; 2:139–50.

reduction posterior annuloplasty, through a standard interatrial groove incision, prior to performing the SVR to avoid the remote possibility of disrupting our ventricular closure.

A word should be mentioned about performing the SVR with the heart beating. One advantage is that poorly functioning, often ischemic, ventricles are not further injured during the period of cardiac arrest. Another is that the degree of mitral regurgitation and the result of mitral repair can be assessed in a beating heart which is felt by some to be advantageous. A final advantage is that it allows the border between contracting and non-contracting segments of the heart to be seen more clearly from within the ventricle and may aid in performing the SVR. The disadvantage is a much more difficult time in placing the sizing device on the mitral annulus and keeping it there to allow accurate placement of sutures. This disadvantage can be partially compensated for by tracing the outline of the margins of the sizer on the endocardium and then deflating the sizer. No good evidence supports any approach, however the novice may be aided with cardiac arrest until experience is gained.

LINEAR CLOSURE WITH SEPTOPLASTY

This technique uses the same anterior ventriculotomy approach to expose the septum and anterior wall. The technique employs a more traditional linear closure to exclude the akinetic or dysinetic areas of the anterior wall. Additionally, the dilated, fibrotic areas of the infracted septum are addressed by either including the septum in the linear closure of the anterior wall or patching the septum. The septum is reconstructed with a patch of Dacron sewn into the scar tissue on the septum along the border zone of infracted and viable tissue. The patch is usually semicircular with the straight part of the patch projecting anteriorly up through the ventriculotomy. The apex of the patch is included in the linear ventriculotomy closure (Fig. 6).

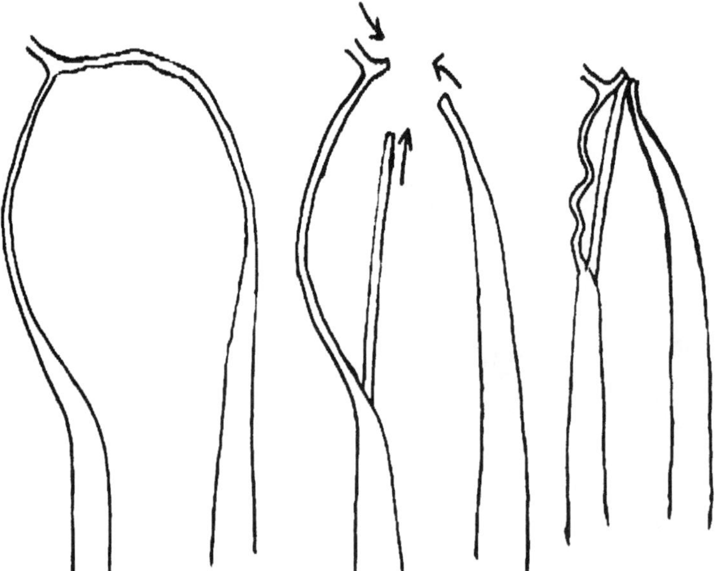

Figure 6 Technique of septal exclusion and linear closure. *Source*: From Mickleborough LL, Merchant N, Provost Y, Carson S, Ivanov J. Ventricular reconstruction for ischemic cardiomyopathy. Ann Thor Surg 2003; 75:S6–12.

MULTIPLE PURSE STRING OR CERCLAGE TECHNIQUE

This technique begins as do the previous two techniques. Once the anterior wall purse string is placed and tied, additional purse strings are placed a few millimeters superficial to the previous purse string. This continues anteriorly until the final remaining defect is small and is closed with a standard linear closure (Fig. 7).

SEPTOPLASTY TECHNIQUE

This technique also begins the same way as other SVR procedures. There is an anterior encircling purse string placed to define the borders of the anterior wall as there is in some of the other SVR techniques. The distinguishing characteristic of this technique is the placement of mattress sutures in the septum to reduce the horizontal length of the septum (Figs. 8 and 9). Once the septal reduction is performed the anterior encircling purse string is tied and the anterior wall is closed primarily or with a patch.

OUTCOMES

It is fair to say there is controversy in the optimal treatment of ischemic cardiomyopathy. Part of the reason for that is that there are no contemporary prospective randomized trials comparing similar groups of patients between medical therapy, coronary artery bypass grafting, and SVR, with or without revascularization. Another issue is that much of the data on SVR often involves large heterogeneous historical groups of patients whose diagnostic studies and evaluation, indications for surgery, surgical procedure, surgeon, follow up and many other factors, may or may not have been the same and the papers themselves do not spell them out very clearly (18). While most of the published data on outcomes from SVR procedures comes from single center studies with a great deal of

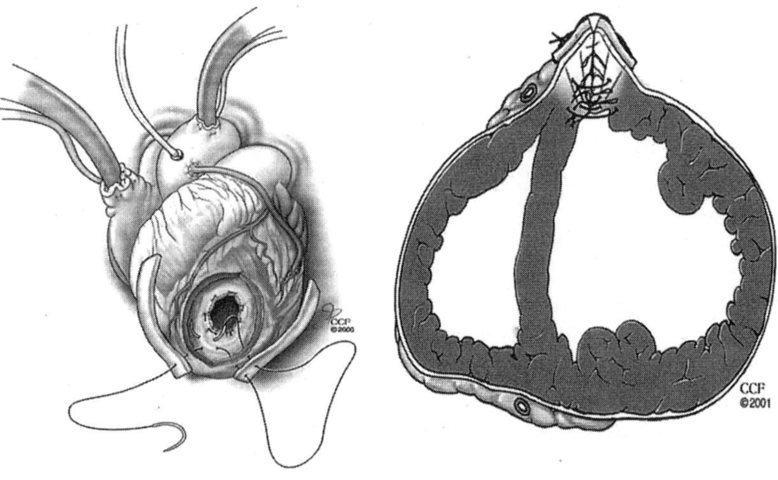

Figure 7 Technique of multiple concentric purse strings or "cerclage" followed by linear closure. *Source*: From Ref. 18.

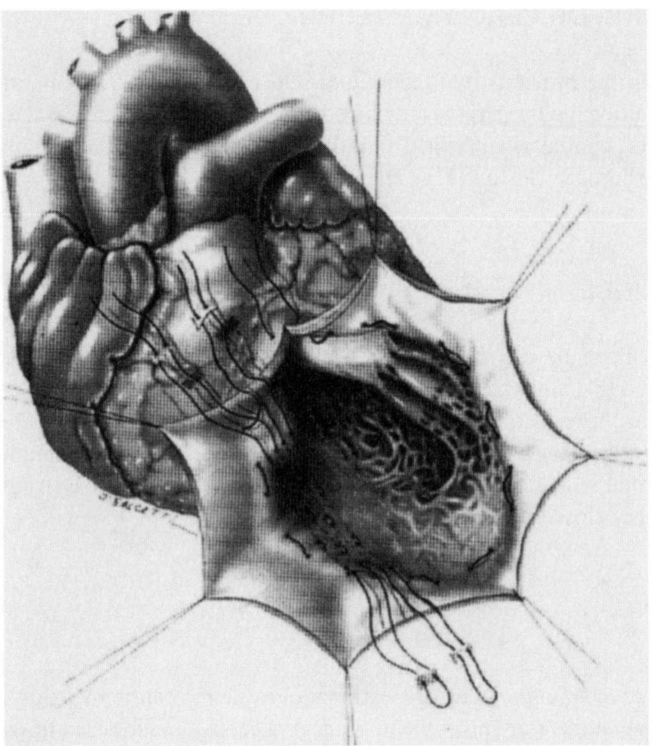

Figure 8 Jatene technique employs a linear septoplasty, concentric purse string suture along the endocardial surface and a modified linear closure to treat post infarction aneurysms. *Source*: From Cox JL. Left atrial isolation. A new technique for the treatment of supraventricular arrhythmias. Semin Thor Cardiovasc Surg 1997; 2:131–8.

experience such as those in Monaco, Milan, and Toronto, there is little published data from multi-center studies. Both types of provide useful clinical information (16,19–22).

The effectiveness of SVR can be assessed from a variety of different perspectives. Survival, morbidity and functional outcomes are the most commonly utilized benchmarks. In a procedure whose functional outcomes are, in part, based on changing the size and shape of the heart, morphological assessments are important considerations.

Menicanti and colleagues from Milan have a large experience of over one thousand patients. The overall experience reflects many of the complicating issues noted above. The overall operative mortality is 7.2% for the group. It is lower (4.8%) in patients who undergo concomitant CABG, higher in patients with a preoperative EF% < 30% (12.3%), with concomitant mitral valve procedures (15%) or NYHA class 4 symptoms (15.2%) (16). What is not easy to discern in this, or any other single institutional experience, is exactly what the interplay among two or three of these factors is. It is logical that the risk is higher. They have identified that factors associated with adverse outcomes include worse NYHA functional class, EF < 20%, age > 70 yr, urgent intervention, mitral valve procedure, pulmonary hypertension (PAS > 60 mmHg, larger ventricles (EDVI > 180 cc/m2), the number and sites of previous myocardial infarctions, and right ventricular dysfunction (16).

The optimal technique for performing SVR has been either implicitly suggested by the surgical technique utilized or studied by direct comparison, usually with a single institutional retrospective study (20,21). The simple fact is that like many areas of this

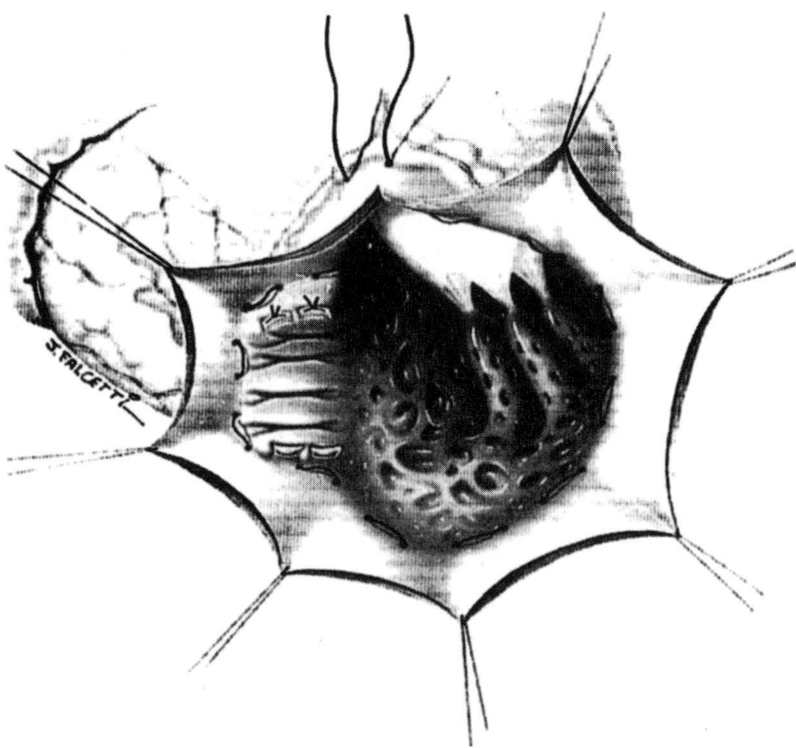

Figure 9 Jatene septoplasty technique demonstrating reduction in volume of septal scar after linear septoplasty sutures are tied, prior to tying the anterior wall purse string. *Source*: From Cox JL. Left atrial isolation. A new technique for the treatment of supraventricular arrhythmias. Semin Thor Cardiovasc Surg 1997; 2:131–8.

emerging field, no study has been studied appropriately to answer this question. Mickleborough and colleagues reported on 285 patients over a 20 yr period utilizing a linear closure technique with (25%) or without septoplasty (75%). The excellent 5 and 10 yr survival was 82% and 62% respectively. As mentioned above, it is unclear if the patient populations are the same. The study group included posterior infarcts and the data is presented together. In the anterior infarct group, (appropriate for SVR) only 62% had CHF of an unknown severity despite having a low EF% (mean $24 \pm 11\%$). Patients had to have a palpably thinned area in the anterior wall, severe MR was an exclusion (only 1% had a valve intervention) and the presence of calcified aneurysms excluded some patients. Despite these differences, the risk factors for poor outcomes were EF<20%, CHF, ventricular tachycardias and hypertension, not too dissimilar to other investigators (23–25).

The RESTORE group is a collection of international centers performing SVR who have combined data to study the outcomes of the SVR procedure. The combined number of patients followed up by this group is 1,198 operated on between the years of 1998 and 2003. Most patients were in NYHA class 3 (40%) and class 4 (29%). Concomitant procedures included coronary artery bypass grafting in 95%, mitral valve repair in 22% and replacement in 1%. This study represents what is probably the best large study to date in performing SVR in a heart failure population.

The RESTORE investigators found that global systolic function increased postoperatively and ventricular size decreased as measured by ventriculography, magnetic resonance imaging, or echocardiography. The ejection fraction increased from 29.6 ± 11% to 39.5 ± 12.3%. The left ventricular end systolic volume index (LVESVI) decreased from 80.4 ± 51.4 ml/m2 to 56.6 ± 34.3 ml/m2.

Survival was excellent in this group. Thirty day mortality was 5.3% and the overall 5 yr survival was 68.6 ± 2.8% (Fig. 4). Logistic regression analysis was performed to identify risk factors for death any time following surgery. These included preoperative EF < 30%, LVESVI > 80 ml/m2 advanced NYHA functional class and age > 75 yr. Patients with and EF > 30% had a survival of 63.8% ± 3.9% compared to 76.7% ± 3.2% 76.7% ± 3.2% for those with an EF > 30% and 83.0 ± 4.0% with an EF of > 40%. The fact that many of these risk factors are the same or similar to those identified by both Menicanti and Mickleborough suggest the ability of a single institution to discover the same findings as seen in multi-center studies (23,24).

Our group at Johns Hopkins has looked at the outcomes of groups of patients with severe advanced CHF. In one study 100% of the patients had class 3 (34%) or class 4 (66%) CHF and an EF% by magnetic resonance imaging of < 20% with 65% having an EF% < 15%. Despite how sick these patients were, 69% improved to NYHA class 1 or 2 with an 1 yr survival of 81% Cox regression analysis demonstrated that pre-operative diabetes, the use of an intra-aortic balloon pump during surgery, incomplete revascularization, and a pre-operative left ventricular end-systolic volume index greater than 130 mL/m^2 were significant predictors of overall mortality (25).

The Hopkins group also looked at the outcomes of SVR in patients who had multi territory infarctions which had been a contraindication in all previously published series. The finding that standard treatment of the anterior wall infarction, along with suture plication of the inferior wall for right coronary artery territory infarctions and the lateral wall for lateral wall infarctions opens the door for a potentially new patient population for this procedure (26).

The group at the Cleveland clinic investigated the impact of ventricular remodeling on the neuroendocrine axis following SVR. Elevations in several markers of the neurohormonal axis are elevated in CHF. They investigated the plasma levels of norepinephrine, rennin, and angiotensin II before and 1 yr following SVR as well as brain natriuretic peptide before and 3 mo following SVR. They found that SVR reduced norepinephrine by 56%, angiotensin II by 60%, rennin activity by 56%, and brain natriuretic peptide by 36% (27).

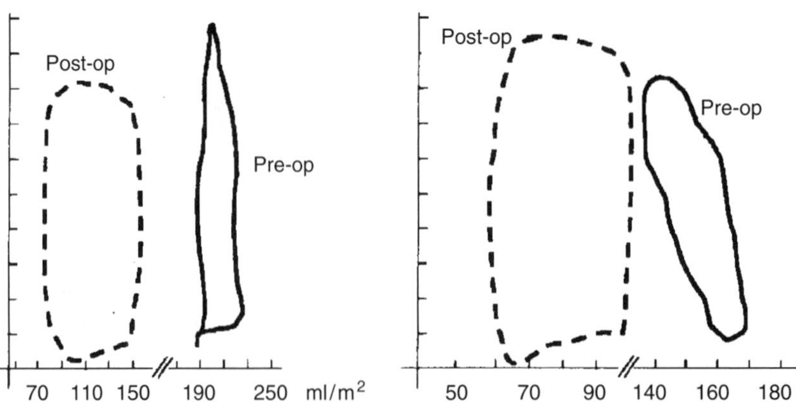

Figure 10 Pressure volume loops in two patients before and following SVR. *Source*: From Ref. 22.

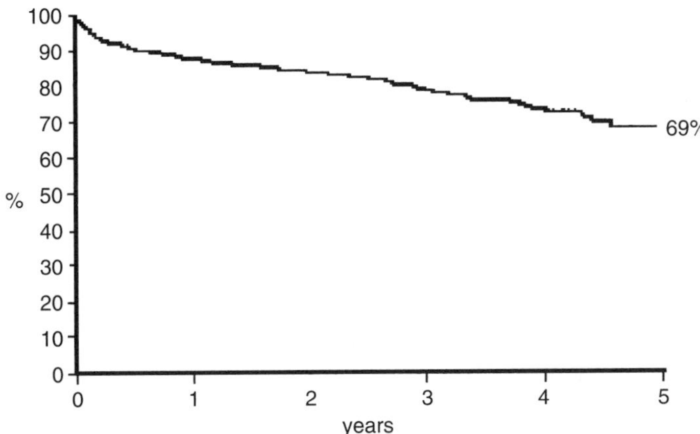

Figure 11 Five year survival in patients following SVR as reported by the RESTORE group. *Source*: From Ref. 23.

One of the most interesting studies of the effectiveness of SVR on cardiac function was performed by DiDonato and colleagues at the Center Cardiothoracique do Monaco. They looked at 30 patients undergoing SVR who did not have electrical asynchrony by QRS definition, but did have mechanical dyssynchrony. Pressure/volume loops (P/V)were obtained with intraventricular micromanometer tipped catheters and pressure/length (P/L) loops were created by analysis of ventriculograms utilizing the Centerline method at 45 discrete intervals. These patients had very abnormal pressure volume loops in size, shape, and orientation with impaired isometric phases with a rightward shift. Endocardial time motion was either early or late yielding P/L loops which were abnormal in size shape and orientation. Postoperatively SVR resulted in a leftward shifting of the P/V loops with a near normalization of P/V loops as well as endocardial motion and P/L loops (Fig. 10). These physiologic results of SVR occurred in concert with improved EF% ($30 \pm 13\%$ to $45 \pm 12\%$), reduced end diastolic and systolic volume indices 202 ± 76 to 122 ± 48 ml/m2 and 144 ± 69 to 69 ± 40 ml/m2 respectively), more rapid peak filling rate (1.75 ± 0.7 to 2.32 ± 0.7 EDV/s), peak ejection rate 1.7 ± 0.07 to $2.6 \pm .09$ Sv/s) and calculated measurements of mechanical efficiency (Figs. 6–11) (22).

In summary, SVR has been shown to improve ventricular size, morphology, EF %, stroke volume index, ventricular energetics, ventricular synchrony and mechanical efficiency. Clinically it results in improved functional capacity (NYHA class) and an excellent 5 yr survival in very sick patients. It is an excellent treatment option in appropriately selected patients with ischemic cardiomyopathy. Where SVR will fit in the armamentarium of a heart failure team will be institution dependent based on their expertise and experience. Further studies are needed to better define the appropriate patients, the basis of the beneficial response ventricular physiology versus relief of ischemia the optimal technique and the appropriate time to perform the procedure.

REFERENCES

1. Buckberg GD. Congestive heart failure: treat the disease, not the symptom—return to normalcy. J Thorac Cardiovasc Surg 2001; 121:628–637.
2. Levy D, Kenchaiah S, Larson MG, et al. Long-term trends in the incidence of and survival with heart failure. N Engl J Med 2002; 347:18.

3. Gheorghiade M, Bonow R. Chronic heart failure in the United States: a manifestation of coronary artery disease. Circulation 1998; 97:282–289.
4. Pfeffer MA, Lamas GA, Vaughan DE, et al. Effect of captopril on progressive ventricular dilation after anterior myocardial infarction. N Engl J Med 1988; 319:80–86.
5. Migrino RQ, Young JB, Ellis SG, et al. End systolic volume index at 90 to 180 minutes into reperfusion therapy for acute myocardial infarction is a strong predictor of early and late mortality. The global utilization of strepti\okinase and t-PA for occluded coronary arteries (GUSTO)-I angiographic investigators. Circulation 1997; 96:116–121.
6. Ghaudron P, Eilles CI, Kugler I, Ertl G. Progressive left ventricular dysfunction and remodeling after myocardial infarction: potential mechanisms and early predictors. Circulation 1993; 87:755–763.
7. White HD, Norris RM, Brown PW, et al. Left ventricular end systolic volume as the major determinant of survival after recovery from myocardial infarction. Circulation 1987; 76:44–51.
8. DiDonato M, Sabatier M, Toso A, et al. Regional myocardial performance of non-ischemic zones remote from anterior wall left ventricularaneurysm. Eur Heart J 1995; 16:1285–1292.
9. Fauchier L, Marie O, Cassett D, et al. Intraventriacular and interventriculaar dyssynchrony in idiopathic dilated cardiomoopathy: a prognostic stuy with fournier phase analysis of radionucleotide angioscintigraphy. J Am Coll Cardiol 2002; 40:2022–2030.
10. Cooley DA, Collins HA, Hall GA, et al. Ventricular aneurysm after myocardial infarction: surgical excision with use of temporary cardiopulmonary bypass. JAMA 1958; 167:557.
11. Mills NL, Everson CT, Hockmuth D, et al. Technical advances in the treatment of left ventricular aneurysm. Ann Thorac Surg 1993; 55:800–972.
12. Jatene AD. Left ventricular aneurysmectomy: resection or reconstruction? J Thorac Cardiovasc Surg 1985; 89:321–331.
13. Dor V, Kreitmann P, Jourdan J. Interest of "physiological" closure of left ventricle after resection and endocardiectomy for aneurysm or akinetic zone comparison with classical technique about a series of 209 left ventricular resections. J Cardiovasc Surg 1985; 26:73 abstract.
14. Cooley D. Ventricular endoaneurysmorrhaphy: a simplified repair for extensive postinfarction aneurysm. J Cardiac Surg 1989; 4:200–205.
15. Cooley DA, Frazier OH, Duncan JM, et al. Intracavitary repair of ventricular aneurysm and regional dyskinesia. Ann Surg 1992; 215:417–423.
16. Menicanti L, DiDonato M. The Dor procedure: what has changed after fifteen years of clinical practice? J Thorac Cardiovasc Surg 2002; 124:886–890.
17. Mickleborough LL. Tech Card Thor Surg 1997; 2:118–131.
18. Caldiera C, McCarthy PM. A simple method of left ventricular reconstruction without patch for ischemic cardiomyopathy. Ann Thorac Surg 2001; 72:2148–2149.
19. Doenst T, Velazquez EJ, Beyersdorf B, et al. To STITCH or not to STITCH: we know the answer, but do we know the question? J Thorac Cardiovasc Surg 2004; 129:246–249.
20. Tavakoli R, Bettex, Webber A, et al. Repair of postinfarction dyskinetic LV aneurysm with either linear or patch technique. Eur J Cardiothorac Surg 2002; 22:129–134.
21. Lunblad R, Abdelnoor M, Svenning JL. Surgery for left ventricular aneurysm: early and late survival after simple linear repair and endoventricular patch plasty. J Thorac Cardiovasc Surg 2004; 128:449–456.
22. DiDonato M, Toso A, Dor V, et al. Surgical ventricular restoration improves mechanical ventricular dyssynchrony in ischemic cardiomyopathy. Circulation 2004; 109:2536–2543.
23. Athanasuleas CL, Buckberg GD, Stanley AW, et al. Surgical ventricular restoration in the treatment of congestive heart failure due to post-infarction ventricular dilation. J Am Coll Card 2004; 44:1439–1445.
24. Mickleborough LL, Merchant N, Ivanov I, et al. Left ventricular reconstruction: early and late results. J Thorac Cardiovasc Surg 2004; 128:127–137.

25. Patel ND, Williams JA, Barreiro CD, et al. Surgical ventricular remodeling for multi territory myocardial infarction: defining a new patient population. J Thorac Cardiovasc Surg 2005; 130:1698–1706.
26. Patel ND, Williams JA, Barreiro CD, et al. Surgical ventricular remodeling for patients with clinically advanced congestive heart failure and severe left ventricular dysfunction (EF < 20%). J Heart Lung Transplant 2005; 24:2022–10.
27. Schenk S, McCarthy PM, Starling RC, et al. Neurohormonal response to left ventricular reduction surgery in ischemic cardiomyopathy. J Thorac Cardiovasc Surg 2003; 128: 38–43.

21 Transmyocardial Laser Revascularization

Keith A. Horvath
Cardiothoracic Surgery Branch, NHLBI, National Institutes of Health, Bethesda, Maryland, U.S.A.

INTRODUCTION

History

Despite the success of medical therapy, percutaneous coronary interventions (PCI), and coronary artery bypass grafting (CABG) in the treatment of coronary artery disease, there are a significant number of patients with refractory angina due to diffuse coronary artery disease that is not amenable to PCI or CABG. This severe coronary artery disease can lead to incomplete revascularization following CABG and is noted to occur in up to 25% of CABG surgery (1). This incomplete revascularization is a powerful independent predictor of operative mortality and perioperative adverse events (1–3). Additionally, the presence of diseased but non-grafted arteries carries a poor prognosis and poses a significant negative influence leading to an increased incidence of death, recurrent angina, myocardial infarction, and the need for repeat CABG (4–6).

Transmyocardial laser revascularization (TMR) was designed to treat patients with end-stage coronary disease. TMR was founded, in part, on previous methods of providing direct perfusion to the myocardium. Prior attempts at direct perfusion were based on Wearn's description of sinusoids that allowed blood to flow directly from the ventricle into the myocardium (7). These arterio-luminal connections provide perfusion in more primitive vertebrate hearts and clinically occur in children with pulmonary atresia, an intact ventricular septum and proximal obstruction of the coronary arteries. Sen and others (8) used myocardial acupuncture to establish direct perfusion and theoretically to recreate a coronary microcirculation similar to that of the reptilian heart. Additional methods of attempting to improve myocardial blood flow include Beck's creation of a form of superficial angiogenesis as a response to epicardial and pericardial inflammation (9). Combining the acupuncture, implantation and inflammation techniques, Boffi (10) as well as Borst (11), used hollow tubes implanted in the myocardium to establish direct perfusion. Results from all of these procedures yielded limited success. The angina relief obtained was not long-lasting, was difficult to replicate, and most importantly, was eventually overshadowed by the ability to perform CABG. The mechanical trauma that resulted in poor long-term patency of myocardial acupuncture was overcome in theory by using a laser to create the channels. Although Mirhoseini et al. (12,13) and Okada et al. (14,15) pioneered the use of a laser to perform this type of revascularization in conjunction with CABG in the early 1980s, the use of a laser as sole therapy to establish its efficacy required advancements in the technology. The carbon dioxide (CO_2) laser used by Mirhoseini had a peak output of 80 W and therefore required a significant amount of time to complete a transmural channel. As a result, to optimally perform TMR, the heart had to be chilled and still. Increasing the output of the laser to 800 W allowed TMR to be performed on a beating heart. This breakthrough lead to the widespread clinical application of TMR. Since then, over 15,000 patients have been treated with TMR around the world and results from individual institutions, multi-center studies and prospective randomized controlled trials have been reported (16–29).

Clinical Trials

The early non-randomized trials demonstrated that sole therapy TMR could be performed safely on patients with severe coronary artery disease who previously had no options. The significant angina relief seen in such patients led to prospective randomized controlled studies to further demonstrate the efficacy of TMR. In these pivotal trials over 1,000 patients were enrolled and randomized to receiving either TMR or medical management as treatment for their severe angina (23–28). The trials employed a 1:1 randomization in which one half of the patients were treated with laser and patients in the control group continued on maximal medical therapy. All patients were followed for 12 mo.

TMR AS SOLE THERAPY

Patients

The entry criteria for these studies, and for sole therapy TMR in general, are as follows: Patients had refractory angina that was not amenable to standard methods of revascularization as verified by a recent angiogram. They had evidence of reversible ischemia based on myocardial perfusion scanning and their left ventricular ejection fractions were greater than 25%.

The typical patient profiles of TMR patients in the randomized controlled trials are listed in Table 1. Because the patients were equally randomized to the medical management group there were no significant demographic differences between the TMR and the control groups for any of these trials. Two different wavelengths of laser light were used. Three studies (23–25) employed a Holmium: yttrium–aluminum–garnett (Ho:YAG) laser and three, (20–28) used a carbon dioxide (CO_2) laser. The average patient age was 62 yr and the majority were male (86%). While there were significant differences in the baseline distribution of patients according to Canadian Cardiovascular Society (CCS) Angina Class, the majority of the patients were in angina Class IV (61%). The ejection fractions for all of the patients were mildly diminished at $48 \pm 10\%$. Many of the patients had suffered at least one previous myocardial infarction and most had some prior revascularization, CABG and/or PCI. Two of the trials, (23,26) permitted a crossover from the medical management group to laser treatment for the presence of unstable angina that necessitated intravenous anti-anginal therapy for which they were unweanable over a period of at least 48 hr. By definition, these crossover patients were less stable and

Table 1 Patient Characteristics in RCTS of Sole Therapy TMR

Characteristic	Allen	Frazier	Burkhoff	Schofield	Aaberge
Patients (N)	275	192	182	188	100
Age (yr)	60	61	63	60	61
Male gender (%)	74	81	89	88	92
EF (%)	47	50	50	48	49
CCS Class III/IV (%)	0/100	31/69	37/63	73/27	66/34
CHF (%)	17	34	NR	9	NR
Diabetes (%)	46	40	36	19	22
Hyperlipidemia (%)	79	57	77	NR	76
Hypertension (%)	70	65	74	NR	28
Prior MI (%)	64	82	70	73	70
Prior CABG (%)	86	92	90	95	80
Prior PCI (%)	48	47	53	29	38

Baseline patient demographics from prospective randomized controlled trials of TMR.
Abbreviations: CABG, coronary artery bypass grafting; CCS, Canadian cardiovascular system angina class; CHF, congestive heart failure; EF, ejection fraction; MI, myocardial infarction; NR, not reported; PCI, percutaneous coronary intervention.

significantly different than those who had been initially randomized to TMR or medical management alone.

Operative Technique

For sole therapy TMR, the patient is placed in a supine position with their left side slightly elevated. General anesthesia is established using a double-lumen endotracheal tube or a bronchial blocker to isolate the left lung. While not mandatory, this facilitates the operation, particularly as most of the patients have pleural and mediastinal adhesions from previous bypass surgery. Additionally, a thoracic epidural catheter can be employed to provide postoperative pain control.

A left anterior thoracotomy in the fifth intercostal space is the usual incision site. Once the ribs are spread by a retractor, the pericardium is opened to expose the epicardial surface of the heart (Fig. 1). Care must be taken to avoid previous bypass grafts. The left anterior descending artery is identified and used as a landmark for the location of the septum. The inferior and posterior lateral portions of the heart can be reached through this incision with a combination of manual traction, placement of packing behind the heart, and, as illustrated, with the use of a right-angled laser handpiece. Channels are created starting near the base of the heart and then serially in a line approximately 1-cm apart toward the apex starting inferiorly and working superiorly to the anterior surface of the heart. As there is some bleeding from the channels, commencement of the TMR inferiorly keeps the anterior area clear and expedites the procedure. The number of channels created depends on the size of the heart and on the size of the ischemic area. Myocardium that is thinned by scar, particularly when the scar is transmural, should be avoided as TMR will be of no benefit to these regions and bleeding from channels in these areas may be problematic. The thoracotomy is then closed after the placement of a chest tube and, in the majority of the cases, the patient is extubated in the operating room.

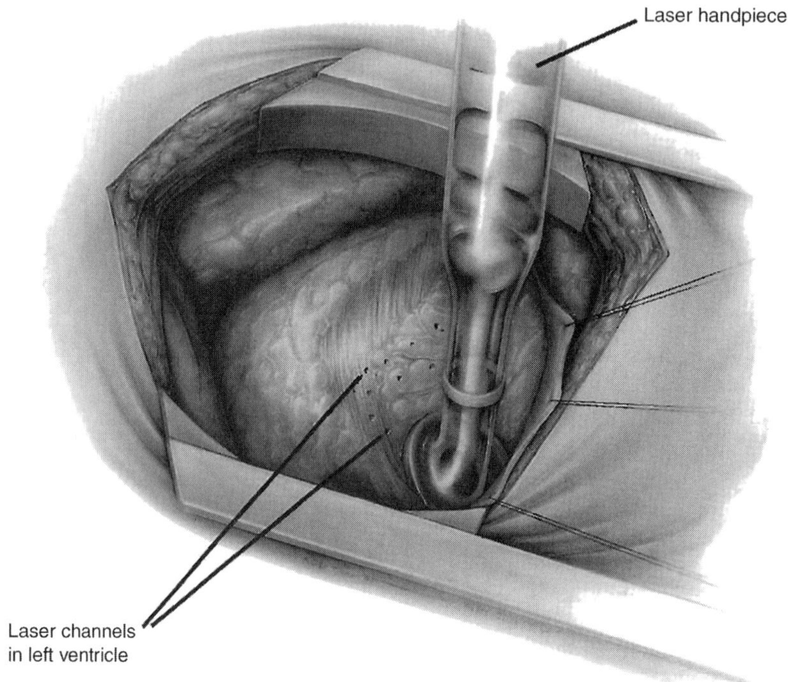

Figure 1 For transmyocardial laser revascularization, channels of one millimeter diameter are created in a distribution of one per square centimeter, starting inferiorly and then working superiorly to the anterior surface of the heart. The number of channels created depends on the size of the heart and on the size of the ischemic area.

The handpiece in Figure 2 is from a CO_2 laser and illustrates one of the differences between the two lasers employed for TMR. The CO_2 laser energy is delivered via hollow tubes and is reflected by mirrors to reach the epicardial surface. 1-mm channels are made with a 15–20 J pulse. The firing of the laser is synchronized to occur on the r wave of the EKG to avoid arrhythmias. The transmural channel is created by a signal pulse in 40 msec and can be confirmed by transesophageal echocardiography (TEE). The vaporization of blood by the laser energy as the laser beam enters the ventricle creates an obvious and characteristic acoustic effect as noted on TEE. The Ho:YAG laser achieves a 1-mm channel by manually advancing a fiber bundle through the myocardium while the laser fires. Typical pulse energies are 2 Jsec for this laser and at a rate of 5 pulses per second, 10–20 pulses are required to traverse the myocardium. Detection of transmural penetration is primarily by tactile and auditory feedback.

Endpoints

The principal subjective endpoint for all of the trials was a change in angina symptoms. This was assessed by the investigator and/or a blinded independent observer. In addition to assigning an angina class, standardized questionnaires such as the Seattle Angina Questionnaire, the Short Form Questionnaire 36 (SF-36), and the Duke Activity Status Index were employed. These tests were used to detect changes in symptoms and quality of life.

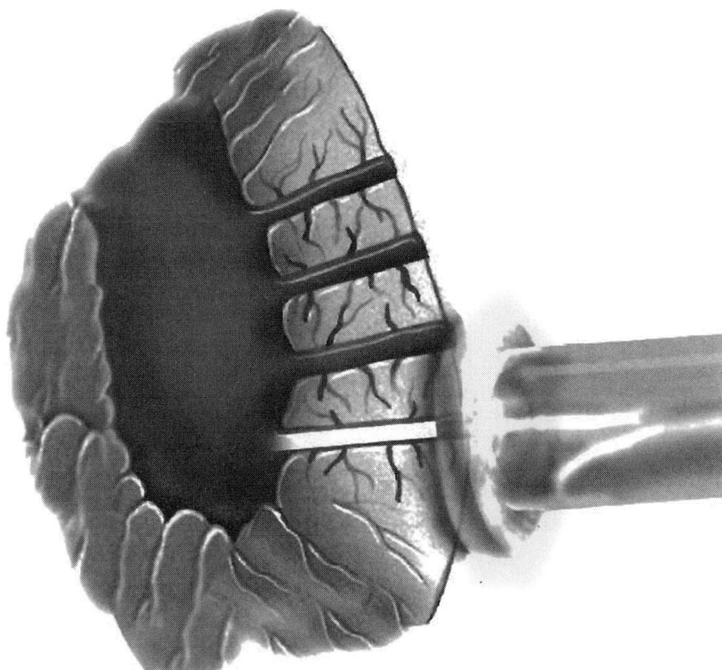

Figure 2 The CO_2 laser creates a transmural channel in a single 20 J pulse. Conceptually direct perfusion may occur via the channel. Evidence indicates the laser stimulates angiogenesis in and around the channel that leads to improved perfusion.

Objective measurements consisted of repeated exercise tolerance testing as well as repeat myocardial perfusion scans. Patients were reassessed at 3, 6, and 12 mo post-randomization.

RESULTS

Mortality

Prior to the randomized studies, mortality rates in the 10%–20% (16–22) range were reported for TMR patients. In the randomized trials, lower perioperative mortality rates were reported ranging from 1%–5% (23–28). One of the important lessons learned from these controlled trials that differ from the earlier studies was a decrease in the mortality when patients taken to the operating room were not unstable, specifically not on IV heparin or nitroglycerin. When patients were allowed to recover from their most recent episode of unstable angina, and were able to be weaned from intravenous medications such that their operation could be performed two weeks later, the mortality dropped to 1% (26). The one-year survival for TMR patients was 84%–95% and for medical management patients was 79%–96%. Meta-analysis of the one-year survival demonstrated no statistically significant difference between the patients treated with a laser to those that continued with their medical therapy (30). Long term survival of the randomized patients from two of these studies has been reported. Four year follow-up from Aaberge et al. in which both the TMR and medical management groups were kept intact demonstrated a 78% survival for TMR versus 76% for medical management ($p = ns$) (31). In a 5-yr follow-up using an intent-to-treat analysis Allen reported a survival for TMR patients at 65% versus 52% for medical management patients ($p=0.05$) (32).

Morbidity

Unlike mortality, the exact definition of various complications varied from one study protocol to the next, and therefore, morbidity data are difficult to pool. Nevertheless, the typical TMR patient's postoperative course had a lower incidence of myocardial infarction, heart failure, and arrhythmias than what has been documented in a similar cohort of patients, those that have reoperative CABG (23–28).

Angina Class

The principal reason for performing TMR is to reduce the patient's anginal symptoms. This can be quantified by assessing the angina class, pre- and post procedure. Angina class assessment was performed by a blinded independent observer in all studies. This was done as the only angina assessment or as comparison with the investigators' assessment. Significant symptomatic improvement was seen in all studies for patients treated with the laser. Using a definition of success as a decrease of two or more angina classes, all of the studies demonstrated a significant success rate after TMR with success rates ranging from 25%–76% (Fig. 3). A meta-analysis of this angina reduction yielded a summary odds ratio of 9.3 (95% CI: 4.6–18.5 $p<0.000001$). Significantly fewer patients in the medical management group experienced symptomatic improvement and the success rate for these patients ranged from 0%–32%. The seemingly broad range of success is due to differences between the baseline characteristics of the studies. It is more difficult to achieve a two

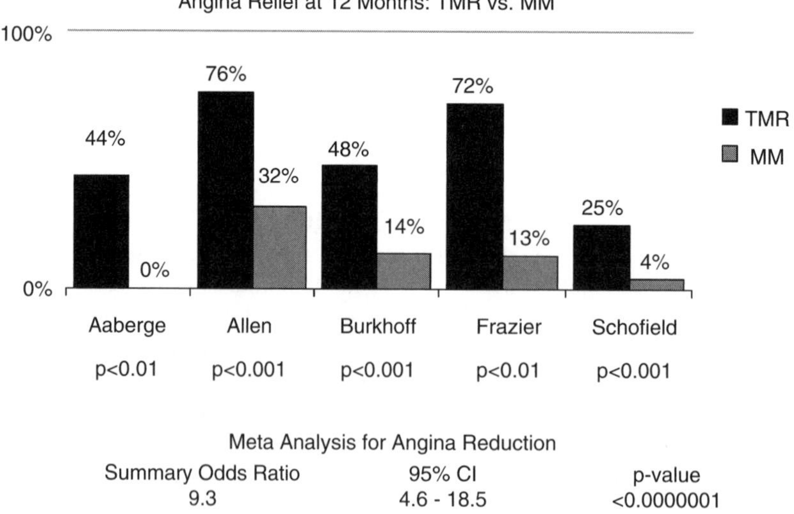

Figure 3 Summary of the angina relief results from five prospective randomized controlled trials comparing transmyocardial laser revascularization (TMR) and medical management (MM). Graph illustrates success rate for TMR or MM as measured by the percentage of patients that had a decrease of two or more angina classes. Meta-analysis of these results documents the significant advantage seen with TMR over MM.

angina class improvement if the baseline angina class is III. Studies that started with most of their patients in angina class III, not surprisingly, showed the lowest success rate. In contrast, the largest success rate for TMR was seen in the trial in which all of the patients were in CCS class IV at enrollment. Of note, the medical management group in this study also showed the largest success rate (23). This underscores some of the baseline differences between the studies.

Quality of Life and Myocardial Function

Quality of life indices as assessed by the Seattle Angina Questionnaire, the SF-36, and Duke Activity Status Index, demonstrated significant improvement for TMR treated patients vs. medical management in every study. Global assessment of myocardial function by ejection fraction using echocardiography or radionuclide multigated acquisition scans showed no significant change in the overall ejection fraction for any of the patients, regardless of group assignment or study.

Hospital Admission

Another indicator of the efficacy of TMR was demonstrated in a reduction in hospital admissions for unstable angina or cardiac related events post-procedure. A meta-analysis of the data provided indicates that the 1 yr hospitalization rate of patients in the laser treated group was statistically significantly less then for those treated medically. Medical management patients were admitted four times more frequently than TMR patients over the year of follow-up (30).

Exercise Tolerance

Additional functional test assessment using exercise tolerance was also performed in three of the trials (24,27,28). While the method of treadmill testing differed between the trials, the results demonstrate an improvement in exercise tolerance for TMR treated patients. Two studies showed an average of 65–70 sec improvement in the TMR group at 12 mo compared to their baseline, while the medical management group had either an average of 5 sec improvement or a 46 sec decrease in exercise time over the same interval (27,28). One additional trial demonstrated that the time to chest pain during exercise increased significantly and fewer patients were limited by chest pain in the TMR group, whereas the medical management group showed no improvement (28).

Medical Treatment

All of the studies employed protocols that continued all of the patients on maximal medical therapy. For each study the frequencies and dosages of antianginal and cardiovascular drugs were similar between the two groups at baseline. TMR patients, as a result of their symptomatic improvement, had a reduction in their medication use over the year of follow-up. As many of these patients used a combination of short and long acting nitrates preoperatively, the trials demonstrated a significant decrease in the use of nitrates in TMR treated patients while the medical management patients showed a slight increase in their nitrate usage. At one year, the overall medication use decreased or remained unchanged in 83% of the TMR patients and, conversely, the use of medications increased or remained unchanged in 86% of the medical management patients (26). The significant angina relief seen following TMR was not due to medication changes or increases for the TMR treated patients.

Myocardial Perfusion

As previously stated, myocardial perfusion scans were obtained preoperatively to verify the extent and severity of reversible ischemia. The four largest randomized trials included follow-up scans as part of their study (23,24,26,27). These results reflect over 800 of the patients randomized. The methodology of recording and analyzing these results differed in each study so it is difficult to pool the data. Nevertheless, review of the results demonstrated an improvement in perfusion for CO_2 TMR treated patients. Fixed (scar) and reversible (ischemic) defects were tallied for both the TMR treated patients and the medical management groups. One CO_2 study demonstrated a significant decrease in the number of reversible defects for both the TMR and the medical management patients (27). This improvement in the reversible defects in the TMR group was seen without a significant increase in the fixed defects at the end of the study. However, the number of fixed defects in the medical management group had nearly doubled over the same 12 mo interval. Similarly, there was a 20% improvement in the perfusion of previously ischemic areas in the CO_2 TMR group of another trial and in that same trial there was a 27% worsening of the perfusion of the ischemic areas in the medical management group at 12 mo (26). There was no difference in the number of fixed defects between the groups at 12 mo, nor was there a significant change in the number of fixed defects for each patient compared with their baseline scans. The remaining two Ho:YAG studies that obtained follow-up scans showed no significant difference between the TMR and the medical management groups at 12 mo and no significant improvement in perfusion in the TMR treated patients over the same interval (23,24).

Non-randomized data had previously demonstrated an improvement in perfusion using dual isotope scanning at one and two years after CO_2 TMR (33). Additionally, using N-13 ammonia position emission tomography (PET) assessment, subendocardial perfusion improved significantly compared to the subpericardial perfusion after CO_2 TMR treatment (34,35).

Long-Term Results

Two reports of long-term follow-up of prospectively randomized patients are available. Similar to the one-year results, intention to treat analyses determined that significantly more TMR than MM patients continued to experience at least two-class angina improvement from basline (88% vs. 44%, $p<0.001$) or were free from angina symptoms altogether (33% vs. 11%, $p=0.02$) at a mean of five years (32). In long-term follow-up of the randomized trial that kept both the TMR and MM groups intact (i.e., no cross-over), it was shown that angina symptoms were still significantly improved (24% vs. 3%, TMR vs. MM, $p=0.001$) and unstable angina hospitalizations were significantly reduced ($p<0.05$) at a mean follow-up of 43 mo (31). Follow-up of a series of nonrandomized patients who received TMR and survived long term, support these findings (36). At a mean of five years and up to seven years post procedure, 81% of these patients improved to Class II or better, 68% were found to have improved at least two angina classes from baseline, 17% were angina-free, and quality of life remained significantly improved. These last two reports reflect the sustained angina relief seen with CO_2 TMR as these patients had no additional procedures to account for their symptom improvement over the long term.

Based on an assessment of the cumulative results from these multiple randomized trials, the recently updated ACC/AHA practice guidelines (37) and STS practice guidelines (38) have determined that the weight of the evidence favors the use of TMR in the treatment of stable, medically refractory, angina patients.

TMR AS AN ADJUNCT TO CABG

Clinical Trials

Owing to its success as sole therapy, TMR has been evaluated in conjunction with CABG in patients with diffuse coronary artery disease who would be incompletely revascularized by CABG alone. The safety and effectiveness of adjunctive TMR have been somewhat difficult to assess due to the influence of coronary bypass grafts and the lack of randomized control arms in some studies (39–41).

Two prospective, randomized, multi-centered controlled trials have been performed using TMR adjunctively with CABG in patients. In these studies patients with one or more viable myocardial target areas served by coronary vessels that were not amenable to bypass grafting received either CABG plus TMR or CABG alone (42,43). Baseline and operative characteristics were similar between groups, including the location and number of bypass grafts placed (3.1 ± 1.2, CABG/TMR; 3.4 ± 1.2, CABG alone, $p=0.07$). Patients were blinded to their treatment group through one-year follow-up.

RESULTS

Mortality

Improved outcomes following TMR+CABG versus CABG alone in terms of a reduced operative mortality rate (1.5% vs. 7.6%, $p=0.02$), reduced postoperative inotropic support requirements (30% vs. 55%, $p=0.001$), increased 30-day freedom from major adverse cardiac events (97% vs. 91%, $p=0.04$), and improved one-year Kaplan–Meier survival (95% vs. 89%, $p=0.05$) have been reported (42). Multivariable predictors of operative mortality were CABG alone (odds ratio 5.3, $p=0.04$) and increased age (odds ratio 1.1, $p=0.03$) (42). A similar trend in operative mortality following TMR+CABG versus CABG alone (9% vs 33%, $p=0.09$) was reported in a study of high-risk patients (43).

Efficacy

The use of TMR adjunctively with CABG has been shown to decrease intensive care unit (ICU) times and length of hospitalization stay (41). In a long-term follow-up of the randomized controlled trial, the effectiveness of TMR+CABG vs CABG alone has been reported (44). At a mean of five years, both groups experienced significant angina improvement from baseline, however, the TMR+CABG group had a lower mean angina-free patients (78% vs. 63%, $p=0.08$), compared to CABG alone patients. Long term survival was similar between randomized groups.

Observational data on the practice of TMR+CABG has been collected in the Society of Thoracic Surgeons National Cardiac Database (45,46). From 1998 to 2003, 5618 patients underwent TMR+CABG. These were compared with 932,715 patients who underwent CABG only operations. The TMR+CABG patients therefore account for 0.6% of the surgical revascularization practice in the Database. Table 2 outlines the significant baseline differences between the CABG only patients and the TMR+CABG patients. The

Table 2 Comparison of CABG Only Versus TMR+CABG Patients

Characteristic	CABG only	TMR+CABG	*P* value
N	932,715	5618	
Body surface area, m^2 (sd)	1.96 (0.24)	1.99 (0.23)	<0.001
Diabetes (all types)	34%	50%	<0.001
Insulin-dependent diabetes	10%	19%	<0.001
Renal failure	5%	7%	<0.001
Dialysis	1%	2%	<0.001
CVA	7%	9%	<0.001
Chronic lung disease	14%	17%	<0.001
Peripheral vascular disease	16%	20%	<0.001
Cerebral vascular disease	12%	17%	<0.001
MI	46%	49%	<0.001
Reoperation	9%	26%	<0.001
3 vessel CAD	71%	80%	<0.001
Hypercholesterolemia	62%	73%	<0.001
Hypertension	72%	80%	<0.001

Baseline demographics of TMR combined with CABG patients enrolled in the Society of Thoracic Surgeons (STS) National Adult Cardiac Database.

Abbreviations: CAD, coronary artery disease; CVA, cerebral vascular accident; MI, myocardial infarction.

Source: STS Adult Cardiac Database 1998–2003.

TMR+CABG patients have an increased incidence of every surrogate marker of diffuse arterial disease and therefore it is not surprising that their observed mortality was higher at (3.8% vs. 2.7% for CABG only patients, $p<0.001$). When unstable angina patients were removed, the observed mortality for TMR+CABG was decreased to 2.7% and the O/E ratio was 0.87. Comparison of use and outcomes from sites that have a TMR laser versus those that do not showed no evidence of overuse of TMR or difference in outcomes (46).

MECHANISMS

Laser–Tissue Interactions

Understanding the mechanism of TMR starts with understanding the laser–tissue interaction. While numerous devices (47,48), including ultrasound (49), cryoablation (50), radio frequency (51,52), heated needles (53,54), as well as the aforementioned hollow and solid needles have been used; none have engendered the same response that is seen with a laser. Additionally, numerous wavelengths of laser light have also been employed. These include xenon-chloride (XeCl) (55,56), Neodymium:YAG (ND:YAG) (57), Erbium:YAG (Er:YAG) (58), and Thulium–Holmium–Chromium:YAG lasers (THC:YAG) (59). All of these devices have been explored experimentally, but have not been pursued on a significant scale clinically. Only CO_2 and Ho:YAG are used for TMR. The result of any laser tissue interaction is dependent on both laser and tissue variables (33,58–60). CO_2 has a wavelength of 10,600-nm, whereas Ho:YAG has a wavelength of 2120 nm. These infrared wavelengths are primarily absorbed in water and therefore rely on thermal energy to ablate tissue. One significant difference however is that the Ho:YAG laser it is pulsed and the arrival of two successive pulses must be separated by time to allow for thermal dissipation, otherwise the accumulated heat will cause the tissue to

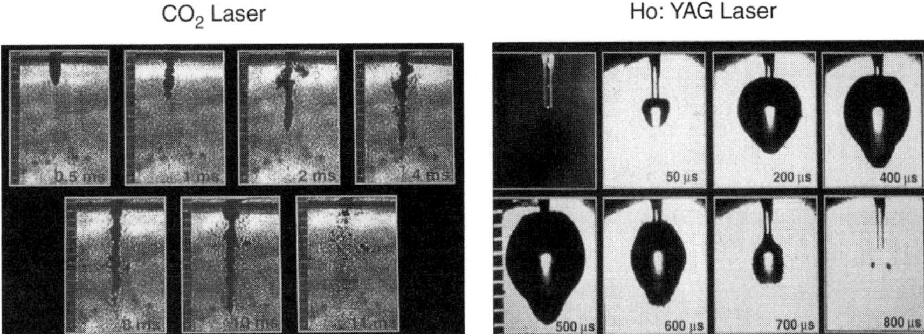

Figure 4 Sequential photography of the firing of a single pulse from a CO_2 laser and a Ho:YAG laser into water. The pulse duration and energy levels are the same as those employed clinically.

explode under pressure. Such explosions create acoustic waves, which travel along the planes of lower resistance between muscle fibers and cause structural trauma as well as thermo-coagulation (60). The standard operating parameters for the Ho:YAG laser, are pulse energies of 1–2 Jsec and 6–8 W/pulse. The energy is delivered at a rate of 5 pulses/sec through a flexible 1-mm optical fiber bundle. Despite the low energy level and short pulse duration, there are very high levels of peak power delivered to the tissue so that with each pulse there is an explosion (Fig. 4). Additionally, the fiber is advanced manually through the myocardium and it is therefore impossible to know whether the channel is being created by the kinetic energy delivered via the mechanical effects of the fiber and whether there has been enough time for thermal dissipation prior to the next pulse.

In contrast the CO_2 was used at an energy level of 15–20 Jsec/pulse with a pulse duration of 25–40 msec. At this level, the laser photons do not cause explosive ablation and the extent of structural damage is limited. Additionally, a transmural channel can be created with a single pulse (Fig. 4). Confirmation of this transmurality is obtained by observing the vaporization of blood within the ventricle using TEE.

Finally the CO_2 laser is synchronized to fire on the r wave and with its short pulse duration arrhythmic complications are minimized. The Ho:YAG device is unsynchronized and due to the motion of the fiber through the myocardium over several cardiac cycles, is more prone to ventricular arrhythmias.

Patent Channels

As noted, the original concept of TMR was to create perfusion via channels connecting the ventricle with the myocardium. Clinical work has demonstrated some evidence of long-term patency (61,62). Additional experimental work showed some evidence of patency as well (63–66). There are also significant reports from autopsy series and laboratories that indicate that the channels do not remain patent (67–71). The consensus is that while channels may occasionally remain patent, this is not the principle mechanism of TMR.

Denervation

In contrast to the open channel mechanism, damage to the sympathetic nerve fibers may explain the angina relief noted in clinical trials. The nervous system of the heart can function independent of inputs from extra cardiac neurons to regulate regional cardiac function by reflex action. This intrinsic system contains afferent neurons, sympathetic efferent, postganglionic neurons, and parasympathetic efferent postganglionic neurons. Because of this complex system, it is difficult to demonstrate true denervation. However, several experimental studies have demonstrated that denervation may indeed play a role in Ho:YAG TMR (72–74). Experimental evidence to the contrary was performed in a nonischemic animal model (75). Although the studies were carefully carried out, it is difficult to isolate the sympathetic afferent nerve fibers and the experiments were in the acute setting and only address short-term effects. Regardless of the methodology employed in the laboratory, there is significant evidence of sympathetic denervation following positron emission tomography of Ho:YAG TMR treated patients (76).

Angiogenesis

The likely underlying mechanism for the clinical efficacy of TMR is the stimulation of angiogenesis. This mechanism fits the clinical picture of significant improvement in symptoms over time as well as a concomitant improvement in perfusion, as seen with the CO_2 laser. Numerous reports have demonstrated a histologic increase in neovascularization as a result of TMR channels (68,70,77–83). More molecular evidence of this angiogenic phenomenon was derived from work that demonstrated an upregulation of vascular endothelial growth factor (VEGF) messenger RNA, expression of FGF2, as well as matrix metalloproteinases following TMR (84–86). Histologically, similar degrees of neovascularization have been noted after mechanical injury of various types. Needle injury has been demonstrated by immunohistochemistry to also stimulate growth factor expression and angiogenesis. The conclusion is that TMR induced angiogenesis is a nonspecific response to injury (87–89). Investigation of this using hot and cold needles, radiofrequency energy, and laser energy to perform TMR clearly demonstrates a spectrum of tissue response to the injury (53). The results in a model of chronic myocardial ischemia to mimic the clinical scenario indicate that indeed neovascularization can occur after mechanical TMR, but if these new blood vessels grow in the midst of a scar, there will be little functional contribution from blood flow through these new vessels. The recovery of function with laser TMR was due to a minimization of scar formation and a maximization of angiogenesis.

This then becomes a critical question: if TMR induces angiogenesis, is there an ensuing improvement in function? Clinically, this has been demonstrated subjectively with quality of life assessments, but more importantly, it has been demonstrated objectively with multiple techniques, including dobutamine stress echocardiography (90), PET (34), and cardiac MRI (91,92). As further evidence of the angiogenic response, experimental data has mirrored the clinical perfusion results noted, with improvements in perfusion in porcine models of chronic ischemia where the ischemic zone was treated with CO_2 TMR (93–96). This improved perfusion did lead to an improvement in myocardial function as well.

PERCUTANEOUS MYOCARDIAL LASER REVASCULARIZATION

Myocardial laser revascularization has been performed percutaneously (97–99), thoracoscopically (100), via thoracotomy (23–29) and via sternotomy (39–42). Aside from the percutaneous (PMR) approach, any of the other surgical approaches have yielded similar symptomatic improvement. Several percutaneous trials have attempted to demonstrate a symptomatic improvement with the creation of 2–3 mm deep subendocardial divots achieved with a laser fiber fed via a peripheral artery into the left ventricle (97–99). Even with the use of electromechanical mapping to verify the position of the fiber and the creation of the channel, the results from PMR have been less favorable than those seen with TMR. A double-blinded randomized controlled trial showed no benefit to the laser treated patients compared to the untreated control group (99). As the patients were blinded to their treatment, the possibility of a significant placebo effect for PMR has been raised. Of note, the morbidity and mortality of PMR is reportedly similar to that seen with TMR. As a result, the United States Food and Drug Administration rendered PMR unapprovable.

The failure of PMR to achieve the same clinical results that have been seen with TMR may be due to several significant limitations. The first of which is the partial thickness treatment of the left ventricle. Even at the maximal estimated depth of 6-mm that has been reported with PMR, this is significantly less than the full thickness treatment of the myocardium that is achieved with an open TMR approach. Furthermore, there are typically fewer of these partial thickness channels created with PMR. The exact location of the channel and the establishment of a wide distribution of the channels from inside a moving ventricle is also problematic. Finally, the limitations of Ho:YAG TMR are also applicable to PMR as that is the wavelength of light that has been employed.

FUTURE USES OF TMR

Other potential applications include the use of TMR in the treatment of cardiac transplant graft atherosclerosis. While performed on a small number of patients, the results have indicated a benefit following TMR (101,102). Finally, the combination of TMR plus other methods of angiogenesis may provide an even more robust response. Experimental work investigating these combinations has verified a synergistic effect with regard to histologic evidence of significant angiogenesis and, perhaps more importantly, an improvement in myocardial function with a combination of TMR and gene therapy versus either therapy alone (103–107).

SUMMARY

Cardiothoracic surgeons are increasingly faced with a more complex patient who has developed a pattern of diffuse coronary artery disease and has exhausted nonsurgical options. Results replicated in multiple randomized, controlled trials augmented by recently available long-term results have validated the safety, effectiveness, and substantially improved health outcomes through the application of TMR for the treatment of selected patients with severe angina due to diffuse disease, when used alone and as adjunctive therapy to achieve a more complete revascularization.

REFERENCES

1. Weintraub WS, Jones EL, Craver JM, et al. Frequency of repeat coronary bypass or coronary angiogplasty after coronary artery bypass surgery using saphenous venous grafts. Am J Cardiol 1994; 73:103–112.
2. Graham MM, Chambers RJ, Davies RF. Angiographic quantification of diffuse coronary artery disease: reliability and prognostic value for bypass operations. J Thorac Cardiovasc Surg 1999; 118:618–627.

3. Osswald B, Blackstone E, Tochtermann U, et al. Does the completeness of revascularization affect early survival after coronary artery bypass grafting in elderly patients? Euro J Cardiothorac Surg 2001; 20:120–126.
4. Lawrie GM, Morris GC, Silvers A, et al. The influence of residual disease after coronary bypass on the 5-year survival rate of 1274 men with coronary artery disease. Circulation 1982; 66:717–723.
5. Schaff H, Gersh B, Pluth J, et al. Survival and functional status after coronary artery bypass grafting: results 10 to 12 years after surgery in 500 patients. Circulation 1983; 68:200–204.
6. Bell MR, Gersh BJ, Schaff HV, et al. Effect of completeness of revascularization on long-term outcomes of patients with three-vessel disease undergoing coronary artery bypass surgery. Circulation 1992; 86:446–457.
7. Wearn J, Mettier S, Klumpp T, et al. The nature of the vascular communications between the coronary arteries and the chambers of the heart. Am Heart J 1933; 9:143–164.
8. Sen P, Udwadia T, Kinare S, et al. Transmyocardial revascularization: a new approach to myocardial revascularization. J Thorac Cardiovasc Surg 1965; 50:181–189.
9. Beck CS. The development of a new blood supply to the heart by operation. Ann Surg 1935; 102:801–813.
10. Massimo C, Boffi L. Myocardial revascularization by a new method of carrying blood directly from the left ventricular cavity into the coronary circulation. J Thorac Surg 1957; 34:257–264.
11. Walter P, Hundeshagen H, Borst HG. Treatment of acute myocardial infarction by transmural blood supply from the ventricular cavity. Eur Surg Res 1971; 3:130–138.
12. Mirhoseini M, Muckerheide M, Cayton MM. Transventricular revascularization by laser. Lasers Surg Med 1982; 2:187–198.
13. Mirhoseini M, Fisher JC, Cayton M. Myocardial revascularization by laser: a clinical report. Lasers Surg Med 1983; 3:241–245.
14. Okada M, Ikuta H, Shimizu OK, et al. Alternative method of myocardial revascularization by laser: experimental and clinical study. Kobe J Med Sci 1986; 32:151–161.
15. Okada M, Shimizu K, Ikuta H, et al. A new method of myocardial revascularization by laser. Thorac Cardiovasc Surg 1991; 39:1–4.
16. Horvath KA, Mannting F, Cummings N, et al. Transmyocardial laser revascularization: operative techniques and clinical results at two years. J Thorac Cardiovasc Surg 1996; 111:1047–1053.
17. Cooley DA, Frazier OH, Kadipasaoglu KA, et al. Transmyocardial laser revascularization: clinical experience with twelve-month follow-up. J Thorac Cardiovasc Surg 1996; 111:791–797.
18. Horvath KA, Cohn LC, Cooley DA, et al. Transmyocardial laser revasculari-zation: results of a multi-center trial using TLR as sole therapy for end stage coronary artery disease. J Thorac Cardiovasc Surg 1997; 113:645–654.
19. Krabatsch T, Tambeur L, Lieback E, et al. Transmyocardial laser revascularization in the treatment of end-stage coronary artery disease. Ann Thorac Cardiovasc Surg 1998; 4:64–71.
20. Hattler BG, Griffith BP, Zenati MA, et al. Transmyocardial laser revascularization in the patient with unmanageable unstable angina. Ann Thor Surg 1999; 68:1203–1209.
21. Milano A, Pratali S, Tartarini G, et al. Early results of transmyocardial revascularization with a holmium laser. Ann Thorac Surg 1998; 65:700–704.
22. Dowling RD, Petracek MR, Selinger SL, et al. Transmyocardial revascularization in patients with refractory, unstable angina. Circulation 1998; 98:II73–II75.
23. Allen KB, Dowling RD, Fudge TL, et al. Comparison of transmyocardial revascularization with medical therapy in patients with refractory angina. N Engl J Med 1999; 341:1029–1036.
24. Burkhoff D, Schmidt S, Schulman SP, et al. Transmyocardial laser revascularization compared with continued medical therapy for treatment of refractory angina pectoris: a prospective randomized trial. Lancet 1999; 354:885–890.

25. Jones JW, Schmidt SE, Richman BW, et al. Holmium: YAG laser transmyocardial revascularization relieves angina and improves functional status. Ann Thorac Surg 1999; 67:1596–1602.
26. Frazier OH, March RJ, Horvath KA. Transmyocardial revascularization with a carbon dioxide laser in patients with end-stage coronary artery disease. N Engl J Med 1999; 341:1021–1028.
27. Schofield PM, Sharples LD, Caine N, et al. Transmyocardial laser revascularization in patients with refractory angina: a randomized controlled trial. Lancet 1999; 353:519–524.
28. Aaberge L, Nordstrand K, Dragsund M, et al. Transmyocardial revascularization with CO_2 laser in patients with refractory angina pectoris. Clinical results from the Norwegian randomized trial. J Am Coll Cardiol 2000; 35:1170–1177.
29. Agarwal R, Ajit M, Kurian VM, et al. Transmyocardial laser revascularization: early results and 1-year follow-up. Ann Thorac Surg 2000; 69:1993–1995.
30. Horvath KA. Results of prospective randomized controlled trials of transmyocardial laser revascularization. Heart Surg Forum 2002; 5:33–40.
31. Aaberge L, Rootwelt K, Blomhoff S, et al. Continued symptomatic improvement three to five years after transmyocardial revascularization with CO_2 laser: a late clinical follow-up of the Norwegian randomized trial with transmyocardial revascularization. J Am Coll Cardiol 2002; 39:1588–1593.
32. Allen KB, Dowling RD, Angell W, et al. Transmyocardial revascularization: five-year follow-up of a prospective, randomized, multicenter trial. Ann Thorac Surg 2004; 77:1228–1234.
33. Horvath KA, Mannting FR, Cummings N, et al. Transmyocardial laser revascularization: operative techniques and clinical results at two years. J Thorac Cardiovasc Surg 1996; 111:1047–1053.
34. Frazier OH, Cooley DA, Kadipasaoglu KA, et al. Myocardial revascularization with laser. Preliminary findings. Circulation 1995; 92:58–65.
35. Kadipasaoglu K, Frazier OH. Transmyocardial laser revascularization: effect of laser parameters of tissue ablation and cardiac perfusion. Semin Thorac Cardiovasc Surg 1999; 11:4–11.
36. Horvath KA, Aranki SF, Cohn LH, et al. Sustained angina relief 5 years after transmyocardial laser revascularization with a CO_2 laser. Circulation 2001; 104:181–184.
37. Gibbons R, Abrams J, Chatterjee K, et al. ACC/AHA 2002 guideline update for the management of patients with chronic stable angina-summary article: a report of the American College of Cardiology/American Heart Association Task Force on Practice Guidelines (Committee on the Management of Patients with Chronic Stable Angina). Circulation 2003; 107:149–158.
38. Bridges CR, Horvath KA, Nugent B, et al. Society of Thoracic Surgeons practice guideline: transmyocardial laser revascularization. Ann Thorac Surg 2004; 77:1484–1502.
39. Trehan J, Mishra M, Bapna R, et al. Transmyocardial laser revascularization combined with coronary artery bypass grafting without cardiopulmonary bypass. Euro J Cardiothorac Surg 1997; 12:276–284.
40. Stamou SC, Boyce SW, Cooke RH, et al. One -year outcome after combined coronary artery bypass grafting and transmyocardial laser revascularization for refractory angina pectoris. J Am Coll Cardiol 2002; 89:1365–1368.
41. Wehberg KE, Julian JS, Todd JC, et al. Improved patient outcomes when transmyocardial revascularization is used as adjunctive revascularization. Heart Surg Forum 2003; 6:1–3.
42. Allen KB, Dowling R, DelRossi A, et al. Transmyocardial revascularization combined with coronary artery bypass grafting: a multicenter, blinded, prospective, randomized, controlled trial. J Thorac Cardiovasc Surg 2000; 119:540–549.
43. Frazier OH, Boyce SW, Griffith BP, et al. Transmyocardial revascularization using a synchronized CO_2 laser as adjunct to coronary artery bypass grafting: results of a prospective, randomized multi-center trial with 12 month follow-up. Circulation 1999; 100:1248.
44. Allen KB, Dowling RD, Schuch D, et al. Adjunctive transmyocardial revascularization: 5-year follow-up of a prospective, randomized, trial. Ann Thorac Surg 2004; 78:458–465.

45. Peterson ED, Kaul P, Kaczmarek RG, et al. From controlled trials to clinical practice: monitoring transmyocardial revascularization use and outcomes. J Am Coll Cardiol 2003; 42:1611–1616.
46. Horvath KA, Ferguson TB, Guyton RA, et al. The impact of unstable angina on outcomes of transmyocardial laser revascularization combined with coronary artery bypass grafting. Ann Thorac Surg 2005, 80:2082–2085.
47. Shawl FA, Kaul U, Saadat V. Percutaneous myocardial revascularization using a myocardial channeling device: first human experience using the AngioTrax system. J Am Coll Cardiol 2000; 35:61A.
48. Malekah R, Reynolds C, Narula N, et al. Angiogenesis in transmyocardial laser revascularization—a nonspecific response to injury. Circulation 1998; 9:62–65.
49. Smith NB, Hynynen K. The feasibility of using focused ultrasound for transmyocardial revascularization. Ultrasound Med Biol 1998; 24:1045–1054.
50. Khairy P, Dubuc M, Gallo R. Cryoapplication induces neovascularization: a novel approach to percutaneous myocardial revascularization. J Am Coll Cardiol 2000; 35:5A–6A.
51. Yamamoto N, Gu AG, Derosa CM, et al. Radio frequency transmyocardial revascularization enhances angiogenesis and causes myocardial denervation in a canine model. Lasers Surg Med 2000; 27:18–28.
52. Dietz U, Darius H, Eick O, et al. Transmyocardial revascularization using temperature controlled HF energy creates reproducible intramyocardial channels. Circulation 1998; 98:3770.
53. Horvath KA, Belkind N, Wu I, et al. Functional comparison of transmyocardial revascularization by mechanical and laser means. Ann Thorac Surg 2001; 72:1997–2002.
54. Whittaker P, Rakusan K, Kloner RA. Transmural channels can protect ischemic tissue. Assessment of long-term myocardial response to laser- and needle-made channels. Circulation 1996; 93:143–152.
55. Hughes GC, Kypson AP, Annex BH, et al. Induction of angiogenesis after TMR: a comparison of holmium: YAG, CO_2, and excimer lasers. Ann Thorac Surg 2000; 70:504–509.
56. Martin JS, Sayeed-Shah U, Byrne JG, et al. Excimer versus carbon dioxide transmyocardial laser revascularization: effects on regional left ventricular function and perfusion. Ann Thorac Surg 2000; 69:1811–1816.
57. Whittaker P, Spariosu K, Ho ZZ. Success of transmyocardial laser revascularization is determined by the amount and organization of scar tissue produced in response to initial injury: results of ultraviolet laser treatment. Lasers Surg Med 1999; 24:253–260.
58. Genyk IA, Frenz M, Ott B, et al. Acute and chronic effects of transmyocardial laser revascularization in the nonischemic pig myocardium by using three laser systems. Lasers Surg Med 2000; 27:438–450.
59. Jeevanandam V, Auteri JS, Oz MC, et al. Myocardial revascularization by laser-induced channels. Surg Forum 1990; 41:225–227.
60. Kadipasaoglu KA, Sartori M, Masai T, et al. Intraoperative arrhythmias and tissue damage during transmyocardial laser revascularization. Ann Thorac Surg 1999; 67:423–431.
61. Cooley DA, Frazier OH, Kadipasaoglu KA, et al. Transmyocardial laser revascularization. Anatomic evidence of long-term channel patency. Tex Heart Inst J 1994; 21:220–224.
62. Mirhoseini M, Shelgikar S, Cayton M. Clinical and histological evaluation of laser myocardial revascularization. J Clin Laser Med Surg 1990; 8:73–77.
63. Hardy RI, James FW, Millard RW, et al. Regional myocardial blood flow and cardiac mechanics in dog hearts with CO_2 laser-induced intramyocardial revascularization. Basic Res Cardiol 1990; 85:179–197.
64. Horvath KA, Smith WJ, Laurence RG, et al. Recovery and viability of an acute myocardial infarct after transmyocardial laser revascularization. J Am Coll Cardiol 1995; 25:258–263.
65. Krabatsch T, Schaper F, Leder C, et al. Histologic findings after transmyocardial laser revasculariza-tion. J Card Surg 1996; 11:326–331.
66. Lutter G, Martin J, Ameer K, et al. Microperfusion enhancement after TMLR in chronically ischemic porcine hearts. Cardiovasc Surg 2001; 9:281–291.

67. Gassler N, Wintzer HO, Stubbe HM, et al. Transmyocardial laser revascularization: histological features in human nonresponder myocardium. Circulation 1997; 95:371–375.
68. Khomoto T, Fisher PE, Gu A, et al. Physiology, histology, and two week morphology of acute myocardial channels made with a CO_2 laser. Ann Thorac Surg 1997; 63:1275–1283.
69. Kohmoto T, Fisher PE, Gu A, et al. Does blood flow through holmium: YAG transmyocardial laser channels? Ann Thorac Surg 1996; 61:861–868.
70. Burkhoff D, Fisher PE, Apfelbaum M, et al. Histologic appearance of transmyocardial laser channels after 4½ weeks. Ann Thorac Surg 1996; 61:1532–1535.
71. Sigel JE, Abramovitch CM, Lytle BW, et al. Transmyocardial laser revascularization: three sequential autopsy cases. J Thorac Cardiovasc Surg 1998; 115:1381–1385.
72. Kwong KF, Kanellopoulos GK, Nikols JC, et al. Transmyocardial laser treatment denervates canine myocardium. J Thorac Cardiovasc Surg 1997; 114:883–890.
73. Kwong KF, Schuessler RB, Kanellopoulos GK, et al. Nontransmural laser treatment incompletely denervates canine myocardium. Circulation 1998; 98:1167–1171.
74. Hirsch GM, Thompson GW, Arora RC, et al. Transmyocardial laser revascularization does not denervate the canine heart. Ann Thorac Surg 1999; 68:460–468.
75. Minisi AJ, Topaz O, Quinn MS, et al. Cardiac nociceptive reflexes after transmyocardial laser revascularization: implications for the neural hypothesis of angina relief. J Thorac Cardiovasc Surg 2001; 122:712–719.
76. Al-Sheikh T, Allen KB, Straka SP, et al. Cardiac sympathetic denervation after transmyocardial laser revascularization. Circulation 1999; 100:135–140.
77. Yamamoto N, Kohmoto T, Gu A, et al. Angiogenesis is enhanced in ischemic canine myocardium by transmyocardial laser revascularization. J Am Coll Cardiol 1998; 31:1426–1433.
78. Fisher PE, Khomoto T, DeRosa CM, et al. Histologic analysis of transmyocardial channels: comparison of CO_2 and Holmium:YAG lasers. Ann Thorac Surg 1997; 64:466–472.
79. Zlotnick AY, Ahmad RM, Reul RM. Neovascularization occurs at the site of closed laser channels after transmyocardial laser revascularization. Surg Forum 1996; 48:286–287.
80. Kohmoto T, Fisher PE, DeRosa C, et al. Evidence of angiogenesis in regions treated with transmyocardial laser revascularization. Circulation 1996; 94:1294.
81. Spanier T, Smith CR, Burkhoff D. Angiogenesis. A possible mechanism underlying the clinical benefits of transmyocardial laser revascularization. J Clin Laser Med Surg 1997; 15:269–273.
82. Mueller XM, Tevaearai HT, Chaubert P, et al. Does laser injury induce a different neovascularization pattern from mechanical or ischemic injuries? Heart 2001; 85:697–701.
83. Hughes GC, Lowe JE, Kypson AP, et al. Neovascularization after transmyocardial laser revascularization in a model of chronic ischemia. Ann Thorac Surg 1998; 66:2029–2036.
84. Horvath KA, Chiu E, Maun DC, et al. Up-regulation of VEGF mRNA and angiogenesis after transmyocardial laser revascularization. Ann Thorac Surg 1999; 68:825–829.
85. Li W, Chiba Y, Kimura T, et al. Transmyocardial laser revascularization induced angiogenesis correlated with the expression of matrix metalloproteinase and platelet-derived endothelial cell growth factor. Eur J Cardiothorac Surg 2001; 19:156–163.
86. Pelletier MP, Giaid A, Sivaraman S, et al. Angiogenesis and growth factor expression in a model of transmyocardial revascularization. Ann Thorac Surg 1998; 66:12–18.
87. Chu V, Kuang J, McGinn A, et al. Angiogenic response induced by mechanical transmyocardial revascularization. J Thorac Cardiovasc Surg 1999; 118:849–856.
88. Chu VF, Giaid A, Kuagn JQ, et al. Angiogenesis in transmyocardial revascularization: comparison of laser versus mechanical punctures. Ann Thorac Surg 1999; 68:301–307.
89. Malekan R, Reynolds C, Narula N, et al. Angiogenesis in transmyocardial laser revascularization: a nonspecific response to injury. Circulation 1998; 98:I62–I66.
90. Donovan CL, Landolfo KP, Lowe JE, et al. Improvement in inducible ischemic during dobutamine stress echocardiography after transmyocardial laser revascularization in patients with refractory angina pectoris. J Am Coll Cardiol 1997; 30:607–612.

91. Laham RJ, Simons M, Pearlman JD, et al. Magnetic resonance imaging demonstrates improved regional systolic wall motion and thickening and myocardial perfusion of myocardial territories treated by laser myocardial revascularization. J Am Coll Cardiol 2002; 39:1–8.
92. Horvath KA, Kim RJ, Judd RM, et al. Contrast enhanced MRI assessment of microinfarction after transmyocardial laser revascularization. Circulation 2000; 102:765–768.
93. Horvath KA, Greene R, Belkind N, et al. Left ventricular functional improvement after transmyocardial laser revascularization. Ann Thorac Surg 1998; 66:721–725.
94. Hughes GC, Kypson AP, St Louis JD, et al. Improved perfusion and contractile reserve after transmyocardial laser revascularization in a model of hibernating myocardium. Ann Thorac Surg 1999; 67:1714–1720.
95. Krabatsch T, Modersohn D, Konertz W, et al. Acute changes in functional and metabolic parameters following transmyocardial laser revascularization: an experimental study. Ann Thorac Cardiovasc Surg 2000; 6:383–388.
96. Lutter G, Martin J, von Samson P, et al. Microperfusion enhancement after TMLR in chronically ischemic porcine hearts. Cardiovasc Surg 2001; 9:281–291.
97. Oesterle SN, Sanborn TA, Ali N, et al. Percutaneous transmyocardial laser revascularization for severe angina: PACIFIC randomized trial. Lancet 2000; 356:1705–1710.
98. Stone GW, Teirstein PS, Rubenstein R, et al. A prospective, multicenter, randomized trial of percutaneous transmyocardial laser revascularization in patients with nonrecanalizable chronic total occlusions. J Am Coll Cardiol 2002; 39:1581–1587.
99. Leon MB, Baim DS, Moses JW, et al. A randomized blinded clinical trial comparing percutaneous laser myocardial revascularization vs. placebo in patients with refractory coronary ischemia. Circulation; 102:II-565.
100. Horvath KA. Thoracoscopic transmyocardial laser revascularization. Ann Thorac Surg 1998; 65:1439–1441.
101. Mehra MR, Uber PA, Prasad AK, et al. Long-term outcome of cardiac allograft vasculopathy treated by transmyocardial laser revascularization early rewards, late losses. J Heart Lung Transplant 2000; 19:801–804.
102. Frazier OH, Kadipasaoglu KA, Radovancevic B, et al. Transmyocardial laser revascularization in allograft coronary artery disease. Ann Thorac Surg 1998; 65:1138–1141.
103. Fleischer KJ, Goldschmidt-Clermont PJ, Fonger JD, et al. One-month histologic response of transmyocardial laser channels with molecular intervention. Ann Thorac Surg 1996; 62:1051–1058.
104. Sayeed-Shah U, Mann MJ, Martin J, et al. Complete reversal of ischemic wall motion abnormalities by combined use of gene therapy with transmyocardial laser revascularization. J Thorac Cardiovasc Surg 1998; 116:763–768.
105. Doukas J, Ma CL, Craig D, et al. Therapeutic angiogenesis induced by FGF-2 gene delivery combined with laser transmyocardial revascularization. Circulation 2000; 102:1214.
106. Lutter G, Dern P, Attmann T, et al. Combined use of transmyocardial laser revascularization with basic fibroblastic growth factor in chronically ischemic porcine hearts. Circulation 2000; 102:3693.
107. Horvath KA, Doukas J, Lu CJ, et al. Myocardial functional recovery after FGF2 gene therapy as assessed by echocardiography and MRI. Ann Thorac Surg 2002; 74:481–487.

22

Percutaneous Left Ventricular Assist Devices

Piotr Sobieszczyk and Andrew C. Eisenhauer
Cardiovascular Division and Cardiac Catheterization Laboratory, Brigham and Women's Hospital, Harvard Medical School, Boston, Massachusetts, U.S.A.

INTRODUCTION

Surgically implanted Left Ventricular Assist Devices (LVADs) are an integral component of managing patients with advanced heart failure awaiting cardiac transplantation (1). Implantable LVADs, despite the recent successes in long-term use of these devices (2), generally continue to function as "bridge to therapy". Mechanical support of left ventricular function results in myocardial unloading, decrease in myocardial oxygen demand and augmentation of coronary and systemic perfusion. It can normalize the hemodynamic derangement of heart failure and serve as a bridge to cardiac transplantation, recovery or even become a destination therapy. Cardiac transplantation remains the destination therapy and patients receive LVADs only after careful planning and patient selection. LVADs are costly, invasive and require considerable surgical expertise for their insertion and management. They remain the domain of specialized centers and are not widely available. They are not practical in situations where circulatory support is needed emergently and transiently.

The aging population and the growing epidemic of cardiovascular risk factors continue to increase the worldwide burden of cardiovascular disease (3). This epidemiological pressure, patient preference for minimally invasive procedures and the constant technological advancement, continue to expand the indications for coronary revascularization. As a result, increasingly complex patient subsets undergo percutaneous coronary revascularization (PCI). Drug-eluting stents, modern antiplatelet therapy and miniaturization of interventional devices allow durable results even in patients too ill for surgical revascularization. Similarly, the field of percutaneous therapy for valvular disease is rapidly expanding. Despite these advances, cardiogenic shock, especially when complicating myocardial infarction, continues to exact high mortality rates (4). There is an increasing need for minimally invasive circulatory support devices which can be inserted percutaneously in any catheterization lab and provide effective support during a high-risk procedure or offer a window of time to consider the next therapy.

In addition to providing periprocedural hemodynamic stability, rapid institution of a simple circulatory support may impart, at least theoretically, some physiological benefits.

The benefit of restoring epicardial flow during acute myocardial infarction, for example, is significantly attenuated if myocardial perfusion remains impaired (5). In animal models of myocardial infarction, mechanical unloading instituted prior to reperfusion has been demonstrated to limit the extent of myocardial damage (6). Myocardial salvage has been shown in experimental models of left ventricular unloading during ischemia using various percutaneous devices. While surgically implanted cardiopulmonary bypass (CPB) during reperfusion therapy is impractical, intra-aortic balloon pump (IABP) support has been shown, albeit inconsistently, to increase myocardial blood flow and myocardial oxygen supply (7). In animal models of cardiogenic shock due to myocardial infarction, left ventricular support using left atrial to femoral artery bypass can restore microvascular coronary flow and reduce the extent of myocardial necrosis (8,9). Transvalvular circulatory support systems have also shown similar benefit (10). There is a growing interest in incorporating simple and minimally invasive circulatory support systems in revascularization strategies for myocardial infarction.

Efforts to develop such circulatory support systems stretch back at least half a century. Much of the impetus for their development was eventually provided by the early coronary balloon angioplasty techniques. Before the advent of coronary stents, prolonged balloon inflation in the coronary arteries was poorly tolerated in patients with depressed LV function, multivessel disease or severe valvular disease. Left ventricular assistance was required in these patients to provide circulatory support during balloon-induced coronary ischemia. In addition to the widely used IABP, clinically evaluated percutaneous systems included the percutaneous CPB as well as transvalvular and left atrial to femoral non-pulsatile flow devices. Despite the procedural success and early survival benefit provided by such combined interventions, balloon angioplasty in these high-risk patients did not provide durable results. As a result, long-term survival remained inferior to that offered by coronary artery bypass graft (CABG) surgery (11). This tempered the enthusiasm for high-risk balloon angioplasty with circulatory support. The introduction of drug-eluting stents with durability comparable to CABG (12) eliminated these early concerns. The devices in development today are a result of innovative technology applied to some of these old ideas. While coronary ischemia is minimal during modern coronary interventions, increasingly complex patients undergo a myriad of percutaneous procedures. The list of potential indications for percutaneous LVAD (Table 1) continues to expand as these devices become smaller and more efficient.

LEFT VENTRICULAR ASSIST DEVICES: PULSATILE AND NON-PULSATILE FLOW

Mechanical circulatory support devices can be divided into nonpulsatile devices, which provide constant flow, and pulsatile displacement devices, which deliver cyclic flow mimicking systole and diastole. Examples of the latter are the pneumatic Thoratec, Medos, Abiomed pumps and the electrical HeartMate I and Novacor pumps. These devices provide a more physiological flow pattern but require surgical implantation of large-bore cannulas and are associated with high bleeding rates and thromboembolic complications. The pulsatile flow they generate requires mechanical valves with their inherent wear-and-tear as well as embolic and infectious complications. The intracorporeal pulsatile devices are large and their use is limited by appropriate body size. Their implantation and maintenance are complicated and not applicable to emergencies but they do offer good long-term durability. The nonpulsatile rotary devices are divided into centrifugal pumps (percutaneous CPB Biomedicus pump, HeartMate III, CorAide) and axial flow pumps

Table 1 Clinical Situations in Which Percutaneous Left Ventricular Assistance May Offer Survival Benefit

Bridge to recovery
Cardiogenic shock
Myocardial ischemia
Acute myocarditis
Decompensated heart failure
Postcardiotomy low output state
Bridge to therapy
End-stage heart failure (pre-surgical LVAD implantation)
Advanced valvular disease
Myocardial ischemia
High-risk PCI (CI $<$2.0 L/min/m^2, systemic hypotension, end-organ hypoperfusion, severely depressed LVEF, treatment of vessel supplying dominant amount myocardial area)
Off-pump CABG
Transplant rejection
Bridge to decision
End-stage heart failure
Cardiogenic shock

(Hemopump, HeartMate II, Jarvik 2000, DeBakey/NASA pump, Impella). These devices are smaller with valveless design, and are easier to implant. Because of the size advantage, all of the percutaneous circulatory assist devices operate on the nonpulsatile principle. Hemolysis has been a major concern in nonpulsatile pumps, especially in those of axial design. The fundamental difference between these devices lies in the nature of the flow pattern they provide. Despite the obvious appeal of the pulsatile design, the clinical outcomes of short-term support with pulsatile or non-pulsatile devices are not significantly different (13). The nonpulsatile pumps assist rather than replace the left ventricle and may be more appropriate as a bridge to recovery where complete LV unloading may be detrimental to eventual recovery.

HISTORICAL PERSPECTIVE

Intra-aortic Balloon Pump

The IABP, first introduced in 1968, has evolved to become a reliable, easily inserted and operated device with decreasing complication rates (14). It reduces left ventricular end diastolic pressure and augments systemic perfusion. Its effect on coronary perfusion is debatable: some studies suggest a 5%–15% augmentation in coronary blood flow in experimental models (15,16), while others have found no effect at all in animals with coronary stenoses (17,18). The increase in cardiac output provided by IABP varies and can be a low as 0.2 L/min (19). IABP was initially used in patients with low cardiac output after cardiac surgery, the so-called post-cardiotomy syndrome. IABP support has been shown to reduce mortality rates in these patients (20). While aortic counter pulsation can improve initial hemodynamics in patients with cardiogenic shock, available data suggest that the benefit of IABP depends on the primary therapy of myocardial ischemia. IABP has been shown to reduce mortality in patients with MI complicated by cardiogenic shock when they are treated with thrombolytics, but it had no benefit when used in conjunction with primary angioplasty (21). Data from larger trials of myocardial infarction confirmed that IABP support has not been independently associated with improvement in LV function or survival (22,23). Mechanical support with IABP has been reported in up to 11% of patients undergoing cardiac transplantation but its utility in this situation is limited due to immobilization imposed by the device.

IABP support can be rapidly initiated without specialized expertise or elaborate supportive infrastructure. It has, however, several major shortcomings. It merely augments the LV function and does not actively replace it. It is only successful in patients with significant degree of residual LV function and cannot be used in patients with complex arrhythmias or in patients with aortic valve disease. The use of IABP for left ventricular support is well established, but its efficacy is limited in many of the sickest patients.

Left Atrial to Femoral Artery Bypass

The first use of circulatory support without the need for thoracotomy was described in 1959 in a canine model (24). In 1962 Dennis et al. (25,26) successfully applied this technique in the clinical arena. The left atrial to femoral artery circuit was established with trans-septal puncture via a jugular approach. A cannula was placed in the left atrium and, with the aid of a roller pump; blood was delivered through a cannula in the femoral artery into the descending aorta without the need for a membrane oxygenator. Left atrial to femoral artery bypass has been proven in animals to decrease infarct size irrespective of treatment of the infarct related artery (9,27). Clinically this design was initially used in patients with postcardiotomy failure who could not be weaned from CPB (28,29). Despite isolated reports of its use in the catheterization laboratory (30–32), technical limitations hindered wider acceptance of this technique. The design was plagued by the lack of adequately sized trans-septal cannula that could provide physiological flow rates and pumps prone to thromboembolism and heating up from high speed and friction. With the advent of intracardiac echo to assist with trans-septal puncture and technical advances in pump design, this technique has gained new life through the development of TandemHeart percutaneous LVAD system.

Percutaneous Cardiopulmonary Bypass

Development of membrane oxygenation and operating room-based CPB technology inevitably led to its transfer into the cardiac catheterization laboratory. Percutaneous cardiopulmonary bypass (pCPB) system (Bard Inc.), capable of producing up to 6 L/min of flow, had a particular appeal in the pre-stent era of percutaneous coronary interventions when the threat of abrupt vessel closure mitigated the enthusiasm for multi-vessel interventions, particularly in patients with impaired LV function or high-risk anatomy. Since both left and right ventricles were supported, CPB was effective in patients with significant pulmonary vascular disease and biventricular failure.

Vogel et al. in 1988 described the first clinical use of CPB in patients undergoing percutaneous coronary and valvular interventions (33). In 1989, Shawl et al., described a fully percutaneous CPB technique (34). The principle of this device was similar to that used in the operating room: unoxygenated blood was aspirated from the mid-right atrium through a percutaneously placed 18- to 20-Fr catheter and passed sequentially through a membrane oxygenator, a heat exchanger, and a pump before being returned to the descending aorta via a catheter in the common femoral artery. Initial clinical experience consisted of 51 patients undergoing non-emergent, high risk percutaneous coronary intervention who were supported for an average of 37 minutes (34). Percutaneous CPB allowed prolonged occlusion of coronary flow (up to 10 minutes) without significant periprocedural complications. There were three in-hospital deaths unrelated to the device and one late death after a mean follow up of 5 months. A single center experience reported by Shawl et al. (35) described 107 patients with severely decreased LVEF who underwent coronary balloon angioplasty with pCPB. The procedural success was 98% with no periprocedural deaths and low (4.7%) in-hospital mortality. These encouraging results were offset by mortality rate of 21% at 21 months after the procedure. One and two year survival was 83% and 77% respectively. Despite a rather complex design, pCPB could be rapidly instituted in victims of cardiogenic shock. Circulatory support was, on average, established in 21 minutes, reducing PCWP to 0–2 mmHg and allowing emergency coronary angioplasty or stabilization until CABG (36,37). Experience from a larger multicenter registry of 105 high-risk patients undergoing non-emergent PCI with pCPB support confirmed high rates of periprocedural success and survival to hospital discharge. This benefit, however came at a price: complication rates reached 39%, mostly as a result of vascular morbidity related to large catheter size (38). There is limited information regarding direct comparison of pCPB and other supportive devices. Schreiber et al., described single institution, non-randomized experience among 149 patients undergoing high risk PCI who were supported with CPB or IABP (19). While there was no difference in major adverse cardiovascular events, pCPB was associated with a significantly higher rate of transfusions (60% vs. 27%) and need for vascular repair, 14% versus 3%. Kaul et al., randomized a similar high-risk group of 40 patients to undergo PCI with IABP or pCPB support (39). In these 40 patients with EF<30% and majority of myocardium supplied by the target vessel, in-hospital mortality was identical at 5% but, again, pCPB was associated with a higher rate of transfusions and vascular complications. Additional drawbacks of the CPB system stemmed from its dependence on the oxygenator. CPB support beyond 6 hours resulted in severe pulmonary and hematological complications and activation of the inflammatory response.

Transvalvular Assist Device—The Hemopump®

The Hemopump® (Medtronic, Inc, Minneapolis, Minnesota, U.S.A.), the first ventricular assist device made specifically for use outside the operating room, was designed by Richard Wampler in 1988 (40). The initial description of this device in an animal model was quickly followed by report of its use in 7 patients with cardiogenic shock (41). After circulatory support for up to 4 days, 5 patients survived to discharge. The design of the Hemopump was quite novel: a catheter-based system was inserted via the femoral artery and advanced through the aorta and across the aortic valve into the left ventricle. A small, turbine-like axial flow pump, located just proximal to the tip of the catheter, rotated at 17,000 to 25,000 rpm and aspirated blood through an inlet port in the catheter resting in the LV. The blood was then expelled distally to the turbine through the catheter's outlet port positioned above the aortic valve in the ascending aorta. The turbine was coupled in the catheter to a 9Fr drive shaft, which exited the body and was powered by an electromechanical coupler. The device was contraindicated in patients with severe aortic valve disease or left ventricular thrombus. It required a functioning right ventricle and was not helpful in patients with pulmonary hypertension. The degree of circulatory support provided by the pump depended on the afterload against which the Hemopump was pumping. The lower the systemic pressure, the higher the pump flow delivered, a relationship, which frequently required the use of pharmacological agents to lower the systemic blood pressure. The original design used a 21F (7 mm in diameter) catheter inserted into the femoral artery with a surgical cut-down and was capable of providing 4 L/min of non-pulsatile flow. The device was designed to provide support for 14 days.

In animal models of myocardial infarction and cardiogenic shock, the Hemopump consistently reduced LV end-diastolic pressure, maintained the mean arterial pressure and cardiac output and increased perfusion in the ischemic territory (42–45). In a sheep model of LAD occlusion, left ventricular unloading and infarct zone reduction achieved with the Hemopump were superior to that provided by IABP counter-pulsation (46).

Clinical experience in 53 patients with cardiogenic shock demonstrated that the 21F Hemopump catheter could be inserted in 77% of patients to provide hemodynamic stabilization and achieve a 30-day survival of 31.7% (47). Smalling et al. quantified the hemodynamic effects of the Hemopump. During the first 24 hr of support in patients with cardiogenic shock, PCWP decreased from 26 ± 4 to 16 ± 4 mmHg ($p=0.01$) and cardiac index increased from 1.6 ± 0.4 to 2.4 ± 0.4 L/min/m^2 (48). Nevertheless, mortality remained high: overall survival in the study group was 4 (36%) of 11 patients. Outside the catheterization laboratory, the Hemopump has been successfully used in postcardiotomy patients (49,50) and as substitute for CPB during CABG (51).

The introduction of a 14F cannula met with considerable enthusiasm. The first application of the 14F system, Hemopump HP 14 was described by Scholz et al. (52) in two hemodynamically compromised patients undergoing high risk PCI. The smaller cannula size provided a somewhat reduced flow rate of 1.5–2.2 L/min but significantly increased the mean arterial pressure and decreased the pulmonary capillary wedge pressure during coronary artery occlusion. Further experience came from several nonrandomized series of patients with cardiogenic shock and those treated with circulatory support during high-risk percutaneous interventions. In a study of 32 patients in cardiogenic shock undergoing high-risk PCI, Hemopump effectively decreased PCWP and maintained cardiac index and systolic blood pressure during balloon inflation and myocardial ischemia at a pre-insertion level (53). Among patients who developed cardiac arrest during balloon occlusion of the coronary artery, Hemopump maintained mean arterial pressure between 40 and 50 mmHg (53). Additional experience with the 14F device was reported by Dubois-Rande in 13 patients undergoing high-risk PTCA. The Hemopump assistance significantly decreased PCWP (23.5 to 18.6 mmHg, $p=0.013$). Applying coronary blood flow velocity measurements, investigators showed that Hemopump had no effect on coronary blood flow velocities before or after the angioplasty. Therefore, while the Hemopump unloaded the left ventricle, it did not alter coronary flow under stable hemodynamic conditions; coronary flow under altered hemodynamics was not assessed (54). Addition of IABP was tested to convert a continuous flow Hemopump system to a pulsatile flow. Meyns et al., demonstrated that this combination reduced the Hemopump output by 11% but increased myocardial blood flow to ischemic regions without additional affect on the perfusion of the peripheral organs (55).

Experience from larger clinical trials did not fulfill the early promise of this device. Despite introduction of a smaller cannula size, bleeding and vascular complications remained quite common, developing in 25% and 16% of patients respectively (53,56). Despite its support, the overall in-hospital mortality after high-risk PCI was 12.5% and hemolysis was frequent (53) In order to prevent thromboembolic events, the Hemopump protocol required a high degree of anticoagulation with ACT above 400 sec, vastly exceeding ACT of 200–300 sec recommended in current percutaneous coronary interventions. Bleeding, transfusion requirement and mild thrombocytopenia developed in 25% of the patients. Despite aggressive anticoagulation, thrombosis remained a concern. The Hemopump never gained the approval of the U.S. Food and Drug Administration.

CONTEMPORARY PERCUTANEOUS LEFT VENTRICULAR ASSIST DEVICES

Impella Recover® System

The Impella device was developed by Impella Cardiosystems GmbH (Aachen, Germany) in the late 1990s and became available in Europe for intraoperative ventricular support in 1999. The Impella pump is a catheter based, transvalvular, microaxial rotary flow pump providing non-pulsatile flow (Fig. 1). This design is a result of the clinical experience with the Hemopump and the technical innovations, which surmounted some of the shortcomings of the Hemopump device. Progressive miniaturization has allowed a less traumatic vascular access while delivering a physiologically adequate flow rate without drive shaft complications. Evolution of the propeller manufacturing technology from hand polished mini-turbine to injection molded impellers has eliminated hemolysis despite high rotational speeds needed to deliver physiological flow.

The device is currently available in a larger, surgically implanted model (Recover® LD) and a smaller, percutaneously implanted design. The larger percutaneous

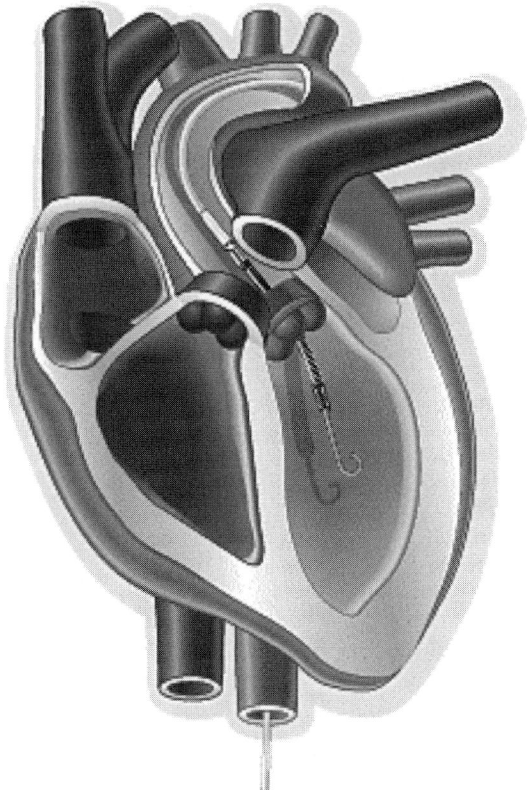

Figure 1 Impella Recover® System. The device is placed over the wire from the femoral artery across the aortic valve.

Recover® LP 5.0 device measures 6.4 mm in diameter (19.5F) and is mounted on a 9F catheter. It is inserted via a femoral artery cut-down and delivers flow of up to 5 L/min at speed of 32,500 rpm for up to 7 days. A thoracotomy-requiring version of this device (Recover LD) is implanted with a trans-thoracic insertion via a 10 mm Dacron conduit sewn into the aorta. Most of the clinical experience with this device comes from surgical patients. The versatility of Recover LD allows direct placement via the ascending aorta into the left ventricle or through the right atrium into the pulmonary artery to establish biventricular support (57). The right ventricular Impella pump (Recover LD) differs in the design of the impeller and the direction of its rotation.

The smaller percutaneous version of this circulatory support, Recover® LP 2.5, measures 4 mm in diameter (12F), is mounted on a 9F pig-tail catheter and can deliver up to 2.5 L/min of non-pulsatile flow (Fig. 2). The principle of insertion is similar to that used for the Hemopump device: the catheter is advanced over a guidewire from the femoral artery into the left ventricle. The suction port is positioned in the LV and the outlet port in the ascending aorta. Once the pump, located at the distal tip of the catheter, is placed across the aortic valve, it aspirates blood from the left ventricle and propels it into the ascending aorta. The pump's performance depends on its rotary speed controlled by an electrical motor, and the afterload facing the pump. The latter, measured as the difference between the aortic and the LV pressure, is sensed by a sensor in the pump, which measures the pressure drop between the tip of the cannula and the end of the pump. This pressure difference and the rotational speed of the pump are monitored by a mobile console, which allows adjustments to provide optimal flow and pump performance. The system is designed for continuous use for up to 5 days and requires relatively low anticoagulation levels.

In animal studies of acute myocardial infarction, ventricular support with the Impella device led to an increase in the diastolic and mean blood pressures and a decrease in the LV end diastolic pressure. While the myocardial blood flow during myocardial ischemia was not affected, it did increase in the reperfusion phase. The myocardial oxygen consumption was reduced, significantly decreasing the infarct size in Impella-supported animals. The reduction in infarct size corresponded to the degree of unloading during reperfusion (58). In animal models of acute mitral regurgitation, Impella pump, when compared to traditional support with IABP, significantly increased cardiac output, coronary and systemic perfusion and lowered left atrial pressure, providing a more

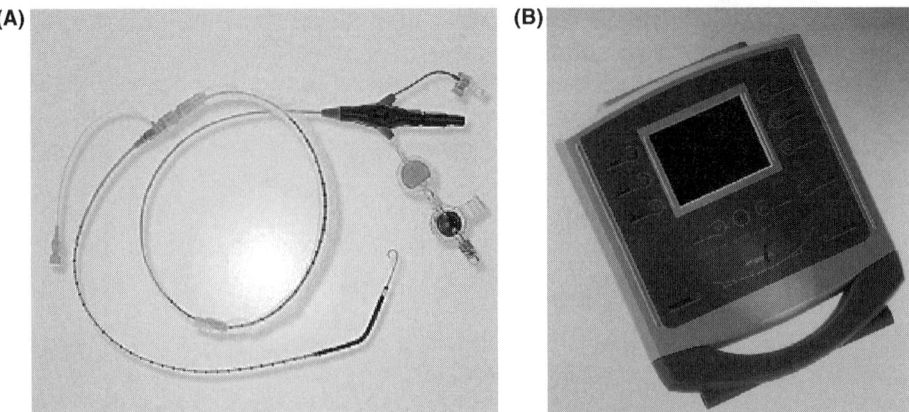

Figure 2 Impella Recover® LP 2.5. The 12F pump is mounted on a 9F catheter (**A**) and is controlled by a mobile console (**B**). *Source*: Photos courtesy of Impella Cardiosystems.

effective LV unloading compared to IABP (59). Moreover, transvalvular placement has not been associated with aortic regurgitation. In animal models of reperfusion injury, Impella supported animals recovered with higher indices of myocardial contractility and higher subendocardial blood flow suggesting a protective effect afforded by the Impella device (60). Despite concerns about the impact of axial pumps on blood cell integrity, animal studies have not shown any significant hemolysis or thrombocytopenia (61).

Early clinical experience with the Impella system came from applications of the Recover LD and Recover LP 5.0 pump. This version has been used extensively in off-pump CABG where it is positioned and monitored with the help of TEE (62,63). The application of mechanical support during off-pump CABG originated from the observation by Grundeman et al. (64) that lifting the heart to expose posterior vessels "flexed" the right ventricle and induced hemodynamic instability. This observation provided an impetus for the development of right ventricular mechanical support. Ultimately changing the operating table position and opening the right pleura overcame this hemodynamic instability. Nevertheless, hemodynamic instability can occur in patients with compromised LV function or in whom heart manipulation provokes myocardial ischemia. Its efficacy as an alternative to extracorporeal circulation has been well documented (65). A randomized comparison of hemodynamic and clinical outcomes in patients undergoing off pump CABG with biventricular Impella support or with standard CPB and traditional CABG, did not show any differences in the intraoperative hemodynamic stability, hemolysis or in the postoperative course (66). In a larger randomized multi-center trial in 199 patients undergoing off-pump CABG with biventricular Impella support or standard CPB supported CABG, Impella supported revascularization was associated with reduced systemic inflammatory response (67). Clinical outcome, myocardial necrosis, end organ function and, more importantly, hemolysis did not differ between the two groups. While routine off-pump CABG does not require additional mechanical support, this device can play a role in more vulnerable patients with decreased LV function.

Additional experience has come from applications of the Impella pump in post-cardiotomy failure, myocarditis and cardiogenic shock. Meyns et al., described their experience in 16 patients with cardiogenic shock supported with the Impella Recover LP 5.0 device. In 6 of these patients the device was implanted via femoral approach and in 10 with direct aortic approach for postcardiotomy heart failure (68). Within 6 hr of deployment, mean flow of 4.24 L/min resulted in a significant improvement in mean arterial pressure, which rose from 57 mmHg to 75 mmHg. There was a significant increase in cardiac output (from 4.1 to 5.5 L/min $p=0.003$) and a decrease in PCWP from 29 to 17 mmHg ($p=0.04$). These hemodynamic changes translated into a decrease in lactate levels. Six patients developed mild hemolysis, which did not require any therapeutic intervention. After 68% of the patients were weaned from the support, 37% survived long-term. Jurmann et al., described successful Impella support in 6 patients with high predicted mortality with postcardiotomy heart failure after CABG (69). Siegenthaler studied 24 patients with postcardiotomy failure with minimal hemolysis and favorable survival in patients with some degree of residual LV function, suggesting that flow provided by the pump may not be sufficient in the absence of some intrinsic myocardial function (70). Outside the operating room, the Impella Recover LP 5.0 has been successful as a "bridge to recovery" in treatment of fulminant myocarditis and cardiogenic shock for up to 18 days(71,72). There is some initial experience with the use of this device as a minimally invasive bridging device in severe mitral and aortic valvular disease as well as patients awaiting transplantation (72).

The clinical experience with the percutaneous Recover LP 2.5 device is growing, especially in Europe where the device has been used in over 200 patients (73). When used during high-risk interventions in the setting of decreased LV function, this device achieved immediate LV unloading and increased the cardiac output by 2.4 L/min without inducing aortic regurgitation (74). The PROTECT I trial will randomize patients undergoing high-risk PCI to Impella LP 2.5 or IABP support to establish safety and efficacy of this device.

There are some physiological limitations to the transvalvular design. It is clearly contraindicated in the presence of significant aortic valve disease and may be difficult to deliver in a diseased aorta. Complete cessation of its function creates the possibility of a back-leak through the pump, thus inducing functional regurgitation into the left ventricle. This has clear implications for weaning the device and can make it difficult to judge the recovery of heart function because of the sudden regurgitant volume load on the left ventricle. This was a particular concern for the Hemopump (75) but can be overcome by Impella's more advanced control system The heart-pump interaction is a reciprocal process where the native heart influences the pump function and vice-versa. Quantifying this interaction may be helpful in identifying optimal timing for weaning. The recovery of left ventricular function and its dynamic contribution to flow creates fluctuation in the pressure head the pump has to face. The increase in aortic pressure and decrease in left ventricular diastolic pressure will increase the gradient of the pressure differential sensed by the pump during the cardiac cycle, offering a determinant of successful weaning (76).

TandemHeart®

TandemHeart® (CardiacAssist, Inc., Pittsburgh, Pennsylvania, U.S.A.) percutaneous ventricular assist device (pVAD) is a centrifugal nonpulsatile flow system, which employs a magnetically driven six-blade propeller pumping blood from the left heart to the femoral artery (Fig. 3). The extra-corporeal pump contains two chambers. The upper housing accommodates the inflow port from the LA and contains an impeller propelling blood out to the outflow port. The lower housing contains a rotor driving the impeller and the anticoagulation infusion port. The low blood contact surface area of the propeller and its free-floating position in the housing generate minimal friction, reducing heat generation, hemolysis and thromboembolism. The pump weighs 280 g and at its maximal speed of 7500 rpm is capable of generating cardiac output up to 4 L/min, independently of the left ventricular function. Under optimal conditions, the pump easily reverses flow in the aorta up to the level of the arch (77). The compact pump size allows very small priming volume of 60 ml. The pump flow is measured by an electromagnetic flow meter and an external power supply unit allows adjustment and monitoring of pump performance (Fig. 4). It operates on an AC current with internal battery back-up support for transportation.

Under ideal conditions an experienced operator can insert TandemHeart VAD in the catheterization laboratory in less than 30 min. The inflow cannula is a 21F polyurethane end and side-hole catheter with 14 side holes. It is placed from the femoral vein into the left atrium via the standard trans-septal technique (78). It must be positioned entirely in the left atrium to avoid right to left shunting (Fig. 5). The cannula aspirates oxygenated blood, which the pump returns to the arterial system via an outflow cannula inserted over a wire from the femoral artery into the abdominal aorta. The outflow cannula size ranges from 14 F to 19F and the size selection depends on the diameter of the iliofemoral arteries and the extent of peripheral arterial disease. The cannula size and the pump speed dictate the magnitude of flow that can be generated. Alternatively, two 12Fr cannulas can be used in both femoral arteries. In the presence of significant peripheral arterial disease, the outflow cannula can become occlusive and cause lower limb ischemia. An additional antegrade catheter may be used to perfuse the leg. Continuous infusion of Heparin (900 U/hr) is

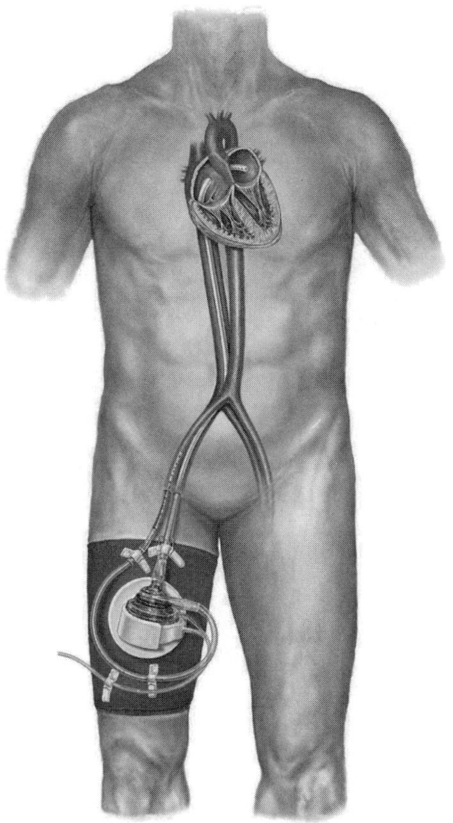

Figure 3 Schematic of TandemHeart® percutaneous left ventricular assist device.

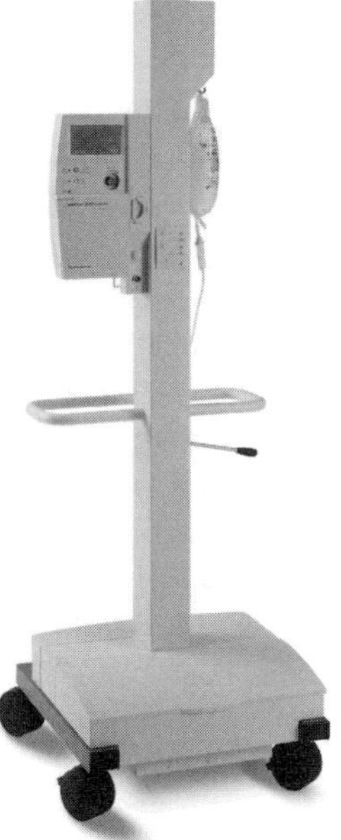

Figure 4 The TandemHeart® mobile control unit. *Source*: Photo courtesy of CardiacAssist Inc.

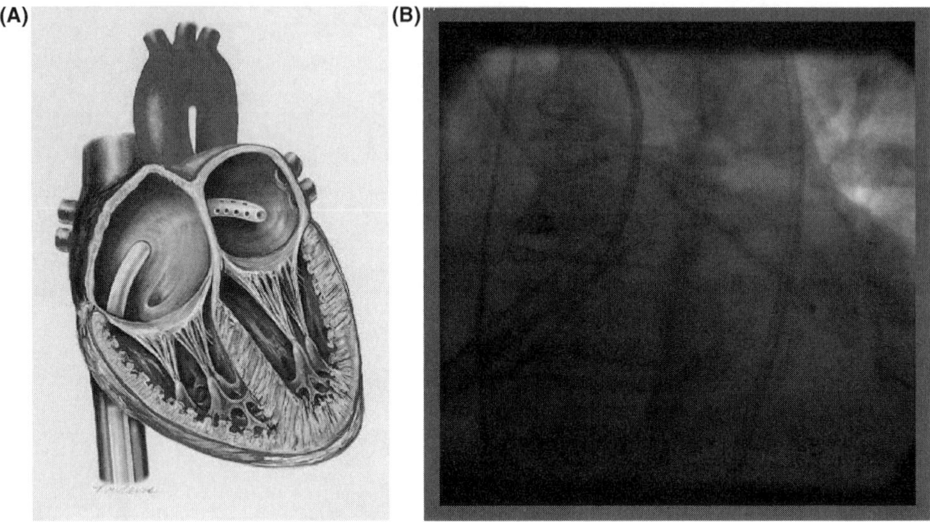

Figure 5 (**A**) The intracardiac position of the inflow cannula. (**B**) TandemHeart® cannula position in a patient undergoing high risk PCI of the left circumflex artery.

required to provide systemic anticoagulation with a target PTT 65–80 (ACT 200 sec). The TandemHeart system is designed for prolonged support of up to 14 days. Weaning protocol involves a stepwise decrease in the flow of the pump: output is decreased in 500 mL/L increments to 0.5 L/min. The device can be removed in patients who can maintain CI > 2.2 L/min/m^2, MAP > 70 mmHg and PCWP < 18 mmHg without inotropic support.

The benefit of a rapidly deployed, percutaneous circulatory assist device should be most obvious in patients with cardiogenic shock due to myocardial ischemia. Thiele et al., supported 18 patients with acute myocardial infarction and cardiogenic shock who also underwent percutaneous revascularization. Maximal duration of TandemHeart support was 7 days with mean pump flow rates of 3.2 L/min. The hemodynamic improvement and reversal of shock was apparent within hours, irrespective of the residual myocardial function. TandemHeart device implantation resulted in a significant increase in cardiac index from1.7 to 2.4 L/min/m^2 ($p < 0.001$), a rise in mean arterial pressure from 63 to 80 mmHg ($p < 0.001$) and a decrease in PCWP from 21 to 14 mmHg ($p < 0.001$). These hemodynamic changes were associated with reversal of metabolic acidosis (77). In five patients who presented with a VSD, the left to right shunt volume was reduced from 4.5 L/min to 2.0 L/min and shunt ratio diminished from 2.6 to 1.6. Despite the left ventricular unloading, there was no evidence of shunt reversal. Four patients died during the support and four more died after weaning from TandemHeart with 10 patients surviving to discharge. Overall, 30-day mortality was 44%. Device implantation was successful in all patients and pump operation did not increase indices of hemolysis measured by haptoglobin and plasma-free hemoglobin. Bleeding complications were limited to access site bleeding and required blood transfusions in 5 patients. The 17F outflow cannula became occlusive in two patients with peripheral arterial disease and required an accessory antegrade perfusion cannula in the common femoral artery. Device associated thromboembolism was not clinically evident: one patient with CT documented infarcts had evidence of a large thrombus at the edge of a VSD.

Multiple case reports describe successful use of TandemHeart pVAD in high-risk percutaneous interventions (79–82). In a series of 7 patients with mean left ventricular ejection fraction of 24%, pVAD has been used for up to 11 days without lower extremity malperfusion or bleeding outside the access site (81). In this small series there was a tendency towards an increase in the mean arterial pressure and decrease in LV filling pressures. Moreover, TandemHeart device has been used successfully in postcardiotomy failure unresponsive to IABP and inotropic support (83). Additional US experience with the TandemHeart system comes from the Phase I study assessing the safety and feasibility of the device. It was conducted in five US centers and enrolled 13 patients mostly in cardiogenic shock due to myocardial infarction. Despite maximal medical therapy 69% of these patients were refractory to IABP support. In this critically ill group, pVAD support increased cardiac index from 2.09 to 2.53 L/min/m^2 ($p=0.017$). The mean arterial pressure rose from 70.6 to 81.7 mmHg ($p=0.014$) with a decrease in PCWP from 27.1 mmHg to 16.5 mmHg ($p=0.013$) (84). Hemolysis, measured by plasma free hemoglobin concentration, and platelet levels were not affected by pVAD operation. There were no device associated deaths or thromboembolic complications. There was no clinically significant ASD after the trans-septal puncture. Six patients were supported as a bridge to surgery or PCI with a 6-wk survival rate of 83%. Three patients expired while being supported while 4 patients were weaned, two of whom were alive at 6 weeks. The subsequent Phase II trial, conducted in US and European centers, randomized 90 patients in cardiogenic shock to conventional therapy or TandemHeart pVAD. The primary end point included sustained reversal of cardiogenic shock while the secondary end point focused on the 30-day survival without permanent neurological dysfunction. Major adverse cardiac events were monitored for a 12-mo period. The results have not been published yet. The THEAMI trial will test the effect of LV support during reperfusion therapy. It is an ongoing multi-center European study randomizing patients undergoing PCI for large anterior MI to IABP or pVAD support. The primary endpoint will be MRI assessment of infarct size and remodeling.

While numerous reports and case series support the use of TandemHeart in ever wider clinical situations, it is not clear whether large-scale use of this device translates into a mortality benefit. To answer this question, Holger et al. (85) conducted a small, randomized trial of 41 patients with acute myocardial infarction complicated by cardiogenic shock who underwent PCI with pVAD support. TandemHeart achieved a superior improvement in hemodynamic and metabolic parameters but at a price of significantly higher rates of bleeding (19% vs. 8% $p=0.002$) and limb ischemia (7% vs. 0, $p=0.009$). Ultimately, survival was identical in both groups with 30-day mortality of 45% versus 43% ($p=0.86$).

Hemolysis, thromboembolism and access site complications were less common in the reported series. Residual ASD at the site of the transseptal puncture closes spontaneously in majority of patients and has not been associated with any clinical significance when it remained open. These observations are similar to the fate of transseptal puncture after mitral valvuloplasty, which is associated with a detectable, although clinically insignificant left-to-right shunt, which decreases or closes after 6 mo. Fonger et al, described animal experience with trans-septal LVAD where the iatrogenic ASD healed by 6 wk (27). Systemic hypothermia has been noted in few patients with prolonged support (81) but can be corrected with shortening of the extracorporeal tubing and active re-warming. Limb loss, vessel injury cannula-associated thrombus and complication of trans-septal puncture are uncommon.

Other Devices in Development

Several other designs are currently in various phases of development. Amed Systems Inc (West Sacramento, CA) has developed a catheter-based intravascular pump for temporary circulatory support. The PUCA pump (PUlsatile CAtheter pump) is a trans-valvular design combining the pulsatile counterpulsation of a balloon pump with the direct unloading effect of the Hemopump. A thin walled catheter of various sizes contains both the in- and out-flow valves and is connected to an external membrane pump. The blood is aspirated from the left ventricle through the tip into the membrane pump and subsequently ejected into the aorta through a valve proximal to the tip. The pump is driven by a variety of commercially available pneumatic driving systems, including those in use for IABP. This system can provide flow rates up to 3.0 L/min when using a 21F cannula and a 40 mL membrane pump (86,87) The results have been promising in animal studies (88,89) but clinical experience is so far limited.

The Cancion CardiacRecovery System (Orqis Medical, Lake Forest CA) is a centrifugal pump system circulating blood from a peripheral artery into the descending aorta. It superimposes this additional continuous flow onto the pulsatile aortic flow. It is designed specifically for treatment of congestive heart failure guided by the principle that increasing the flow in the aorta will unload the left ventricle and subsequently increase the renal flow and beneficially modulate the neurohormonal axis. Evidence from animal models of heart failure suggests that this device can be effective in restoring hemodynamic homeostasis (90). This "rest to recovery" application will be investigated in a multi-center MOMENTUM trial enrolling patients with heart failure unresponsive to standard medical therapy. The limited clinical experience so far suggests that the device can unload the left ventricle by lowering the capillary wedge pressure, increasing the cardiac output and improving renal function (91,92).

CONCLUSION

The existing and contemplated percutaneous ventricular assist devices have validated the concept of the value of left ventricular support. However, existing devices, though improved, carry with them cannula sizes that engender vascular complications and are more difficult to insert than an intra-aortic balloon pump. The challenge for the future will be to apply the principles learned from the first generations of these devices to the development a system as easy to insert and monitor as the existing intra-aortic balloon pump.

REFERENCES

1. Stevenson LW, et al. Mechanical cardiac support 2000: current applications and future trial design: June 15–16, 2000 Bethesda, Maryland. Circulation 2001; 103:337–342.
2. Rose EA, et al. Long-term mechanical left ventricular assistance for end-stage heart failure. N Engl J Med 2001; 345:1435–1443.
3. Bonow RO, et al. World Heart Day 2002: the international burden of cardiovascular disease: responding to the emerging global epidemic. Circulation 2002; 106:1602–1605.

4. Hochman JS, et al. Early revascularization in acute myocardial infarction complicated by cardiogenic shock. SHOCK Investigators. Should we emergently revascularize occluded coronaries for cardiogenic shock. N Engl J Med 1999; 341:625–634.
5. De Luca G, et al. Impaired myocardial perfusion is a major explanation of the poor outcome observed in patients undergoing primary angioplasty for ST-segment-elevation myocardial infarction and signs of heart failure. Circulation 2004; 109:958–961.
6. Nanas JN, Moulopoulos SD. Counterpulsation: historical background, technical improvements, hemodynamic and metabolic effects. Cardiology 1994; 84:156–167.
7. Nanas JN, et al. Myocardial salvage by the use of reperfusion and intraaortic balloon pump: experimental study. Ann Thorac Surg 1996; 61:629–634.
8. Catinella FP, et al. Left atrium-to-femoral artery bypass: effectiveness in reduction of acute experimental myocardial infarction. J Thorac Cardiovasc Surg 1983; 86:887–896.
9. Laschinger JC, et al. Adjunctive left ventricular unloading during myocardial reperfusion plays a major role in minimizing myocardial infarct size. J Thorac Cardiovasc Surg 1985; 90:80–85.
10. Achour H, et al. Mechanical left ventricular unloading prior to reperfusion reduces infarct size in a canine infarction model. Catheter Cardiovasc Interv 2005; 64:182–192.
11. Ferrari M, Scholz KH, Figulla HR. PTCA with the use of cardiac assist devices: risk stratification, short- and long-term results. Catheter Cardiovasc Diagn 1996; 38:242–248.
12. Serruys, PW, ARTS-2: 1 year follow up. in American College of Cardiology, Scientific Sessions. (2005) Orlando, FL.
13. Mesana TG. Rotary blood pumps for cardiac assistance: a "must"? Artif Organs 2004; 28:218–225.
14. Cohen M, et al. Sex and other predictors of intra-aortic balloon counterpulsation-related complications: prospective study of 1119 consecutive patients. Am Heart J 2000; 139:282–287.
15. Powell WJ, Jr., et al. Effects of intra-aortic balloon counterpulsation on cardiac performance, oxygen consumption, and coronary blood flow in dogs. Circ Res 1970; 26:753–764.
16. Shaw J, Taylor DR, Pitt B. Effects of intraaortic balloon counterpulsation on regional coronary blood flow in experimental myocardial infarction. Am J Cardiol 1974; 34:552–556.
17. Kimura A, et al. Effects of intraaortic balloon pumping on septal arterial blood flow velocity waveform during severe left main coronary artery stenosis. J Am Coll Cardiol 1996; 27:810–816.
18. Toyota E, et al. Evaluation of intramyocardial coronary blood flow waveform during intraaortic balloon pumping in the absence or presence of coronary stenosis. Artif Organs 1996; 20:166–168.
19. Norman JC, et al. Prognostic indices for survival during postcardiotomy intra-aortic balloon pumping. Methods of scoring and classification, with implications for left ventricular assist device utilization. J Thorac Cardiovasc Surg 1977; 74:709–720.
20. McGee MG, et al. Retrospective analyses of the need for mechanical circulatory support (intrasortic balloon pump/abdominal left ventricular assist device or partial artificial heart) after cardiopulmonary bypass. A 44 month study of 14,168 patients. Am J Cardiol 1980; 46:135–142.
21. Barron HV, et al. The use of intra-aortic balloon counterpulsation in patients with cardiogenic shock complicating acute myocardial infarction: data from the National Registry of Myocardial Infarction 2. Am Heart J 2001; 141:933–939.
22. Stone GW, et al. A prospective, randomized evaluation of prophylactic intraaortic balloon counterpulsation in high risk patients with acute myocardial infarction treated with primary angioplasty. Second Primary Angioplasty in Myocardial Infarction (PAMI-II) Trial Investigators. J Am Coll Cardiol 1997; 29:1459–1467.
23. Berger PB, et al. Impact of an aggressive invasive catheterization and revascularization strategy on mortality in patients with cardiogenic shock in the Global Utilization of Streptokinase and Tissue Plasminogen Activator for Occluded Coronary Arteries (GUSTO-I) trial. An observational study. Circulation 1997; 96:122–127.
24. Salisbury PF, et al. Effects of partial and of total heart-lung bypass on the heart. J Appl Physiol 1959; 14:458–463.

25. Dennis C, et al. Left atrial cannulation without thoracotomy for total left heart bypass. Acta Chir Scand 1962; 123:267–279.
26. Dennis C, et al. Clinical use of a cannula for left heart bypass without thoracotomy: experimental protection against fibrillation by left heart bypass. Ann Surg 1962; 156:623–637.
27. Fonger JD, et al. Enhanced preservation of acutely ischemic myocardium with transseptal left ventricular assist. Ann Thorac Surg 1994; 57:570–575.
28. Killen DA, et al. Bio-medicus ventricular assist device for salvage of cardiac surgical patients. Ann Thorac Surg 1991; 52:230–235.
29. Pavie A, et al. Left centrifugal pump cardiac assist with transseptal percutaneous left atrial cannula. Artif Organs 1998; 22:502–507.
30. Glassman E, et al. Percutaneous left atrial to femoral arterial bypass pumping for circulatory support in high-risk coronary angioplasty. Catheter Cardiovasc Diagn 1993; 29:210–216.
31. Satoh H, et al. Clinical application of percutaneous left ventricular support with a centrifugal pump. Asaio J 1993; 39:153–155.
32. Edmunds LH, Jr., et al. Left ventricular assist without thoracotomy: clinical experience with the Dennis method. Ann Thorac Surg 1994; 57:880–885.
33. Vogel RA, Tommaso CL, Gundry SR. Initial experience with coronary angioplasty and aortic valvuloplasty using elective semipercutaneous cardiopulmonary support. Am J Cardiol 1988; 62:811–813.
34. Shawl FA, et al. Percutaneous cardiopulmonary bypass support in high-risk patients undergoing percutaneous transluminal coronary angioplasty. Am J Cardiol 1989; 64:1258–1263.
35. Shawl FA, et al. Percutaneous cardiopulmonary bypass-supported coronary angioplasty in patients with unstable angina pectoris or myocardial infarction and a left ventricular ejection fraction $<$ or $=25\%$. Am J Cardiol 1996; 77:14–19.
36. Shawl FA, et al. Emergency cardiopulmonary bypass support in patients with cardiac arrest in the catheterization laboratory. Catheter Cardiovasc Diagn 1990; 19:8–12.
37. Shawl FA, et al. Emergency percutaneous cardiopulmonary bypass support in cardiogenic shock from acute myocardial infarction. Am J Cardiol 1989; 64:967–970.
38. Vogel RA, et al. Initial report of the National Registry of Elective Cardiopulmonary Bypass Supported Coronary Angioplasty. J Am Coll Cardiol 1990; 15:23–29.
39. Kaul U, et al. Coronary angioplasty in high risk patients: comparison of elective intraaortic balloon pump and percutaneous cardiopulmonary bypass support—a randomized study. J Interv Cardiol 1995; 8:199–205.
40. Wampler RK, et al. In vivo evaluation of a peripheral vascular access axial flow blood pump. ASAIO Trans 1988; 34:450–454.
41. Frazier OH, et al. First human use of the Hemopump, a catheter-mounted ventricular assist device. Ann Thorac Surg 1990; 49:299–304.
42. Merhige ME, et al. Effect of the hemopump left ventricular assist device on regional myocardial perfusion and function. Reduction of ischemia during coronary occlusion. Circulation 1989; 80:III158–III166.
43. Scholz KH, et al. Left-ventricular unloading by transvalvular axial flow pumping in experimental cardiogenic shock and during regional myocardial ischemia. Cardiology 1994; 84:202–210.
44. Scholz KH, et al. Protective effects of the Hemopump left ventricular assist device in experimental cardiogenic shock. Eur J Cardiothorac Surg 1992; 6:209–214.
45. Hering JP, et al. Myocardial support and protection during regional myocardial ischemia using the Hemopump assist device. Thorac Cardiovasc Surg 1991; 39:257–262.
46. Smalling RW, et al. Improved regional myocardial blood flow, left ventricular unloading, and infarct salvage using an axial-flow, transvalvular left ventricular assist device. A comparison with intra-aortic balloon counterpulsation and reperfusion alone in a canine infarction model. Circulation 1992; 85:1152–1159.

47. Wampler RK, et al. Treatment of cardiogenic shock with the Hemopump left ventricular assist device. Ann Thorac Surg 1991; 52:506–513.
48. Smalling RW, et al. Transvalvular left ventricular assistance in cardiogenic shock secondary to acute myocardial infarction. Evidence for recovery from near fatal myocardial stunning. J Am Coll Cardiol 1994; 23:637–644.
49. Lonn U, et al. Hemopump treatment in patients with postcardiotomy heart failure. Ann Thorac Surg 1995; 60:1067–1071.
50. Meyns BP, et al. Left ventricular assistance with the transthoracic 24F Hemopump for recovery of the failing heart. Ann Thorac Surg 1995; 60:392–397.
51. Lonn U, et al. Coronary artery operation with support of the Hemopump cardiac assist system. Ann Thorac Surg 1994; 58:519–522; discustion 523.
52. Scholz KH, et al. Mechanical left ventricular unloading during high risk coronary angioplasty: first use of a new percutaneous transvalvular left ventricular assist device. Catheter Cardiovasc Diagn 1994; 31:61–69.
53. Scholz KH, et al. Clinical experience with the percutaneous hemopump during high-risk coronary angioplasty. Am J Cardiol 1998; 82:1107–1110 see also p. A6.
54. Dubois-Rande JL, et al. Effects of the 14F hemopump on coronary hemodynamics in patients undergoing high-risk coronary angioplasty. Am Heart J 1998; 135:844–849.
55. Meyns B, et al. Organ perfusion with Hemopump device assistance with and without intraaortic balloon pumping. J Thorac Cardiovasc Surg 1997; 114:243–253.
56. Scholz KH, et al. Transfemoral placement of the left ventricular assist device "Hemopump" during mechanical resuscitation. Thorac Cardiovasc Surg 1990; 38:69–72.
57. Christiansen S, et al. A new right ventricular assist device for right ventricular support. Eur J Cardiothorac Surg 2003; 24:834–836.
58. Meyns B, et al. Left ventricular support by catheter-mounted axial flow pump reduces infarct size. J Am Coll Cardiol 2003; 41:1087–1095.
59. Reesink KD, et al. Miniature intracardiac assist device provides more effective cardiac unloading and circulatory support during severe left heart failure than intraaortic balloon pumping. Chest 2004; 126:896–902.
60. Meyns B, et al. Micropumps to support the heart during CABG. Eur J Cardiothorac Surg 2000; 17:169–174.
61. Mueller XM, et al. Bi-ventricular axial micropump: impact on blood cell integrity. Swiss Surg 2001; 7:213–217.
62. Catena E, et al. Echocardiographic evaluation of patients receiving a new left ventricular assist device: the Impella recover 100. Eur J Echocardiogr 2004; 5:430–437.
63. Ender J, et al. Epicardial echocardiography for correct placement of the intracardial biventricular assist device (Impella). Thorac Cardiovasc Surg 2002; 50:92–94.
64. Grundeman PF, et al. Exposure of circumflex branches in the tilted, beating porcine heart: echocardiographic evidence of right ventricular deformation and the effect of right or left heart bypass. J Thorac Cardiovasc Surg 1999; 118:316–323.
65. Lonn U, et al. Beating heart coronary surgery supported by an axial blood flow pump. Ann Thorac Surg 1999; 67:99–104.
66. Autschbach R, et al. A new intracardiac microaxial pump: first results of a multicenter study. Artif Organs 2001; 25:327–330.
67. Meyns B, et al. Coronary artery bypass grafting supported with intracardiac microaxial pumps versus normothermic cardiopulmonary bypass: a prospective randomized trial. Eur J Cardiothorac Surg 2002; 22:112–117.
68. Meyns B, et al. Initial experiences with the Impella device in patients with cardiogenic shock—Impella support for cardiogenic shock. Thorac Cardiovasc Surg 2003; 51:312–317.
69. Jurmann MJ, et al. Initial experience with miniature axial flow ventricular assist devices for postcardiotomy heart failure. Ann Thorac Surg 2004; 77:1642–1647.
70. Siegenthaler MP, et al. The Impella Recover microaxial left ventricular assist device reduces mortality for postcardiotomy failure: a three-center experience. J Thorac Cardiovasc Surg 2004; 127:812–822.

71. Colombo T, et al. First successful bridge to recovery with the Impella Recover 100 left ventricular assist device for fulminant acute myocarditis. Ital Heart J 2003; 4:642–645.
72. Garatti A, et al. Impella recover 100 microaxial left ventricular assist device: the Niguarda experience. Transplant Proc 2004; 36:623–626.
73. www.Impella.com, Impella Cardiosystems.
74. Valgimigli M, et al. Left ventricular unloading and concomitant total cardiac output increase by the use of percutaneous impella recover LP 2.5 assist device during high-risk coronary intervention. Catheter Cardiovasc Interv 2005.
75. Wulff J, et al. Flow characteristics of the Hemopump: an experimental in vitro study. Ann Thorac Surg 1997; 63:162–166.
76. Stolinski J, et al. The heart-pump interaction: effects of a microaxial blood pump. Int J Artif Organs 2002; 25:1082–1088.
77. Thiele H, et al. Reversal of cardiogenic shock by percutaneous left atrial-to-femoral arterial bypass assistance. Circulation 2001; 104:2917–2922.
78. Brockenbrough EC, Braunwald E, Ross J, Jr., Transseptal left heart catheterization. A review of 450 studies and description of an improved technic. Circulation 1962; 25:15–21.
79. Kar B, et al. Hemodynamic support with a percutaneous left ventricular assist device during stenting of an unprotected left main coronary artery. Tex Heart Inst J 2004; 31:84–86.
80. Vranckx P, et al. Clinical introduction of the Tandemheart, a percutaneous left ventricular assist device, for circulatory support during high-risk percutaneous coronary intervention. Int J Cardiovasc Interv 2003; 5:35–39.
81. Lemos PA, et al. Usefulness of percutaneous left ventricular assistance to support high-risk percutaneous coronary interventions. Am J Cardiol 2003; 91:479–481.
82. Ramondo A, Tarantini G, Chioin R. Refractory angina with severe left ventricular dysfunction: a case for percutaneous transseptal ventricular assistance supported revascularization. Ital Heart J 2002; 3:673–675.
83. Pitsis AA, et al. Temporary assist device for postcardiotomy cardiac failure. Ann Thorac Surg 2004; 77:1431–1433.
84. Cohen ??. New devices for hemodynamic support: Clinical results with a percutaneous LVAD. inTranscatheter Cardiovascular Therapeutics 2003. Washington, DC.
85. Thiele H, et al. Randomized comparison of intra-aortic balloon support with a percutaneous left ventricular assist device in patients with revascularized acute myocardial infarction complicated by cardiogenic shock. Eur Heart J 2005.
86. Verkerke B, et al. The PUCA pump: a left ventricular assist device. Artif Organs 1993; 17:365–368.
87. Vandenberghe S, et al. In vitro evaluation of the PUCA II intra-arterial LVAD. Int J Artif Organs 2003; 26:743–752.
88. Mihaylov D, et al. Evaluation of the optimal driving mode during left ventricular assist with pulsatile catheter pump in calves. Artif Organs 1999; 23:1117–1122.
89. Reitan O, Steen S, Ohlin H. Hemodynamic effects of a new percutaneous circulatory support device in a left ventricular failure model. ASAIO J 2003; 49:731–736.
90. Tuzun E, et al. Evaluation of a new cardiac recovery system in a bovine model of volume overload heart failure. ASAIO J 2004; 50:557–562.
91. Wasler A, et al. First use of the Cancion cardiac recovery system in a human. ASAIO J 2003; 49:136–138.
92. Zile MR, Van Bakel A, et al. Cancion recovery system: hemodynamic and renal effects. J Am Coll Cardiol 2004; 43:A190–A191.

23
Selecting Patients for Durable Support with Ventricular Assist Devices

Lynne Warner Stevenson
Cardiovascular Division, Brigham and Women's Hospital, Harvard Medical School, Boston, Massachusetts, U.S.A.

THE CURRENT PICTURE

The progress in medical therapy for heart failure has allowed many patients to remain stable with adequate resting perfusion and good quality of life despite low left ventricular ejection fraction. Systematic, serial adjustment of recommended medications and, in some cases, pacing devices is required before patients can be considered to have moved "beyond medical therapy"(1). At this stage, some patients are evaluated for definitive options such as cardiac transplantation and/or mechanical cardiac support devices, while the majority should partner in decisions regarding end-of-life care. The selection of patients for implantable ventricular assist devices, as with any therapy, centers on the expected improvement of outcome offered by the intervention (2). Currently, there are only a small number of patients for whom benefit is anticipated from left ventricular assist devices, but relatively minor improvements in current device outcomes could dramatically increase the candidate population. While the majority of left ventricular assist devices are implanted with intent for a bridge to transplantation, many transplant candidates now survive beyond 6 mo and sometimes 1–2 yr on VAD before transplantation, which for some patients may never occur. The boundary between devices for bridge and for permanent "destination" is increasingly blurred, both for the initial selection decision and for the collection of outcomes. This chapter will focus on selection of patients for "destination" VAD, but it may soon be most appropriate to consider for "durable" VAD support, without pre-specification of ultimate transplant status.

BEYOND "OPTIMAL" MEDICAL THERAPY

The components of appropriate medical and reconstructive surgical therapy for heart failure have been reviewed in the preceding chapters (1,3). The expertise and diligence with which these must be pursued for optimal results once heart failure has progressed to advanced stages defines effective heart failure management programs, which are difficult to access in many communities (4). Resources of even greater intensity and higher cost are required, however, for maintenance of successful outpatient VAD programs (Table 1) (5). Patients with advanced heart failure should traverse through the highest level of heart failure management before any consideration of ventricular support device therapy.

Neurohormonal antagonism with beta adrenergic blocking agents and ACEI or ARB form the foundation of the medical regimen, as shown in Figure 1 (1). Loop diuretics are added as needed for fluid retention. Once decompensation has occurred, increasing adjustments are needed in the regimen for fluid balance, which may include multiple diuretics and repeated education regarding salt and fluid intake. Nitrates with or without hydralazine may be added for patients with persistent symptoms (6). Bi-ventricular pacing offers significant benefit in both symptoms and survival for selected patients with marked dysynchrony as evidenced by QRS > 150 msec (7), but should not be attempted as "rescue therapy" for patients who have deteriorated to develop renal dysfunction or requirement for intravenous inotropic therapy.

Patients may "fail" optimal medical therapy with either recurrent or refractory decompensation. With "recurrent" decompensation, patients can be stabilized close to normal volume status but experience frequent relapses into fluid retention. These patients should be carefully considered for more intensive management and surveillance programs. Some of these patients may be found to have poor compliance with their medical regimen that would compromise their outcomes with any therapy. For others it may be possible to maintain stability by more sensitive monitoring to guide intervention for early evidence of fluid retention.

With refractory decompensation, patients usually cannot be restored to optimal volume status, but remain severely volume overloaded with accompanying congestive symptoms of dyspnea and/or abdominal discomfort. For some, cardiac output remains at levels too low to adequately support organ function and nutrition. These patients are unlikely to benefit from additional outpatient management. In some cases, reduction or withdrawal of neurohormonal antagonists may allow higher perfusion pressure and better renal function for the short term. The long-term outcome is unfavorable, however, after withdrawal of either beta blockers or ACEI for patients in whom these neurohormonal antagonists were previously tolerated (Fig. 2)(8). Intravenous inotropic agents are often instituted as temporary therapy in hopes of re-establishing stability on oral agents. Failure to wean inotropic agents successfully has frequently been considered a milestone in progression to truly end-stage disease. Dependence on these infusions has been defined as the repeated inability to reduce or discontinue without symptomatic deterioration (9). For patients demonstrated to be inotrope-dependent in the REMATCH trial, 30% met criteria for weaning despite ongoing inotropic support (10). In 12% of patients, weaning failed during discontinuation of 1 of 2 agents administered together. In the remaining patients, inability to the wean was documented by symptomatic

Table 1 Requirements of VAD Center to Provide Destination Therapy

(1) Experience with evaluation and management of end-stage heart failure, including selection for cardiac transplantation and provision of end-of-life care
(2) A team of cardiologists, cardiac surgeons, anesthetists, perfusionists, nurses, and other health care professionals who have been properly trained and equipped to perform the VAD implantation and all subsequent follow-up device management, patient training, and long-term care
(3) Formal plan to evaluate, select, and follow patients with VADs for destination therapy
(4) Outpatient facilities for chronic care of VAD patients and surveillance for VAD malfunction

Abbreviation: VAD, ventricular assist device.
Source: From Ref. 5.

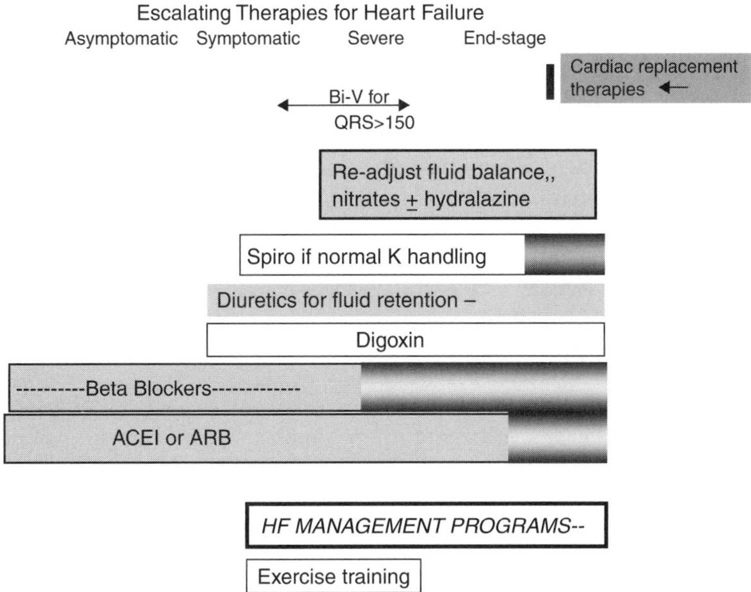

Figure 1 Steps of escalating therapies for stages of heart failure from asymptomatic (Stage A) to refractory, end-stage (Stage D). Cardiac transplantation and mechanical circulatory assist devices represent a tiny proportion of the overall therapy provided for patients with heart failure. *Source*: Adapted from Ref. 1.

hypotension in over half of the patients (average systolic blood pressure 73mmHg), progressively deteriorating renal function, or worsening dyspnea at rest. For eight other REMATCH patients without distinct worsening of symptoms, inotrope withdrawal was accompanied by mean cardiac indices 1.0–1.5 L/min/m^2. When weaning is not possible, continuous intravenous inotropic therapy is sometimes employed as a "bridge" to transplantation. It is occasionally provided as palliation of symptoms during the final weeks of life to some patients with good resources at home, but is associated with

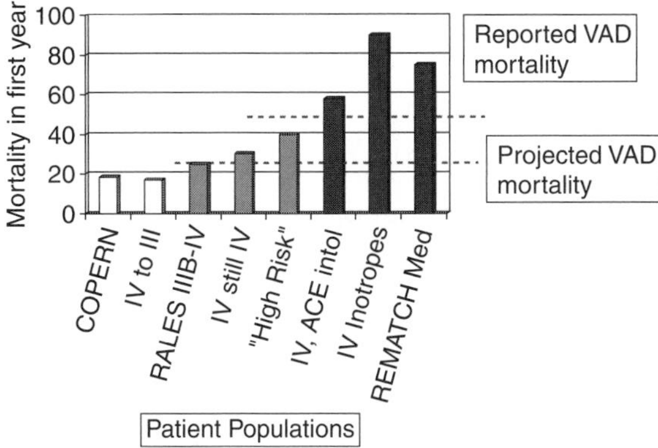

Figure 2 Bar graph comparing the estimated 1-year mortality of different heart failure populations in relation to the current reported mortality with left ventricular assist devices. The populations of patients with expected benefit from the device will extend into lower-risk populations as the projected ventricular assist device mortality declines.

multiple complications and re-admissions (11). Before commitment to continuous intravenous inotropic infusions, all other options, such as support with mechanical devices, should be considered in eligible patients. However, it is important to retain perspective for the majority of patients with end-stage heart failure, who are over 75 yr of age with multiple co-morbidities (12). As patients move beyond the reach of optimal medical therapy to relieve resting symptoms, the emphasis of care should shift increasingly toward palliative interventions to provide comfort and support for those in whom definitive device therapy is not appropriate (Figure 3).

BENEFIT OF VAD FOR DURABLE SUPPORT

Benefit of a therapy is the improvement in predicted outcomes with the device compared to predicted outcomes without the device. Benefit can be dominated by either survival or quality of life, as long as the other factor is sufficient to render the improvement clinically significant. For current LVAD populations, the major benefit demonstrated has been for survival (13). For survivors, the quality of life is clearly improved and sufficient to make the additional survival time meaningful.

Survival Benefit with VAD

Survival with LVAD

Survival with left ventricular assist devices is currently approximately 50% at one year. The REMATCH trial demonstrated 52% one-year survival in the 69 patients undergoing implantation as part of a randomized trial (13). Subsequent one-year survival in the Thoratec Registry of the HeartMate device approved for permanent "destination" therapy remains in the range of 50%. One-year data from patients surviving with the Novacor pulsatile device and other pulsatile and non-pulsatile investigational devices used as bridge to transplant is also in the range of 50%. Survival from the MCSD (Mechanical Cardiac Support Database), which includes 655 patients receiving multiple types of implanted devices for bridge and destination therapy, indicates one-year survival of about 50%. (www.ishlt.org/registries/). There is relatively little data about longer-term survival, but two-year survival for REMATCH device recipients was 29%, in selected centers with particular emphasis on preventing device infection up to 40%.

The major causes of death with LVAD during the REMATCH trial were infection and device failure. In the MCSD, the major causes of death reported were multiple organ failure in 35%, hemorrhage in 15%, stroke in 10%, and infection in 8%(14).

Would VAD survival have been better if patients were less severely ill at the time of implantation? Detailed analysis from REMATCH is limited by the small number of patients receiving LVAD, but was performed in relation to baseline inotropic use (10). One-year survival with LVAD was 57% for patients not on inotropic infusions at baseline compared to 49% with LVAD for all patients on inotropic infusions, who had lower systolic blood pressure and lower serum sodium at baseline. While the patients on baseline inotropic therapy had slightly worse survival with LVAD than patients on oral therapy, their survival on medical therapy was much worse, such that the benefit derived from the device was greater. Survival with LVAD at one year was 41% for patients who demonstrated inotropic dependence as described above, compared to 19% for those patients on medical therapy. The best survival with LVAD was 62% at 1 yr, seen in patients who were on inotropic therapy at randomization without documented weaning attempt, qualifying for the trial based on peak oxygen consumption (mean 9 ml/kg/min). Further data are needed to understand the degree to which LVAD outcomes are determined by the patient characteristics versus the characteristics inherent to the device. Overall a one-year survival of 50% represents a synthesis of current experience with implantable LVADs.

Death with Heart Failure

It is assumed that patients considered for VAD have been considered for all other reconstructive surgical intervention and undergone aggressive medical therapy supervised by an experienced heart failure program, as described above, prior to serious consideration of VAD therapy. (Fig. 3) In order to derive survival benefit from ventricular assist devices, these patients would have an anticipated 1-yr mortality of over 50%.

Survival after the initial diagnosis of heart failure remains in the range of 50% at 5 yr. No single descriptor is adequate to identify a sub-population with a one-year mortality over 50%. Patients from the general community hospitalized for heart failure in the United States, Canada, and Scotland as a group have a one-year mortality of 30–50%(15), but these patients have an average age of 74–75 yr with multiple attendant co-morbidities, some of which contribute to death within the next year (16).

For otherwise healthy patients with heart failure, Class IV symptoms alone are not enough to predict 50% 1 yr mortality. Prognosis is best determined after an intensive hospitalization for re-evaluation and re-design of therapy. The majority of patients who

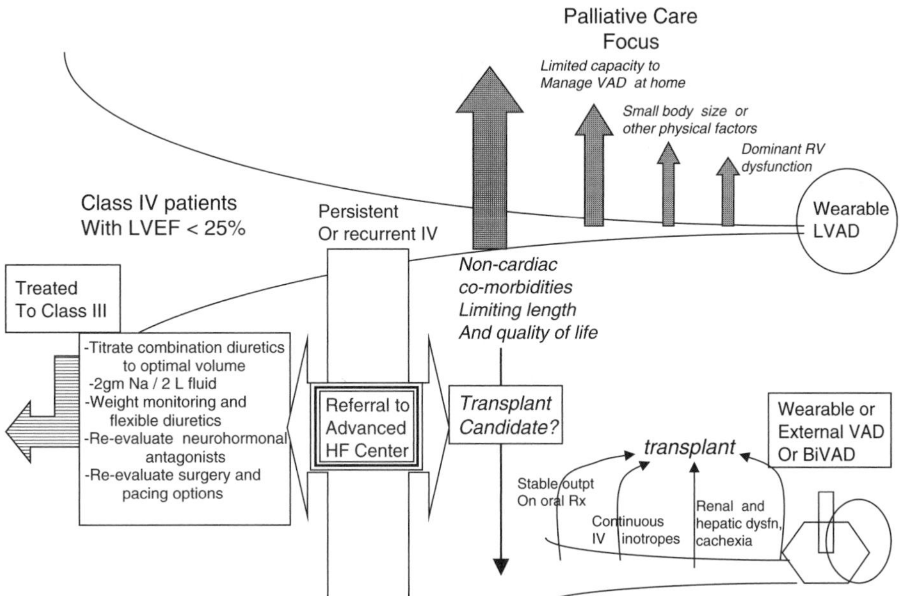

Figure 3 Stream diagram demonstrating the sequence of evaluation for the small number of patients who are not eligible for transplant but are nonetheless eligible for the current wearable ventricular assist device approved as permanent therapy. Patients with recurrent or refractory Class IV symptoms initially undergo intensive evaluation, therapy, and outpatient heart failure management at advanced heart failure centers. The majority of contraindications for transplantation are also contraindications for the current wearable left ventricular assist device. Although the population of transplant candidates is small, they represent the majority of patients currently receiving both approved and investigational ventricular assist devices.

have had Class IV heart failure symptoms can be restored to Class III status and its expected 1-year mortality of 10%–25% within a heart failure program of the intensity required at programs offering VAD's for discharge to home (17).

Continuous outpatient inotropic therapy confers a mortality that approaches 50% at six months (9). Patients in whom ACEI have to be discontinued permanently due to symptomatic hypotension or progressive renal dysfunction have a one year mortality exceeding 50%(8). For other patients, previous risk scores from earlier eras of therapy have limited relevance. The increasing prevalence of implantable defibrillators has decreased sudden death and the use of bi-ventricular pacing for patients with QRS > 150 has also prolonged survival (7). Peak oxygen consumption < 14 ml/kg/min once indicated very high risk in transplant candidates, but in the age of beta blocker use is now often lower, without the same ominous portent (18). From data such as that in the recent ESCAPE trial of patients hospitalized with advanced heart failure, risk models for high early mortality are being constructed based on the profile at hospital discharge, including blood urea nitrogen, serum sodium, systolic blood pressure, six-minute walk distance, B-type natriuretic peptide levels, diuretic dose and ability to take neurohormonal antagonists.

Current Indications for LVAD to Lengthen Survival in Non-transplant Candidates

It is generally agreed that the population receiving LVAD therapy in REMATCH represented the most compromised patients who would ever be considered. It is important to note, however, that compromise of this severity was neither mandated nor anticipated when that trial was designed (19). The entry criteria would have encompassed a broader population with lower mortality on medical therapy than what was actually observed. Nonetheless, as a starting point, the currently accepted indications for LVAD use in non-transplant candidates are derived from the REMATCH criteria (Table 2).

From an operational standpoint, it is clear from the REMATCH experience, and from cumulative other experience, that patients in whom inotrope dependence is demonstrated should be considered for VAD placement before further deterioration. For other patients, Class IV status is currently required to be supported by peak oxygen consumption < 12 ml/kg/min. It is hoped that combinations of risk factors, including functional indices, laboratory parameters, and therapies tolerated such as those above, will be validated that could identify patients who have low likelihood of one-year survival but have not yet deteriorated to the level where multi-organ failure is imminent and perioperative outcomes are jeopardized. As survival with devices improves, the relevant range within which updated survival statistics for heart failure are critical will move in concert with it, to patients with less imminent compromise and risk.

Function and Quality with LVAD

The current pulsatile left ventricular assist devices can provide stroke volume up to 85 cc and cardiac output up to 10 l/min when venous return is high, as during exercise. This is generally adequate to support activity at a Class II–III level after physical rehabilitation. Some patients have returned to golfing, bowling, bicycling, skiing, and various employments (20).

The currently approved devices for long-term use are large pulsatile devices that are placed in the left upper quadrant, with tunneling of the drive-line site to exit on the right side of the abdomen. Each pulsation is associated with strong torque initially felt intensely by the patient, and a significant noise that limits attendance at public places such as movie theatres and concert halls. Many patients have loss of appetite and experience early satiety

Table 2 Patient Selection for LVAD as Destination Therapy

Indications	All of the following conditions should be met: (1) New York Heart Association Class IV symptoms for at least 60 of 90 days (2) Optimal medical therapy as tolerated with ACEI, beta-blockers, spironolactone, digoxin, and titration of high-dose combination diuretics to relieve congestion, compliance with salt and fluid restriction and weight monitoring, supervised in advanced heart failure management program (3) LVEF $\leq$25% AND: (a) Dependence on intravenous inotropic infusions despite multiple weaning attempts, limited by symptomatic hypotension, progressively declining renal function, or worsening symptoms (usually dyspnea) OR: (b) Peak oxygen consumption $\leq$10–12 ml/kg/min during exercise testing with demonstrated achievement of cardiac limitation (usually anaerobic metabolism indicated by respiratory quotient $\geq$1.1) OR: (c) Imminent risk profile, undergoing definition
Contraindications	(1) Heart failure with obstructive hypertrophic cardiomyopathy or potentially reversible cause of cardiomyopathy (2) Technical obstacles that pose high surgical risk for successful LVAD implantation and maintenance (3) Co-existing terminal condition (e.g., advanced metastatic cancer or clinically significant co-morbidities that might limit functional survival, such as severe lung, liver, peripheral vascular disease or intrinsic kidney disease.) (4) Active systemic infection or major chronic risk for infection (5) Fixed pulmonary hypertension (generally $\geq$8 Wood units) (6) Severe right ventricular dysfunction out of proportion to left ventricular failure, deemed unlikely to resolve after LVAD implantation (7) Presence of mechanical valve that will not be converted to bioprosthetic valve at the time of LVAD implantation (8) Abdominal aortic aneurysm $\geq$5 cm (9) Body surface area $<$1.5 M^2, inadequate transverse abdominal dimension or other physical restriction to device placement (10) Body mass index $>$40 kg/m^2 (11) Patient inability to understand and provide informed consent (12) Inability of patient and companions to maintain the VAD in operating condition (change batteries, recognize alarms, hand pump)

Many of these are derived from the design of the randomized trial of LVAD as destination therapy and may evolve with subsequent clinical experience.
Abbreviations: LVAD, left ventricular assist devices; VAD, ventricular assist devices.

due to the loss of abdominal space. When away from the bedside console, the batteries are worn in a vest that is inconspicuous for most men, but burdensome for some women. Other concerns voiced by patients are the dependence on community power sources and batteries with limited capacity.

Neurological events can compromise clinical function and quality of life after implantation. Most neurological events occur transiently in the early post-operative period, attributed to toxic-metabolic and other factors. Strokes can occur from emboli and/or cerebral hemorrhage. In the REMATCH trial, 16% of LVAD patients had a stroke, for a rate of 0.19 per year (21).

Despite the physical presence of the device and the concern regarding infections and device function, quality of life is improved for most device recipients (Fig. 4). The level achieved, as measured by the Minnesota Living with Heart Failure questionnaire, is comparable to that for patients with less severe initial compromise who underwent bi-ventricular pacing in the pivotal trials (22).

Both survival and quality of life are important to patients facing imminent death. In studies examining patient utilities with heart failure, the majority of patients with advanced heart failure in the Class IV range express willingness to trade more than half of remaining time, or risk more than 50% chance of death, in order to feel better (23).

CONTRAINDICATIONS FOR CURRENT VADs

After the approval of VAD for "destination" therapy, it was anticipated that several thousand would be implanted yearly for this purpose. In the past 3 yr, fewer than 200 VAD have been implanted in the United States for "destination". This is in part due to the blurred distinction between bridge and destination intent. Many patients undergo long-term VAD placement due not to ineligibility for transplantation, but due to large body size, multiple pre-formed antibodies or other factors that predict a long or futile wait for a donor heart. Contra-indications initially considered temporary such as recent malignancy or renal dysfunction may lead to VAD support that becomes final.

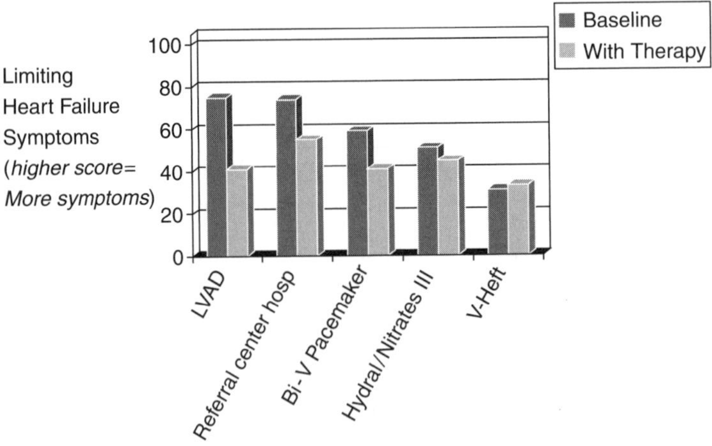

Figure 4 Bar graph showing the impact of interventions on heart failure symptoms in relation to the initial symptom severity. The largest benefit is shown for patients with the most severe symptoms receiving left ventricular assist devices. The impact of hospitalization at a referral heart failure center is shown for symptoms at 6 mo after discharge, from the ESCAPE trial. Symptomatic improvement is shown from the bi-ventricular pacing trial, the trial of the hydralazine-nitrate combination in African Americans, and the original V-Heft II trial in mild-moderate heart failure. *Source*: From Refs. 6, 13, 22, 24, and 25.

Transplant Status

There are, however, few reasons that make a person ineligible for a transplant without compromising their eligibility for a good outcome after a ventricular assist device (Fig. 5). Issues such as pulmonary disease, peripheral vascular disease, infection, and psychosocial status affect both. (Fig. 3) A relative exception is renal dysfunction, which when related to poor cardiac output often improves after VAD placement, and often worsens on the calcineurin inhibitors for immunosuppression after transplant. Nonetheless, a high creatinine is a risk factor for worse outcome with VAD as well as with transplantation and with continued medical therapy (14). Another potential candidate for direct VAD is a patient with a recently treated malignancy for which survival is expected to exceed 2 yr, but might be worsened by immunosuppression.

Age

The target population for VAD for permanent support is anticipated to be comprised largely of people in their sixties and seventies. Further data will be required on outcomes beyond one year with the current and new investigational devices. The current limited data suggests that the best outcome with support devices is in patients under 65 yr, who from the MCSD sample had a one year survival of 83% with destination LVAD compared to 52% for older patients (14a).

Body Size

The current implantable VADs require a body surface area of at least 1.5 m^2 but often are not well accommodated unless the BSA is at least 1.7 m^2. Some abdominal cavity shapes are also inhospitable. Approximately half of women are too small for implantable VAD's. They have to receive the external Thoratec pumps that lie next to the body and can be powered by a portable driver on wheels, which is currently approved as therapy prior to transplantation but not for permanent therapy.

Right Ventricular Failure

Right ventricular function is a major determinant of compensation in chronic heart failure. Most patients with good right ventricular function are able to maintain fluid balance and modest daily activity and thus do not often present the profile of refractory

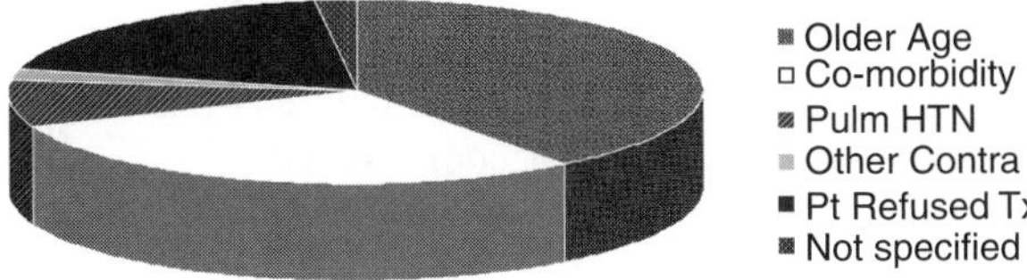

Mechanical Cardiac Support Database
2005 N = 129

Figure 5 Pie chart showing the reasons listed for ineligibility for heart transplantation in patients found to be candidates for left ventricular assist device therapy in end-stage heart failure. *Source*: From Ref. 14.

decompensation. Chronically elevated left ventricular and pulmonary artery pressures can eventually lead to secondary right heart failure. At that time, patients usually present with a profile of biventricular failure, with pulmonary venous and systemic venous pressures severely elevated. The symptoms and signs of systemic venous congestion may dominate the clinical picture.

Implantable ventricular assist devices are currently available only for the left ventricle. Unloading the left-sided pressures, consequently the pulmonary artery pressures and the right ventricular afterload, often leads to marked improvement of right ventricular function. While rapid, this improvement may take days, during which right ventricular failure can persist (26). During this time, VAD flows may be marginal or inadequate due to lack of sufficient return from the pulmonary veins. In addition, increased left-sided output can aggravate the clinical picture of right ventricular failure. Compromise of hepatic function and nutrition can jeopardize the post-operative recovery.

Right heart failure can be improved by pulmonary vasodilators, such as inhaled nitric oxide, nitroglycerin, or nesiritide. Intravenous inotropic therapy often helps provide support for the right ventricle during this transition period. Temporary right ventricular support devices have also been used. Outcomes have not been favorable with current combinations of right and left ventricular support devices, which likely reflects not only the complexity of two devices, but also worse pre-existing organ dysfunction. The 6-month survival after simultaneous right and left ventricular assist device placement in the Mechanical Cardiac Support Database is only 40%, compared to 74% with LVAD alone (14). Additionally, there can be a penalty of trying to "ride it out" using pharmacologic support during right ventricular failure in the early post-operative period.

The frequency of right ventricular failure requiring right ventricular support is estimated be approximately 20% of patients after LVAD placement. Considerable effort has been devoted to identifying those patients most at risk (26). Looking at the relative elevation of right atrial and pulmonary capillary wedge pressures is qualitatively helpful. If both are high, when right atrial pressure exceeds about 2/3 of the left-sided filling pressures, it becomes less likely that right ventricular function can recover solely from unloading of left-sided filling pressures. Paradoxically, high pulmonary artery pressures in the setting of high left sided pressures are a favorable sign for this situation, as the right ventricle is performing substantial work that can be reduced. On the other hand, if the pulmonary artery pressures are very high (over 60 mmHg) with pulmonary capillary wedge pressure <22 mmHg, it is likely that there is intrinsic pulmonary hypertension (27) that will not completely reverse with left ventricular support and secondary right heart dysfunction may persist. It should be noted that current estimates of 20% significant right heart failure after LVAD derive only from patients for whom LVAD was selected with the expectation that right heart function would be adequate. Patients with apparently dominant right heart failure have rarely undergone isolated LVAD placement. As more patients survive to late-stage heart failure, the prevalence of right ventricular failure is expected to increase, and more sophisticated modes of assessment will become crucial.

The Face and Pace of Progress

The limited number of patients who have undergone destination therapy since REMATCH have not provided adequate data to demonstrate encouraging evolution of outcomes. Sites with the most experience have the best outcomes, as more is learned about infection prophylaxis and device surveillance. Newer VAD's will offer decreased rates of known complications, but will likely bring new facets of concern. During device development, it

Table 3 Comparing New Wearable Devices

Global outcomes	% survival to and after transplant % 6 and 12 mo actuarial survival with device # patients followed > 1 yr on device Causes of death
Size of device and eligible recipients	
Device control	Mode of response to increased demand Possibility of negative intravascular pressure Peak output of device in clinical settings Level of activity demonstrated in patient series
Reliability	Frequency of component malfunction per patient-year Mode of monitoring for malfunction What happens if device stops?
Adverse events	
Thromboembolic	Type of anticoagulation recommended Rate of clinical neurologic event (reversible or permanent) in 30 days, 90 days, per patient-year
Hematologic	Evidence of hemolysis
Infectious	Rate of drive line site infection in first 90 days, then per patient-year Rate of systemic infection with positive blood cultures per patient-year

is critical to compare similar parameters across devices, as suggested in Table 3. The basis of evidence for new devices will likely include a range of patients and follow-up with the destination intent, the intent to bridge mechanically to transplant, and the intent to follow for potential transplant eligibility. Outcomes with devices for all of these patients may be aggregated as "durable support."

As devices become more versatile, they may be used across a wider spectrum of patients and purposes. Patients not yet afflicted with end-stage heart failure may receive partial circulatory support from unobtrusive devices implanted to prevent later decompensation. Patients with end-stage non–ischemic heart failure may receive devices in order to support "recovery," either as a result of adjusted loads and neurohormonal modulation (28), or specific reconstructive therapy with genes or progenitor cells and supporting matrices. For the present, however, recovery occurs in less than 5% of patients implanted with left ventricular assist devices for the therapy of truly chronic heart failure (29).

Mechanical circulatory support devices currently offer major benefit to only a sliver of the overall pie of the heart failure population. Even as they evolve, it is unlikely that devices to supplement cardiac output will eclipse other medical and surgical therapies. The complexity of the patient population and the varied therapeutic options mandate that patients undergo careful evaluation to identify the right therapy for each. For some patients, meticulous heart failure management can restore a level of compensation commensurate or better than achievable with mechanical support. For many others, the best option will be to connect with an end-of-life care team who will bring comfort and dignity (Fig. 3). The technological and human resources required to offer all the options represent a multi-faceted commitment (Table 1), which should appropriately be focused at dedicated centers.

REFERENCES

1. Nohria A, Lewis E, Stevenson LW. Medical management of advanced heart failure. JAMA 2002; 287:628–640.
2. Stevenson LW, Rose EA. Left ventricular assist devices: bridges to transplantation, recovery, and destination for whom? Circulation 2003; 108:3059–3063.
3. Hunt SA, Baker DW, Chin MH, et al. ACC/AHA guidelines for the evaluation and management of chronic heart failure in the adult: executive summary. A report of the american college of cardiology/american heart association task force on practice guidelines (Committee to revise the 1995 guidelines for the evaluation and management of heart failure). J Am Coll Cardiol 2001; 38:2101–2113.
4. McAlister FA, Stewart S, Ferrua S, McMurray JJ. Multidisciplinary strategies for the management of heart failure patients at high risk for admission: a systematic review of randomized trials. J Am Coll Cardiol 2004; 44:810–819.
5. Deng MC, Young JB, Stevenson LW, et al. Destination mechanical circulatory support: proposal for clinical standards. J Heart Lung Transplant 2003; 22:365–369.
6. Taylor AL, Ziesche S, Yancy C, et al. Combination of isosorbide dinitrate and hydralazine in blacks with heart failure. N Engl J Med 2004; 351:2049–2057.
7. Bristow MR, Saxon LA, Boehmer J, et al. Cardiac-resynchronization therapy with or without an implantable defibrillator in advanced chronic heart failure. N Engl J Med 2004; 350:2140–2150.
8. Kittleson M, Hurwitz S, Shah MR, et al. Development of circulatory-renal limitations to angiotensin-converting enzyme inhibitors identifies patients with severe heart failure and early mortality. J Am Coll Cardiol 2003; 41:2029–2035.
9. Stevenson LW. Clinical use of inotropic therapy for heart failure: looking backward or forward? Part II: chronic inotropic therapy. Circulation 2003; 108:492–497.
10. Stevenson LW, Miller LW, Desvigne-Nickens P, et al. Left ventricular assist device as destination for patients undergoing intravenous inotropic therapy: a subset analysis from Randomized Evaluation of Mechanical Assistance in Treatment of Chronic Heart Failure (REMATCH). Circulation 2004; 110:975–981.
11. Hershberger R, Nauman D, Walker T, Dutton D, Burgess D. Care processes and clinical outcomes of continuous outpatient inotropic therapy in patients with refractory endstage heart failure. J Cardiac Fail 2003; 9:180–187.
12. Fonarow GC, Adams KF, Jr, Abraham WT, Yancy CW, Boscardin WJ. Risk stratification for in-hospital mortality in acutely decompensated heart failure: classification and regression tree analysis. JAMA 2005; 293:572–580.
13. Rose EA, Gellijns AC, Moskowitz AJ, et al. Long-term use of a left ventricular assist device for end-stage heart failure. N Engl J Med 2001; 345:1435–1443.
14. Deng MC, Edwards LB, Hertz MI, et al. Mechanical Circulatory Support Device Database of the International Society for Heart and Lung Transplantation: second annual report. J Heart Lung Transplant 2004; 23:1027–1034.

14a. www.ishlt.org/registries/

15. MacIntyre K, Capewell S, Stewart S, et al. Evidence of improving prognosis in heart failure: trends in case fatality in 66,547 patients hospitalized between 1986 and 1995. Circulation 2000; 102:1126–1131.
16. Lee DS, Austin PC, Rouleau JL, Liu PP, Naimark D, Tu JV. Predicting mortality among patients hospitalized for heart failure: derivation and validation of a clinical model. JAMA 2003; 290:2581–2587.
17. Lucas C, Johnson W, Hamilton MA, et al. Freedom from congestion predicts good survival despite previous class IV symptoms of heart failure. Am Heart J 2000; 140:840–847.
18. Shakar SF, Lowes BD, Lindenfeld J, et al. Peak oxygen consumption and outcome in heart failure patients chronically treated with beta-blockers. J Card Fail 2004; 10:15–20.

19. Rose EA, Moskowitz AJ, Packer M, et al. The REMATCH trial: rationale, design, and end points. Randomized Evaluation of Mechanical Assistance for the Treatment of Congestive Heart Failure. Ann Thorac Surg 1999; 67:723–730.
20. Jaski BE, Lingle RJ, Kim J, et al. Comparison of functional capacity in patients with end-stage heart failure following implantation of a left ventricular assist device versus heart transplantation: results of the experience with left ventricular assist device with exercise trial. J Heart Lung Transplant 1999; 18:1031–1040.
21. Lazar RM, Shapiro PA, Jaski BE, et al. Neurological events during long-term mechanical circulatory support for heart failure: the Randomized Evaluation of Mechanical Assistance for the Treatment of Congestive Heart Failure (REMATCH) experience. Circulation 2004; 109:2423–2427.
22. Abraham WT, Fisher WG, Smith AL, et al. Cardiac resynchronization in chronic heart failure. N Engl J Med 2002; 346:1845–1853.
23. Lewis EF, Johnson PA, Johnson W, Collins C, Griffin L, Stevenson LW. Preferences for quality of life or survival expressed by patients with heart failure. J Heart Lung Transplant 2001; 20:1016–1024.
24. Shah MR, O'Connor CM, Sopko G, Hasselblad V, Califf RM, Stevenson LW. Evaluation Study of Congestive Heart Failure and Pulmonary Artery Catheterization Effectiveness (ESCAPE): design and rationale. Am Heart J 2001; 141:528–535.
25. Cohn JN, Johnson G, Ziesche S, et al. A comparison of enalapril with hydralazine-isosorbide dinitrate in the treatment of chronic congestive heart failure. N Engl J Med 1991; 325:303–310.
26. Kavarana MN, Pessin-Minsley MS, Urtecho J, et al. Right ventricular dysfunction and organ failure in left ventricular assist device recipients: a continuing problem. Ann Thorac Surg 2002; 73:745–750.
27. Drazner MH, Hamilton MA, Fonarow G, Creaser J, Flavell C, Stevenson LW. Relationship between right and left-sided filling pressures in 1000 patients with advanced heart failure. J Heart Lung Transplant 1999; 18:1126–1132.
28. Yacoub MH. A novel strategy to maximize the efficacy of left ventricular assist devices as a bridge to recovery. Eur Heart J 2001; 22:534–540.
29. Mancini DM, Beniaminovitz A, Levin H, et al. Low incidence of myocardial recovery after left ventricular assist device implantation in patients with chronic heart failure. Circulation 1998; 98:2383–2389.

24
Ventricular Assist Devices

Jason A. Williams and John V. Conte
Division of Cardiac Surgery, The Johns Hopkins Hospital, Baltimore, Maryland, U.S.A.

HISTORY OF MECHANICAL VENTRICULAR ASSISTANCE

Gibbon's creation of a bubble oxygenator not only allowed for the surgical treatment of complex cardiovascular diseases, it also hailed the beginning of mechanical cardiopulmonary assistance (1). However, it became clear to pioneers in the field of cardiac surgery that certain patients would not easily be weaned from cardiopulmonary bypass (CPB), indicating the necessity of having mechanical devices that assist with native cardiac function until the heart recovers. The first successful use of a mechanical bridge to recovery was reported in 1963, when four patients suffering from postcardiotomy heart failure were maintained on femoral–femoral bypass until their hearts recovered adequate function to support them (2).

Advancements in the field of mechanical ventricular assistance then led to the development of intra-thoracic devices such as the device introduced by DeBakey in 1963, which drew blood from the left atrium and ejected it into the descending thoracic aorta. The complex pneumatic controller and blood chamber was modified a few years later to yield the first successful mechanical bridge to recovery in a patient suffering from acute heart failure after double valve replacement (3).

The development of ventricular mechanical assistance was further advanced after the National Heart Institute formed the Artificial Heart Program in 1964 (4). Once a national effort was in place to fund research in this field, investigators were able to successfully produce different devices for different heart failure indications. Devices were then developed for use not only as a bridge to recovery, but also as a bridge to transplantation (5,6).

The first left ventricular assist device (LVAD) implantation as a bridge to transplantation occurred in 1982 (7). As experience with this indication for LVAD use grew, clinicians began to envision a new indication for LVAD use: permanent cardiac assistance. The term "destination therapy" has been applied to devices used in such a fashion. The REMATCH trial in 2001 demonstrated improved outcomes in patients with end-stage CHF receiving LVADs when compared to patients treated with optimal medical management (8). The success of these devices in bridging patients to recovery and transplantation, as well as the success of patients treated with LVADs as destination therapy, provides tremendous hope for patients with end-stage CHF who would otherwise have little hope for survival.

Throughout the 1980s and 1990s, advances in the technology of mechanical ventricular assistance has improved outcomes and broadened the indications for the use of these devices. This chapter will address these indications, as well as the issues of patient and device selection. Finally, a discussion of individual devices will conclude with current research in this field and the prospects for mechanical assist devices in the future.

OVERVIEW OF VENTRICULAR ASSIST DEVICES

Short-Term Indications

The development of mechanical ventricular assistance has led to two separate types of indications. The first set of indications encompasses patients that should only require mechanical ventricular assistance for a short period of time. Patients with acute left ventricular failure who will likely recover from their heart failure event may only require support for a few days to weeks. These patients often have ventricular assist devices (VADs) placed as a bridge to recovery, which can be implanted as a right ventricular assist device (RVAD), LVAD, or bilateral ventricular assist device (BiVAD). Patients with acute myocarditis, postcardiotomy syndrome, myocardial infarction (with revascularization), and post-transplant reperfusion injury often fit into this category (9).

Certain patients originally designated as bridge to recovery will fail to regain adequate cardiac function after device placement. In these patients who have undergone short term LVAD placement, the LVAD may become a bridge to the placement of a longer term device (i.e., bridge to bridge). Many LVADs implanted on a short term basis are not able to sustain patients over a longer period of time. Therefore, in patients receiving some of these short term devices, the device needs to be replaced within a few days to weeks by an LVAD that is able to sustain patients over the long term. This bridge to bridge function of certain LVADs becomes a very important option for patients undergoing cardiac surgery at non-transplant centers. Once it becomes clear that patients require mechanical circulatory assistance, surgeons can place a short term device that sustains the patient until they are transported to a quaternary center for definitive treatment.

Long-Term Indications

Certain types of heart failure will require long term mechanical ventricular assistance in order to sustain the patient. Long term goals for the use of LVADs include bridge to transplantation, destination therapy, and bridge to recovery in special circumstances or under experimental protocol. As technology improves so that devices are becoming smaller and more manageable for patients, many of the devices can be used for either indication. Table 1 indicates the most common causes of heart failure necessitating the placement of a long term LVAD.

Devices used as a bridge to transplantation may be in place for a number of months to years. They can enable patients to recover function of other end-organs that may have sustained damage from poor circulation (10). Patients who do not qualify for transplantation may still benefit from the placement of a long term LVAD as destination therapy. The benefit of this use of LVADs was first shown in the REMATCH Trial, which demonstrated a significant survival benefit for non-transplantable end-stage CHF patients receiving LVAD compared to optimal medical therapy (8). However, whenever possible, patients who are transplant candidates should be listed for transplantation, because long

Table 1 Most Common Indications for the Placement of a Long-Term LVAD for Use as a Bridge to Transplantation or Destination Therapy

Acute decompensation of chronic heart failure
Myocarditis
Chronic heart failure
Ventricular arrhythmias
High-risk reparative cardiac operations (LVAD used as back-up)

Abbreviation: LVAD, left ventricular assist device.
Source: From Ref. 7.

term outcomes in transplant recipients are still better than patients who have current generation long-term LVADs in place (11).

PATIENT SELECTION

Optimal patient selection is critical to the success of LVAD implantation. While different centers have adopted their own criteria for patient selection and eligibility for LVAD placement, certain universal guidelines should be followed in most cases to ensure optimal outcomes in this very fragile patient population. Table 2 indicates the patient considerations necessary when selecting a patient for mechanical circulatory assistance.

Cardiac Considerations

Right ventricular dysfunction is often reported to be the primary cause of unsuccessful placement of a LVAD (12,13). Chronic left heart failure leads to elevated pulmonary vascular resistance, which can result in right ventricular decompensation. Although placement of a LVAD often unloads the left ventricle and relieves pulmonary congestion, acute decompensation can occur after device placement, which may lead to patient demise. In the setting of elevated pulmonary pressures, patients should be considered for biventricular support, or biventricular support should be available as a back-up in case LVAD support fails. However, because concomitant placement of RVAD increases mortality, considerable clinical judgment is required to determine which patients will benefit from this therapy and which patients should avoid RVAD placement (14).

Patients with valvular disease require special consideration, as well. Many types of valve pathology are circumvented by the LVAD circuit and have little effect on flows or function of the device. However, in patients that have LVADs placed as bridge to recovery, valvular pathology must be corrected at the time of device implantation so that this pathology does not interfere with cardiac function after the device is removed. Aortic stenosis and mitral regurgitation should affect device function very little, and are not normally an issue in patients undergoing long-term LVAD implantation. However, aortic insufficiency can present a significant challenge and may require valvuloplasty during LVAD implantation to prevent regurgitant flow postoperatively. Mitral stenosis can impede device filling and should be addressed at the time of device implantation to optimize LVAD function. Patients with a mechanical aortic prosthesis should have this valve changed to a bioprosthesis, or the mechanical prosthesis should be oversewn with a patch to prevent thrombotic complications.

Coronary artery disease not amenable to surgical or medical therapy is a growing indication for LVAD placement. However, even after the decision to place a LVAD has

Table 2 Left Ventricular Assist Device Patient Selection

Transplant candidate (FDA criteria for LVAD insertion)
Hemodynamic variables
Cardiac index < 2 L/min/m^2
Systolic blood pressure < 80 mm Hg
Pulmonary capillary wedge pressure > 20 mm Hg
On maximized medical therapy
Cardiac consideration
Right ventricular function
Valvular disease
Ischemia
Intracardiac shunts (i.e., PFO)
Arrhythmias
Non-cardiac considerations
Neurologic function
Infectious diseases
Prothrombin time > 16 s
Urine output
Blood urea nitrogen
Bilirubin
Pulmonary disease
Patient preference
Technical considerations
Body surface area < 1.5 m^2
Prosthetic valves
Reoperation
Left ventricular thrombus

Abbreviation: LVAD, left ventricular assist device.
Source: From Ref. 9.

been made, every effort should be made to revascularize as much myocardium as possible. This will serve two purposes for the patient. First, revascularization can minimize angina and improve quality of life (9). In addition, patients undergoing LVAD implantation still require adequate right ventricular function, so optimal revascularization of the right coronary circulation should be performed whenever possible.

Non-cardiac Considerations

The function of non-cardiac organ systems is very important in determining outcomes following LVAD insertion. The timing of device insertion can be a critical factor for the health of these non-cardiac organ systems. Ideally, device insertion should be considered prior to distant organ failure and dysfunction, so it is paramount to assess the preoperative status of each organ system.

In many patients with acute cardiac arrest leading to the need for LVAD insertion, the central nervous system can be damaged during the acute event or during resuscitative efforts. Often, due to the patients overall health status prior to device insertion, it is difficult to fully assess neurologic status prior to making the decision to proceed with LVAD insertion. Therefore, neurologic evaluation should occur as often as possible to ensure that the patient's clinical status has not deteriorated beyond recovery. If, at any point after LVAD insertion the patient is deemed to have sustained devastating neurologic damage, withdrawal of LVAD support should be considered. Furthermore, detailed discussions with patients' families regarding these issues should occur prior to LVAD insertion so that family members are educated about the process and are not taken by surprise once a patient's neurologic status is determined to be unrecoverable.

Infection is one of the most common and devastating complications that patients may develop following LVAD insertion, with as many as half of all LVAD recipients reported to acquire some type of infection postoperatively (15,16). To complicate the issue, controversy exists in the literature regarding specific risk factors for developing postoperative LVAD-related infections (17–20). Given the consequences of post-insertion infections, most clinicians agree that patients should have no evidence of active infection for at least seven days prior to device insertion. Furthermore, after implantation, strict surveillance and swift action are mandatory to prevent the devastating complications that can occur after infection arises.

Renal dysfunction requiring dialysis is one of the strongest predictors of mortality in patients undergoing LVAD insertion (9). Elevated blood urea nitrogen (BUN) >40 mg/dL and depressed urine output <30 mL/hr despite the use of diuretics have both been shown to be independent predictors of mortality in separate series (19,20). However, most patients suffering from renal dysfunction following acute and chronic heart failure tend to recover most function during the support period (21–23). Therefore, prompt insertion of left ventricular mechanical support is warranted in patients with heart failure accompanied by deteriorating renal function in order to salvage the kidneys and prevent increased risk of death later in the course of the disease.

Hepatic dysfunction, as evidenced by elevated bilirubin levels and increased serum coagulopathy (PT$>$16 sec), portends worse outcomes in LVAD recipients (9,24). Since synthetic dysfunction in the form of coagulopathy has the greatest potential acute impact following surgery, strict attention should be paid to this issue in the immediate preoperative period. Prothrombin time should be corrected by the aggressive administration of vitamin K and fresh frozen plasma in an effort to prevent significant bleeding complications and right heart dysfunction in the early postoperative period.

Preoperative pulmonary function can also have a significant impact on outcomes following LVAD insertion. Pulmonary edema should be expected to resolve after LVAD insertion and unloading of the left ventricle. However, significant underlying pulmonary disease such as chronic obstructive pulmonary disease (COPD) or other interstitial processes are relative contraindications to LVAD insertion given the low likelihood that patients will recover from these disorders after LVAD placement (9).

PATIENT MANAGEMENT

Preoperative Management

In order to ensure optimal patient outcomes following LVAD implantation, aggressive efforts should be made to optimize the patient's preoperative medical condition prior to surgery. Cardiac function, especially right ventricular function, should be optimized using diuretics, systemic and pulmonary vasodilation, and intra-aortic balloon counterpulsation, when indicated. By increasing perfusion, these maneuvers may also improve the function of other vital end-organs, such as the CNS, kidneys, and liver. Echocardiography should be performed to determine the presence of intracardiac shunts, such as septal defects or patent foramen ovales. These anatomic problems can cause significant postoperative physiologic alterations if they are not corrected during LVAD insertion.

Patients with known systemic infections must be adequately treated, with appropriate laboratory and radiologic evidence of clearance of the infection prior to insertion of mechanical ventricular assistance. Routine screening for bloodstream infections, pneumonia, and urinary tract infections should occur prior to LVAD insertion in all patients, regardless of a history of infection.

As mentioned previously, hemodialysis should commence, when necessary, to support patients prior to LVAD insertion. In patients requiring dialysis, every effort should be made to obtain optimal creatinine clearance immediately prior to LVAD insertion. However, optimizing renal function without the need for dialysis is preferred, when possible. This may include the use of diuretics, inotropic support, or placement of an LVAD prior to the need for dialysis in the appropriate setting. In addition, any coagulopathies should be corrected and monitored prior to LVAD insertion, as previously discussed.

Strict attention should be paid to the patient's preoperative pulmonary status. For patients who are intubated, elevating the head to 45° accompanied by frequent suctioning and turning of the patients can reduce secretions and prevent pulmonary infections postoperatively. Patients who do not require mechanical ventilatory support should undergo aggressive pulmonary toilet with incentive spirometry and flutter valves prior to surgery.

Operative Technique

The technique for inserting LVADs has been well described in the literature (25–28). Each device is slightly different, so the technique for their insertions may also vary. However, the basic concept for device insertion is the same for most devices used as left ventricular mechanical support. Although some devices may be implanted without the use of CPB, most procedures require CPB for successful completion.

After sternotomy and careful exposure of the heart, the patient is prepared for the institution of CPB. This can be accomplished with aorto–caval or femoral–femoral CPB, depending on the clinical scenario. Once placed on bypass, a ventriculotomy is made at the apex of the left ventricle. This is the site for insertion of the inflow cannula to the device. Interrupted sutures are placed around the circumference of the ventriculotomy, and these sutures are then passed through the sewing ring on the inflow cannula. Variations of this technique exist, with some investigators choosing to secure the inflow cannula to the left atrium, depending on the device being used.

Once the inflow cannula is secured, the outflow cannula is connected to the ascending aorta using a running, polypropylene suture in an end-to-side anastomosis. Prior to use, the device must undergo a series of de-airing maneuvers to ensure that air emboli will not cause catastrophic events after insertion.

Some devices are partially implantable and others are external. For devices that are implantable, a pocket must be created in the peritoneum, thorax, or pre-peritoneal space to house the device after insertion. For these devices, the drive line is generally the only external component. Paracorporeal devices that have most components external to the patient require tunnels to be created so that the inflow and outflow cannulae can travel from the device to their respective locations on the heart or great vessels. These devices are generally more cumbersome and are fraught with higher infection rates due to the amount of external components. However, they are also more versatile and can be used for a wide range of clinical scenarios.

Postoperative Management

Successful outcomes following LVAD insertion often depend on meticulous, aggressive care in the immediate and short-term postoperative period. Patients often leave the operating room coagulopathic, which can lead to significant bleeding complications in the initial 24–48 hr after surgery. Anterior and posterior mediastinal drainage tubes, along with bilateral chest tubes, can indicate the amount of bleeding that is occurring postoperatively. However, these tubes can often become clotted, so meticulous drain care is paramount for determining whether or not significant bleeding is ongoing. Many centers have adopted a routine, planned second-look operation within 24 hr of device implantation in order to monitor bleeding, evacuate clot, and inspect all anastomoses prior to final closure of the sternotomy.

Early postoperative anticoagulation is required for most VADs. Typically, heparin infusion is started within 24 hr in low doses and is slowly increased to a goal partial thromboplastin ratio (PTTr) of 2–3. Antiplatelet agents are added after 48 hr and heparin is transitioned to coumadin once patients have stabilized.

As previously discussed, right ventricular failure can seriously impact patient outcomes after LVAD insertion. The most accurate predictor of right heart failure after LVAD insertion is the amount of blood transfused, so achieving meticulous hemostasis intraoperatively is essential (29,30). In addition, avoiding the right ventricle, septum, and left anterior descending coronary artery during placement of the apical cannulation stitches may help to prevent right ventricular dysfunction. Invasive pulmonary artery catheter monitoring is used to continuously assess pulmonary artery pressures and right ventricular function. If dysfunction of the right ventricle is suspected, emergent echocardiography is indicated. If maneuvers to reduce pulmonary artery pressures and improve right ventricular function fail (e.g., inhaled nitric oxide, intravenous inotropes, and intravenous nitric oxide synthase agonists), then emergent placement of a RVAD is indicated.

Following the resolution of any acute post-surgical issues, attempts should be made to wean ventilatory support, optimize nutrition, and institute rehabilitation and physical therapy as soon as possible. As always, strict infection surveillance and aggressive therapy once infections are suspected can prevent serious complications that may hinder patients' recovery. These procedures afford patients their best opportunities for good outcomes following the insertion of mechanical ventricular assistance.

Weaning and Recovery

Certain devices are implanted with the idea that patients will recover sufficient native myocardial performance to allow device removal. Laboratory and clinical studies have shown that hearts supported with mechanical ventricular assistance have improvement in histology, myocardial performance, and clinical function, even years after device removal (31–34). Therefore, determining patients that may be candidates for device removal and the appropriate timing for weaning mechanical ventricular support is an important part of surgical practice in any center that routinely implants VADs. Recognizing patients that may recover native myocardial function requires considerable clinical experience, but patients with the best chance for recovery include those with postcardiotomy acute heart failure, acute myocarditis, patients with a relatively short history of congestive heart failure, and patients with acute graft failure following cardiac transplantation (35).

The first step to myocardial recovery after LVAD implantation is resuming optimal medical therapy for congestive heart failure. These treatments include, β-blockers, angiotensin converting enzyme (ACE) inhibitors, diuretics, vitamin supplements, and digoxin (35). Once patients recover from surgery, aggressive rehabilitation should be instituted.

Patients usually require complete unloading of the left ventricle for 2–3 mo. During this time, patients undergo weekly echocardiography studies to evaluate myocardial functional improvement. These improvements can be determined by improvements in ejection fraction and left ventricular end-diastolic dimensions. Once clinicians note normalization of myocardial performance during maximal LVAD support, the pump is slowly weaned by adjusting the rate and mode of the pump to increase the circulatory load on the native heart. By changing pumps to a fill-to-empty mode or by increasing the ejection delay in these pumps (decreasing the rate), the patients must rely more heavily on his or her own cardiac function. Demonstration of near normal myocardial performance on echocardiography during minimal LVAD support, coupled with normalization of mixed venous oxygen saturation, cardiac index, mean arterial pressure, and decreases in atrial pressures, are reasonable predictors of good outcomes following LVAD explantation (36).

Investigators are developing new strategies which may enhance myocardial recovery over time. The use of stem cells to treat damaged and scarred myocardium has shown great potential in clinical and laboratory studies (37–39). Recent reports of combining stem cell treatment with LVAD implantation have demonstrated the ease and feasibility of combining these two modalities (40).

Agents with β-adrenergic properties (e.g., clenbuterol) are also being tested for their ability to induce myocardial hypertrophy, which may aid in recovery by allowing viable areas of myocardium to compensate for areas that have sustained more damage. Clenbuterol has shown promise in two separate studies which demonstrate enhanced myocardial recovery after left ventricular unloading with mechanical assistance (41,42). However, long term clinic follow-up will be needed before definitive conclusions can be made regarding the efficacy of these treatments.

DEVICE SELECTION

Selection of the appropriate device to use in each individual patient's situation requires considerable clinical judgment. Very few studies have been performed which compare outcomes of different devices for the same indication. Therefore, device availability, clinician preference, cost, and patient preference all play roles in the selection of which device to use in any given scenario. To complicate matters, many devices can be used for multiple indications, and some devices can be used for short term or long term support, depending on the clinical situation and the issues surrounding the patient's need for mechanical assistance. The following discussion will give an overview of individual devices, their major strengths and weakness, and the most common indications for which each are used.

BRIDGE TO RECOVERY DEVICES

ABIOMED BVS 5000® (ABIOMED, Danvers, Massachusetts, U.S.A.)

The ABIOMED BVS 5000® was approved by the FDA in 1992 as a bridge to recovery for all types of recoverable heart failure. The device is an external, pulsatile VAD capable of supporting either or both ventricles for a period of days to weeks. The device is a pneumatically driven, asynchronous, pulsatile, polycarbonate housed dual chamber pump (Fig. 1). The "atrial" chamber acts as a reservoir and is passively filled by gravity. The atrial chamber is separated from the "ventricular" chamber by a tri-leaflet valve. The ventricular chamber contains an internal bladder comprised of flexible polyurethane which holds a volume of approximately 100 mL. Surrounding this bladder is air, which is displaced as the bladder fills with blood from the atrial chamber. Once the drive console senses a displacement of 70 mL of air, indicating that the bladder is full, compressed air is sent back into the chamber surrounding the bladder, forcing blood into the patient via pneumatic pressure.

The entire pump and the console are paracorporeal. A single pump is able to support one ventricle, and patients requiring biventricular support can have both pumps supported by one external drive console. The pump is capable of delivering a maximal output of 6 L/min, at a constant stroke volume of 70–80 mL. The right sided inflow cannula is placed in the mid-right atrium or at the ventricular free wall. The left sided inflow cannula is either placed in the right superior pulmonary vein, left atrium, or the ventricular apex. The advantage of left ventricular apical cannulation is that it allows complete decompression of the left ventricle, making it advantageous for left ventricular recovery. It is also desirable to have left ventricular apical inflow drainage in the presence of a mechanical mitral prosthesis, since this positioning allows functioning of the leaflets and avoids complications due to thrombus formation.

The ABIMOED BVS 5000 is easy to manage and operate after implantation. It automatically adjusts its output based on the preload and afterload of the patient. The drive console works on an alternating current and battery. In addition, a foot operated manual pump is available in case of power failure or device malfunction.

The limitations of this device include limited mobility and restricted flow capability. This limited flow capability can become problematic during situations requiring increased flow such as fulminant infections and patients with large body mass indices. Furthermore, the device requires full systemic anticoagulation. Because it is a paracorporeal device with an extended amount of inflow and outflow tubing, systemic anticoagulation must be

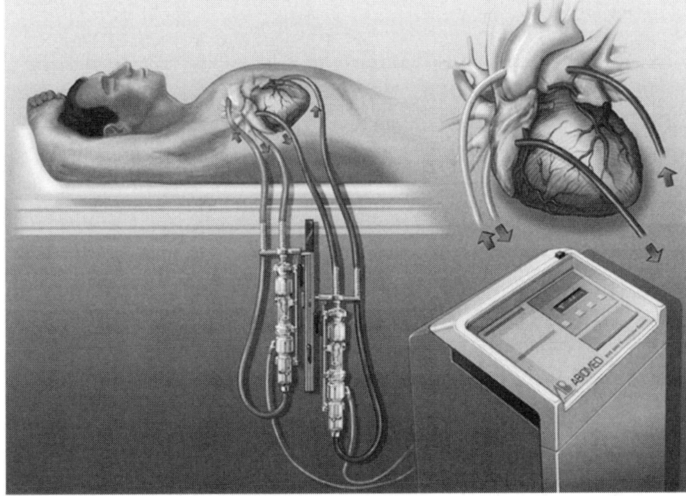

Figure 1 The ABIOMED BVS 5000®. *Source*: Photo courtesy of ABIOMED, Danvers, Massachusetts, U.S.A.

closely monitored in order to avoid the complications of thromboembolism that plague devices of this type.

In one retrospective review, the BVS 5000 was implanted in 47 patients as a bridge to recovery (38 patients) or bridge to transplantation (9 patients) (43). Twenty-five patients (66%) in the bridge-to-recovery group were weaned off of mechanical support, and 16 patients (42%) were ultimately discharged from the hospital. In the bridge-to-transplantation group, one patient recovered myocardial function and one died while awaiting transplantation. Seven patients (77%) underwent successful cardiac transplantation with post-transplant survival of 66%. The device was used for left ventricular support in 28%, biventricular support in 45%, and right ventricular support in 28%. Other centers have reported similar, cost effective results with the ABIOMED BVS 5000, with wean and discharge rates of approximately 60% and 40%, respectively (44,45).

ABIOMED AB 5000® (ABIOMED, Danvers, Massachusetts, U.S.A.)

The ABIOMED AB 5000 circulatory support system is the newer model from ABIOMED (Fig. 2). This paracorporeal device contains a pneumatically driven ventricle which can support either of the patient's native ventricles. Placement of two AB 5000 devices can be performed if biventricular support is required. Blood fills the bladder of the ventricle (approximately 100 mL) with the assistance of vacuum technology, which augments passive filling and improves the efficiency of the device. Once the bladder is full, pneumatic pressure empties the bladder contents into the patient's circulation to augment cardiac function.

The AB 5000 was designed with the intention to allow patients easier freedom of movement so that rehabilitation can take place during myocardial recovery. A single or

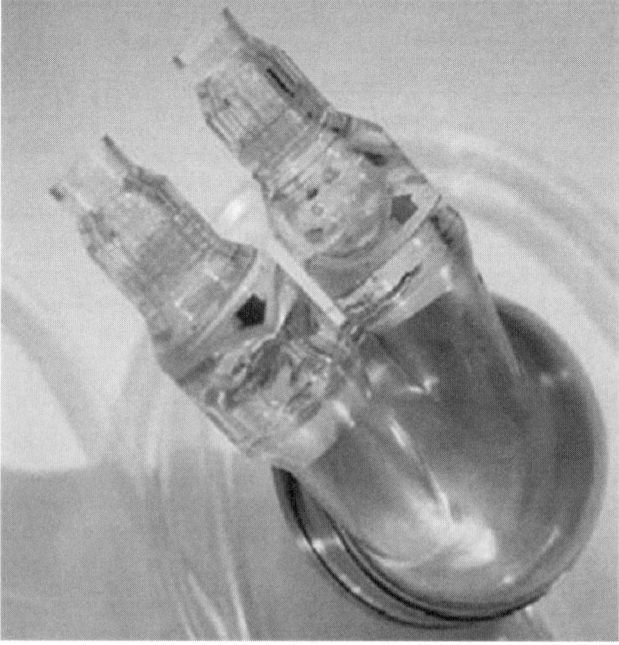

Figure 2 ABIOMED AB 5000® ventricle. *Source*: Photo courtesy of ABIOMED, Danvers, Massachusetts, U.S.A.

double device set-up can be driven by the same device console, which is lightweight and can be used by patients to assist with ambulation. Like its predecessor, strict attention to systemic anticoagulation must be paid in order to prevent thromboembolic complications. This device is new to the market, so only anecdotal reports of its use are available. However, the device seems to function well and patients have had good outcomes after its limited use in the United States.

Centrifugal Pumps

Centrifugal pumps are the cheapest and most easily available assist devices for short term support lasting hours to days. These devices work using rotating blades which propel blood forward and draw blood in from the venous system. Alternatively, pumps can use impellers and concentric cones with inflow and outflow connectors (46). They do not have valves or multiple moving or occluding parts which, in theory, can reduce hemolysis. This simple technology provides high flow rates with low pressure rises.

Centrifugal pumps are most commonly employed for short term use after post-cardiotomy failure and failure to wean from CPB (Fig. 3). Other indications for use include left heart bypass for thoracic aortic surgery, institution of ECMO, bridge to transplantation, or bridge to another VAD if myocardial recovery is unlikely within a few days. Various devices that are available for use in the United States include the Sarns centrifugal pump (3-M Health Care, Ann Arbor, MI), the St. Jude Medical Lifestream centrifugal pump (St. Jude Medical, Inc, Chelmsford, MA), the BioMedicus BioPump (Medtronic BioMedicus, Inc., Eden Prairie, MN), and the Carmeda BioMedicus BioPump (Medtronic BioMedicus, Inc., Eden Prairie, MN).

Systemic anticoagulation is necessary after device insertion and needs to be monitored closely. These devices are usually easily managed by nurses in the cardiac surgical intensive care units. However, care must be taken to secure the external cannulae in order to avoid any movement of these tubes. The majority of the hemorrhagic complications encountered with centrifugal pumps result from movement of unsecured cannulae.

Criteria for removal of these pumps include recovery of myocardial performance, return of hemodynamic stability, and overall improvement of whatever physiologic process necessitated initial device placement. If after 96 hr the myocardium has not shown significant signs of recovery, consideration should be given to instituting a longer term

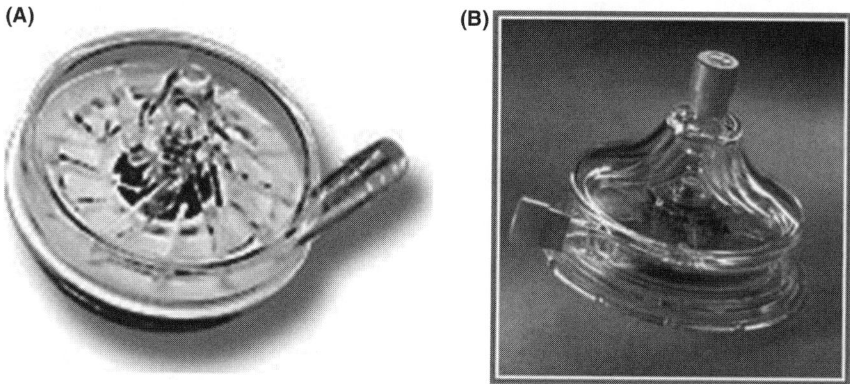

Figure 3 (**A**) Sarns centrifugal pump. *Source*: Photo courtesy of 3-M Health Care, Ann Arbor, Michigan, U.S.A. (**B**) BioMedicus BioPump®. *Source*: Photo courtesy of Medtronic BioMedicus, Inc., Eden Prairie, Minnesota, U.S.A.

cardiac assist device. Centrifugal pumps usually fail by breakage of the seal in the pump head, which eventually causes fluid entry into the magnetic chamber (47).

Clinical experience has shown that these pumps are especially well suited for left heart bypass and for short term support during post-cardiotomy left ventricular failure. In one study, 62 patients were supported using centrifugal pumps after failure to wean from CPB. Twenty-two patients required left ventricular support, 9 patients required right ventricular support, and 31 patients required biventricular support. Forty-two patients were weaned successfully and 27 patients were ultimately discharged home. Of these, 18 patients survived more than a year (48). Other studies have reported similar results for short term support using centrifugal pumps, with over one half of patients being weaned from support and 20%–40% discharged home (46,49–51).

Levitronix CentriMag® Blood Pumping System (Levitronix, Waltham, Massachusetts, U.S.A.)

Levitronix has applied contact free, friction free technology to mechanical ventricular support in order to prevent the complications of hemolysis and reduce some of the complications of thromboembolism. The CentriMag ventricular assist system (VAS) is a paracorporeal system that is implanted in similar fashion to other devices in this category (Fig. 4). The inflow and outflow cannulae are connected in series to a small drive console positioned at the patient's bedside. This console contains a centrifugal pump that uses an electromagnetic suspended impeller to propel blood through the circuit in a manner similar to standard centrifugal pumps. However, because the technology uses magnetic bearings, there is no contact between the bearings and other surfaces.

Theoretically, the magnetic levitation centrifugal pump eliminates moving parts such as seals, bearings, valves, diaphragms, and sacs (bladders) which can cause thrombotic complications, hemolytic complications, or which can fail over time. This technology minimizes hemolysis and reduces the need for anticoagulation, although low-dose anticoagulation may still be required for these patients. Furthermore, magnetic levitation offers the ability to more precisely vary flows through the device at wider ranges

(A)

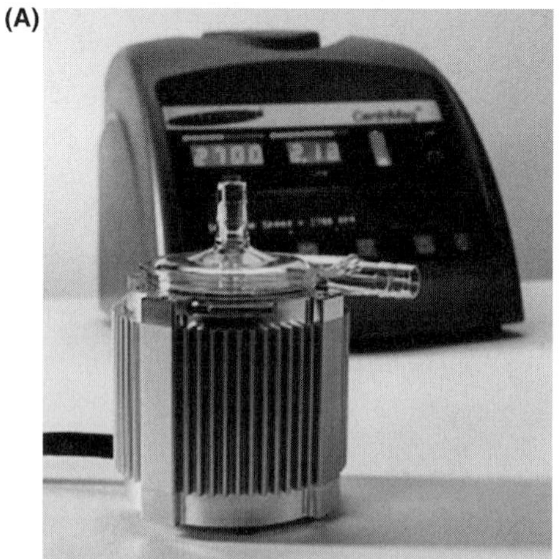

(B)

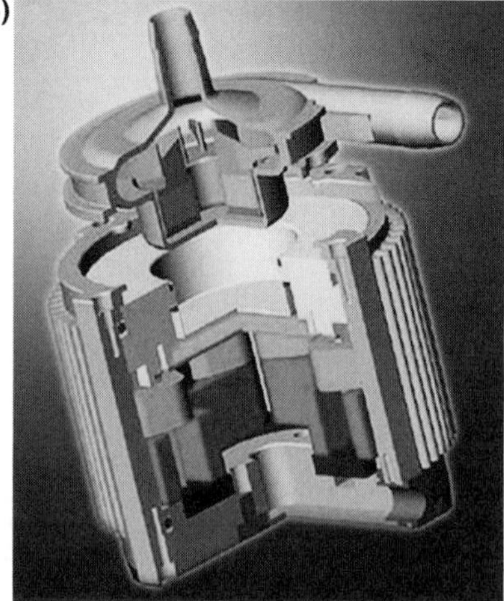

Figure 4 (A) Levitronix CentriMag® blood pumping system. (B) Internal schematic of magnetic levitation technology that powers the centrifugal pump. *Source*: Photos courtesy of Levitronix, Waltham, Massachusetts, U.S.A.

of flows (up to 10 L/min). This can improve weaning off of the device and can offer better support to patients requiring higher flows.

Currently, the CentriMag VAS is commercially available only in Europe, but is undergoing investigational trials in the United States. One study of this technology in standard CPB circuits of 11 patients undergoing CABG demonstrated no pump dysfunction, minimal hemolysis, and no internal thrombus formation despite the use of only low-dose heparin (52).

BRIDGE TO BRIDGE DEVICES

The development of short term devices and the advances that have been made in long-term devices have enabled a new indication for mechanical assistance to emerge. In some situations, adequate function fails to return to hearts supported temporarily by devices that were implanted with the intention of bridge to recovery. Manufacturing strategies of these short-term devices do not allow for their long-term use. In these situations, short-term devices need to be replaced by devices that can support the failed myocardium for months at a time.

This "bridge to bridge" role of short-term devices has enabled non-transplant centers to become active in the acute management for heart failure. Most long-term devices can only be placed and managed in centers capable of performing cardiac transplantation. Unfortunately, patients suffering acute post-cardiotomy heart failure in non-transplant centers had relatively few options, leaving them with very poor outcomes. However, short-term mechanical assist devices such as the centrifugal pumps and the BVS 5000 are relatively easy to implant and are quite portable. This allows cardiac surgeons at non-transplant centers the ability to place these devices into patients with failing hearts so that they can be transferred to transplant centers for definitive management (46,53). This definitive management may include support until the myocardium recovers, transplantation, or placement of long-term mechanical assistance as a bridge to transplantation or as destination therapy. Regardless of the ultimate therapy, these short-term devices provide clinicians with flexibility while trying to manage very complex medical issues.

BRIDGE TO TRANSPLANT AND DESTINATION THERAPY

Like short-term devices, mechanical circulatory support designed for long-term use has interchangeable indications. As previously mentioned, the REMATCH trial demonstrated that patients who do not qualify for heart transplantation can still benefit from the long-term mechanical assistance used in patients awaiting heart transplantation (8). To that end, manufacturers no longer simply target patients awaiting heart transplant when they are designing new LVAD technology. Instead, designers are now creating devices that can be comfortably used by patients awaiting transplantation or as destination therapy. Because of these design considerations, devices are becoming smaller, more manageable, and more easily implantable. Older generation devices still have a place in the management of certain patients with heart failure, but these newer devices hope to change the landscape of heart failure treatment permanently.

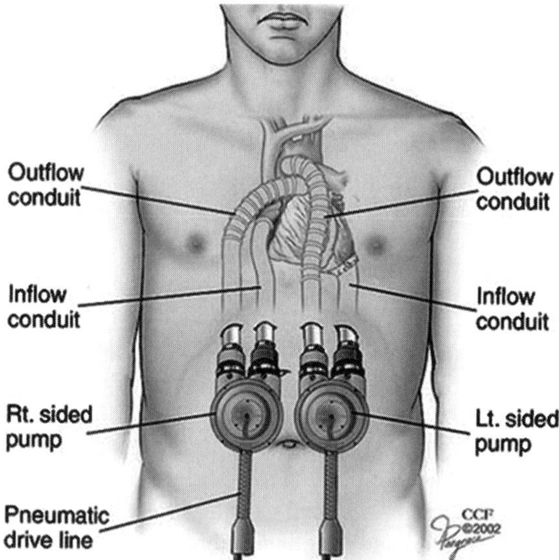

Figure 5 Thoratec® VAD. *Source*: Photo courtesy of Thoratec Corporation, Pleasanton, California, U.S.A.

First Generation Devices

Thoratec® VAD (Thoratec Corporation, Pleasanton, California, U.S.A.)

The Thoratec® VAD is a paracorporeal device that was first used clinically in 1982 for post-cardiotomy failure (Fig. 5). By 1996, the FDA had approved this device for use as a bridge to cardiac transplantation and as a bridge to recovery. The Thoratec VAD remains the only device on the market that is approved for these dual uses, and its paracorporeal design make it available for use in patients of all sizes.

The VAD pumps are pneumatically driven, prosthetic ventricles consisting of a smooth, seamless pumping chamber enclosed in a rigid polysulfone case. The blood sac contains a surface modifying additive which is thrombo-resistant, improves blood and tissue compatibility, and maintains long-term in vivo stability. Two mechanical tilting disc valves maintain unidirectional flow through the blood pump. A sensor detects when the VAD is full of blood and automatically signals the console to eject blood ($\approx$65 mL) from the pump at a rate of 20 to 110 beats per minute, for a total output of 1.3 to 7.2 L/min. Alternatively, the device can be set at a fixed rate or synchronous to the EKG, depending on physician preference and the clinical scenario.

Inflow and outflow cannulae are composed of Dacron and are coated with a thrombo-resistant coating to help prevent thrombo-embolic complications. The dual drive console offers two independent drive modules for left and right ventricular support. The drive line works via alternating pulses of vacuum and pressure to fill and empty the VAD, which provides pulsatile flow to the patient.

The device is cumbersome and is limited by the need for strict anti-coagulation. The console is quite large and limits patient mobility, forcing patients to stay in the hospital until a donor heart can become available.

To date more than 2500 patients have undergone Thoratec VAD implantation for left, right, and biventricular support. The device has been found to be especially useful as a bridge to transplantation in patients who require biventricular support (54). In an analysis of 828 bridge to transplant patients, the Thoratec VAD was used for biventricular support in 472 cases, left ventricular support in 326 cases, and right ventricular support in 30 cases (up to 515 days of support) (54). Sixty percent of the 828 patients underwent transplantation, and the post-transplant survival rate was 86%. In the 195 patients who needed post-cardiotomy support, the device was used for up to 80 days until myocardial recovery. Thirty-eight percent of patients were weaned from the device, and 59% of patient who were weaned were ultimately discharged from the hospital. Forty-nine post-cardiotomy patients were considered for transplantation; of these, 32 received a transplant and 23 were discharged. Other groups have reported transplant rates of over 60%–70%, with post-transplant survival of 90% after bridging with the Thoratec VAD. These results indicate the enormous success this device has had in bridging patients to transplantation and allowing for meaningful survival after transplantation (55,56).

HeartMate® LVAD (Thoratec Corporation, Pleasanton, California, U.S.A.)

The HeartMate® IP LVAD was originally designed in 1975 to be an implantable, pulsatile, pneumatically actuated (IP), intracorporeal device (57). The device was first implanted in 1986, and in 1994 it received FDA approval as the first commercially available LVAS to be used as a bridge to transplantation.

The HeartMate IP LVAD is a pneumatically driven unit that is manufactured from sintered titanium and houses a flexible, textured, polyurethane diaphragm (Fig. 6). The console controls a pusher plate mechanism which compresses air, causing blood to flow into the aorta via the outflow cannula. The inflow and outflow cannulae utilize porcine xenograft valves (Medtronic-Hancock, Minneapolis, MN) to ensure unidirectional flow through the device. The HeartMate IP is able to generate a maximum stroke volume of approximately 85 mL with a maximum output of up to 11 L/min.

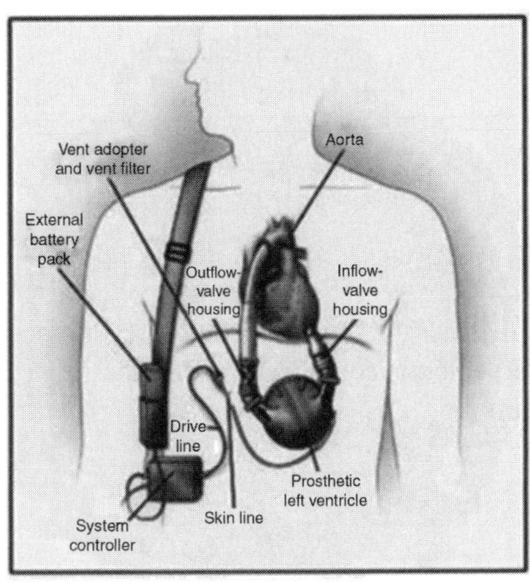

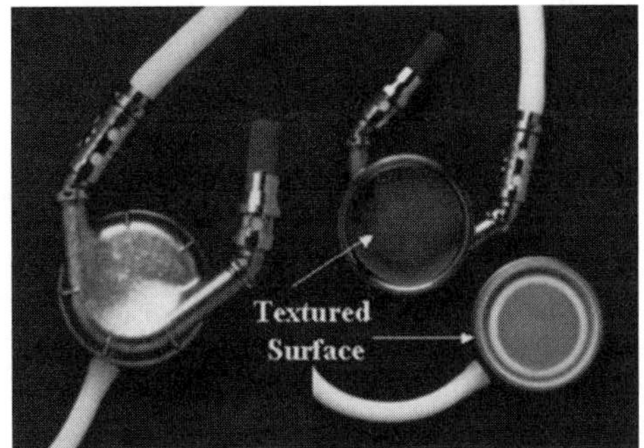

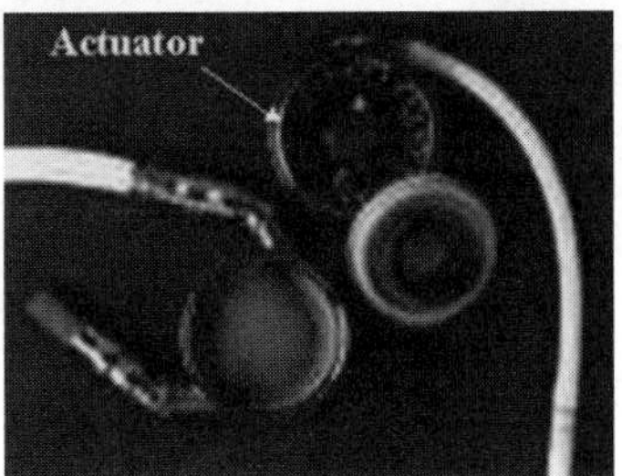

Figure 6 HeartMate® LVAD. *Source*: Photos courtesy of Thoratec Corporation, Pleasanton, California, U.S.A.

The blood contacting portion of the HeartMate IP, unlike other devices, is made of textured titanium which incorporates titanium microspheres, and a polyurethane diaphragm that is specially treated with textured polyurethane. These materials encourage deposition of a fibrin-collagen matrix, forming a pseudo-intimal layer. This, in turn, reduces the device's thrombogenicity and the amount of anticoagulation that is required.

Because the device is implantable, patients must have a body surface area of at least 1.5 m^2 in order to be candidates for HeartMate IP implantation. The pump is connected to the left ventricle and aorta in standard fashion, and a pre–peritoneal or intra-peritoneal pocket is then created which houses the device. The only external component is the drive line, which connects to a console that drives the unit. The console can be programmed in either a fixed mode, which delivers a pre–set amount of output at a predetermined rate, or auto mode, which pumps at a responsive rate determined by the hemodynamic requirements of the patient.

The major drawback of the HeartMate IP LVAD is the large, cumbersome console that drives the device. This led to the development of an electrically vented HeartMate VE in 1991, which has a much smaller console and affords patients considerably more mobility (58). This device received FDA approval in 1998 for use as a bridge to transplantation. Subsequently, Thoratec Corporation expanded upon the HeartMate VE concept to create the HeartMate XVE LVAS, which contains a new inflow valve conduit that has much longer durability than previous models. This latest device received FDA approval as a bridge to transplant in 2002. In April of 2003, the HeartMate XVE LVAS received FDA approval to be used for destination therapy. The HeartMate XVE's miniaturized, wearable components include the system controller (worn on the patient's belt) and two rechargeable batteries which provide about 6 hr of mobile patient support. This compact system allows patients to return to an active, productive lifestyle while on the device.

Presently, more than 1300 patients have undergone implantation with the HeartMate IP LVAS, while close to 2500 have had the HeartMate VE LVAS implanted. Experience in 95 patients from Columbia University receiving a total of 100 devices over a 7 yr period demonstrated a survival rate of 75% and a transplantation rate of 70%. The mean duration of support during this period was 108 days (59,60).

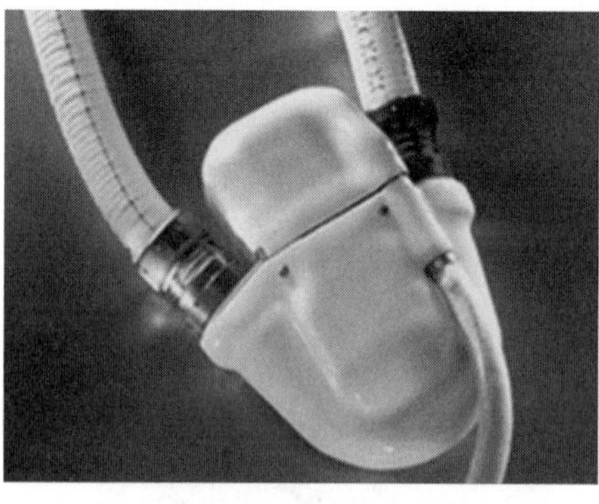

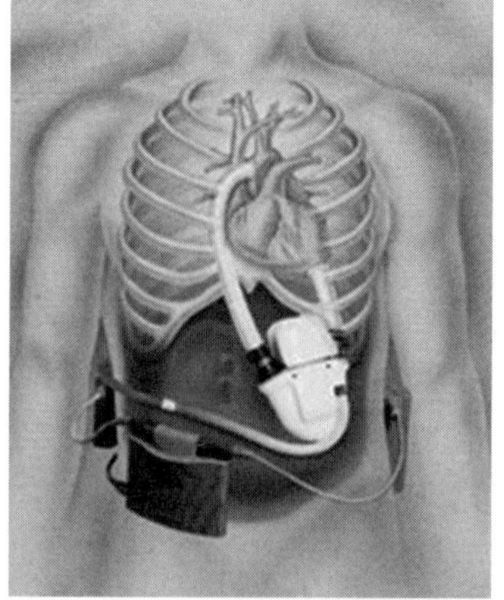

Figure 7 Novacor® LVAS. *Source*: Photos courtesy of World Heart Corporation, Oakland, California, U.S.A.

Novacor® LVAS (World Heart Corporation, Oakland, California, U.S.A.)

The Novacor® LVAS was first tested as a bridge to transplantation in 1984. The device was originally designed as a totally implantable system, developed in collaboration with Stanford University. Over the years it has evolved into a console based VAD.

This device is an abdominally implanted, electromagnetically driven pump (Fig. 7). The ventricle is a seamless, ultra-smooth, polyurethane pump sac that incorporates dual pusher plates to drive the pump output. The polyester inflow and outflow cannulae each contain a porcine valve to maintain unidirectional flow. The pump itself uses a high efficiency linear motor with a pulsed solenoid energy converter, so it requires no gears, cams, or intermediate hydraulic conversion, which ensures an extremely low mechanical failure rate. This pump can provide a stroke volume of approximately 70 mL.

The system contains an external controller that is connected to the implanted pump by a percutaneous lead. The controller and two rechargeable power packs (with 6 hr of work life apiece) may be worn on a belt or carried in a shoulder bag, vest, or back pack for ease of movement. The system is completely self-regulating, automatically adjusting its beat rate and stroke volume in response to the recipient's changing circulatory requirements. Patients using the Novacor LVAS do require strict monitoring of anticoagulation. The main mode of mechanical failure of this device is from wear-out of the energy converter, but this usually can be detected at least 3 mo in advance of the failure (61).

The Novacor LVAS has been successfully used in over 1600 patients over the past two decades as a bridge to cardiac transplantation. In one report of an institutional experience with this device, 53 patients with a mean support time of 56 days (range of 1 to 374) underwent device implantation. Sixty-six percent of the supported patients were successfully bridged to cardiac transplantation (62). Another recent study demonstrated that Novacor reliability at 2 yr (98.3%) exceeded the HeartMate VE at 2 mo (93.5%). The Novacor durability at 3 yr was 85.9%, with 78% surviving to transplantation in this series (63). The majority of the complications related to thromboembolism occur within the first 3 mo (64).

To date, 152 patients undergoing device implantation as a bridge to transplant have been supported for more than 1 yr, 42 patients have been supported for more than 2 yr, 22 patients for more than 3 yr, and 7 for more than 4 yr. This is the first device reported to support a patient for more than 6 yr. Only 1.4% of the pumps have needed replacement due to mechanical failure.

In 2004, the FDA approved the RELIANT trial (Randomized Evaluation of the Novacor LVAS in A Non-Transplant population) to evaluate the use of this device as destination therapy. The conditional approval permits immediate enrollment of up to 40 centers and up to 50 patients in the United States. Total enrollment is expected to be at least 225 patients.

Second Generation Devices

DeBakey VAD® (MicroMed Technology, Inc., Houston, Texas, U.S.A.)

The DeBakey VAD® is an axial flow system that was developed as a result of collaboration between Baylor College of Medicine and Johnson Space Research, NASA (47). The device is a small, hermetically sealed, titanium flow tube that is 30 mm in diameter, 76 mm in length, with a weight of 95 g. Because of its small size, the DeBakey VAD can be implanted in smaller adult patients and in children, which is an improvement upon first generation implantable devices (Fig. 8).

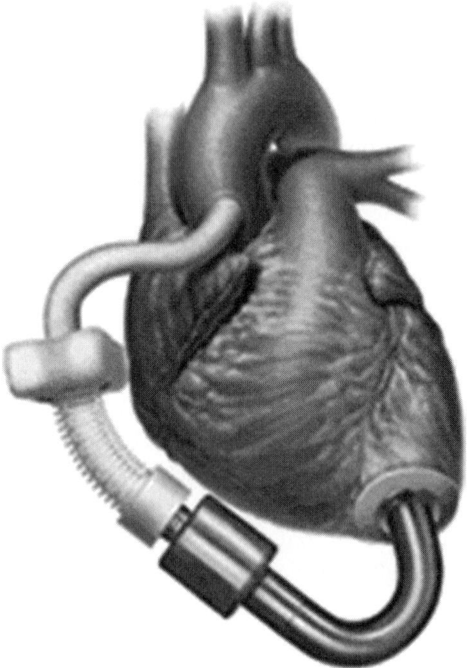

Figure 8 DeBakey VAD®. *Source*: Photo courtesy of MicroMed Technology, Inc., Houston, Texas, U.S.A.

Within the titanium flow tube is one moving part, a titanium inducer/impeller that spins at 7500 to 12,500 rpm and is powered by eight magnets that are hermetically sealed in each blade (Fig. 9). This system is capable of generating flows in excess of 10 L/min. The flow generated is non-pulsatile, and laboratory indices have shown that the device causes no significant hemolysis or changes in plasma free hemoglobin.

The pump is attached to a titanium inlet cannula that is placed into the left ventricle. The outflow cannula connects to a graft that can be anastomosed to the ascending or descending aorta. The pump is driven by a brushless, direct current motor that is contained in the stator housing. This motor is powered by a percutaneous cable that connects to an

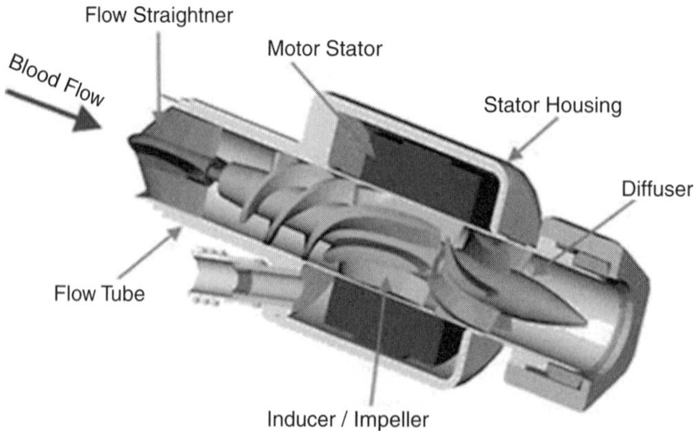

Figure 9 Schematic of DeBakey VAD® axial flow system technology.

external power supply and control console. The device does require systemic anticoagulation, with a goal INR of 2.0–2.5.

In early 2005, the DeBakey VAD was implanted in the 300th patient to receive this device. A report of 150 patients who underwent placement of the DeBakey VAD as a bridge to transplantation demonstrated that 82 patients (55%) were either successfully bridged to transplantation, recovered, or continue to be supported by this device (65). Sixty-eight patients (45%) in this series died. In the United States, the FDA has recently approved the DELTA trial (Destination Evaluation Long-Term Assist) (66). DELTA is a randomized control trial to evaluate the DeBakey VAD and the HeartMate XVE in a patient randomization scheme of 2:1. The current enrollment goal is 360 patients, with plans to perform an interim patient review after 152 patient implants.

Jarvik 2000® (Jarvik Heart, Inc., New York, New York, U.S.A.)

The Jarvik 2000® is a titanium based rotor pump (axial flow technology) that is 25 mm in diameter, 51 mm in length, and weighs 90 g (Fig. 10). It is implanted in the apico-aortic position with the pump being inserted in the left ventricular cavity and the outflow cannula anastomosed to the descending aorta (50). This affords the advantage of being able to implant the device through a left thoracotomy without the need for a sternotomy.

The Jarvik 2000 works in much the same way as the DeBakey pump (51). Although incredibly small, the rotary pump is capable of augmenting the native cardiac function to produce flows of 7 L/min at 8000 to 12,000 rpm. This pump also has the advantage of adjusting the flow rate manually in times of increased activity. Patients using the Jarvik 2000 require systemic anticoagulation, and the system is powered by a small external battery pack that connects to the device through a percutaneous cable.

The device is currently approved in the United States and Europe for use as a bridge to transplantation. However, in 2005 the European Union gave its approval to use the Jarvik 2000 as destination therapy. Plans are underway to begin trials in the United States for destination therapy, as well. Over 100 patients have received this device to date, with dozens of patients being maintained for 3 yr or longer. One series of 35 patients who

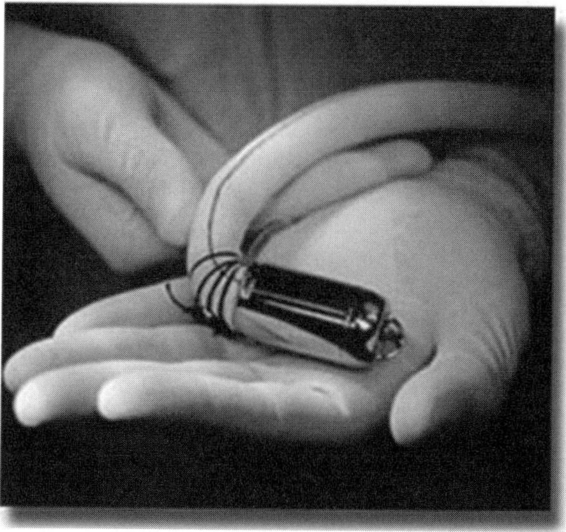

Figure 10 Jarvik 2000®. *Source*: Photo courtesy of Jarvik Heart, Inc., New York, New York, U.S.A.

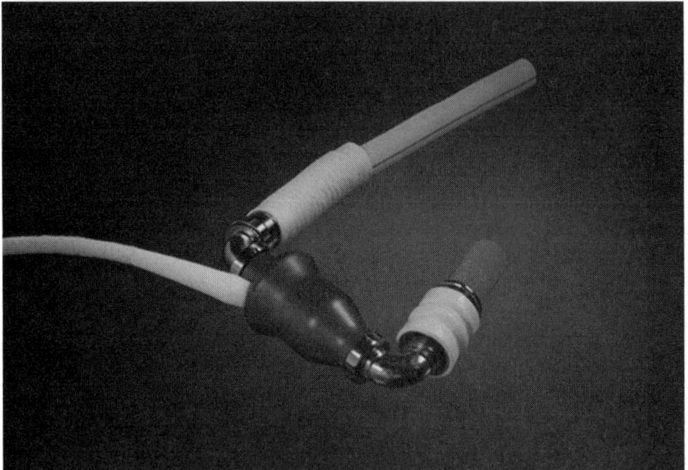

Figure 11 HeartMate II®. *Source*: Photo courtesy of Thoratec Corporation, Pleasanton, California, U.S.A.

received the device demonstrated an average support period of 67 days. Eighteen patients in this series underwent successful transplantation, and 12 patients died during the support period (53).

HeartMate II® (Thoratec Corporation, Pleasanton, California, U.S.A.)

The HeartMate II® is the next generation, axial flow device in the HeartMate family of mechanical ventricular assistance (Fig. 11). Like other pumps in this class, it is quite small, with a diameter of 40 mm, a length of 70 mm, and a weight of 176 g (67). The pumping mechanism is similar to the DeBakey VAD and the Jarvik 2000. Using this same axial flow technology, it is able to achieve a flow rate of up to 10 L/min at speeds between 6000 and 13,000 rpm.

The inflow cannula inserts in the left ventricular apex, with the outflow cannula anastomosed to the ascending aorta. The pump itself is placed in the pre–peritoneal space. A percutaneous cable connects the device to a portable controller and battery pack. The controller allows the system to operate in manual or auto modes.

The HeartMate II was designed for use as destination therapy, which affords patients the opportunity to use the device as a bridge to transplantation, as well. The first human implant of the HeartMate II took place in 2000 (68). Currently, clinical trials of this device are underway in Europe and the United States. In May 2003, Thoratec received conditional approval from the FDA for a pilot study in the United States. This study will enroll up to 25 patients at 10 centers and is for bridge-to-transplant patients only. A multi-center trial in Europe is currently evaluating the use of the HeartMate II as destination therapy for end-stage heart failure. To date 21 patients in the US and 6 patients in Europe have received the device.

DEVICES IN DEVELOPMENT (THIRD GENERATION DEVICES)

HeartMate III® (Thoratec Corporation, Pleasanton, California, U.S.A.)

The HeartMate III® is currently being developed as a 3rd generation HeartMate device. This system is an implantable miniature centrifugal LVAD that features a magnetically levitated, bearingless motor designed to provide extended life to the device. The pump also contains the same textured surface as the HeartMate XVE LVAS, which encourages the formation of a tissue layer within the LVAD to minimize thromboembolic complications and reduce the need for anticoagulation.

Novacor II® (World Heart Corporation, Oakland, California, U.S.A.)

World Heart Corporation is expanding on its design of the Novacor LVAS to create a totally implantable device without external drive lines or percutaneous power lines. The Novacor II®, currently under development, utilizes similar pump technology to the Novacor LVAS. However, this device also contains a Transcutaneous Energy Transmission System (TETS) which utilizes electromagnetic energy to power the system. A receiver is embedded subcutaneously with a wire that connects the receiver to the device. An external power source placed over the subcutaneous receiver can then inductively transmit power transcutaneously to the device. This promises to eliminate many of the infectious complications related to mechanical assist devices because there will be no percutaneous components.

CorAide® (Arrow International, Reading, Pennsylvania, U.S.A.)

The CorAide® LVAS was originally developed at the Cleveland Clinic. It is a small, continuous flow, centrifugal pump that has a magnetically levitated rotor. The device is small, weighing 293 g, and can generate blood flow up to 6 L/min. Clinical trials are underway in Europe to test this device. To date 5 patients have received the device with good results.

HeartQuest® (World Heart Corporation, Oakland, California, U.S.A.)

The HeartQuest® was originally designed by MedQuest Products, Inc., which was awarded a 4 yr NIH contract for developing the device. World Heart Corporation has taken over the design and production of this system, which is an abdominally implantable centrifugal device with magnetic levitation technology. The original configuration calls for a percutaneous lead to connect the device to an external controller and power pack. However, plans are underway to add TETS technology to this device, making it completely implantable. The physiologic control system is currently under development, and plans are underway for feasibility trials to begin in 2006.

OUTCOMES

Outcomes using mechanical ventricular assistance continue to improve with advances in technology. A large series that studied a combined registry of VAD patients receiving support as a bridge to recovery demonstrated acceptable results. In 965 patients who underwent device implantation, 433 (45%) were able to be weaned off of support, and 237 (25%) were ultimately discharged home. Of the patients who were discharged, the 2 yr actuarial survival was 82%.

The most significant report of outcomes in patients receiving LVAD support came with the REMATCH trial (8). This trial randomized patients with end-stage CHF who were not transplant candidates to receive either left VAD therapy (HeartMate

LVAD) or maximal medical therapy. One hundred twenty nine patients were randomized. At 1 yr, the mortality rate was 48% lower in the LVAD group than the medical therapy group. At 2 yr, nearly all patients in the medical therapy group had died, although 23% of the LVAD patients were still alive. While this landmark study demonstrated tremendous survival benefit and improved quality of life in patients receiving mechanical ventricular assistance, these results did not come without complications. Forty one percent of the LVAD patients ultimately died of sepsis and 17% died from device failure.

Realizing the limitations of early model devices in clinical use, investigators have begun to evaluate the newer device technology. In a multi-institution study of 42 patients receiving the HeartMate XVE LVAS for destination therapy, investigators compared outcomes in this group to the group of patients that underwent HeartMate implantation during the REMATCH study (69). XVE patients demonstrated a 40% lower mortality rate than REMACTH patients at 1 yr, with death rates due to sepsis being 8.3 times lower in the XVE group. These results demonstrate that improvements in technology continue to lead to improvements in outcomes. However, with a 1 yr survival of 61%, there is clearly more room for improvement.

Most 1st generation devices currently in use as bridges to transplantation are able to support approximately 70% of patients until successful transplantation can be performed. Survival after transplantation in this group often exceeds 85%, and studies have shown that patients receiving LVADs as a bridge to transplantation have better post-transplant outcomes than patients treated with maximal medical therapy prior to transplantation (70). More importantly, studies have shown that this group of patients reports significant improvements in quality of life after device implantation prior to transplantation, indicating the positive effects that LVAD therapy has not only on longevity, but also on quality of life (71,72).

Bleeding is the most common complication in the immediate postoperative period after device implantation, with a reported incidence as high as 50% (56). Technical factors that lead to this complication include the creation of large pockets for device placement, device related leakage from connectors and conduits, and leakage from cannulation sites. Other factors responsible for bleeding include coagulopathy due to liver failure, prior anti-platelet and anti-thrombotic treatment, and CPB related platelet consumption. The management involves meticulous hemostasis, a low threshold for re-exploration, and judicious use of blood products and clotting factors in the early postoperative period.

As previously stated, thromboembolic complications continue to plague recipients of mechanical ventricular assistance. However, improvements in device components and anticoagulation management have improved the incidence of stroke in LVAD patients. In the REMATCH trial, 16% of LVAD patients suffered a stroke, which was significantly more than the 4 patients in the medical group who suffered this complication (73). However, patients in the LVAD group still had a 44% reduction in major complications or death compared to the medically managed group.

Infectious complications also lead to significant morbidity and mortality in LVAD patients (8). Studies demonstrate that 20%–60% of patients receiving LVADs will suffer infectious complications depending on which device is used (74,75). The majority of these infections occur on the drive line, although LVAD pocket infections and infections of the device itself leading to sepsis are also significant contributors to this complication (74–76). Completely implantable devices will be required to significantly reduce this complication, but strict surveillance and prompt action to treat the infection can certainly reduce morbidity.

THE FUTURE OF VENTRICULAR ASSIST DEVICES

As technology improves and devices become more reliable, ventricular assistance will become a bigger part of the treatment for end-stage congestive heart failure. The next step in design and development of these devices involves the implementation of a totally implantable system that uses TETS technology to help avoid the infectious complications that result from having percutaneous device components. In addition, better design of the internal components of these devices should lead to the development of systems that do not require anticoagulation, which will dramatically improve the quality of life that these patients already enjoy.

A new (and old) frontier of mechanical ventricular assistance also lies in the development and use of total artificial hearts (TAH), which can replace the function of the failing heart and totally support patients until transplantation. Current TAH systems under investigation and development include the CardioWest TAH (SynCardia Systems, Inc., Tucson, AZ); AbioCor TAH (ABIOMED, Danvers, MA); Jarvik-7 TAH (Jarvik Heart, Inc., New York, NY); and the VentrAssist TAH (Ventracor Limited, Chatswood, NSW, Australia). While these systems can certainly be used as bridges to transplantation, the ultimate goal for their use lies in destination therapy, which will offer thousands of heart failure patients the opportunity to thrive when donor hearts would otherwise be unavailable.

As technology continues to improve, more and more patients will enjoy the benefits of mechanical ventricular assistance for end-stage CHF. However, given the current prevalence of device related complications, such as thromboembolism, bleeding, and infection, considerable work still needs to be accomplished in developing devices that are universally safe and applicable to a wide range of patients.

REFERENCES

1. Gibbon JH. Application of a mechanical heart and lung apparatus in cardiac surgery. Minn Med 1954; 37:171–185.
2. Spencer FC, Eiseman B, Trinkle JK, Rodd NP. Assisted circulation during and after cardiac or aortic surgery. Am J Cardiol 1963; 12:399–405.
3. DeBakey ME. Left ventricular bypass pump for cardiac assistance. Clinical experience. Am J Cardiol 1971; 27:3–11.
4. Frazier OH, Fuqua JM, Helman DN. Clinical left heart assist devices: a historical perspective. In: Goldstein DJ, Oz MC, eds. Cardiac Assist Devices. Armonk, NY: Futura Publishing Co, 2000.
5. Norman JC, Brook MI, Cooley DA, et al. Total support of the circulation of a patient with postcardiotomy stone-heart syndrome by a partial artificial heart (ALVAD) for 5 days followed by heart and kidney transplantation. Lancet 1978; 1:1125–1127.
6. Cooley DA, Akutsu T, Norman JC, et al. Total artificial heart in two-staged cardiac transplantation. Tex Heart Inst J 1981; 8:305–319.
7. Kanter KR, McBride LR, Pennington DG, et al. Bridging to cardiac transplantation with pulsatile ventricular assist devices. Ann Thorac Surg 1988; 46:134–140.
8. Rose EA, Gelijns AC, Moskowitz AJ, et al. Long-term use of a left ventricular assist device for end-stage heart failure. N Eng J Med 2001; 345:1435–1443.
9. Williams MR, Oz MC. Indications and patient selection for mechanical ventricular assistance. Ann Thorac Surg 2001; 71:S86–S91 discussion S114–S115. Review.
10. Sun BC, Catanese KA, Spanier TB, et al. 100 long-term implantable left ventricular assist devices: the Columbia Presbyterian interim experience. Ann Thorac Surg 1999; 68:688–694.

11. United Network for Organ Sharing. The Organ Procurement and Transplant Network page, 2005. (Accessed September 19, 2005, at: www.optn.org.)
12. Levin H, Burkhoff D, Oz M, et al. Preoperative right ventricular stroke work is a major determinant of right heart failure in patients after left ventricular assist device implantation. J Heart Lung Transplant 1994; 13:S73.
13. Nakatane S, Thomas J, Savage R, et al. Predication of right ventricular dysfunction after left ventricular assist device implantation. Circulation 1996; 94:II-216–II-221.
14. McCarthy PM. HeartMate implantable left ventricular assist device: bridge to transplantation and future applications. Ann Thorac Surg 1995; 59:S146–S151.
15. Malani PN, Dyke DB, Pagani FD, Chenoweth CE. Nosocomial infections in left ventricular assist device recipients. Clin Infect Dis 2002; 34:1295–1300.
16. Simon D, Fischer S, Grossman A, et al. Left ventricular assist device-related infection: treatment and outcome. Clin Infect Dis 2005; 40:1108–1115.
17. Swartz MT, Votapka TV, McBride LR, et al. Risk stratification in patients briddged to cardiac transplantation. Ann Thorac Surg 1994; 58:1142–1145.
18. Pennington DG, McBride LR, Peigh PS, et al. Eight years' experience with briding to cardiac transplantation. J Thorac Cardiovasc Surg 1994; 107:472–481.
19. Farrar DJ. Preoperative predictors of survival in patients with thoratec ventricular assist devices as a bridge to heart transplantation. Thoratec Ventricular Assist Device Principle Investigators. J Heart Lung Transplant 1994; 13:93–101.
20. Oz MC, Goldstein DJ, Pepino P, et al. Screening scale predicts successfully receiving long-term implantable left ventricular assist devices. Circulation 1995; 92:II-169–II-173.
21. Gracin N, Hohnson MR, Spokas D, et al. The use of APACHE II scores to select candidates for left ventricular assist device placement. J Heart Lung Transplant 1998; 17:1017–1023.
22. Friedel N, Viazis P, Schiessler A, et al. Recovery of end-organ failure during mechanical circulatory support. Eur J Cardiothorac Surg 1992; 6:519–523.
23. Frazier OH, Macris MP, Myers TJ, et al. Improved survival after extended bridge to cardiac transplantation. Ann Thorac Surg 1994; 57:1416–1422.
24. Reinhartz O, Farrar DJ, Hershon JH, et al. Importance of preoperative liver function as a predictor of survival in patients supported with thoratec ventricular assist devices as a bridge to transplantation. J Thorac Cardiovasc Surg 1998; 116:633–640.
25. Parnis SM, McGee MG, Ido SR, et al. Anatomic considerations for abdominally placed permanent left ventricular assist devices. ASAIO Trans 1989; 35:728–730.
26. Oz MC, Goldstein DJ, Rose EA. Preperitoneal placement of ventricular assist devices: an illustrated stepwise approach. J Card Surg 1995; 10:288–294.
27. Scheld HH, Hammel D, Schmid C, et al. Beating heart implantation of a wearable NOVACOR left-ventricular assist device. Thorac Cardiovasc Surg 1996; 44:62–66.
28. McCarthy PM, Smedira NG. Implantable LVAD insertion in patients with previous heart surgery. J Heart Lung Transplant 2000; 19:S95–S100.
29. Goldstein DJ, Seldomridge JA, Chen JM, et al. Use of aprotinin in LVAD recipients reduces blood loss, blood use, and perioperative mortality. Ann Thorac Surg 1995; 59:1063–1067 discussion 1068.
30. Cryer HG, Mavroudis C, Yu J, et al. Schock, transfusion, and pneumonectomy, Death is due to right heart failure and increased pulmonary vascular resistance. Ann Surg 1990; 212:197–201.
31. Liang H, Muller J, Wen Y, et al. Changes in myocardial collagen content before and after left ventricular assist device application in dilated cardiomyopathy. Chin Med J (Engl) 2004; 117:401–407.
32. Nakamura T, Hayashi K, Seki J, et al. Chronic effects of a cardiac assist device on the bulk and regional mechanics of the failed left ventricle in goats. Artif Organs 1993; 17:350–361.
33. Dandel M, Weng Y, Sinjawaski H, et al. Long-term results in patients with idiopathic dilated cardiomyopathy after weaning from left ventricular assist devices. Circulation 2005; 112:I37–I45.
34. Hetzer R, Muller J, Weng Y, et al. Cardiac recovery in dilated cardiomyopathy by unloading with a left ventricular assist device. Ann Thorac Surg 1999; 68:742–749.

35. Meuller J, Hetzer R. Left ventricular recovery during left ventricular assist device support. In: Goldstein DJ, Oz MC, eds. Cardiac Assist Devices. Armonk, NY: Futura Publishing Co, 2000.
36. Termuhlen DF, Swartz MT, Pennington DG, et al. Predictors for weaning patients from ventricular assist devices. ASAIO Trans 1988; 34:131–139.
37. Tran N, Marie PY, Nloga J, et al. Autologous cell based therapy for treating chronic infarct myocardium. Clin Hemorheol Microcirc 2005; 33:263–268.
38. Leor J, Guetta E, Feinberg MS, et al. Human umbilical cord blood-derived CD133+ cells enhance function and repair of the infarcted myocardium. Stem Cells 2005; Oct. Epub ahead of print.
39. Limbourg FP, Ringes-Lichtenberg S, Schaefer A, et al. Haematopoietic stem cells improve cardiac function after infarction without permanent cardiac engraftment. Eur J Heart Fail 2005; 7:722–729.
40. Dib N, McCarthy P, Campbell A, et al. Feasibility and safety of autologous myoblast transplantation in patients with ischemic cardiomyopathy. Cell Transplant 2005; 14:11–19.
41. Tsunevoshi H, Oriyanhan W, Kanemitsu H, et al. Does the beta2-agonist clenbuterol help to maintain myocardial potential to recover during mechanical unloading? Circulation 2005; 112:I51–I56.
42. Barton PJ, Felkin LE, Birks EJ, et al. Myocardial insulin-like growth factor-I gene expression during recovery from heart failure after combined left ventricular assist device and clenbuterol therapy. Circulation 2005; 112:I46–I50.
43. Dekkers RJ, FitzGerald DJ, Couper GS. Five-year clinical experience with ABIOMED BVS 5000 as a ventricular assist device for cardiac failure. Perfusion 2001; 16:13–18.
44. Samuels LE, Holmes EC, Thomas MP, et al. Management of acute cardiac failure with mechanical assist: experience with the ABIOMED BVS 5000. Ann Thorac Surg 2001; 71:S67–S72 discussion S82–S85.
45. Couper GS, Dekkers RJ, Adams DH. The logistics and cost-effectiveness of circulatory support: advantages of the ABIOMED BVS 5000. Ann Thorac Surg 1999; 68:646–649.
46. Curtis JJ, Walls JT, Wagner-Mann CC, et al. Centrifugal pumps: description of devices and surgical techniques. Ann Thorac Surg 1999; 68:666–671.
47. Curtis JJ, Boley TM, Walls JT, et al. Frequency of seal disruption with the sarns centrifugal pump in postcardiotomy circulatory assist. Artificial Organs 1994; 18:235–237.
48. Hoy FBY, Mueller DK, Geiss DM, et al. Bridge to recovery for postcardiotomy failure: is there still a role for centrifugal pumps? Ann Thorac Surg 2000; 70:1259–1263.
49. Magovern GJ, Jr. The biopump and postoperative circulatory support. Ann Thorac Surg 1993; 55:245–249.
50. Noon GP, Ball JW, Jr., Papaconstantinou HT. Clinical experience with BioMedicus centrifugal ventricular support in 172 patients. Artificial Organs 1995; 19:756–760.
51. Joyce LD, Kasler JC, Frasier L, et al. Experience with generally accepted centrifugal pumps: personal and collective experience. Ann Thorac Surg 1996; 61:287–290.
52. Mueller JP, Kuenzli A, Reuthebuch O, et al. The CentriMag: a new optimized centrifugal blood pump with levitating impeller. Heart Surg Forum 2004; 7:E477–E480.
53. Morgan JA, Stewart AS, Lee BJ, et al. Role of the ABIOMED BVS 5000 device for short-term support and bridge to transplantation. ASAIO J 2004; 50:360–363.
54. Farrar DJ. The Thoratec ventricular assist device: a paracorporeal pump for treating acute and chronic heart failure. Semin Thorac Cardiovasc Surg 2000;243–250.
55. El-Banayosy A, Korfer R, Arusoglu L, et al. Bridging to cardiac transplantation with the thoratec ventricular assist device. Thorac Cardiovasc Surg 1999; 47:307–310.
56. Minami K, El-Banayosy A, Sezai A, et al. Morbidity and outcome after mechanical ventricular support using thoratec. Novacor, and heartmate for bridging to heart transplantation. Artif Organs 2000; 24:421–426.
57. DeRose JJ, Jr., Umana JP, Argenziano M, et al. Implantable left ventricular assist devices provide an excellent outpatient bridge to transplantation and recovery. J Am Coll Cardiol 1997; 30:1773–1777.

58. Frazier O. First use of an untethered, vented electric left ventricular assist device for long-term support. Circulation 1995; 89:2908–2914 published erratum appears in Circulation Jun 15;91(12):3026.
59. Morgan JA, John R, Rao V, et al. Bridging to transplant with the heartmate left ventricular assist device: The Columbia Presbyterian 12-yr experience. J Thorac Cardiovasc Surg 2004; 127:1309–1316.
60. Sun BC, Catanese KA, Spanier TB, et al. 100 long-term implantable left ventricular assist devices: the Columbia Presbyterian interim experience. Ann Thorac Surg 1999; 68:688–694.
61. Wheeldon DR, LaForge DH, Lee J, et al. Novacor left ventricular assist system long-term performance: comparison of clinical experience with demonstrated in vitro reliability. ASAIO J 2002; 48:546–551.
62. Robbins RC, Kown MH, Portner PM, Oyer PE. The totally implantable novacor left ventricular assist System. Ann Thorac Surg 2001; 71:162S–165S.
63. Pasque MK, Rogers JG. Adverse events in the use of heartmate vented electric and novacor left ventricular assist devices: Comparing apples and oranges. J Thorac Cardiovasc Surg 2002; 124:1063–1067.
64. Di Bella I, Pagani F, Banfi C, et al. Results with the novacor assist system and evaluation of long-term assistance. Eur J Cardiothorac Surg 2000; 18:112–116.
65. Goldstein DJ. Worldwide experience with the micromed DeBakey ventricular assist device as a bridge to transplantation. Circulation 2003; 108:II272–II277.
66. Noon GP, Morley DL, Irwin S, et al. Clinical experience with the MicroMed DeBakey ventricular assist device. Ann Thorac Surg 2001; 71:133S–138S.
67. Burke DJ, Burke E, Parsaie F, et al. The Heartmate II: design and development of a fully sealed axial flow left ventricular assist system. Artif Organs 2001; 25:380–385.
68. Griffith BP, Kormos RL, Borovetz HS, et al. HeartMate II left ventricular assist system: from concept to first clinical use. Ann Thorac Surg 2001; 71:116S–120S.
69. Long JW, Kfoury AG, Slaughter MS, et al. Long-term destination therapy with the heartmate XVE left ventricular assist device: improved outcomes since the REMATCH study. Congest Heart Fail 2005; 11:133–138.
70. Bank AJ, Mir SH, Nguyen DQ, et al. Effects of left ventricular assist devices on outcomes in patients undergoing heart transplantation. Ann Thorac Surg 2000; 69:1369–1374 discussion 1375.
71. Grady KL, Meyer PM, Mattea A, et al. Change in quality of life from before to after discharge following left ventricular assist device implantation. J Heart Lung Transplant 2003; 22:322–333.
72. Grady KL, Meyer P, Mattea A, et al. Improvement in quality of life outcomes 2 weeks after left ventricular assist device implantation. J Heart Lung Transplant 2001; 20:657–669.
73. Lazar RM, Shapiro PA, Jaski BE, et al. Neurological events during long-term mechanical circulatory support for heart failure: the randomized evaluation of mechanical assistance for the treatment of congestive heart failure (REMATCH) experience. Circulation 2004; 109:2423–2427. Epub 2004 May 3.
74. Bentz B, Hupcey JE, Polomano RC, et al. A retrospective study of left ventricular assist device-related infections. J Cardiovasc Manag 2004; 15:9–16.
75. Siegenthaler MP, Martin J, Pernice K, et al. The Jarvik 2000 is associated with less infections than the heartmate left ventricular assist device. Eur J Cardiothorac Surg 2003; 23:748–754 discussion 754-755.
76. Sivaratnam K, Duggan JM. Left ventricular assist device infections: three case reports and a review of the literature. ASAIO J 2002; 48:2–7. Review.

25
Total Artificial Heart (AbioCor™)

Laman A. Gray Jr.
Division of Thoracic and Cardiovascular Surgery, Department of Surgery, University of Louisville, Louisville, Kentucky, U.S.A.

BACKGROUND

The AbioCor™ Total Implantable Replacement Heart (Fig. 1) has been developed by ABIOMED, Inc. (Danvers, Massachusetts, U.S.A.) over the past twenty years. Initial preclinical trials were conducted at the Texas Heart Institute under the direction Dr. O. H. Frazier (1). Additional work at the University of Louisville involving the implantation of all components of the device demonstrated consistent survival in the bovine model. Approval for a multi-center trial for the use of the AbioCor in humans was granted by the FDA in early 2001 (2). On July 2, 2001, the device was implanted for the first time in Robert Tools. This marked the first time that a total implantable system had been used in a human to provide complete support for the circulation.

DEVICE DESCRIPTION

The AbioCor Implantable Replacement Heart has both internal and external components (Fig. 2). It does not require percutaneous lines or the need for any percutaneous access to run or control the device. The internal components consist of the thoracic unit, battery, controller, and transcutaneous energy transfer (TET) coil. The thoracic unit is placed in the orthotopic position after excluding the native ventricles. The thoracic unit consists of an energy converter and two pumping chambers that function as a right and left ventricle. The energy converter is situated between the two ventricles and contains a high-efficiency miniature centrifical pump that rotates between 6000–8000 RPMs (Fig. 3). The motor speed of this pump can be varied to account for the different resistances in the systemic and pulmonary vascular systems and the systolic ejection duration. A two-position switching valve is used to alternate the direction of the hydraulic flow between the left and right pumping chambers, thus resulting in alternate left and right systole. The rate of the switching valve determines the beat rate of the device and can vary between 75 and 150 beats per minute, resulting in a range of flows from 4–8 L/min. There is a 1–1 correspondence between blood and hydraulic fluid displacement. Displacement of hydraulic fluid to one side results in the creation of a negative pressure in the opposite

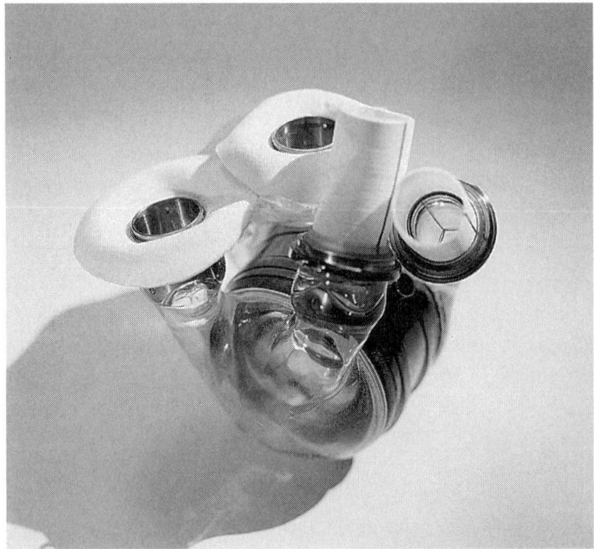

Figure 1 AbioCor™ total implantable replacement heart. *Source*: Photo courtesy of ABIOMED, Inc., Danvers, Massachusetts, U.S.A.

ventricle, thus the device is considered an active fill device. An atrial balance chamber is present and allows for decreased right-sided stroke volumes to maintain right and left fluid balance (3,4). A portion of the hydraulic fluid is shunted into a balance chamber, which is associated with the left atrium, allowing displacement of the hydraulic fluid rather than into the right pumping chamber. The amount of fluid that is shunted into the balance chamber can be adjusted manually or automatically on the basis of relative left and right filling pressures. All blood-containing surfaces of the AbioCor thoracic unit, including the

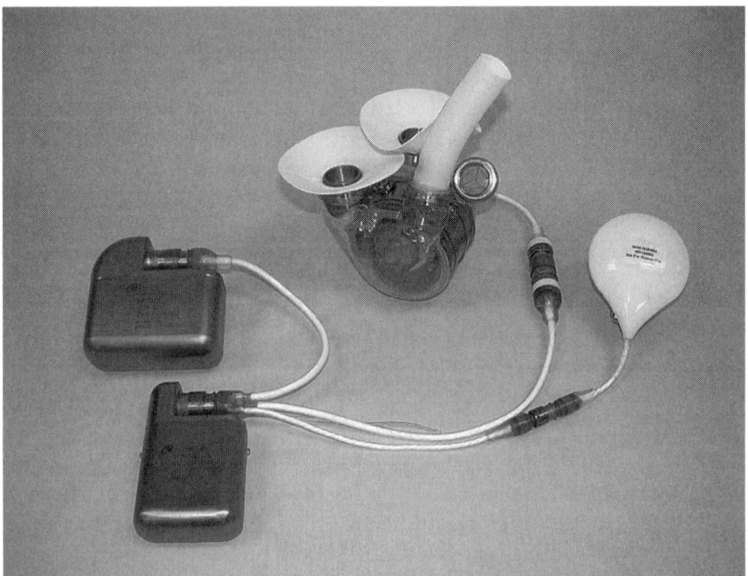

Figure 2 Internal components of the AbioCor™ total implantable replacement heart. *Source*: Photo courtesy of ABIOMED, Inc., Danvers, Massachusetts, U.S.A.

(A) 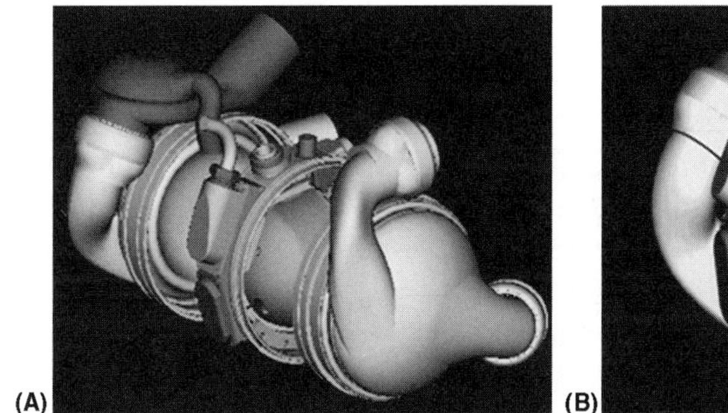

(B) 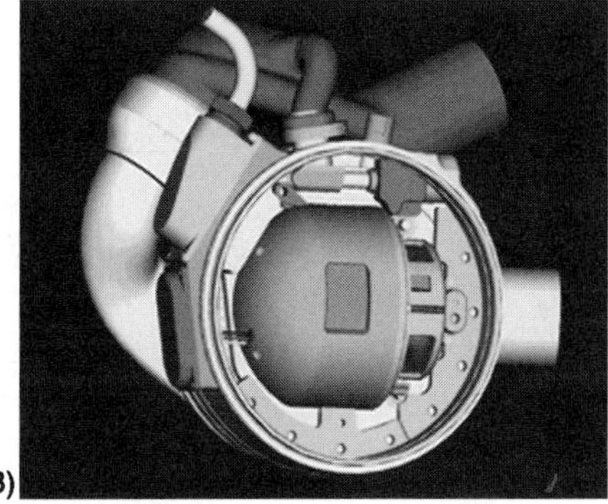

Figure 3 Energy converter and right and left pumping chambers.

tri-leaflet valves (20 mm internal diameter) are made of polyurethane (angioflex), resulting in a smooth, continuous blood contacting surface from the inflow to the outflow grafts.

The internal battery is lithium ion-based and is able to energize the thoracic unit for approximately 20 min. The internal controller drives the energy converter in the thoracic unit, monitors the implant components and transmits device performance data to the bedside by means of radio frequency telemetry. The radio frequency transmissions from the internal controller to the external controller convey information including continuous real-time telemetry, hydraulic wave forms, systemic operating parameters, battery status, component temperatures, and alarm information. This information is in real-time and is stored for later retrieval and analysis. The internal TET coil receives high-frequency power that is transmitted across the skin from the external TET coil. The internal TET system electronically converts this oscillating current into direct current that is used to power the thoracic unit and recharge the internal battery.

The external components consist of an external TET coil, a TET module, a bedside console, and batteries. The external TET coil transfers energy across the skin to the internal coil and is secured over the internal TET coil with an adhesive dressing. The external TET coil can be connected to either the bedside console or a portable TET module. The bedside console is used during implantation, recovery, and when the patient is in his primary residence. The bedside console provides clinicians with a graphic user interface for control and monitoring of the implant system through RF communication in real time. The console can be remotely monitored through the internet. A rechargeable battery in the console allows it to be disconnected from AC power for brief periods of time without discharging the patient's internal battery. When the patient is ambulatory, the external TET coil is connected to a portable TET module (Fig. 4). This module delivers energy to the TET from external batteries and contains basic alarms that are activated if there is a misalignment of the TET coil, low external battery voltage, or general alarm indicating a potential problem with the system. The external batteries are lithium-based and are able to provide up to one hour of support per pound of battery. The external batteries can be carried in a vest or a handbag or attached to a Velcro® belt.

PREOPERATIVE CONSIDERATIONS

Since the AbioCor Total Artificial Replacement Device is large, it is extremely important to ensure that the device will fit within the chest cavity. A computer software program

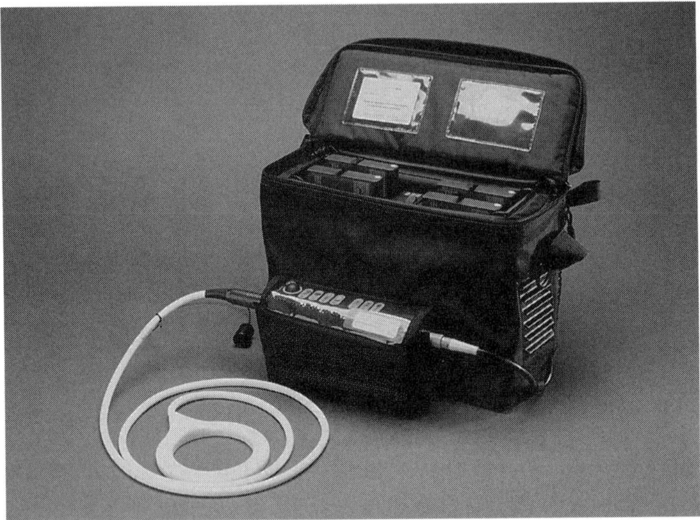

Figure 4 Ambulatory power supply and controller.

allows for the virtual surgical implantation of the AbioCor thoracic unit. All potential candidates undergo a computerized tomography scan of the chest. The virtual surgery program (AbioFit®) is then performed. The native ventricles are then "removed" and the thoracic unit is implanted as would be performed in an operation. This virtual model is designed to determine whether the AbioCor can be positioned in the chest without impinging vital structures, such as the superior or inferior vena cava or pulmonary veins. Since the device fits mostly within the left lower chest cavity, the left lower lobe bronchus can be compromised leading to atelectolesis in the left lower lobe. AbioFit is used by the surgical team to assist in determining whether the artificial heart will have a high degree of certainty of fitting within the chest cavity without obstructing vital structures before the actual operative surgery.

Anatomical fit studies of the total artificial heart demonstrate that one of the most critical dimensions is the distance between the pulmonary bifurcation and the level of the diaphragm. If this distance is too short, then there may be compression of the left pulmonary veins. At the time of surgery, one way to assess compression of the pulmonary veins is through the use of a transesophogeal echocardiogram (5). The pulmonary vein velocity can be easily obtained. If the pulmonary vein blood flow velocities are greater than 60–100 mL/s, there is some obstruction to the inflow to the left side of the heart and the AbioCor must be repositioned. Despite the use of AbioFit, in one case the chest was difficult to close because of obstruction to the left pulmonary veins. This was remedied by placing a large Gortex patch in the central tendon of the diaphragm. This allowed the AbioCor device to be displaced into the abdomen, reducing the pulmonary vein obstruction and allowing the chest to be closed.

OPERATIVE TECHNIQUE

A median sternotomy incision is performed and extended halfway to the umbilicus. The sternum is opened with a sternal saw. A pocket is then formed beneath both the right and left costal margins for the battery and controller. In addition, a pocket is formed beneath the right or left clavicle. The TETs coil is placed in this pocket and the lead tunneled to the controller. After hepranization, a standard arch cannula is inserted high up in the aortic arch. A right angle catheter is then inserted into the SVC and tapes placed around the SVC and IVC. Simultaneously, another incision is made over the groin and dissection is carried down to the femoral vein. A long femoral vena cannula is then placed in the femoral vein and, with transesophogeal guidance, positioned just below the right atrium.

The patient is placed on cardiopulmonary bypass, tapes are tightened around the SVC and IVC, and the aorta is cross-clamped. The right and left ventricles are then removed at the site of the atrial ventricular groove, leaving the mitral and tricuspid veins intact. The mitral and tricuspid valve leaflets are fully excised. The left atrial appendage is ligated; the coronary sinus is over sewn with 4-0 Prolene® and the patent foramen ovalve (PFO) over sewn if present. The left atrial cuff is then trimmed to the appropriate size and sewn to the native left annulus, using a running 4-0 prolene suture which is reinforced with Teflon® felt. A second layer of 4-0 prolene is used to reinforce the anastomosis. Similarly, the right atrial cuff is trimmed in place and sewn to the tricuspid annulus with a running 4-0 prolene suture reinforced by Teflon felt strips. The two reinforced suture layers are designed to prevent both bleeding and the entrapment of air. A Mylar® transducer is then placed in the left atrium through the right superior vein and let out below the main incision. Both the right and left atrial suture lines are checked for any bleeding by injecting saline into the respective atrium.

An AbioCor dummy heart is then placed in the chest cavity and attached to the left and right atrial cuffs. This allows for the determination of the length and orientation of the right and left outflow grafts. These grafts are cut to appropriate lengths; the dummy is removed from the chest cavity and the outflow grafts are sewn to the pulmonary artery and aorta with running 4-0 prolene sutures, which are again reinforced with Teflon strips. These two suture lines are tested for hemostasis. The AbioCor thoracic unit is connected to the left atrium, aorta, and pulmonary artery (Fig. 5). Saline is then injected through the right inflow valve of the thoracic unit to remove air from the right ventricle. The tape is removed from the inferior vena cava and the right atrium is connected to the AbioCor right ventricle, removing as much air as possible.

The second caval tape is removed from the SVC and the cannula removed from the SVC. The primary reason for having the femoral venus cannula is to allow weaning from the cardiopulmonary bypass without allowing any air into the device when the cannula is removed. The thoracic unit is then connected to the internal controller which, in turn, is hard wire connected to the external console. The external console is used to control the AbioCor Implantable Replacement Heart during the weaning process. There are large de-airing ports on the outflow grafts to the pulmonary artery and to the aorta. These are initially left unclamped to allow egress of any air in the device as the pump is started (Fig. 6). Once the right side of the heart is de-aired, a clamp is placed over the de-airing port on the pulmonary outflow graft. Blood is forced through the lungs and into the left atrium and through the left ventricle. During this time, the aortic outflow graft remains totally clamped and all the blood is exiting the de-airing port. After the left side of the device has been completely de-aired, the de-airing port is clamped at the same time the cross clamp is removed from the aorta. The patient is weaned from cardiopulmonary bypass over a one to two minute period of time. During this time, there is continuous monitoring of the right and left atrial pressures and systemic pressure. Any imbalance between the left and right filling pressures is corrected by making appropriate adjustments to the atrial balance chamber. If the right filling pressures are low, this is treated by a volume infusion. If the pressures are high, the beat rate of the AbioCor device is decreased.

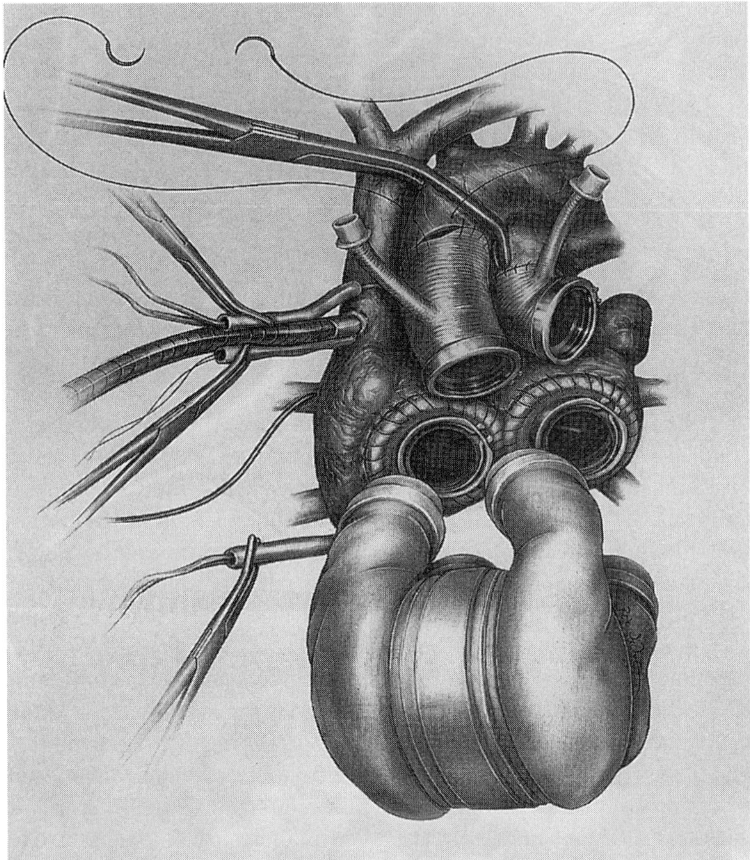

Figure 5 Right and left atrial cuffs and outflow grafts have been sewn into place. *Source:* From Ref. 6.

After hemostasis is assured, the patient is decannulated and protamine is administered.

A sterile external TETs secondary coil is then placed and the internal battery connected. The external console continues to control the heart through RF telemetry. The chest is then temporarily closed. It is extremely important to measure the flows in the pulmonary veins using a transesophogeal cardiogram. If the flows are too high, indicating stenosis of the pulmonary vein, then the device is repositioned. Once a satisfactory position of the device is assured, chest tubes are placed and the chest closed in a routine fashion (6).

CLINICAL TRIAL

The AbioCor Implantable Replacement Heart clinical trial is designed to assess the device's use as destination therapy, although, future uses could include bridge to transplant (7). The purpose of this study is to extend an acceptable quality of life for heart failure patients who are at immediate risk of death with no alternative therapy (Fig. 7). Patients who can benefit from AbioCor support are those patients with idiopathic or

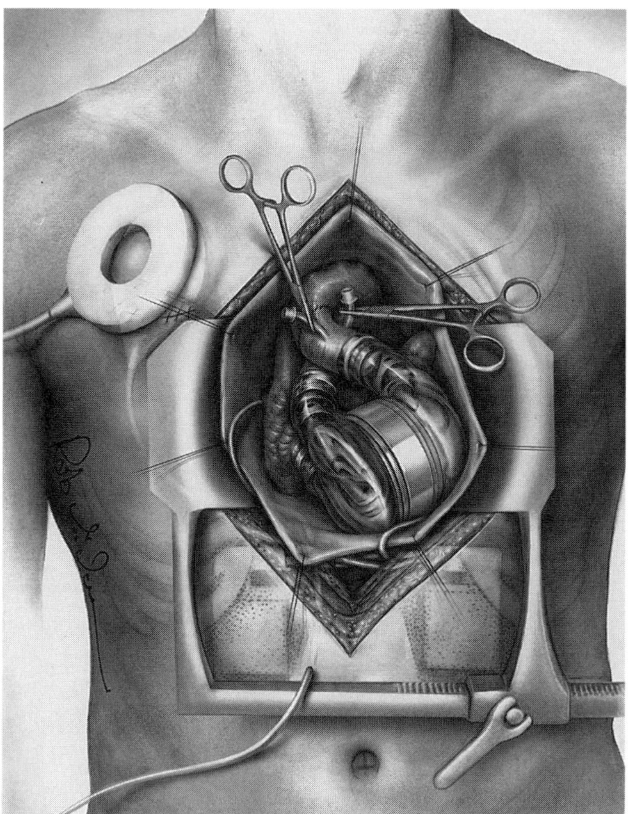

Figure 6 AbioCor™ is connected and being de-aired. *Source:* From Ref. 6.

ischemic cardiomyopathy who are in biventricular failure (Table 1). The trial includes patients who have had heart transplant rejection, severe but reversible liver or renal failure, reversible chronic pulmonary disease, or severe arrhythmias which cannot be treated medically. Common pre-operative conditions include bed-bound patients at immediate risk of dying who are dependent upon two or more inotropes, IABP, significant pulmonary hypertension, hepatic failure, or renal insufficiencies and severe right ventricular failure.

AbioCor patients have multiple co-morbidities. These patients are much sicker than those patients receiving left ventricular assist devices. The mean time to death in the REMATCH medically-controlled group of patients was twenty weeks compared to a mean time of survival of two weeks for the AbioCor control patients who did not receive the device (8). Of the fourteen patients in the initial trial, ten patients had previous surgeries; ten patients had prior pacemakers or AICDs; ten were on intra-aortic balloon pumps; four patients were on ventilator support at the time of surgery; nine patients had renal dysfunction; four patients had liver dysfunction; and six patients had diabetes.

Inclusion criteria for the trial are adult patients who are not transplant candidates (Table 2). All patients were in biventricular failure, on multiple inotropes, or if on temporary assist device, unweanable and on optimal medical management. These patients have a greater than 70% chance of dying (AbioScore) within thirty days on maximum medical treatment. A fit study (AbioFit) is performed on all patients pre-operatively in order to insure the device will lie properly in the chest cavity. Patients and family undergo

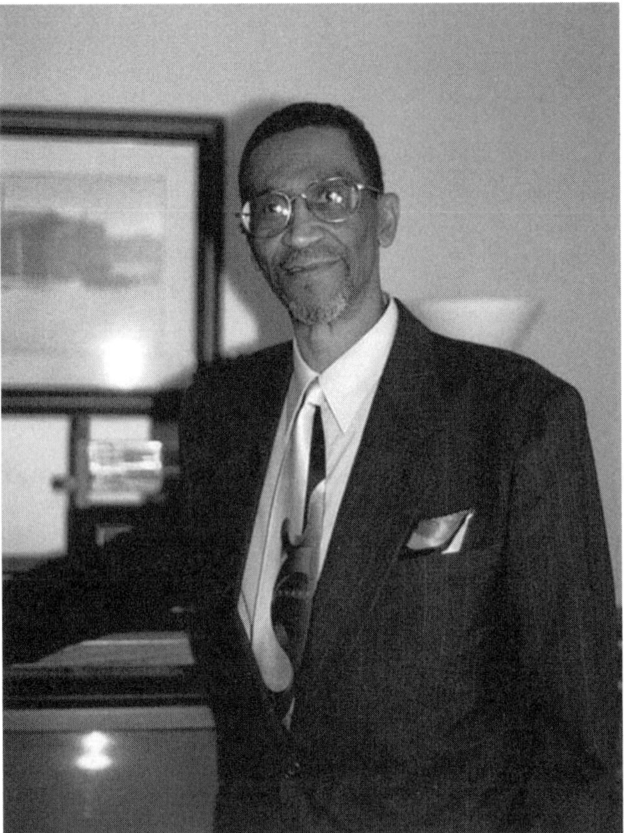

Figure 7 Robert Tools—first recipient of the AbioCor™ total implant.

social and psychological evaluation pre-implant to make sure they can handle the stress of the post-implant. Although the majority of patients had hepatic and renal dysfunction, it was felt in all patients that these would be recoverable with proper circulatory support. The reasons patients were not transplant candidates include pulmonary hypertension (5); age (6); malignancy (2); diabetes, neuropathy and organ dysfunction (9). All patients were in severe biventricular failure.

Fourteen patients were enrolled at four centers (Table 3). There were two perioperative deaths. Twelve patients were successfully supported, five of whom were ambulatory after

Table 1 Conditions of End-Stage Heart Failure Patients That Can Benefit from AbioCor™ Support

Heart transplant rejection
Severe but reversible liver failure
Chronic pulmonary disease
Severe rhythm disorders
Biventricular failure
AMI—cardiogenic shock
Chronic—idiopathic or ischemic

Abbreviation: AMI, acute myocardial infarction.

Table 2 Inclusion and Exclusion Criteria

Inclusion criteria
Adult, non-transplant candidate
Biventricular failure
On optimal medical management (OMM)
High likelihood of dying within the next 30 days
Not weanable if on a temporary assist device
Pre-surgical fit assessment
Exclusion criteria
Predicted 30-day mortality $<70\%$
Inadequate psychosocial support
Non–recoverable end organs that may compromise survival and recovery

surgery and four had out-of-hospital trips. Two patients were discharged and one returned home and lived 512 days. The support duration varied from 53 to 512 days, with a mean 5.4 mo. There was a cumulative support of five patient years.

Several AbioCor patients survived conditions that are lethal to a native heart. These include extreme acidosis (PH less than 7); severe fiberile conditions (106–107°F); chronic high systemic pulmonary artery pressures; and severe liver dysfunction (Table 4). The majority of patients (thirteen) required tracheostomy for pulmonary management; six of eight patients recovered renal function following dialysis; six of seven patients recovered from hepatic failure; two patients had malignant neuroleptic syndrome; two had acute cholecystectomy requiring acute cholecystectomy; three had recurring GI bleeding; one patient had respiratory failure requiring ECMO. All but two patients required reoperation due to bleeding or tamponade.

The device functioned extremely well throughout the clinical trials. There were no device-related infections, device-related clinical hemolyisis, and significant tissue injury. The TET coils were easy to use. There was one battery that required replacement, which was a routine, uncomplicated procedure. There was one hydraulic membrane wear out that occurred at fifteen months post-implant. This was detectable approximately one month prior to wear out. The situation was discussed with the family and patient and it was decided not to change out the device. There was one console failure due to a battery overcharging. There was one motor-bearing failure secondary to running the device outside of assigned parameters; this caused a catastrophic device failure.

Anticoagulation management is extremely important in the postoperative care of the total artificial heart patients. It is important to achieve proper balance between the risk for bleeding and thrombosis. Heparin therapy, with a target PTT being around 2.5 times normal, is initiated after physical hemostasis has been verified and the chest tube drainage is less than 30 cc/hr for approximately 24 hr. It is withheld if the platelet count is less than 100,000 μl. The thromboelastogram (TEG) is monitored daily to make sure the patient

Table 3 Fourteen Patients Enrolled at Four Centers

Two perioperative deaths
Twelve successfully supported
• One patient not ambulatory
• Five patients were ambulatory after surgery
• Four patients had out-of-hospital trips
• Two were discharged, one returned home and lived 512 days

Table 4 Extremely Sick Cohort of Patients

Majority of patients (13) required tracheostomy for pulmonary management
Six of eight patients recovered renal function following dialysis
Six of seven patients recovered hepatic failure
Malignant neuroleptic syndrome (2), acute cholecystitis (3), recurrent GI bleeding (3), respiratory failure requiring ECMO (1)
All but two patients required reoperation due to bleeding or tamponade

Abbreviation: ECMO, extracorporeal membrane oxygenation.

maintains a normal coagulable state and does not become hypercoagulable. Patients with total artificial hearts tend to be hypercoaguluable as indicated by TEGs using the sample with heparinase in recalcified whole blood. A balance state can be achieved with the TEG showing normal coaguluability. Antiplatelet therapy is begun once the platelet count is over 100,000 per microliter. This is achieved with the use of aspirin, dipyridamole, and/or Plavix and is monitored daily by platelet aggravation or TEG. The platelet activity should be maintained below 50% of normal. Warfarin therapy is initiated when renal and hepatic function improves, and the patient is stable and begins to ambulate (Table 5).

The patients' quality of life after recovering from the initial surgery was very good. Patients attended movies, shows, sporting events, participated in religious services, visited parks, dined in restaurants, and had close interactions with friends and families. Six recipients celebrated a next birthday and one recipient welcomed a great-grandchild. The patients and families adapted very well to the TETs coil and found this very easy to manage. They had no difficulties in changing from the console to the portable electronics so the patient could fully ambulate.

As anticipated, because of the very sick cohort of patients in the trial, there were multiple morbidities. The primary problem has been strokes. In reviewing the early autopsy findings, there was thrombus on the left and right atrial cage struts (Fig. 8). The pumps themselves were clean with no evidence of thrombosis or clotting. There was no evidence of any significant tissue injury or infection. It was felt that the strokes were secondary to thrombus forming on the struts of the inflow cages on the right and left atria. Therefore, the inflow configuration was redesigned. Of the first five patients supported, all had inflow cages and cuffs sutured to the annulas. There were three CVAs in this first group. A second group of six patients had no inflow cages. There was one inflow obstruction, secondary to the right atrium obstructing the right-sided inflow valve; this patient died in transfer to the recovery room. There was one intraoperative CVA and two

Table 5 Anticoagulation Strategy for the AbioCor™

Start anticoagulation slowly to avoid swings
Heparin after chest drainage <30 cc/hr
Coumadin INR 2.5–3.5
Use proper antiplatelet therapy based on platelet activity level
ASA, Persantine®, Plavix®
Monitor
PT, PTT, platelet aggregation
TEG invaluable

Abbreviations: INR, international normalized ratio; ASA, aspirin; PT, prothrombin time; PTT, partial thromboplastin time; TEG, thrombelastograph.

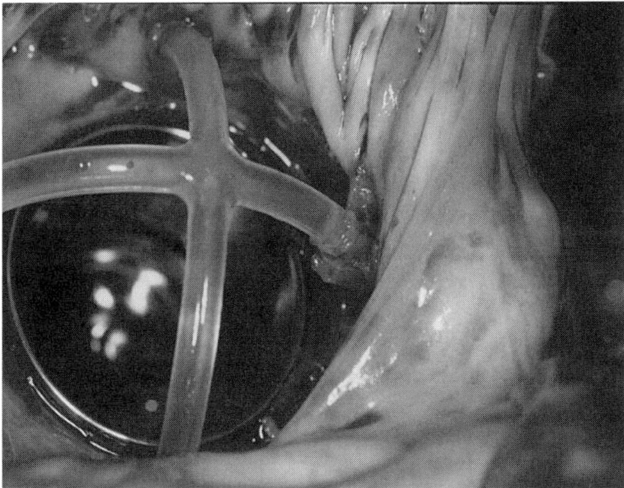

Figure 8 Thrombus on left atrial cage.

embolic CVA post-implants. A third group of three patients had modified connectors. All of these had inflow cages but the atrial connector was moved, separating the left atrial wall from the cage and connector. None of these patients had any evidence of embolism while on anticoagulation (Fig. 9). It is the current feeling that the modified atrial connectors will ensure there is no tissue contact with the struts which would lead to formation of a thrombus. With this modified connector, the incidence of thrombo embolisms will be greatly reduced. The expanded multi-center use of the AbioCor Total Replacement Heart

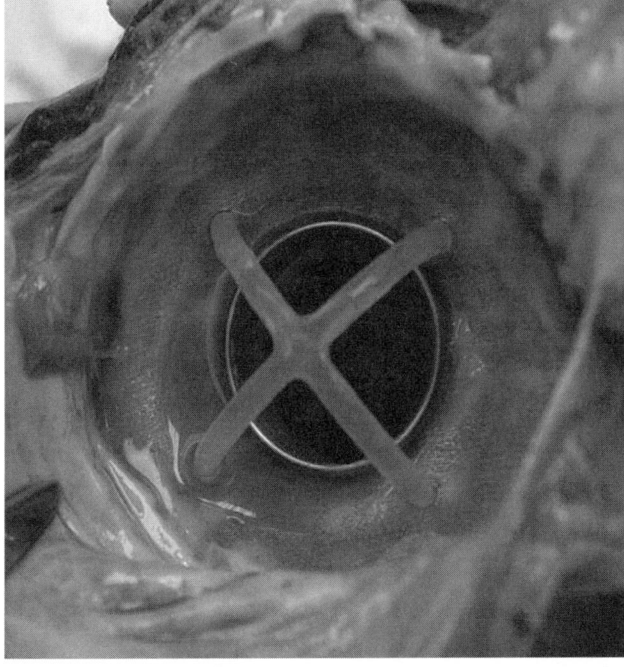

Figure 9 Revised connector showing good ingrowth of tissue and no evidence of thrombosis.

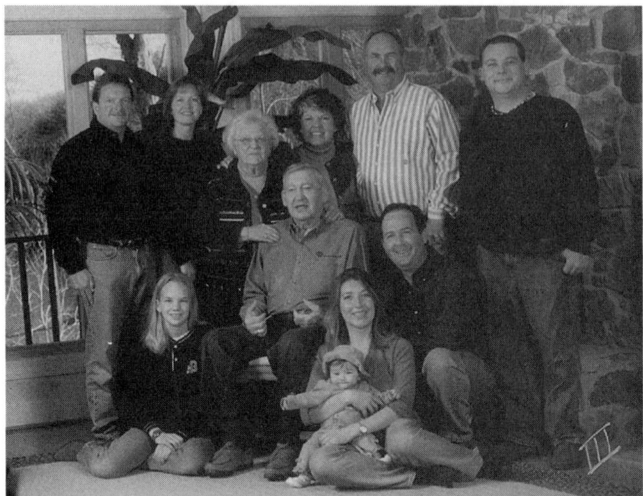

Figure 10 Mr. Tom Christerson living a normal lifestyle with his family—he survived 512 days.

under an humanitarian device exemption (HDE) offers an exciting new way to treat end-stage biventricular failure (Fig. 10).

NEW DEVICES

A second generation AbioCor heart is currently under development by ABIOMED. This device called the AbioHeart™ is a hybrid design using the strengths of the Penn State electrical total artificial heart and the current generation AbioCor. The AbioHeart is an electromechanical heart using a jack screw motor with pusher plates to alternately direct the right and left systole. The compliance chamber has been removed from the thoracic unit and placed in the chest cavity. One major advantage of this new device is that it is approximately 30% smaller in size than the current AbioCor Replacement Heart. This will allow implantation in both men and women and will reduce the chances of inflow obstruction of the pulmonary veins or cava. Additionally, the advantages of the AbioHeart include improved membrane durability and decreased membrane trauma. The inflow and outflow valves are valves consisting of tri-leaflet valves that are fabricated from polyurethane. The device is passive and filled from both the right and left atria, which will make the device more physiological. The AbioHeart includes automatic controls for beat rate control, stroke volume, and right/left balance. Initial preclinical trials are being conducted at the University of Louisville. The initial results are very promising. Initial clinical trials are scheduled for late 2006 or early 2007.

REFERENCES

1. Parnis S, Yu LS, Ochs BD, Macris MP, Frazier OH, Kung RT. Chronic in vivo evaluation of an electrohydraulic total artificial heart. ASAIO J 1994; 40:M489–M493.
2. Dowling RD, Etoch SW, Stevens KA, Johnson AC, Gray LA, Jr. Current status of the AbioCor Implantable Replacement Heart. Ann Thorac Surg 2001; 71:S147–S149.
3. Kung RT, Yu LS, Ochs B, Parnis S, Frazier OH. An atrial hydraulic shunt in a total artificial heart. A balance mechanism for the bronchial shunt. ASAIO J 1993; 39:M213–M217.

4. Kung RT, Ochs BD, Singh PI. A unique left–right flow balance compensation scheme for an Implantable Total Artificial Heart. ASAIO J 1989; 35:468–470.
5. Theilmeier KA, Pank JR, Dowling RD, Gray LA. Anesthetic and perioperative considerations in patients undergoing placement of totally Implantable Replacement Hearts. Semin Cardiothorac Vasc Anesth 2001; 5:335–344.
6. Dowling RD, Etoch SW, Gray LA, Jr. Operative techniques for implantation of the AbioCor total Artificial Heart. Oper Tech Thorac Cardiovasc Surg 2002; 7:139–151.
7. Dowling RD, Gray LA, Jr, Etoch SW, et al. Initial experience with the AbioCor Implantable Replacement Heart System. J Thorac Cardiovasc Surg 2004; 127:131–141.
8. Rose E, Gelijns AC, Moskowitz AJ, et al. N Engl J Med 2001; 345:1435–1443.

26

The SynCardia CardioWest™ Total Artificial Heart

Marvin J. Slepian
Department of Medicine (Cardiology), University of Arizona Sarver Heart Center, Tuscon, Arizona, U.S.A.

Richard G. Smith
Artificial Heart Program, University Medical Center–Tucson, Tucson, Arizona, U.S.A.

Jack G. Copeland
Department of Cardiothoracic Surgery, University of Arizona Sarver Heart Center, Tucson, Arizona, U.S.A.

INTRODUCTION

Congestive heart failure (CHF) is commonly regarded as the "final common pathway" of cardiovascular decline resulting from all forms of heart disease. Despite advances in the prevention and treatment of many forms of cardiovascular disease, CHF continues to exist as a major and, unfortunately, growing form of morbidity and mortality in the United States and around the world. As myocardial function declines and systemic compensatory systems are activated to support blood pressure and organ perfusion, patients progress through increasingly severe stages of CHF, each with increasing morbidity and mortality.

The past decade has seen significant advances in our understanding of the pathophysiology and pharmacologic approach to the treatment of CHF. These developments have lead to a "shift to the right" of the mortality curve for CHF, with patients living longer with improved quality of life. Unfortunately once patients reach the steep or rapidly declining phase of the mortality curve, i.e. being classified as AHA/ACC Class D and NYHA Class IV CHF, their decline continues in an accelerating fashion. Patients with Class IV CHF face a greater than 75% two-year mortality risk. At that point in their natural history, medical therapy is of limited value.

It is exactly for this group of maximally medically managed patients with persistent and worsening CHF that the field of mechanical circulatory support has emerged (Fig. 1). Over the years, devices have been developed with progressively increasing hemodynamic support capabilities. However, when complete bi-ventricular failure occurs, replacement of total heart pump function is needed. It is for this situation that the Total Artificial Heart has been developed.

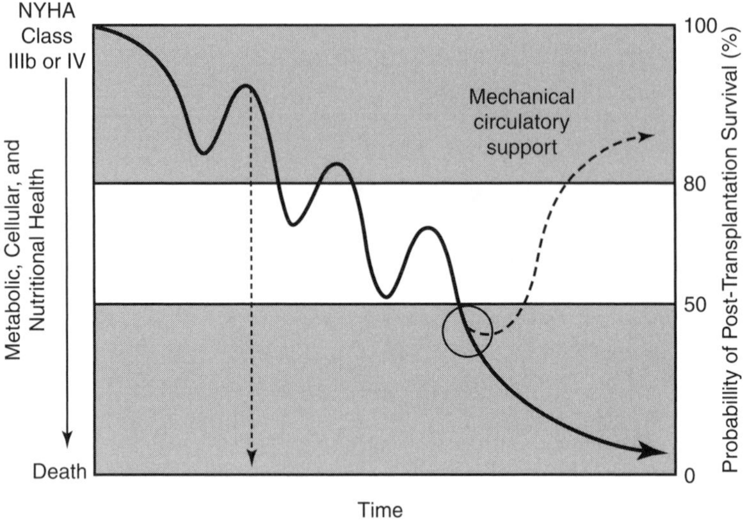

Figure 1 Natural history of New York Heart Association class III/IV chronic heart failure.

In this chapter the background, technical, and clinical experience with the SynCardia CardioWest™ Total Artificial Heart (TAH), the first and only TAH to be approved by the U.S. Food and Drug Administration, is reviewed. Specifically we discuss: (1) the rationale for the TAH, (2) the history of artificial heart technology, (3) technical and operational details of the CardioWest TAH, (4) indications for use of the TAH, (5) clinical experience with the CardioWest TAH, and (6) future applications of the TAH.

RATIONALE FOR THE TOTAL ARTIFICIAL HEART

The artificial heart arose from the unmet clinical need for a device or system capable of completely restoring systemic and pulmonary blood circulation and organ perfusion pressure in patients with failed circulatory systems due to irreversible biventricular dysfunction. Early in the history of TAH development the vision was for the creation of such a device as a long-term permanent cardiac replacement. While this was a laudable initial goal, it proved to be too big a technical, clinical, and social leap in the early days of TAH development (1). With the eventual parallel take-off of heart transplantation, as a result of the advent of effective anti-rejection pharmacology, a new unforeseen rationale for the TAH arose. The growth of transplantation, with inadequate instant donor heart availability created the need for a "bridge," rather than permanent device, capable of sustaining the life of a patient until a donor heart might be procured. Today with advances in TAH development both of these visions, i.e., short term "bridge" and long term "destination therapy," are back in the minds of the medical and technical community and are being actively addressed.

Additional rationale exist for the TAH. These may be categorized as being medical/technical, humanitarian, and economic. On the medical level, the TAH obviates many limitations, which are associated with ventricular assist device (VAD)-mediated cardiac support. Leaving the ventricles intact in the end-stage CHF patient often turns out to be a major liability for the patient. With time it has been demonstrated that the major cause of cardiac failure of patients supported with LVADs is eventual right heart failure.

In this scenario, placement of a second VAD as an RVAD carries a high morbidity and mortality with dramatically reduced bridge-to-transplant success. The TAH provides a complete cardiac solution for this scenario. Further, the minimally contracting myocardium often is a nidus for endoventricular thrombus formation. Placement of VADs in this situation has lead to significant embolization and stroke. Removing the ventricles with orthotopic placement of a TAH significantly reduces this embolic risk. Cardiac arrhythmias, frequent in the end-stage heart, undermine ventricular contractile performance and further reduce VAD function. Cardiac removal and replacement with the TAH overcomes this limitation. The presence of a prosthetic valve in a heart supported by a VAD increases the risk of thrombosis and embolization from the valve. This too is obviated through TAH use. Presence of ventricular septal defects and other structural derangements, which further compromise cardiac output in ventricles supported with VADs, are overcome with the use of a TAH. Finally, use of a device, which occupies the same anatomic location, without the need for violating other body cavities or further crowding the thoracic cavity, has motivated the development of an effective cardiac replacement device.

On the humanitarian level, the clear rationale for the TAH is that it may save lives. The majority of patients that have been recipients of such a device to date have been young to middle-aged patients in the prime of life. While their lives have unfortunately been compromised by devastating cardiovascular disease, they frequently are otherwise fairly healthy. Complete organ replacement in these patients, either with eventual cardiac transplantation or through continued destination therapy support, has the potential to afford them the chance for life with quality. Further, the TAH allows these patients the opportunity to recover from the devastating systemic effects of low circulatory output. Hence the rationale exists to salvage and recover the patient, reducing edema and congestion and increasing vital organ perfusion through the TAH.

Additional rationale for the TAH exists from an economic perspective. In the bridge scenario, allowing patients to recover prior to transplantation has the possibility of reducing the cost of hospitalization through reduced ICU stay and lower acute care levels for patients. Further, in the future, in the United States and presently in Europe, the possibility of recovery and waiting at home prior to transplantation is a reality with a TAH. This has the potential of saving the cost of 60 to 270 days of hospitalization, the duration post-acute recovery that patients wait on average, in the United States and Europe, respectively, for a transplant.

In the "destination therapy" scenario, even greater cost savings are possible. Presently CHF represents the leading cause of hospitalization in the United States and carries a price tag exceeding $27 billion (2). As patients worsen and progress to more advanced stages of CHF, their frequency of hospitalization and the length of stay and associated costs increase. As such, the TAH has the potential of radically improving the quality of life of patients with end-stage CHF, reducing their frequency and extent of hospitalization and their overall cost of care.

HISTORICAL OVERVIEW OF ARTIFICIAL HEART TECHNOLOGY

The artificial heart has had a greater than forty-year development history (Table 1). Initial efforts at creating a complete cardiac replacement artificial organ began as one of several scientific initiatives advocated during the Kennedy administration in the 1960s. In 1964, the National Institutes of Health launched an artificial heart program, fostering the development of partial and full cardiac replacement devices. Parallel efforts began in Texas and in Cleveland on circulatory replacement systems. Reflecting back on the early beginnings of this field differing visions and perceptions of the TAH are recalled.

Table 1 Total Artifical Heart (TAH) Timeline

1964	U.S. Government National Heart Initiative to produce a TAH
1969	Cooley at the Texas Heart Institute performs first human artificial heart implant to bridge a patient for 64 hr until a donor heart is transplanted
1981	Kolff, DeVries, and Jarvik at the University of Utah receive FDA approval to implant a TAH into a human for permanent application
1982	Dr. Barney Clark receives the Jarvik-7 device, lives 112 days
1983	Symbion acquires rights to manufacture Jarvik-7
1985	Copeland at UMC[a] implants the Phoenix TAH, opening the door for the FDA to approve the TAH as a bridge-to-transplant, rather than a permanent implant. He later performs the first successful bridge to transplant with a TAH using the Jarvik-7
1986	The smaller Jarvik-7-70 TAH is first implanted, expanding the use of the TAH into most adults (including women)
1990	The FDA withdraws the study of the Symbion Jarvik TAHs because of quality issues
1991	Symbion transfers all the TAH assets to CardioWest™/UMC
1992	CardioWest receives FDA approval to begin a new study with a modified Jarvik-7-70 design—The Multi-Center PMA Trial
1993	First CardioWest TAH is implanted in a women at UMC. She was successfully transplanted after 186 days
1999	CardioWest receives CE mark approval for clinical use of the TAH in Europe
2001	SynCardia Systems Inc. (Tucson, AZ) was founded to obtain FDA approval and commercialize the TAH
2004	SynCardia CardioWest™ TAH becomes the first TAH to receive FDA approval for use as a bridge-to-transplant in patients with irreversible bi-ventricular failure

[a]UMC, University Medical Center, Tucson, Arizona.
Abbreviations: FDA, food and drug administration; PMA, pre-market approval.

An initial clear memory is that of the dramatic first attempts by Dr. Denton Cooley to save dying patients who could not be weaned from the heart–lung machine after routine cardiac procedures in 1969 with the Liotta TAH (3) and then in 1981 with the Akutsu TAH (4). Next we remember, primarily from extensive media coverage, the use of the Jarvik-7 TAH as a permanent cardiac replacement by DeVries and his team in four patients in Salt Lake City and Louisville (5). The initial attempt at destination therapy led to the first long-term survival (112 days in Dr. Barney Clark) of humans on any type of mechanical circulatory device. Unfortunately, public expectations far exceeded the realities of that era. This was reminiscent of the era when heart transplantation had been banned in nearly every hospital in the world after a shaky but well-publicized start. In reality the goal of complete cardiac replacement was too extensive for the level of scientific, clinical, and social maturation of the era.

In 1985, the authors utilized a TAH for a different indication, that of "bridge to tranplantation," rather than permanent cardiac replacement. The team utilized an unapproved Phoenix TAH as a bridge device, in a desperate situation of a patient who had rejected his heart transplant. After failing at this and preparing for the next experience, the team was fortunate to have the first successful bridge to transplant with a TAH (Jarvik-7) in August 1985 (6).

The Jarvik-7 TAH was designed and tested preclinically in animals by Drs. Kolff, Olsen, Jarvik as well as others from the 1950s through the 1970s (7). The device was specifically designed and durability tested to permanently replace the heart. Dr. William DeVries and his team in the United States implanted four and Dr. Bjarne Semb in Stockholm implanted one Jarvik-7 TAH, with 100-mL ventricles, in the early 1980s. All five implants were in chronically ill patients. Early postoperative complications included hemorrhage and renal failure. There was one death from hemorrhage occurring 10 days post-implantation. The other four patients died of sepsis, living as long as 620 days (mean survival of 291 days). Two of DeVries' patients suffered thrombo-embolic strokes (8). Dr. Semb's patient was photographed on numerous occasions walking around Stockholm supported by a portable briefcase-sized pneumatic driver. In summary, given the complete absence of long-term human experience with such devices at that time, the results seemed extraordinarily good. Yet, in many ways, the medical profession was not prepared for this technology. Most of the preclinical experience was in healthy growing calves that were resistant to infection, had little if any evidence of stroke, and, unfortunately, had to be euthanized within a few months of implantation as they "outgrew" the device. The major complications of mechanical circulatory devices in humans—bleeding, thromboembolism with stroke, and infection—had not been major problems in calves. Consequently, expectations were high, and the media was disappointed with the early clinical results in man.

Two major changes were made in the Jarvik-7 based upon that experience (9): Medtronic-Hall valves were substituted for Bjork-Shiley and the rate of pressure rise (dp/dt) by the pneumatic driver was lowered to about 4500 mmHg/sec. The authors began to understand many of the major problems of the total artificial heart in the bridge-to-transplant scenario. After their first implant in August 1985, 37 other centers implanted a total of 198 Jarvik-7 TAHs between 1985 and 1992. Seventy percent of these implants were done between 1986 and 1988. More than 75% of them occurred in eight centers. The remaining centers accounted for less than five cases per center. Thirty-nine of the hearts were the 100-mL size (the last one implanted in 1992) and 159 were with the smaller 70-mL ventricles that are currently used. The last registry of this experience (10) reported that 143 implant patients (72% of those implanted) were transplanted and that 89 (59% of transplants and 43% of the total) were discharged. More than 60% of these patients had the device for less than 2 wk. The rush to transplantation might explain why only 59% of those transplanted were discharged. The average patient age was 42 and the average duration of implantation was 24 days (range 1–603), resulting in 13 patient-years of experience. The cause of patients dying while on device support was: multiple organ failure (17 patients), sepsis (16), neurologic (6), and respiratory (6). Complications included infection (37%), hemorrhage (26%), renal failure (20%), stroke (5%), and transient ischemic attack (4%). A variety of experiences and impressions from this early period have been previously summarized. Among the most compelling publications from that era was a 60-case series from La Pitie Hospital in Paris in which no neurologic adverse events were reported. They used a multicomponent coagulation monitoring and anticoagulant therapy protocol developed by Szefner and colleagues (11).

In 1991, the Jarvik-7 (then called Symbion) study was halted by the FDA. At that point, the technology was licensed to a new start-up company known as CardioWest and the heart was renamed the CardioWest C-70 TAH. A new FDA study was started in 1993. Changes were made in manufacturing and the previous skin button was replaced with Dacron velour attached directly to the air conduits. Only one size (70 mL) was continued in production. In 2001 SynCardia, a company organized to complete the ongoing U.S. clinical trial, proceeded with regulatory submission to the FDA and initiated device commercialization, and renaming the device the SynCardia CardioWest™ TAH. As of June 2005, 612 TAHs of all types had been implanted worldwide. Ninety percent (554 of 612) have been of the CardioWest–type design, accounting for 77 patient-years, or about 91% of the worldwide TAH experience. There have been more than 350 actual CardioWest implants to date, accounting for over 60 patient-years or more than 70% of the worldwide TAH experience.

Presently the only other TAH under clinical investigation is the AbioCor® fully implantable TAH, an electrohydraulic pump that has been implanted in fourteen patients as of June 2005. The size and pumping characteristics are very different from the CardioWest™ TAH. Clinical experience with the AbioCor has thus far been limited and results, including survival and adverse events, have not been published. In May 2005 the US FDA Advisory Panel rejected Abiomed's request for a humanitarian device exemption to market the AbioCor.

TECHNICAL AND OPERATIONAL DETAILS OF THE CARDIOWEST™ TAH

The SynCardia CardioWest™ TAH is a biventricular orthotopic pneumatic pulsatile pump with two separate artificial ventricles that take the place of the native ventricles (Fig. 2A). The two artificial ventricles, although differing in the spacing and angulations of the inflow and outflow valves and the entry sites for the conduits for the left and right sides, are basically the same in construction. Each has a rigid spherical outer "housing" that supports a seamless blood-contacting diaphragm, two intermediate diaphragms, and an air diaphragm, all made of segmented polyurethane, separated by thin coatings of graphite (Fig. 2B). The inflow (27-mm) and outflow (25-mm) Medtronic-Hall valves are mounted on the housing. The diaphragm excursion is essentially from one wall of the housing to the

(A)

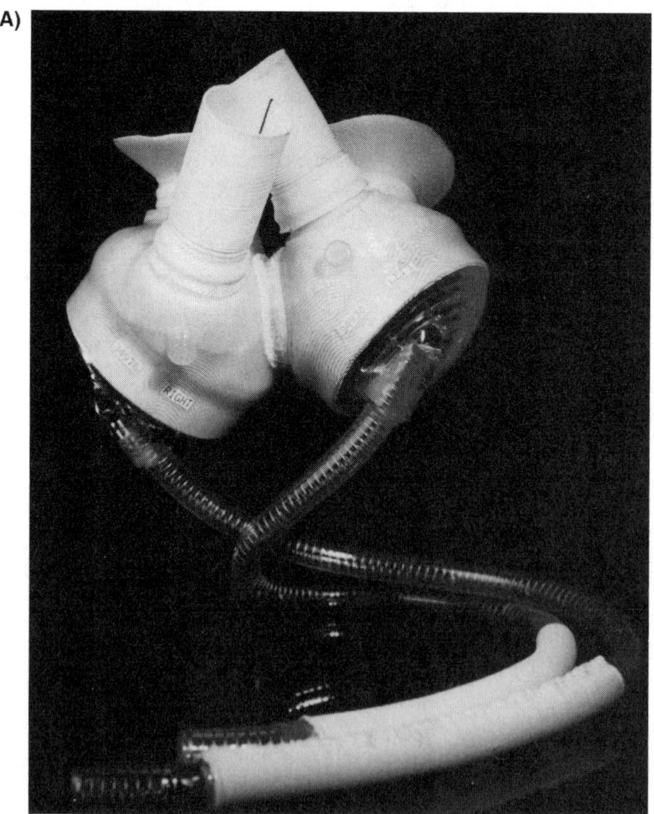

Figure 2 (**A**) SynCardia CardioWest™ Total Artificial Heart. (**B**) Total Artificial Heart ventricle. *Abbreviation*: SPUS, segmented polyurethane solution. (*Continued*)

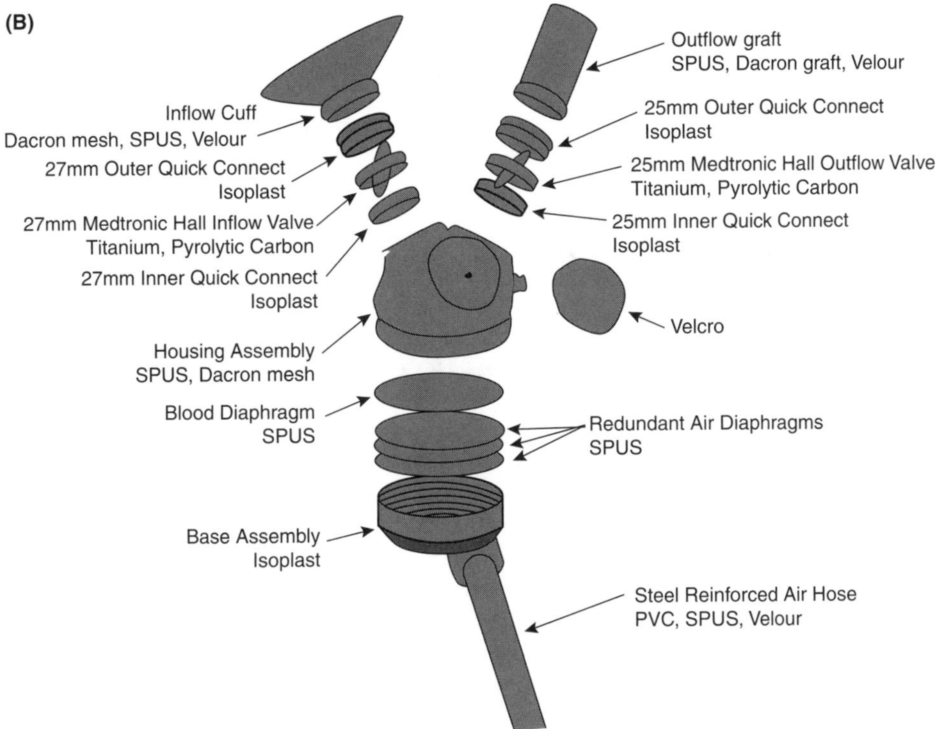

Figure 2 *(Continued from previous page)*

other, allowing the ventricle to fully fill and fully eject nearly 70 mL per beat. A flexible polyurethane lined inflow connector called a "quick connect" is sewn to the atrial cuff of the recipient heart and then snapped on to the inflow valve mount of the artificial ventricle. On the outflow side, the Dacron outflow connectors are snapped on to the outflow valve mounts of the artificial ventricles after the distal connector anastomoses have been completed.

Wire-reinforced air conduits covered with Dacron in the transabdominal wall pathway connect to longer drivelines and to an external console (Fig. 3). This console is mobile by virtue of batteries and compressed air tanks, allowing the patient freedom to move about the hospital or other care facility. With the current configuration, patients are able to ambulate within the confines of the medical center (e.g., going to the cafeteria, or outdoors). Further, they perform most cardiac rehabilitation exercises, a necessary step toward their full recovery.

Portable pneumatic driver/consoles that provide pneumatic power have been developed and tested and will soon be available (Fig. 4A and B). These will provide increased mobility and, most importantly, discharge from the hospital. A "wearable" disposable driver/console is being developed and will be the third generation of drive power for the CardioWest™, further improving the quality of life of implanted patients.

The external console consists of two pneumatic drivers, one primary and one backup, transport batteries, air tanks, and an alarm and computer monitoring system. Beat rate, % systole (% of cardiac cycle occupied by systole), and left and right driving pressure are manually controlled. Once set, it is rare for these parameters to need resetting. Cardiac

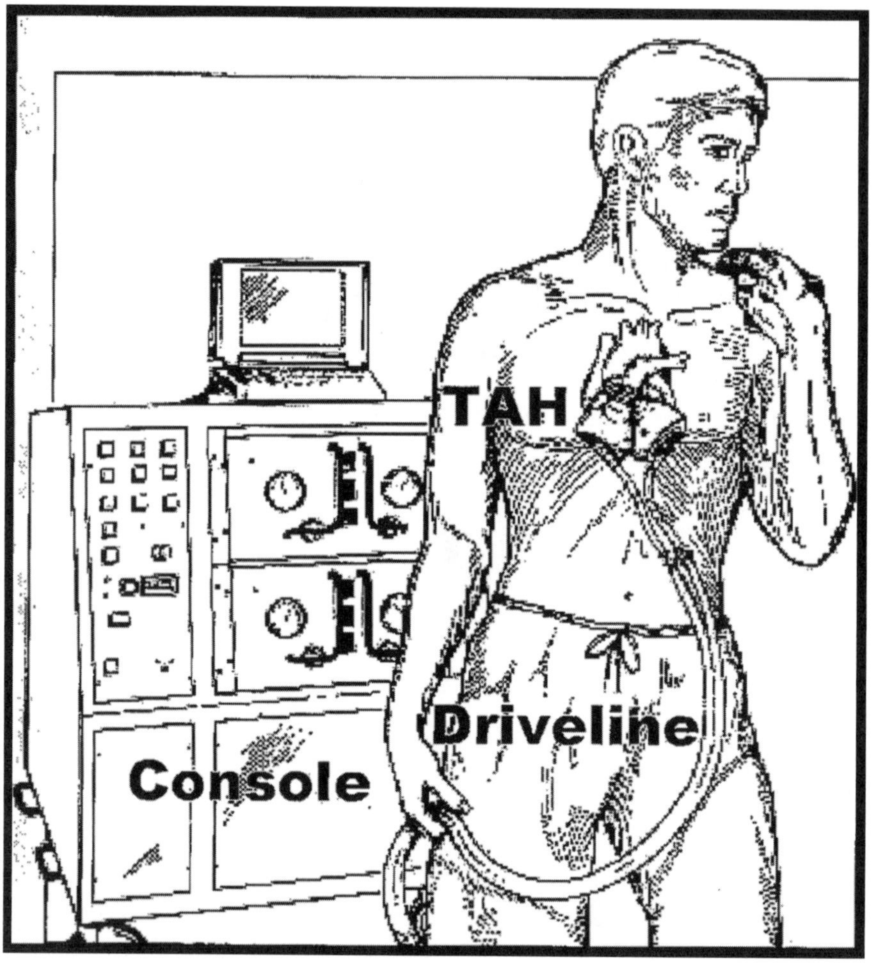

Figure 3 SynCardia CardioWest™ Total Artificial Heart (TAH) System. Note three components: TAH, existing pneumatic driveline, and driver console.

(A)

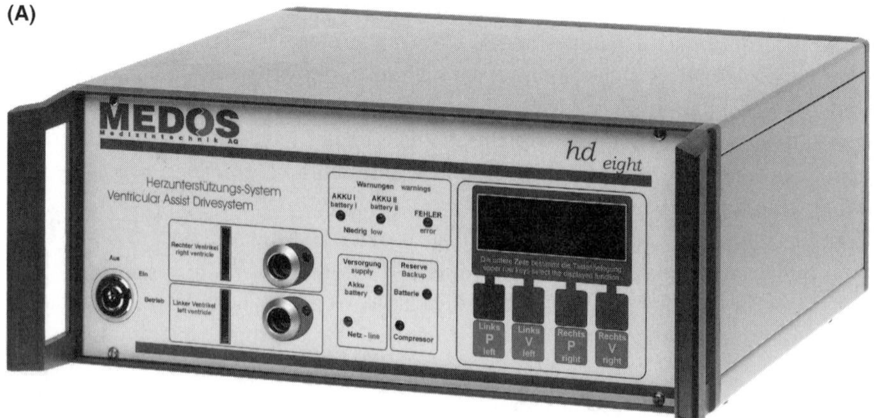

Figure 4 (**A**) SynCardia MEDOS HD8™ Mobile Driver. (**B**) Berlin Heart EXCOR™ Portable Driver. *(Continued)*

(B)

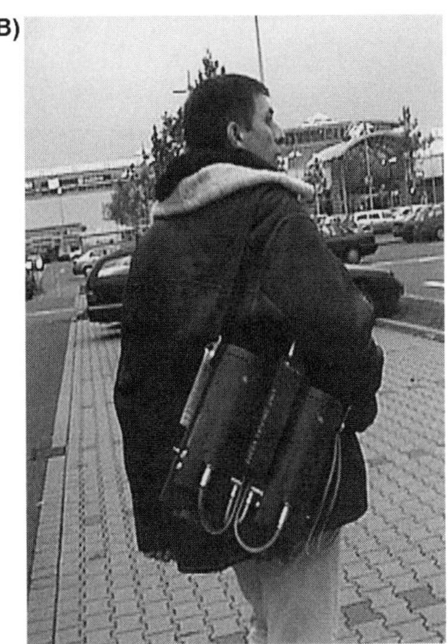

Figure 4 *(Continued from previous page)*

output based on volume of airflow out of the drivelines as well as trend plots of left-sided and right-sided cardiac output are continuously displayed as is drive pressure for each artificial ventricle. Separate ventricular fill volumes are also continuously displayed.

The primary driver is set to fully eject blood (Fig. 5) from each artificial ventricle with each beat. This is achieved by setting the ejection pressures for the right ventricle 30 mmHg higher than the pulmonary artery pressure and the systemic drive pressure 60 mmHg higher than the systemic pressure. The driver, however, is not set to allow the artificial ventricle to fully fill. Filling of 50 to 60 mL per beat by initial adjustment of the beat rate and % systole is optimal. Thus, within the 70-mL artificial ventricle on the air-side of the diaphragm is a "cushion" of 10 to 20 mL (Fig. 6). In the event of increased venous return, as in the cases of exercise or volume loading, some of this air is displaced and cardiac output automatically increases as occurs with the Starling mechanism in a normal heart. Using this protocol coupled with a negative intraventricular pressure at the onset of diastole of 10 to 15 mmHg and a central venous pressure of 8 to 15 mmHg, the cardiac output generated by the CardioWest™ TAH is generally 7 to 8 L/min. Mean arterial pressures are usually in the 70 to 90 mmHg range, resulting in a perfusion pressure of 55 to 80. Delivery of this magnitude of pressure and flow has resulted in consistent return of renal, hepatic, and other end-organ function to normal even in the sickest of patients. Needless to say, there is no concern about right heart failure, pulmonary hypertension, valve issues, or arrhythmias as with LVADs. Further, the flow limitation, always seen with extra corporeal BVADS (Thoratec provides a maximum flow of 5 to 6 L/min), and seen in cases of RV failure with LVADs, is not present with the CardioWest. In a study of CardioWest, Novacor (World Heart Corporation, Ottawa, Ontario, Canada), and Thoratec (Thoratec Corporation, Pleasanton, California, U.S.A.) in very sick deteriorating patients (12) we found that during the first 24 hr post-implant a cardiac index of 2.5 L/min/M^2 correlated positively with survival in all groups. For many American patients with BSAs of $>2\ M^2$ an output of at least 5 to 6 L/min early after implant would be the minimally acceptable value. Our approach at all times with the CardioWest™ TAH has been to maximize cardiac output not only for improved pressure and flow to end organs, but also as

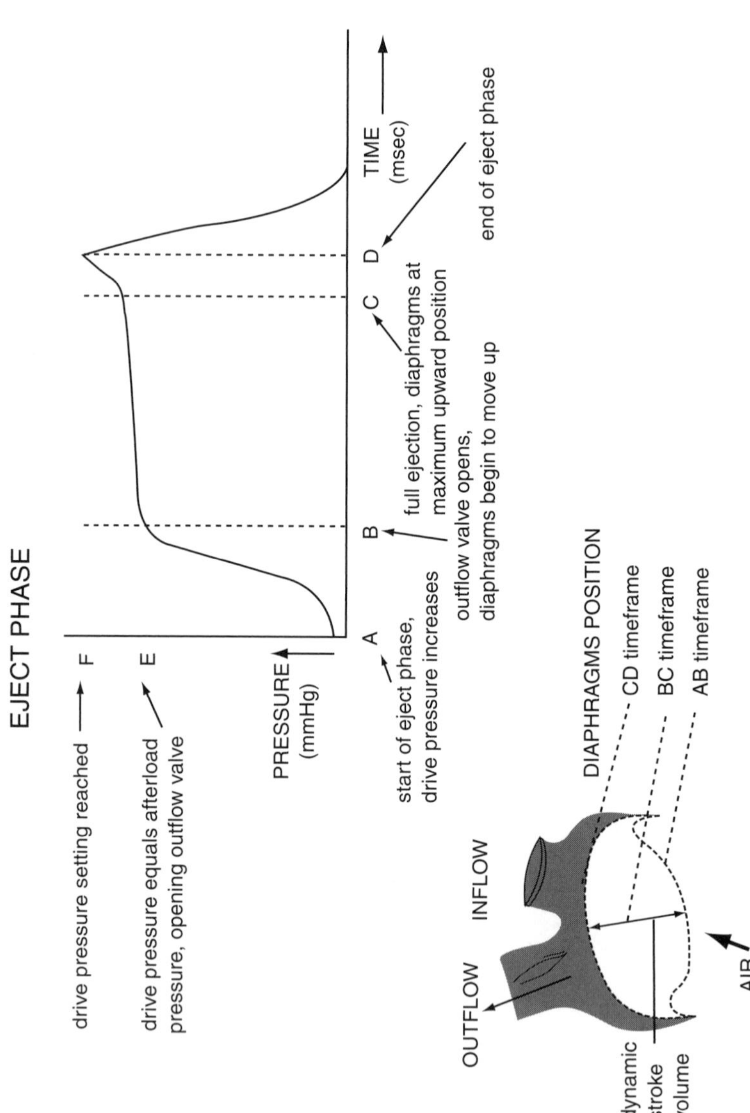

Figure 5 TAH pressure waveform.

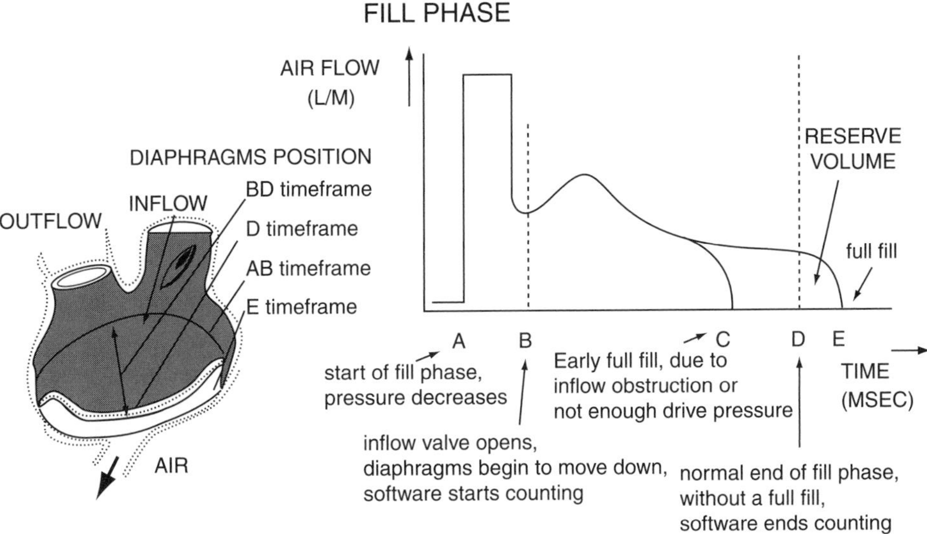

Figure 6 TAH flow waveform.

a strategy to increase "washing" of the device's blood-contacting surface as well, thus reducing the risk of thromboembolism.

INDICATIONS FOR USE OF THE CARDIOWEST™ TAH

The TAH is presently indicated for use in the United States as an in-hospital bridge for patients with end-stage biventricular heart failure awaiting heart transplantation (Table 2). Outside the United States, the TAH has been used for broader indications. In Europe the TAH has been used as a means of bridging patients, though allowing them to be discharged, residing at home while awaiting transplantation. The TAH has also been used outside of the United States as an acute bailout device for patients with irreversible cardiogenic shock associated with acute myocardial infarction. The TAH has further been indicated in cases of post-cardiotomy heart failure, with an inability to wean patients off cardio-plumonary bypass. Recently the TAH has begun initial trial use in Europe for "destination therapy," i.e., as a permanent cardiac replacement device utilizing a new portable mobile driver.

CLINICAL EXPERIENCE WITH THE CARDIOWEST™ TAH

As outlined above, the bulk of the world's TAH experience has occurred with TAH devices built on the technology platform common to the present SynCardia CardioWest™ TAH. The largest recent single center experiences to date have been described in Arizona, Paris, and at Bad Oeyenhausen, Germany.

From 1993–2002 patients, 62 patients (51 men and 11 women) with irreversible bi-ventricular failure underwent implantation with the TAH at Arizona (13). Mean LV ejection fraction and CVP pre-implant were $20 \pm 8\%$ and 20 ± 7 mmHg, respectively. The mean time on TAH support was 92 ± 11 days (range 1–413 d). Seventy-seven percent of

Table 2 Current and Future Applications of the SynCardia CardioWest™ Total Artificial Heart

Applications	Candidate patients
Current (FDA approved)	
Bridge-to-transplantation in cardiac transplant-eligible patients at risk of imminent death from bi-ventricular failure (in hospital use)	NYHA Class IV, AHA/ACC Class D CHF—Transplant-eligible with bi-ventricular failure refractory to medical therapy Ischemic, myopathies, intra-op, adult congential heart disease Contraindications to VAD support such as refractory arrhythmias, aortic regurgitation, stenosis or prosthesis, ventricular thrombus or VSD Unresuscitatable cardiac arrest Massive myocardial infarction or direct myocardial injury that affects technical insertion of a VAD through the left ventricle Failure to wean from cardiopulmonary bypass with bi-ventricular injury
Future (not presently FDA approved)	
Bridge-to-transplantation in transplant-eligible patients with bi-ventricular failure with anticipated hospital discharge and-out-of hos-pital use	Same as above
Long-term destination therapy TAH with hospi-tal discharge to the home setting	NYHA Class IV, AHA/ACC Class D CHF—Not transplant-eligible with bi-ventricular failure refractory to medical therapy

Abbreviations: FDA, Food and Drug Administration; NYHA, New York Heart Association; AHA/ACC, American Heart Association/American College of Cardiology; CHF, chronic heart failure; VAD, ventricular assist device; VSD, ventricular septal defect.

patients survived to transplantation, with the TAH. Sixty-eight percent of the total group survived to discharge post-transplantation. Twenty-three percent of patients died during device support. Multi-organ failure caused 50% of these deaths. Adverse events included bleeding (20%), device malfunction (5%), fit complications (3%), mediastinal infections (5%), visceral embolus (1.6%), and stroke (1.6%). The linearized stroke rate was 0.068 events per patient-year.

A similar experience was reported by the group from Paris (14). To date, this group at Hospital La Pitie-Salpetriere has the largest experience with the TAH. Between 1986 and 2001, 127 patients (108 males, mean age 38 ± 13) underwent bridge to transplantation with the TAH. Mean arterial blood pressure and CVP pre-implant were 70 ± 8 mmHg and CVP 27 ± 8 mmHg, respectively. The duration of support increased progressively in the French experience, averaging 2 mo after 1997 with a range from 5–271 days. One patient in their early experience was maintained on the TAH for 602 days, due to pre-implantation pre-formed anti-HLA antibodies. Overall 64% of patients survived to transplantation, with the TAH. Twenty-three percent of patients died during device support. Multi-organ failure caused 67% of these deaths. The clinical thromboembolic event rate they observed was low, with no incidence of CVA and only

2 TIAs. In all, they reported on a total experience of 3606 implant days with only one instance of mechanical dysfunction.

Recently the surgical group at Bad Oeyenhausen reported on their experience as well. Between February 2001 and December 2003, forty-two patients (37 men and 5 women, mean age 51 ± 13 yr) received a TAH. All patients were in persistent cardiogenic shock in spite of maximum inotropic support. Interestingly, ten of the forty-two patients were in cardiogenic shock as a result of massive acute myocardial infarction. Mean duration of support was 86 ± 81 days (range 1 ± 291 d). Eleven of 42 patients (26%) underwent successful cardiac transplantation, with 10 patients being discharged home. Twenty-two patients (52%) died under support, 13 of them from multi-organ failure after 1–68 days of support. They too observed low thromboembolic complication rates, with only one CVA and two TIAs noted.

All of these centers used the TAH for patients with biventricular failure, with adequate thoracic cavity volume to successfully fit the device in the resident space left by excision of the native heart ventricles and valves. Other devices were used for left ventricular dysfunction and biventricular failure in smaller patients who could not fit the TAH.

Overall, all these single center experiences, in medical centers utilizing the TAH for many years or new to the device as of late, demonstrate successful salvage of patients in imminent risk of death utilizing the TAH. Through meticulous attention to anticoagulation, as outlined in these studies, a low thromboembolic event rate was reported.

The most robust experience reported with the TAH to date was the recently published multi-center PMA trial experience (15). In this trial the hypothesis tested was that use of the TAH in patients with irreversible bi-ventricular failure would saves lives by allowing for effective subsequent transplantation. Inclusion criteria for the study were: patients eligible for transplant, NYHA CHF Class IV, BSA range 1.7–2.5 m^2, and severe hemodynamic insufficiency. From 1993–2002 the TAH was implanted in 95 patients (81 protocol, 15 out-of protocol) with irreversible biventricular failure in imminent danger of death. Major efficacy endpoints included rates of survival to transplantation, overall survival, survival after transplantation and "treatment success," defined as alive, NYHA Class I or II, not on dialysis or a ventilator and ambulating. A control cohort of patients matched with those in the protocol group, without receiving a TAH, was used for contextual comparison.

In this study overall survival to transplantation was achieved in 79% of patients receiving the TAH versus 46% of the controls, $p < 0.001$. Treatment success was achieved in 69% of the implant patients versus 37% of of controls, $p = 0.002$. The mean time from entry into the study to transplantation or death was 79.1 days for the implant group versus 8.5 days among the controls, $p < 0.001$. The overall survival rate at one year was 70% (95% confidence limit, 63 to 77%) in the group receiving an implant as per protocol compared with 31% in the control group, $p < 0.001$ (Fig. 7). Survival at one and five years after heart transplantation was 86% and 64%, respectively, compared with 69% and 34%, respectively in the controls. This data compares favorably with the reported overall UNOS survival data of 84.7% and 69.8%, at one and five years, respectively (16).

In the multi-center trial significant improvement in secondary endpoints was noted as well for the TAH group. Patient's hemodynamic status immediately improved following placement of the TAH, with increased systemic pressure, reduced central vesnous pressure, and increased organ perfusion pressure observed. Cardiac index rose from a baseline pre-implant of 1.9 L/min/m^2 to 3.2 L/min/m^2. Renal and hepatic function and the levels of BUN, creatinine, bilirubin, and transaminases returned to normal within three weeks of implantation. Electrolyte levels, white count, and platelet count also normalized

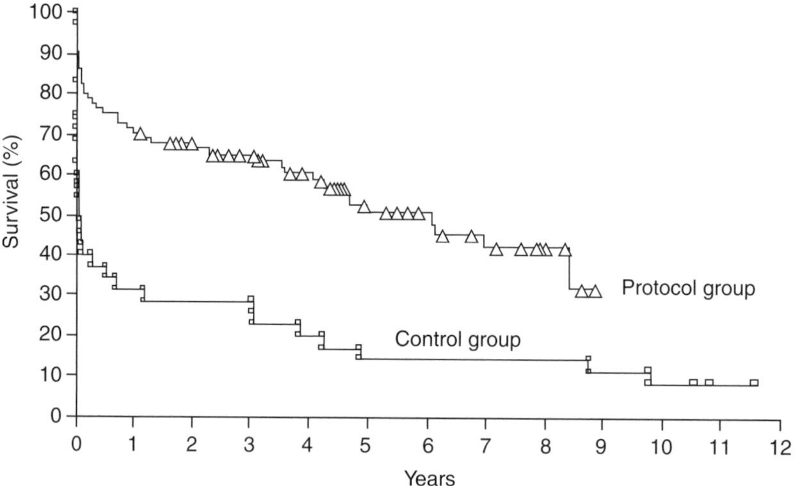

Figure 7 U.S. multi-center trial overall survival curve.

by three to four weeks post-TAH implantation. Quality of life also improved for the TAH group. One week post-implant, 75% of these patients were ambulating. More than 60% of patients were able to walk more than 100 ft. two weeks following implantation.

Seventeen of the eighty-one patients (21%) in the treatment group died before transplantation, compared with nineteen of the thirty-five control patients (54%). Causes of death in the treatment group were: multi-organ failure (in seven patients), procedural or technical complications (4 patients), bleeding (in two), sepsis (in two), CHF (one) and pulmonary edema (one). Causes of death in the control group prior to transplantation were: cardiac arrest (in seven patients), heart failure (seven patients), multi-organ failure (three), acute rejection (one), and pulmonary edema (one).

Detailed records of numerous potential adverse events were taken in this trial. The major adverse events reported, in addition to death, were: bleeding, infection neurologic dysfunction and device malfunction. In the implant group there were 102 bleeding events, fifty-five of which occurred after implantation requiring "takeback" to the operating room for control. All but one of these procedures occurred within the first 21 days of implantation. Only two patients in this series died from bleeding. There were 125 infections recorded in the trial during use of the TAH, fifty being respiratory, 28 GU, 17 involving the driveline, 12 GI, 7 blood borne, six involving indwelling catheters and five mediastinal infections. In sixty eight of the eight one protocol patients (84%) these infections did not delay transplantation or contribute to death. All driveline infections were superficial, with none ascending to the mediastinum. Twenty-six neurologic events were noted in the protocol group, including stroke [11 events in 10 patients (12%)], transient ischemic attacks (4 events), anoxic encephalopathy (5 events), seizure (4 events), and syncope (1 event). Of the strokes observed six of the eleven completely resolved without detectable residua after 48 hr, and four had mild residua with one having persistent hemiplegia. The linearized rate of stroke was 0.05 events per month. One serious device malfunction was observed in the entire experimental cohort, that of a perforation of the pumping membrane. This occurred on day 124 post-implant resulting in a patient death. No other serious device malfunctions have occurred during more than 12,000 patient-days of use of the TAH.

FUTURE APPLICATIONS OF THE CARDIOWEST™ TAH

We are on the verge of a paradigm shift in the field of mechanical circulatory support. It appears clear that as the myriad of devices currently being studied find their nitches, a general rationale is developing for patients with varying degrees of Class IV CHF. In the field of bridge-to-transplant what is becoming clear is that for patients with more mild, typically single, i.e. left ventricular failure, they are well served with LVADs. However as the degree of cardiac failure worsens, with either severe left ventricular failure or the development of bi-ventricular failure, more robust cardiac support and frank replacement systems are needed. It is in this role of complete hemodynamic support where the TAH is emerging as clearly demonstrating its therapeutic superiorty. Of all devices presently available it stands alone in terms of an ability to provide the highest degree of cardiac output of any prosthetic device, up to 9.5 L/min. This type of extensive support is needed to salvage and recover truly end-stage patients. As such the TAH has the potential to emerge as the standard of care for irreversible bi-ventricular failure patients, the indication for which it is presently approved. With time its application to severe single ventricular failure, inadequately supported by a VAD may emerge.

In addition to bridge applications the TAH has the potential of providing therapeutic benefit to several other groups of patients. One group that would benefit from the TAH is the group of patients with persistent cardiogenic shock following acute myocardial infarction, despite attempted percutaneous or surgical revascularization. This group presently carries a greater than 50% mortality with no viable therapeutic option save for emergency heart transplantation, which is logistically very difficult. Other future applications for the TAH include use for post-cardiotomy cardiogenic shock, rescue of patients failing on VAD devices, patients with cardiogenic shock placed on ECMO and for failed transplants.

In addition to bridge-to-transplantation and other bail-out applications, the CardioWest™ TAH has an even greater long-term potential use—that of serving as a "destination therapy" device. Today CHF is an epidemic that is growing in the United States and world-wide. There are over 100,000 patients per year with NYHA Class IV CHF. As such for these patients their imminent mortality is certain. While many patients have significant co-morbidities or are elderly and many not be considered appropriate candidates for, or for that matter capable of accommodating to, a life-extending technology, there are many patients that would benefit from such a therapy. By conservative estimates upwards of 30,000 patients per year may be candidates for total cardiac replacement with a long-term, i.e., permanent, artificial heart. We must recall that the CardioWest™ TAH was built based on a technology platform aimed for permanent implantation. As mentioned in an earlier section that vision was too big a leap at the outset of clinical use with this device. Now based on over 550 implants and 60 patient-years of experience the time has come to seriously consider utilizing this TAH, with new portable mobile driver technology, as destination therapy for these patients in dire therapeutic need.

CONCLUSION

The CardioWest™ TAH was created and initially tested at the same time as the Thoratec, Novacor, and HeartMate devices. It was designed as a permanent artificial heart and was the first-ever mechanical circulatory device to be used as destination therapy. Several decades have passed since that early experience. Pneumatic technology is still current and being developed, as in existing or new implantable Thoratec VADs the pneumatic

Heart-Mate and the Abiomed BVS 5000 pumps. Portable pneumatic drivers have been available since 1982, and in recent times have allowed discharge to home of substantial numbers of patients, thus reducing the length of hospital stays and making mechanical device support less expensive to society and more tolerable to patients. Within months, portable drivers for the CardioWest™ will be available. The CardioWest™ TAH has had a long and progressive development path. In its present status it has evolved as a successful and robust bridge to transplant device and is the only FDA approved TAH for this indication.

The documented benefits of the CardioWest TAH include the rescue of: critically ill patients with advanced heart failure; patients with biventricular failure, especially those with significant right heart failure, elevated pulmonary vascular resistance, or pulmonary edema; patients with renal or hepatic failure secondary to low cardiac output; patients with massive myocardial damage such as those with post-infarction VSD or irreversible cardiac graft rejection; patients with mechanical valves or native valve disease; and patients with intractable arrhythmias and heart failure. High device outputs with restoration of normal filling pressures result in high perfusion pressures that have led to dramatic recoveries, convalescence, and return to levels of activity compatible with normal life. The average device output with the CardioWest TAH is higher than any other approved or investigational device. The reason for this resides in design simplicity as this device has the shortest and largest inflow pathway.

Stroke, in the authors' own series, is rare with a linearized rate of 0.068 events per patient year using a tailored protocol (17). If the experiences of La Pitie and the University of Arizona are combined, there has been one stroke in 25 patient years (0.04 events/patient year).

Serious infections have been rare. To date there has been only one case of clinical mediastinitis, which contributed to patient death. Drivelines have "healed in" tightly and never caused "ascending" infection. There has not been a case of device endocarditis. Using a broad definition of bleeding, including takeback re-operation for bleeding, bleeding more than 8 units in the first postoperative 24 hr or 5 units over any other 48-hr period, a 25% to 36% incidence has been documented. No cases of fatal exsanguination have resulted. The incidence of bleeding as an adverse event is about 17% lower than the rate reported for the HeartMate VE LVAD, and it is about the same as that reported for Novacor and for Thoratec.

Implantation of this device is not technically difficult. If one follows the guidelines for fitting the device, and takes the recommended advice for implantation, hemostasis is excellent and restoration of immediate cardiac function with high flows is nearly automatic (18). Use of a neopericardium of 0.1 mm EPTFE at the time of implantation (19) assures atraumatic and relatively quick re-entry for transplantation and prevents the normal inflammatory mediastinal reaction that might be desirable in a destination application.

In selected patients the CardioWest™ TAH is the device of choice for bridge to transplantation. When a portable driver becomes available, out-of-hospital management of CardioWest™ TAH patients will be feasible and consideration of this device for long-term applications (e.g., "destination therapy,") will be reasonable. A wearable driver, even smaller than a portable, will improve quality of life and expand the patient population that may be therapeutically served with this system.

In short, the CardioWest™ TAH has come nearly full circle. It was first used as a destination device. It has since been used as a bridge to transplantation in nearly 200 patients as the Jarvik-7/Symbion TAH and, since 1993, in over 350 patients as CardioWest™. The results have improved with time. Thromboembolism and infection rates have been competitive with currently available devices. Device reliability and durability have been excellent. Survival rates have been very high in a group of perhaps the sickest patients to be supported with any pulsatile device. Pneumatic technology has improved with portability and miniaturization, and there is reason to believe that it will become even better. Application of modern manufacturing techniques to this very simple device raises the possibility of significant manufacturing cost reduction in an era of prohibitive cost for other devices. All of this establishes the CardioWest™ as a valuable device for any program that is seriously interested in end-stage heart disease and a likely device for permanent use in appropriately selected patients.

Increases in CardioWest™ TAH implantations worldwide and expansion of the number of implanting centers will provoke more interest in the uses of this device as well as in its comparison, with other technologies. Portable drivers that are currently used primarily in Germany expand the applicability and practicality of the TAH while reducing the cost by allowing out-of-hospital care. This, in addition to the high pump flows and control of the entire circulation, may have already led to shifts in patient and device selection philosophies. We believe there could well be a paradigm shift underway with regard to TAH use, as the advantages of this technology become apparent in the hands of a greater number of users.

REFERENCES

1. Hogness JR, VanAntwerp M. The artificial heart prototypes, policies, and patients. Washington, D.C.: Institute of Medicine, National Academy Press, 1991.
2. Heart Disease and Stroke Statistics—2005 Update page 26 AHA.
3. Cooley DA, Liotta D, Hallman GL, et al. Orthotopic cardiac prosthesis for two-stage cardiac replacement. Am J Cardiol 1969; 24:723–730.
4. Cooley DA, Akutsu T, Norman JC, et al. Total artificial heart in two-staged cardiac transplantation. Cardiovas Dis Bull Texas Heart Inst 1981; 8:305–319.
5. DeVries WC, Anderson JH, Joyce LD, et al. Clinical use of the total artificial heart. N Engl J Med 1984; 310:273–278.
6. Copeland JG, Levinson MM, Smith R, et al. The total artificial heart as a bridge to transplantation. A report of two cases. JAMA 1986; 256:2991–2995.
7. Copeland JG, Smith RG, Cleavinger MR. Development and current status of the CardioWest C-70 (Jarvik-7) total artificial heart. In: Lewis T, Graham TR, eds. Mechanical circulatory support. Great Britain: Edward Arnold, 1995:186–198.
8. DeVries WC. The permanent artificial heart. Four case reports. JAMA 1988; 259:849–859.
9. Kolff WJ, DeVries WC, Joyce LD, et al. Lessons learned from the barney clark in the first patient with an artificial heart. Int J Artif Organs 1983; 1:165–174.
10. Johnson KE, Prieto M, Joyce LD, et al. Summary of the clinical use of the symbion total artificial heart: a registry report. J Heart Lung Transplant 1992; 11:103–116.
11. Szefner J, Cabrol C. Control and treatment of hemstasis in patients with a total artificial heart: the experience at la pitie. In: Piffare R, ed. Anticoagulation, hemostasis, and blood preservation in cardiovascular surgery. Philadelphia: Hanley and Belfus, 1993:237–264.
12. Copeland JG, Smith RG, Arabia FA, et al. Comparison of the CardioWest total artificial heart, the novacor left ventricular assist system and the thoratec ventricular assist system in bridge to transplantation. Ann Thorac Surg 2001; 71:S92–S97.
13. Copeland JG, Smith RG, Arabia FA, et al. Total artificial heart bridge to transplantation: a 9-year experience with 62 patients. J Heart Lung Transplant 2004; 23:823–831.
14. Leprince P, Bonnet N, Rama A, et al. Bridge to transplantation with the Jarvik-7 (CardioWest) total artificial heart: a single center 15-year experience. J Heart Lung Transplant 2003; 22:1296–1303.

15. Copeland JG, Smith RG, Arabia FA, et al. Cardiac replacement with a total artificial heart as a bridge to transplantation. N Engl J Med 2004; 351:859–867.
16. 2001 Annual report of the U.S. Organ Procurement and Transplantation Network and the scientific Registry of Transplantation Recipients. Vol. 1. Washington, D.C.: Department of Health and Human Services. N Engl J 2001: 439–483
17. Copeland JG, Arabia FA, Tsau PH, et al. Total artificial hearts: bridge to transplantation. Cardiol Clin 2003; 21:101–113.
18. Arabia FA, Copeland JG, Pavie A, et al. Implantation technique for the CardioWest total artificial heart. Ann Thorac Surg 1999; 68:698–704.
19. Copeland JG, Arabia FA, Smith RG, et al. Synthetic membrane neo-pericardium facilitates total artificial heart explantation. J Heart Lung Transplant 2001; 20:654–656.

27

Selection and Management of Cardiac Transplantation Candidates

Christopher Newton-Cheh and Marc J. Semigran
Heart Failure and Transplantation Section, Massachusetts General Hospital, Harvard Medical School, Boston, Massachusetts, U.S.A.

INTRODUCTION

Patients with heart failure refractory to medical, surgical, and device therapy who have a high risk of mortality in one year can have both their survival and functional status improved by orthotopic heart transplantation. Advances in the care of the advanced heart failure patient prior to and following transplantation have improved both the quality and duration of life of cardiac transplant recipients; however, the limited number of available donor organs remains a major constraint on the utilization of this therapy. Thus, the recognition of the heart failure patient sick enough to require referral for transplantation, the evaluation of the potential transplantation candidate and the management of the patient awaiting transplantation are important skills for the cardiologist caring for heart failure patients.

GENERAL INDICATIONS FOR CARDIAC TRANSPLANTATION

Acute Decompensation

Heart failure patients who are candidates for cardiac transplantation can broadly be classified by the duration of their heart failure into acutely and chronically ill patients. With the broader utilization of inotropic and mechanical support, more patients can be stabilized from an acutely decompensated state. Moreover, because many causes of new-onset heart failure can show significant clinical improvement in the time span of 3 to 6 mo, efforts to avoid transplantation in the early period may often be warranted (1–3). Previously healthy patients with an abrupt development of severe heart failure such as culminant myocarditis, in general have a better prognosis for recovery of myocardial function, if patients can be supported through the initial period of hemodynamic embarrassment (1,4). Other causes of acute cardiomyopathy include peripartum cardiomyopathy and hypertensive and alcoholic cardiomyopathy, all of which may be associated with dramatic improvements in myocardial performance if the underlying source of myocardial injury can be treated or removed.

It has been observed that approximately 4% of chronic heart failure patients admitted with acute decompensation will die during hospitalization. Recursive partitioning analysis of over 33,000 heart failure hospitalizations found that the presence on admission of a BUN $\geq$43 mg/dl, a creatinine $\geq$2.75 mg/dl, and a systolic blood pressure $<$115 mmHg identified patients with a ten-fold greater risk of mortality compared with those in whom these findings were absent (5). It is reasonable that patients with these characteristics on admission should be considered for evaluation for transplantation, particularly if all three of these parameters are present.

Patients with known pre-existing left ventricular dysfunction who undergo cardiac surgery (e.g. coronary revascularization, valvular repair/replacement) may have significant difficulty weaning from extracorporeal cardiopulmonary bypass either due to limited left ventricular myocardial reserve or due to right ventricular failure (a particular issue in patients with fixed pulmonary hypertension). In such patients, placement of a ventricular assist device may allow separation from cardiopulmonary bypass and ultimately cardiac transplantation after adequate recovery from surgery. Consideration of the possible need for mechanical support, either as a bridge to transplantation or to recovery or as destination therapy, is an essential component of the cardiologist's evaluation of the high-risk cardiomyopathy patient in whom cardiac surgery is contemplated.

Chronic Severe Heart Failure

All patients with chronic advanced heart failure should receive medical therapy including maximum-tolerated doses of neurohormonal antagonists and a flexible diuretic program to maintain a euvolemic weight range. Implantation of an implantable cardiac defibrillator and/or a biventricular pacemaker should be performed when indicated. Surgical relief from coronary artery disease or significant valvular disease should also be employed, if appropriate, with consideration of the need for postoperative mechanical cardiac support entering into the pre-operative decision-making process.

In the patient who continues to have severe heart failure symptoms despite optimal medical management, and whose one-year survival is limited, consideration of cardiac transplantation is appropriate. Inability to avoid recurrent hospitalizations for intravenous inotropic or vasodilator support or inability to wean from these agents should similarly prompt such evaluation. Unlike the patient with new-onset heart failure, who has a reasonable chance of significant improvement in myocardial performance, functional status and prognosis, when the patient with chronic severe heart failure presents with an acute decompensation, it is unlikely that long-term recovery will occur, and consideration of cardiac transplantation should proceed. Of course, if the acute decompensation is a result of a preventable intercurrent precipitant, transplant evaluation should not replace approaches such as patient education regarding dietary and medication compliance, or adjustment of medical therapy.

Across the world, the highest percentage of heart transplants are necessitated by idiopathic cardiomyopathy (46%), coronary artery disease (45%), and valvular heart disease (3%) (6).

Less Common Indications for Transplantation

Although refractory heart failure is the most common indication for cardiac transplantation, some with other cardiac diseases and symptoms may be considered for transplantation. Some have been transplanted for refractory angina despite adequate attempts at medical therapy and percutaneous or surgical revascularization. Some patients have been transplanted for refractory ventricular tachycardia or ventricular fibrillation in the absence of severe heart failure. Patients with primary cardiac tumors without metastasis such as sarcomas have been treated with transplantation successfully (7,8). Endocarditis refractory to medical and surgical therapy may result in sufficient undermining of cardiac integrity that orthotopic heart transplantation is necessary, despite obvious infectious risk from immunosuppression (9–11).

EVALUATION OF SEVERITY AND PROGNOSIS OF CHRONIC HF: IS THIS PATIENT'S PROGNOSIS POOR ENOUGH TO REQUIRE TRANSPLANTATION?

Patients undergoing heart transplantation in the current era experience a survival to one year of 83% with a median survival of 9.4 yr (96) (6). The selection of patients for cardiac transplantation requires a comparable mortality risk in the absence of transplantation. Given the shortage of available donors and the allocation scheme of the United Network for Organ Sharing (www.unos.org), the mortality risk of individuals transplanted is higher in the short term (3–6 mo) (see discussion in "Outcomes on waitlist for TXP" and Fig. 5 below). The severity of disease in a patient with heart failure can be assessed by symptoms or objective non-invasive and invasive testing.

Symptoms

All patients undergoing heart transplantation for heart failure have advanced symptoms. The most recent revision of the New York Heart Association functional classification scheme of cardiac symptomatology (12) classified patients based on the presence of limiting symptoms of cardiac disease with ordinary (II), less than ordinary (III), and minimal exertion or at rest (IV). While subjective, and with modest inter-observer reproducibility (13), the NYHA classification scheme is predictive of mortality and is frequently used by cardiologists to classify the functional limitation experienced by a patient (14). Most patients undergoing transplantation have advanced NYHA class III or IV heart failure symptoms. Alternative systems have been developed to quantify functional limitation or quality of life (13,15). In addition, the joint American College of Cardiology/American Heart Association consensus guideline from 2002 proposed a new classification scheme of the stages of heart failure ranging from A through D (16). Those patients evaluated for cardiac transplantation fall into stage C (symptomatic heart failure managed with medication) and stage D (advance heart failure symptoms leading to frequent hospitalizations for inotropic or mechanical support) (16). Beyond the patient's "baseline" functional capacity, the development of acutely decompensated heart failure requiring admission has been used as a correlate of symptom status and may contribute to the overall mortality risk assessment (17–19).

Resting Echocardiography

Resting left ventricular ejection fraction can be determined non-invasively by echocardiography, as well as radionuclide ejection fraction and magnetic resonance imaging. While its quantification can be imprecise, it stands as a powerful predictor of mortality in patients with heart failure (20–26). Generally, severe symptoms of heart failure refractory to medical therapy do not result unless the ejection fraction is less than 20–25% in predominantly systolic dysfunction patients. However, many patients with low ejection fractions have excellent functional capacities or a very stable pattern of heart failure despite lack of improvement in ejection fraction with maximal medical and device therapy. The resting ejection fraction does not quantify the limitation to exertion that a patient's symptoms may suggest.

Beyond left ventricular ejection fraction, left ventricular end-diastolic dimension or volume has been shown to predict mortality in some heart failure studies (27–31). In a study by Grayburn et al. of multiple echocardiographic predictors of mortality in patients with left ventricular systolic dysfunction, only left ventricular end-diastolic volume indexed to body surface area $>120\ mL/m^2$ was a significant predictor of mortality on multivariable analysis (27).

Additionally, echocardiography right ventricular function and estimated pulmonary arterial systolic pressure can be assessed with severe mitral regurgitation and evidence of aneurysmal dilation of the left ventricular apex may identify individuals whose clinical state can be significantly improved with surgery.

Cardiopulmonary Exercise Testing

Cardiopulmonary exercise testing allows the quantification of functional limitation and the assessment of hemodynamic derangements that contribute to exercise limitation. In addition, cardiopulmonary exercise testing can distinguish a cardiac, pulmonary and skeletal muscular limit to exercise. At a minimum, cardiopulmonary exercise involves bicycle or treadmill exercise in a continuous incremental fashion until a functional limit is reached with electrocardiographic, non-invasive blood pressure and arterial pulse oxygen saturation monitoring. Additional analysis of inspired oxygen and expired carbon dioxide allows assessment of the peak oxygen consumption (VO_2 maximum) at the anaerobic threshold and at peak exercise, and the relative contribution of respiratory limitation to exercise. Maximum oxygen consumption is most significantly limited in patients with heart failure by the ability to augment cardiac output, although disordered skeletal muscle energy utilization and restrictive, obstructive, and diffusion limitations to pulmonary function may contribute to effort intolerance. As shown originally by Mancini et al., a maximum VO_2 achieved during graded exercise is a strong independent predictor of mortality in patients with heart failure (Fig. 1) (32).

Historically, maximum VO_2 levels less than 10–14 cc/kg/min have portended a significantly increased risk of dying in the intermediate term, although specific cut-offs are not clearly supported by the literature (14,20,24,25,32–34). However, in the current era of medical therapy including beta adrenergic blocking agents, cut-offs developed in heart failure patients at earlier times may be inappropriate (34,35). As shown by O'Neill et al. in 2105 patients with ejection fraction less than 35% and symptomatic heart failure referred for cardiopulmonary exercise testing, peak oxygen consumption less than 14 cc/kg/min continues to predict increased mortality in the patients using beta blocking agents (34). However, the absolute mortality risk in these patients is lower, suggesting that using a lower threshold of peak oxygen consumption in the decision to list a patient as a transplant recipient may be appropriate in patients treated with beta blockers (Fig. 2) (34). Some studies have also examined the percentage of predicted VO_2 maximum achieved, adjusted for gender, age, height and weight, as a prognostic factor, which may be more important in women and individuals at the extremes of body mass distribution (36,37).

Pulmonary arterial catheter use during cardiopulmonary excercise testing allows assessment of right and left ventricular filling pressures, pulmonary pressures, and cardiac

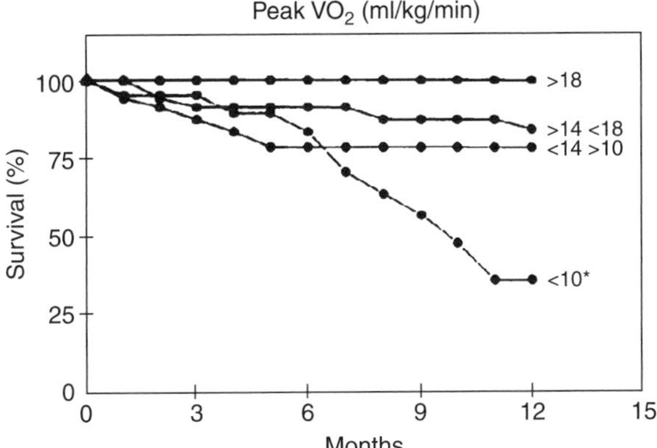

Figure 1 Survival in 114 patients not listed for cardiac transplantation stratified by maximum oxygen consumption (peak VO_2 in ml/kg/min). Note the incremental decrease in survival with declining exercise capacity and the dramatic reduction in survival of those with peak oxygen consumption less than 10 ml/kg/min. *Source*: Adapted from Ref. 32.

output during exercise. Significant increases in pulmonary pressures during exercise may suggest the functional importance of mitral regurgitation and candidacy for mitral valve surgery. First-pass radionuclide imaging or simultaneous echocardiography allows the quantification of right and left ventricular ejection fraction at rest and during exercise. In a study by DiSalvo et al. of 67 patients with severe heart failure due to *left* ventricular systolic dysfunction undergoing cardiopulmonary exercise testing with radionuclide imaging, a right ventricular ejection fraction less than 35% was a strong predictor of

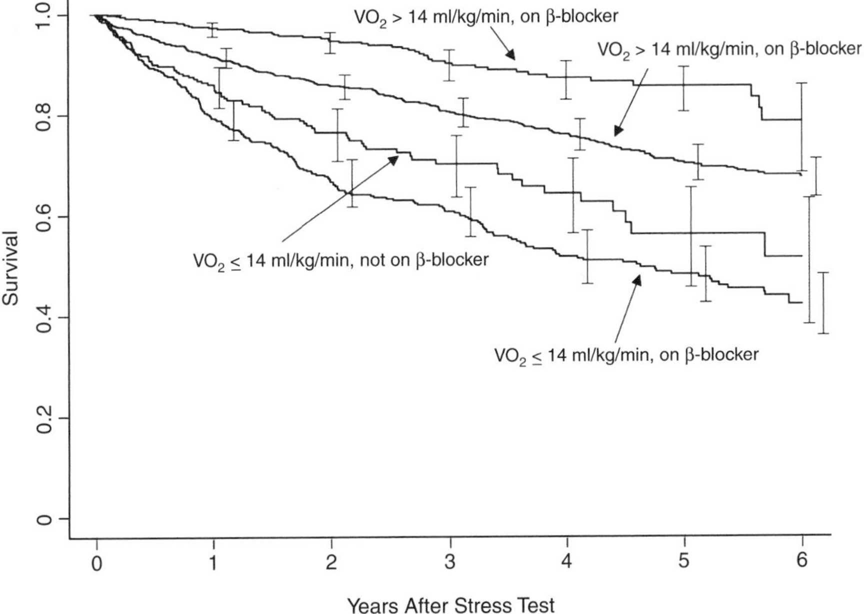

Figure 2 Survival free of transplantation in 2105 patients with heart failure and ejection fraction less than 35%, stratified by beta-blocker use and peak VO_2 $>$ or ≤ 14 ml/kg/min on cardio-pulmonary exercise testing. *Source*: Adapted from Ref. 34.

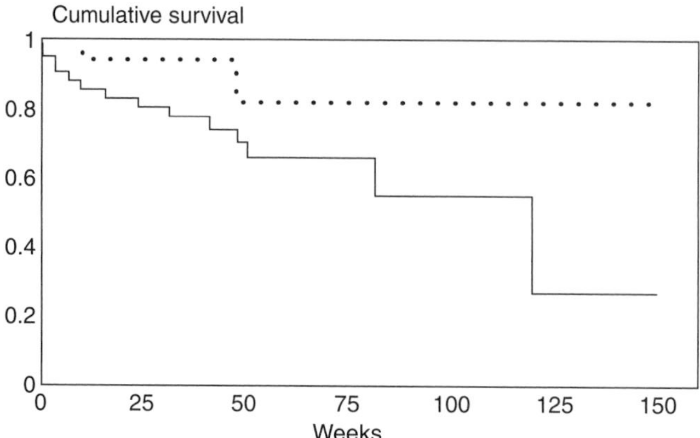

Figure 3 Survival in 67 patients with advanced heart failure undergoing cardiopulmonary exercise testing stratified by right ventricular ejection fraction $<35\%$ (*solid*) or $\geq 35\%$ (*dotted*). *Source*: Adapted from Ref. 3.

mortality (Fig. 3) (38). Lastly, arterial cannulation can allow for monitoring of blood gas and lactate generation during cardiopulmonary exercise testing.

Cardiac Catheterization

Pulmonary arterial catheterization allows quantification of right and left ventricular filling pressures, cardiac output, and severity of pulmonary hypertension and pulmonary vascular resistance. Because of their strong dependence on volume status, pharmacotherapy and device therapy, no discrete cut-offs of resting cardiac output or filling pressures exist to suggest greater benefit of cardiac transplantation. However, Stevenson et al. have shown that patients attaining a pulmonary capillary wedge pressure (PCWP) less than or equal to 16 mmHg after maximal medical intervention have a one-year survival of 83% compared to 38% in those with PCWP greater than 16 mmHg (39). In addition, pulmonary hypertension can adversely influence intermediate term prognosis. However, pulmonary hypertension when irreversible is more important as a marker of increased risk of peri-operative mortality in the patient undergoing transplantation and thus can represent a cardiac contraindication to transplantation in a patient in whom it might otherwise be indicated (*vide infra*).

Risk Prediction in the Individual Patient

The estimation of short- and intermediate-term mortality risk without cardiac transplantation most commonly includes incorporation of subjective and quantitative information about functional capacity, objective resting left ventricular performance, and hemodynamics measured at right heart catheterization, as well as other biochemical and epidemiological data (5,40–45). However, the estimation of mortality risk in an individual is different than the identification of statistically significant predictors in multi-variable modeling in large numbers of patients. The discrimination between high-risk and low-risk can be imprecise; but the development of predictive algorithms to allow more informed discussion with patients of risks and benefits would be welcome. Ultimately, the patient's cardiologist must integrate disparate pieces of clinical data to make an informed determination of the relative risks and potential benefits of cardiac transplantation.

TIMING OF REFERRAL TO TRANSPLANT CENTER

A cardiologist should consider referral of the patient with severe heart failure symptoms whose functional capacity has worsened to NYHA late class III or class IV, or who experiences repeated exacerbations of acutely decompensated heart failure despite maximal medical, surgical, and device therapy. Evaluation of an outpatient's candidacy for cardiac transplantation takes time and effort on the part of the patient and the transplant team evaluating each patient. Many transplant centers have active research protocols for patients with advanced heart failure that may be considered for patients waiting for transplant as the wait for a suitable donor can be prolonged. Furthermore, the patient should have the opportunity to learn about the rigors of life while awaiting and following transplantation, allowing them to make an informed decision regarding their treatment.

Cardiologists and cardiac surgeons should consider involving a transplant cardiologist in the preoperative assessment of a patient at high risk for right ventricular or left ventricular failure complicating surgery. While most such patients can be supported through the peri-operative period with drug and mechanical therapies, the patient who fails to wean from cardiopulmonary bypass because of right or left heart failure may be a candidate for cardiac transplantation. Typically, only limited pre-operative testing for absolute contraindications to cardiac transplantation is appropriate. As more patients with left ventricular assist devices can go home with the device as destination therapy, the importance of assessing candidacy for transplantation in the pre-operative setting may decline (46).

CONTRAINDICATIONS TO CARDIAC TRANSPLANTATION

As the survival of patients undergoing cardiac transplantation has improved owing to improved surgical and immunosuppressive approaches, many patients with historical contraindications to transplantation have successfully undergone transplantation. Most contraindications to transplantation can therefore be viewed as relative and the patient's overall burden of comorbidities must be considered in its entirety for each individual patient. Some comorbid conditions may complicate the immediate peri-operative period, some may progress more rapidly as a side effect of the medical regimens in the post-transplant patient, and some may introduce a major non-cardiac limit to the functional status of the transplant recipient. Absolute contraindications to transplantation include any advanced non-cardiac disease with a high risk of mortality within one year. We consider in turn below the major relative contraindications to cardiac transplantation (Table 1).

Infections

Uncontrolled chronic infections with agents such as the human immunodeficiency virus, hepatitis C virus, and tuberculosis may have an explosive progression under the marked immunosuppression of the early post-transplant period and pose a significant risk of early mortality. HIV-positive patients treated with highly-active antiretroviral therapy have progressively improving prognoses and may develop non-opportunistic causes of morbidity and mortality including coronary artery disease or dilated cardiomyopathy. While some have considered the transplantation of patients with very low viral loads and high T-cell counts, most transplantation programs in the United States consider HIV infection a strong contraindication to heart transplantation (47).

Table 1 Relative Contraindications to Transplantation

Chronic infection
Pulmonary hypertension
Respiratory insufficiency
Peripheral vascular disease
Hepatic dysfunction
Renal dysfunction
Diabetes
Obesity
Recent malignancy
Osteoporosis, severe
Substance abuse, active or recent
Inadequate cognitive and social support
Advanced age

Some patients with chronic hepatitis C have been successfully transplanted, but total mortality may be increased (48–51). Patients require attention to liver function tests and hepatitis C viral loads and may benefit from therapy with ribavirin and interferon. Liver transplant recipients with hepatitis C infection have comparable 5 year graft and individual survival rates to the non-hepatitis C population, although increased rates of viremia, graft injury, and cirrhosis have been reported (52). Candidacy of HCV-infected patients varies by transplant program, but it appears that some individuals with evidence of suppressed viral replication either with or without antiviral therapy may be successfully transplanted (48–51).

Heart transplant recipients have an increased risk of primary or reactivation tuberculosis. Experience transplanting patients with a history of active, treated tuberculosis is limited. Testing of individuals from endemic areas with intradermal tuberculin and chest x-ray and antibiotic prophylaxis or preemptive treatment of individuals with evidence of prior exposure is prudent. Close surveillance in the post-transplant period is also clearly warranted. Thus, the advent of highly active treatments for chronic infections has improved the candidacy of many patients with viral and mycobacterial disease that were previously thought not eligible to be cardiac transplant recipients.

Chagas disease, caused by infection with the parasite *Trypanosoma cruzi* transmitted by the reduviid bug, can cause an acute myocarditis and later chronic congestive heart failure. The treatment of severe chagasic cardiomyopathy with transplantation remains controversial. Recurrent chagasic myocarditis, increased rates of rejection, and possibly higher rate of post-transplant malignancy have all been reported (53–55). The role of specific antiparasitic therapy has not been defined but is commonly employed in patients undergoing transplantation.

History of exposure to cytomegalovirus, *Toxoplasma gondii*, *Treponema pallidum*, varicella zoster virus, or Ebstein-Barr virus as detected by positive serology may alter the risk for complications of transplantation. However, they are not relative contraindications to transplantation as effective prophylactic and therapeutic treatments exist for some and the likelihood of reactivation after transplantation for others is limited.

Pulmonary Hypertension

The donor heart, which undergoes an ischemic time from explantation to implantation in the recipient, often experiences an acute decline in right and left myocardial performance. Elevated pulmonary vascular resistance in the recipient may present an intolerable afterload to the post-ischemic right ventricle resulting in right ventricular failure in the peri-transplant period. Many patients with elevated left atrial pressure have "reactive" pulmonary hypertension with increased pulmonary vascular resistance, which falls with a reduction in left atrial pressure, as occurs with diuresis or following transplantation. A patient whose pulmonary vascular resistance remains elevated despite an optimized left ventricular filling pressure has a higher likelihood of early mortality in the peri-transplant period (56,57).

Vasodilator agents can be useful both prognostically and therapeutically in the peri-operative period. Pulmonary vascular resistance of greater than 5 Wood units (>400 dyne*sec/cm^{-5}) that fails to fall below 2.5 Wood units with intravenous nitroprusside or that falls only with excessive systemic hypotension (systolic arterial pressure <85 mmHg) identifies an individual with a significantly increased peri-operative mortality and thus represents a strong contraindication to transplantation (58). Inhaled nitric oxide is particularly useful both in evaluation of the potential transplant candidate and in their peri-operative care because of its minimal effect on systemic blood pressure (by contrast to nitroprusside), although it is important to recognize its potential to increase left ventricular filling pressures, likely related to selective pulmonary vasodilation without a reduction in left ventricular afterload (Fig. 4) (59,60).

Pulmonary Disease

Patients with respiratory insufficiency may have difficulty weaning from the ventilator in the peri-operative period and may have a sustained functional limitation, despite receipt of a functioning allograft. Intrinsic lung disease, due to chronic obstructive pulmonary disease or less commonly amiodarone toxicity, can be found in many patients evaluated for transplantation (61). Distinguishing intrinsic pulmonary dysfunction from that due to increased pulmonary fluid in chronic heart failure is crucial. Increased lung water can contribute to restrictive and obstructive patterns as well as a diffusion abnormality (61). Ideally, pulmonary function testing is performed after left atrial pressure has been optimized with diuresis. Computed tomographic chest radiography can assist

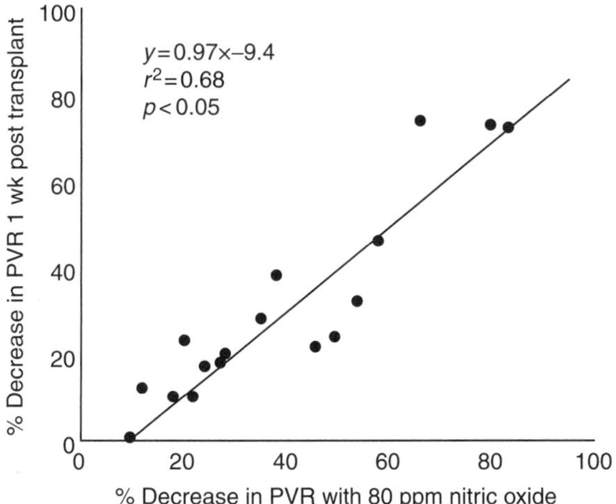

Figure 4 Relationship of the percentage change in pulmonary vascular resistance in response to 80 ppm inhaled nitric oxide to the change in pulmonary vascular resistance one week after cardiac transplantation. The preoperative response to inhaled nitric oxide is strongly predictive of the early post-transplant pulmonary vascular resistance ($r^2=0.68$, $p<0.05$). *Source*: Adapted from Ref. 59.

in the qualitative assessment of the burden of pulmonary fibrosis or emphysema. In general, patients can tolerate a decline in FEV_1 to below 40–50% predicted and still wean successfully from the ventilator, making pulmonary insufficiency only a modest relative contraindication to transplantation (62). Consultation with a pulmonologist and repeating pulmonary function testing after appropriate therapy with bronchodilators and anti-inflammatory agents can be important in the apparently marginal candidate. Lastly, recent pulmonary embolism requires aggressive pursuit and treatment of the underlying thrombotic risk and, in the case of infarction, postponement of transplantation, because of the risk of hemorrhage on cardiopulmonary bypass or abscess formation in the immunocompromised post-transplant patient (63).

Non-cardiac Vascular Disease

Given the large fraction of patients referred for transplantation with end-stage atherosclerotic coronary disease, the identification of peripheral vascular disease is an important consideration in the patient being evaluated for transplantation. Moreover, immunosuppressive regimens including calcineurin inhibitors, such as cyclosporine and tacrolimus, and chronic steroid use can contribute to progression of atherosclerotic disease diffusely. Severe cerebrovascular disease must be corrected surgically or percutaneously before transplantation to reduce the risk of peri-operative stroke. Severe lower extremity vascular disease can result in impaired healing of lower extremity trauma and result in chronic infection in the immunosuppressed patient. Adequate vascular supply to the lower extremities should be restored prior to transplantation. A history of revascularization surgery does not contraindicate cardiac transplantation.

Hepatic Dysfunction

Passive hepatic congestion may result in abnormal liver function that is readily reversible after the restoration of normal hemodynamics following transplantation. However, primary liver dysfunction, as may occur with hemochromatosis or chronic severe right heart failure, may result in irreversible cirrhosis. The presence of cirrhosis on biopsy with abnormal liver function is a contraindication to cardiac transplantation because of the risk of peri-operative hemorrhage from porto-systemic varices and represents a major barrier to adequate nutrition and resistance to infection in the post-transplant period. Whether patients with compensated cirrhosis have good outcomes following cardiac transplantation is not known. Combined heart-liver transplantation has been carried out in select patients (64). Additional risks exist of abnormal metabolism of medications following transplantation, such as cyclosporine (65), in patients with abnormal liver function.

Renal Dysfunction

Historically, renal dysfunction was considered a strong contraindication to cardiac transplantation because of the risk of progressive renal functional deterioration on long-term calcineurin inhibitors and the infection risks associated with frequent vascular access (66,67). However, simultaneous cardiac and heterotopic kidney transplantation has removed the barrier to transplant of renal dysfunction (68). A creatinine clearance less than 20–30 mL/min is considered an indication for combined heart-kidney transplantation. Lesser degrees of renal insufficiency are associated with increased risk of end-stage renal disease and of mortality following transplantation (6,66,67). Predictors of progression to end-stage renal disease include glomerular filtration rate less than 50 ml/min, older age at transplantation and elevated early cyclosporine levels, and diabetes (66,67,69–72).

Diabetes

As a major contributor to clinical atherosclerosis and owing to the rise in obesity in industrialized nations, diabetes is present in 19.3% of recent heart transplant recipients (6). While calcineurin inhibitors and prednisone can increase insulin resistance, well-controlled diabetes is not a significant barrier to successful cardiac transplantation. End-organ dysfunction, such as severe retinopathy or neuropathy, is a relative contraindication to transplantation but the major concern is for severe small vessel disease contributing to poorly healing lower extremity ulcers. Diabetic transplant recipients are at higher risk of serious infection, especially in the early post-operative period when immunosuppression is most intense (73). Consultation of a diabetologist can be invaluable in the management of the diabetic patient awaiting and following cardiac transplantation.

Obesity

Given the consistent trend of increasing in body mass index throughout the developed and developing worlds, it is no surprise that overweight or obesity are found in 25% patients considered for heart transplant (74). No clear thresholds exist at which transplantation is not performed but a minority of patients with body mass index greater than 35 kg/m^2 are transplanted at programs in the United States. Weight gain following cardiac transplantation, in part secondary to chronic steroid use, is common and is a potent risk factor for the development of diabetes. Pre-operative obesity is associated with increased rates of infection and mortality post-transplant (74,75). Moreover, the identification of a heart from a donor of adequate size can increase time on the waitlist and donor-recipient size mismatch can impair post-operative outcomes. An undersized heart (donor body weight less than $\approx$80% that of recipient) may result in a restrictive hemodynamic pattern, requiring higher heart rates and filling pressures to maintain a normal cardiac index, but it is not clear that this translates into a significant limitation to exercise (57,76,77). An undersized heart poses a particular risk in the presence of significant pulmonary hypertension in the peri-operative period, as the post-ischemic right ventricle faces significant afterload and the need for an adequate stroke volume. Weight loss while awaiting transplantation can significantly reduce the risk of morbidity following transplantation.

Age

There is no clear age above which cardiac transplantation is not performed. Age is both a surrogate for many of the degenerative disorders that can complicate transplantation and a strong risk factor for death. The median survival by age group in the most recent registry data from the International Society for Heart and Lung Transplantation was 11.5 years for those 18–34 years old, 10.1 years for those 35–49 years old, 8.9 years for those 50–64 years old, 8.1 years for those 65–69 years old and 5.9 years for those 70 years and older (96) (6). Historically, programs rarely transplant patients over age 65 years. However, patients older than 65 years with few other comorbidities have been increasingly transplanted in the past several years and represent a large pool of potential transplant recipients. In the ISHLT registry data from 2000–2003 the age distribution among adult transplant recipients was 18–34 (10.1%), 35–49 (25.6%), 50–64 (54.8%), and 65+(9.5%) (96) (6).

Malignancy

Immunosuppression removes an important check on the proliferation of potentially malignant cells. Patients with active malignancy are not transplanted. Patients with apparent cure from a malignancy in the past five years have a relative contraindication to transplantation. The risk of relapse for certain cancers such as Hodgkin's lymphoma or non-melanomatous skin cancers may decline earlier than five years, while for other cancers such as breast cancer later relapses may be more common. Active screening for malignancy is an important part of the pre- and post-transplantation evaluation. Aggressive efforts to biopsy suspicious lesions should be carried out to avoid early death in the period immediately after transplantation during which immunosuppression is most intense.

Amyloidosis

Historically, cardiac amyloidosis, most commonly secondary to a sporadic plasma cell dyscrasia (light chain disease), has been considered a strong contraindication to cardiac transplantation (78,79). Because the underlying plasma cell dyscrasia and production of amyloidogenic light chain are not corrected by cardiac transplantation, increased intermediate term mortality from recurrent cardiac and or progressive of systemic amyloid have been limiting factors (80,81). Systemic amyloidosis has been treated with chemotherapy and autologous stem cell rescue, but this treatment is poorly tolerated in patients with cardiac amyloid at presentation because of its rapid progression and the patients' inability to tolerate anti-plasma cell treatment (82). Some centers, including our own, have begun staged cardiac transplantation in an attempt to stabilize the patient for potentially curative eradication of the underlying plasma cell dyscrasia with subsequent chemotherapy and autologous stem cell rescue (83). In our consecutive series of 5 patients with light-chain amyloid and one with a transthyretin mutation, cardiac transplantation was followed by chemotherapy and stem cell rescue (or liver transplantation for the patient with transthyretin mutation) a median of 7.5 mo later (84). In median follow-up of 21 mo (3–53 mo), all patients are alive with New York Heart Association functional class I symptoms, without extracardiac amyloid-related organ dysfunction or cardiac amyloid on routine right ventricular biopsies. Reactivation of cytomegalovirus in those with pre-transplant exposure was common following chemotherapy (84). Longer follow-up is required. Interestingly, the recent treatment of a patient with cardiac amyloid with successful heart transplantation followed by allogeneic bone marrow transplantation to induce mixed chimerism and a graft-versus-plasma-cell response may further expand therapeutic options for a disease with an otherwise dismal prognosis (85).

Ability to Comply with Complex Medical Care

Several social and inadequate cognitive factors must be in place for the care of the pre- and post-transplant patient. The transplant recipient must understand a complex medical regimen and bring to the attention of the transplant team worrisome symptoms that often require thorough evaluation. Failure to comply with the complex post-transplant regimen can result in rejection or overwhelming opportunistic infection. Patients must have a support system in place to assist in their care at times of illness. Uncontrolled psychiatric disease or substance abuse can lead to an impaired ability to participate actively in the self-care required of a transplant recipient. Full evaluation by a psychiatrist and social worker is important in order to identify the at-risk patient. Active dependence on mind-altering substances (such as alcohol or cocaine) is a strong contraindication to transplantation. Active tobacco use, because of its strong interaction with immunosuppression and tumorigenesis, is also a strong contraindication to transplant.

Osteoporosis

Cardiac transplant candidates have a high rate of osteopenia and osteoporosis (86–88). The combination of lack of weight-bearing exercise, chronic calcium wasting from loop diuretics, and renal insufficiency are likely contributors (89). Moreover, chronic glucocorticoid and cyclosporine use contribute to further bone demineralization post--transplant. Identification of the at-risk patient prior to transplant allows for the prophylactic administration of calcium, vitamin D, and bisphosphonates as appropriate (90). Osteoporosis, unless associated with multiple fractures, is rarely a major barrier to transplantation.

Diagnostic tests to identify potential contraindications to transplantation are listed in Table 2.

IMPLICATIONS OF THE SYSTEM FOR ORGAN ALLOCATION

The number of potential organ recipients far exceeds the number of available organs. As improvements in the surgical and medical care of the transplant patient continue, the number of patients who would experience a functional and mortality benefit with transplantation can only increase. The United Network for Organ Sharing (UNOS), a private non-profit organization under contract with the federal government, provides a uniform set of standards for the allocation of organs in the United States. UNOS policies are open for public review and comment and are under federal oversight. This system prioritizes the distribution of organs by blood group to the sickest heart failure patients preferentially over those with chronic more compensated heart failure. UNOS status 1A

Table 2 Pre-transplant Evaluation for Potential Contraindications

Complete blood count
Prothrombin, activated partial thromboplastin time
BUN, creatinine
24 hour urine for protein, creatinine
Liver function tests
Fasting glucose, Hgb A1c if diabetic
HCV antibody
HBV surface antibody, surface antigen
HIV Ab
Pulmonary function testing, including DLCO
Carotid duplex ultrasound if clinical atherosclerosis, or age >40 years old
Abdominal ultrasound
PPD
Bone mineral density
PSA >40 years old
Mammogram >45 years old
Colonoscopy >50 years old (younger with 1st degree relative)
Psychiatry consultation
Social work consultation

Abbreviations: BUN, blood urea nitrogen; HCV, hepatitis C virus; HBV, hepatitis B virus; DLCO, diffusing capacity of the lung for carbon monoxide; PPD, purified protein derivative; PSA, prostate-specific antigen.

patients are hospitalized patients on a high dose of one or any doses of multiple vasoactive medications with a pulmonary artery catheter, on an intra-aortic balloon pump or mechanical ventilator, or who have had a ventricular assist device for less than 30 days (may be home on a ventricular assist device). Status 1B patients are on a vasoactive medication or have a ventricular assist device longer than 30 days. Status 2 patients include all others. Organs are allocated in order of time on each category waitlist starting with 1A patients by geographic region. The net effect of this allocation scheme and the limited number of donor organs is that patients must become severely decompensated to have a good chance of receiving a heart. Many patients die on the list despite not being "sick" enough to be allocated an organ under this scheme. Other schemes might include prioritization of transplanting patients who are less ill and who will potentially have a lower morbidity or mortality following transplantation.

OUTCOMES ON WAITLIST FOR TRANSPLANT

The shortage of donor organs results in lengthy periods on the waitlist for cardiac transplantation. Outcomes on the waitlist have been compared to outcomes after transplantation to guide the development of the donor organ allocation scheme described above. Recent data compiled by the United Network for Organ Sharing highlights the gap between the improved survival following transplantation compared to continued medical management (Fig. 5). While Status 1A patients receive an immediate survival benefit from transplantation relative to continued "waiting," Status 2 patients do not achieve this

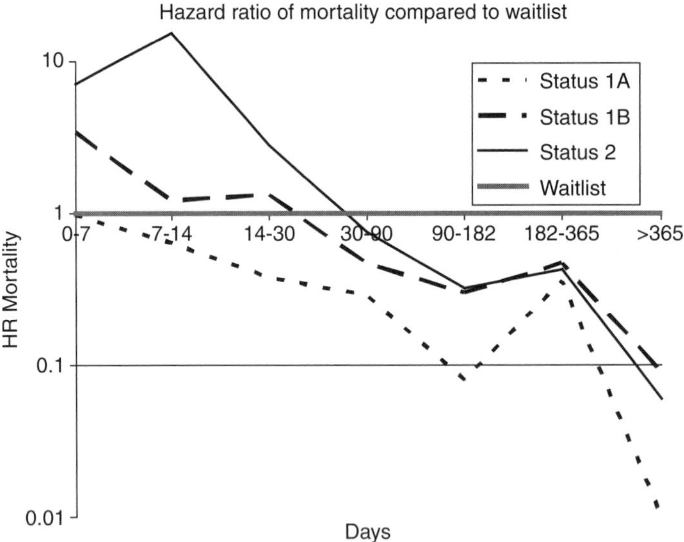

Figure 5 Hazard ratio for mortality for time periods after transplant compared to time on the waitlist. A hazard ratio of less than 1.0 (*gray line*) represents a survival advantage of transplantation compared to continued waiting. Note that status 1A transplant candidates (N = 1796) show a statistically significant survival advantage starting at 2–4 wk ($p < 0.05$). Status 1B candidates (N = 1672) show a significant survival advantage at 1–3 mo. Status 2 candidates (N = 1105) do not demonstrate a survival advantage until 3–6 mo and show significantly worse survival through the first month. Time periods extend from 0–7, 7–14, 14–30, 30–90, 90–182, 182–365, >365 days. Hazard ratios are plotted on a logarithmic scale. *Source*: Adapted from UNOS Public Comment Notice, March 15, 2005.

relative benefit until they have survived approximately 90 days after transplantation. Thus, although Status 1 patients derive a more immediate survival benefit from transplantation, there is little question that lower status patients also benefit and this must be taken into account as organ allocation schemes are designed.

MANAGEMENT PRIOR TO TRANSPLANT

Patients waiting on the list for cardiac transplantation should receive optimal medical, surgical and device therapies as reviewed elsewhere. In addition, patients should have regular surveillance for the potential complications of heart failure or other comorbidities that might preclude transplantation entirely. Right heart catheterization to screen for the development of significant pulmonary hypertension should be performed periodically in the stable outpatient or guided by change in clinical status. Patients require periodic assessment of renal function to identify irreversible changes that might require simultaneous kidney transplantation. Additionally, patients should be screened for the development of antibodies to major histocompatability complex antigens, especially after ventricular assist device implantation. The period after listing and prior to transplantation is risky and cardiologists must approach such patients with vigilance.

CONCLUSION

The early identification of potential transplant candidates and referral for evaluation at a transplant center, combined with improvements in medical and device therapies for those awaiting transplant should continue to improve the functional status and survival of the sickest heart failure patients.

APPENDIX A: DONOR IDENTIFICATION AND MANAGEMENT

At the time of determination of brain death, an individual who has previously expressed a desire to be an organ donor or whose proxy consents to organ donation must be screened for the appropriateness of organ donation. The ideal organ donor is young, free of systemic disease, and has no structural heart disease. Major contraindications to organ donation include infection with HIV, hepatitis C or hepatitis B virus, the presence of malignancy, or of severe infection (91). Structural heart disease such as severe left ventricular hypertrophy, coronary artery disease, intractable ventricular tachycardia and severe left ventricular dysfunction absolutely preclude use of the organ (91). Relative contraindications include prolonged CPR, carbon monoxide poisoning, modest left ventricular hypertrophy and donor age greater than 55 yr old. Because of the severe shortage of donors, some have advocated the use of a marginal recipient list to whom hearts are allocated from marginal donors with relative contraindications (92,93).

In some potential donors the left ventricular ejection fraction is depressed because of the release of neurohumoral factors in the brain-dead patient. To improve the salvage of hearts with an ejection fraction less than 45%, protocols have been developed to try to reverse the neurohumoral derangements that contribute to reduced myocardial performance (94). Administration of intravenous triiodothyroxine, arginine vasopressin, steroids, and insulin can result in a significant improvement in ejection fraction allowing the successful harvest and transplantation of these organs (95).

REFERENCES

1. Keogh AM, Baron DW, Hickie JB. Prognostic guides in patients with idiopathic or ischemic dilated cardiomyopathy assessed for cardiac transplantation. Am J Cardiol 1990; 65:903–908.
2. Steimle AE, Stevenson LW, Fonarow GC, Hamilton MA, Moriguchi JD. Prediction of improvement in recent onset cardiomyopathy after referral for heart transplantation. J Am Coll Cardiol March 1994; 23:553–559.
3. Cross AM, Jr., Steenbergen C, Higginbotham MB. Recovery of left ventricular function in acute nonischemic congestive cardiomyopathy. Am Heart J 1995; 129:24–30.
4. McCarthy RE, III, Boehmer JP, Hruban RH, et al. Long-term outcome of fulminant myocarditis as compared with acute (nonfulminant) myocarditis. N Engl J Med 2000; 342:690–695.
5. Fonarow GC, Adams KF, Jr., Abraham WT, Yancy CW, Boscardin WJ. Risk stratification for in-hospital mortality in acutely decompensated heart failure: classification and regression tree analysis. JAMA 2005; 293:572–580.
6. Taylor DO, Edwards LB, Boucek MM, Trulock EP, Keck BM, Hertz MI. The Registry of the International Society for Heart and Lung Transplantation: twenty-first official adult heart transplant report. J Heart Lung Transplant 2004; 23:796–803.
7. Koerner MM, Tenderich G, Minami K. Results of heart transplantation in patients with preexisting malignancies. Am J Cardiol 1997; 79:988–991.
8. Rodriguez-Cruz E, Cintron-Maldonado RM, Forbes TJ. Treatment of primary cardiac malignancies with orthotopic heart transplantation. Bol Asoc Med P R 2000; 92:65–71.
9. Blanche C, Freimark D, Valenza M, Czer LS, Trento A. Heart transplantation for Q fever endocarditis. Ann Thorac Surg 1994; 58:1768–1769.
10. DiSesa VJ, Sloss LJ, Cohn LH. Heart transplantation for intractable prosthetic valve endocarditis. J Heart Transplant 1990; 9:142–143.
11. Pulpon LA, Crespo MG, Sobrino M. Recalcitrant endocarditis successfully treated by heart transplantation. Am Heart J 1994; 127:958–960.
12. The Criteria Committee of the New York Heart Association.. 9th ed Nomenclature and Criteria for Diagnosis of Diseases of the Heart and Great Vessels. Boston, MA: Little, Brown & Co, 1994.
13. Goldman L, Hashimoto B, Cook EF, Loscalzo A. Comparative reproducibility and validity of systems for assessing cardiovascular functional class: advantages of a new specific activity scale. Circulation 1981; 64:1227–1234.
14. Costanzo MR, Augustine S, Bourge R, et al. Selection and treatment of candidates for heart transplantation. A statement for health professionals from the Committee on Heart Failure and Cardiac Transplantation of the Council on Clinical Cardiology, American Heart Association. Circulation 1995; 92:359–612.
15. Konstam V, Salem D, Pouleur H, et al. Baseline quality of life as a predictor of mortality and hospitalization in 5025 patients with congestive heart failure. SOLVD Investigations. Studies of Left Ventricular Dysfunction Investigators. Am J Cardiol 1996; 78:890–895.
16. Hunt SA, Baker DW, Chin MH, et al. ACC/AHA Guidelines for the Evaluation and Management of Chronic Heart Failure in the Adult: Executive Summary A Report of the American College of Cardiology/American Heart Association Task Force on Practice Guidelines (Committee to Revise the 1995 Guidelines for the Evaluation and Management of Heart Failure): Developed in Collaboration With the International Society for Heart and Lung Transplantation; Endorsed by the Heart Failure Society of America. Circulation 2001; 104:2996–3007.
17. Felker GM, Leimberger JD, Califf RM, et al. Risk stratification after hospitalization for decompensated heart failure. J Card Fail 2004; 10:460–466.
18. Cleland JG, Swedberg K, Follath F, et al. The EuroHeart Failure survey programme—a survey on the quality of care among patients with heart failure in Europe. Part 1: patient characteristics and diagnosis. Eur Heart J 2003; 24:442–463.

19. Graff L, Orledge J, Radford MJ, Wang Y, Petrillo M, Maag R. Correlation of the Agency for Health Care Policy and Research congestive heart failure admission guideline with mortality: peer review organization voluntary hospital association initiative to decrease events (PROVIDE) for congestive heart failure. Ann Emerg Med 1999; 34:429–437.
20. Likoff MJ, Chandler SL, Kay HR. Clinical determinants of mortality in chronic congestive heart failure secondary to idiopathic dilated or to ischemic cardiomyopathy. Am J Cardiol 1987; 59:634–638.
21. Gottdiener JS, McClelland RL, Marshall R, et al. Outcome of congestive heart failure in elderly persons: influence of left ventricular systolic function. The Cardiovascular Health Study. Ann Intern Med 2002; 137:631–639.
22. Juilliere Y, Barbier G, Feldmann L, Grentzinger A, Danchin N, Cherrier F. Additional predictive value of both left and right ventricular ejection fractions on long-term survival in idiopathic dilated cardiomyopathy. Eur Heart J 1997; 18:276–280.
23. Bourassa MG, Gurne O, Bangdiwala SI, et al. Natural history and patterns of current practice in heart failure. The Studies of Left Ventricular Dysfunction (SOLVD) Investigators. J Am Coll Cardiol 1993; 22:9A–14A.
24. van den Broek SA, van Veldhuisen DJ, de Graeff PA, Landsman ML, Hillege H, Lie KI. Comparison between New York Heart Association classification and peak oxygen consumption in the assessment of functional status and prognosis in patients with mild to moderate chronic congestive heart failure secondary to either ischemic or idiopathic dilated cardiomyopathy. Am J Cardiol 1992; 70:359–363.
25. Cohn JN, Johnson GR, Shabetai R, et al. Ejection fraction, peak exercise oxygen consumption, cardiothoracic ratio, ventricular arrhythmias, and plasma norepinephrine as determinants of prognosis in heart failure. The V-HeFT VA Cooperative Studies Group. Circulation 1993; 87:V15–V16.
26. Bart BA, Shaw LK, McCants CB, Jr., et al. Clinical determinants of mortality in patients with angiographically diagnosed ischemic or nonischemic cardiomyopathy. J Am Coll Cardiol 1997; 30:1002–1008.
27. Grayburn PA, Appleton CP, DeMaria AN, et al. Echocardiographic predictors of morbidity and mortality in patients with advanced heart failure: the Beta-blocker Evaluation of Survival Trial (BEST). J Am Coll Cardiol 2005; 45:1064–1071.
28. White HD, Norris RM, Brown MA, Brandt PW, Whitlock RM, Wild CJ. Left ventricular end-systolic volume as the major determinant of survival after recovery from myocardial infarction. Circulation 1987; 76:44–51.
29. St John SM, Pfeffer MA, Plappert T, et al. Quantitative two-dimensional echocardiographic measurements are major predictors of adverse cardiovascular events after acute myocardial infarction. The protective effects of captopril. Circulation 1994; 89:68–75.
30. St John SM, Pfeffer MA, Moye L, et al. Cardiovascular death and left ventricular remodeling two years after myocardial infarction: baseline predictors and impact of long-term use of captopril: information from the Survival and Ventricular Enlargement (SAVE) trial. Circulation 1997; 96:3294–3299.
31. Koelling TM, Semigran MJ, Mijller-Ehmsen J, et al. Left ventricular end-diastolic volume index, age, and maximum heart rate at peak exercise predict survival in patients referred for heart transplantation. J Heart Lung Transplant 1998; 17:278–287.
32. Mancini DM, Eisen H, Kussmaul W, Mull R, Edmunds LH, Jr., Wilson JR. Value of peak exercise oxygen consumption for optimal timing of cardiac transplantation in ambulatory patients with heart failure. Circulation 1991; 83:778–786.
33. Roul G, Moulichon ME, Bareiss P, et al. Prognostic factors of chronic heart failure in NYHA class II or III: value of invasive exercise haemodynamic data. Eur Heart J 1995; 16:1387–1398.
34. O'Neill JO, Young JB, Pothier CE, Lauer MS. Peak oxygen consumption as a predictor of death in patients with heart failure receiving beta-blockers. Circulation 2005; 111:2313–2318.
35. Shakar SF, Lowes BD, Lindenfeld J, et al. Peak oxygen consumption and outcome in heart failure patients chronically treated with beta-blockers. J Card Fail 2004; 10:15–20.

36. Aaronson KD, Mancini DM. Is percentage of predicted maximal exercise oxygen consumption a better predictor of survival than peak exercise oxygen consumption for patients with severe heart failure? J Heart Lung Transplant 1995; 14:981–989.
37. Osada N, Chaitman BR, Miller LW, et al. Cardiopulmonary exercise testing identifies low risk patients with heart failure and severely impaired exercise capacity considered for heart transplantation. J Am Coll Cardiol 1998; 31:577–582.
38. Di Salvo TG, Mathier M, Semigran MJ, Dec GW. Preserved right ventricular ejection fraction predicts exercise capacity and survival in advanced heart failure. J Am Coll Cardiol 1995; 25:1143–1153.
39. Stevenson LW, Tillisch JH, Hamilton M, et al. Importance of hemodynamic response to therapy in predicting survival with ejection fraction less than or equal to 20% secondary to ischemic or nonischemic dilated cardiomyopathy. Am J Cardiol 1990; 66:1348–1354.
40. Myers J, Gullestad L, Vagelos R, et al. Clinical, hemodynamic, and cardiopulmonary exercise test determinants of survival in patients referred for evaluation of heart failure. Ann Intern Med 1998; 129:286–293.
41. Lee DS, Austin PC, Rouleau JL, Liu PP, Naimark D, Tu JV. Predicting mortality among patients hospitalized for heart failure: derivation and validation of a clinical model. JAMA 2003; 290:2581–2587.
42. Bouvy ML, Heerdink ER, Leufkens HG, Hoes AW. Predicting mortality in patients with heart failure: a pragmatic approach. Heart 2003; 89:605–609.
43. De MT, Goldman L. Predicting outcomes in severe heart failure. Circulation 1997; 95:2597–2599.
44. Cowie MR, Wood DA, Coats AJ, et al. Survival of patients with a new diagnosis of heart failure: a population based study. Heart 2000; 83:505–510.
45. Mudge GH, Goldstein S, Addonizio LJ, et al. 24th Bethesda conference: Cardiac transplantation. Task Force 3: Recipient guidelines/prioritization. J Am Coll Cardiol 1993; 22:21–31.
46. Rose EA, Gelijns AC, Moskowitz AJ, et al. Long-term mechanical left ventricular assistance for end-stage heart failure. N Engl J Med 2001; 345:1435–1443.
47. Freudenberger RS, Boruchoff SE, Anderson MB. Policies of U.S. heart transplant programs regarding transplantation of human immunodeficiency-positive patients. J Heart Lung Transplant 2004; 23:785.
48. Lake KD, Smith CI, Milfred-La Forest SK, Pritzker MR, Emery RW. Outcomes of hepatitis C positive (HCV+) heart transplant recipients. Transplant Proc 1997; 29:581–582.
49. Lake KD, Smith CI, LaForest SK, Allen J, Pritzker MR, Emery RW. Policies regarding the transplantation of hepatitis C-positive candidates and donor organs. J Heart Lung Transplant 1997; 16:917–921.
50. Lunel F, Cadranel JF, Rosenheim M, et al. Hepatitis virus infections in heart transplant recipients: epidemiology, natural history, characteristics, and impact on survival. Gastroenterology 2000; 119:1064–1074.
51. Castella M, Tenderich G, Koerner MM, et al. Outcome of heart transplantation in patients previously infected with hepatitis C virus. J Heart Lung Transplant 2001; 20:595–598.
52. Gane EJ, Portmann BC, Naoumov NV, et al. Long-term outcome of hepatitis C infection after liver transplantation. N Engl J Med 1996; 334:815–820.
53. de CV, Sousa EF, Vila JH, et al. Heart transplantation in Chagas' disease 10 years after the initial experience. Circulation 1996; 94:1815–1817.
54. Bocchi EA, Bellotti G, Mocelin AO, et al. Heart transplantation for chronic Chagas' heart disease. Ann Thorac Surg 1996; 61:1727–1733.
55. Bocchi EA, Higuchi ML, Vieira ML, et al. Higher incidence of malignant neoplasms after heart transplantation for treatment of chronic Chagas' heart disease. J Heart Lung Transplant 1998; 17:399–405.
56. Griepp RB, Stinson EB, Dong E, Jr., Clark DA, Shumway NE. Determinants of operative risk in human heart transplantation. Am J Surg 1971; 122:192–197.

57. Young JB, Naftel DC, Bourge RC, et al. Matching the heart donor and heart transplant recipient. Clues for successful expansion of the donor pool: a multivariable, multiinstitutional report. The Cardiac Transplant Research Database Group. J Heart Lung Transplant 1994; 13:353–364.
58. Costard-Jackle A, Hill I, Schroeder JS, Fowler MB. The influence of preoperative patient characteristics on early and late survival following cardiac transplantation. Circulation 1991; 84:III329–III337.
59. Semigran MJ, Cockrill BA, Kacmarek R, et al. Hemodynamic effects of inhaled nitric oxide in heart failure. J Am Coll Cardiol 1994; 24:982–988.
60. Loh E, Stamler JS, Hare JM, Loscalzo J, Colucci WS. Cardiovascular effects of inhaled nitric oxide in patients with left ventricular dysfunction. Circulation 1994; 90:2780–2785.
61. Wright RS, Levine MS, Bellamy PE, et al. Ventilatory and diffusion abnormalities in potential heart transplant recipients. Chest 1990; 98:816–820.
62. Bussieres LM, Cardella CJ, Daly PA, David TE, Feindel CM, Rebuck AS. Relationship between preoperative pulmonary status and outcome after heart transplantation. J Heart Transplant 1990; 9:124–128.
63. Young JN, Yazbeck J, Esposito G, Mankad P, Townsend E, Yacoub M. The influence of acute preoperative pulmonary infarction on the results of heart transplantation. J Heart Transplant 1986; 5:20–22.
64. Tazbir JS, Cronin DC. Indications, evaluations, and postoperative care of the combined liver-heart transplant recipient. AACN Clin Issues 1999; 10:240–252.
65. Burckart GJ, Venkataramanan R, Ptachcinski RJ, et al. Cyclosporine pharmacokinetic profiles in liver, heart, and kidney transplant patients as determined by high-performance liquid chromatography. Transplant Proc 1986; 18:129–136.
66. Lindelow B, Bergh CH, Herlitz H, Waagstein F. Predictors and evolution of renal function during 9 years following heart transplantation. J Am Soc Nephrol 2000; 11:951–957.
67. Rubel JR, Milford EL, McKay DB, Jarcho JA. Renal insufficiency and end-stage renal disease in the heart transplant population. J Heart Lung Transplant 2004; 23:289–300.
68. Narula J, Bennett LE, DiSalvo T, Hosenpud JD, Semigran MJ, Dec GW. Outcomes in recipients of combined heart-kidney transplantation: multiorgan, same-donor transplant study of the International Society of Heart and Lung Transplantation/United Network for Organ Sharing Scientific Registry. Transplantation 1997; 63:861–867.
69. Parameshwar J, Schofield P, Large S. Long-term complications of cardiac transplantation. Br Heart J 1995; 74:341–342.
70. van GT, Balk AH, Zietse R, Hesse C, Mochtar B, Weimar W. Renal insufficiency after heart transplantation: a case-control study. Nephrol Dial Transplant 1998; 13:2322–2326.
71. Sehgal V, Radhakrishnan J, Appel GB, Valeri A, Cohen DJ. Progressive renal insufficiency following cardiac transplantation: cyclosporine, lipids, and hypertension. Am J Kidney Dis 1995; 26:193–201.
72. Tinawi M, Miller L, Bastani B. Renal function in cardiac transplant recipients: retrospective analysis of 133 consecutive patients in a single center. Clin Transplant 1997; 11:1–8.
73. Marelli D, Laks H, Patel B, et al. Heart transplantation in patients with diabetes mellitus in the current era. J Heart Lung Transplant 2003; 22:1091–1097.
74. Grady KL, White-Williams C, Naftel D, et al. Are preoperative obesity and cachexia risk factors for post heart transplant morbidity and mortality: a multi-institutional study of preoperative weight–height indices. Cardiac Transplant Research Database (CTRD) Group. J Heart Lung Transplant 1999; 18:750–763.
75. Lietz K, John R, Burke EA, et al. Pretransplant cachexia and morbid obesity are predictors of increased mortality after heart transplantation. Transplantation 2001; 72:277–283.
76. Hosenpud JD, Pantely GA, Morton MJ, Norman DJ, Cobanoglu AM, Starr A. Relation between recipient: donor body size match and hemodynamics three months after heart transplantation. J Heart Transplant 1989; 8:241–243.

77. Morley D, Boigon M, Fesniak H, et al. Posttransplantation hemodynamics and exercise function are not affected by body-size matching of donor and recipient. J Heart Lung Transplant 1993; 12:770–778.
78. Falk RH, Comenzo RL, Skinner M. The systemic amyloidoses. N Engl J Med 1997; 337:898–909.
79. Merlini G, Bellotti V. Molecular mechanisms of amyloidosis. N Engl J Med 2003; 349:583–596.
80. Hosenpud JD, DeMarco T, Frazier OH, et al. Progression of systemic disease and reduced long-term survival in patients with cardiac amyloidosis undergoing heart transplantation. Follow-up results of a multicenter survey. Circulation 1991; 84:III338–III343.
81. Dubrey SW, Burke MM, Khaghani A, Hawkins PN, Yacoub MH, Banner NR. Long term results of heart transplantation in patients with amyloid heart disease. Heart 2001; 85:202–207.
82. Saba N, Sutton D, Ross H, et al. High treatment-related mortality in cardiac amyloid patients undergoing autologous stem cell transplant. Bone Marrow Transplant 1999; 24:853–855.
83. Mohty M, Albat B, Fegueux N, Rossi JF. Autologous peripheral blood stem cell transplantation following heart transplantation for primary systemic amyloidosis. Leuk Lymphoma 2001; 41:221–223.
84. Sudhakar SS, Bimalangshu DR, Falk RH, et al. Orthotopic heart transplantation in patients with cardiac amyloidosis. J Heart Lung Transplant 2005; 24:S122–S123.
85. Thaunat O, Alyanakian MA, Varnous S, et al. Long-term successful outcome of sequential cardiac and allogeneic bone marrow transplantations in severe AL amyloidosis. Bone Marrow Transplant 2005; 35:419–420.
86. Lee AH, Mull RL, Keenan GF, et al. Osteoporosis and bone morbidity in cardiac transplant recipients. Am J Med 1994; 96:35–41.
87. Berguer DG, Krieg MA, Thiebaud D, et al. Osteoporosis in heart transplant recipients: a longitudinal study. Transplant Proc 1994; 26:2649–2651.
88. Glendenning P, Kent GN, Adler BD, et al. High prevalence of osteoporosis in cardiac transplant recipients and discordance between biochemical turnover markers and bone histomorphometry. Clin Endocrinol (Oxf) 1999; 50:347–355.
89. Kerschan-Schindl K, Strametz-Juranek J, Heinze G, et al. Pathogenesis of bone loss in heart transplant candidates and recipients. J Heart Lung Transplant 2003; 22:843–850.
90. Braith RW, Magyari PM, Fulton MN, Aranda J, Walker T, Hill JA. Resistance exercise training and alendronate reverse glucocorticoid-induced osteoporosis in heart transplant recipients. J Heart Lung Transplant 2003; 22:1082–1090.
91. Baldwin JC, Anderson JL, Boucek MM, et al. Twenty fourth Bethesda conference: Cardiac transplantation. Task Force 2: Donor guidelines. J Am Coll Cardiol 1993; 22:15–20.
92. Marelli D, Laks H, Patel B, et al. Heart transplantation in patients with diabetes mellitus in the current era. J Heart Lung Transplant 2003; 22:1091–1097.
93. Johannes L. Double standard: For some transplant patients, diseased hearts are lifesavers. Surgeons enlist elderly, sick to receive inferior organs; the new ethical issues facing a risk of hepatitis C. Wall Street J 2005; 14:A1.
94. Wood KE, Becker BN, McCartney JG, D'Alessandro AM, Coursin DB. Care of the potential organ donor. N Engl J Med 2004; 351:2730–2739.
95. Zaroff JG, Rosengard BR, Armstrong WF, et al. Consensus conference report: maximizing use of organs recovered from the cadaver donor: cardiac recommendations, March 28–29, (2001), Crystal City, Va. Circulation 2002; 106:836–841.
96. www.ishlt.org/registries.

PART V: PSYCHOSOCIAL ISSUES

28
Education, Psychosocial Issues, and Sociodemographic Barriers in Heart Failure Disease Management

Aileen Aponte, Norma Osborn, Joanne R. Weintraub, and Michelle A. Young
Advanced Heart Disease Section, Cardiovascular Division, Brigham and Women's Hospital, Boston, Massachusetts, U.S.A.

INTRODUCTION

Key components in heart failure management include education, strategies for outpatient follow up, recognition of significant comorbidities, and barriers to care. This chapter reviews the importance of different learning styles and strategies, components of outpatient heart failure management, and the effect of depression and anxiety in this patient population. Sociodemographic barriers related to individual patients, providers, health care, and health care systems will also be discussed.

PATIENT EDUCATION

Patient education can be defined as an ongoing process of influencing patient behavior and producing the changes in knowledge, attitudes, and skills necessary to maintain or improve health (1). It is a professional responsibility of health care providers to be involved in the education of patients, families, and their communities to achieve optimal states of health. Nurses have become more aware of the potential benefits of educating patients with chronic diseases to become more independent with their self-care needs. Through health education, nurses can encourage the practice of healthy lifestyle behaviors, especially in patients with heart failure. As heart failure progresses, it becomes more difficult for patients to adapt to the lifestyle changes necessary to maintain health. The most important goal for patients with heart failure is to improve their self-care abilities such as restricting fluid and salt intake, adhering to their medication regimen, exercising, monitoring symptoms, and seeking assistance when symptoms worsen (2). Patients who are educated in self-care management to optimize their heart failure condition have fewer hospital admissions and improved quality of life (3).

CHALLENGES IN HEALTH EDUCATION

Health care providers need to communicate in a way to promote understanding, which requires open communication between the health care provider and their patient at all times. But this does not come without challenges. One of the more striking challenges is the knowledge deficit of both the patient and the educator. Nurses are the primary providers of patient education in most health care settings. A review of the literature found that no research has been done investigating specific learning needs of nurses who provide health education and care for patients with heart failure (3). "Heart failure nurses need to have experience in cardiac care and have the ability to work independently. They need to have a deeper understanding of the heart failure syndrome and its treatment, as well as a psychosocial aspect of being chronically ill and how to adapt to self-care behavior." (2) In the United States, this level of practice suggests advanced training at a university level where the nurse's training focuses on clinical decision-making, research, and skills. The nurses are Masters degree prepared and are trained as advanced practice nurses or clinical nurse specialists. Because the availability of advanced practice nurses is not always possible, it may benefit patients to have a multidiscipline team approach to education (2).

In addition, very little research has been done to assess the patient's knowledge of heart failure. Ni and colleagues assessed knowledge of and adherence to self-care among patients with heart failure in 1999. Of the 113 patients surveyed, he found that approximately 40% of patients did not recognize the importance of daily weights, only 80% knew they should limit salt intake, and 64% knew to limit fluid intake (4). Although knowledge alone does not ensure self-care compliance, we must remember that education is ongoing and encouragement and reinforcement are necessary for all.

Interpretation of medical information is another challenge in health education. Interpretation of information and educational level are individual. People have difficulty understanding health information for a variety of reasons including literacy, age, disability, language, culture, and emotion (5). Nearly 20% of Americans are functionally illiterate and lack the reading skills necessary for basic daily activities (6). *Healthy People 2010*, a United States public health initiative, stated "health literacy is the degree to which individuals have the capacity to obtain, process, and understand basic health information and services needed to make appropriate health decisions." (7) There are formal health literacy tests available to help assist in determining the needs of patients. Two formal health literacy tests are the REALM and TOFHLA. The REALM (Rapid Estimate of Adult Literacy in Medicine) is a reading recognition test that asks patients to pronounce 66 words commonly seen in medical settings, ranging in difficulty. This test provides grade level scores for people who read below the ninth-grade level. The TOFHLA (Test of Functional Health Literacy in Adults) is a series of health-related reading tasks that measure numeric and reading comprehension (5,8).

Barriers to health education include readiness to learn, fear that the illness cannot be cured, fear of being burdened by others, fear of dying, and fear of cost of hospitalization (1). The patients' needs must be considered before education can begin. In 1950, the Health Belief Model was developed to describe why people did not participate in educational programs to help treat or prevent diseases. Factors that contribute to a patient's perceived state of health and the probability of taking appropriate health care actions are (1) believing that they are susceptible to the ill-health condition in question, (2) believing that the condition would seriously affect their lives if they should contract it, (3) believing that the benefits of action outweigh the barriers to action, and, (4) they are confident that they can perform the action (9). "The Health Belief Model is used to assess whether the patient holds these beliefs, and if not, guides teaching at missing skills or information." (9).

Learning Strategies

To be an effective educator, one must be enthusiastic, have clinical competence, and provide a safe, nonjudgmental, non-threatening learning environment (10). This helps to motivate the patient and promotes a readiness to learn. It is important for the educator to also try to customize teaching to suit the patient's needs. The Joint Commission on Accreditation of Healthcare Organizations (JCAHO) states that a "patient receives education and training specific to patient's assessed needs, abilities, learning preferences, and readiness to learn as appropriate to the care and services provided by the hospital" (11).

Patient educators need to be aware of their patients' preferred learning style. The three most common learning styles used to gather and process information are visual, auditory, and kinesthetic (12). Highly visual learners prefer pictures, videos, anatomical charts, pamphlets, and drawings, while auditory learns prefer hearing new information through listening and reading, and highly kinesthetic people need to feel and be physically involved with their hands (12). Adapting individual learning styles to patient education can increase motivation and enhance learning.

In addition to learning styles, educators must be aware of individuals who are at higher risk of low literacy. This group may include people with less education, the elderly, certain racial or ethnic groups, and low socioeconomic populations (8). More than 90 million people do not understand the health information provided to them (13). People with less than 12 yr of education have an increase in mortality compared with people who have more than 13 yr of education. The elderly, racial, and ethnic minority population groups, as well as low-income families, have an increased risk of hospitalization with poor outcomes. Much of this is due to limited access to resources and the inability to possess health insurance (8,14).

Up to two thirds of hospital admissions for heart failure are attributed to problems with patient compliance. Educating patients and helping them take an active role in their self-care abilities can decrease hospitalizations and improve outcomes (15). To do this, health care providers need to be aware of several strategies when educating individuals and their families about their health. One must start by creating an environment that facilitates learning. A room where the temperature, sounds, lighting, furniture, supplies, and people involved provide comfort for each individual establishes the correct environment. A teachable moment, when the learner asks a question or a skill is being performed, allows for an appropriate time to educate. Whenever possible involve family members and use interpreters for foreign languages. It is important to individualize teaching to the patient's learning preferences. Use videotapes, verbal teaching, and demonstration as educational tools. Written teaching materials should be at a sixth-grade reading level or lower. Written grafts, charts, tables, and diagrams are best when simplified. Most importantly, try to evenly distribute information given to patients and families starting upon hospital admission through discharge and continue in the outpatient setting. Using a multidisciplinary approach to educating patients has also been shown to have better outcomes (8,11,12,16,17).

Health Educational Programs

An English philosopher Herbert Spencer once stated, "The great aim of education is not knowledge but action." (11) In order to motivate patients to learn about their health and become more independent with self-care, quality patient educational programs need to be established. Educational programs should "provide current information on such topics as health care issues, medications, and equipment; attempt to change inappropriate attitudes, beliefs and perceptions, when warranted; meet individual needs; be easy to access; facilitate evaluation; allow program changes to be made easily; and provide a framework that may be suitable for adaptation" (11). Creating educational materials for the targeted population should be done using the strategies mentioned above. An example of a heart failure patient educational program is seen in Table 1 (18).

Table 1 Heart Failure Patient Education Program

Teaching content	Self-care behaviors	Educational tips
Sodium restriction	Monitors sodium intake Reads nutritional labels and limits sodium intake	Recommend 2–3 g sodium diet Educate patient and family on food and preparation choices Teach the importance of sodium restrictions and how it affects fluid balance
Fluid restriction	Measures and records daily fluid intake Manages thirst without consuming excess fluid	Recommend 2–3 L fluid restriction according to patient's needs Encourage the use of lozenges, mints, or gum to quench one's thirst
Daily weights	Has scale and weighs each morning after voiding and before breakfast Limit amount of clothing when weighing self	Teach patient the connection between increased "water" weight and congestive heart failure Increase in more than 2 lbs overnight or 5 lbs in a week should be reported to RN/MD Some patients may be able to titrate diuretics based on daily weights
Medication compliance	Consistently follows prescribed medication schedule Monitors supply and plans for refills Has system (pill box, routine time) for monitoring own compliance Adjusts supplement diuretic dose based on weight	Medication education should include a written schedule with medication dose and frequency Simplify regimen to enhance adherence. Instruct patients when and how much supplemental diuretics to take according to increased weight
Exercise	Walks or participates in supervised program Avoids strenuous exercise, extreme temperatures, and heavy lifting	Teach the importance and benefit of aerobic exercise in patients with heart failure Enforce the importance of the balance of rest and activity
Sign and symptoms to be reported to health care provider	Call RN/MD with any change in severity of symptoms: weight gain >2 lbs overnight or 5 lbs in a week, shortness of breath or cough, chest pain, edema, abdominal bloating, dizziness, nausea, fatigue, using more pillows at night when sleeping, racing heart beat	Teach/counsel regarding signs and symptoms of heart failure Reinforcement of teaching information as needed

Evaluation of Health Education Programs

After implementing an educational program, it is essential to evaluate the effectiveness of the program. Learning can be evaluated at four different levels by asking a simple question at each level (1). The first level is the patient and family involvement during the interventions. "*Did they like it*?" Did the learners participate in discussion, ask questions and show interest. Second level is the patient performance immediately after the learning experience. "*Did they learn it?*" Did the learners meet the objectives? Were they able to return demonstration? The third level is the patient performance at home. "*Did they use it?*" Were they able to apply what they learned at home? The fourth level is the patient's overall self-care and health management. "*Was teaching worth it in the long run?*" Was there an improvement in health care outcomes? Was the patient's health maintained or improved? (1) Gathering feedback can be a useful tool in evaluating the educational program and implementing changes when necessary.

Heart failure patient education is a continuum. Patient education needs to start during the initial hospitalization and continue as an outpatient. A patient's condition often changes over time and learning needs may change, requiring additional teaching. Education should also be done as a multidisciplinary approach involving nurses, physicians, dieticians, physical therapists, and any other specialists involved in patient care. This allows for expert knowledge to be given to each patient by the most appropriate provider. Nevertheless, the most important goal in heart failure education is to assist patients in improving their self-care abilities such as dietary restriction, daily weights, medication compliance, exercise, and knowing symptoms of worsening heart failure and when to seek health care (2).

OUTPATIENT HEART FAILURE DISEASE MANAGEMENT

Transition from Inpatient to Outpatient Management

The heart failure patient's transition from inpatient care into the outpatient setting should involve careful discharge planning. The patient and family members need to be part of the multidisciplinary team and to begin the planning process shortly after admission to the hospital. The goal of integrating inpatient heart failure care with outpatient care is to maintain clinical stability and decrease the need for hospital readmission. Many patients may require multiple costly admissions for acute decomposition with 20% of hospitalized patients needing readmission within one month and up to 44% within 6 mo (19). Heart failure disease management tools have resulted in clinical benefit (20).

Participation in an HF management program may include comprehensive patient and family education, dietary assessment and instruction, social services consultation for discharge planning, clinical medication review, and intensive follow-up care. Patients who were randomized to receive intensive HF management services benefited from a 56.2% reduction of hospital readmissions compared with controls, with an overall cost savings of $460 per patient (20).

JCAHO, the nation's predominant source for healthcare accreditation, has developed core performance measures based on existing heart failure care guidelines. They include adequate discharge instructions which should address activity level, diet, discharge medication, follow-up appointment, weight monitoring, and what to do if symptoms worsen (21). Compliance with these expectations was assessed by using the data from Medicare beneficiaries and data acquired by the Acute Decompensated Heart Failure Registry (ADHERE) (22,23). During the hospitalization with acute decompensated heart failure, only 32% of patients were documented as having received instructions based on these heart failure guidelines (23).

The ACC/AHA Guidelines for the Evaluation and Management of Chronic Heart Failure in the Adult indicates that multidisciplinary disease-management programs for patients at high risk for hospital admission or clinical deterioration is a Class I recommendation: conditions for which there is evidence and/or general agreement that a given procedure therapy is useful and effective (24).

Strategies for Outpatient Disease Management

There are several strategies used for outpatient disease management of heart failure. The goal of most programs is to reduce re-hospitalization rates and costs and improve quality of life. Cardiovascular nurses play an integral role in implementing each of these strategies.

Specialty Heart Failure Clinics

Cardiologists and nurses with heart failure expertise direct care in a specialty clinic setting. The focus is outpatient care and continuous follow-up to maintain clinical stability. Heart failure cardiologists and nurses work together to manage patients after discharge by optimizing pharmacological therapy, providing hemodynamic monitoring, and continued teaching. A heart failure management team at the University of California, Los Angeles, Medical Center followed 214 patients who were in New York Heart Association functional class III or IV (25) and demonstrated during the 6 mo after referral to the clinic, there was a 85% reduction in hospital readmissions, improved functional status, and estimated savings in hospital readmission costs (after subtracting the initial hospital costs of $9800 per patient). This was accomplished by optimization of medications, education of patients and family members, telephone contact with patients in their homes, and frequent adjustment of diuretics for weight gain or postural hypotension.

Patient Management

Medications

Several medications are used in the treatment of heart failure that require careful titration based on physiologic data collected from the patient at each visit. Current medications should be reviewed at each visit. This may include the need for some patients to bring all their medications in the original containers to ensure compliance. The review of current medication should include over-the-counter medication that may exacerbate heart failure or cause dangerous drug–drug interactions.

The use of a wallet-sized card with the patient's current list of medications/allergies is encouraged. Strategies to increase compliance include utilizing once-a-day dosing when possible, devising a medication chart with times of administration, and filling pill containers with a week's worth of medicine. It is important to adopt a nonjudgmental attitude about medicine compliance to allow the patient to verbalize reasons for noncompliance. Many patients complain that the need for frequent urination interferes with their daily activities and helping the patient adjust their medication schedule in order to avoid unnecessary interruptions in their day should help compliance. Asking about a medication's cost is also helpful in ensuring compliance. Patients may need help with information about drug assistance programs or changing prescriptions to lower cost but effective medications. Asking for assistance from family members to help administer or remind patients to take medications is an effective strategy to increase adherence with medications (26).

Laboratory Testing

The use of diuretics and other medications used in heart failure necessitates laboratory monitoring. Renal and liver function, electrolyte monitoring, along with complete blood count to identify anemia that may aggravate a patient's heart failure, are important components in the heart failure management. Increased diuretic use may mandate more frequent monitoring and careful repletion of both potassium and magnesium to prevent dangerous dysrhythmias. Routine monitoring of digoxin levels is not indicated unless the patient has demonstrated clinical signs of toxicity or there is a concern for drug–drug interactions; however, digoxin levels above 0.8 may increase mortality (27). Brian natriuretic peptide (BNP) is secreted primarily from the ventricles of the heart in response to stretching and increased volume. BNP levels may be obtained to assess the severity of heart failure disease (28,29) and used to guide therapy (30).

Lifestyle Modifications

Daily Monitoring of Weight. Each clinic visit should include a carefully obtained weight measurement using the same scale and approximately the same amount of clothing without shoes. At each visit, patients should be asked for their concurrent home weights and be encouraged use a calendar at home to record serial weights.

Monitoring of Sodium and Fluid Restriction. Patients are queried about the adherence to sodium and fluid restriction (if applicable) and barriers to compliance are explored. Nutrition consultation may be necessary in refractory patients.

Exercise/Activity Level. Moderate exercise can produce sustained improvements in functional status and quality of life in patients with heart failure (31). Patient's activity level and regular participation in exercise are assessed at each visit. Patients in compensated heart failure are encouraged to stay active and participate in regular aerobic exercise. Barriers to exercise are also explored and referrals to cardiac rehabilitation programs, when indicated, may be helpful to overcome a patient's reticence to begin an exercise program.

Issues surrounding concerns about sexual activity also need to be addressed. Practitioners need to create an environment in which the patient/partner feels comfortable discussing difficulties/concerns over sexual activity and heart failure.

Home-Based Monitoring/Telemonitoring

Special care devices are connected through telephone lines, cable networks, or broadband technology to allow monitoring of physiologic markers such as weight, blood pressure, and heart rate on a daily basis. The information obtained is used to make adjustments to therapy and reduces the needs for office visits (32). The current data from telemanagement studies for heart failure patients suggest that telemonitoring might be most useful as an adjunct to specialized home-based disease management in order to quickly identify worsening signs/symptoms that require intervention (33,34).

DEPRESSION IN HEART FAILURE PATIENTS

Incidence of Depression

Heart failure, a major cause of disability and morbidity, often hinders the ability of patients to perform activities of daily living and support their families (35). Due to the development of heart failure symptoms and the physical limitations patients are at significant risk for the development of depression.

Depression is a relatively common condition among individuals with heart failure, with rates reported from 24% (36) to >40% (37) in patients with stable ambulatory heart failure (38) and has been linked to adverse outcomes. Depressive symptoms in patients with heart failure are strongly associated with a decline in health status (39,40) and an increase in the risk of hospitalization and death (38,40,41).

Symptoms of Depression in Heart Failure Patients

Chronic cardiac illness evokes depression through narcissistic injury, object loss, and guilt. Narcissistic injury occurs through the loss or threat of loss of functions, including limitations on occupational, recreational, and sexual activities. Death is the ultimate catastrophe for the self, but the losses associated with premature death carry different meaning depending on the person's particular emotional investments. A patient may feel robbed of seeing children grow up, providing for dependents, finishing a life's work or reaching a hard-earned retirement. Each of these real and feared losses is another blow to the individual's narcissism, and produces feelings of depression (42).

Heart failure causes symptoms that may be misinterpreted as representing a primary psychiatric disorder. Mild to moderate heart failure produces insomnia, anorexia, fatigue, weakness, and constipation, symptoms that may be mistakenly attributed to depression (42). In severe heart failure, patients may develop subtle or overt encephalopathy, including confusion, cognitive dysfunction, drowsiness, and apprehension (42).

Depression is suggested by pronounced feelings of guilt or worthlessness, suicidal ideation, anhedonia, and functional disability and affective disturbance that are out of proportion to the degree of heart failure (42). Depressed patients have difficulties adhering to their medical regimen and are unable to modify their lifestyle appropriately. These factors increase the probability of recurrent cardiac events and death.

Predictors of Development of Depression

Four predictors of the development of depressive symptoms in heart failure patients have been noted in a recent study. They include: living alone, alcohol abuse, financial burden from medical care, and worse baseline heart failure–specific health status (40). All patients with heart failure should be screened for depression, especially those who have one of the above risk factors. By knowing the risk factors for the development of depression, clinicians will be able to recognize and provide appropriate treatment for depressed heart failure patients.

Treatment of Depression in Heart Failure Patients

Patients with the depression risk factors may need psychosocial interventions, such as case management, social worker evaluation, cognitive therapy for social isolation, or alcohol abuse intervention (40).

Pharmacologic treatment of depression in cardiac patients has been studied. Most of the newer antidepressants such as the selective serotonin reuptake inhibitors do not have quinidine-like type 1 antiarrhythmic effects, which may cause prolongation of the Q-T and QRS interval, nor have they been associated with increases in heart rate, and most do not cause orthostatsis (42). The selective serotonin reuptake inhibitors have rarely been associated with bradycardia or sinus node dysfunction. Studies of the efficacy and safety of selective serotonin reuptake inhibitors appear to indicate they cause fewer adverse cardiac effects than tricyclic antidepressants (42).

Selective serotonin reuptake inhibitors should be the first line of pharmacologic therapy in the appropriate cardiac patient. Heart failure patients who elicit signs and symptoms of moderate to severe depression should be referred to psychiatry for further evaluation and treatment.

ANXIETY IN HEART FAILURE PATIENTS

Incidence of Anxiety

Psychiatric disorders frequently occur as complications or as comorbid conditions in individuals with cardiovascular disease. Surveys of ambulatory cardiology practice patients with documented heart disease show a 5% to 10% prevalence of anxiety disorders, predominantly panic attacks and phobias (43). The onset of symptomatic cardiac disease is a potent provocation for anxiety symptoms. Angina, arrhythmias, and acute heart failure produce anxiety caused by fears of heart attacks, disability, and sudden death (42).

Anxiety has been characterized as a strongly negative emotion with a component of fear. It is associated with cognitive, neurobiological, and behavioral manifestations and often is concurrently present with depression, especially in the elderly and in medically ill populations. Although anxiety and depression are highly correlated in heart failure patients, depression alone predicts a significantly worse prognosis for these patients (44,45).

Manifestations of Anxiety Disorders

Anxiety can be defined as a subjective sense of unease, dread, or foreboding. It can indicate a primary psychiatric condition or can be a component of, or reaction to, a primary medical disease (46).

When evaluating an anxious patient, it is important for the clinician to first determine whether the anxiety antedates or postdates a medical illness or if it is due to a medication side effect. Approximately one-third of patients presenting with anxiety have a medical etiology for their psychiatric symptoms (46).

The most common anxiety disorders associated with cardiac patients are: panic attacks, phobias, and post-traumatic stress disorder (PTSD). Panic attacks are episodes of distinct, intense fear and discomfort associated with several physical symptoms, including shortness of breath, palpitations, chest pain or discomfort, dizzy or light-headedness, abdominal distress or nausea, shaking or trembling, sweating, and a fear of impending doom or death (46). Since the symptoms of panic attacks are similar to those of heart failure and other cardiac conditions, a careful history will usually lead to a correct diagnosis. Once any medical etiology for the panic attack has been excluded, only then, can the diagnosis of panic disorder be made.

Phobic disorders are characterized by fear of objects or situations, which results immediately in an anxiety reaction (46). The stimulation of this phobia usually causes a panic attack. Some common phobias which cardiac patients experience are: fear of hospitals, blood, needles, and sudden cardiac death.

It is important for clinicians to be sensitive to various phobias and fears that patients may have. By providing appropriate psychotherapeutic interventions and reassurance it is possible to establish a stronger clinician-patient relationship.

PTSD is the development of anxiety after exposure to an extreme traumatic event such as the threat of personal death or injury or the death of a loved one (46). It is characterized by the re-experiencing of the traumatic event accompanied by symptoms of increased arousal and by avoidance of stimuli associated with the trauma (47). Patients who suffer from PTSD are preoccupied by negative health beliefs, and they exhibit more somatic complaints than patients without PTSD (47). PTSD is commonly seen in cardiac patients who have survived cardiac arrest, cardiac surgery, and those with implanted cardiac defibrillators. It is important for clinicians to identify patients suffering from PTSD early and refer them for appropriate treatment.

Treatment of Anxiety Disorders

Acute anxiety disorders are usually self-limited, and treatment typically involves the short-term use of benzodiazepines (46). Given orally, benzodiazepines are essentially free of cardiovascular side effects (42). Buspirone has no recognized cardiovascular side effects and may have a place in treatment of cardiac patients with anxiety disorders (42). Psychotherapeutic interventions such as cognitive behavioral therapy, desensitization therapy, and supportive/expressive psychotherapy (46) also play an important role in the treatment of anxiety disorders.

Due to the chronic and recurrent nature of PTSD, a more complex approach employing drug and behavioral treatments (46) must be implemented. The use of serotonin reuptake inhibitors has been effective in reducing symptoms of anxiety and avoidance behaviors in these patients. Psychotherapeutic strategies for PTSD help the patient overcome avoidance behaviors (46). Therapies that encourage the patient to dismantle avoidance behaviors through focusing stepwise on the experience of the traumatic event are most effective (46).

SOCIODEMOGRAPHIC BARRIERS TO CARE

Persistent health inequalities put people at risk for poor health outcomes. Racial, ethnic, and cultural differences can cause patients to be at risk for suboptimal health and health care. The elimination of health inequalities is described in Healthy People 2010 as a critical public health goal for the United States (7). Levine and colleagues believe that fundamental changes are needed to emphasize preventive care if the U.S. is to achieve current national health goals, based on their research showing that black-white age adjusted mortality and life expectancy at birth had "no sustained decrease" since 1945 (48). Among African Americans between 1960 and 2000, despite income and high school drop out rate disparities as compared to European Americans, mortality rates showed little improvement (49). The National Conference on Cardiovascular Disease Prevention concluded in 1999 that, while coronary heart disease mortality rates had decreased in the U.S. population as a whole, black Americans had the highest rates of stroke and coronary heart disease as compared to non-Hispanic whites, Native Americans, Asians, and Hispanics (50). Health care system and geodemographic characteristics can generate obstacles to optimal health care. An examination of cardiovascular mortality variances between groups in areas of high and low socioeconomic characteristics from 1969–1998 demonstrated continuing and growing inequalities. Mortality dropped in high socioeconomic group areas while increasing in deprived socioeconomic group areas. Twenty-one wide ranging socioeconomic status indicators included the following variables in men and women age 25–64 yr studied: education, income, occupation, unemployment and poverty rates, single-parent household rate, home ownership and home value, rent, mortgage, household crowding, English language proficiency, divorce rate, percent urban, percent immigrants, and the percent of households without access to phone, plumbing, and motor vehicle (51). Individual providers and patient profiles can also create impediments to ideal health care.

Sociodemographic barriers may be grouped into 4 overlapping categories: those related to individual patients, a health care provider, individual health care, and the health care system in general. Barriers related to individual patients include race, nationality/ethnicity, insurance, language, affordability of medicines, access to specialists, socioeconomic status, transportation, living environment/neighborhood, homelessness, telephone access, competing demands, education, and trust. Barriers related to a health care provider include lack of provider–patient concordance, bias/prejudice, and contrasting decision-making models or family structure. Barriers related to individual health care include perception of disease, health beliefs/attitudes, and diet. Finally, barriers related to a health care system include lack of interpreters, waiting time for providers, provider–patient concordance, and accessibility of health care delivery sites and specialists.

Barriers Related to Individual Patients

There is evidence of disparities in the cardiovascular care and health of African Americans versus European Americans as demonstrated in cardiovascular mortality (52), recommendation for cardiac catheterization (50,53–55), coronary artery bypass grafting (56,57), and diagnosis of hypercholesterolemia (59). Hill describes black males under age 50 yr as the "age-race-gender group" with the "least well diagnosed, treated and controlled hypertension" (59). In 1990 the Council on Ethical and Judicial Affairs of the American Medical Association published a call to decrease racial disparities in health care through greater access for blacks The report also called for increased black Americans in medical schools as faculty and students, and elimination of discriminatory clinical decision making through the use of treatment parameters eliminating racial criteria.

Lillie-Blanton has found that while people of color represent 34% of the U.S. population they compromise 52% of the uninsured. Compared to whites, Hispanics were less likely to have a "usual source of care" (60). This finding would make it more likely that Hispanics were also less likely to have a usual source of cardiovascular care. Lack of health insurance accounted for a significant segment of the disparity with income, education, family status citizenship, employment status, and health status accounting for small parts of the discrepancy (60). Undiagnosed hypertension in uninsured adults was found by Ayanian and colleagues to be more likely in Hispanics (58).

Immigrants categorized as noncitizens have been shown by Ku to be more likely than citizens to be uninsured and to have worse access to outpatient and emergency care (61). Differing ethnicity or national origin between a patient and a provider may set the stage for misunderstandings. Kagawa-Singer, et al., have stated that cultural insensitivity can contribute to inappropriate clinical outcomes and poor interactions with patients (62). Cohen has proposed that an increase in the racial and ethnic diversity of the health care workforce would improve health care access to minorities (63).

The equanimity in benefits in the federal Medicare program for those over age sixty-five has contributed greatly to decreasing barriers in access to health care due to lack of insurance in that age group. Prior to 1966 when Medicare coverage began, access to care for uninsured non-white elderly and disabled patients was severely limited. However, as a condition of Medicare reimbursement, hospitals were required to desegregate. The uninsured near-elderly (<65 yr) remains a population with substantial risk due to rises in health care costs with the onset of health problems typical at those ages—heart, lung, and cerebrovascular diseases, breast and colorectal cancers (64,65).

Desegregation of participating hospitals was a major step in improving access to care for racial and ethnic minorities (66). Ongoing work is being done by the United States Department of Health and Human Services (HHS) and the Centers for Medicare and Medicaid Services (CMS) to diminish remaining inequalities in care such as improving the Social Security Administration database on race and ethnicity, requiring fee-for-service health plans to implement initiatives to reduce "factors contributing to racial, ethnic, or rural disparities," (67) and using the Civil Rights Act (68) and court decisions to require providers to eliminate barriers to those not fluent in English. National standards for health care organizations published in December 2000 by the Office for Minority Health of HHS require the provision of linguistically competent services (69). The Director of Interpreter Services at Brigham and Women's Hospital in Boston, Massachusetts states that it is now possible to access via telephone or in person competent interpreter services for patients in more than 150 different languages from American Sign Language to Cambodian to Macedonian to Zulu. Spanish-speaking patients with a Spanish-speaking doctor have been shown to better follow medical treatment plans and have fewer emergency room visits than those patients without a doctor competent in their language (70).

A study by Federman and colleagues based on Medicare claims showed that elders with Medicare insurance but no supplemental drug coverage were less likely to be using statin therapy than elders with Medicare and supplemental drug coverage and elders with Medicaid coverage. This result was hypothesized to be due to the increased cost of statins with non-generic equivalents over other cardiovascular medications such as diuretics and beta-blockers (71).

Care by specialists can influence outcomes. Ayanian studied 35,520 patients post–myocardial infarction aged 65 yr or older in seven states in the United States to find that patients seeing cardiologists as opposed to internists or family practice physicians were more likely to be white, have undergone an invasive cardiac procedure, and had a lower 2 yr mortality rate (72). Evidenced-based care and improved outcomes in the treatment of coronary disease and heart failure are thought to be more likely with care by cardiologists (73). Geographic area may influence access to specialists. Improvement in implantation of internal cardiac defibrillators (ICD) for blacks versus whites occurred between 1990–2000 in part because more varied geographic locations began to provide ICD implantation in areas of larger black populations (74).

Low socioeconomic status (SES) as defined by education and income has been found to negatively impact health. A review of the literature by (75) Blair et al found that only 8 clinical studies addressed the connection between congestive heart failure and SES. Low SES was found to have a negative effect on health status on hospital admission, and being listed for cardiac transplant.

In people aged 25 yr or older in the United States, House et al. (76) found that preventable health problems are more prevalent in lower socioeconomic groups during their thirties and forties while higher socioeconomic groups are able to postpone morbidity and health decline to their sixties and seventies. Williams and Jackson (77) state that cardiovascular mortality in low-income black women is 65% higher than their white counterparts.

Poor access to transportation may create another obstacle to good health care by preventing a person from being able to get to appointments. In households in 12 rural western North Carolina counties, patients able to drive had more than double the chronic care health appointments than non-drivers. Also, those who had friends or family who could drive the patient to an appointment had 1.58 more chronic health care check ups than those who had no transportation support (78).

Lower socioeconomic groups may live in neighborhoods with characteristics that create barriers to optimal health. Cheadle and colleagues (79) in 1991 found correlation between the availability of healthy food in grocery stores and the healthy dietary practices of residents. In 2001 Perry (80) found that low-income neighborhoods in Philadelphia had 30% fewer supermarkets than high-income neighborhoods and had higher diet related deaths in 3 areas: neoplasms (stomach, other digestive disorders, breast); endocrine, nutritional, and immunity disorders (diabetes mellitus); and circulatory system diseases (hypertension, myocardial infarction, heart disease). Fulp (81) and colleagues described the inability of 2 groups of women (aged 65 yr and older living alone, and less than 65 yr with children 18 yr and younger living at home) to purchase a nutritionally adequate diet in their community. Demographic descriptors of this community include the following data: 52% blacks, 22% Hispanic, 29% of residents living below the federal poverty level, mean household income in 1999 of $26,515, 29% with less than a high school education or general equivalence degree, 51% overweight or obese, 29% MD-diagnosed hypertension, 38.4% diabetes mortality. Proposals to increase access to healthy food through food stamps for farmers' markets, increase healthy selections at local convenience stores, schools and workplaces, and development of supermarkets in low income areas may lessen this problem.

One could hypothesize that homelessness would also be a substantial barrier to positive health outcomes. Though there were no studies found of the relationship between heart failure and homelessness, Dewan (82) and colleagues found that both homelessness and congestive heart failure were independent risk factors for mortality in a study of tuberculosis treatment in Orel, Russia. Lack of a telephone could easily be suspected of being a barrier to care by causing or increasing isolation, and lack of or difficult communication with health care resources. Competing demands in an individual's life such as child or elder care, schooling or work, life-maintenance activities (grocery shopping, laundry, legal business, vehicle maintenance, or other tasks deemed essential), and health care visits could easily cause a person to put off a health care visit.

Lack of education can also be a barrier to health. In an examination of data on cause of death from longitudinal mortality studies between 1990–1997 Huisman et al. (83) found that all causes of death at age 75 or older except prostate cancer in men and lung cancer in women, showed increased mortality in the less educated as compare to the more educated groups. Cardiovascular death accounted for differences of 39% for men and 60% for women.

Trust is an essential component in breaching potential cross-cultural barriers just as it is key to a positive patient–provider relationship within similar cultural contexts. Racism exemplified by the Tuskegee syphilis study and segregation in hospitals is well known as a health care barrier to older African-Americans. The syphilis study, The Tuskegee Study of Untreated Syphilis in the Negro Male, conducted by the United States Public Health Service from 1932–1972 withheld treatment for syphilis for up to 40 yr (84). Approximately 250 men received military exemptions in 1941 during World War II, and local physicians agreed not to treat study subjects despite the availability of penicillin in 1943. In 1972 a Senate investigation stopped the study after a United States Public Health Service officer questioned the ethics of the study. In recent times patient trust in research physicians and health care systems, particularly managed care, has eroded with concerns about denial of therapeutic or diagnostic procedures and emergency care, and financial incentives for minimal care (84,85). Trust in a specialist after an initial visit has been found to be greater in whites than in blacks and Hispanics (86).

Barriers Related to a Health Care Provider

Provider concordance may influence trust in the patient-provider relationship. Race and gender discordance are associated with less satisfaction in participative decision making during visits with physicians. African American and minority patients perceive their physician appointments as less participatory than whites in an analysis of physicians' participatory decision-making style ratings by their patients (87). Suspicion of race or gender bias may influence patient perceptions of a discordant provider. Evidence of poorer outcomes in non-white patients has been discussed earlier. Language discordance between provider and patient as a socioeconomic variable associated with poorer health outcomes has been a significant factor, influencing the United States Department of HHS to require competent interpreters in health care facilities (7).

Differences in health care decision-making style can create dissonance between provider and patient. Blackhall et al. (88), in a study of 200 subjects from four differing ethnicities found that patients of Korean American and Mexican American families may prefer a family centered decision-making model instead of the patient autonomy model of African-American or European-American families. Decisions studied included whether or not a patient should be told of a terminal diagnosis, and whether a patient should make decisions about life support. A physician who urges a family or patient to make an autonomous decision in the above family would risk alienating the patient and family.

Barriers Related to Individual Health Care

In patients with heart failure, women have been shown to have more positive perceptions about their own health than men in research examining physical impairment (decreased functional ability and vitality, symptom distress), role limitation (personal and professional, change in self concept), loss (independence, control), and emotional burden (fear of death, hopelessness, depression, anger, anxiety) (89). Perception of and adjustment to illness may be a substantially large barrier to males. Horowitz (90) and colleagues studied patient perception and health behavior finding that patients in an urban hospital perceived congestive heart failure as only an acute condition and therefore did not try to imbed heart failure self-care into their daily routines. These findings suggest that emphasis should be on describing heart failure as a chronic condition. Ayanian et al. (91) found that in 3 different regions of the U.S. patients who believed that lowering cholesterol was very important were more likely to be women and ironically, patients without diabetes mellitus or heart failure. Males and smokers put a lower value on cholesterol treatment and may require more education to adjust their health beliefs.

Dietary habits are deeply ingrained cultural behaviors. When dietary habits conflict with the best clinical advice for heart failure, cultural sensitivity is required to negotiate optimum health. A typical day in a heart failure management clinic may include interactions with a Russian elder who cherishes sausage and occasional caviar, a Thai homemaker cooking with fish sauce on a daily basis, a retired Greek businessman who eats feta and olives for breakfast, and several Caucasian American men who eat out or use packaged microwave foods exclusively because of lack of cooking skills. Abundant time, counseling, creativity, and nutrition consults may be necessary to convert patients to eating patterns that more closely resemble a low sodium diet.

Barriers Related to a Health Care System

Current Medicare and Medicaid guides provide a benefit of 12 wk participation in a cardiac rehabilitation program for patients who "within the preceding 12 mo have had acute myocardial infarction, coronary artery bypass, or have stable angina pectoris." (92) Unfortunately, there is no benefit for patients with congestive heart failure, angioplasty, or transplantation without the above inclusion criteria. Patients with heart failure would benefit greatly from an insured benefit for cardiac rehabilitation. Presently, such programs are only available if the individual patient is willing to pay for the program at great expense or if a private insurer provides such a benefit.

Solutions

Creative, persistent, targeted long-term and short-term solutions are required by a coalition of the concerned to achieve health care equity in the United States as well as the world community. Thankfully, citizens, clinicians, academics, and policy makers believe that solutions such as those below will bring the goal of optimal health care for all closer to reality. Kennedy (93) proposes an increase in minority population access to care through expansion of Medicare, improved cultural competence and diversity of providers, expansion of health data collection by race and ethnicity, and investment in the entire public health infrastructure. Development of geocoding databases using race, ethnicity, and socioeconomic status characteristics to specifically identify health disparities by area and neighborhood, and create area-specific interventions has been suggested by Fremont (94). A "state minority health care report card" developed by Trivedi (95) and colleagues would include analysis of non-elderly low-income insurance coverage, physician workforce diversity, promotion of minority health by agencies of state government, and mortality by race and ethnicity to focus attention on areas in need of health care intervention. Grass roots efforts in the corporate sector are underway such as diabetes chronic disease management, Breast Health Initiative programs and African American Preterm Labor Prevention and Breastfeeding programs at the health care insurer, Aetna (96). Verizon Communications is contributing to the elimination of health disparities by implementing 3 recommendations of the Institute of Medicine of the Department of HHS. These include increasing health disparities awareness among Verizon employees and the public, creating employee education programs on access to care and treatment decision-making, and health care access data collection involving sociodemographic characteristics (97).

Focus, diligence, funding, and imaginative programs such as those described will contribute greatly to eradicating health disparities in this decade. Optimal health for all can be accomplished.

REFERENCES

1. Rankin SH, Stallings KD, London F. Patient Education in Health and Illness. Philadelphia: Lippincott, 2005.
2. Stromberg A. Educating nurses and patients to manage heart failure. Eur J Cardiovasc Nurs 2002; 1:33–40.

3. Albert NM, Collier S, Sumodi V, et al. Nurses' knowledge of heart failure education principles. Heart & Lung: The Journal of Acute and Critical Care. Elsevier. ISSN#01479653. 2002.
4. Ni H, Nauman D, Burgess D, Wise K, Crispell K, Hershberger RE. Factors influencing knowledge of and adherence to self-care among patients with heart failure. Arch Intern Med 1999; 159:1613–1619.
5. Osborne H. Health Literacy from A to Z. Jones and Bartlett. 2005. Sudbury, MA.
6. Vanderberg-Dent S. Part II. Challenges in educating patients. Dis Mon 2000; 46:798–810.
7. Services UDoHaH. Healthy People 2010: Understanding and Improving Health. Washington: US GPO, 2000.
8. International R. Literacy and Health Outcomes. North Carolina: University of North Carolina Evidence Bases Practice Center. Agency for Healthcare Research and Quality, 2004.
9. Redman BK. The Practice of Patient Educaion. St. Louis, Missouri: Mosby, 2001.
10. Buchel TL, Edwards FD. Characteristics of effective clinical teachers. Fam Med 2005; 37:30–35.
11. Organizations TJCoAoH. The Joint Commission Guide to Patient and Family Education. Illinois: Joint Commission Resources, 2003.
12. Chase TM. Learning styles and teaching strategies: enhancing the patient education experience. SCI Nurs 2001; 18:138–141.
13. Academies IoMotN. Health Literacy: A prescription to End Confusion. Washington, DC: National Academies Press, 2004.
14. Rudd K, Yamamoto K. Literacy and Health in America. Princeton, NJ: Center for Global Assessment Educational Testing Services, 2004.
15. Koelling TM, Johnson ML, Cody RJ, Aaronson KD. Discharge Education Improves Clinical Outcomes and Adherence to Self-Care Measures in Patients with Chronic Heart Failure. American Heart Association Scientific Sessions 2003 AOP.62.1.
16. London F. No Time To Teach. Philadelphia: Lippincott, 1999.
17. Jaarsma T, Halfens R, Tan F, Abu-Saad HH, Dracup K, Diederiks J. Self-care and quality of life in patients with advanced heart failure: the effect of a supportive educational intervention. Heart Lung 2000; 29:319–330.
18. Rutledge DND, Nancy E, Pravikoff, Diane S. Patient Education in Disease and Symptom Management: Congestive Heart Failure. ONline J Clin Innovations 2001; 4:1–52.
19. Krumholz HM, Parent EM, Tu N, et al. Readmission after hospitalization for congestive heart failure among Medicare beneficiaries. Arch Intern Med 1997; 157:99–104.
20. Rich MW, Beckham V, Wittenberg C, Leven CL, Freedland KE, Carney RM. A multidisciplinary intervention to prevent the readmission of elderly patients with congestive heart failure. N Engl J Med 1995; 333:1190–1195.
21. Joint Commission on Accreditation of Healthcare Organizations D-SCHFEP. Disease-specific care standardized heart failure measure set. On-line http://www.jcaho.org/dscc/dsc/performance+measures/heart+failure+measure+set.htm: http//www.jcaho.org/dscc/dsc/performance+measures/heart+failure+measure+set.htm, 1997:Vol. 2004.
22. Adams KF, Fonarow GC, Emerman CL. Characteristics and outcomes of patients hospitalized for heart failure in the United states (2001–2003): rationale, design and preliminary observations from the Acute Decompensated Heart Failure National Registry (ADHERE). Am Heart J, In Press.
23. Fonarow GC, Yancy CW, Chang SF. Variation in heart failure quality of care indicators among U.S. hospitals: analysis of 230 hospitals in the ADHERE registry. J Card Fail 2003;S82.
24. ACC/AHA Guidelines for the Evaluation and Management of Chronic Heart Failure in the Adult. A Report of the American College of Cardiology/American Heart Association Task Force on Practice Guidelines, 2001.
25. Fonarow GC, Stevenson LW, Walden JA, et al. Impact of a comprehensive heart failure management program on hospital readmission and functional status of patients with advanced heart failure. J Am Coll Cardiol 1997; 30:725–732.

26. Grady KL, Dracup K, Kennedy G, et al. Team management of patients with heart failure: A statement for healthcare professionals from The Cardiovascular Nursing Council of the American Heart Association. Circulation 2000; 102:2443–2456.
27. Beller GA, Smith TW, Abelmann WH, Haber E, Hood WB, Jr. Digitalis intoxication. A prospective clinical study with serum level correlations. N Engl J Med 1971; 284:989–997.
28. Lee SC, Stevens TL, Sandberg SM, et al. The potential of brain natriuretic peptide as a biomarker for New York Heart Association class during the outpatient treatment of heart failure. J Card Fail 2002; 8:149–154.
29. Group DI. The Effect of Digoxin on Mortality and Morbidity in Patients with Heart Failure. N Engl J Med 1997; 336:525–533.
30. Troughton RW, Frampton CM, Yandle TG, Espiner EA, Nicholls MG, Richards AM. Treatment of heart failure guided by plasma aminoterminal brain natriuretic peptide (N-BNP) concentrations. Lancet 2000; 355:1126–1130.
31. Belardinelli R, Georgiou D, Cianci G, Purcaro A. Randomized, controlled trial of long-term moderate exercise training in chronic heart failure: effects on functional capacity, quality of life, and clinical outcome. Circulation 1999; 99:1173–1182.
32. Louis AA, Turner T, Gretton M, Baksh A, Cleland JG. A systematic review of telemonitoring for the management of heart failure. Eur J Heart Fail 2003; 5:583–590.
33. Cordisco ME, Benjaminovitz A, Hammond K, Mancini D. Use of telemonitoring to decrease the rate of hospitalization in patients with severe congestive heart failure. Am J Cardiol 1999; 84:860–862 see also p. A8.
34. Knox D, Mischke L. Implementing a congestive heart failure disease management program to decrease length of stay and cost. J Cardiovasc Nurs 1999; 14:55–74.
35. Garg R, Packer M, Pitt B, Yusuf S. Heart failure in the 1990s: evolution of a major public health problem in cardiovascular medicine. J Am Coll Cardiol 1993; 22:3A–5A.
36. Havranek EP, Ware MG, Lowes BD. Prevalence of depression in congestive heart failure. Am J Cardiol 1999; 84:348–350 see also p. A9.
37. Skotzko CE, Krichten C, Zietowski G, et al. Depression is common and precludes accurate assessment of functional status in elderly patients with congestive heart failure. J Card Fail 2000; 6:300–305.
38. Vaccarino V, Kasl SV, Abramson J, Krumholz HM. Depressive symptoms and risk of functional decline and death in patients with heart failure. J Am Coll Cardiol 2001; 38:199–205.
39. Rumsfeld JS, Havranek E, Masoudi FA, et al. Depressive symptoms are the strongest predictors of short-term declines in health status in patients with heart failure. J Am Coll Cardiol 2003; 42:1811–1817.
40. Havranek EP, Spertus JA, Masoudi FA, Jones PG, Rumsfeld JS. Predictors of the onset of depressive symptoms in patients with heart failure. J Am Coll Cardiol 2004; 44:2333–2338.
41. Jiang W, Alexander J, Christopher E, et al. Relationship of depression to increased risk of mortality and rehospitalization in patients with congestive heart failure. Arch Intern Med 2001; 161:1849–1856.
42. Levenson JL, Dwight M. Cardiology. In: Stoudemire A, Fogel B, Greenberg D, eds. Psychiatric Care of the Medical Patient. New York: Oxford University Press, 2002:717–731.
43. Shapiro P. In: Sadock B, Sadock V, eds. Cardiovascular disorders. In: Comprehensive Textbook of Psychiatry, Vol. 2. Philadelphia: Lippincott Williams & Wilkins, 2005:2136–2148.
44. Conwell Y. Suicide in elderly patients. In: Schneider LS, Reynolds CT, Lebowitz BD, eds. Diagnosis and Treatment of Depression in Late Life. Washington, D.C.: American Psychiatric Press, 1996:397–418.
45. Jiang W, Kuchibhatla M, Cuffe MS, et al. Prognostic value of anxiety and depression in patients with chronic heart failure. Circulation 2004; 110:3452–3456.
46. Reus V. In: Kasper D, Braunwald E, Fauci A, Longo D, Hauser S, Jameson L, eds. Mental Disorders. In: Harrison's Principles of Internal Medicine, Vol. 2. New York: McGraw-Hill, 2005:2547–2561.
47. Ladwig KH, Schoefinius A, Dammann G, Danner R, Gurtler R, Herrmann R. Long-acting psychotraumatic properties of a cardiac arrest experience. Am J Psychiatry 1999; 156:912–919.

48. Levine RS, Foster JE, Fullilove RE, et al. Black–white inequalities in mortality and life expectancy, 1933–1999: implications for healthy people 2010. Public Health Rep 2001; 116:474–483.
49. Satcher D, Fryer GE, Jr, McCann J, Troutman A, Woolf SH, Rust G. What if we were equal? A comparison of the black-white mortality gap in 1960 and 2000 Health Aff (Millwood) 2005; 24:459–464.
50. Cooper R, Cutler J, Desvigne-Nickens P, et al. Trends and disparities in coronary heart disease, stroke, and other cardiovascular diseases in the United States: findings of the national conference on cardiovascular disease prevention. Circulation 2000; 102:3137–3147.
51. Singh GK, Siahpush M. Increasing inequalities in all-cause and cardiovascular mortality among US adults aged 25–64 yr by area socioeconomic status, 1969–1998. Int J Epidemiol 2002; 31:600–613.
52. Fang J, Madhavan S, Alderman MH. The association between birthplace and mortality from cardiovascular causes among black and white residents of New York City. N Engl J Med 1996; 335:1545–1551.
53. Schulman KA, Berlin JA, Harless W, et al. The effect of race and sex on physicians' recommendations for cardiac catheterization. N Engl J Med 1999; 340:618–626.
54. Chen J, Rathore SS, Radford MJ, Wang Y, Krumholz HM. Racial differences in the use of cardiac catheterization after acute myocardial infarction. N Engl J Med 2001; 344:1443–1449.
55. Ferguson JA, Tierney WM, Westmoreland GR, et al. Examination of racial differences in management of cardiovascular disease. J Am Coll Cardiol 1997; 30:1707–1713.
56. Wenneker MB, Epstein AM. Racial inequalities in the use of procedures for patients with ischemic heart disease in Massachusetts. Jama 1989; 261:253–257.
57. Peterson ED, Shaw LK, DeLong ER, Pryor DB, Califf RM, Mark DB. Racial variation in the use of coronary-revascularization procedures. Are the differences real? Do they matter? N Engl J Med 1997; 336:480–486.
58. Ayanian JZ, Zaslavsky AM, Weissman JS, Schneider EC, Ginsburg JA. Undiagnosed hypertension and hypercholesterolemia among uninsured and insured adults in the Third National Health and Nutrition Examination Survey. Am J Public Health 2003; 93:2051–2054.
59. Hill MN, Bone LR, Hilton SC, Roary MC, Kelen GD, Levine DM. A clinical trial to improve high blood pressure care in young urban black men: recruitment, follow-up, and outcomes. Am J Hypertens 1999; 12:548–554.
60. Lillie-Blanton M, Hoffman C. The role of health insurance coverage in reducing racial/ethnic disparities in health care. Health Aff (Millwood) 2005; 24:398–408.
61. Ku L, Matani S. Left out: immigrants' access to health care and insurance. Health Aff (Millwood) 2001; 20:247–256.
62. Kagawa-Singer M, Chung R. A paradigm for culturally based care for minority populations. J Community Psychol 1994;192–208.
63. Cohen JJ, Gabriel BA, Terrell C. The case for diversity in the health care workforce. Health Aff (Millwood) 2002; 21:90–102.
64. McWilliams JM, Zaslavsky AM, Meara E, Ayanian JZ. Impact of medicare coverage on basic clinical services for previously uninsured adults. JAMA 2003; 290:757–764.
65. US Department of Health and Human Services OoDPaHP. Clinicians Handbook of Preventive Services: Putting Prevention into Practice. Washington: US GPO, 1994.
66. Smith DB. Racial and ethnic health disparities and the unfinished civil rights agenda. Health Aff (Millwood) 2005; 24:317–324.
67. Eichner J, Vladeck BC. Medicare as a catalyst for reducing health disparities. Health Aff (Millwood) 2005; 24:365–375.
68. Title VI of the 1964 Civil Rights Act, 42 U.S.C. Sec. 2000d (1964).
69. Services UDoHaH. Assuring cultural competence in health care: recommendations for national standards and an outcome-focused research agenda. In: 80865 FR, ed, 2000.

70. Brach C, Fraser I, Paez K. Crossing the language chasm. Health Aff (Millwood) 2005; 24:424–434.
71. Federman AD, Adams AS, Ross-Degnan D, Soumerai SB, Ayanian JZ. Supplemental insurance and use of effective cardiovascular drugs among elderly medicare beneficiaries with coronary heart disease. Jama 2001; 286:1732–1739.
72. Ayanian JZ, Landrum MB, Guadagnoli E, Gaccione P. Specialty of ambulatory care physicians and mortality among elderly patients after myocardial infarction. N Engl J Med 2002; 347:1678–1686.
73. Go AS, Rao RK, Dauterman KW, Massie BM. A systematic review of the effects of physician specialty on the treatment of coronary disease and heart failure in the United States. Am J Med 2000; 108:216–226.
74. Groeneveld PW, Heidenreich PA, Garber AM. Trends in implantable cardioverter-defibrillator racial disparity: the importance of geography. J Am Coll Cardiol 2005; 45:72–78.
75. Blair AS, Lloyd-Williams F, Mair FS. What do we know about socioeconomic status and congestive heart failure? A review of the literature J Fam Pract 2002; 51:169.
76. House JS, Lepkowski JM, Kinney AM, Mero RP, Kessler RC, Herzog AR. The social stratification of aging and health. J Health Soc Behav 1994; 35:213–234.
77. Williams DR, Jackson PB. Social sources of racial disparities in health. Health Aff (Millwood) 2005; 24:325–334.
78. Arcury TA, Preisser JS, Gesler WM, Powers JM. Access to transportation and health care utilization in a rural region. J Rural Health 2005; 21:31–38.
79. Cheadle A, Psaty BM, Curry S, et al. Community-level comparisons between the grocery store environment and individual dietary practices. Prev Med 1991; 20:250–261.
80. Perry D. The need for more supermarkets in Philadelphia: Food for every child. Philadelphia: The Food Trust, 2001.
81. Fulp RS, McManus KD, Johnson PA. Food stamps benefits are inadequate to purchase heart-healthy, culturally appropriate foods in a low-income African American Community. Circulation 2004; 110:800.
82. Dewan PK, Arguin PM, Kiryanova H, et al. Risk factors for death during tuberculosis treatment in Orel, Russia. Int J Tuberc Lung Dis 2004; 8:598–602.
83. Huisman M, Kunst AE, Bopp M, et al. Educational inequalities in cause-specific mortality in middle-aged and older men and women in eight western European populations. Lancet 2005; 365:493–500.
84. Francis CK. The medical ethos and social responsibility in clinical medicine. J Natl Med Assoc 2001; 93:157–169.
85. Kassirer JP. Managed care and the morality of the marketplace. N Engl J Med 1995; 333:50–52.
86. Keating NL, Gandhi TK, Orav EJ, Bates DW, Ayanian JZ. Patient characteristics and experiences associated with trust in specialist physicians. Arch Intern Med 2004; 164:1015–1020.
87. Cooper-Patrick L, Gallo JJ, Gonzales JJ, et al. Race, gender, and partnership in the patient-physician relationship. JAMA 1999; 282:583–589.
88. Blackhall LJ, Murphy ST, Frank G, Michel V, Azen S. Ethnicity and attitudes toward patient autonomy. JAMA 1995; 274:820–825.
89. Evangelista LS, Kagawa-Singer M, Dracup K. Gender differences in health perceptions and meaning in persons living with heart failure. Heart Lung 2001; 30:167–176.
90. Horowitz CR, Rein SB, Leventhal H. A story of maladies, misconceptions and mishaps: effective management of heart failure. Soc Sci Med 2004; 58:631–643.
91. Ayanian JZ, Landon BE, Landrum MB, Grana JR, McNeil BJ. Use of cholesterol-lowering therapy and related beliefs among middle-aged adults after myocardial infarction. J Gen Intern Med 2002; 17:95–102.
92. Article for what are covered diagnoses for Cardiac Rehabilitation Programs? (A14132) Medicare Coverage Database. www.cms.hhs.gov.access. 5/25/2005.
93. Kennedy EM. The role of the federal government in eliminating health disparities. Health Aff (Millwood) 2005; 24:452–458.

94. Fremont AM, Bierman A, Wickstrom SL, et al. Use of geocoding in managed care settings to identify quality disparities. Health Aff (Millwood) 2005; 24:516–526.
95. Trivedi AN, Gibbs B, Nsiah-Jefferson L, Ayanian JZ, Prothrow-Stith D. Creating a state minority health policy report card. Health Aff (Millwood) 2005; 24:388–396.
96. Hassett P. Taking on racial and ethnic disparities in health care: the experience at Aetna. Health Aff (Millwood) 2005; 24:417–420.
97. Izair AC. Verizon works to eliminate disparities in health care for its divers workforce. Health Aff 2005; 24:421–423.

29

Prognosis Assessment and End of Life Issues

Eldrin F. Lewis
Advanced Heart Disease Section, Cardiovascular Division, Brigham and Women's Hospital, Harvard Medical School, Boston, Massachusetts, U.S.A.

Carol M. Flavell
Advanced Heart Disease Section, Cardiovascular Division, Brigham and Women's Hospital, Boston, Massachusetts, U.S.A.

INTRODUCTION

Heart failure is a complex, progressive disease with unexpected acute exacerbations and decreased functional status, marked symptom burden due to dyspnea and fatigue, and impaired quality of life (1,2). Although there are various etiologies for the disease, the development of heart failure is associated with a dramatic worsening of the prognosis of the patient (3). Despite the improvement in outcomes of heart failure patients over the past few decades, survival following the diagnosis of heart failure remains poor with a median survival of 8 years and an estimated median survival of 1.64 years after a discharge for decompensated heart failure (4). Given the poor prognosis overall in heart failure patients, there have been intense efforts to identify those patients at particularly high risk of early mortality to aid in counseling and medical decision making. Therefore, many factors have been identified as markers of short- and long-term poor prognosis (5–7). These prognostic factors are often identified through clinical experience, epidemiologic cohorts, and large, clinical trials, and they can be grouped into several categories including clinical, hemodynamic, electrophysiological, and biochemical markers. A detailed discussion of prognostic factors in heart failure patients is found elsewhere in this text.

Most of the prognostic factors that have been identified are more specific for progressive pump failure death. Clinicians often have an idea of the *long-term* prognosis of patients after a detailed history and physical examination, routine laboratory tests, echocardiography, and right- and left-heart cardiac catheterization. Although a cross-sectional assessment of this information may provide insight into the patient's prognosis, longitudinal follow-up of patients gives additional information about the trajectory of the natural history in an individual patient. This is particularly important after the initial patient referral. For example, patients may present with advanced symptoms at the time of initial therapy. If their symptom status and functional status can be improved with therapy, that patient's prognosis is much better than the patient who remains in an advanced heart failure state despite medical management (5). Moreover, discussion of long-term prognosis is challenging in that one must give the patient optimism about the ability to maximize survival with advancing medical therapies while ensuring that they have a realistic understanding of their shortened life expectancy. Therefore, clinicians often *think* of prognosis and incorporate this prognostic information into medical decision making more frequently than they actually *discuss* prognosis with the patient and their families.

CLINICAL USE OF PROGNOSTIC FACTORS

Healthcare providers use prognostic factors in many ways. First, recognizing the patients with poor prognostic markers allows targeting of the population most likely to benefit from a medical therapy (8). Secondly, patients and families often seek an estimate of prognosis to address fears that are associated with the diagnosis of heart failure and for reassurance that they do not need immediate transplantation. Clinicians may use prognostic factors to assist in determining the optimal targets of therapy. The timing of transplant evaluation or referral to an advanced heart failure provider is often guided by the short-term prognosis. Finally, prognostic factors can be followed serially to determine if a patient is responding to treatment. These prognostic factors are used both in the acute management of patients hospitalized with decompensated heart failure and in the chronic ambulatory management of patients.

Inpatient Management

In the inpatient setting, negative prognostic markers such as progressive oliguria, worsening serum creatinine, hypotension, low pulse–pressure proportion, and tachycardia may signify particularly high-risk patients (9). These patients may require invasive hemodynamic monitoring and clinicians may be more likely to use intravenous vasodilators or inotropes to facilitate diuresis. Other poor markers for the decompensated heart failure patient include low cardiac index, high systemic vascular resistance, and high pulmonary vascular resistance. These patients may require more aggressive therapies such as intravenous vasodilators or inotropes and consideration of urgent evaluation and listing for cardiac transplantation. Patients who are inotrope-dependent are particularly high-risk (10,11) and should signal consideration of intra-aortic balloon pump insertion and implantation of a ventricular assist device to improve hemodynamics to bridge to transplant. In patients with these markers who are not suitable candidates for more intensive therapy, conversations with patients and their families often occur to explain the lack of further medical therapeutic options and to define code status.

Ambulatory Management

Clinicians use prognostic markers more frequently in the management of ambulatory heart failure patients. Although a crude estimate, New York Heart Association (NYHA) classification remains one of the most powerful predictors of mortality. NYHA is a physician's estimate of the patient's functional limitations due to the dyspnea and fatigue associated with heart failure. It is an enduring method of characterizing disease severity. As a result of its universal acceptance and clinical simplicity, it has been used in randomized clinical trials to help define patient populations and disease severity. As a result, NYHA guides the choice of therapy, partly based upon the evidence available from the clinical trial data. For example, beta-blockers have been demonstrated to be effective in improving survival of heart failure patients with NYHA Class II through IV (12–15). However, beta-blockers have not been demonstrated to be efficacious to date with routine use in NYHA Class I patients and may be used in special circumstances such as in the treatment of concomitant coronary artery disease, supraventricular and ventricular arrhythmias, refractory hypertension, and/or peri-operative management. Based upon the excellent one-year survival of NYHA Class I patients, the goals of therapy are to prevent progression of disease, identify those patients at high risk for sudden cardiac death, educate patients on the clinical signs of disease progression, consider revascularization options, and encourage health behavior modifications. As the patient's NYHA functional class worsens, the aggressiveness of medical therapy also increases and may include adding spironolactone, (16) combining angiotensin receptor blockers with ACE-inhibitors, (17) or considering cardiac resynchronization therapy (CRT) (18,19). In other populations, such as African-Americans with advanced NYHA class, the addition of a nitrate and hydralazine to ACE-inhibitors and beta-blockers may have an incremental benefit on survival (20).

Assessment of the left ventricular ejection fraction (LVEF) is one of the first stratification steps after assessment of the patient's functional status. Those patients with preserved systolic function may have a better prognosis than patients with low LVEF (21–24). However, LVEF is most useful when characterizing patients into broad categories and not as useful as a linear variable in clinical practice. The prognostic impact of 5% points may not be as clinically significant as classifying a patient as having "mild" versus "severe" left ventricular dysfunction. Clinicians use the LVEF as commonly as NYHA in deciding the therapies offered for patients, in part driven by the enrollment criteria of Phase 3 clinical trials. For example, CRT and spironolactone are generally reserved for patients with low LVEF. Implantable cardioverter defibrillator (ICD) insertion for primary prevention of sudden cardiac death is also not recommended if the LVEF is $>35\%$ based upon the relatively low risk of sudden death (25). An increasingly recognized important echocardiographic parameter is the right ventricular (RV) systolic function. Patients with RV dysfunction have more symptom burden, may be less tolerant of vasodilators, may have more pulmonary hypertension, and may have a worse peri-operative mortality following valve and revascularization surgeries. These patients may not be referred for left ventricular assist device (LVAD) alone, given the frequent need for RV support. Left ventricular dimensions are also used to estimate the duration of heart failure in a patient who presents with newly diagnosed heart failure and to decide the timing and risk of valve repair and coronary artery bypass graft surgeries.

Another useful prognostic factor is exercise capacity. Although there are many ways to assess exercise capacity, including 6-minute walk test, patient's self-assessment of their abilities, and various exercise testing protocols, one of the more enduring ways to measure exercise capacity is the cardiopulmonary exercise test (26). Irrespective of predictive models (with or without beta-blocker use), peak VO_2 remains one of the strongest prognostic factors (27). Patients with peak VO_2 less than 14 ml/kg/min at a level of exercise above anaerobic threshold have a worse prognosis than those patients with peak VO_2 above that threshold, (26) and these patients are often considered for cardiac transplantation. Patients are also encouraged to enroll in cardiac rehabilitation and are considered for CRT, both of which have been associated with improved peak VO_2. Clinicians often follow the peak VO_2 longitudinally to assess response to therapies, to identify patients with progressive heart failure, and to determine the threshold for more aggressive therapies such as transplantation. Often, the peak VO_2 may be re-assessed after stabilization following hospitalization for decompensated heart failure (5).

Neurohormonal activation has been recognized as an important marker of poor prognosis in heart failure for decades (28,29). However, the clinical application of these markers made it challenging to incorporate them into routine clinical practice.

The reliability of assays measuring brain natriuretic peptide (BNP) and pro-BNP has allowed the growth of the clinical applications of this biomarker in heart failure management as a powerful prognostic marker (30,31). Patients with elevated BNP have a worse prognosis irrespective of ejection fraction. These patients may be targeted for more aggressive diuresis or vasodilator therapy, earlier referral for cardiac transplantation, or discussions about their elevated risk of mortality and transitioning to palliation. The clinical impact of serial BNP-guided strategies is still debatable.

Older age is a strong predictor of outcomes following cardiac surgery and the recovery time and morbidity is also likely to be higher. Clinicians often are less likely to consider aggressive therapies in older patients. Compared with patients <50 years old, those patients >80 years are approximately 60% less likely to receive surgery, 40% less likely to receive a right heart catheterization, and 80% less likely to receive dialysis (32). Some clinicians believe that older patients should not receive ICD for primary, and even secondary, prevention of sudden cardiac death. Cardiac transplantation is also less likely to be offered in older patients.

There are many other poor prognostic factors that are used by clinicians, often without thinking of its prognostic significance. For example, patients who develop progressive renal dysfunction may be referred for early transplantation consideration to avoid irreversible chronic renal insufficiency becoming an absolute contraindication to transplant. Patients with syncope of uncertain etiology are referred for an ICD.

Patient vs. Physician Assessment of Prognosis

The estimate of a patient's short-term and long-term prognosis is likely to be related to their medical decision making about therapies (33). However, both patients and physicians are not accurate at predicting short-term prognosis (34). In heart failure patients who died within 6 months, 70% of the patients estimated a >6 months survival between 3–6 months prior to death. At 1–3 months prior to death, 65% of patients felt that they had >6 months survival. Strikingly, up to 3 days-1 month before death, over 50% of patients still estimated their survival to be >6 months (34). Physicians are not much better at predicting short-term prognosis.

The estimated prognosis of the patient has major implications in medical decision making for heart failure patients. Given the limited supply of donors, the number of cardiac transplants in the United States has remained stable over the last 5–10 years (35,36). It is reserved for those with poor prognosis who also do not have contraindications for transplanation (37). Moreover, the 1-year survival following transplantation is approximately 85%. Thus, if a patient's estimated prognosis is better than 85% one-year survival, then transplant is often deferred. It appears that in carefully screened patients who are followed closely in a pre-transplant center, there does not appear to be worse outcomes in those patients in whom clinicians delay the timing of listing for cardiac transplantation. However, the clinician is often faced with balancing a patient's prognosis with the slow deterioration of other organs, which may impact their future transplant candidacy (38). For example, progressive renal dysfunction may lead to earlier listing for transplant prior to irreversible chronic renal insufficiency. In regards to cardiac surgery, often patients are offered surgical revascularization and valve surgery despite a high operative risk given a worse prognosis without surgery. Patients with a very poor short-term prognosis may opt for high-risk revascularization, valve surgery, or left ventricular remodeling surgery such as the Dor procedure. With improving surgical techniques, including mitral valve repair, the surgical limits continue to be pushed to operate on more advanced heart failure patients with worse prognoses.

Patient Preference for Quality vs. Quantity

One of the challenging aspects of the management of heart failure patients is assessing patient preferences for treatment options. In hypothetical situations, patients tend to favor conditions that they consider better than death and reject treatments that are perceived as worse than death (39). Also, as their perceived prognosis worsens, the patient's willingness to endure invasive procedures decreases. However, patients are willing to endure invasive therapies if there is a chance for cure and improvement of their status (40). Heart failure patients, as a group, have a poorer quality of life than patients with any other chronic disease. However, the variability of quality of life perception is great among individual patients. Those patients with excellent quality of life often have less signs of congestion, better exercise capacity, and better NYHA functional class. When asked about their willingness to trade time for perfect health, patients with NYHA class III and IV functional status were willing to trade over 30% and 80% of their remaining time to achieve perfect health, respectively (41). Those patients with NYHA class I would trade less than 10% of their time as a group. A patient's perception of poor quality of life was strongly correlated to an increased preference to trade remaining time for perfect health (correlation coefficient 0.64). Moreover, when patients were stratified by quartiles of quality of life scores, there was a linear association between worse quality of life and increased willingness to trade time, ranging from 5% in the best quality of life quartile to 60% in the worst quartile. Ironically, patient preferences for better quality over quantity of life were associated with worse mortality over the next 12 months (42). Among patients who subsequently died, three-quarters were willing to trade most of their remaining time, suggesting that longevity was not as important.

Implementing patient preferences into medical decision-making is quite complex. As patient responses to hypothetical situations have not been correlated to actual medical decisions, clinicians are not currently able to reliably ensure that therapies offered are consistent with an individual patient's preference. The patient should always play a role in the medical decision process. In the setting of uncertainty of the best therapeutic approach, patient preference should play an even larger role. For example, mitral valve repair is a growing option for patients with advanced heart failure (43,44). A patient who is a suitable cardiac transplant candidate and mitral valve repair candidate may favor a high-risk valve surgery with hopes of improving outcomes without the need for immediate listing for transplant. However, this approach may create a relative contraindication to transplantation if there are major complications. Another common scenario is the consideration of ICD for NYHA Class II and III heart failure patients for the primary prevention of sudden cardiac death. Although there is an improved survival rate, heart failure symptoms are worse and patients are often concerned about the pain of receiving an inappropriate shock and are willing to risk sudden death to avoid this complication (45). These situations require careful discussions with patients and their families to delineate the risks and benefits of the management strategy. Given time limitations in the outpatient setting and limited attendance of family in the ambulatory areas, these discussions often occur in the hospitalized patient. Another common scenario in the heart failure patient is the discussion of code status. In the SUPPORT (Studies to Understand Prognoses and Preferences for Outcomes and Risks of Treatment) experience, independent predictors of a preference NOT to want cardiopulmonary resuscitation (CPR) included older age, worse functional status, patient's estimate of a poor 2-month survival, and higher income (46). Preferences for CPR are not stable in one-quarter of patients, possibly reflecting uncertainty of preference, change in patient's perspective or estimate of prognosis, or initial misclassification of code status (47). This finding illustrates the importance of constant communication with the family and patient about code status.

TARGETS OF THERAPY

There are five main goals of therapy in heart failure management: (1) to increase survival, (2) to reduce hospitalizations, (3) to reduce progression of disease, (4) to improve functional status, and (5) to improve quality of life. In the early stages of heart failure, it is reasonable to attempt to achieve all 5 goals with medical management. Historically, the focus of clinical investigation has been on achieving the first 4 goals with little emphasis on improving quality of life. Moreover, clinicians and patients may rank the importance of these goals differently. Clinicians may focus on improving survival, reducing progression of disease, and reducing hospitalizations; patients may be less interested in the physiologic changes that occur with progressive heart failure, but are more focused on symptom burden, the impact of their disease on daily activities, as well as overall survival. Nevertheless, therapies such as ACE-inhibitors, beta-blockers, and spironolactone have been demonstrated to dramatically improve survival without having a consistent improvement in quality of life. This is reasonable in the early stages of heart failure. However, as patients progress to more advanced heart failure stages, the magnitude of survival benefit is attenuated and the clinician must weigh the actual benefit of using a therapy with the impact of the side effect profile on the patient's sense of well-being. For example, ACE-intolerant patients due to cardio-renal limitations have a much worse survival compared with patients who are not intolerant (10). If a patient tolerates minimal doses of ACE-inhibitors due to significant dizziness and hypotension, it is unclear if they will have a significant improvement in their longevity, but their health status has been dramatically worsened. Thus, although we should aim to optimize patients with therapies that improve survival in heart failure, we must also individualize the management strategies as patients have more advanced disease.

As the 5 goals of therapy are not often congruent, it is difficult to predict what is the most important goal of therapy for an individual patient and their family. For example, many elderly patients (>65 years old) are quite interested in living longer and would endure major morbidity such as high-risk surgery in order to increase longevity. Conversely, many young patients prefer to avoid ICDs despite the possibility of prolonging life. It is possible that quality of life is not as important in earlier stages of heart failure, but gains importance as the patient becomes more limited due to their disease (8). However, little is known about which goals should be the principal targets in various stages of heart failure and this needs further study.

Transition Point for Quality vs. Quantity of Life

One of the more difficult decisions as a clinician is to identify the patient with advanced heart failure who is transitioning to end-stage disease. Identifying the "transition point" will allow clinicians and patients to set reasonable targets of therapy. Some signals of this transition point include refractory symptoms despite aggressive care, inotrope dependency, cardiac cachexia, rapid decline in functional status, progressive hypotension and renal insufficiency, and decreasing serum sodium (34,48,49). Cardiologists often focus on using advanced technologies and aggressive medical management even as the patient is transitioning to a stage in which few interventions will change the natural history. Thus, heart failure patients often are treated with aggressive therapy up until 3 days prior to death. Based upon REMATCH (11), therapies such as "Destination" (LVAD) are available for those patients who are poor candidates for transplant, which further blurs the boundaries between aggressively improving survival to improving the quality and dignity of death. Patients are often very hesitant to inactivate ICDs and may seek the implantation of these devices even if they have a miserable quality of life with intractable symptoms. CRT also offers an invasive approach to the management of advanced heart failure patients, although one-third of patients will not respond. As we move forward, careful research needs to explore the appropriate roles for these advanced and invasive therapies. Finally, there are therapies that improve quality of life, but at the expense of worsening survival such as oral phosphodiesterase inhibitors and intermittent intravenous dobutamine (50,51). Current pressures to enhance survival may limit the availability of drugs that improve quality of life in the end-stage patient, unless the mortality risk is neutral. However, if a patient is interested in improving quality of life, they may be willing to accept excess mortality to achieve better health status.

Considering therapies that improve well-being at the expense of worsening survival would require a change in the paradigm of heart failure management. Prior to implementation, several steps need to occur. First, we need to reliably identify factors that signal the "transition point" at which time quality of life is more important than quantity of life for individual patients. Some of these factors may include improved precision of "short-term" prognostic markers signaling a $>50\%$ chance of mortality in the subsequent few months. A clear understanding by the family of limitations in current therapies or intolerable quality of life or symptom burden may lead the family to seek more palliation. A tool that measures the patient preference for quality vs. quantity of life in a simple, quick, and reliable way will further aid identifying the transition point. Secondly, patients and families must completely understand and accept the significance of therapies with potential excess mortality that may improve or maximize the patient's sense of well-being. Finally, insurers, clinicians, and regulators must be willing to accept therapies without survival benefit that improve the patient's symptom burden for the management of the advanced heart failure patient.

Clinicians can involve the patient and family in the decision-making during this transition period. It is important to understand the likely trajectory of the heart failure course in the short-term and the likely impact of any therapeutic options. Discussing the possible health states that may result from any intervention or lack of intervention will help patients decide on the appropriate strategy. For example, many patients fear the loss of independence due to functional or cognitive impairment (52). Heart failure patients are not willing to undergo a treatment with little risk or discomfort if it negatively impacts this aspect of health status, but would endure a high-burden intervention if it restores their quality of life (52). Next, an understanding of the patient's goals of therapy as well as the consequences of therapies that they will find unbearable will allow the clinician to frame the discussion, including the likely outcomes of any intervention. Finally, a multidisciplinary approach to discussions with patients and families that includes the physician, nurse, social worker, and faith-based staff may help them with difficult decisions as the patient realizes their own mortality.

CLINICAL ISSUES IN END OF LIFE CARE OF HEART FAILURE

Identifying End of Life in Heart Failure

The success of heart failure treatment has shifted the trajectory of the disease from an acute and rapidly fatal course to a chronic and slowly fatal one. In 2001, there were 52,828 deaths recorded with a primary diagnosis of heart failure and 206,000 additional deaths with heart failure as a secondary cause (53). On average, one in 5 patients dies within a year of diagnosis. To date there has been little research to understand the process of dying with heart failure, what kinds of end of life care would best achieve a "good death", and how to allocate appropriate resources to support patients and their families.

Planning for end of life care in heart failure is complicated by the inherent problem of predicting just when the process of dying is occurring in a disease characterized by a rollercoaster of exacerbations and resurrections. Most previous efforts have focused on identifying predictors of long-term prognosis. However, it is equally important to patients and families to identify those patients who are transitioning to dying. While attempts at defining predictors of the transition period may help to identify when the process of dying has begun, they are not useful in establishing a timeline for any particular patient (34,48,49). The SUPPORT study shows that neither physicians nor patients were able to predict impending death (34). In fact, this prognostic uncertainty may explain why 40% of hospitalized heart failure patients undergo a major intervention in the last 3 days of life and explain the low numbers of heart failure patients referred for hospice care (49). Given the current limitations, prognostic measures for patients are best given as a range estimate (48).

Dying with Heart Failure

There are two main modes of death in heart failure. Between 33–50% of heart failure patients die suddenly with a higher proportion in the lower NYHA functional classes (54,55). Greater utilization of ICD's may lead to a reduction in this number. However, worsening of arrhythmias parallels worsening pump failure and decreasing the rate of sudden death may simply shift the mechanism of death to progressive heart failure (8). Heart failure patients have been shown to know less about their prognosis and are less involved in the decision-making process than cancer patients (56). At present, there are no data specific to heart failure patients examining their understanding of heart failure as a fatal disease or how critically they perceive their role as decision-maker in their care. Among patients dying of progressive heart failure, 70% described their quality of life as fair to poor in the last month of life. Moderate to severe dyspnea is reported by 63%, and 50% describe moderate to severe pain in the last days of life (57). Other distressing symptoms included lack of energy, weakness and fatigue, insomnia, and depression (57). Family members described 64% of these heart failure patients as "extremely ill" or "very ill" (58). Therefore, for patients dying of progressive heart failure, end of life decision-making and care planning are critical.

Studies looking at patient decision-making at end of life have identified significant problems in patient-family-physician communication around end of life issues. In one study of seriously ill, hospitalized patients, a majority had not discussed preferences in end of life care and had no wish to do so despite having preferences regarding interventions (46). Twenty-five percent of these patients wished to forego CPR and 87% did not wish prolonged ventilation (59). Among hospitalized patients, 70% preferred having their family and physician make decisions for them if they were unable and only 22% wanted their own stated preferences followed. Physicians, nurses, and surrogates understanding of patient preferences was only moderately better than chance in correctly predicting patient wishes (60). In the SUPPORT study, 20% of patients changed their resuscitation preference within 2 months of hospital discharge (61). These data reflect both patient ambivalence about the decision-making process and caregiver uncertainty in interpreting patient wishes.

End of life discussions are difficult and time consuming. They require care providers to offer reassurance and support while realistically answering difficult questions about end of life, resuscitation measures, and likely outcomes of those efforts. Patients and families move through the dying process at different rates and in different ways that can lead to disagreement in the planning of care and may even require involvement of the clergy or social workers to help facilitate a plan that will be acceptable to everyone. Since patient preferences may change, these discussions must be viewed as an ongoing process and not a one-time event.

Advance Directives

Advance directive planning is being strongly encouraged by healthcare institutions to communicate patients' preferences to all providers. These directives, consisting of a Health Care Proxy and a Living Will Declaration, record a patient's wishes regarding medical care and decision-making. The Health Care Proxy is legally recognized as the surrogate decision maker if the patient is unable to make health care decisions. A Living Will Declaration outlines patient preferences regarding medical care to sustain life. Advance Directives are intended to provide direction in case of future emergencies and as a way of relieving physicians, and surrogates, of the burden of decision-making. Because medical status and therapy are highly variable, living wills are often used as guidelines for medical interventions rather than specific directives and are not considered legally binding. The SUPPORT study found that even when specific instructions were documented in advance directives, care was inconsistent with those wishes nearly half the time and 50% of patients who requested no CPR never had DNR orders written (8). The investigators suggest that inconsistencies in care may be associated with factors other than preferences or prognosis and may require systematic changes (46,62).

Ideally, general discussions about advance directives and end of life care should begin as soon as the patient and physician have established a relationship and preferably before the patient becomes too sick to participate in the discussion. Since primary care providers or internists care for three-quarters of heart failure patients, (63) these providers are often in the best position to address these issues. Review of the patient's choices and advance directives should occur periodically throughout the patient-provider relationship including at diagnosis, annual visits, a decline in function, or a hospitalization. These discussions are emotionally challenging for patients, families and physicians, all bringing their own cultural and spiritual beliefs and personal values to the table. It is difficult to address death and end of life issues given the typical time constraints of an ambulatory visit and these discussions may need to be scheduled separately.

Palliative Care and Hospice

Despite patient descriptions of distressing symptoms at end of life, and the endorsements of the American Heart Association, the American College of Cardiology, and the World Health Organization, only 10% of heart failure patients are enrolled in hospice care (57). This may be due to the difficulty of trying to "diagnose dying" or due to physician concerns about the accuracy of a <6 months prognosis for hospice benefits under Medicare (64). Statistics showing hospice use by heart failure patients indicate that less than 3% of heart failure patients used more then 6 months of hospice benefits (8) and 37% of patients referred to hospice survived for only 1 week or less, (57) indicating probable underutilization of this service.

Because distressing symptoms often begin before dying is diagnosed, referral to hospice programs may seem premature to patients and providers. Palliative care programs, which help to gradually transition the focus from cure to care, can be integrated into heart failure care as soon as symptom management becomes an issue. Early involvement of palliative care may make the shift toward specific end of life issues and hospice care easier as further decline occurs. Palliative and hospice care are intended as complementary treatments to be added to the routine medical management of heart failure, not in place of medical care, and can be integrated into disease management programs. Reassuring patients that palliative care provides more care, not less, enhances patient acceptance and relieves concerns of being "abandoned to strangers" at the end of life. Preliminary data is inconclusive but both palliative and hospice care may also help to reduce costs by decreasing hospital readmissions that constitute the largest health care expenditure for heart failure (57).

Managing the Dying Patient

Goals of care for the dying heart failure patient begin with comfort. Blood tests and intravenous therapies should be evaluated and discontinued if inappropriate (64,65). Current medications need to be assessed and non-essential medications, or those with greater burden than benefit, should be discontinued. A multidisciplinary consensus panel consisting of experts in advanced heart failure, palliative medicine, geriatrics, outcomes, research, and health care improvement examined the current evidence available for interventions to relieve symptoms, improve quality of life, and support patients and families. The panel recommended that medical therapy be optimized for all patients with advanced heart failure according to the guidelines established by the American Heart Association and the American College of Cardiology. Ace inhibitors, diuretics, and beta-blockers have been shown to reduce rates of hospitalization and death and were the only therapies with sufficient evidence to support recommendation (8). The panel did not make any recommendations on how to adjust doses or withdraw medications near the end of life. In practice, diuretics produce the greatest symptom relief and should be continued regardless of renal function. ACE-inhibitor and beta-blocker doses often need to be reduced due to hypotension. If beta-blockers are used for heart rate control or in ischemic patients, reduction in dose or withdrawal may result in increased palpitations or angina and may increase symptom burden. Decisions about medication adjustments need to be individualized to each patient and situation.

Small studies in end-stage heart failure suggest that intravenous inotropes may reduce readmissions and symptoms in some patients even though mortality remains high (51,66–69). However, inotropic infusions may exclude patients from hospice care due to the high cost or because specific hospice organizations are unfamiliar with their use. They may be useful in situations where a patient wishes to achieve a specific personal or family goal.

Sleep-disordered breathing is reported in nearly 50% of heart failure patients and is associated with fatigue, worsening functional capacity, and arrhythmias. Continuous positive airway pressure (CPAP), and possibly supplemental oxygen, were reported by the panel to be beneficial in reducing symptoms (8). However, CPAP is often not tolerated in anxious patients near end of life and patients may prefer supplemental oxygen that may provide psychological relief from dyspnea.

Table 1 Medication Options for Pain and Symptom Management in End of Life from Heart Failure

Symptom	Medication	Considerations
Pain	First line—mild pain Aspirin Tylenol	NSAIDs should be avoided, may worsen heart and renal failure
	Second line—moderate pain Codeine Hydrocodone Tramadol	Used infrequently in heart failure
	Third line—severe pain	Use liquid or patch for best absorption and to prevent problems with swallowing
	Morphine	Morphine may also relieve respiratory distress thereby treating 2 symptoms with 1 medication
	Fentanyl	In opiate naïve patients, begin with small oral dose and increase as needed Add patch only when patient tolerates opioids and smoother pain/symptom control is needed Consider non-pharmacological strategies such as touch, relaxation exercises and breathing, music
Constipation	Initial regime	
	Senna and/or lactulose at HS Bisacodyl and/or lactulose at HS	Prophylactic laxatives must be given with opioids
	Second line	
	Increase dose and/or frequency of above	Increasing fiber may cause bloating Use osmotic or stimulating agents
	Obstipation MOM Magnesium citrate Lactulose QID Mineral oil	
	Impaction Disimpaction and enemas More aggressive prophylactic regimen	
Anxiety	Benzodiazepines	Do not withdraw abruptly
Dyspnea	Benzodiazepines	Most frightening symptom to patients
	Morphine	Also responds to non-pharmacologic measures such as open windows, use of fans
Depression	Serotonin reuptake inhibitors	Full effect may take months Counseling may be helpful
Insomnia	Benzodiazipines Antidepressants Morphine	Consider etiology of insomnia (i.e., anxiety, depression, pain) and choose agent which helps to treat underlying cause
	Hypnotics	Assess sleep hygiene

(Continued)

Table 1 Medication Options for Pain and Symptom Management in End of Life from Heart Failure (*Continued*)

Symptom	Medication	Considerations
Emergency medications	Benzodiazepines Morphine Scopalamine or atropine Haldol Compazine suppositories	Consider giving a small supply of medications to be used in emergency situations for symptom management with professional direction Kit should contain medications for anxiety, pain, nausea and vomiting, and to reduce oral secretions
Final days		
Delirium or agitaion	Benzodiazepines Haloperidol Chlorpromazine	Reassurance, physical presence are often helpful Assess for reversible physical problems such as impaction, urinary retention, or pain Educate family about the death process and what actions they need to take
Death rattle	Scoplamine Atropine	Position patient in side-lying position

Abbreviation: NSAIDs, nonsteroidal anti-inflammatory drugs.
Source: Adapted from Ref. 75.

Many symptoms are difficult to treat and evaluate. Fatigue is a frequent problem, but psychostimulants (used in other chronic illnesses) are unstudied in heart failure and may increase the risk of arrhythmias. Depression is reported in up to 50% of patients with end-stage heart failure and anecdotally has been shown to respond to antidepressant medications if treated early. All patients should be assessed for pain. The pain of many comorbid conditions worsens at the end of life and should be treated to optimize function and without fear of addiction. Drugs to treat pain, agitation, excess oral secretions, nausea, and vomiting should be on hand in small quantities for use in acute situations. Families and patients should be instructed on when and how to use them. Drug choices and recommendations are indicated in Table 1.

Communication between care providers, the patient, and family is essential and complex. Failure to communicate honestly with a patient or family may lead to a lack of trust in the physician and care team and often to distress, dissatisfaction, and bereavement problems for the family (65). Do Not Resuscitate (DNR) orders as well as discussions about inactivating defibrillators and pacemakers should occur when end of life preferences are reviewed at the transition point to hospice or palliative care. ICD shocks are described by patients as moderately uncomfortable, but are tolerated because they offer a lifesaving benefit earlier in the course of heart failure (70). Single and multiple shocks have been reported in patients near death when the burden of treatment may be greater than the likelihood of benefit. Proposed inactivation of devices has generated ethical concerns among practitioners. However, ethics committees agree that patients who have these devices should have the opportunity to discuss disabling the device as death approaches (71–73). Consonance between DNR orders and defibrillator deactivation is a reasonable goal.

Palliative and hospice care provide multidisciplinary support to patient and family throughout the dying process and across all settings ranging from home to hospital to in-patient hospice or nursing home care. Integrating the support of palliative care or hospice with careful medical management can provide patients with the best end of life care. Although there is much to be learned about end of life in heart failure, we must remember, "The terminally ill fear the unknown more than the known, professional disinterest more than professional ineptitude, the process of dying rather than death itself" (74).

REFERENCES

1. Gorkin L, Norvell NK, Rosen RC, et al. Assessment of quality of life as observed from the baseline data of the Studies of Left Ventricular Dysfunction (SOLVD) trial quality-of-life substudy. Am J Cardiol 1993; 71:1069–1073.
2. Dracup K, Walden JA, Stevenson LW, Brecht ML. Quality of life in patients with advanced heart failure. J Heart Lung Transplant 1992; 11:273–279.
3. Ho KK, Anderson KM, Kannel WB, Grossman W, Levy D. Survival after the onset of congestive heart failure in Framingham Heart Study subjects. Circulation 1993; 88:107–115.
4. MacIntyre K, Capewell S, Stewart S, et al. Evidence of improving prognosis in heart failure: trends in case fatality in 66,547 patients hospitalized between 1986 and 1995. Circulation 2000; 102:1126–1131.
5. Lund LH, Aaronson KD, Mancini DM. Validation of peak exercise oxygen consumption and the Heart Failure Survival Score for serial risk stratification in advanced heart failure. Am J Cardiol 2005; 95:734–741.
6. Aaronson KD, Schwartz JS, Chen TM, Wong KL, Goin JE, Mancini DM. Development and prospective validation of a clinical index to predict survival in ambulatory patients referred for cardiac transplant evaluation. Circulation 1997; 95:2660–2667.
7. Lee DS, Vasan RS. Novel markers for heart failure diagnosis and prognosis. Curr Opin Cardiol 2005; 20:201–210.
8. Goodlin SJ, Hauptman PJ, Arnold R, et al. Consensus statement: palliative and supportive care in advanced heart failure. J Card Fail 2004; 10:200–209.
9. Tokmakova MP, Skali H, Kenchaiah S, et al. Chronic kidney disease, cardiovascular risk, and response to angiotensin-converting enzyme inhibition after myocardial infarction: the survival and ventricular enlargement (SAVE) study. Circulation 2004; 110:3667–3673.
10. Kittleson M, Hurwitz S, Shah MR, et al. Development of circulatory-renal limitations to angiotensin-converting enzyme inhibitors identifies patients with severe heart failure and early mortality. J Am Coll Cardiol 2003; 41:2029–2035.
11. Rose EA, Gelijns AC, Moskowitz AJ, et al. Long-term mechanical left ventricular assistance for end-stage heart failure. N Engl J Med 2001; 345:1435–1443.
12. The Cardiac Insufficiency Bisoprolol Study II (CIBIS-II): a randomised trial. Lancet 1999; 353:9–13.
13. Effect of metoprolol CR/XL in chronic heart failure: Metoprolol CR/XL Randomised Intervention Trial in Congestive Heart Failure (MERIT-HF). Lancet 1999; 353:2001–2007.
14. A trial of the beta-blocker bucindolol in patients with advanced chronic heart failure. N Engl J Med 2001; 344:1659–1667.
15. Packer M, Coats AJ, Fowler MB, et al. Effect of carvedilol on survival in severe chronic heart failure. N Engl J Med 2001; 344:1651–1658.
16. Pitt B, Zannad F, Remme WJ, et al. The effect of spironolactone on morbidity and mortality in patients with severe heart failure. Randomized Aldactone Evaluation Study Investigators. N Engl J Med 1999; 341:709–717.
17. McMurray JJ, Ostergren J, Swedberg K, et al. Effects of candesartan in patients with chronic heart failure and reduced left-ventricular systolic function taking angiotensin-converting-enzyme inhibitors: the CHARM-Added trial. Lancet 2003; 362:767–771.
18. Cleland JG, Daubert JC, Erdmann E, et al. The effect of cardiac resynchronization on morbidity and mortality in heart failure. N Engl J Med 2005; 352:1539–1549.

19. Abraham WT, Fisher WG, Smith AL, et al. Cardiac resynchronization in chronic heart failure. N Engl J Med 2002; 346:1845–1853.
20. Taylor AL, Ziesche S, Yancy C, et al. Combination of isosorbide dinitrate and hydralazine in blacks with heart failure. N Engl J Med 2004; 351:2049–2057.
21. Rodeheffer RJ, Jacobsen SJ, Gersh BJ, et al. The incidence and prevalence of congestive heart failure in Rochester, Minnesota. Mayo Clin Proc 1993; 68:1143–1150.
22. Redfield MM, Jacobsen SJ, Burnett JC, Jr., Mahoney DW, Bailey KR, Rodeheffer RJ. Burden of systolic and diastolic ventricular dysfunction in the community: appreciating the scope of the heart failure epidemic. JAMA 2003; 289:194–202.
23. Philbin EF, Rocco TA, Jr., Lindenmuth NW, Ulrich K, Jenkins PL. Systolic versus diastolic heart failure in community practice: clinical features, outcomes, and the use of angiotensin-converting enzyme inhibitors. Am J Med 2000; 109:605–613.
24. Smith GL, Masoudi FA, Vaccarino V, Radford MJ, Krumholz HM. Outcomes in heart failure patients with preserved ejection fraction: mortality, readmission, and functional decline. J Am Coll Cardiol 2003; 41:1510–1518.
25. Hunt SA, Baker DW, Chin MH, et al. ACC/AHA guidelines for the evaluation and management of chronic heart failure in the adult: executive summary. A report of the American College of Cardiology/American Heart Association Task Force on Practice Guidelines (Committee to revise the 1995 Guidelines for the Evaluation and Management of Heart Failure). J Am Coll Cardiol 2001; 38:2101–2113.
26. Mancini DM, Eisen H, Kussmaul W, Mull R, Edmunds LH, Jr., Wilson JR. Value of peak exercise oxygen consumption for optimal timing of cardiac transplantation in ambulatory patients with heart failure. Circulation 1991; 83:778–786.
27. Lund LH, Aaronson KD, Mancini DM. Predicting survival in ambulatory patients with severe heart failure on beta-blocker therapy. Am J Cardiol 2003; 92:1350–1354.
28. Cohn JN, Levine TB, Olivari MT, et al. Plasma norepinephrine as a guide to prognosis in patients with chronic congestive heart failure. N Engl J Med 1984; 311:819–823.
29. Givertz MM, Braunwald E. Neurohormones in heart failure: predicting outcomes, optimizing care. Eur Heart J 2004; 25:281–282.
30. Hartmann F, Packer M, Coats AJ, et al. Prognostic impact of plasma N-terminal pro-brain natriuretic peptide in severe chronic congestive heart failure: a substudy of the Carvedilol Prospective Randomized Cumulative Survival (COPERNICUS) trial. Circulation 2004; 110:1780–1786.
31. Latini R, Masson S, Anand I, et al. The comparative prognostic value of plasma neurohormones at baseline in patients with heart failure enrolled in Val-HeFT. Eur Heart J 2004; 25:292–299.
32. Hamel MB, Phillips RS, Teno JM, et al. Seriously ill hospitalized adults: do we spend less on older patients? Support investigators. Study to understand prognoses and preference for outcomes and risks of treatments. J Am Geriatr Soc 1996; 44:1043–1048.
33. Coppola KM, Bookwala J, Ditto PH, Lockhart LK, Danks JH, Smucker WD. Elderly adults' preferences for life-sustaining treatments: the role of impairment, prognosis, and pain. Death Stud 1999; 23:617–634.
34. Levenson JW, McCarthy EP, Lynn J, Davis RB, Phillips RS. The last six months of life for patients with congestive heart failure. J Am Geriatr Soc 2000; 48:S101–S109.
35. Bennett LE, Keck BM, Daily OP, Novick RJ, Hosenpud JD. Worldwide thoracic organ transplantation: a report from the UNOS/ISHLT International Registry for Thoracic Organ Transplantation. Clin Transpl 2000;31–44.
36. Costanzo MR, Augustine S, Bourge R, et al. Selection and treatment of candidates for heart transplantation. A statement for health professionals from the Committee on Heart Failure and Cardiac Transplantation of the Council on Clinical Cardiology, American Heart Association. Circulation 1995; 92:3593–3612.
37. Mudge GH, Goldstein S, Addonizio LJ, et al. 24th Bethesda conference: Cardiac transplantation. Task Force 3: Recipient guidelines/prioritization. J Am Coll Cardiol 1993; 22:21–31.

38. Lewis EF, Tsang SW, Fang JC, et al. Frequency and impact of delayed decisions regarding heart transplantation on long-term outcomes in patients with advanced heart failure. J Am Coll Cardiol 2004; 43:794–802.
39. Patrick DL, Pearlman RA, Starks HE, Cain KC, Cole WG, Uhlmann RF. Validation of preferences for life-sustaining treatment: implications for advance care planning. Ann Intern Med 1997; 127:509–517.
40. Emanuel LL, Barry MJ, Stoeckle JD, Ettelson LM, Emanuel EJ. Advance directives for medical care–a case for greater use. N Engl J Med 1991; 324:889–895.
41. Lewis EF, Johnson PA, Johnson W, Collins C, Griffin L, Stevenson LW. Preferences for quality of life or survival expressed by patients with heart failure. J Heart Lung Transplant 2001; 20:1016–1024.
42. Lewis EFTS, Stevenson LW. Patients with preference to trade time for better health or poorer quality of life have a higher mortality rate. J Cardiac Failure 2002; 8:S14.
43. Bolling SF, Pagani FD, Deeb GM, Bach DS. Intermediate-term outcome of mitral reconstruction in cardiomyopathy. J Thorac Cardiovasc Surg 1998; 115:381–386 discussion 387–8.
44. Mehta RH, Eagle KA, Coombs LP, et al. Influence of age on outcomes in patients undergoing mitral valve replacement. Ann Thorac Surg 2002; 74:1459–1467.
45. Stevenson LW. Rites and responsibility for resuscitation in heart failure: tread gently on the thin places. Circulation 1998; 98:619–622.
46. Krumholz HM, Phillips RS, Hamel MB, et al. Resuscitation preferences among patients with severe congestive heart failure: results from the SUPPORT project. Study to understand prognoses and preferences for outcomes and risks of treatments. Circulation 1998; 98:648–655.
47. Rosenfeld KE, Wenger NS, Phillips RS, et al. Factors associated with change in resuscitation preference of seriously ill patients. The SUPPORT investigators. Study to understand prognoses and preferences for outcomes and risks of treatments. Arch Intern Med 1996; 156:1558–1564.
48. Pantilat SZ, Steimle AE. Palliative care for patients with heart failure. JAMA 2004; 291:2476–2482.
49. Christakis NA, Escarce JJ. Survival of Medicare patients after enrollment in hospice programs. N Engl J Med 1996; 335:172–178.
50. Cohn JN, Goldstein SO, Greenberg BH, et al. A dose-dependent increase in mortality with vesnarinone among patients with severe heart failure. Vesnarinone Trial Investigators. N Engl J Med 1998; 339:1810–1816.
51. Felker GM, O'Connor CM. Inotropic therapy for heart failure: an evidence-based approach. Am Heart J 2001; 142:393–401.
52. Fried TR, Bradley EH, Towle VR, Allore H. Understanding the treatment preferences of seriously ill patients. N Engl J Med 2002; 346:1061–1066.
53. Heart Disease and Stroke Statistics–2005 Update. Dallas: American Heart Association.
54. Stevenson WG, Stevenson LW. Prevention of sudden death in heart failure. J Cardiovasc Electrophysiol 2001; 12:112–114.
55. Stevenson WG, Epstein LM. Predicting sudden death risk for heart failure patients in the implantable cardioverter-defibrillator age. Circulation 2003; 107:514–516.
56. Formiga F, Chivite D, Ortega C, Casas S, Ramon JM, Pujol R. End-of-life preferences in elderly patients admitted for heart failure. QJM 2004; 97:803–808.
57. Zambroski CH. Hospice as an alternative model of care for older patients with end-stage heart failure. J Cardiovasc Nurs 2004; 19:76–83 quiz 84–5.
58. Hauptman PJ, Havranek EP. Integrating palliative care into heart failure care. Arch Intern Med 2005; 165:374–378.
59. La Rovere MT, Pinna GD, Maestri R, et al. Short-term heart rate variability strongly predicts sudden cardiac death in chronic heart failure patients. Circulation 2003; 107:565–570.
60. Weissman DE. Decision making at a time of crisis near the end of life. JAMA 2004; 292:1738–1743.

61. Puchalski CM, Zhong Z, Jacobs MM, et al. Patients who want their family and physician to make resuscitation decisions for them: observations from SUPPORT and HELP. Study to understand prognoses and preferences for outcomes and risks of treatment. Hospitalized elderly longitudinal project. J Am Geriatr Soc 2000; 48:S84–S90.
62. Teno JM, Licks S, Lynn J, et al. Do advance directives provide instructions that direct care? SUPPORT Investigators. Study to understand prognoses and preferences for outcomes and risks of treatment J Am Geriatr Soc 1997; 45:508–512.
63. Philbin EF, Jenkins PL. Differences between patients with heart failure treated by cardiologists, internists, family physicians, and other physicians: analysis of a large, statewide database. Am Heart J 2000; 139:491–496.
64. Ellershaw J, Ward C. Care of the dying patient: the last hours or days of life. BMJ 2003; 326:30–34.
65. Ward C. The need for palliative care in the management of heart failure. Heart 2002; 87:294–298.
66. Young JB, Moen EK. Outpatient parenteral inotropic therapy for advanced heart failure. J Heart Lung Transplant 2000; 19:S49–S57.
67. Lopez-Candales A, Vora T, Gibbons W, Carron C, Simmons P, Schwartz J. Symptomatic improvement in patients treated with intermittent infusion of inotropes: a double-blind placebo controled pilot study. J Med 2002; 33:129–146.
68. Oren RM, Cotts WG, Pies CJ, Duncan ML. Difficult cases in heart failure: Importance of patient selection in the use of intermittent inotrope infusions for advanced heart failure. Congest Heart Fail 1999; 5:86–90.
69. Hershberger RE, Nauman D, Walker TL, Dutton D, Burgess D. Care processes and clinical outcomes of continuous outpatient support with inotropes (COSI) in patients with refractory endstage heart failure. J Card Fail 2003; 9:180–187.
70. Ahmad M, Bloomstein L, Roelke M, Bernstein AD, Parsonnet V. Patients' attitudes toward implanted defibrillator shocks. Pacing Clin Electrophysiol 2000; 23:934–938.
71. Goldstein NE, Lampert R, Bradley E, Lynn J, Krumholz HM. Management of implantable cardioverter defibrillators in end-of-life care. Ann Intern Med 2004; 141:835–838.
72. Mueller PS, Hook CC, Hayes DL. Ethical analysis of withdrawal of pacemaker or implantable cardioverter-defibrillator support at the end of life. Mayo Clin Proc 2003; 78:959–963.
73. Braun TC, Hagen NA, Hatfield RE, Wyse DG. Cardiac pacemakers and implantable defibrillators in terminal care. J Pain Symptom Manage 1999; 18:126–131.
74. Doyle D, Denton T. Pain and Symptom Control in Terminal Care. Edinburgh: St. Columba's Hospice, 1986.
75. Abrahm J. A Physician's Guide to Pain and Symptom Management in Cancer Patients. Baltimore: The Johns Hopkins University Press, 2000.

PART VI: RESEARCH

30

Regenerative Medicine: The Promise of Cellular Cardiomyoplasty

Anastasios P. Saliaris, Luciano C. Amado, Karl H. Schuleri, and Joshua M. Hare
Institute for Cell Engineering and Cardiology Division, Department of Medicine, Johns Hopkins University School of Medicine, Baltimore, Maryland, U.S.A.

INTRODUCTION

The incidence of congestive heart failure (HF) is increasing with epidemic proportions, occurring most frequently in patients with structural heart disease resulting from myocardial infarction (MI). The process of cardiac remodeling, which provides a substrate for HF, results from fibrotic scar formation that replaces regions of myocyte necrosis coupled with insufficient endogenous repair responses. In addition, surviving myocytes undergo hypertrophy, which may be initially beneficial but transitions to a maladaptive process in which myocytes become vulnerable to apoptosis. The heart dilates due to infarct expansion, with wall thinning and dilatation, hyperplasia of fibroblasts, and scar formation, changes its geometry and loses contractile function—the defining features of ventricular remodeling (1). While cardiomyocytes may not be terminally differentiated and endogenous cardiac stem cells are now identified within the heart (2–5), it is clear from these clinical sequellae that endogenous repair mechanisms are insufficient to adequately allow the heart to heal structurally and functionally from MI.

The desire to harness novel cellular regenerative approaches for preventing or reversing remodeling and progression to HF following MI has sparked two parallel and closely related avenues of research. First, much attention has been paid to the biology of endogenous stem or precursor cells that may participate in healing of adult organs (6–10), and second, translational attempts to utilize exogenous cells for myocardial repair (11,12) have prompted early human studies (13,14). The latter has aroused substantial enthusiasm (15) and transplantation of a variety of progenitor cells into a region of myocardium damaged by MI, termed cellular cardiomyoplasty (14,16), is currently under active investigation in small trials. In experimental models the cell types and/or strategies which have been investigated include fetal and neonatal cardiomyocytes (17–30), embryonic stem cell derived myocytes (ES) (31–34), tissue engineered contractile grafts (35–40), skeletal myoblasts (SM) (41–52), several cell types derived from adult bone marrow (53–58), and cardiac stem cells resident within the heart itself (3,8,59,60).

REPAIR MECHANISMS

While the mechanism by which cellular therapy improves myocardial function remains highly controversial, three general mechanisms have been proposed which appear alone or in combination to explain the cardiac reparative properties of cellular cardiomyoplasty: differentiation of the administered stem cells into various cellular constituents of the heart—myocytes, endothelial cells and smooth muscle cells (12,61), fusion between the stem cell and endogenous cardiac myoctyes (62), and release of paracrine factors that stimulate endogenous cardiac repair mechanisms (Fig. 1) (63,64).

Differentiation of transplanted precursor cells into cardiac myocytes has long been held as the central mechanism of a stem cell reparative effect, and therefore one of the primary areas of ongoing investigation is the differentiation potential of various stem cell sources. There is experimental support for the differentiation of endothelial progenitor cells (EPCs), mesenchymal stem cells (MSCs), and embryonic stem cells (ESs), whereas that of hematopoetic stem cells (HSCs) and SM remains highly controversial (Table 1).

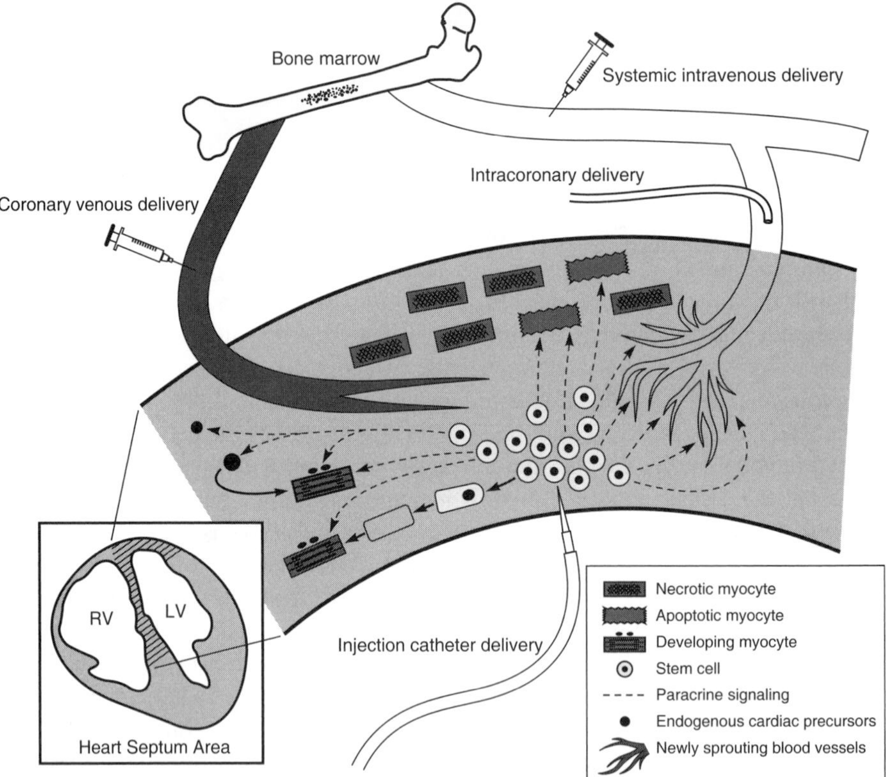

Figure 1 Myocardial loss and chamber remodeling results from ischemic myocyte necrosis. Endogenous stem cells or therapeutically administered cell preparations traffic to the injured area through the bloodstream or directly if injected into myocardium. Successful cardiomyoplasty results from growth of new cardiac myocytes capable of generating electomechanically coupled contraction, reduction of scar formation, or a combination of both. Stem cells may either differentiate into cellular constituents necessary for new muscle or vacular formation, fuse with existing cells, or exert paracrine effects capable of recruiting additional cells (i.e., cardiac stem cells) or stimulate other protective effects such as reducing apoptotic cell loss or collagen deposition. See text for details.

Table 1 Mechanisms and Effects of Stem Cell Types

	Differentiation	Neovascularization	Decreased apoptosis	Fusion	Cardiac function
Endothelial progenitor cells (183)	+(111,112)	+(110,114)	+(72,73)	+(184) −(112)	+(72,73, 110,114)
Hematopoetic progenitor cells	+(9,102) −(62,103,104)	+(102)	?	+(62)	+(102) −(185)
Mesenchymal stem cells (186)	+(11,53,79,82, 86,97,187–194)	+(57,75, 91,93)	+(57)	+(69,189) −(195)	+(11,74,75, 91,92)
Skeletal myoblasts (47,196)	+(51,52,132, 197,197–199) −(200)	?	?	+(184) −(198)	+(51,52,132, 201,202)
Embryonic stem cells (130,203)	+(31,33,204, 205)	+(206)	?	+(65,207)	+(31,33,208)

Controversy over differentiation has stimulated investigation of alternative hypotheses that include fusion, whereby donor cells fuse with recipient cells, subsequently adopting the recipients phenotype (8,65), and paracrine signaling involving the secretion of protective factors or factors stimulating cell–cell interactions. Indeed, studies demonstrating fusion of bone marrow–derived cells with cardiac myocytes and other cell types have lead to doubt regarding the role of cell differentiation in stem cell therapy (62,66), while still other studies have argued against a substantial role for cell fusion (67,68). There is growing support for paracrine signaling characterized by upregulation of angiogenic factors (VEGF-A, HGF, bFGF, angiopoietin-1 and -2, and PDGF-B), cardiac transcription factors (GATA-4, Nkx2.5, and MEF2C), as well as IGF-1 and stromal cell-derived factor-1α in stem cell transplanted hearts (69). The net effect of paracrine signaling may be improved neovascularization and perfusion (70,71), reduced myocyte apoptosis and remodeling of failing myocardium, (72) and perhaps most importantly stimulation of proliferation of endogenous cardiomyocytes (73). A recent study demonstrating cytoprotective effects of genetically modified MSCs suggests that improved cardiac function associated with MSC therapy may be due to reduced myocyte loss rather than myocyte regeneration (64). In summary, the exact mechanism of stem cell effect still remains to be fully clarified and likely involves interplay between transdifferentiation, fusion, and paracrine signaling.

Macroscopic Mechanisms

While most attention has focused on the above cellular and molecular mechanisms, there is very clearly a need to understand how cellular cardiomyoplasty affects the heart at a gross level. Given an effective cell source, will its application replace fibrotic scar or regenerate myocardium independent of the scar? A tightly linked question relates to delivery of the cell, i.e., by direct injection into the scar or via a vascular approach. To address these important translational studies, there are emerging studies utilizing large animal preclinical models and early human trials. Together these studies demonstrate that cellular cardiomyoplasty has the potential to decrease infarct size and improve myocardial contractility, although much more work is needed to define some of these key issues (55,67,74–77). For example, in a study utilizing the direct myocardial injection of allogeneic MSCs (Fig. 2), engrafted MSCs dramatically reduced the extent of necrotic myocardium, promoted regeneration of new contractile myocardium along the subendocardial surface of the MI and led to the recovery of cardiac energy metabolism,

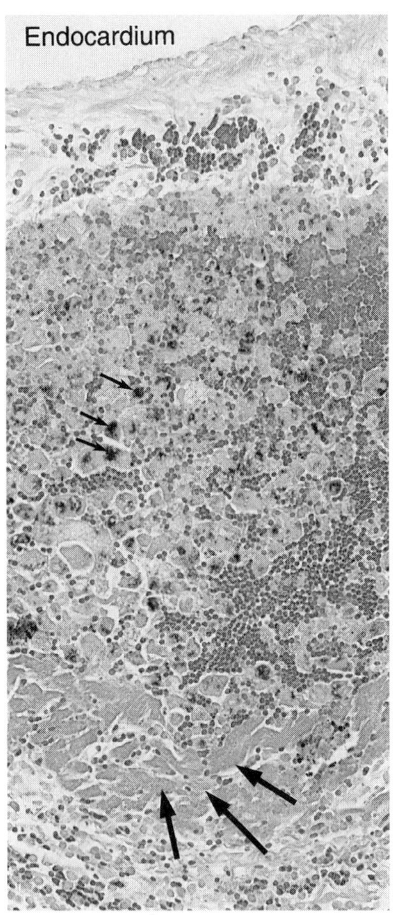

Figure 2 Sixty-four times magnification of Prossian Blue section of myocardium. Injected Feridex labeled mesenchymal stem cells (*small arrows*) can be seen along the subendocardial border of myocardium adjacent to necrotic myocytes (*large arrows*).

systolic and diastolic cardiac function, and global cardiac performance (Fig. 3). Importantly this effect took approximately 2 mo (78).

CELL TYPES INVOLVED IN CARDIAC REGENERATION AND REPAIR

Bone Marrow Cells

In general, bone marrow cells have been prepared on the basis of being (1) MSCs purified on the basis of their fibroblast morphology and ability to divide in culture and to differentiate into mesodermal lineages (79), and (2) HSCs that express the stem cell factor (SCF) receptor, c-Kit (Fig. 4). While much controversy exists on how these cells relate to each other at fundamental biological levels, their use in translational experiments has proceeded at a rapid pace.

Mesenchymal Stem Cells

MSCs, derived from bone marrow or processed lipoaspirates, are a highly promising cell type for cardiomyoplasty as they are a true adult stem cell possessing the ability to

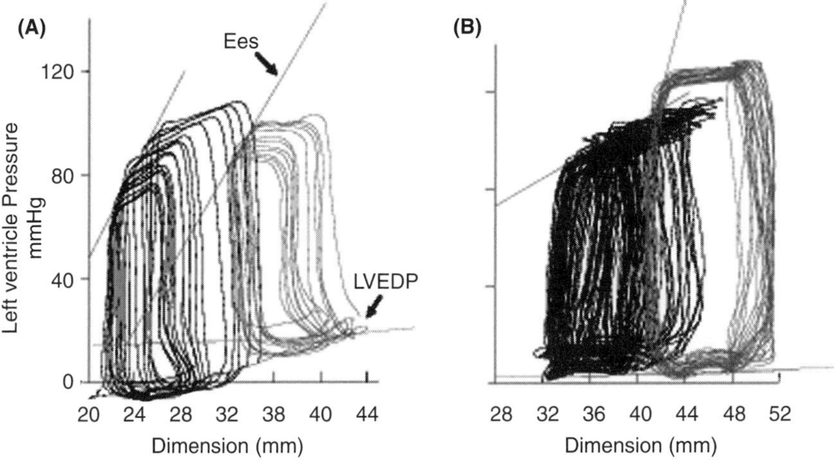

Figure 3 Physiologic impact of mesenchymal stem cell therapy following anterior myocardial infarction (MI) in pigs. Pressure-dimension (PD) data from a placebo (**A**) and a MSC-trehated (**B**) pig obtained 3 days (*dark black loops*) and 8 wk (*grey loops*) following MI. Placebo animals exhibit an increase in left-ventricular end-diastolic pressure (LVEDP) and dimension. Both myocardial contractility, measured by the slope of the end systolic pressure-dimension relationship (ventricular elastance, Ees), and ventricular stroke work, pressure-dimension loop area, decline in controls. In MSC-treated animals, Ees and stroke work increase to normal.

replicate and differentiate into various mesodermal lineages, (79–81) including spontaneously beating cardiomyocytes (82). Though the isolation of MSCs from peripheral blood has been reported (83,84), their identification and clinical potential remain poorly defined. In terms of cell surface markers, MSCs (85) are reported by some (86) but not all (87) investigators to express c-kit, the 145 KD tyrosine kinase receptor for SCF (Table 2) (88–90).

Studies on MSC engraftment in rodent and swine models of MI have shown: (i) functional benefit in post-MI recovery with MSC administration (11,74,75,91,92), (ii) evidence of neoangiogenesis at the site of the infarct (57,75,91,93), (iii) decrease in collagen deposition in the region of the scar, and (iv) evidence of cells with a myocyte-like phenotype, expressing contractile and sarcomeric proteins but lacking functional organization (11,12). Indeed, our group has found that allogeneic MSCs delivered to a region of damaged myocardium, engraft and express proteins typically restricted to cardiac myocytes, vascular endothelium, and smooth muscle (78). Further, engrafted MSCs reduce the extent of necrotic myocardium, promoting regeneration of new contractile myocardium along the subendocardial surface of the infarct, thereby restoring cardiac energy metabolism and subsequently normalizing systolic and diastolic cardiac function and performance. Finally, MSC's exhibit minimal MHC class II and ICAM expression and lack of MHC class I and B-7 costimulatory molecules necessary for T-cell mediated immune response (94) making them candidates for allogeneic transplantation.

In addition to potential differentiation capacity, MSCs participate in a coordinated program of cytokine and growth factor release following MI, marshalling both MSC and non-MSC cells such as cardiac stem cells to participate in cardiac repair. Injury signals, such as SDF-1, released from ischemic myocardium recruit MSCs to the area which then release other chemoattractants including SDF-1, G-CSF, and VEGF, recruiting other cells,

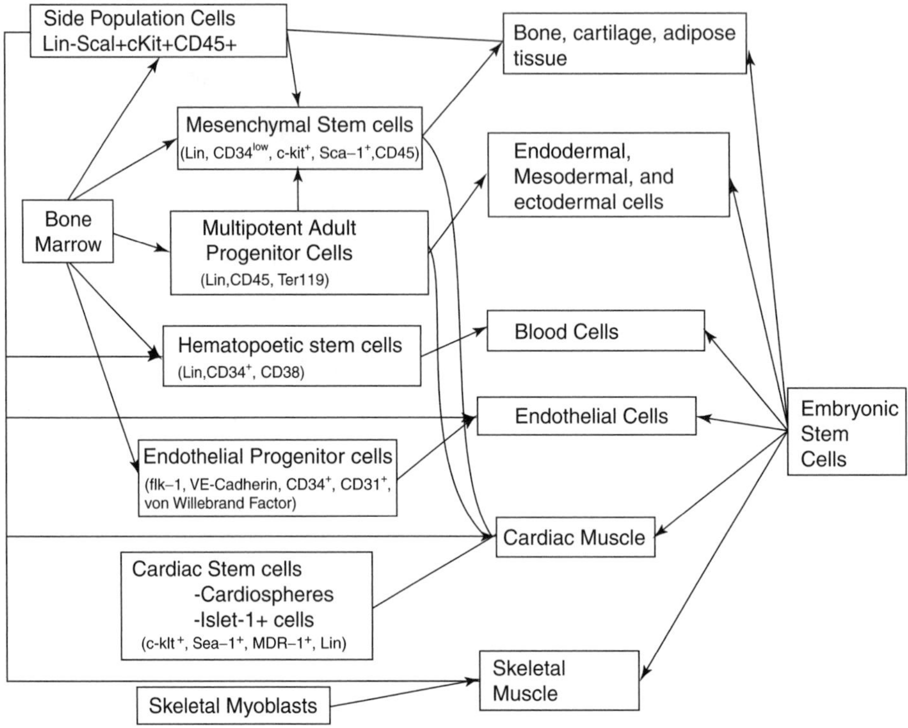

Figure 4 Depiction of stem cell types with their characteristic surface markers.

stimulating endogenous cardiac precursor cells to traffic and differentiate, and enhancing neovascularization (57,95,96). MSCs also reduce inflammation, collagen deposition, and cardiomyocyte hypertrophy and have been shown to regenerate up to 80–90% of lost myocardium after ischemic insult (11,12). Further, MSCs may provide anti-apoptotic stimuli as evidenced by studies demonstrating that MSC transplantation increases vascular density and blood flow, resulting in decreased apoptosis of hypertrophied myocytes (57).

Table 2 Human Mesenchymal Stem Cells Surface Markers

Positive			Negative		
CD13	CD102	CD140a	CD3	CD21	CD62E,L,S
CD29	CD105	CD166	CD4	CD25	CD80
CD44	CD106	P75	CD6	CD31	CD86
CD49a,b,c,d,e,f	CDw119	TGFb1R	CD9	CD34	CD95
CD51	CD120a	TGFbIIR	CD10	CD36	CD117
CD54	CD120b	HLA-A,B,C	CD11a	CD38	CD133
CD58	CD123	SSEA-3	CD14	CD45	SSEA-1
CD71	CD124	SSEA-4	CD15	CD49d	
CD73	CD126	D7	CD18	CD50	
CD90	CD127				

The letters a, b, c, d, e, f signify different subtypes of the CD49 molecule and are part of the standard nomenclature.
Source: From Ref. 186.

Finally, genetically engineered MSCs overexpressing the anti-apoptotic protein Akt1 lead to dramatic improvements in structure and function when transplanted into ischemic myocardium (12), suggesting that improved survival of transplanted MSCs is associated with increased cardiac repair.

Other investigators have identified cell populations with similar potential that appear to be closely related to MSCs. Jiang et al. (97) identified a population of multipotent adult progenitor cells (MAPCs) from the marrow of mice, which were found to purify along with MSCs. When injected into early blastocysts, MAPCs contributed to the formation of virtually all cell types, including myocardium. It has been postulated that MAPCs represent a precursor to MCSs that are capable of forming a variety of tissues, including myocytes and blood vessels thought to be essential for myocardial regeneration. In addition, side-population cells (SP), defined by their ability to exclude the fluorescent DNA-binding dye Hoechst 33342 via the verapamil sensitive ATP binding cassette (ABC) half-transporter, Abcg2 (98,99), obtained both from embryos and adult bone marrow have been shown to differentiate into both cardiac muscle (9) and bone (100) suggesting that they may be similar or related to MSC precursors. Finally, there exists a recently discovered cell type referred to as human BM-derived multipotent stem cells, distinct from MSCs and capable of differentiating into cardiomyocytes, endothelial cells, and smooth muscle cells (69). When injected into an area of ischemic myocardium these cells exert paracrine effects on the host myocardium, preventing apoptosis and stimulating proliferation of host tissue thereby preserving cardiac function.

Hematopoetic Precursor Cells

The defining properties of HSCs are their ability for radioprotection, self renewal, and differentiation. Their phenotype is characterized as being $CD34^+$, stem cell antigen $(SCA\text{-}1)^+$, $c\text{-}kit^+$, and Lin^- (101). Early reports indicated that when they engrafted into infarcted myocardium they form new myocytes, smooth muscle, and endothelial cells, (102). Moreover, developing myocytes express cytoplasmic and nuclear proteins typical of adult cardiomyocytes, including connexin 43 necessary for gap junction formation. Interestingly, although the HSCs were transplanted into the border zone of the infarct, new myocardium was formed within the infarct, suggesting that the donor cells migrated to the damaged area (102). The net result was a striking improvement in functional competence with significant increases in indices of contractility and lower left ventricular end-diastolic pressures (102). However, these early reports have been contradicted by more recent studies showing that engraftment of HSC in infarcted myocardium is transient in nature and results only in the development of hematopoietic cells rather than cardiomyocytes (62,103,104).

Peripheral Blood–Derived Cells

Endothelial Progenitor Cells

EPCs may play an important role in endothelial maintenance and their use for cardiomyoplasty is based on the notion that they will induce revascularization of the ischemic area through a process known as postnatal vasculogenesis. EPCs can be identified in the peripheral blood by the expression of several cell surface antigens including CD34, Flk-1, a receptor for vascular endothelial growth factor (VEGF), (105,106) and CD133 (107–109). The contribution of these cells to vasculogenesis has been demonstrated by studies showing that this population of cells circulates in the peripheral blood, expresses CD34 antigen and Flk-1, and can differentiate into endothelial cells in vitro and incorporate into sites of active angiogenesis in in vivo animal models of ischemia (105).

Experimental evidence demonstrates potential salutary effects of EPC administration in MI. Human EPCs injected intravenously into rats after MI home to ischemic areas of myocardium, differentiate into mature endothelial cells, and incorporate into a vascular network (110). Other studies suggest that EPCs may differentiate into a cardiomyocyte-like phenotype, expressing myocyte proteins including α-sarcomeric actinin, troponin I, and atrial natriuretic peptide and exhibiting synchronized calcium transients and gap junction–mediated communication with adjacent cardiomyocytes (111,112). On the other hand, endothelial cells derived from the embryonic mouse aorta can differentiate in vivo into myosin-positive cardiomyocytes and contribute to myocardial repair and new tissue repair in postischemic myocardium (113). Functional studies of EPC cardiomyoplasty demonstrate smaller ventricular dimensions, improved LV function, decreased size of the ischemic area, increased capillary density and coronary collateralization, and significantly decreased extent of left ventricular scarring (110,114).

The use of these cells in humans is still in the early stages of investigation though initial results are quite promising. The number and migratory activity of circulating EPCs inversely correlates with risk factors for coronary artery disease (115) and the number of circulating CD34+EPC precursors increases significantly in patients with acute MI (116). Interestingly, the clinical benefit of hydroxymethyl glutaryl coenzyme A reductase inhibitor therapy in patients with coronary artery disease may be partially due to inhibition of senescence (117) and increases in number, functional activity (118), and migration (119) of EPCs. Other interventions that stimulate EPC mobilization, such as erythropoietin supplementation (120), are currently under investigation.

Endogenous Cardiac Stem Cells

Cardiac myocytes have been traditionally considered to withdraw permanently from the cell cycle shortly following birth (7). Recent findings from several laboratories now challenge this notion. First, given that myocyte apoptotic death occurs in normal hearts during aging, (121) it has become clear that, in the absence of myocyte regeneration, the normal heart would lose most of its mass in few decades and would not support the human life span (7). Second, (4,122) mitotic bodies were demonstrated in the myocardium of individuals with MI that increase in MI border zones and, to a lesser extent, in distant myocardium (3). Finally, studies of female hearts transplanted into male recipients have revealed the presence of integrated cardiomyocytes containing the Y chromosome (123,124) as well as an increase in the number of putative progenitor cells as indicated by the cell surface markers, c-kit, MDR1, or Sca-1 (5).

In 2003, a seminal report described the existence of Lin^{-}, c-kit positive cardiac progenitor cells which possessed the properties of self-renewal, clonogenicity, and multipotency (59). When injected into ischemic rat myocardium in vivo, these cells led to the formation of bands of reconstituted myocardium strongly resembling neonatal myocardium in arteriolar and capillary density. When isolated, regenerated myocytes were functionally competent, exhibiting sarcomeric shortening and calcium cycling. Several laboratories subsequently described endogenous cardiac progenitor cells capable of homing to injured myocardium and differentiating into a cardiac phenotype (8). Notably, Oh and coworkers described a CPC that was characterized by Sca1 positivity (8), Messina et al. isolated undifferentiated clonogenic cells expressing stem cell and endothelial progenitor cell markers that grow as contractile cardiospheres comprising 100–1000 cells (125). More recently, Laugwitz and colleagues identified $isl1^{+}$ cardiac progenitor cells in rat, mouse, and human myocardium capable, in the absence of cell fusion, of developing into a mature cardiac phenotype with intact Ca^{2+}-cycling, action potentials, and expression of myocytic markers (126). Interestingly, the SP cells described above have also been isolated from the myocardium (99) indicating that multiple sources of precursor cells reside in the heart.

To date limited in vivo data exist describing the functional effects of endogenous cardiac stem cell transplantation. However, a recent report of intra-aortic injection of cardiac stem cells in a rat MI model revealed preservation of left ventricular wall thickness, mass, volume, and function as well as evidence of myocardial regeneration and infarct size reduction in the absence of cell fusion (67). Thus, this cell type holds great promise and awaits further study to document its in vivo characteristics.

Skeletal Muscle–Derived Cells

Skeletal muscle precursors with the capacity to regenerate injured muscle have long been postulated to be of potential value as a cardiac reparative agent. Myoblasts or satellite cells are easy to obtain and autografts can be used to avoid immunorejection, making these cells a potentially useful source for cardiomyoplasty (41). When co-cultured with beating cardiomyocytes, skeletal muscle derived cells differentiate into cardiomyocyte-like cells, and express cardiac specific proteins, connexin 43 and cadherin (127). In addition, in vivo transplantation of skeletetal myoblasts into ischemic myocardium causes them to align in the cardiac fiber direction and switch to low-twitch fiber phenotype (128). However, enthusiasm over this cell type has been curbed by the demonstration that the transplanted SM lack α-myosin heavy chain, cardiac troponin I, and ANP, indicating incomplete trans-differentiation and are functionally isolated from the host tissue, raising significant concerns of the potential arrythmogenic implications of skeletal myoblast transplantation (129). Indeed, as outlined below, there is already evidence suggesting that the use of this cell type may be limited by the development of ventricular tachyarrythmia.

Embryonic Stem Cells

ESs, derived from the inner cell mass of the blastocyst-stage of early mammalian embryos, can proliferate indefinitely and be differentiated into derivates of the three primary germ layers in vitro. These cells can survive in damaged rat myocardium without immunorejection, differentiate into rod-shaped, striated myocytes and stimulate increased capillary density (32). Further, they have been shown to functionally couple with host cardiac myocytes and express connexin 43, supporting the notion that transplanted cardiac myocytes form a functional syncytium with the host myocardium in vitro (23). Finally, ES injection into acutely infarcted myocardium results in increased wall thickness and improved fractional shortening (31). However, the potential for teratoma formation (130) and ethical concerns over their use has limited their application in the United States.

DELIVERY ROUTES

The ideal route of delivery for stem cell therapy remains to be established. However, the ideal delivery system should be safe and ensure that adequate numbers of cells are delivered to and retained in the myocardium. To date, systemic intravenous (72,110), intracoronary (14,74,76,131–139), percutaneous endomyocardial (13,140–144), transepicardial (46,49,145–149), and even retrograde coronary venous (50,150) administration of stem cells have been used. Most animal and early human studies have examined the impact of direct injection of stem cells into the myocardium during open chest surgery. While this seems to be a relatively safe and somewhat effective means of delivery, clinically it is limited to patients undergoing thoracotomy. Percutaneous endomyocardial delivery of cells involves the use of specialized injection catheters to introduce cells directly into the myocardium. This technique ensures that the cells are delivered to the area of interest while avoiding the need for open chest surgery. Other studies have examined the safety and efficacy of intracoronary artery infusion of stem cells. In these studies the cells are typically infused through the central lumen of an angioplasty balloon catheter which is inflated for short periods of time during infusion in order to maximize the exposure time, and theoretically the engraftment of the stem cells to the host myocardium. The least invasive method of cell delivery is the systemic intravenous approach whereby cells are delivered via a peripheral vein. The feasibility of this approach is based on studies demonstrating the ability of stem cells to home to areas of ischemia (see below).

HOMING AND MIGRATION OF STEM CELLS

There is accumulating evidence that stem cell homing is directed by injury signal(s) emanating from the area within or surrounding the infarct. For example, stromal-cell-derived factor 1 (SDF-1), a chemokine that is a natural ligand for the CXCR4 receptor, is crucial for bone marrow retention of hematopoietic stem cells (151,152), cardiogenesis (92), recruitment of EPCs to sites of ischemic tissue (153) and, perhaps, migration of tissue-committed stem/progenitor cells (154). Interestingly, it was recently shown that the CXCR4 receptor is strongly expressed by a proportion of MSCs and that it plays an important role in MSC mobilization (155). Expression of SDF-1 dramatically increases over the first week following infarction and exogenous expression of SDF-1 increases the numbers of mobilized BMCs homing to the heart at time periods remote from infarction (156). Furthermore, tissue ischemia results in upregulation of angiogenic factors, including VEGF, which through its interaction with its receptors VEGFR2 and VEGFR1 expressed on bone marrow–derived EPCs, circulating EPCs (CEP), HSCs, and hematopoietic progenitor cells (HPC), promotes migration of these cells to the site of injury (157).

Several studies of MSC transplantation have further solidified the evidence for stem cell migration. For instance, mice pretreated with recombinant rat SCF and recombinant human G-CSF for 5 days (90) prior to MI demonstrate myocardial regeneration with formation of myocytes, arterioles, and capillaries and significantly decreased infarct size and mortality compared to control animals. These results demonstrate that exogenous cytokines have the potential to induce stem cell mobilization and migration to the infarct, regenerating functionally integrated myocardium. Also, transplantation of MSCs into the MI borderzone results in new myocardium formation within the infarct, suggesting MSC migration to the damaged area (102). Finally, detection of Y chromosome–containing cells in male recipients of female donor hearts has solidified the evidence for stem cell migration (5).

HUMAN TRIALS

Based on the above described preclinical work, a variety of cell-based therapies have entered early clinical studies. As described below, the results, to date, offer cautious optimism regarding the future of cellular cardiomyoplasty but also raise cautionary notes about pro-arrhythmia.

Skeletal Myoblasts

There have been several case reports and very small phase I clinical trials investigating the feasibility of autologous skeletal myoblast transplantation (46,147,158,159) for ischemic cardiomyopathy as well as the ability of transplanted cells to survive and differentiate in human myocardium. Though limited by extremely small numbers of patients (typically less than 10 to 15) as well as a lack of blinding, control groups and randomization, these studies suggest potential improvements in left ventricular ejection fraction (147,160), increased wall thickening (143), and New York Heart Association functional class(46,160). However, the lack of electromechanical coupling between engrafted SM and cadiac myocytes in vivo (129,161) has raised serious concerns over the likelihood of an increase in ventricular tachyarrhythmias secondary to the formation of re-entry circuits (15,46,143). Indeed, reports of increased arrhythmias in these patients have mandated the use of ICD placement for enrolled patients (162).

Autologous Mononuclear Bone Marrow Cells (AMBMC)

Based on growing awareness that BM contains a variety of stem cells, preliminary clinical studies have been conducted using autologous mononuclear bone marrow cells (AMBMC). The Therapeutic Angiogenesis using Cell Transplantation Study investigators (163) injected bone marrow mononuclear cells into the gastrocnemius of patients with lower extremity ischemia and demonstrated significant improvement in ankle-brachial pressure index, rest pain, and pain-free walking time, concluding that the efficacy of implantation of these cells is due to the supply of EPCs (Table 3).

Acute MI

As with SM, there have been several small studies evaluating the safety and feasibility of AMBMC cardiomyoplasty in patients in the peri-infarct period. Although these studies are also limited by similarly small numbers of patients, lack of blinding, control groups, and randomization, they do offer promising insights into the potential of AMBMC transplantation. In the earliest such study, Strauer and colleagues performed a clinical trial randomizing 20 patients with transmural MI to receive either intracoronary AMBMC injection 12 hr after acute MI or standard medical therapy. The IC AMBMC decreased infarct size from $30 \pm 13\%$ to $12 \pm 7\%$ and also decreased the size of perfusion defects as assessed by ^{201}thallium scintigraphy by 26% ($174 \pm 99\ cm^2$ to $128 \pm 71\ cm^2$) compared to baseline values (14). Subsequently, Stamm and colleagues demonstrated similar improvements in perfusion, LV dimensions, and EF in an uncontrolled, non–blinded phase I study in 12 patients with transmural MI and LV dysfunction (EF of $39.7 \pm 9\%$). These patients had infarct areas not amenable to surgical or interventional revascularization and received intraoperative AMBMC injection during elective CABG performed to bypass occlusions of coronary arteries other than the infarct vessel in the first 3 mo post-MI (148,149). In the TOPCARE-AMI (135) trial,

Table 3 Human Trials of Cellular-Based Therapies

Study	N	Cell type	Delivery	Timing	Effect
Strauer (14)	10 treated, 10 controls	Bone marrow	IC	Acute MI	Improved regional wall motion and perfusion, decreased infarct size
TOPCARE-AMI (135)	29 Bone marrow patients, 30 EPC patients, 11 controls	Bone marrow, EPC	IC	Acute MI	Improved regional wall motion, coronary flow, LVEF, and decreased infarct size
Fernandez-Aviles (137)	20 treated, 13 controls	Bone marrow	IC	Acute MI	Improved regional wall motion and LVEF
Kuethe (210)	5 treated	Bone marrow	IC	Acute MI	No change in regional wall motion or LVEF
BOOST (134)	30 treated, 30 controls	Bone marrow	IC	Acute MI	Improved regional wall motion and LVEF
Chen (139)	34 treated, 35 controls	MSC	IC	Acute MI	Improved regional wall motion and LVEF, decreased infarct size, decreased left ventricular end diastolic volume
Hamano (146)	5 treated	Bone marrow	Transepicardial	Chronic	Increased perfusion

Tse (144)	8 treated	Bone marrow	Transendocardial	Chronic	Increased perfusion, increased regional wall motion
Fuchs (141)	10 treated	Bone marrow	Transendocardial	Chronic	Increased perfusion
Perin (13,142)	14 treated, 7 controls	Bone marrow	Transendocardial	Chronic	Improved regional wall motion and LVEF, perfusion
Menasche (46)	10 treated	Myoblasts	Transepicardial	Chronic	Improved regional wall motion and LVEF
Herreros (147)	11 treated	Myoblasts	Transepicardial	Chronic	Improved regional wall motion and LVEF, incresed viability in infarct scar
Siminiak (49)	10 treated	Myoblasts	Transepicardial	Chronic	Improved regional wall motion and LVEF
Chachques (211)	20 treated	Myoblasts	Transepicardial	?	Improved regional wall motion and LVEF, incresed viability in infarct scar
Smits (143)	5 treated	Myoblasts	Transendocardial	Chronic	Improved regional wall motion and LVEF
Stamm (148,149)	12 treated	Bone marrow	Transepicardial	Chronic	Improved LVEF, perfusion, decresead left ventricular end diastolic volume

Abbreviations: EPC, endothelial progenitor cell; MI, myocardial infarction; IC, intracardial; LVEF, left ventricular ejection fraction.
Source: Adapted from Ref. 209.

patients post-MI were randomized to receive either AMBMC (n=9) or peripheral blood derived progenitor cells (n=11) into the infarct artery approximately four days after reperfusion with coronary stenting. Over 90% of the cells derived from peripheral blood exhibited endothelial cell characteristics including VEGF receptor (KDR), von Willebrand factor, CD31, and VE-Cadherin while those derived form bone marrow included cells exhibiting CD34 and CD133. The results demonstrated a ~9% absolute increase in LV ejection fraction (from 51.6±9.6% at baseline to 60.1±8.6% after 4 mo) as well as improvement in wall motion abnormalities in the infarct area, and reduction in end-systolic LV volume. Furthermore there was complete normalization of coronary flow reserve in the infarct artery and a significant increase in myocardial viability within the infarcted segments. Importantly, these improvements did not differ between patients receiving bone marrow or peripheral blood–derived progenitor cells. Though this was a pilot trial, limited by the lack of a control group and only four months of follow-up, the results were quite promising, supporting larger, controlled clinical trials.

In the recent randomized controlled Intracoronary autologous bone marrow cell transfer after myocardial infarction; the BOOST randmized controlled clinical trial. Patients received either intracoronary transfer of AMBMC (n=30) or standard post-infarct medical therapy 4 to 8 days after percutaneous coronary intervention for their first acute ST segment elevation MI. They demonstrated a 6.7±9.5% absolute improvement in global LV EF in the cell group (46.3±10.6% at baseline to 53.0±15.5% at 6 mo) as compared to only a 1.1±11.8% increase in the control group (47.8±9.7% at baseline to 48.9±15.2%) (p=0.0026). Furthermore, stem cell transplantation was also associated with increased systolic wall motion in the MI border zone. Interestingly, there was no difference between the control and AMBMC-treated groups with respect to the number of premature ventricular complexes or ventricular tachyarrythmias as assessed by Holter monitoring for up to 6 mo of follow-up (134), reassuring data suggesting that AMBMC therapy did not increase risk for arrhythmias. Importantly, infarct size as measured by late enhancement MRI was not reduced compared to placebo in BOOST. Recently, in a clinical study of stem cell homing, Hoffmann and colleagues demonstrated that, when administered using an intracoronary technique, unselected bone marrow cells engraft in the infarct center and border zone, while CD34 enriched bone marrow cells preferentially home to the border zone (164).

In addition to cell therapy there is emerging clinical data regarding the use of bone marrow–stimulating cytokine cocktails, alone or in combination with cell administration. The MAGIC cell clinical trial randomized 27 patients undergoing percutaneous coronary intervention for acute and chronic MI to receive granulocyte-colony stimulating factor (G-CSF) (n=10), G-CSF plus peripheral blood mononuclear cell infusion (n=10) or standard medical therapy alone (n=7). They demonstrated after 6 mo of follow-up that peripheral blood mononuclear cells stimulated by G-CSF and infused into the infarct related artery resulted in improved exercise capacity, myocardial perfusion (6.3% absolute decrease in the areas of hypoperfusion as measured by SPECT (11.6±9.6% at baseline vs. 5.3±5% at 6 mo; p=0.004)), and improved LV EF as measured by SPECT [6.7% absolute increase (48.7±8.3% at baseline vs. 55.1±7.4% at 6 mo; p=0.020)] compared to baseline (131). Unfortunately, an unexpectedly high rate of in-stent restenosis was noted in the patients receiving G-CSF, prompting early termination of the trial (131). Despite the limitations stated above, these data (n~100 patients) offer promising but not conclusive data regarding the potential of cardiomyoplasty as a therapy in acute MI. It is clear that properly randomized controlled clinical trials are needed to elucidate the mechanisms and benefits of the therapeutic modality.

Chronic Ischemia

Though multiple studies have investigated the safety and feasibility of autologous bone marrow cell transplantation for ischemic heart disease these too are small and often not controlled (13,54,141,144,146,165).

Hamano and colleagues performed a non-randomized study of direct injection of AMBMC into the ungraftable or peri-infarct myocardium during CABG in 5 patients and found improved perfusion to the treated areas up to one year after surgery (146). Ozbaran and colleagues injected peripheral blood stem cells mobilized with G-CSF into the myocardium of 6 patients with severe ischemic cardiomyopathy (EF<25%) demonstrating significant improvements in NYHA functional class and quality of life (166). However, it is important to note that it is difficult to determine how much of the improvement in perfusion is secondary to the stem cells as opposed to the surgical revascularization.

Several small non-randomized studies of sample sizes less than 20 using catheter based injections of AMBMC into chronically ischemic myocardium have demonstrated improvement in myocardial function and perfusion as well as symptoms (13,141,144). Perin and colleagues performed a nonrandomized, open-labeled study comparing AMBMC injection (n=14) to standard therapy (n=7) in 21 patients with severe ischemic HF. They used a NOGA catheter to percutaneously inject AMBMC into the hibernating myocardium of patients with severe ischemic HF. They showed a 73% reduction in the total reversible perfusion defect, improved mechanical function of injected segements as determined by electromechanical mapping, improved EF (9%) and global LV function, as well as improved New York Heart Association functional class and Canadian Cardiovascular Society Angina score (13). Together these results support ongoing research into AMBMC transplants for chronic ischemic cardiomyopathy (167).

Mesenchymal Stem Cells

Early studies have also investigated the use of MSCs in Acute MI. Chen and colleagues (139) randomized patients (n=69) who had undergone coronary catheterization within 12 hr after onset of acute MI to receive intracoronary injection of autologous MSCs or saline ~18 days after the acute event. Using positron emission tomography, cardiac catheterization, and cardiac echocardiography they demonstrated significantly improved left ventricular function in the MSC-treated patients. Other, non-cardiac, uses of MSC transplantation include their administration for the prevention of lethal graft versus host disease in bone marrow transplant patients (168–170) and osteogenesis imperfecta (171–175).

POTENTIAL COMPLICATIONS

As outlined above, multiple studies have safely delivered stem cells to patients. However, concerns remain regarding the potential complications of cellular cardiomyoplasty. While systemic delivery of cells appears safe, it may be limited by trapping substantial numbers of cells in the lungs and other tissues (176,177). While intracoronary delivery offers better localization of cells to the myocardium there is evidence suggesting that this technique may cause myocardial microinfarctions (133). Direct intramyocardial delivery of cells may lead to the stimulation of arrhythmias during the injection procedure or puncture of the myocardium with resultant tamponade. However, there is emerging experience that these techniques have acceptable safety (13,44,74,133,142).

Adult stem cells may evolve spontaneous genetic changes leading to tumorigenicity (178–180). Indeed, it has been shown that bone marrow cells can migrate and integrate into gliomas after intravascular delivery (181) and play an important role in the angiogenesis and progression of neuroblastomas (182). These in vivo reports highlight the need for long-term preclinical studies and phase I safety studies with candidate cell types before entry into clinical trials.

CONCLUSION

The field of stem cell–mediated myocardial repair has advanced rapidly over the past few years, with early studies being performed in humans. Emerging results suggest that this therapeutic approach may hold substantial promise for the treatment of a host of diseases of the myocardium. While this field is at an early stage, both basic and translational research approaches are proceeding at a rapid pace. The performance of clinical trials with rigorous design informed by appropriate pre-clinical and mechanistic studies will clarify the role for this new therapy in the armamentarium of approaches to structural heart disease.

REFERENCES

1. Pfeffer MA, Braunwald E. Ventricular remodeling after myocardial infarction. Experimental observations and clinical implications. Circulation 1990; 81:1161–1172.
2. Anversa P, Kajstura J. Ventricular myocytes are not terminally differentiated in the adult mammalian heart. Circ Res 1998; 83:1–14.
3. Beltrami AP, Urbanek K, Kajstura J, et al. Evidence that human cardiac myocytes divide after myocardial infarction. N Engl J Med 2001; 344:1750–1757.
4. Kajstura J, Leri A, Finato N, et al. Myocyte proliferation in end-stage cardiac failure in humans. Proc Natl Acad Sci USA 1998; 95:8801–8805.
5. Quaini F, Urbanek K, Beltrami AP, et al. Chimerism of the transplanted heart. N Engl J Med 2002; 346:5–15.
6. Anversa P, Nadal-Ginard B. Myocyte renewal and ventricular remodelling. Nature 2002; 415:240–243.
7. Nadal-Ginard B, Kajstura J, Leri A, et al. Myocyte death, growth, and regeneration in cardiac hypertrophy and failure. Circ Res 2003; 92:139–150.
8. Oh H, Bradfute SB, Gallardo TD, et al. Cardiac progenitor cells from adult myocardium: homing, differentiation, and fusion after infarction. Proc Natl Acad Sci USA 2003; 100:12313–12318.
9. Jackson KA, Majka SM, Wang H, et al. Regeneration of ischemic cardiac muscle and vascular endothelium by adult stem cells. J Clin Invest 2001; 107:1395–1402.
10. Aicher A, Heeschen C, Mildner-Rihm C, et al. Essential role of endothelial nitric oxide synthase for mobilization of stem and progenitor cells. Nat Med 2003; 9:1370–1376.
11. Shake JG, Gruber PJ, Baumgartner WA, et al. Mesenchymal stem cell implantation in a swine myocardial infarct model: engraftment and functional effects. Ann Thorac Surg 2002; 73:1919–1925.
12. Mangi AA, Noiseux N, Kong D, et al. Mesenchymal stem cells modified with akt prevent remodeling and restore performance of infarcted hearts. Nat Med 2003; 9:1195–1201.
13. Perin EC, Dohmann HF, Borojevic R, et al. Transendocardial, autologous bone marrow cell transplantation for severe, chronic ischemic heart failure. Circulation 2003; 107:2294–2302.

14. Strauer BE, Brehm M, Zeus T, et al. Repair of infarcted myocardium by autologous intracoronary mononuclear bone marrow cell transplantation in humans. Circulation 2002; 106:1913–1918.
15. Couzin J, Vogel G. Cell therapy. Renovating the heart. Science 2004; 304:192–194.
16. Chiu RC, Zibaitis A, Kao RL. Cellular cardiomyoplasty: myocardial regeneration with satellite cell implantation. Ann Thorac Surg 1995; 60:12–18.
17. Reffelmann T, Leor J, Muller-Ehmsen J, et al. Cardiomyocyte transplantation into the failing heart-new therapeutic approach for heart failure? Heart Fail Rev 2003; 8:201–211.
18. Huwer H, Winning J, Vollmar B, et al. Long-term cell survival and hemodynamic improvements after neonatal cardiomyocyte and satellite cell transplantation into healed myocardial cryoinfarcted lesions in rats. Cell Transplant 2003; 12:757–767.
19. Etzion S, Battler A, Barbash IM, et al. Influence of embryonic cardiomyocyte transplantation on the progression of heart failure in a rat model of extensive myocardial infarction. J Mol Cell Cardiol 2001; 33:1321–1330.
20. Leor J, Patterson M, Quinones MJ, et al. Transplantation of fetal myocardial tissue into the infarcted myocardium of rat. A potential method for repair of infarcted myocardium? Circulation 1996; 94:II332–II336.
21. Li RK, Jia ZQ, Weisel RD, et al. Cardiomyocyte transplantation improves heart function. Ann Thorac Surg 1996; 62:654–660.
22. Li RK, Mickle DA, Weisel RD, et al. Natural history of fetal rat cardiomyocytes transplanted into adult rat myocardial scar tissue. Circulation 1997; 96:II-86.
23. Rubart M, Pasumarthi KBS, Nakajima H, et al. Physiological coupling of donor and host cardiomyocytes after cellular transplantation. Circ Res 2003; 92:1217–1224.
24. Ruhparwar A, Tebbenjohanns J, Niehaus M, et al. Transplanted fetal cardiomyocytes as cardiac pacemaker. Eur J Cardiothorac Surg 2002; 21:853–857.
25. Scorsin M, Marotte F, Sabri A, et al. Can grafted cardiomyocytes colonize peri-infarct myocardial areas? Circulation 1996; 94:II337–II340.
26. Scorsin M, Hagege AA, Marotte F, et al. Does transplantation of cardiomyocytes improve function of infarcted myocardium? Circulation 1997; 96:II-93.
27. Scorsin M, Hagege AA, Dolizy I, et al. Can cellular transplantation improve function in doxorubicin-induced heart failure? Circulation 1998; 98:II151–II155.
28. Skobel E, Schuh A, Schwarz ER, et al. Transplantation of fetal cardiomyocytes into infarcted rat hearts results in long-term functional improvement. Tissue Eng 2004; 10:849–864.
29. Yamamoto M, Sakakibara Y, Nishimura K, et al. Improved therapeutic efficacy in cardiomyocyte transplantation for myocardial infarction with release system of basic fibroblast growth factor. Artif Organs 2003; 27:181–184.
30. Yokomuro H, Li RK, Mickle DA, et al. Transplantation of cryopreserved cardiomyocytes. J Thorac Cardiovasc Surg 2001; 121:98–107.
31. Min JY, Yang Y, Converso KL, et al. Transplantation of embryonic stem cells improves cardiac function in postinfarcted rats. J Appl Physiol 2002; 92:288–296.
32. Min JY, Yang Y, Sullivan MF, et al. Long-term improvement of cardiac function in rats after infarction by transplantation of embryonic stem cells. J Thorac Cardiovasc Surg 2003; 125:361–369.
33. Hodgson DM, Behfar A, Zingman LV, et al. Stable benefit of embryonic stem cell therapy in myocardial infarction. Am J Physiol Heart Circ Physiol 2004; 287:H471–H479.
34. Klug MG, Soonpaa MH, Koh GY, et al. Genetically selected cardiomyocytes from differentiating embronic stem cells form stable intracardiac grafts. J Clin Invest 1996; 98:216–224.
35. Zimmermann WH, Eschenhagen T. Cardiac tissue engineering for replacement therapy. Heart Fail Rev 2003; 8:259–269.
36. Eschenhagen T, Didie M, Munzel F, et al. 3D engineered heart tissue for replacement therapy. Basic Res Cardiol 2002; 97:I146–I152.
37. Mann BK, West JL. Tissue engineering in the cardiovascular system: progress toward a tissue engineered heart. Anat Rec 2001; 263:367–371.

38. Remppis A, Pleger ST, Most P, et al. S100A1 gene transfer: a strategy to strengthen engineered cardiac grafts. J Gene Med 2004; 6:387–394.
39. Shimizu T, Yamato M, Isoi Y, et al. Fabrication of pulsatile cardiac tissue grafts using a novel 3-dimensional cell sheet manipulation technique and temperature-responsive cell culture surfaces. Circ Res 2002; 90:e40.
40. Zimmermann WH, Didie M, Wasmeier GH, et al. Cardiac grafting of engineered heart tissue in syngenic rats. Circulation 2002; 106:I151–I157.
41. Thompson RB, Emani SM, Davis BH, et al. Comparison of intracardiac cell transplantation: Autologous skeletal myoblasts versus bone marrow cells. Circulation 2003; 108:264–271.
42. Dib N, McCarthy P, Campbell A, et al. Feasibility and safety of autologous myoblast transplantation in patients with ischemic cardiomyopathy. Cell Transplant 2005; 14:11–19.
43. Gulbins H, Schrepfer S, Uhlig A, et al. Myoblasts survive intracardiac transfer and divide further after transplantation. Heart Surg Forum 2002; 5:340–344.
44. Ince H, Petzsch M, Rehders TC, et al. Transcatheter transplantation of autologous skeletal myoblasts in postinfarction patients with severe left ventricular dysfunction. J Endovasc Ther 2004; 11:695–704.
45. Menasche P, Vilquin J-T, Desnos M, et al. Early results of autologous skeletal myoblast transplantation in patients with severe ischemic heart failure. Circulation 2002; 104:II-598.
46. Menasche P, Hagege AA, Vilquin JT, et al. Autologous skeletal myoblast transplantation for severe postinfarction left ventricular dysfunction. J Am Coll Cardiol 2003; 41:1078–1083.
47. Menasche P. Skeletal myoblast transplantation for cardiac repair. Expert Rev Cardiovasc Ther 2004; 2:21–28.
48. Murtuza B, Suzuki K, Bou-Gharios G, et al. Transplantation of skeletal myoblasts secreting an IL-1 inhibitor modulates adverse remodeling in infarcted murine myocardium. Proc Natl Acad Sci USA 2004; 101:4216–4221.
49. Siminiak T, Kalawski R, Fiszer D, et al. Autologous skeletal myoblast transplantation for the treatment of postinfarction myocardial injury: phase I clinical study with 12 months of follow-up. Am Heart J 2004; 148:531–537.
50. Siminiak T, Fiszer D, Jerzykowska O, et al. Percutaneous trans-coronary-venous transplantation of autologous skeletal myoblasts in the treatment of post-infarction myocardial contractility impairment: the POZNAN trial. Eur Heart J 2005.
51. Tambara K, Sakakibara Y, Sakaguchi G, et al. Transplanted skeletal myoblasts can fully replace the infarcted myocardium when they survive in the host in large numbers. Circulation 2003; 108:II259–II263.
52. Taylor DA, Atkins BZ, Hungspreugs P, et al. Regenerating functional myocardium: improved performance after skeletal myoblast transplantation. Nat Med 1998; 4:929–933.
53. Davani S, Marandin A, Mersin N, et al. Mesenchymal progenitor cells differentiate into an endothelial phenotype, enhance vascular density, and improve heart function in a rat cellular cardiomyoplasty model. Circulation 2003; 108:II253–II258.
54. Galinanes M, Loubani M, Davies J, et al. Autotransplantation of unmanipulated bone marrow into scarred myocardium is safe and enhances cardiac function in humans. Cell Transplant 2004; 13:7–13.
55. Kudo M, Wang Y, Wani MA, et al. Implantation of bone marrow stem cells reduces the infarction and fibrosis in ischemic mouse heart. J Mol Cell Cardiol 2003; 35:1113–1119.
56. Lopes OE, Ribeiro VP, Castro JP SW, et al. Bone marrow stromal cells improve cardiac performance in healed infarcted rat hearts. Am J Physiol Heart Circ Physiol 2004.
57. Tang YL, Zhao Q, Zhang YC, et al. Autologous mesenchymal stem cell transplantation induce VEGF and neovascularization in ischemic myocardium. Regul Pept 2004; 117:3–10.
58. Zhang S, Guo J, Zhang P, et al. Long-term effects of bone marrow mononuclear cell transplantation on left ventricular function and remodeling in rats. Life Sci 2004; 74:2853–2864.
59. Beltrami AP, Barlucchi L, Torella D, et al. Adult cardiac stem cells are multipotent and support myocardial regeneration. Cell 2003; 114:763–776.

60. Beltrami AP, Urbanek K, Kajstura J, et al. Evidence that human cardiac myocytes divide after myocardial infarction. N Engl J Med 2001; 344:1750–1757.
61. Kajstura J, Rota M, Whang B, et al. Bone marrow cells differentiate in cardiac cell lineages after infarction independently of cell fusion. Circ Res 2004.
62. Nygren JM, Jovinge S, Breitbach M, et al. Bone marrow-derived hematopoietic cells generate cardiomyocytes at a low frequency through cell fusion, but not transdifferentiation. Nat Med 2004; 10:494–501.
63. Fraidenraich D, Stillwell E, Romero E, et al. Rescue of cardiac defects in Id knockout embryos by injection of embryonic stem cells. Science 2004; 306:247–252.
64. Gnecchi M, He H, Liang OD, et al. Paracrine action accounts for marked protection of ischemic heart by Akt-modified mesenchymal stem cells. Nat Med 2005; 11:367–368.
65. Terada N, Hamazaki T, Oka M, et al. Bone marrow cells adopt the phenotype of other cells by spontaneous cell fusion. Nature 2002; 416:542–545.
66. Alvarez-Dolado M, Pardal R, Garcia-Verdugo JM, et al. Fusion of bone-marrow-derived cells with Purkinje neurons, cardiomyocytes and hepatocytes. Nature 2003; 425:968–973.
67. Dawn B, Stein AB, Urbanek K, et al. Cardiac stem cells delivered intravascularly traverse the vessel barrier, regenerate infarcted myocardium, and improve cardiac function. Proc Natl Acad Sci USA 2005; 102:3766–3771.
68. Quesenberry PJ, Abedi M, Aliotta J, et al. Stem cell plasticity: an overview. Blood Cells Mol Dis 2004; 32:1–4.
69. Yoon YS, Wecker A, Heyd L, et al. Clonally expanded novel multipotent stem cells from human bone marrow regenerate myocardium after myocardial infarction. J Clin Invest 2005; 115:326–338.
70. Kamihata H, Matsubara H, Nishiue T, et al. Implantation of bone marrow mononuclear cells into ischemic myocardium enhances collateral perfusion and regional function via side supply of angioblasts, angiogenic ligands, and cytokines. Circulation 2001; 104:1046–1052.
71. Kamihata H, Matsubara H, Nishiue T, et al. Improvement of collateral perfusion and regional function by implantation of peripheral blood mononuclear cells into ischemic hibernating myocardium. Arterioscler Thromb Vasc Biol 2002; 22:1804–1810.
72. Kocher AA, Schuster MD, Szabolcs MJ, et al. Neovascularization of ischemic myocardium by human bone-marrow-derived angioblasts prevents cardiomyocyte apoptosis, reduces remodeling and improves cardiac function. Nat Med 2001; 7:430–436.
73. Schuster MD, Kocher AA, Seki T, et al. Myocardial neovascularization by bone marrow angioblasts results in cardiomyocyte regeneration. Am J Physiol Heart Circ Physiol 2004; 287:H525–H532.
74. Chen SL, Fang WW, Qian J, et al. Improvement of cardiac function after transplantation of autologous bone marrow mesenchymal stem cells in patients with acute myocardial infarction. Chin Med J (Engl) 2004; 117:1443–1448.
75. Nagaya N, Fujii T, Iwase T, et al. Intravenous administration of mesenchymal stem cells improves cardiac function in rats with acute myocardial infarction through angiogenesis and myogenesis. Am J Physiol Heart Circ Physiol 2004; 287:H2670–H2676.
76. Schachinger V, Assmus B, Britten MB, et al. Transplantation of progenitor cells and regeneration enhancement in acute myocardial infarction. Final one-year results of the TOPCARE-AMI trial. J Am Coll Cardiol 2004; 44:1690–1699.
77. Jain M, DerSimonian H, Brenner DA, et al. Cell therapy attenuates deleterious ventricular remodeling and improves cardiac performance after myocardial infarction. Circulation 2001; 103:1920–1927.
78. Amado LC, Saliaris AP, Schuleri KH, et al. Cardiac repair with intra-myocardial injection of allogeneic mesenchymal stem cells following myocardial infarction. Proc Natl Acad Sci USA 2005; 102:11474–11479.
79. Pittenger MF, Mackay AM, Beck SC, et al. Multilineage potential of adult human mesenchymal stem cells. Science 1999; 284:143–147.
80. Zuk PA, Zhu M, Ashjian P, et al. Human adipose tissue is a source of multipotent stem cells. Mol Biol Cell 2002; 13:4279–4295.

81. Zuk PA, Zhu M, Mizuno H, et al. Multilineage cells from human adipose tissue: implications for cell-based therapies. Tissue Eng 2001; 7:211–228.
82. Rangappa S, Fen C, Lee EH, et al. Transformation of adult mesenchymal stem cells isolated from the fatty tissue into cardiomyocytes. Ann Thorac Surg 2003; 75:775–779.
83. Zvaifler NJ, Marinova-Mutafchieva L, Adams G, et al. Mesenchymal precursor cells in the blood of normal individuals. Arthritis Res 2000; 2:477–488.
84. Fernandez M, Simon V, Herrera G, et al. Detection of stromal cells in peripheral blood progenitor cell collections from breast cancer patients. Bone Marrow Transplant 1997; 20:265–271.
85. Deans RJ, Moseley AB. Mesenchymal stem cells: biology and potential clinical uses. Exp Hematol 2000; 28:875–884.
86. Gojo S, Gojo N, Takeda Y, et al. In vivo cardiovasculogenesis by direct injection of isolated adult mesenchymal stem cells. Exp Cell Res 2003; 288:51–59.
87. Peister A, Mellad JA, Larson BL, et al. Adult stem cells from bone marrow (MSCs) isolated from different strains of inbred mice vary in surface epitopes, rates of proliferation, and differentiation potential. Blood 2003; 103:1662–1668.
88. Ashman LK. The biology of stem cell factor and its receptor C-kit. Int J Biochem Cell Biol 1999; 31:1037–1051.
89. Heissig B, Werb Z, Rafii S, et al. Role of c-kit/Kit ligand signaling in regulating vasculogenesis. Thromb Haemost 2003; 90:570–576.
90. Orlic D, Kajstura J, Chimenti S, et al. Mobilized bone marrow cells repair the infarcted heart, improving function and survival. Proc Natl Acad Sci USA 2001; 98:10344–10349.
91. Silva GV, Litovsky S, Assad JA, et al. Mesenchymal stem cells differentiate into an endothelial phenotype, enhance vascular density, and improve heart function in a canine chronic ischemia model. Circulation 2005; 111:150–156.
92. Tomita S, Mickle DA, Weisel RD, et al. Improved heart function with myogenesis and angiogenesis after autologous porcine bone marrow stromal cell transplantation. J Thorac Cardiovasc Surg 2002; 123:1132–1140.
93. Ma J, Ge J, Zhang S, et al. Time course of myocardial stromal cell-derived factor 1 expression and beneficial effects of intravenously administered bone marrow stem cells in rats with experimental myocardial infarction. Basic Res Cardiol 2005; 100:217–223.
94. Klyushnenkova E, Shustova V, Mosca J, et al. Human mesenchymal stem cells induce unresponsiveness in preactivated but not naive alloantigen specific T cells. Exp Hematol 1999; 27:122.
95. Zhu GR, Zhou XY, Lu H, et al. Human bone marrow mesenchymal stem cells express multiple hematopoietic growth factors. Zhongguo Shi Yan Xue Ye Xue Za Zhi 2003; 11:115–119.
96. Al Khaldi A, Eliopoulos N, Martineau D, et al. Postnatal bone marrow stromal cells elicit a potent VEGF-dependent neoangiogenic response in vivo. Gene Ther 2003; 10:621–629.
97. Jiang Y, Jahagirdar BN, Reinhardt RL, et al. Pluripotency of mesenchymal stem cells derived from adult marrow. Nature 2002; 418:41–49.
98. Meeson AP, Hawke TJ, Graham S, et al. Cellular and molecular regulation of skeletal muscle side population cells. Stem Cells 2004; 22:1305–1320.
99. Martin CM, Meeson AP, Robertson SM, et al. Persistent expression of the ATP-binding cassette transporter. Abcg2, identifies cardiac SP cells in the developing and adult heart. Dev Biol 2004; 265:262–275.
100. Olmsted-Davis EA, Gugala Z, Camargo F, et al. Primitive adult hematopoietic stem cells can function as osteoblast precursors. Proc Natl Acad Sci USA 2003; 100:15877–15882.
101. Huss R. Isolation of primary and immortalized CD34-hematopoietic and mesenchymal stem cells from various sources. Stem Cells 2000; 18:1–9.
102. Orlic D, Kajstura J, Chimenti S, et al. Bone marrow cells regenerate infarcted myocardium. Nature 2001; 410:701–705.
103. Balsam LB, Wagers AJ, Christensen JL, et al. Haematopoietic stem cells adopt mature haematopoietic fates in ischaemic myocardium. Nature 2004; 428:668–673.

104. Murry CE, Soonpaa MH, Reinecke H, et al. Haematopoietic stem cells do not transdifferentiate into cardiac myocytes in myocardial infarcts. Nature 2004; 428:664–668.
105. Asahara T, Murohara T, Sullivan A, et al. Isolation of putative progenitor endothelial cells for angiogenesis. Science 1997; 275:964–967.
106. Asahara T, Masuda H, Takahashi T, et al. Bone marrow origin of endothelial progenitor cells responsible for postnatal vasculogenesis in physiological and pathological neovascularization. Circ Res 1999; 85:221–228.
107. Gehling UM, Ergun S, Schumacher U, et al. In vitro differentiation of endothelial cells from AC133-positive progenitor cells. Blood 2000; 95:3106–3112.
108. Peichev M, Naiyer AJ, Pereira D, et al. Expression of VEGFR-2 and AC133 by circulating human CD34(+) cells identifies a population of functional endothelial precursors. Blood 2000; 95:952–958.
109. Schmeisser A, Strasser RH. Phenotypic overlap between hematopoietic cells with suggested angioblastic potential and vascular endothelial cells. J Hematother Stem Cell Res 2002; 11:69–79.
110. Kawamoto A, Gwon HC, Iwaguro H, et al. Therapeutic potential of ex vivo expanded endothelial progenitor cells for myocardial ischemia. Circulation 2001; 103:634–637.
111. Badorff C, Brandes R, Popp R, et al. Human endothelial progenitor cells can transdifferentiate into functionally active cardiomyocytes. Eur Heart J 2002; 23:16.
112. Badorff C, Brandes RP, Popp R, et al. Transdifferentiation of blood-derived human adult endothelial progenitor cells into functionally active cardiomyocytes. Circulation 2003; 107:1024–1032.
113. Condorelli G, Borello U, De Angelis L, et al. Cardiomyocytes induce endothelial cells to trans-differentiate into cardiac muscle: implications for myocardium regeneration. Proc Natl Acad Sci USA 2001; 98:10733–10738.
114. Kawamoto A, Tkebuchava T, Yamaguchi J, et al. Intramyocardial transplantation of autologous endothelial progenitor cells for therapeutic neovascularization of myocardial ischemia. Circulation 2003; 107:461–468.
115. Vasa M, Fichtlscherer S, Aicher A, et al. Number and migratory activity of circulating endothelial progenitor cells inversely correlate with risk factors for coronary artery disease. Circ Res 2001; 89:E1–E7.
116. Shintani S, Murohara T, Ikeda H, et al. Mobilization of endothelial progenitor cells in patients with acute myocardial infarction. Circulation 2001; 103:2776–2779.
117. Assmus B, Urbich C, Aicher A, et al. HMG-CoA reductase inhibitors reduce senescence and increase proliferation of endothelial progenitor cells via regulation of cell cycle regulatory genes. Circ Res 2003; 92:1049–1055.
118. Vasa M, Fichtlscherer S, Adler K, et al. Increase in circulating endothelial progenitor cells by statin therapy in patients with stable coronary artery disease. Circulation 2001; 103:2885–2890.
119. Landmesser U, Engberding N, Bahlmann FH, et al. Statin-induced improvement of endothelial progenitor cell mobilization, myocardial neovascularization, left ventricular function, and survival after experimental myocardial infarction requires endothelial nitric oxide synthase. Circulation 2004.
120. Heeschen C, Aicher A, Lehmann R, et al. Erythropoietin is a potent physiologic stimulus for endothelial progenitor cell mobilization. Blood 2003; 102:1340–1346.
121. Olivetti G, Giordano G, Corradi D, et al. Gender differences and aging: effects on the human heart. J Am Coll Cardiol 1995; 26:1068–1079.
122. Olivetti G, Melissari M, Balbi T, et al. Myocyte nuclear and possible cellular hyperplasia contribute to ventricular remodeling in the hypertrophic senescent heart in humans. J Am Coll Cardiol 1994; 24:140–149.
123. Muller P, Pfeiffer P, Koglin J, et al. Cardiomyocytes of noncardiac origin in myocardial biopsies of human transplanted hearts. Circulation 2002; 106:31–35.
124. Laflamme MA, Myerson D, Saffitz JE, et al. Evidence for cardiomyocyte repopulation by extracardiac progenitors in transplanted human hearts. Circ Res 2002; 90:634–640.

125. Messina E, De Angelis L, Frati G, et al. Isolation and expansion of adult cardiac stem cells from human and murine heart. Circ Res 2004; 95:911–921.
126. Laugwitz KL, Moretti A, Lam J, et al. Postnatal isl1+ cardioblasts enter fully differentiated cardiomyocyte lineages. Nature 2005; 433:647–653.
127. Iijima Y, Nagai T, Mizukami M, et al. Beating is necessary for transdifferentiation of skeletal muscle-derived cells into cardiomyocytes. FASEB J 2003; 17:U253–U268.
128. Al Attar N, Carrion C, Ghostine S, et al. Long-term (1 year) functional and histological results of autologous skeletal muscle cells transplantation in rat. Cardiovasc Res 2003; 58:142–148.
129. Leobon B, Garcin I, Menasche P, et al. Myoblasts transplanted into rat infarcted myocardium are functionally isolated from their host. Proc Natl Acad Sci USA 2003; 100:7808–7811.
130. Foley A, Mercola M. Heart induction: embryology to cardiomyocyte regeneration. Trends Cardiovasc Med 2004; 14:121–125.
131. Kang HJ, Kim HS, Zhang SY, et al. Effects of intracoronary infusion of peripheral blood stem-cells mobilised with granulocyte-colony stimulating factor on left ventricular systolic function and restenosis after coronary stenting in myocardial infarction: the MAGIC cell randomised clinical trial. Lancet 2004; 363:751–756.
132. Suzuki K, Murtuza B, Suzuki N, et al. Intracoronary infusion of skeletal myoblasts improves cardiac function in doxorubicin-induced heart failure. Circulation 2001; 104:I213–I217.
133. Vulliet PR, Greeley M, Halloran SM, et al. Intra-coronary arterial injection of mesenchymal stromal cells and microinfarction in dogs. Lancet 2004; 363:783–784.
134. Wollert KC, Meyer GP, Lotz J, et al. Intracoronary autologous bone-marrow cell transfer after myocardial infarction: the BOOST randomised controlled clinical trial. Lancet 2004; 364:141–148.
135. Assmus B, Schachinger V, Teupe C, et al. Transplantation of progenitor cells and regeneration enhancement in acute myocardial infarction (TOPCARE-AMI). Circulation 2002; 106:3009–3017.
136. Britten MB, Abolmaali ND, Assmus B, et al. Infarct remodeling after intracoronary progenitor cell treatment in patients with acute myocardial infarction (TOPCARE-AMI): mechanistic insights from serial contrast-enhanced magnetic resonance imaging. Circulation 2003; 108:2212–2218.
137. Fernandez-Aviles F, San Roman JA, Garcia-Frade J, et al. Experimental and clinical regenerative capability of human bone marrow cells after myocardial infarction. Circ Res 2004; 95:742–748.
138. Taylor DA, Silvestry SC, Bishop SP, et al. Delivery of primary autologous skeletal myoblasts into rabbit heart by coronary infusion: A potential approach to myocardial repair. Proc Assoc Am Phys 1997; 109:245–253.
139. Chen SL, Fang WW, Ye F, et al. Effect on left ventricular function of intracoronary transplantation of autologous bone marrow mesenchymal stem cell in patients with acute myocardial infarction. Am J Cardiol 2004; 94:92–95.
140. Fuchs S, Baffour R, Zhou YF, et al. Transendocardial delivery of autologous bone marrow enhances collateral perfusion and regional function in pigs with chronic experimental myocardial ischemia. J Am Coll Cardiol 2001; 37:1726–1732.
141. Fuchs S, Satler LF, Kornowski R, et al. Catheter-based autologous bone marrow myocardial injection in no-option patients with advanced coronary artery disease—A feasibility study. J Am Coll Cardiol 2003; 41:1721–1724.
142. Perin EC, Dohmann HF, Borojevic R, et al. Improved exercise capacity and ischemia 6 and 12 months after transendocardial injection of autologous bone marrow mononuclear cells for ischemic cardiomyopathy. Circulation 2004; 110:II213–II218.
143. Smits PC, van Geuns RJ, Poldermans D, et al. Catheter-based intramyocardial injection of autologous skeletal myoblasts as a primary treatment of ischemic heart failure: clinical experience with six-month follow-up. J Am Coll Cardiol 2003; 42:2063–2069.
144. Tse HF, Kwong YL, Chan JK, et al. Angiogenesis in ischaemic myocardium by intramyocardial autologous bone marrow mononuclear cell implantation. Lancet 2003; 361:47–49.

145. Atkins BZ, Lewis CW, Kraus WE, et al. Intracardiac transplantation of skeletal myoblasts yields two populations of striated cells in situ. Ann Thorac Surg 1999; 67:124–129.
146. Hamano K, Nishida M, Hirata K, et al. Local implantation of autologous bone marrow cells for therapeutic angiogenesis in patients with ischemic heart disease: clinical trial and preliminary results. Jpn Circ J 2001; 65:845–847.
147. Herreros J, Prosper F, Perez A, et al. Autologous intramyocardial injection of cultured skeletal muscle-derived stem cells in patients with non–acute myocardial infarction. Eur Heart J 2003; 24:2012–2020.
148. Stamm C, Westphal B, Kleine HD, et al. Autologous bone-marrow stem-cell transplantation for myocardial regeneration. Lancet 2003; 361:45–46.
149. Stamm C, Kleine HD, Westphal B, et al. CABG and bone marrow stem cell transplantation after myocardial infarction. Thorac Cardiovasc Surg 2004; 52:152–158.
150. Thompson CA, Nasseri BA, Makower J, et al. Percutaneous transvenous cellular cardiomyoplasty. A novel nonsurgical approach for myocardial cell transplantation. J Am Coll Cardiol 2003; 41:1964–1971.
151. Levesque JP, Hendy J, Takamatsu Y, et al. Disruption of the CXCR4/CXCL12 chemotactic interaction during hematopoietic stem cell mobilization induced by GCSF or cyclophosphamide. J Clin Invest 2003; 111:187–196.
152. Petit I, Szyper-Kravitz M, Nagler A, et al. G-CSF induces stem cell mobilization by decreasing bone marrow SDF-1 and up-regulating CXCR4. Nat Immunol 2002; 3:687–694.
153. Yamaguchi J, Kusano KF, Masuo O, et al. Stromal cell-derived factor-1 effects on ex vivo expanded endothelial progenitor cell recruitment for ischemic neovascularization. Circulation 2003; 107:1322–1328.
154. Ratajczak MZ, Kucia M, Reca R, et al. Stem cell plasticity revisited: CXCR4-positive cells expressing mRNA for early muscle, liver and neural cells 'hide out' in the bone marrow. Leukemia 2004; 18:29–40.
155. Wynn RF, Hart CA, Corradi-Perini C, et al. A small proportion of mesenchymal stem cells strongly express functionally active CXCR4 receptor capable of promoting migration to bone marrow. Blood 2004.
156. Askari AT, Unzek S, Popovic ZB, et al. Effect of stromal-cell-derived factor 1 on stem-cell homing and tissue regeneration in ischaemic cardiomyopathy. Lancet 2003; 362:697–703.
157. Rafii S, Lyden D. Therapeutic stem and progenitor cell transplantation for organ vascularization and regeneration. Nature Medicine 2003; 9:702–712.
158. Pagani FD, DerSimonian H, Zawadzka A, et al. Autologous skeletal myoblasts transplanted to ischemia-damaged myocardium in humans. Histological analysis of cell survival and differentiation. J Am Coll Cardiol 2003; 41:879–888.
159. Siminiak T, Fiszer D, Jerzykowska O, et al. Percutaneous autologous myoblast transplantation in the treatment of post-infarction myocardial contractility impairment—report on two cases. Kardiol Pol 2003; 59:492–501.
160. Menasche P, Hagege AA, Scorsin M, et al. Myoblast transplantation for heart failure. Lancet 2001; 357:279–280.
161. Reinecke H, MacDonald GH, Hauschka SD, et al. Electromechanical coupling between skeletal and cardiac muscle. Implications for infarct repair. J Cell Biol 2000; 149:731–740.
162. Makkar RR, Lill M, Chen PS. Stem cell therapy for myocardial repair: is it arrhythmogenic? J Am Coll Cardiol 2003; 42:2070–2072.
163. Tateishi-Yuyama E, Matsubara H, Murohara T, et al. Therapeutic angiogenesis for patients with limb ischaemia by autologous transplantation of bone-marrow cells: a pilot study and a randomised controlled trial. Lancet 2002; 360:427–435.
164. Hofmann M, Wollert KC, Meyer GP, et al. Monitoring of bone marrow cell homing into the infarcted human myocardium. Circulation 2005; 111:2198–2202.
165. Li TS, Hamano K, Hirata K, et al. The safety and feasibility of the local implantation of autologous bone marrow cells for ischemic heart disease. J Card Surg 2003; 18:S69–S75.

166. Ozbaran M, Omay SB, Nalbantgil S, et al. Autologous peripheral stem cell transplantation in patients with congestive heart failure due to ischemic heart disease. Eur J Cardiothorac Surg 2004; 25:342–350.
167. Mathur A, Martin JF. Stem cells and repair of the heart. Lancet 2004; 364:183–192.
168. Maitra B, Szekely E, Gjini K, et al. Human mesenchymal stem cells support unrelated donor hematopoietic stem cells and suppress T-cell activation. Bone Marrow Transplant 2004; 33:597–604.
169. Chung NG, Jeong DC, Park SJ, et al. Cotransplantation of marrow stromal cells may prevent lethal graft-versus-host disease in major histocompatibility complex mismatched murine hematopoietic stem cell transplantation. Int J Hematol 2004; 80:370–376.
170. Lazarus HM, Koc ON, Devine SM, et al. Cotransplantation of HLA-identical sibling culture-expanded mesenchymal stem cells and hematopoietic stem cells in hematologic malignancy patients. Biol Blood Marrow Transplant 2005; 11:389–398.
171. Horwitz EM, Prockop DJ, Fitzpatrick LA, et al. Transplantability and therapeutic effects of bone marrow-derived mesenchymal cells in children with osteogenesis imperfecta. Nat Med 1999; 5:309–313.
172. Pelled G, Turgeman G, Aslan H, et al. Mesenchymal stem cells for bone gene therapy and tissue engineering. Curr Pharm Des 2002; 8:1917–1928.
173. Millington-Ward S, Allers C, Tuohy G, et al. Validation in mesenchymal progenitor cells of a mutation-independent ex vivo approach to gene therapy for osteogenesis imperfecta. Hum Mol Genet 2002; 11:2201–2206.
174. Chamberlain JR, Schwarze U, Wang PR, et al. Gene targeting in stem cells from individuals with osteogenesis imperfecta. Science 2004; 303:1198–1201.
175. Pochampally RR, Horwitz EM, Digirolamo CM, et al. Correction of a mineralization defect by overexpression of a wild-type cDNA for COL1A1 in marrow stromal cells (MSCs) from a patient with osteogenesis imperfecta: a strategy for rescuing mutations that produce dominant-negative protein defects. Gene Ther 2005.
176. Barbash IM, Chouraqui P, Baron J, et al. Systemic delivery of bone marrow-derived mesenchymal stem cells to the infarcted myocardium: feasibility, cell migration, and body distribution. Circulation 2003; 108:863–868.
177. Chin BB, Nakamoto Y, Bulte JW, et al. ^{111}In oxine labelled mesenchymal stem cell SPECT after intravenous administration in myocardial infarction. Nucl Med Commun 2003; 24:1149–1154.
178. Burns JS, Abdallah BM, Guldberg P, et al. Tumorigenic heterogeneity in cancer stem cells evolved from long-term cultures of telomerase-immortalized human mesenchymal stem cells. Cancer Res 2005; 65:3126–3135.
179. Rubio D, Garcia-Castro J, Martin MC, et al. Spontaneous human adult stem cell transformation. Cancer Res 2005; 65:3035–3039.
180. Serakinci N, Guldberg P, Burns JS, et al. Adult human mesenchymal stem cell as a target for neoplastic transformation. Oncogene 2004; 23:5095–5098.
181. Nakamizo A, Marini F, Amano T, et al. Human bone marrow-derived mesenchymal stem cells in the treatment of gliomas. Cancer Res 2005; 65:3307–3318.
182. Jodele S, Chantrain CF, Blavier L, et al. The contribution of bone marrow-derived cells to the tumor vasculature in neuroblastoma is matrix metalloproteinase-9 dependent. Cancer Res 2005; 65:3200–3208.
183. Szmitko PE, Fedak PWM, Weisel RD, et al. Endothelial progenitor cells—New hope for a broken heart. Circulation 2003; 107:3093–3100.
184. Matsuura K, Wada H, Nagai T, et al. Cardiomyocytes fuse with surrounding noncardiomyocytes and reenter the cell cycle. J Cell Biol 2004; 167:351–363.
185. Deten A, Volz HC, Clamors S, et al. Hematopoietic stem cells do not repair the infarcted mouse heart. Cardiovasc Res 2005; 65:52–63.
186. Pittenger MF, Martin BJ. Mesenchymal stem cells and their potential as cardiac therapeutics. Circ Res 2004; 95:9–20.

187. Liechty KW, MacKenzie TC, Shaaban AF, et al. Human mesenchymal stem cells engraft and demonstrate site-specific differentiation after in utero transplantation in sheep. Nat Med 2000; 6:1282–1286.
188. Min JY, Sullivan MF, Yang Y, et al. Significant improvement of heart function by cotransplantation of human mesenchymal stem cells and fetal cardiomyocytes in postinfarcted pigs. Ann Thorac Surg 2002; 74:1568–1575.
189. Spees JL, Olson SD, Ylostalo J, et al. Differentiation, cell fusion, and nuclear fusion during ex vivo repair of epithelium by human adult stem cells from bone marrow stroma. Proc Natl Acad Sci USA 2003; 100:2397–2402.
190. Moscoso I, Centeno A, Lopez E, et al. Differentiation "in vitro" of primary and immortalized porcine mesenchymal stem cells into cardiomyocytes for cell transplantation. Transplant Proc 2005; 37:481–482.
191. Shim WS, Jiang S, Wong P, et al. Ex vivo differentiation of human adult bone marrow stem cells into cardiomyocyte-like cells. Biochem Biophys Res Commun 2004; 324:481–488.
192. Kawada H, Fujita J, Kinjo K, et al. Nonhematopoietic mesenchymal stem cells can be mobilized and differentiate into cardiomyocytes after myocardial infarction. Blood 2004; 104:3581–3587.
193. Xu W, Zhang X, Qian H, et al. Mesenchymal stem cells from adult human bone marrow differentiate into a cardiomyocyte phenotype in vitro. Exp Biol Med (Maywood) 2004; 229:623–631.
194. Toma C, Pittenger MF, Cahill KS, et al. Human mesenchymal stem cells differentiate to a cardiomyocyte phenotype in the adult murine heart. Circulation 2002; 105:93–98.
195. Pochampally RR, Neville BT, Schwarz EJ, et al. Rat adult stem cells (marrow stromal cells) engraft and differentiate in chick embryos without evidence of cell fusion. Proc Natl Acad Sci USA 2004; 101:9282–9285.
196. Menasche P. Skeletal myoblast for cell therapy. Coron Artery Dis 2005; 16:105–110.
197. Murry CE, Wiseman RW, Schwartz SM, et al. Skeletal myoblast transplantation for repair of myocardial necrosis. J Clin Invest 1996; 98:2512–2523.
198. Winitsky SO, Gopal TV, Hassanzadeh S, et al. Adult murine skeletal muscle contains cells that can differentiate into beating cardiomyocytes in vitro. PLoS Biol 2005; 3:e87.
199. Hagege AA, Carrion C, Menasche P, et al. Viability and differentiation of autologous skeletal myoblast grafts in ischaemic cardiomyopathy. Lancet 2003; 361:491–492.
200. Reinecke H, Poppa V, Murry CE. Skeletal muscle stem cells do not transdifferentiate into cardiomyocytes after cardiac grafting. J Mol Cell Cardiol 2002; 34:241–249.
201. Scorsin M, Hagege A, Vilquin JT, et al. Comparison of the effects of fetal cardiomyocyte and skeletal myoblast transplantation on postinfarction left ventricular function. J Thorac Cardiovasc Surg 2000; 119:1169–1175.
202. Atkins BZ, Hueman MT, Meuchel JM, et al. Myogenic cell transplantation improves in vivo regional performance in infarcted rabbit myocardium. J Heart Lung Transplant 1999; 18:1173–1180.
203. Kumar D, Kamp TJ, LeWinter MM. Embryonic stem cells: differentiation into cardiomyocytes and potential for heart repair and regeneration. Coron Artery Dis 2005; 16:111–116.
204. Kawai T, Takahashi T, Esaki M, et al. Efficient cardiomyogenic differentiation of embryonic stem cell by fibroblast growth factor 2 and bone morphogenetic protein 2. Circ J 2004; 68:691–702.
205. Kehat I, Kenyagin-Karsenti D, Snir M, et al. Human embryonic stem cells can differentiate into myocytes with structural and functional properties of cardiomyocytes. J Clin Invest 2001; 108:407–414.
206. Yang Y, Min JY, Rana JS, et al. VEGF enhances functional improvement of postinfarcted hearts by transplantation of ESC-differentiated cells. J Appl Physiol 2002; 93:1140–1151.
207. Ying QL, Nichols J, Evans EP, et al. Changing potency by spontaneous fusion. Nature 2002; 416:545–548.
208. Kehat I, Khimovich L, Caspi O, et al. Electromechanical integration of cardiomyocytes derived from human embryonic stem cells. Nat Biotechnol 2004; 22:1282–1289.

209. Wollert KC, Drexler H. Clinical applications of stem cells for the heart. Circ Res 2005; 96:151–163.
210. Kuethe F, Richartz BM, Sayer HG, et al. Lack of regeneration of myocardium by autologous intracoronary mononuclear bone marrow cell transplantation in humans with large anterior myocardial infarctions. Int J Cardiol 2004; 97:123–127.
211. Chachques JC, Herreros J, Trainini J, et al. Autologous human serum for cell culture avoids the implantation of cardioverter-defibrillators in cellular cardiomyoplasty. Int J Cardiol 2004; 95:S29–S33.

31
Gene Therapy for Heart Failure

Shi Yin Foo and Anthony Rosenzweig
Program in Cardiovascular Gene Therapy, Cardiovascular Research Center and Cardiology Division, Massachusetts General Hospital, Harvard Medical School, Boston, Massachusetts, U.S.A.

INTRODUCTION

Pharmacological and device-based therapies described in detail elsewhere in this text continue to provide significant benefits for heart failure patients. However, heart failure remains a growing cause of morbidity and mortality, prompting exploration of novel therapeutic approaches, including genetic therapies which facilitate highly specific and local manipulation of molecular pathways for which often no pharmacologic reagent exists. In the process, the contributions of particular pathways to disease pathogenesis can be assessed and mechanistic hypotheses tested, thereby validating potential targets for intervention through a variety of approaches including traditional pharmaceutical development. Thus, gene transfer offers not only an opportunity for therapy but also an experimental tool that can facilitate a range of treatment approaches.

While the ability to reprogram the heart genetically represents an exciting and innovative approach, it is vital to remember that these procedures carry a risk of serious (1) or even fatal consequences (2) that may be difficult to anticipate fully. Therefore, we believe that until the safety of a particular formulation has been definitively established, it should be reserved for investigational use in patients with a compelling clinical need for whom conventional therapeutic options have been exhausted. Despite these legitimate concerns, we also believe there is reason to explore gene therapy as an option in selected clinical settings and that advanced heart failure is one of these. As discussed below, this cautious enthusiasm is prompted by recent developments that suggest such effective therapy for heart failure may be feasible. These include improved vector and delivery systems, as well as a growing understanding of the pathophysiological mechanisms of heart failure that help guide the choice of molecular targets.

In addition to these considerations, several features of the target population support further investigation of this approach. First, the poor prognosis of specific subsets of heart failure patients provides a clinical imperative for creative approaches. Second, genetic intervention in the heart is likely a more feasible target than the widely distributed targets in genetic conditions being considered for gene therapy. Undoubtedly the wealth of catheter-based interventional experience that has accumulated in cardiology will provide an important advantage in the development of delivery strategies. Finally, the advanced age of many heart failure patients enhances the feasibility of genetic therapy. For example, the technical requirements for durability of transgene expression may be more modest in this setting than in treating inborn errors of metabolism where the hope would be for early delivery and lifelong expression. In heart failure, even months to years of improved function could have a significant benefit on patient quality of life or perhaps even favorably influence disease evolution. In this population, concerns about reproductive risks after gene therapy are also generally alleviated.

These features of the target population, in combination with the scientific advances noted above, prompt careful consideration of genetic interventions for heart failure. Clinical success of this approach in any context depends on an appropriate combination of three essential components: a vector (or packaging system for the genetic material), a delivery system to get this material to the target organ, and (perhaps most important) a validated molecular target for intervention. In this chapter, we review the status of these three components with a focus on approaches most relevant to heart failure.

VECTORS FOR CARDIAC GENE TRANSFER

Vectors provide the packaging for the therapeutic genetic material. While a variety of systems are available (Table 1) (3–5), many of these are not applicable to the heart, which necessitates gene transfer in vivo and usually targets cardiomyocytes which generally are not replicating. The vectors most relevant to the heart are discussed briefly below.

Plasmid DNA

Simple DNA expression plasmids, termed "naked DNA" since they are not clothed in a more elaborate packaging system, can be internalized after injection into the heart to mediate transgene expression. An appeal of this approach is that it minimizes biosafety concerns. On the other hand, these vectors produce low-level and relatively inefficient transgene expression. Whether this expression suffices will obviously depend on the context and biological goals. For example, muscle injection of plasmid vectors encoding secreted angiogenesis factors has demonstrated significant biological effects in animal models (6–8), presumably because of the cascade of paracrine effects these growth factors can mediate. In contrast, improving cardiac function through expression of genes that act only in the transduced cells (*cell autonomous transgenes*) likely requires a more robust expression vector. It may be possible to modify plasmid vectors chemically to improve their effectiveness without invoking substantial biosafety concerns. For example, liposomal preparations use an artificial lipid bilayer to surround the DNA that facilitates cell internalization (9). In the heart, liposomal gene transfer is still relatively inefficient but engenders less of an inflammatory reaction in comparison to adenoviral vectors (10), leading to an enhanced biological efficacy. Liposomal-plasmid DNA micelles can be used in combination with gas-filled microbubbles, similar to those used in echocardiography for contrast. After intravenous injection, ultrasound can be used to stimulate uptake of the plasmid into the myocardium (11). Other strategies include the incorporation of proteins into the liposomal shell that enhance cellular entry (such as the HIV *tat* protein) (10,12). It is hoped that these ongoing efforts will ultimately yield chemical reagents capable of mediating highly effective cardiac gene transfer with minimal biosafety concerns. However, currently most efforts targeting cardiac dysfunction have utilized viral vectors because of their ability to achieve high-level and highly efficient cardiac gene transfer. Viral vectors useful for cardiac gene transfer are discussed below.

Table 1 Vectors for Cardiac Gene Transfer

Vector	Duration of expression	Advantages	Disadvantages
Plasmid DNA	4–7 days	Favorable bio safety profile	Low efficiency, low level expression
Adenovirus	7–28 days, longer with new generation	High efficiency and high level of expression; minimal concerns about insertional effects	Transient expression; host immune and inflammatory response—particularly with early generation vectors
Adeno-associated virus	Months to years	Durable expression Little host cellular immune or inflammatory response	Unable to package large constructs. Delayed onset of transgene expression. Possibility of insertional mutagenesis and/or adverse activation of neighboring genes. Large-scale production of clinical grade vectors remains challenging
Lentivirus (pseudo-typed virus)	Months to years	Durable expression High efficiency	Large-scale production of clinical grade vectors remains challenging Integration can cause insertional mutagenesis and/or adverse activation of neighboring genes Derivative of HIV family raises some biosafety issues
Herpesvirus/ amplicon	Weeks	Ability to package large transgenes	Complex construction Tropism for neurons

Adenoviral Vectors

Adenoviruses are double-stranded DNA viruses that have significant advantages for cardiac gene transfer. First, they can be prepared at extremely high titers, typically in the range of 10^{12} particles/ml. Second, they can efficiently infect non-replicating cells, yielding high-efficiency and high-level transduction of cardiomyocytes in vitro and in vivo (13). However, these advantages are counterbalanced by disadvantages, most importantly transient expression and a potent host immune and inflammatory response. After vascular gene transfer, this inflammatory response is marked by upregulation of adhesion molecules, increased leuckocytes infiltration, and the development of neointimal hyperplasia (14). Cardiac gene transfer with original (*first generation*) adenoviral vectors usually achieves high-level transgene expression lasting approximately one week in animal models in vivo (13,15–17). Expression is then terminated or markedly attenuated by the host cellular immune response.

Several approaches are being investigated in hopes of overcoming these disadvantages while retaining the beneficial features of these vectors. Mutation or deletion of additional early adenoviral genes in *second generation* vectors can significantly attenuate viral gene expression and therefore the host immune response to the vectors, resulting in more durable expression (18). Newer *gutless* adenoviral vectors have also been engineered through recombination that lack virtually all viral genes, not only further eliminating viral gene expression but increasing the size of the transgene that can be encoded (19). These approaches also further reduce the chance of generating wild-type adenovirus through recombination events. In contrast, retaining some specific adenoviral genes can paradoxically also mitigate the host response by co-opting natural viral defenses that have evolved to escape the host immune system. Inclusion of the E3 region in adenoviral vectors reduced vascular inflammation and neointimal hyperplasia after arterial gene transfer in vivo (20). Additional study is needed to clarify the long-term effects of these modified vectors in the heart.

Adeno-Associated Viruses

Recombinant adeno-associated viruses (rAAV) are single-stranded DNA viruses derived from parvoviruses not known to be pathogenic in human disease and do not elicit a significant cellular immune response (3,21,22). rAAV effect durable transgene expression that can last months to years in many systems (21,23,24). rAAV cardiac gene transfer generally confers lower levels of initial but more sustained transgene expression when compared to the adenoviral vectors described above (3,21,22). For these reasons, rAAV may be particularly well suited for sustained expression of secreted gene products. Whether rAAV can mediate enough transgene expression to favorably alter heart function as has been achieved with adenovirus (25), is less clear. Production of large amounts of clinical grade rAAV remains challenging with current generation and purification techniques.

Recently, Samulski and colleagues have developed a promising approach to improving the relatively low-level and delayed initial expression seen with traditional AAV vectors. Utilizing a single-stranded, self-complementary DNA molecule, they have demonstrated accelerated and enhanced transgene expression (26). These differences could be critical in clinical settings where early and robust transgene expression is needed. The application of this system to cardiac gene transfer has not been reported as of this writing. Of note, however, is that the use of self-complementing DNA constructs further reduces the already stringent packaging constraints of AAV vectors and thus is reserved for small expression constructs (<2 kb), excluding many of the molecular targets being considered in heart failure. More recently identified serotypes may prove useful as well. AAV8 appears to have a robust tropism for striated muscle, including the heart (27). This particular serotype outperforms AAV1 in cardiac muscle transduction after intravenous administration, but not after intramuscular injection in mice, suggesting that an additional barrier to successful gene transfer for these vectors is the ability to traverse the blood vessel wall (27).

Lentiviruses

Although related to retroviruses, lentiviruses (in contrast to traditional retroviruses) can effectively infect nondividing cells and thus are potentially useful for cardiac gene transfer. Lentiviruses encode an RNA genome which is reverse-transcribed to DNA in the host cell that subsequently integrates into the host chromosome. Pseudotyping the lentiviral envelope by employing the envelope of vesicular stomatitis virus (VSV) generates lentiviral vectors with a much broader host cell range (28). Lentiviral gene vectors have been successfully employed in a wide variety of cell types, including cardiomyocytes (28–33). Chromosomal insertion increases the durability of transgene expression but also raises concerns about the risk of insertional mutagenesis or activation of neighboring oncogenes, as seen in recent clinical trials using retroviral vectors (34,35).

Herpesvirus/Amplicons

Vectors derived from herpes simplex 1 (HSV-1) infect both dividing and non-dividing cells, and manifest a broad host cell range (though with a predilection favoring neuronal infection). HSV-1-derived vectors can encode relatively large transgenes (>35 kb), and this characteristic has been used to advantage in studies of large transgenes of interest to cardiac function such as the ryanodine receptors and titin (36). Such studies would not be possible with most other vectors. In addition to HSV-1-derived vectors which insert transgenes into the viral backbone, plasmids engineered to contain the HSV origin of replication and packaging signal, known as HSV amplicons, can also be used to produce infective virions. These amplicon plasmids can only incorporate up to 8 kb of exogenous DNA. Amplicon HSV vectors have been used to efficiently transduce cardiomyocytes in vitro and cardiac tissues ex vivo (37), although their in vivo efficacy has not been demonstrated for cardiac gene transfer.

Adverse Effects

As discussed above, none of the currently available vectors is ideal and all carry some risk of adverse side effects. Although no deaths attributable to gene transfer have occurred in cardiac gene therapy trials, fatal and serious complications have occurred in other such trials and provide an important cautionary note as cardiac gene therapy efforts move forward. In one instance, a 17 yr-old volunteer with mild ornithine transcarbamylase (OTC) deficiency, which can cause neurological symptoms, died after hepatic infusion of large quantities of a second-generation adenoviral vector (38). In retrospect, the patient likely developed the systemic inflammatory response syndrome with activation of the complement cascade, culminating in his demise despite intensive medical efforts (2,39). In another case, retroviral gene transfer to bone marrow stem cells from children afflicted with X-linked severe combined immunodeficiency syndrome (X-SCID) produced durable disease remission (40) but was complicated by a leukemia-like syndrome marked by clonal T-cell proliferation (1). Analyses linked this complication to construct insertion leading to increased levels of proto-oncogene expression. Though the theoretical risk of such insertional events had been well recognized, the alarmingly high frequency (occurring in two of the ten patients) (1) was entirely unanticipated. These cases should serve as humbling reminders of how limited our understanding remains and underscore the importance of considering these approaches only after exhausting conventional therapeutic options and carefully weighing the potential risks and benefits of genetic intervention.

DELIVERY SYSTEMS

A large number of systems have been investigated in animal models (32,41–45), although clinical experience with these systems is limited. Some systems employed with healthy animals may not be readily translatable to ill cardiac patients who are the intended recipients. Importantly, different technical approaches produced dramatically different levels and patterns of transgene expression and thus must be chosen in the context of the disease and biological targets being considered. In general, direct myocardial injection (whether at surgery or via a catheter) produces high-level though focal transgene expression. In contrast, perfusion techniques tend to confer more diffuse and homogeneous, though lower-level expression. In addition, they carry a higher risk of systemic dissemination of vector.

Myocardial Injection

Direct myocardial injection was one of the first techniques utilized clinically (46) and has several advantageous characteristics. Injection can be targeted to specific areas likely to benefit from gene transfer, simultaneously enhancing the effect in these regions while mitigating potentially adverse effects in regions where it is not needed. Genes delivered in this way are also less likely to be disseminated into the systemic circulation. In addition, direct injection avoids barriers to vascular access presented by pre-existing coronary stenoses or other vascular abnormalities. However, the highly focal nature of transgene expression will generally not be appropriate when gene transfer to a majority of the heart is required. Even covering a significant subsection of myocardium may require many injections, and thus could increase the risk of mechanical complications, such as myocardial rupture. This may be a particular concern for patients with advanced heart failure whose general debilitation in combination with thinned myocardial walls could increase these risks.

Perfusion-Based Approaches

An alternative to direct myocardial injection is perfusion of vector solution through the vascular system of the heart. Intracoronary infusion of vector has been reported to produce efficient myocardial transduction (47–49), although systemic vector dissemination with this technique remains a concern. Gene transfer to the entire heart in animal models can be enhanced by using whole heart perfusion with cross-clamping of the aorta alone or in combination with the pulmonary artery (42,50). The technique produces relatively homogeneous and diffuse cardiac transgene expression but, more importantly, can alter the intrinsic contractile function of the heart (42,51). Possible approaches to extending this conceptual approach to clinical applications include whole-heart perfusion during cardiopulmonary bypass (52) or retroperfusion via catheters (53). Perfusion-based approaches generally confer more widely distributed but lower levels of transgene expression than the direct injection approaches. The optimal choice will obviously directly depend on the target and biological goals.

BIOLOGICAL TARGETS IN HEART FAILURE

Given the diverse etiologies of clinical heart failure, one strategy is to target genetic interventions to characteristics common to many forms of heart failure. Targets that appear particularly promising include cardiomyocyte apoptosis, abnormalities in cardiomyocyte calcium handling, and dysfunctional adrenergic signaling (Table 2). These are discussed below.

Table 2 Potential Targets for Gene Therapy in Heart Failure

Targeted process	Molecular targets	Status	Comments
Cardiomyocyte death	Anti-apoptotic transgenes [Bcl-2 overexpression (56), overexpression of Akt or other pro-survival kinases]	Demonstrated acute and mid-term benefits in animal models of acute ischemic injury (64) and/or remodeling (56) post-infarction	Greater than expected benefit in vivo may reflect combined effects on cardiomyocyte survival and function Complexity of signaling pathways raises possibility of ligand expression (69)
Calcium handling	SERCA2a overexpression (51)	Strongest pre-clinical data in a variety of animal models and human cells in vitro support SERCA2a overexpression	Clinical trial will utilize rAAV vectors
	Phospholamban inhibition (80)	Clinical trial being initiated for LVAD patients (74)	
Adrenergic receptors and downstream signaling	β2-AR overexpression (71); βARKct expression (72)	Strong pre-clinical data in a variety of models	Clinical trial will utilize an adenoviral vector
	Adenylyl cyclase VI overexpression (49)	Ongoing clinical trial for heart failure patients (74)	

Abbreviation: LVAD, left ventricular assist device.

Cardiomyocyte Apoptosis

Cardiomyocyte apoptosis has been documented in many forms of cardiac disease, including heart failure of diverse etiologies [reviewed in (54)]. Although the prevalence of apoptotic cardiomyocytes in human heart failure is low, studies in transgenic mice suggest that comparably low levels of programmed cell death or apoptosis in cardiomyocytes can cause a lethal cardiomyopathy (55). Despite the conceptual importance of this finding, it still leaves open the critical clinical question as to the extent of anatomic and functional benefit to be gained in common varieties of heart failure through inhibition of apoptosis. For example, would cardiomyocytes simply go on to die through another mechanism or, perhaps, survive but function poorly? Despite these concerns, recent animal studies activating anti-apoptotic pathways in models of myocyte loss and/or dysfunction suggest these approaches may yield substantial benefits. These benefits likely reflect the role of convergent signaling pathways in controlling both cardiomyocyte survival and function. Because of this, highly specific interventions can, in fact, promote overall survival and improved function of cardiomyocytes, thus mediating what we would consider "meaningful rescue." Representative anti-apoptotic targets being explored are discussed below.

Bcl-2

Bcl-2 is a mitochondrial-associated protein with anti-apoptotic effects in many cell systems. In the heart, injection of an adenoviral vector encoding Bcl-2 *after* transient coronary ligation had significant favorable effects on left ventricular remodeling six weeks after ischemic injury despite comparable initial infarcts (56). These cardiac effects were associated with a reduction in the apoptotic index at 6 weeks from 2.77 to 1.01% (56). Since even lower levels of apoptosis can cause a cardiomyopathy over time (55), it seems plausible that this reduction in apoptosis contributes to the favorable effects on ventricular function and geometry observed after Bcl-2 gene transfer. Given the clinical importance of adverse ventricular remodeling to the development of heart failure, as well as the clinically relevant time-frame of vector infusion, this strategy warrants further investigation.

The potential importance of Bcl-family proteins is also illustrated in studies that model the heart failure that develops in patients treated with the chemotherapeutic agent, trastuzumab (herceptin). Mice in which ErbB2, the receptor target of trastuzumab, has been genetically deleted in cardiomyocytes, develop a dilated cardiomyopathy (57,58) which can be prevented by gene transfer of another anti-apoptotic Bcl-family protein, Bcl-xL (58) even though there is little apparent apoptosis in these hearts. While it may be that small changes in cardiomyocyte apoptosis account for these functional effects, we have recently proposed an alternative explanation based on our finding that antibodies to ErbB2 cause mitochondrial dysfunction and reduced ATP levels in association with apoptotic signaling, without inducing substantial apoptosis (59). It seems likely that mitochondrial dysfunction contributes to cardiomyocyte dysfunction, and that this, in combination with the cardiomyocyte death, results in the observed overall cardiac dysfunction. Interestingly, antibody treatment dramatically increased the ratio of pro-apoptotic Bcl-xs to anti-apoptotic Bcl-xL (59). The significance of these changes was demonstrated by protein transduction using the BH4 domain of Bcl-xL which both restored ATP levels and prevented mitochondrial dysfunction in cardiomyocytes. This "interrupted apoptosis" may contribute to heart failure both by impairing cardiomyocyte energetics and function, as well as by making cardiomyocytes more susceptible to apoptosis after additional stresses. Interestingly, failing human hearts similarly demonstrate widespread activation of apoptotic signaling and a relative paucity of frankly apoptotic cardiomyocytes (60). These observations suggest that the benefits of anti-apoptotic signaling may be even greater than would be predicted based simply on the number of overtly apoptotic cardiomyocytes.

Phosphoinositide 3-Kinase/Akt Signaling

Cantley and colleagues first identified this pathway as a key arbiter of cell survival in a variety of settings (61,62). In the heart, numerous cardioprotective peptides including insulin, gp130-dependent cytokines, and Insulin-like Growth Factor I (IGF-I), activate this signaling pathway, which prompted evaluation of the role of phosphoinositide 3-kinase (PI 3-kinase) and Akt (also known as Protein Kinase B) in the heart. These studies lend further support to the concept that anti-apoptotic interventions hold promise in cardiac dysfunction because of their dual ability to influence cardiomyocyte survival and function favorably. Adenoviral expression of activated mutant of PI 3-kinase or Akt inhibits apoptosis in cardiomyocytes (63). Importantly, adenoviral activation of Akt also prevents cardiomyocyte dysfunction in vitro and in vivo, while expression of a dominant-negative Akt construct increases hypoxia-induced cardiomyocyte dysfunction (64). Thus Akt represents an important node in cardiomyocyte signaling that controls both survival and function, and these two effects likely underlie the dramatic in vivo benefits of acute Akt activation (64).

Long-Term Effects of Akt Activation

Although these studies demonstrate that acute Akt activation mediates potent pro-survival and functional benefits in cardiomyocytes, paradoxically Akt phosphorylation is actually increased in the hearts of chronic heart failure patients (65). This finding suggested to us that chronic Akt activation could become maladaptive over time. To address this issue, we engineered transgenic mice with cardiac-specific expression of the same activated Akt shown previously to protect cardiomyocytes acutely (66). These mice have concentric hypertrophy, preserved systolic function, and no overt cardiac disease at baseline (66). However, in a Langendorff isolated heart model of ischemia and reperfusion, functional recovery of these hearts is dramatically impaired in association with a substantial increase in infarct size and CPK release (67). Biochemical analyses revealed no change in downstream or parallel signaling pathways that appeared to account for these dramatic adverse consequences of chronic Akt activation. However, chronic Akt activation did lead to impressive feedback inhibition of upstream signaling in the same pathway. Specifically, levels of the adaptor proteins, IRS-1 and-2 (which link tyrosine kinase receptors to PI3-kinase) were significantly reduced, thereby inhibiting activation of PI3-kinase (67). Adenoviral cardiac gene transfer of a PI 3-kinase mutant that functions independently of IRS-proteins restored functional recovery and reduced injury after ischemia-reperfusion, thus establishing the importance of PI3-kinase-*dependent* but Akt-*independent* pathways in regulating cardiomyocyte survival and function. Intriguingly, a similar reduction in IRS-1 was evident in cardiac tissue from patients with heart failure suggesting that chronic Akt activation may lead to a similar feedback inhibition of upstream signaling in heart failure patients as well (67). We hypothesize that multiple parallel pathways downstream of PI 3-kinase control cardiomyocyte survival and function. In addition to Akt, serum and glucocorticoid-responsive kinase-1 (SGK1), another PI3-kinase-dependent kinase with homology to Akt, also appears to be an important regulator of cardiomyocyte survival (68). Interestingly, SGK1 phosphorylation (activation) is reduced by chronic Akt activation in the heart (67). One approach to dealing with the evident complexity of this system would be the gene transfer of a cardioprotective ligand, such as IGF-I (69), capable of simultaneously activating all these downstream pathways (Fig. 1). We have recently shown that this can mediate autocrine and paracrine cardioprotection after gene transfer in the heart without elevating systemic IGF-I levels (69). Whichever construct ultimately proves optimal, these studies lend support to the strategy of targeting survival signaling and illustrate the utility of gene transfer as an experimental tool that will likely contribute to a more complete understanding of the signals controlling cardiomyocyte survival essential to exploiting the therapeutic potential of this approach fully.

Preserving Cardiomyocyte Function

In both animal models and clinical heart failure, calcium handling and adrenergic signaling are consistently impaired, providing an impetus to target these pathways in the hope of preventing or reversing cardiomyocyte contractile dysfunction.

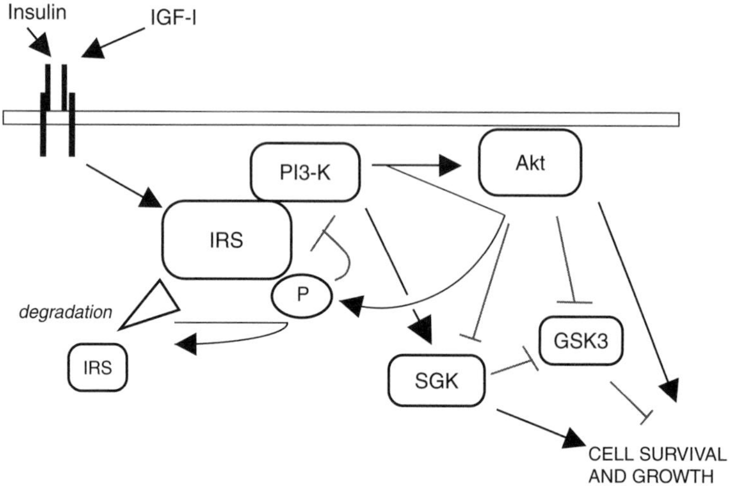

Figure 1 Schematic of P13K signaling pathways. Multiple P13K-dependent pathways modulate cell survival and growth, including Akt and SGK. There is feedback inhibition is this system, as well as convergent downstream targets, although Akt and SGK likely also signal through distinct downstream effectors.

β-Adrenergic Signaling

β-Adrenergic signaling initiated by catecholamine binding to cell-surface receptors is a critical determinant of myocardial contractility. β-adrenergic receptors are downregulated in chronic heart failure (70). Several approaches have been explored to restore adrenergic signaling in heart failure through gene transfer. Cardiac gene transfer of the β2-adrenergic receptor (β2-AR) improves left ventricular contractility both at baseline and in response to isoproterenol in rabbits (71). Inactivation of βAR occurs at least in part through phosphorylation mediated by the βAR kinase (βARK1) prompting efforts to inhibit βARK1 through expression of a peptide inhibitor (βARKct) (72). Adenoviral gene transfer of βARKct preserves β2-AR density and signaling in a rabbit model of post-infarction heart failure thereby mitigating cardiac dysfunction (73). cAMP mediates many of the effects of adrenergic signaling, and improved cardiac function in a pig model of pacing-induced cardiac dysfunction has recently been demonstrated after gene transfer of type VI adenylyl cyclase (49). A Phase I/II clinical trial is currently underway using this approach in heart failure patients (74). Although these approaches appear quite promising, their long-term consequences are incompletely understood. Moreover, the concept of amplifying adrenergic signaling at any of these levels (receptor, its kinase, or downstream signaling) appears to counter the well-documented clinical benefits of β-adrenergic antagonists in heart failure (75). Particularly in heart failure patients, it is worth remembering that there is historical precedent for the improved cardiac function seen with some inotropes to be offset by an increase in mortality (76).

Calcium Handling

Strategies to improve the cardiac calcium handling are actively being pursued in a variety of models. The sarcoplasmic reticulum (SR) plays a critical role in taking calcium into the SR during diastole through the action of the SR calcium adenosine triphosphatase pump (SR-ATPase), SERCA2a. Phospholamban binds to SERCA2a and inhibits its activity.

SERCA2a and SR Ca^{2+}-ATPase activity are reduced in heart failure (77,78). Rational strategies to restoring SR ATPase activity include overexpression of SERCA2a as well as inhibition of phospholamban. The latter can be effected through the introduction of antisense RNA to bind to and prevent the translation of the phospholamban mRNA, or through dominant negative constructs encoding mutant phospholamban proteins that interfere with the function of the endogenous gene products. Adenoviral expression of SERCA2a improves the dysfunction seen in failing human cardiomyocytes in vitro (79), while in vivo cardiac gene transfer of SERCA2a improves both systolic and diastolic function, as well as survival in a rat heart failure model (51). These studies provide important conceptual support for the hypothesis that SR ATPase abnormalities are critical contributors to the pathophysiology of heart failure and suggest that gene transfer of SERCA2a could well be beneficial in heart failure patients. Similarly, overexpression of dominant negative phospholamban using rAAV in a hamster model of cardiomyopathy led to long-term functional improvement in vivo (80). Importantly, there is reason to believe that these approaches will not incur the same adverse effects seen with other positive inotropes. First, SERCA2a gene transfer increases contractility without increasing cAMP or energy requirements. Moreover, survival is actually improved by this intervention in preclinical animal models (81). Nevertheless, these concepts will require rigorous clinical validation and a clinical trial of SERCA2a gene therapy for end-stage heart failure patients requiring ventricular assist devices is being initiated at the time of this writing (74).

SUMMARY AND CONCLUSIONS

The persistently poor prognosis in specific subsets of heart failure patients prompts careful consideration of novel therapeutic approaches, including targeted genetic therapies. Exploration of such approaches is warranted not only by this clinical need but also because recent improvements in vectors, catheter-based delivery systems, as well as our understanding and validation of potential molecular targets have increased the feasibility of this strategy. Nevertheless, the risks associated with gene therapy remain significant and difficult to fully anticipate. For these reasons, we advocate clinical studies of this approach proceed first in patients with significant cardiac impairment and in whom conventional therapeutic options have already been fully explored. Potential strategies under active investigation include inhibition of cardiomyocyte programmed cell death, as well as targeted approaches to improve myocyte contraction. While it is hoped that ongoing investigations will generate viable and clinically validated genetic therapies, an under-appreciated benefit of this work is the insight it provides into disease pathogenesis. Thus gene transfer offers both a novel therapeutic modality as well as an experimental tool, allowing us to validate targets for intervention whether through genetic or more traditional pharmaceutical means.

REFERENCES

1. Hacein-Bey-Abina S, Von Kalle C, Schmidt M, et al. LMO2-associated clonal T cell proliferation in two patients after gene therapy for SCID-X1. Science 2003; 302:415–419.
2. Marshall E. Gene therapy death prompts review of adenovirus vector. Science 1999; 286:2244–2245.
3. Gao GP, Wilson JM, Wivel NA. Production of recombinant adeno-associated virus. Adv Virus Res 2000; 55:529–543.

4. Cemazar M, Sersa G, Wilson J, et al. Effective gene transfer to solid tumors using different nonviral gene delivery techniques: electroporation, liposomes, and integrin-targeted vector. Cancer Gene Ther 2002; 9:399–406.
5. Rosenzweig A, Dracopoli N, Haines J et al, eds. Vectors for gene therapy. In: Current Protocols in Human Genetics, Vol. 3, NY: John Wiley & Sons, 2001.
6. Isner JM. Myocardial gene therapy. Nature 2002; 415:234–239.
7. Marban E. Cardiac channelopathies. Nature 2002; 415:213–218.
8. Towbin JA, Bowles NE. The failing heart. Nature 2002; 415:227–233.
9. Zhang JS, Li S, Huang L. Cationic liposome-protamine-DNA complexes for gene delivery. Methods Enzymol 2003; 373:332–342.
10. Sen L, Hong YS, Luo H, et al. Efficiency, efficacy, and adverse effects of adenovirus vs. liposome-mediated gene therapy in cardiac allografts. Am J Physiol Heart Circ Physiol 2001; 281:H1433–H1441.
11. Chen S, Shohet RV, Bekeredjian R, et al. Optimization of ultrasound parameters for cardiac gene delivery of adenoviral or plasmid deoxyribonucleic acid by ultrasound-targeted microbubble destruction. J Am Coll Cardiol 2003; 42:301–308.
12. Gratton JP, Yu J, Griffith JW, et al. Cell-permeable peptides improve cellular uptake and therapeutic gene delivery of replication-deficient viruses in cells and in vivo. Nat Med 2003; 9:357–362.
13. Hajjar RJ, Schmidt U, Matsui T, et al. Modulation of ventricular function through gene transfer in vivo. Proc Natl Acad Sci USA 1998; 95:5251–5256.
14. Newman KD, Dunn PF, Owens JW, et al. Adenovirus-mediated gene transfer into normal rabbit arteries results in prolonged vascular cell activation, inflammation, and neointimal hyperplasia. J Clin Invest 1995; 96:2955–2965.
15. del Monte F, Williams E, Lebeche D, et al. Improvement in survival and cardiac metabolism following gene transfer of SERCA2a in a rat model of heart failure. Circulation 2001; (in press).
16. Del Monte F, Butler K, Boecker W, et al. Novel technique of aortic banding followed by gene transfer during hypertrophy and heart failure. Physiol Genomics 2002; 9:49–56.
17. del Monte F, Harding SE, Dec GW, et al. Targeting phospholamban by gene transfer in human heart failure. Circulation 2002; 105:904–907.
18. Engelhardt JF, Ye X, Doranz B, et al. Ablation of E2A in recombinant adenoviruses improves transgene persistence and decreases inflammatory response in mouse liver. Proc Natl Acad Sci USA 1994; 91:6196–6200.
19. Kochanek S, Clemens PR, Mitani K, et al. A new adenoviral vector: replacement of all viral coding sequences with 28 kb of DNA independently expressing both full-length dystrophin and beta-galactosidase. Proc Natl Acad Sci USA 1996; 93:5731–5736.
20. Wen S, Driscoll RM, Schneider DB, et al. Inclusion of the E3 region in an adenoviral vector decreases inflammation and neointima formation after arterial gene transfer. Arterioscler Thromb Vasc Biol 2001; 21:1777–1782.
21. Ng P, Evelegh C, Cummings D, et al. Cre levels limit packaging signal excision efficiency in the Cre/loxP helper-dependent adenoviral vector system. J Virol 2002; 76:4181–4189.
22. Gao G, Qu G, Burnham MS, et al. Purification of recombinant adeno-associated virus vectors by column chromatography and its performance in vivo. Hum Gene Ther 2000; 11:2079–2091.
23. Ng P, Parks RJ, Cummings DT, et al. A high-efficiency Cre/loxP-based system for construction of adenoviral vectors. Hum Gene Ther 1999; 10:2667–2672.
24. Cordier L, Gao GP, Hack AA, et al. Muscle-specific promoters may be necessary for adeno-associated virus-mediated gene transfer in the treatment of muscular dystrophies. Hum Gene Ther 2001; 12:205–215.
25. Svensson EC, Marshall DJ, Woodard K, et al. Efficient and stable transduction of cardiomyocytes after intramyocardial injection or intracoronary perfusion with recombinant adeno-associated virus vectors. Circulation 1999; 99:201–205.

26. Fu H, Muenzer J, Samulski RJ, et al. Self-complementary adeno-associated virus serotype 2 vector: global distribution and broad dispersion of AAV-mediated transgene expression in mouse brain. Mol Ther 2003; 8:911–917.
27. Wang Z, Zhu T, Qiao C, et al. Adeno-associated virus serotype 8 efficiently delivers genes to muscle and heart. Nat Biotechnol 2005; 23:321–328.
28. MacKenzie TC, Kobinger GP, Kootstra NA, et al. Efficient transduction of liver and muscle after in utero injection of lentiviral vectors with different pseudotypes. Mol Ther 2002; 6:349–358.
29. Naldini L, Blomer U, Gallay P, et al. In vivo gene delivery and stable transduction of nondividing cells by a lentiviral vector. Science 1996; 272:263–267.
30. Naldini L, Blomer U, Gage FH, et al. Efficient transfer, integration, and sustained long-term expression of the transgene in adult rat brains injected with a lentiviral vector. Proc Natl Acad Sci USA 1996; 93:11382–11388.
31. Sakoda T, Kasahara N, Hamamori Y, et al. A high-titer lentiviral production system mediates efficient transduction of differentiated cells including beating cardiac myocytes. J Mol Cell Cardiol 1999; 31:2037–2047.
32. Peng KW, Pham L, Ye H, et al. Organ distribution of gene expression after intravenous infusion of targeted and untargeted lentiviral vectors. Gene Ther 2001; 8:1456–1463.
33. Zhao J, Pettigrew GJ, Thomas J, et al. Lentiviral vectors for delivery of genes into neonatal and adult ventricular cardiac myocytes in vitro and in vivo. Basic Res Cardiol 2002; 97:348–358.
34. Check E. Second cancer case halts gene-therapy trials. Nature 2003; 421:305.
35. Hacein-Bey-Abina S, von Kalle C, Schmidt M, et al. A serious adverse event after successful gene therapy for X-linked severe combined immunodeficiency. N Engl J Med 2003; 348:255–256.
36. Goins WF, Krisky DM, Wolfe DP, et al. Development of replication-defective herpes simplex virus vectors. Methods Mol Med 2002; 69:481–507.
37. Ferrera R, Cuchet D, Zaupa C, et al. Efficient and non-toxic gene transfer to cardiomyocytes using novel generation amplicon vectors derived from HSV-1. J Mol Cell Cardiol 2005; 38:219–223.
38. Hollon T. Researchers and regulators reflect on first gene therapy death. Nat Med 2000; 6:6.
39. Bostanci A. Gene therapy. Blood test flags agent in death of Penn subject. Science 2002; 295:604–605.
40. Hacein-Bey-Abina S, Le Deist F, Carlier F, et al. Sustained correction of X-linked severe combined immunodeficiency by ex vivo gene therapy. N Engl J Med 2002; 346:1185–1193.
41. Guzman RJ, Lemarchand P, Crystal RG, et al. Efficient gene transfer into myocardium by direct injection of adenovirus vectors. Circ Res 1993; 73:1202–1207.
42. Hajjar RJ, Schmidt U, Matsui T, et al. Modulation of ventricular function through gene transfer in vivo. Proc Natl Acad Sci USA 1998; 95:5251–5256.
43. Donahue JK, Kikkawa K, Thomas AD, et al. Acceleration of widespread adenoviral gene transfer to intact rabbit hearts by coronary perfusion with low calcium and serotonin. Gene Ther 1998; 5:630–634.
44. Fromes Y, Salmon A, Wang X, et al. Gene delivery to the myocardium by intrapericardial injection. Gene Ther 1999; 6:683–688.
45. Ikeda Y, Gu Y, Iwanaga Y, et al. Restoration of deficient membrane proteins in the cardiomyopathic hamster by in vivo cardiac gene transfer. Circulation 2002; 105:502–508.
46. Rosengart TK, Lee LY, Patel SR, et al. Angiogenesis gene therapy: phase I assessment of direct intramyocardial administration of an adenovirus vector expressing VEGF121 cDNA to individuals with clinically significant severe coronary artery disease. Circulation 1999; 100:468–474.
47. Giordano FJ, Ping P, McKirnan MD, et al. Intracoronary gene transfer of fibroblast growth factor-5 increases blood flow and contractile function in an ischemic region of the heart. Nat Med 1996; 2:534–539.
48. Kaspar BK, Roth DM, Lai NC, et al. Myocardial gene transfer and long-term expression following intracoronary delivery of adeno-associated virus. J Gene Med 2005; 7:316–324.

49. Lai NC, Roth DM, Gao MH, et al. Intracoronary adenovirus encoding adenylyl cyclase VI increases left ventricular function in heart failure. Circulation 2004; 110:330–336.
50. Champion HC, Georgakopoulos D, Haldar S, et al. Robust adenoviral and adeno-associated viral gene transfer to the in vivo murine heart: application to study of phospholamban physiology. Circulation 2003; 108:2790–2797.
51. Miyamoto MI, del Monte F, Schmidt U, et al. Adenoviral gene transfer of SERCA2a improves left-ventricular function in aortic-banded rats in transition to heart failure. Proc Natl Acad Sci USA 2000; 97:793–798.
52. Davidson MJ, Jones JM, Emani SM, et al. Cardiac gene delivery with cardiopulmonary bypass. Circulation 2001; 104:131–133.
53. Boekstegers P, von Degenfeld G, Giehrl W, et al. Myocardial gene transfer by selective pressure-regulated retroinfusion of coronary veins. Gene Ther 2000; 7:232–240.
54. Foo RS, Mani K, Kitsis RN. Death begets failure in the heart. J Clin Invest 2005; 115:565–571.
55. Wencker D, Chandra M, Nguyen K, et al. A mechanistic role for cardiac myocyte apoptosis in heart failure. J Clin Invest 2003; 111:1497–1504.
56. Chatterjee S, Stewart AS, Bish LT, et al. Viral gene transfer of the antiapoptotic factor Bcl-2 protects against chronic postischemic heart failure. Circulation 2002; 106:I212–I217.
57. Ozcelik C, Erdmann B, Pilz B, et al. Conditional mutation of the ErbB2 (HER2) receptor in cardiomyocytes leads to dilated cardiomyopathy. Proc Natl Acad Sci USA 2002; 99:8880–8885.
58. Crone SA, Zhao YY, Fan L, et al. ErbB2 is essential in the prevention of dilated cardiomyopathy. Nat Med 2002; 8:459–465.
59. Grazette LP, Boecker W, Matsui T, et al. Inhibition of ErbB2 causes mitochondrial dysfunction in cardiomyocytes Implications for herceptin-induced cardiomyopathy. J Am Coll Cardiol 2004; 44:2231–2238.
60. Narula J, Pandey P, Arbustini E, et al. Apoptosis in heart failure: release of cytochrome c from mitochondria and activation of caspase-3 in human cardiomyopathy. Proc Natl Acad Sci USA 1999; 96:8144–8149.
61. Franke TF, Cantley LC. Apoptosis. A bad kinase makes good. Nature 1997; 390:116–117.
62. Cantley LC. The phosphoinositide 3-kinase pathway. Science 2002; 296:1655–1657.
63. Matsui T, Li L, del Monte F, et al. Adenoviral gene transfer of activated PI 3-kinase and Akt inhibits apoptosis of hypoxic cardiomyocytes in vitro. Circulation 1999; 100:2373–2379.
64. Matsui T, Tao J, del Monte F, et al. Akt activation preserves cardiac function and prevents injury after transient cardiac ischemia in vivo. Circulation 2001; 104:330–335.
65. Haq S, Choukroun G, Lim H, et al. Differential activation of signal transduction pathways in human hearts with hypertrophy versus advanced heart failure. Circulation 2001; 103:670–677.
66. Matsui T, Li L, Wu JC, et al. Phenotypic spectrum caused by transgenic overexpression of activated Akt in the heart. J Biol Chem 2002; 277:22896–22901.
67. Nagoshi T, Matsui T, Aoyama T, et al. Phosphoinositide 3-kinase rescues the detrimental effects of chronic Akt activation in the heart during ischemia-reperfusion injury. J Clin Invest 2005; (in press).
68. Aoyama T, Matsui T, Novikov M, et al. Serum and glucocorticoid-responsive kinase-1 regulates cardiomyocyte survival and hypertrophic response. Circulation 2005; 111:1652–1659.
69. Chao W, Matsui T, Novikov MS, et al. Strategic advantages of insulin-like growth factor-I expression for cardioprotection. J Gene Med 2003; 5:277–286.
70. Bristow MR, Hershberger RE, Port JD, et al. Beta-adrenergic pathways in nonfailing and failing human ventricular myocardium. Circulation 1990; 82:I12–I25.
71. Maurice JP, Hata JA, Shah AS, et al. Enhancement of cardiac function after adenoviral-mediated in vivo intracoronary beta2-adrenergic receptor gene delivery. J Clin Invest 1999; 104:21–29.
72. Koch WJ, Rockman HA, Samama P, et al. Cardiac function in mice overexpressing the beta-adrenergic receptor kinase or a beta ARK inhibitor. Science 1995; 2685:1350–1353.

73. White DC, Hata JA, Shah AS, et al. Preservation of myocardial beta-adrenergic receptor signaling delays the development of heart failure after myocardial infarction. Proc Natl Acad Sci USA 2000; 97:5428–5433.
74. www.wiley.co.uk/genmed. Clinical trials—charts and statistics [WWW]. September 1, 1999. Available at: www.wiley.co.uk/genmed.
75. Packer M, Bristow MR, Cohn JN, et al. The effect of carvedilol on morbidity and mortality in patients with chronic heart failure. U.S. Carvedilol Heart Failure Study Group. N Engl J Med 1996; 334:1349–1355.
76. Packer M, Carver JR, Rodeheffer RJ, et al. Effect of oral milrinone on mortality in severe chronic heart failure. The PROMISE study research group. N Engl J Med 1991; 325:1468–1475.
77. Beuckelmann DJ, Nabauer M, Erdmann E. Intracellular calcium handling in isolated ventricular myocytes from patients with terminal heart failure. Circulation 1992; 85:1046–1055.
78. Hasenfuss G. Calcium pump overexpression and myocardial function. Implications for gene therapy of myocardial failure. Circ Res 1998; 83:966–968.
79. del Monte F, Harding SE, Schmidt U, et al. Restoration of contractile function in isolated cardiomyocytes from failing human hearts by gene transfer of SERCA2a. Circulation 1999; 100:2308–2311.
80. Hoshijima M, Ikeda Y, Iwanaga Y, et al. Chronic suppression of heart-failure progression by a pseudophosphorylated mutant of phospholamban via in vivo cardiac rAAV gene delivery. Nat Med 2002; 8:864–871.
81. del Monte F, Williams E, Lebeche D, et al. Improvement in survival and cardiac metabolism after gene transfer of sarcoplasmic reticulum Ca(2+)-ATPase in a rat model of heart failure. Circulation 2001; 104:1424–1429.

32

Genetics and Heart Failure: Hypertrophic Cardiomyopathy

Carolyn Y. Ho and Christine E. Seidman
Cardiovascular Division, Brigham and Women's Hospital, Harvard Medical School, Boston, Massachusetts, U.S.A.

INTRODUCTION

Cardiomyopathies are disorders of the myocardium that arise from a variety of etiologies and culminate in hypertrophic or dilated remodeling of the heart. Over the past two decades, there have been significant scientific advances in the study of primary cardiomyopathies—disorders of cardiac myocytes that remodel the myocardium in the absence of other underlying or contributing disease process. Inherited gene defects are increasingly recognized as the most common cause of hypertrophic cardiomyopathy (HCM) and a frequent cause of dilated cardiomyopathy. Elucidation of the molecular pathways that lead from gene mutation to clinical phenotype will have profound effects not only on our fundamental understanding of broader issues of basic myocyte structure and function, but will also importantly influence our practical approach to the management of disease.

HYPERTROPHIC CARDIOMYOPATHY

Although HCM was initially described over 100 years ago, the modern characterization dates to 1959, and the molecular genetic basis was determined in the early 1990s. The diagnosis of HCM is typically based on the finding of unexplained left ventricular hypertrophy (LVH) that develops in the absence of other systemic or cardiac conditions (such as hypertension or valvular heart disease) (Fig. 1).

The histopathologic hallmarks of this condition are myocyte hypertrophy with myocardial disarray and fibrosis (Fig. 2). The distribution of disarray may be patchy and typically affects the deeper myocardial layers; therefore, catheter-based endomyocardial biopsy is often non-diagnostic. Although small amounts of myocyte disarray may be seen in other forms of cardiac disease, the higher degree of disarray present in HCM is distinctive. Genetic studies have defined HCM to be a disease of the sarcomere, caused by dominant mutations in genes encoding different components of the contractile apparatus (Fig. 3).

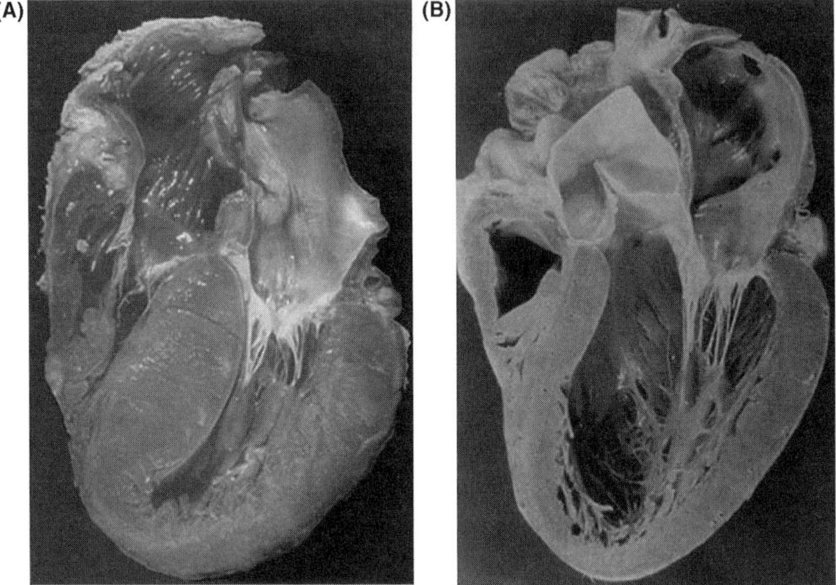

Figure 1 Gross cardiac pathology showing hypertrophic cardiomyopathy (HCM) (**A**) and normal morphology (**B**). Note the marked increase in left ventricular wall thickness associated with HCM.

The prevalence of unexplained LVH in the general population is estimated to be one in 500 (1). The prevalence of sarcomere mutations in different populations is unclear, but a small number of genetic epidemiological studies have been performed to attempt to address this. No specific racial or ethnic predilections have been identified. Direct DNA sequencing of six sarcomere genes (MYH7, TNNT2, TNNI3, TPM1, ACTC, MYBPC3) performed on a cohort of 389 unrelated probands referred to a single center for management of symptomatic HCM identified sarcomere mutations in 147/389 (38%) individuals, most commonly involving MYH7 and MYBPC3 (87% of mutation positive individuals) (2–5). In a separate study, direct DNA sequencing of eight sarcomere proteins (above plus myosin essential and regulatory light chains) was performed on probands with symptomatic and asymptomatic HCM. 187/249 (75%) of these probands were found to

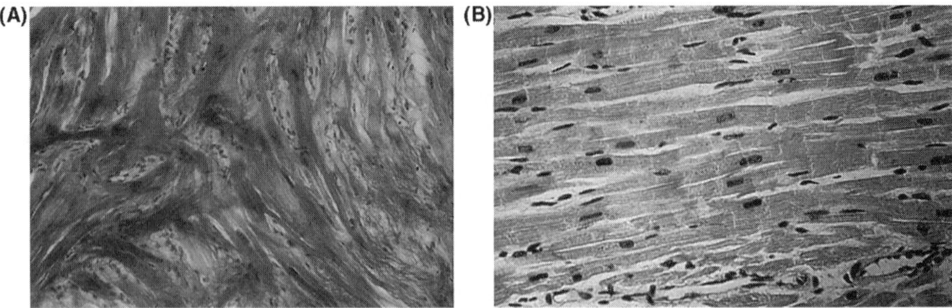

Figure 2 Histologic section from a patient with hypertrophic cardiomyopathy (HCM) (**A**) stained with Masson's trichrome shows characteristic myocyte disarray, hypertrophy, and increased interstitial fibrosis. This is in contrast to the orderly arrangement of myocytes and scant interstitial fibrosis characteristic of normal myocardium, stained with hematoxylin and eosin (**B**).

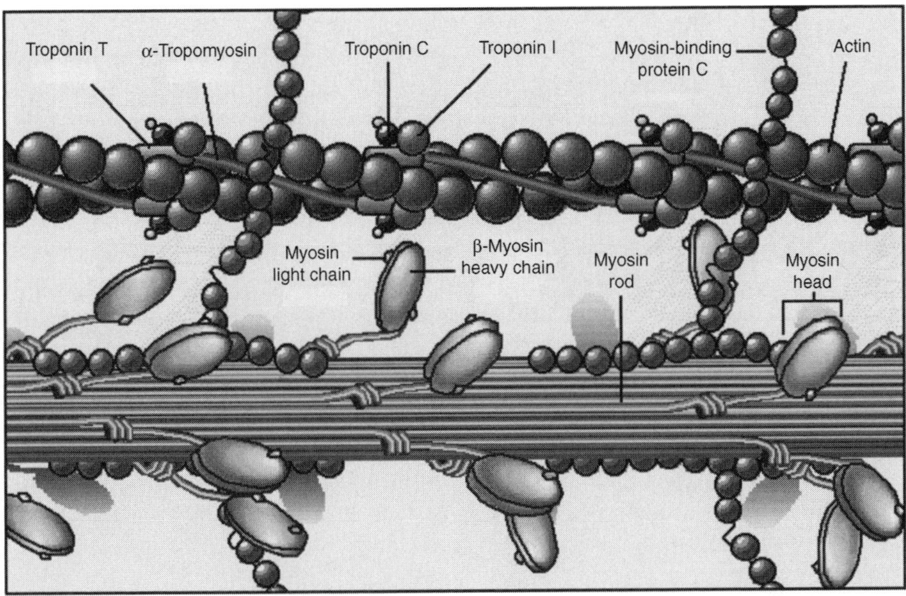

Figure 3 Hypertrophic cardiomyopathy is a disease of the sarcomere, caused by dominantly inherited mutations in the different constituents of the contractile apparatus. The thick filament is composed of myosin heavy chain and myosin essential and regulatory light chains. The thin filament is composed of actin, the troponin complex, and α-tropomyosin. Cardiac myosin binding protein C provides structural support by binding myosin heavy chain and titin. *Source*: Adapted from Spirito PSC, McKenna WJ, Maron BJ. Medical progress: the management of hypertrophic cardiomyopathy. N Eng J Med, 1997; 336(11):775–785.

carry sarcomere gene mutations, 73% in MYH7 and MYBPC3 (5a). Overall, sarcomere gene mutations may account for up to 75% of unexplained LVH that fulfills clinical criteria for HCM, making HCM the most common genetic cardiovascular disorder (6). The prevalence of HCM in the general population contributes to why this diagnosis leads all other causes of sudden death among competitive athletes in the United States (7,8).

PHENOTYPE AND NATURAL HISTORY

Phenotype

Hypertrophic cardiomyopathy has been traditionally characterized by unexplained LVH. LV wall thickness greater than two standard deviations above normal or greater than 13 mm in the adult population are widely accepted as diagnostic echocardiographic criteria for HCM. However, LVH is not present in all individuals with sarcomere gene mutations, particularly early in life (age-dependent penetrance) (9,10). Although a pattern of asymmetric septal hypertrophy is most common, any pattern of LVH may be seen, including isolated apical hypertrophy, concentric hypertrophy, or asymmetric hypertrophy involving other myocardial segments (Fig. 4) (11,12).

The clinical spectrum of HCM is extremely diverse. While some individuals experience no or only minor symptoms and are diagnosed incidentally or in the course of family screening, others may develop refractory symptoms of pulmonary congestion or end stage heart failure requiring cardiac transplantation. In a small subset of patients,

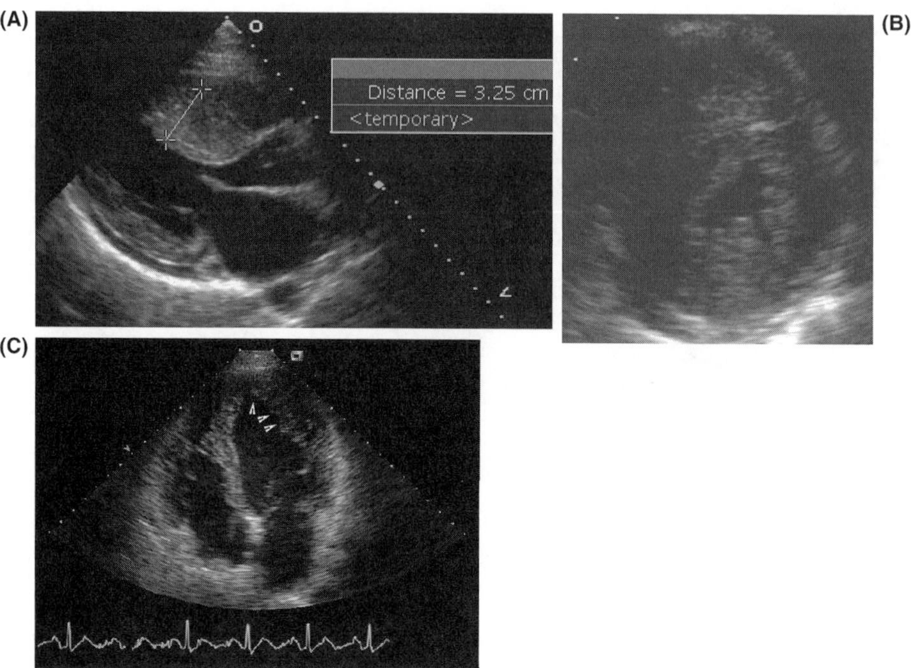

Figure 4 Morphologic variants of hypertrophic cardiomyopathy. Asymmetric septal hypertrophy is most common; however, all variations are seen with respect to distribution, extent, and site of hypertrophy. (**A**) Asymmetric septal hypertrophy; (**B**) concentric hypertrophy; (**C**) apical hypertrophy.

sudden cardiac death is the presenting event (13–16). Shortness of breath, particularly on exertion, is the most common symptom of HCM, occurring in approximately 90% of patients. Other manifestations include chest pain (~30%, often exertional), palpitations, atrial fibrillation (20–25% with associated risk of stroke), orthostatic lightheadedness, presyncope and syncope (15–25%), orthopnea/paroxysmal nocturnal dyspnea, and fatigue (13,16). There is limited correlation between specific morphologic findings and the clinical manifestations of disease. The magnitude of LVH is not closely predictive of the severity of symptoms associated with HCM (13,15). The clinical impact of outflow tract obstruction has been debated with more recent studies suggesting that the presence of outflow tract obstruction (>30 mmHg) may be correlated with increased disease-related morbidity and mortality (17).

Left ventricular systolic function is typically preserved in HCM, however abnormal diastolic function is well described. Diastolic dysfunction may largely account for symptoms of pulmonary congestion and exercise intolerance (18,19). Animal models and recent human studies indicate that diastolic dysfunction precedes the development of LVH and is therefore a more fundamental representation of the HCM phenotype and an earlier manifestation of the underlying sarcomere gene mutation (20–22).

Natural History

The natural history of HCM is highly variable, even between family members who have inherited the same causal mutation. It is unusual for obvious manifestations of HCM to be detected in infancy or early childhood; development of LVH commonly occurs in adolescence in conjunction with the pubertal growth spurt. The specific underlying gene defect may significantly influence the age of onset of detectable LVH (10,23). Disease caused by mutations in the β-myosin heavy chain (β-MHC) gene is typically associated with clinically obvious and early HCM with development of LVH by the 2nd decade of life in 90% of MHC mutation carriers. In contrast, clinically evident hypertrophy may not be present until the 4 or 5th decade of life in disease caused by mutations in the cardiac myosin binding protein C (MyBPC) gene. MyBPC mutations have also been associated with elderly-onset HCM (Fig. 5) (23).

Estimates of annual mortality attributable to HCM are not clearly defined. Early data from specialized referral centers suggested a substantial annual mortality rate of 4–6%. In contrast, community-based studies which may be less influenced by selection bias indicate a considerably more benign course with a projected annual mortality rate of 1–2% (24). Sudden cardiac death (accounting for approximately half of HCM-related deaths), progressive heart failure, atrial fibrillation associated with an increased risk of thromboembolism and stroke, and heart failure are common causes of the morbidity and mortality associated with HCM. Sudden death is the most feared complication of HCM. Accurately estimating an individual's risk for sudden death is imprecise and remains a considerable clinical challenge. The annual risk for sudden death in the overall HCM population varies from 1–5% with approximately 10–20% of patients at highest risk (13,14,25). A higher risk for SCD has been associated with a family history of sudden death, recurrent syncope, an abnormal fall in blood pressure with exercise, ventricular ectopy on Holter monitoring, and massive LVH (>30 mm) (13,14).

Heart failure may develop in patients with HCM and is associated with an annual mortality rate of 0.5%. Less than 10–20% of patients progress to the "burnt-out" or end stage phase of HCM, marked by worsening symptomatic heart failure, left ventricular systolic dysfunction, progressive LV wall thinning, and chamber dilatation (13–15).

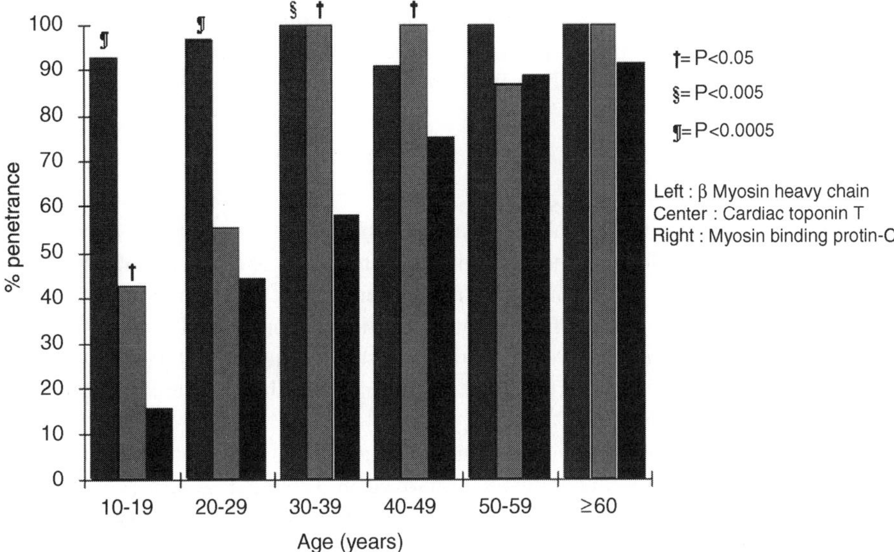

Figure 5 The penetrance (expression of a gene mutation) of left ventricular hypertrophy in hypertrophic cardiomyopathy (HCM) is dependent on age. HCM caused by mutations in myosin heavy chain is clinically evident early in life (by the second decade). In contrast, individuals with mutations in myosin binding protein C may not have clinically evident hypertrophy until after the fourth decade of life. *Source*: Adapted from Ref. 10.

Table 1 Screening Strategy for Family Members in Hypertrophic Cardiomyopathy Kindreds

First degree relatives
PE Echo EKG
Under age 12: Definitive findings rare
Screening optional unless
(1) Malignant FH
(2) Competitive athlete
(3) Suspicion of early onset LVH
Consider q5 yr screening
Age 12–22: q12–24 mo screening
Over age 23: q5 yr (or until genetic testing confirms diagnosis)
If mutation (+): continue serial clinical evaluation
If mutation (−): no further clinical evaluation is required

These patients may ultimately require cardiac transplantation for management of end-stage heart failure.

Hypertrophic cardiomyopathy is inherited in an autosomal dominant manner; therefore, clinical screening of first-degree relatives of affected individuals is recommended. This consists of history, physical examination, 12-lead EKG, and echocardiography. Since the penetrance of LVH is age-dependent, the lack of clinical findings on a single initial assessment does not exclude the possibility of future disease development or the inheritance of an underlying sarcomere mutation. Serial screening and longitudinal follow-up are required to evaluate for the development of phenotypic manifestations with aging. The strategy outlined in Table 1 has been proposed for familial HCM (26). Recently available clinical genotyping (Laboratory for Molecular Mechanism, Harvard-Partners Center for Genetics and Genomics, Cambridge, M.A; http://www.hpcgg.org) should assist in restricting longitudinal clinical evaluation to individuals who are identified to carry a sarcomere mutation. In genotyped families, family members who have not inherited the mutation are not at risk for developing HCM or transmitting the condition to their offspring. Serial clinical evaluation is not required.

GENETIC ASPECTS

Hypertrophic cardiomyopathy is inherited as a Mendelian autosomal dominant trait. Linkage analysis and candidate gene screening of large kindreds with HCM identified discrete mutations in genes which encode different elements of the contractile apparatus, including cardiac β and α myosin heavy chain, cardiac troponins T, I, and C, cardiac myosin binding protein C, α-tropomyosin, actin, the essential and regulatory myosin light chains, and titin (Table 2) (27–31). Thus genetic studies established the paradigm of HCM as a disease of the sarcomere (Fig. 3).

To date, more than 300 individual mutations have been identified in 12 different components of the contractile apparatus, summarized in Table 2 (32–35). A variety of types of mutations have been described, including missense, nonsense, short insertions and deletions, and alteration of splice donor or acceptor sites. There is no predominant common mutation and no significant founder effect in HCM. Mutations tend to be "private"—unique from family to family with rare recurrences in unrelated kindreds. De novo or sporadic mutations are also well described.

The sarcomere is the functional unit of contraction of the myocyte. Proteins are organized into thick (myosin heavy and light chains) and thin (actin, the troponin complex

Table 2 Gene Mutations That Cause Unexplained Left Ventricular Hypertrophy

	Gene	Designation	Chromosome	Frequency	No. of mutations	Phenotypic correlation
HCM-sarcomere proteins	β-Myosin heavy chain	β-MHC	14q1	~30–40%	>80	Obvious disease with significant LVH; several severe phenotypes (end-stage heart failure and sudden death) described
	α-Myosin heavy chain	α-MHC	14q1	Rare	<5	
	Cardiac myosin binding protein C	cMYBPC	11q1	~30–40%	>50	More mild disease but severe phenotypes have been described; elderly-onset HCM
	Cardiac troponin T	cTnT	1q3	~15–20%	>20	Mild LVH but increased association with sudden death severe benign phenotype described
	Cardiac troponin I	cTnI	19p1	<5%	>10	
	Cardiac troponin C	CTnC	3p	Rare	1	
	α-Tropomyosin	α-TM	15q2	<5%	8	
	Myosin essential light chain	MLC-1	3p	Rare	2	Skeletal myopathy
	Myosin regulatory light chain	MLC-2	12q	Rare	8	Skeletal myopathy
	Actin		11q	Rare	5	
	Titin		2q3	Rare	1	
Inherited left ventricular hypertrophy	γ-Subunit AMP kinase	PRKAG2	7q3	?	4	Preexcitation and conduction disease
	Lysosome associted membrane protein	LAMP2	X	?	6	Preexcitation and conduction disease
	Muscle LIM protein	CRP3	11p	?	3	

Abbreviations: HCM, hypertrophic cardiomyopathy; LVH, left ventricular hypertrophy.
Source: Adapted from Refs. 21, 32, and 33 and http://cardiogenomics.med.harvard.edu/project-detail?project_id=230.

and α-tropomyosin) filaments that interdigitate during muscle fiber shortening and lengthening. The detachment and attachment of actin and the myosin head drive contraction and relaxation at the molecular level. The hydrolysis of adenosine triphosphate (ATP) powers this motor and carefully orchestrated fluxes in intracellular Ca^{2+} concentration coordinate thick and thin filament interaction (Fig. 6) (reviewed in Ref. 36).

Mutations in cardiac β myosin heavy chain, cardiac myosin binding protein C, and cardiac troponin T, and cardiac troponin I account for approximately 80% of described cases of HCM caused by sarcomere gene mutations (32,33,35). Clinical correlates for mutations in different HCM genes are broadly outlined in Table 2, however numerous exceptions to these themes have been documented (2,37). A discrete number of mutations identified via family studies have been characterized as "benign" or "malignant," but in isolation, the specific identity of the gene mutation is insufficiently predictive of outcome and integration of this information with clinical risk assessment is appropriate. Further identification of causal mutations and more accurate definition of genotype-phenotype correlations remain a work in progress, but the wide genetic and clinical spectrum of HCM challenges this task. It remains unclear why some sarcomere mutations cause more severe disease than others and why individuals with the same mutation have a wide range of clinical features. Mutations in α and β-MHC as well as titin, cMyBPC, and thin filament components troponin T and actin have also been associated with genetic dilated cardiomyopathy. Description of wider genetic and environmental factors that shape the expression of the underlying mutation is an active area of investigation.

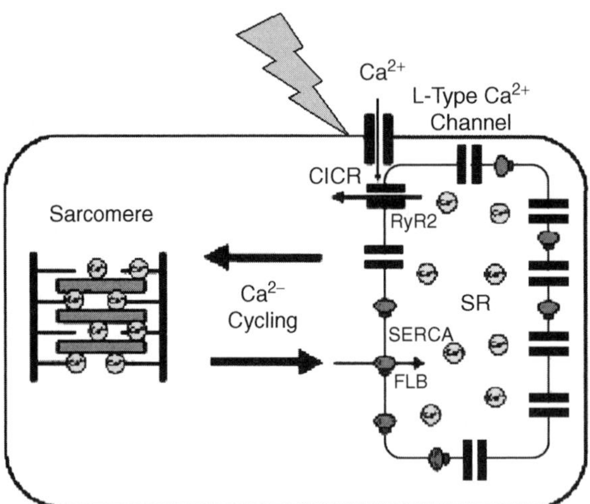

Figure 6 Membrane depolarization by the action potential elicits calcium influx through cell membrane L-type calcium channels. Ryanodine receptors (RyR2) on the sarcoplasmic reticulum (SR) are then activated to trigger calcium-induced calcium release. The resultant rise in intracellular Ca^{2+} concentration leads to calcium binding of troponin C and causes conformational changes in the troponin complex, releasing troponin I inhibition of actin and allowing actin–myosin crossbridge formation. Myosin then hydrolyzes ATP and undergoes conformational changes that allow the myosin head to be propelled against the thin filament. Activation of the sarcoplasmic/endoplasmic Ca^{2+} ATPase membrane pump, SERCA, causes sequestration of cytosolic Ca^{2+} back into the SR. The myosin head detaches from actin, troponin I inhibition of actomyosin interaction is reestablished, and myocyte relaxation ensues. *Source*: Adapted from Ref. 65.

Cardiac β-Myosin Heavy Chain Mutations (β-MHC)

Myosin heavy chains account for approximately 1% of total myocyte protein. They are large molecules of >200,000 kDa, organized into two functional domains: an amino terminal globular head that interacts with actin and a carboxyl terminal rod (38,39). Force is transduced via a hinge region between these two domains. There are two cardiac-specific myosin heavy chain isoforms, α-cardiac MHC (MYH6) and β-cardiac MHC (MYH7), encoded in tandem on chromosome 14. The α-isoform predominates in fetal life and in the adult atria; the β-isoform predominates in the adult, accounting for more than 70% of total ventricular myosin (40). The majority of HCM-causing mutations are of the missense variety and clustered within the globular head of β-MHC.

Over 80 different β-MHC missense mutations have been reported in both familial and sporadic disease and β-MHC mutations are thought to account for ~30–40% of cases of HCM (32,33,35). The phenotypic expression of these mutations is usually obvious with significant degrees of LVH apparent by late adolescence. Although heterogeneous, the clinical course of certain MHC mutations is often quite severe, associated with an increased risk of sudden death or development of end-stage heart failure. The precise determinants of the relationship between prognosis and underlying gene mutation are likely multifactorial and currently poorly understood. Mutations that result in a change in the charge of the substituted amino acid may result in more severe disease, presumably due to more dramatic effects on protein structure and function.

Cardiac α-Myosin Heavy Chain (α-MHC)

Although β-MHC is the predominant isoform expressed by the adult human ventricular myocardium, the α-isoform may account for up to 30% of adult ventricular myosin heavy chain (41). Expression is developmentally regulated such that the α-isoform is abundant in the atria and ventricles during fetal development. After birth, the ventricles express predominantly the β-isoform (42,43). Mutations in α-MHC have been associated with sporadic cases of elderly-onset HCM (23). Although highly speculative, it is possible that the lower expressed amounts of this isoform in the adult ventricle may account for the delayed onset of hypertrophy.

Myosin Light Chains

The regulatory (MYL2, chromosome 12) and essential (MYL3, chromosome 19) myosin light chains may be involved in determining the speed and force of actomyosin sliding by interacting with the head-rod junction of MHC (44,45). Mutations in myosin light chains are rarely reported genetic etiologies of HCM, accounting for <1% of disease (46).

Cardiac Myosin Binding Protein C (cMyBPC)

The cardiac myosin binding protein C gene (MYBPC3) spans 24 kb of chromosome 11 and encodes a 1274 amino acid (137 kDa) protein. Functionally, MyBPC may provide structural integrity to the sarcomere (binding MHC and titin) as well as modulate myosin ATPase activity and cardiac contractility in response to adrenergic stimulation (47). Missense, splice site, and deletion/insertion mutations in cMyBPC likely account for ~30–40% of cases of HCM (32,33,35). In a significant subset of individuals with cMyBPC mutations, the development of clinically apparent LVH is delayed until age 50 yr or above (10,23). cMyBPC mutations have also been identified in 20% of a cohort of individuals with elderly-onset of HCM which is distinguished by late-onset hypertrophy and often absence of family history (23).

Cardiac Troponin T (cTnT)

Troponin T links the troponin complex to α-TM and thus plays a central role in the regulation of contractile function. The cardiac troponin T gene (TNNT2) spans 17 kb of DNA on chromosome one and encodes a 288 amino acid peptide (36–39 kDa). Approximately 5% of HCM is thought to be attributable to cTnT mutations.

Cardiac Troponin I (cTnI)

Troponin I is the inhibitory subunit of the troponin complex, acting to inhibit actin–myosin interaction. When Ca^{2+} binds to troponin C, conformational changes occur in TnI which release the inhibition of TnT and α-TM, allowing actomyosin crossbridge formation to occur. The cardiac-specific isoform of troponin I (TNNI3) spans eight exons on chromosome 19 and encodes a 210 amino acid (27–31 kDa) protein (48). Direct DNA sequence analysis of cTnI in patients with HCM suggests that mutations in this gene account for at least 3% of disease (5a).

Cardiac Actin

Cardiac actin is a 375 amino acid protein (41 kilodaltons; kDa) encoded by the cardiac actin gene (ACTC) and organized into six exons on chromosome 15 (49). Mutations in actin typically located in proximity to the putative myosin binding site and are a rare cause of HCM (50,51). Actin mutations have also been identified as a rare cause of familial dilated cardiomyopathy (52).

α-Tropomyosin (α-TM)

The α-tropomyosin gene (TPM1) is organized into 15 exons on chromosome 15 (53) and encodes a 284 amino acid protein expressed in both fast skeletal and cardiac muscle (54). α-TM forms a complex with troponin T that regulates actin–myosin interaction in response to intracellular Ca^{2+} concentration. Calcium binding to troponin C causes conformational changes in troponins I and T that ultimately allow actin–myosin crossbridge formation. Mutations in TPM1 are thought to account for a small proportion (<2%) of familial and sporadic HCM, including a potential founder effect in the Finnish population (28,31,55–58).

Although α-tropomyosin is expressed in both cardiac and skeletal muscle, the clinical expression of TPM1 mutations is dominated by HCM, rather than skeletal myopathy. The cardiac specificity of phenotype may be due to the fact that the identified mutations alter the portions of the α-TM molecule that interact with the cardiac-specific isoform of troponin T. Alterations in calcium sensitivity may also play a role in the tissue-specificity of TPM1 mutations (59).

NEW PARADIGMS OF INHERITED CARDIAC HYPERTROPHY

Deficits of Energy Production and Regulation

Hypertrophic cardiomyopathy is caused by mutations in genes that encode sarcomere proteins. More recently, mutations have been described in non-sarcomere proteins that mimic the gross clinical phenotype of HCM. Genetic studies of families and sporadic cases of unexplained LVH with conduction abnormalities (progressive atrioventricular block, atrial fibrillation, ventricular pre-excitation/Wolff–Parkinson–White syndrome) have identified a novel disease caused by mutations in the $\gamma 2$ regulatory subunit (PRKAG2) of adenosine monophosphate (AMP)-activated protein kinase, an enzyme involved with glucose metabolism, as well as mutations in the X-linked lysosome-associated membrane protein (LAMP2) gene (6,60–62).

In these patients, ventricular pre-excitation typically occurs early in life and is often symptomatic. Progressive conduction disease occurs with increasing age such that permanent pacemaker implantation was required in 30% of affected individuals. This higher prevalence of conduction system disease helps to discriminate disease caused by PRKAG2 mutations from HCM caused by sarcomere mutations (62). Severe clinical outcomes were noted in a subset of patients with PRKAG2 mutations, including progression to end-stage heart failure or transplantation and sudden cardiac death. X-linked LAMP2 mutations may be distinguished from HCM due to the presence of ventricular pre-excitation, male-predominance, earlier age of presentation, more severe prognosis, and more striking EKG and echocardiographic manifestations of LVH (typically concentric; Fig. 7) (6). LAMP2 mutations are also the genetic etiology of Danon disease, a multisystem disorder with cardiac, neurologic, skeletal muscle, and hepatic involvement.

Inherited LVH caused by PRKAG2 or LAMP2 mutations define a new paradigm of glycogen storage cardiomyopathies. This is a disease entity distinct from HCM caused by

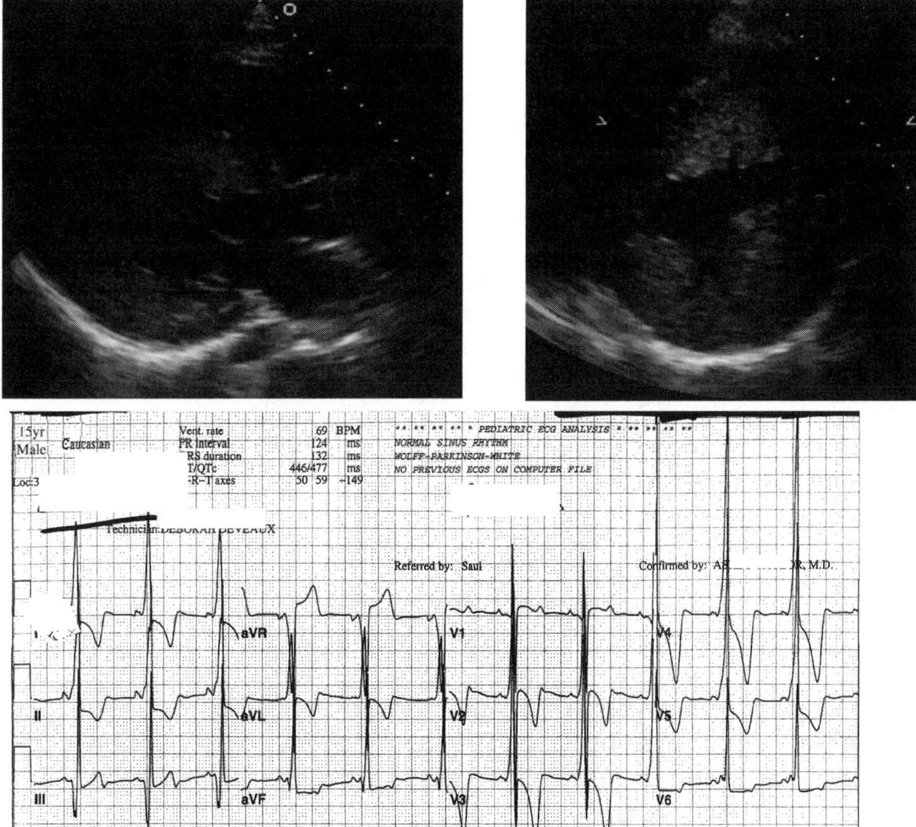

Figure 7 Typical cardiac manifestations of LAMP2 mutations are demonstrated by this 16-year-old male. LAMP2 mutations are associated with striking evidence of left ventricular hypertrophy on echocardiography and EKG.

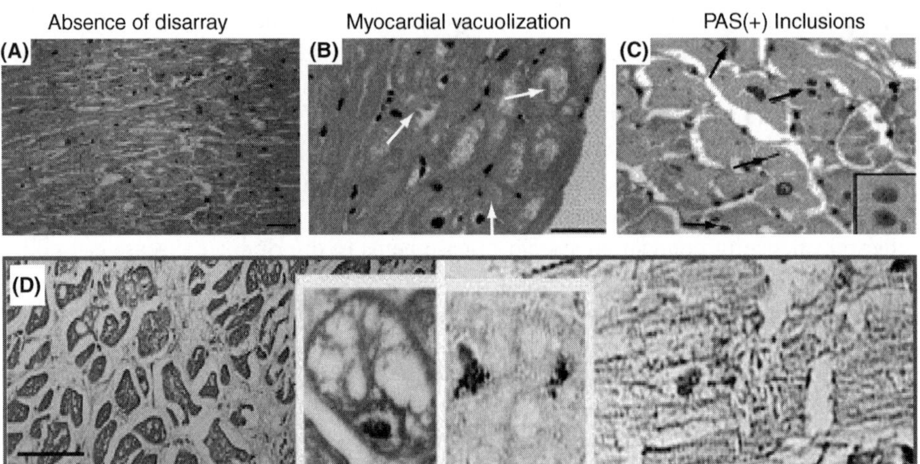

Figure 8 Histopathology of glycogen storage cardiomyopathies. (**A–C**) Patients with mutations in PRKAG2 show non-membrane bound vacuoles in myocytes (*arrows*) that stain for glycogen and amylopectin. There is only mild fibrosis and no myocyte disarray. (**D**) Mutations in LAMP2 show vacuoles with large periodic acid-Schiff positive (PAS+) inclusions. As with PRKAG2 mutations, myocyte size is increased, not due to classic hypertrophy, but rather due to the presence of glycogen-filled vacuoles.

sarcomere protein mutations. Despite the shared finding of cardiac hypertrophy, there are marked differences in other pathologic manifestations associated with PRKAG2 and LAMP2 mutations as compared to HCM. Histopathologically, PRKAG2 and LAMP2 mutations do not display either the myocardial disarray or interstitial fibrosis characteristic of HCM, but rather show prominent non-membrane bound vacuoles that, if appropriately handled and stained, are demonstrated to show glycogen and amylopectin accumulation (Fig. 8). Although incompletely defined, the molecular signaling pathways triggered by PRKAG2 and LAMP2 mutations are almost certainly different from those produced by sarcomere gene mutations (Fig. 9). These differences suggest that the clinical approach to individuals with PRKAG2 and LAMP2 mutations should not be predicated on management tenets for HCM. An algorithm to distinguish HCM from glycogen storage cardiomyopathies is illustrated in Figure 10.

CONTEMPORARY DIAGNOSIS OF HCM

The identification of unexplained LVH, typically via echocardiographic imaging, is the traditional basis for diagnosing HCM. However, since LVH is not universally present throughout life or detectable in all individuals with sarcomere gene mutations, the presence of unexplained LVH is not the most specific or sensitive manifestation of HCM. Further definition of the full spectrum of the HCM phenotype is required. Animal and human studies have indicated that diastolic abnormalities are present prior to the development of LVH (20–22,63). Biochemical abnormalities, namely alterations in intracellular calcium handling, may represent an even more fundamental manifestation of sarcomere gene mutations (64,65). Describing the early HCM phenotype is crucial to better understanding disease pathophysiology.

Genetic testing allows for precise identification of individuals at risk for developing HCM independently of age and clinical manifestations and should be incorporated into

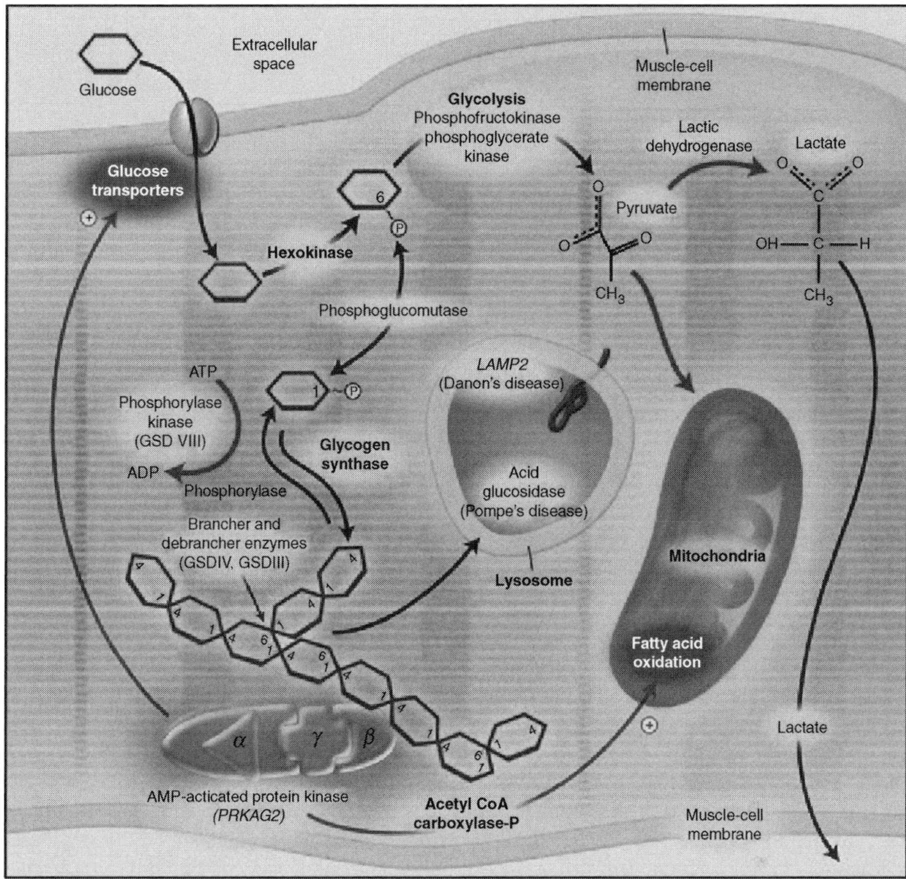

Figure 9 Pathways of muscle glycogen metabolism: proteins implicated in glycogen storage diseases associated with cardiomyopathy are shown. Glucose enters the myocyte through transmembrane transport proteins and undergoes phophorylation by hexokinase. It then enters pathways for glycolysis or glycogen synthesis by glycogen synthase. Glycogen, a branched glucose polymer, is a dynamic energy reservoir for muscles, as dictated by enzyme activity to change phosphorylation state. Glycogen metabolism is also influenced by AMP-activated protein kinase (regulates glucose uptake and fatty acid oxidation via acetyl CoA carboxylase) and by lysosome activity. Defects in pathways of glycogen degradation (phosphorylase, phosphorylase kinase, phosphoglucomutase, phosphofructokinase, phosphoglycearate kinase, lactic dehydrogenase, and brancher/debrancher enzymes) result in glycogen accumulation. Mutations in PRKAG2 (the regulatory γ subunit of AMP kinase) or LAMP2 may cause glycogen accumulation resulting in cardiac hypertrophy and electrophysiological abnormalities. *Source*: Adapted from Ref. 62.

the contemporary diagnosis of this disorder. This is currently accomplished by bidirectional DNA sequence analysis of the exons and intron/exon boundaries of sarcomere genes to identify potential disease-associated sequence variants. This is a daunting task that underscores the need for more efficient yet reliable techniques for screening large stretches of DNA.

The identification of a sarcomere gene mutation in the appropriate clinical setting allows the definitive diagnosis of HCM and establishes the exact genetic etiology. Mutation confirmation can then be performed in family members in a simple and straightforward manner. Individuals found to carry the family-specific mutation despite

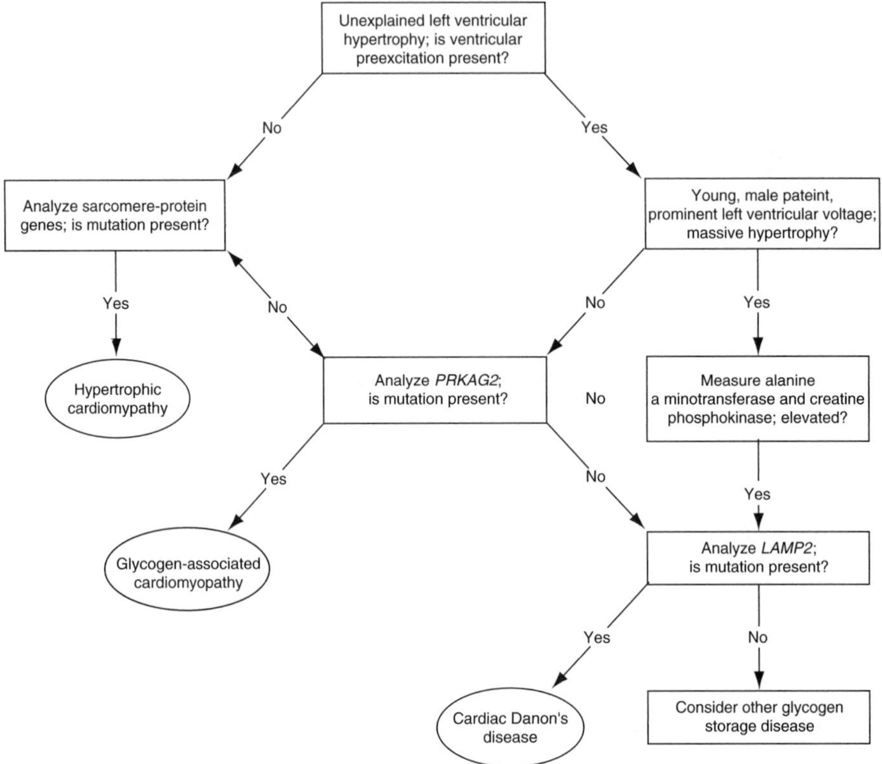

Figure 10 The diagnosis of hypertrophic cardiomyopathy is suggested by an autosomal dominant pattern of inheritance of left ventricular hypertrophy (LVH) unaccompanied by systemic manifestations or evidence of ventricular preexcitation. This diagnosis can be confirmed by the identification of a sarcomere gene mutation. Glycogen storage cardiomyopathy is suggested by the presence of preexcitation in conjunction with unexplained LVH. Disease due to PRKAG2 mutations is suggested by autosomal dominant inheritance and the absence of systemic manifestations. Danon disease is suggested by male gender and abnormalities in liver, musculoskeletal, or neurologic function. Cardiac manifestations are typically present at a young age and have particularly striking echocardiographic and EKG manifestations. *Source*: Adapted from Ref. 26.

the absence of clinical manifestations are at risk for developing HCM and require longitudinal clinical follow up as described earlier in this chapter. Such individuals should also be counseled of the 50% chance of transmission of the mutation to offspring. Family members who do not carry the mutation have no risk for developing HCM or transmitting the condition. Longitudinal clinical follow up is not necessary.

There are limitations to this strategy of genetic diagnosis. Mutations in sarcomere genes are thought to account for 60–75% of cases of inherited LVH; expanding the screen to include PRKAG2 and LAMP2 will further increase diagnostic yield. Nonetheless, mutations will not be detected in all individuals with unexplained LVH. Therefore a negative result from this method of screening does not exclude a genetic etiology. Continued efforts to determine how gene mutations lead to HCM will ultimately inspire new strategies of disease management designed to alter phenotype rather than merely palliating symptoms. Genetic diagnosis will play a crucial role in this endeavor by allowing the identification of individuals with gene mutations prior to the development of clinically detectable disease. A better understanding of the biochemical and clinical features of early stage disease will ultimately allow development of novel treatment strategies designed to change the phenotypic expression of these gene defects rather than merely palliating symptoms.

REFERENCES

1. Maron BJ, Gardin JM, Flack JM, Gidding SS, Kurosaki TT, Bild DE. Prevalence of hypertrophic cardiomyopathy in a general population of young adults—echocardiographic analysis of 4111 subjects in the CARDIA study. Circulation 1995; 92:785–789.
2. Van Driest SL, Ackerman MJ, Ommen SR, et al. Prevalence and severity of "benign" mutations in the beta-myosin heavy chain, cardiac troponin T, and alpha-tropomyosin genes in hypertrophic cardiomyopathy. Circulation 2002; 106:3085–3090.
3. Van Driest SL, Ellsworth EG, Ommen SR, Tajik AJ, Gersh BJ, Ackerman MJ. Prevalence and spectrum of thin filament mutations in an outpatient referral population with hypertrophic cardiomyopathy. Circulation 2003; 108:445–451.
4. Van Driest SL, Jaeger MA, Ommen SR, et al. Comprehensive analysis of the beta-myosin heavy chain gene in 389 unrelated patients with hypertrophic cardiomyopathy. J Am Coll Cardiol 2004; 44:602–610.
5. Van Driest SL, Vasile VC, Ommen SR, et al. Myosin binding protein C mutations and compound heterozygosity in hypertrophic cardiomyopathy. J Am Coll Cardiol 2004; 44:1903–1910.

5a. http://cardiogenomics.med.harvard.edu

6. Arad M, Maron BJ, Gorham JM, et al. Glycogen storage diseases presenting as hypertrophic cardiomyopathy. N Engl J Med 2005; 352:362–372.
7. Maron BJ, Mitten MJ, Quandt EF, Zipes DP. Competitive athletes with cardiovascular disease—the case of Nicholas Knapp. N Engl J Med 1998; 339:1632–1635.
8. Maron BJ. Sudden death in young athletes. N Engl J Med 2003; 349:1064–1075.
9. Rosenzweig A, Watkins H, Hwang DS, et al. Preclinical diagnosis of familial hypertrophic cardiomyopathy by genetic analysis of blood lymphocytes [see comments]. N Engl J Med 1991; 325:1753–1760.
10. Niimura H, Bachinski LL, Sangwatanaroj S, et al. Mutations in the gene for cardiac myosin-binding protein C and late-onset familial hypertrophic cardiomyopathy [see comments]. N Engl J Med 1998; 338:1248–1257.
11. Wigle ED, Sasson Z, Henderson MA, et al. Hypertrophic cardiomyopathy. The importance of the site and the extent of hypertrophy. A review. Prog Cardiovasc Dis 1985; 28:1–83.
12. Klues HG, Schiffers A, Maron BJ. Phenotypic spectrum and patterns of left ventricular hypertrophy in hypertrophic cardimoypathy: morphologic observations and significance as assessed by two-dimensional echocardiography in 600 patients. J Am Coll Cardiol 1995; 26:1699–1708.
13. Maron BJ. Hypertrophic cardiomyopathy: a systematic review. JAMA 2002; 287:1308–1320.
14. McKenna WJ, Behr ER. Hypertrophic cardiomyopathy: management, risk stratification, and prevention of sudden death. Heart 2002; 87:169–176.
15. Elliott P, McKenna WJ. Hypertrophic cardiomyopathy. Lancet 2004; 363:1881–1891.
16. Nishimura RA, Holmes DR, Jr. Clinical practice. Hypertrophic obstructive cardiomyopathy. N Engl J Med 2004; 350:1320–1327.
17. Maron MS, Olivotto I, Betocchi S, et al. Effect of left ventricular outflow tract obstruction on clinical outcome in hypertrophic cardiomyopathy. N Engl J Med 2003; 348:295–303.
18. Briguori C, Betocchi S, Losi MA, et al. Noninvasive evaluation of left ventricular diastolic function in hypertrophic cardiomyopathy. Am J Cardiol 1998; 81:180–187.
19. Briguori C, Betocchi S, Romano M, et al. Exercise capacity in hypertrophic cardiomyopathy depends on left ventricular diastolic function. Am J Cardiol 1999; 84:309–315.
20. Geisterfer-Lowrance AA, Christe M, Conner DA, et al. A mouse model of familial hypertrophic cardiomyopathy. Science 1996; 272:731–734.

21. Nagueh SF, Bachinski LL, Meyer D, et al. Tissue Doppler imaging consistently detects myocardial abnormalities in patients with hypertrophic cardiomyopathy and provides a novel means for an early diagnosis before and independently of hypertrophy. Circulation 2001; 104:128–130.
22. Ho CY, Sweitzer NK, McDonough B, et al. Assessment of diastolic function with Doppler tissue imaging to predict genotype in preclinical hypertrophic cardiomyopathy. Circulation 2002; 105:2992–2997.
23. Niimura H, Patton KK, McKenna WJ, et al. Sarcomere protein gene mutations in hypertrophic cardiomyopathy of the elderly. Circulation 2002; 105:446–451.
24. Maron BJ, Casey SA, Hauser RG, Aeppli DM. Clinical course of hypertrophic cardiomyopathy with survival to advanced age. J Am Coll Cardiol 2003; 42:882–888.
25. Elliott PM, Poloniecki J, Dickie S, et al. Sudden death in hypertrophic cardiomyopathy: identification of high risk patients. J Am Coll Cardiol 2000; 36:2212–2218.
26. Maron BJ, Seidman JG, Seidman CE. Proposal for contemporary screening strategies in families with hypertrophic cardiomyopathy. J Am Coll Cardiol 2004; 44:2125–2132.
27. Thierfelder L, MacRae C, Watkins H, et al. A familial hypertrophic cardiomyopathy locus maps to chromosome 15q2. Proc Natl Acad Sci U.S.A. 1993; 90:6270–6274.
28. Thierfelder L, Watkins H, MacRae C, et al. Alpha-tropomyosin and cardiac troponin T mutations cause familial hypertrophic cardiomyopathy: a disease of the sarcomere. Cell 1994; 77:701–712.
29. Jarcho JA, McKenna W, Pare JA, et al. Mapping a gene for familial hypertrophic cardiomyopathy to chromosome 14q1. N Engl J Med 1989; 321:1372–1378.
30. Watkins H, MacRae C, Thierfelder L, et al. A disease locus for familial hypertrophic cardiomyopathy maps to chromosome 1q3. Nat Genet 1993; 3:333–337.
31. Watkins H, McKenna WJ, Thierfelder L, et al. Mutations in the genes for cardiac troponin T and alpha-tropomyosin in hypertrophic cardiomyopathy. N Engl J Med 1995; 332:1058–1064.
32. Seidman JG, Seidman C. The genetic basis for cardiomyopathy: from mutation identification to mechanistic paradigms. Cell 2001; 104:557–567.
33. Marian AJ, Roberts R. The molecular genetic basis for hypertrophic cardiomyopathy. J Mol Cell Cardiol 2001; 33:655–670.
34. Charron P, Heron D, Gargiulo M, et al. Genetic testing and genetic counselling in hypertrophic cardiomyopathy: the French experience. J Med Genet 2002; 39:741–746.
35. Richard P, Charron P, Carrier L, et al. Hypertrophic cardiomyopathy: distribution of disease genes, spectrum of mutations, and implications for a molecular diagnosis strategy. Circulation 2003; 107:2227–2232.
36. Fatkin D, Graham RM. Molecular mechanisms of inherited cardiomyopathies. Physiol Rev 2002; 82:945–980.
37. Ackerman MJ, VanDriest SL, Ommen SR, et al. Prevalence and age-dependence of malignant mutations in the beta-myosin heavy chain and troponin T genes in hypertrophic cardiomyopathy: a comprehensive outpatient perspective. J Am Coll Cardiol 2002; 39:2042–2048.
38. Rayment I, Holden HM, Whittaker M, et al. Structure of the actin–myosin complex and its implications for muscle contraction. Science 1993; 261:58–65.
39. Sata M, Stafford WF, Mabuchi K, Ikebe M. The motor domain and the regulatory domain of myosin solely dictate enzymatic activity and phosphorylation-dependent regulation, respectively. Proc Natl Acad Sci U.S.A. 1997; 94:91–96.
40. Saez LJ, Gianola KM, McNally EM, et al. Human cardiac myosin heavy chain genes and their linkage in the genome. Nucleic Acids Res 1987; 15:5443–5459.
41. Nakao K, Minobe W, Roden R, Bristow MR, Leinwand LA. Myosin heavy chain gene expression in human heart failure. J Clin Invest 1997; 100:2362–2370.
42. Schiaffino S, Reggiani C. Molecular diversity of myofibrillar proteins: gene regulation and functional significance. Physiol Rev 1996; 76:371–423.
43. Nadal-Ginard B, Mahdavi V. Molecular basis of cardiac performance. Plasticity of the myocardium generated through protein isoform switches. J Clin Invest 1989; 84:1693–1700.
44. Lowey S, Waller GS, Trybus KM. Skeletal muscle myosin light chains are essential for physiological speeds of shortening. Nature 1993; 365:454–456.

45. VanBuren P, Waller GS, Harris DE, Trybus KM, Warshaw DM, Lowey S. The essential light chain is required for full force production by skeletal muscle myosin. Proc Natl Acad Sci U.S.A. 1994; 91:12403–12407.
46. Poetter K, Jiang H, Hassanzadeh S, et al. Mutations in either the essential or regulatory light chains of myosin are associated with a rare myopathy in human heart and skeletal muscle. Nat Genet 1996; 13:63–69.
47. Freiburg A, Gautel M. A molecular map of the interactions between titin and myosin-binding protein C. Implications for sarcomeric assembly in familial hypertrophic cardiomyopathy. Eur J Biochem 1996; 235:317–323.
48. Mogensen J, Kruse TA, Borglum AD. Assignment of the human cardiac troponin I gene (TNNI3) to chromosome 19q13.4 by radiation hybrid mapping. Cytogenet Cell Genet 1997; 79:272–273.
49. Hamada H, Petrino MG, Kakunaga T. Molecular structure and evolutionary origin of human cardiac muscle actin gene. Proc Natl Acad Sci U.S.A. 1982; 79:5901–5905.
50. Mogensen J, Klausen IC, Pedersen AK, et al. Alpha-cardiac actin is a novel disease gene in familial hypertrophic cardiomyopathy. J Clin Invest 1999; 103:R39–R43.
51. Olson TM, Doan TP, Kishimoto NY, Whitby FG, Ackerman MJ, Fananapazir L. Inherited and de novo mutations in the cardiac actin gene cause hypertrophic cardiomyopathy. J Mol Cell Cardiol 2000; 32:1687–1694.
52. Olson TM, Michels VV, Thibodeau SN, Tai YS, Keating MT. Actin mutations in dilated cardiomyopathy, a heritable form of heart failure. Science 1998; 280:750–752.
53. Mogensen J, Kruse TA, Borglum AD. Refined localization of the human alpha-tropomyosin gene (TPM1) by genetic mapping. Cytogenet Cell Genet 1999; 84:35–36.
54. Schultheiss T, Lin ZX, Lu MH, et al. Differential distribution of subsets of myofibrillar proteins in cardiac nonstriated and striated myofibrils. J Cell Biol 1990; 110:1159–1172.
55. Watkins H, Anan R, Coviello DA, Spirito P, Seidman JG, Seidman CE. A de novo mutation in alpha-tropomyosin that causes hypertrophic cardiomyopathy. Circulation 1995; 91:2302–2305.
56. Yamauchi-Takihara K, Nakajima-Taniguchi C, Matsui H, et al. Clinical implications of hypertrophic cardiomyopathy associated with mutations in the alpha-tropomyosin gene. Heart 1996; 76:63–65.
57. Coviello DA, Maron BJ, Spirito P, et al. Clinical features of hypertrophic cardiomyopathy caused by mutation of a "hot spot" in the alpha-tropomyosin gene. J Am Coll Cardiol 1997; 29:635–640.
58. Jaaskelainen P, Soranta M, Miettinen R, et al. The cardiac beta-myosin heavy chain gene is not the predominant gene for hypertrophic cardiomyopathy in the finnish population. J Am Coll Cardiol 1998; 32:1709–1716.
59. Bottinelli R, Coviello DA, Redwood CS, et al. A mutant tropomyosin that causes hypertrophic cardiomyopathy is expressed in vivo and associated with an increased calcium sensitivity. Circ Res 1998; 82:106–115.
60. Blair E, Redwood C, Ashrafian H, et al. Mutations in the gamma(2) subunit of AMP-activated protein kinase cause familial hypertrophic cardiomyopathy: evidence for the central role of energy compromise in disease pathogenesis. Hum Mol Genet 2001; 10:1215–1220.
61. Gollob MH, Green MS, Tang AS, et al. Identification of a gene responsible for familial Wolff-Parkinson-White syndrome. N Engl J Med 2001; 344:1823–1831.
62. Arad M, Benson DW, Perez-Atayde AR, et al. Constitutively active AMP kinase mutations cause glycogen storage disease mimicking hypertrophic cardiomyopathy. J Clin Invest 2002; 109:357–362.
63. Nagueh SF, Kopelen HA, Lim DS, et al. Tissue Doppler imaging consistently detects myocardial contraction and relaxation abnormalities, irrespective of cardiac hypertrophy, in a transgenic rabbit model of human hypertrophic cardiomyopathy. Circulation 2000; 102:1346–1350.
64. Fatkin D, McConnell BK, Mudd JO, et al. An abnormal Ca(2+) response in mutant sarcomere protein-mediated familial hypertrophic cardiomyopathy. J Clin Invest 2000; 106:1351–1359.
65. Semsarian C, Ahmad I, Giewat M, et al. The L-type calcium channel inhibitor diltiazem prevents cardiomyopathy in a mouse model. J Clin Invest 2002; 109:1013–1020.

33

Genetics and Heart Failure: Dilated, Restrictive, and Right Ventricular Cardiomyopathies

Nicole M. Johnson and Daniel P. Judge
Division of Cardiology, Johns Hopkins University School of Medicine, Baltimore, Maryland, U.S.A.

INTRODUCTION

Although the most common type of inherited cardiomyopathy is hypertrophic cardiomyopathy (HCM), there are several other genetic forms of cardiomyopathy which are less frequently recognized as having a familial component. Identifying a genetic or familial etiology as the primary cause of a patient's cardiomyopathy may aide in prognosis, management, and risk assessment for the individual patient and their family members.

This chapter reviews the genetic forms of dilated, restrictive, and right ventricular cardiomyopathies. Each is associated with considerable genetic heterogeneity, and therefore the ability to identify the specific genetic cause of an individual patient's cardiomyopathy through current clinical genetic testing is lower than for HCM. However, even if clinical genetic testing options do not yield a specific pathogenic mutation, familial forms of cardiomyopathy can still be identified through thorough assessment of the patient's clinical history and imaging studies, as well as screening of family members. Continued investigation of both the molecular causes and phenotypic manifestations of heritable forms of cardiomyopathy should lead to improvements in recognition of these conditions, and better understanding of disease pathogenesis.

FAMILIAL DILATED CARDIOMYOPATHY

Nonischemic DCM affects 36.5 per 100,000 in the United States (1). There are numerous causes of nonischemic DCM, including valvular heart disease, viral infection, endocrine disorders, and toxins (2,3). In addition to the numerous acquired causes of DCM, primary disorders of the myocardium also occur, such as familial dilated cardiomyopathy (FDC).

In 1999, Mestroni, and colleagues proposed criteria for the diagnosis of FDC (4). For a proband, DCM is diagnosed with an ejection fraction less than 45% (or fractional shortening less than 25%) with left ventricular enlargement (greater than 117% predicted, based on age and body surface area). In the absence of standard exclusion criteria, familial disease is established on the basis of one similarly affected family member or the presence of a first-degree relative of a proband with documented unexplained sudden death at age less than 35 years.

Prior to the early 1990s, the incidence of FDC was thought to be somewhat rare. Over the past 15 years, several epidemiologic investigations have led to our current recognition that 20–35% of idiopathic DCM cases may be classified as FDC (5–7). In fact, using simply the criterion of left ventricular enlargement in family members of individuals with idiopathic DCM, one trial found the prevalence to be as high as 48% (8). The true incidence of FDC is often under-appreciated due to incomplete pedigrees, lack of knowledge about the health of family members among probands, de novo mutations, variable expressivity, and incomplete penetrance of this disorder. Despite these limitations, multiple genomic loci and genes have been identified in association with FDC (Table 1). In light of the frequency of FDC, current guidelines regarding evaluation of a patient with idiopathic DCM recommend echocardiographic screening of all first-degree relatives to identify presymptomatic family members (9).

As one would anticipate in the setting of widespread genetic heterogeneity, clinical phenotypes are widely varied and may provide some clue as to the responsible genetic mutation. However, among family members with the identical pathogenic mutation, variable expressivity may be prominent including age of onset and clinical presentation.

Patients tend to present late in the course of this disease unless screened prior to symptoms. Age at onset varies from neonatal to elderly, and intrafamilial variation is common. Most patients are first seen between the ages of 20 and 50 years, but some present in childhood and others in later years (10). In contrast to acquired DCM, initial manifestations are typically vague, such as mild exertional dyspnea, fatigue, and palpitations. Dyspnea in young individuals is often confused with more common respiratory disorders, such as asthma. Mild symptoms may occur in the setting of profound ventricular enlargement and elevation of pulmonary pressures.

In an analysis of a population of 350 consecutive patients with idiopathic DCM screened for familial disease, the Heart Muscle Disease Study Group found only a younger age of onset, and perhaps a higher ejection fraction on in initial presentation could distinguish FDC from sporadic DCM (11).

Molecular Genetics: Autosomal Dominant FDC

To date, many genes have been identified with mutations resulting in FDC, including both common and rare examples. We will highlight some of these examples, though others currently exist, and undoubtedly, additional genes will be identified in the near future. Clinical genetic testing is available for many of the genes that are discussed in this section.

Multiple patterns of inheritance have been described in association with FDC. The most common is autosomal dominant, such that all offspring of an affected individual have a fifty percent chance of inheriting a genetic predisposition to DCM (5). Reduced penetrance and variable expressivity can mask an autosomal dominant pattern of inheritance. The phenotype is age-dependent, and one investigation cites 90% penetrance at age greater than 40 years, but only 10% penetrance at age less than 20 years (11). Genetic anticipation (progressively earlier onset with successive generations) is not currently thought to play a role in familial forms of dilated cardiomyopathy. However, individuals in a family may be diagnosed at a younger age than previous generations due

Table 1 Genes and Genomic Loci Associated with Familial Dilated Cardiomyopathy

Locus	Gene	Protein	Additional features
1p1–q21	*LMNA*	Lamin A/C	CD, SkM, others
1q32	*TNNT2*	Troponin T, cardiac	None
1q42–q43	*ACTN2*	Alpha-actinin-z	None
2q35	*DES*	Desmin	CD, SkM
2q31	*TTN*	Titin	None
2q11–q22	?	?	CD
3p21	*SCN5A*	Cardiac sodium channel, type Vα	CD, AF
5q33	*SGCD*	Delta-sarcoglycan	None
6q22.1	*PLN*	Phospholamban	None
6q23	?	?	SkM
6q23–q24	*EYA4*	Eyes absent-4	SNHL
9q13–q22	?	?	None
10q21–q23	*VCL*	Vinculin/metavinculin	None
10q22.2	*ZASP (LDB3)*	Cypher/LIM domain binding 3	LVNC, SkM
11p11.2	*MYBPC3*	Cardiac myosin-binding protein C	None
11p15.1	*MLP*	Cardiac LIM domain protein	None
12p12.1	*ABCC9*	Sulfonylurea receptor-2	VT
14q11	*MYH7*	Beta-myosin heavy chain	None
14q12	*MYH6*	Alpha-myosin heavy chain	None
15q14	*ACTC*	Alpha-cardiac actin	None
15q22	*TPM1*	Alpha-tropomyosin	None
17q12	*TCAP*	Telethonin	SkM
19q13.4	*TNNI3*	Troponin I, Cardiac	CD
Xp21	*DYS*	Dystrophin	SkM
Xq28	*EMD*	Emerin	SkM
Xq28	*TAZ*	Tafazzin	SS, NP

Abbreviations: CD, conduction disease; SkM, skeletal myopathy; AF, atrial fibrillation; SNHL, sensorineural hearing loss; LVNC, left ventricular noncompaction; VT, ventricular tachycardia, SS, short stature; NP, neutropenia.

either to normal variability in the age of onset or to increased familial awareness that leads to pre-symptomatic screening of at-risk family members.

Genes with mutations resulting in autosomal dominant FDC can be divided into those encoding sarcomere proteins, cytoskeletal elements/intermediate filaments, components of the nuclear envelope, elements of the sarcoplasmic reticulum, ion channels, and transcription factors.

Sarcomere

As in HCM, mutations in genes encoding elements of the cardiac sarcomere may also cause DCM (12). Approximately 10% of cases of FDC appear to be caused by a mutation in one of these genes. In contrast to HCM, dramatic myocyte disarray is not typically present, and hypertrophy of the left ventricular wall does not precede dilatation. Typically, the histopathologic findings in this form of FDC are nonspecific, including myocyte hypertrophy, and fibrosis. Late conduction abnormalities, such as left bundle branch block or nonspecific intraventricular conduction delay, may occur as a consequence of ventricular dilatation, but typically patients with FDC due to a mutation in a component of the cardiac sarcomere do not display primary conduction block, skeletal myopathy, or other features. An exception to this is seen in patients with Laing distal myopathy, in which affected individuals have distal skeletal myopathy, neuropathy, and may have dilated cardiomyopathy, caused by mutations in *MYH7*, encoding cardiac beta myosin heavy chain (13,14).

To date, at least eight elements of the cardiac sarcomere have been described with mutations resulting in FDC. These include cardiac actin, α-tropomyosin, β-myosin heavy chain, troponin T, myosin-binding protein-C, titin, telethonin, and troponin I (12,15–20). Mutation in each of these has also been described causing HCM.

The mechanism whereby mutations in the same gene result in either DCM or HCM remains unknown. Animal models, such as the naturally occurring Syrian hamster with deletion of the delta-sarcoglycan gene, provide some insight (21). This model develops DCM or HCM depending on the background strain, suggesting that modifier genes determine the development of different phenotypes in a single spectrum of disease (22). Similarly, in mice harboring a heterozygous mutation in the predominant murine cardiac myosin heavy chain develop HCM, whereas mice homozygous for this mutation develop early onset DCM (23).

In contrast, humans with mutation in genes encoding elements of the cardiac sarcomere develop DCM or HCM with remarkable consistency. No family has been identified with a single mutation in a sarcomere gene resulting in DCM or HCM in different affected members sharing the identical mutation. Rare individuals with homozygous mutation in an element of the cardiac sarcomere have severe HCM, not DCM (24). Although these two forms of cardiomyopathy may represent different points on the same spectrum, it is perhaps more likely that specific mutations result in different functional consequences, and stimulate different neurohormonal cascades, resulting in ventricular wall thickening or dilation.

Genotype-phenotype correlations have identified specific residues in proteins such as cardiac beta myosin heavy chain that correspond to DCM in contrast to, at times, remarkably nearby residues in which mutations correspond to HCM. Pathophysiology by which mutations in sarcomere proteins lead to DCM includes both alteration in force production and impaired transmission of force by the cardiac sarcomere. Reviewing many of the known sarcomere genes with mutations resulting in FDC, one may speculate that mutations in interacting proteins or those with similar roles in the cardiac sarcomere might also result in FDC.

Cytoskeletal Elements/Intermediate Filaments

As a direct lesson learned from work in patients with dystrophin deficiency resulting in Duchenne muscular dystrophy (DMD), additional components of the dystrophin-glycoprotein complex and cytoskeleton have been implicated in FDC. Mutations in *SGCD*, encoding delta-sarcoglycan, result in DCM with or without limb-girdle skeletal myopathy (25,26). Similarly, alteration in desmin results in isolated FDC in some families, and FDC with skeletal myopathy in others (27,28). Again, choosing a candidate gene based on its function of force transmission in the sarcomere-cytoskeletal interface, Olson, and colleagues investigated 350 unrelated patients with DCM for mutations in the portion of *VCL* that is specific to cardiac metavinculin (exon 19) (29). They identified two individuals with mutations disrupting conserved functional domains, confirming the hypothesis that alterations in cytoskeletal elements which transmit contractile force may lead to FDC.

Nuclear Envelope

The first component of the nuclear envelope found to be involved with FDC was emerin, encoded by EMD (30). Emerin is localized to the inner nuclear membrane in many cell types, and appears to be involved in anchoring the cytoskeleton to the nuclear membrane. Mutations in emerin, which is on the X chromosome, typically result in Emery-Dreiffus muscular dystrophy (EDMD) (30). This disorder consists of weakness and atrophy of skeletal muscle, flexion contractures, and mental retardation (31). Cardiac manifestations typically involve atrioventricular conduction block and DCM (32). Female carriers of EDMD may develop cardiac conduction abnormalities or DCM (33).

In 1999, Fatkin, and colleagues first reported that mutations in *LMNA* can cause FDC (34). *LMNA* encodes the nuclear envelope proteins lamins A and C through alternate splicing of the same gene. Mutations in this gene result in a wide variety of different phenotypes collectively referred to as "laminopathies." This includes FDC, autosomal dominant EDMD, Hutchinson-Gilford progeria, Charcot-Marie-Tooth disease, familial partial lipodystrophy, limb-girdle muscular dystrophy type 1B, atypical Werner syndrome, and mandibuloacral dysplasia (34–41). To date, the mechanism whereby mutations in *LMNA* result in disease remains unknown, though clues exist. Analysis in *Lmna*-deficient murine cells demonstrated increased nuclear deformation, defective mechanotransduction, and impaired viability under mechanical strain (42). Additional analyses in lamin A/C-deficient mice revealed abnormalities in myocyte calcium transients, as well as disorganization of the desmin filaments and of the Z disc cross-striation pattern, which likely leads to the loss of myocyte contractile force transmission (43). This remains consistent with the data implicating similar loss of force mechanotransduction in the pathogenesis of other forms of FDC. However, the mechanism whereby profoundly different phenotypes, including those with segmental progeroid manifestations, result from mutations in lamin A/C remains unknown at this time.

Arrhythmia is an issue of particular relevance for probands and family members with *LMNA* mutations. Several reports highlight conduction block, tachyarrhythmias, and bradyarrhythmias cosegregating with mutations in this gene (44–46). A meta-analysis of 299 individuals with lamin A/C mutations reports that 25% died at a mean age of 46 years, predominantly from tachyarrhythmias (46). The age-dependent incidence of arrhythmia was greater than that of heart failure among all mutation carriers.

Sarcoplasmic Reticulum

Development of force within the cardiac myocyte relies on complex regulation of calcium cycling. Contraction is initiated by release of calcium from the sarcomplasmic reticulum (SR) into the cytosol, and relaxation is mediated by calcium reuptake into the SR through calcium ATPase, SERCA2a. Rare mutations in a negative regulator of the SERCA2a pump, phospholamban, have been described resulting in FDC (47,48). Curiously, ablation of the phospholamban gene in mice leads to increased SERCA2a function, and cross breeding experiments have shown that loss of phospholamban rescues the DCM phenotype in mice without muscle-specific LIM protein (49).

Ion Channels

Typically, arrhythmia is the cardiac phenotype associated with mutations that alter ion channel function. However, mutations in at least two ion channel genes are associated with FDC. First, a portion of the K_{ATP} channel subunit encoded by *ABCC9* was recognized as important for maintenance of cellular homeostasis under stress. Its encoded protein binds sulfonylureas, and it is called SUR2 for sulfonylurea receptor-2. Bienengraeber and colleagues screened 323 unrelated probands with idiopathic DCM for mutations in *ABCC9*, finding two with mutations in the C-terminal portion (50). Both individuals had severely dilated hearts and ventricular arrhythmias. Both mutations resulted in distortion of the ATP-dependent potassium pore regulation (50).

A second ion channel gene associated with FDC is *SCN5A*, encoding a voltage-gated sodium channel, type 5, alpha subunit. Mutations in this gene had previously been reported in association with Long QT syndrome, Type 3 (51). More recently, two groups reported mutations in this gene in association with DCM and cardiac arrhythmia (52,53). One of these groups also described a high incidence of atrial fibrillation among *SCN5A*-mutation carriers (53).

Transcription Factors

One of the most interesting genes recently identified opens the door to additional candidate genes in remaining loci where typical candidate genes have been excluded. In 2000, Schonberger, and colleagues described two families with cosegregation of sensorineural hearing loss and DCM, with linkage to a 2.8 cM genomic interval at 6q23–q24 (54). Subsequent fine mapping and exclusion of genes not expressed in heart or cochlea led to identification of three genes, none of which were recognized to be involved in development, regulation, or transmission of force within the heart. A truncated transcript from the *EYA4* gene was identified from one affected individual, and found to be caused by a genomic deletion (55). The protein product of this gene, eyes absent-4 or eya4, is one of four vertebrate orthologs of the drosophila eya protein which function as transcriptional activators. A cardiac role was not previously recognized.

Molecular Genetics: Other Forms of FDC

Autosomal recessive FDC also occurs, and is more commonly associated with inborn errors of metabolism, such as disorders of fatty acid oxidation which typically present in childhood (56). One report describes homozygous mutation in *TNNI3* in two siblings with DCM. The unaffected parents were suspected to have remote consanguinity by haplotype analysis (19). Limb Girdle Muscular Dystrophy Type 2I has also been associated with a recessive form of dilated cardiomyopathy caused by mutations in the gene encoding fukutin related protein *(FKRP)*. In one family, dilated cardiomyopathy was identified in three adult siblings prior to the onset of skeletal muscle weakness (57).

Several genetic disorders have so far been associated with X-linked forms of dilated cardiomyopathy. Barth syndrome consists of dilated cardiomyopathy, skeletal myopathy, short stature, and neutropenia (58). Elevated levels of urinary organic acids (3-methylglutaconate, 3-methylglutarate, and 2-ethylhydracrylate) occur and may be diagnostic for this condition (59). It is caused by mutations in the gene encoding taffazin, *TAZ*, which is also known as G4.5 (60). The X-linked form of Emery-Dreifuss muscular dystrophy is associated with dilated cardiomyopathy, skeletal myopathy, and cardiac conduction block (61). Mutations in the dystrophin gene, *DYS*, are responsible for Duchenne (DMD) and Becker (BMD) muscular dystrophies, and for X-linked dilated cardiomyopathy (XLDC) (62–65). Female carriers with any of these conditions may manifest DCM later in life as a consequence of skewed X-inactivation. Finally, McLeod syndrome is a rare X-linked systemic disorder which involves acanthocytosis, hemolytic anemia, dilated cardiomyopathy, neuropsychiatric disease, and mild skeletal myopathy (66). Mutations in the gene encoding the XK membrane transport protein result in this condition (67).

Matrilinear (mitochondrial) inheritance of FDC also occurs. Because the heart relies prominently on mitochondria for energy production, mutations in mitochondrial genes sometimes lead to dilated cardiomyopathy (68). Affected patients may present with isolated DCM, or associated skeletal myopathy, hearing loss, ocular disease, and/or neuropathy (69). Serologic studies may reveal elevations in lactate or pyruvate, or reduced carnitine.

FAMILIAL RESTRICTIVE CARDIOMYOPATHY

A few families have been described with heart failure segregating without ventricular dilatation or hypertrophy, classified as familial restrictive cardiomyopathy (FRC; Table 2). Genome-wide linkage analysis of one large family with FRC resulted in identification of mutations in *TNNI3*, encoding cardiac troponin I (70). Subsequent analysis of nine additional unrelated probands with restrictive cardiomyopathy revealed mutations in *TNNI3* in six of them (70). Mutations in *DES* encoding desmin have also been associated with FRC. Dalakas and colleagues reported their analysis of eight families with dominantly inherited skeletal and cardiac myopathy and two patients with sporadic disease (71). They identified mutations in *DES* in four of the eight families and both individuals with sporadic disease. Among the probands and family members with *DES* mutations, seven of twelve had cardiomyopathy, typically restrictive (71). Although these numbers are small, mutations in the troponin I and desmin genes appear to play a prominent role in FRC. Another group described a four-generation family segregating FRC without skeletal myopathy, and linked this phenotype to 10q23.3 after excluding the desmin and troponin I genes (72).

Despite familial involvement, consensus opinions support the use of endomyocardial biopsy in the evaluation of patients with this condition, as histopathologic findings may be diagnostic (9). For instance, mutations in *DES* encoding desmin, result in particular ultrastructural abnormalities, although these histopathologic findings are not specific to mutations in *DES* (71). Cardiac biopsies that identify amyloid deposits should prompt further staining to determine if transthyretin (TTR) is present. Amyloid cardiomyopathy may segregate in families with mutations in the gene encoding prealbumin, also known as transthyretin *(TTR)*.

Familial amyloid cardiomyopathy may be mistaken for senile systemic amyloidosis due to the late onset of this condition in some families. Often these patients will have systemic manifestations, including polyneuropathy, carpal tunnel syndrome, or pulmonary deposition of amyloid fibrils. Jacobson and colleagues described a variant *TTR* allele in which isoleucine is substituted for valine at position 122 (Val122Ile), present among 3.9% of African Americans, and disproportionately represented among African Americans with late-onset cardiac amyloid (73). For patients who are eligible, consideration should be

Table 2 Genes and Genomic Loci Associated with Familial Restrictive Cardiomyopathy

Locus	Gene	Protein	Additional features
2q35	*DES*	Desmin	CD, SkM
10q23.3	?	?	None
18q11.2	*TTR*	Transthyretin	Systemic amyloidosis
19q13.4	*TNNI3*	Troponin I	CD

Abbreviations: CD, conduction disease; SkM, skeletal myopathy.

given to dual organ transplant (heart and liver) as the liver is the site where the abnormal protein is synthesized.

RIGHT VENTRICULAR CARDIOMYOPATHY

Arrhythmogenic right ventricular dysplasia/cardiomyopathy (ARVD/C) is a curious form of familial cardiomyopathy characterized by fibrofatty replacement of ventricular myocytes and prominent ventricular arrhythmias (74). In contrast to more typical forms of FDC, this disorder preferentially affects the right ventricle, though may proceed to left ventricular involvement. A list of genes and genomic loci associated with this condition is in Table 3. Detailed criteria for diagnosis of ARVD/C have been proposed and are shown in Table 4 (75).

A variant of ARVD/C, known as Naxos syndrome, was first reported by Protonotarios in 1986 (76). It is an autosomal recessive disorder that includes palmoplantar keratoderma, wooly hair, and ARVD/C. Mutations in *JUP*, encoding junctional plakoglobin, result in this rare phenotype (77). To date, mutations in this gene have not been described in nonsyndromic ARVD/C. Another desmosomal protein, desmoplakin, was subsequently described with mutations resulting in dominantly inherited palmoplantar keratoderma and wooly hair, without evident ARVD/C (78). Patients with homozygous or compound heterozygous mutations in this gene manifest the same skin and hair disease, as well as left ventricular cardiomyopathy (Carvajal syndrome) (79). An isolated family dominantly segregating ARVD/C without evident skin or hair abnormalities, has since been described with a *DSP* mutation that disrupts binding of desmoplakin to plakoglobin (80). A recent report described the clinical features of thirty-eight subjects from four separate families segregating ARVD/C and *DSP* mutations (81).

Gerull and colleagues described widely prevalent mutations in *PKP2*, encoding plakophilin-2 among a large cohort of probands with ARVD/C (82). The incidence of *PKP2* mutations was 29% among 120 patients screened, and a separate report describes 43% of 58 probands with ARVD/C with *PKP2* mutations (82,83). The report by Gerull and colleagues also suggests that a prior report of linkage of ARVD/C to 2q32.1–q32.3 was incorrect (82,84). An affected member of one of these families linked to this locus was found to have a pathogenic mutation in *PKP2* on 12p11. Segregation of ARVD/C within

Table 3 Genes and Genomic Loci Associated with Arrhythmogenic Right Ventricular Dysplasia/Cardiomyopathy

Designation	Locus	Gene	Protein
ARVD1	14q23–q24	*TGFB3*	Transforming growth factor-beta-3
ARVD2	1q42–q43	*RYR2*	Cardiac ryanodine receptor
ARVD3	14q12–q22	?	?
ARVD4	2q32.1–q32.3	?	?
ARVD5	3p23	?	?
ARVD6	10p14–p12	?	?
ARVD7	10q22.3	?	?
ARVD8	6p24	*DSP*	Desmoplakin
Naxos disease	17q21	*JUP*	Plakoglobin
ARVD9	12p11	*PKP2*	Plakophilin-2

Table 4 Diagnostic Criteria for Arrhythmogenic Right Ventricular Dysplasia/Cardiomyopathy

		Major criteria	Minor criteria
I	Structural or functional RV abnormality	Severe RV dilation and reduction of RV EF with little or no LV involvement Localized RV aneurysm, or Severe segmental dilation of the RV	Mild global RV dilation and/or EF reduction with normal LV Mild segmental dilation of the RV, or Regional RV hypokinesia
II	Tissue characterization	Infiltration of RV myocardium by fibro-fatty replacement tissue	(None)
III	ECG depolarization/ conduction abnormality	Epsilon waves or localized prolongation (> 110 ms) of the QRS complex in right precordial leads (V1–V3)	Late potentials on signal-averaged ECG
IV	ECG repolarization abnormality	(None)	Inverted T waves in ECG leads V1–V3, aged > 12 years, without RBBB
V	Arrhythmias	(None)	LBBB-type VT (sustained or nonsustained), or Frequent PVCs (> 1000/24 hours)
VI	Family history	Family history of ARVD/C confirmed on autopsy or surgery	Family history of ARVD/C clinically and independently diagnosed Familial history of premature sudden death (< 35 years) due to suspected ARVD/C

These criteria are fulfilled in the setting of two major criteria, one major and two minor criteria, or four minor criteria. The criteria must come from different groups.
Abbreviations: EF, ejection fraction; RBBB, right bundle branch block; LBBB, left bundle branch block; VT, ventricular tachycardia; PVC, premature ventricular contraction.

this family was consistent with segregation of the *PKP2* mutation, excluding 2q32.1–q32.3 as the locus for ARVD/C for this family.

Plakophilin-2 is the third component of the cardiac desmosome implicated in this disorder, suggesting that it is a disease of the cardiac desmosome. However, the mechanism whereby mutations in components of the desmosome result in right ventricular cardiomyopathy with fibrofatty infiltration remains unknown. Some have suggested that an impaired cardiac desmosome results in deficient contact between myocytes, and that stress, such as that imparted by athletic activity, worsens this adherence (82). Fibrofatty degeneration of myocytes results first in areas of highest physiologic stress, and consequently ventricular arrhythmia follows this pattern of scarring.

An atypical form of ARVD/C without significant right ventricular dilation or mechanical dysfunction is associated with mutations in *RYR2*, encoding the cardiac ryanodine receptor (85). Mutations in this gene cause catecholaminergic polymorphic ventricular tachycardia (CPVT) (86), and most consider this to be a different disease than ARVD/C. Finally, a recent report describes sequence variants in the 5′ and 3′ untranslated regions of the gene encoding transforming growth factor-beta-3 (*TGFB3*) in association with ARVD/C (87). Transient transfections with luciferase reporter constructs harboring these alterations suggest increased *TGFB3* mRNA abundance, implicating this cytokine in the pathogenesis of ARVD/C.

CLINICAL IMPLICATIONS

There are several important clinical points to emphasize from this chapter. First, many patients initially labeled as "idiopathic DCM" will be found to have a familial form of disease if proper screening within their family can be arranged. Second, recognition of the pattern of inheritance of familial cardiomyopathy can lead to appropriate pre-symptomatic screening of those at risk. Third, some genetic forms of cardiomyopathy have a particularly high incidence of fatal or life-threatening ventricular arrhythmias, supporting early and aggressive monitoring for this manifestation among those who have inherited this genetic predisposition.

Clinical genetic testing is currently available for several forms of familial dilated, restrictive, and right ventricular cardiomyopathy. Due to the genetic heterogeneity of FDC, the chance that a pathogenic mutation will be identified for a particular patient is much lower than for HCM. However, pursuing a specific genetic etiology may have important clinical implications for the patient and their family members. Identification of specific genetic mutations, such as mutations in *LMNA* or *PKP2* may provide an additional piece of information when evaluating the patient's risk for sudden cardiac death and discussion of preventative interventions.

Identification of a familial cardiomyopathy should also prompt a discussion with the patient about the importance of communicating cardiac screening recommendations to at-risk family members. At-risk family members should undergo cardiac evaluation that includes an echocardiogram and an electrocardiogram every three to five years. At-risk family members should only be offered pre-symptomatic genetic testing once a pathogenic mutation has been identified in an affected family member. If at-risk family members are found not to have the primary pathogenic mutation that has previously been found in the family, then their risk to develop cardiomyopathy is greatly reduced.

It is important to note that due to incomplete penetrance, variable expressivity, and age-dependence of the phenotypes, the presence of a predisposing mutation does not indicate absolutely that an individual will develop cardiomyopathy. However, an individual with a genetic predisposition to develop cardiomyopathy who never shows evidence of the disease, can still pass this predisposition down to their offspring, who may in turn go on to develop cardiomyopathy. Similarly, despite thorough analysis for a mutation in all genes known to be associated with a familial cardiomyopathy, the absence of a discernible mutation does not exclude that there is a genetic or familial component to the patient's cardiomyopathy. Therefore, genetic testing should not yet be undertaken to "rule out" that there is a genetic component to an individual's cardiomyopathy. The reduced penetrance and variable expressivity associated with familial cardiomyopathy is most likely due to yet unidentified environmental and genetic modifiers. Given the complexity of multiple patterns of inheritance, multiple associated genes, reduced penetrance, variable expressivity, results of uncertain clinical significance, unexpected results, and issues related to genetic discrimination, genetic counseling, provided by a genetic counselor or a physician knowledgeable in genetics, is recommended prior to diagnostic, pre-symptomatic, or research genetic testing.

As in any genetic disorder, some families will choose not to pursue genetic testing. Other families may pursue a genetic diagnosis with current technology but not identify a mutation. In such cases, clinical DNA banking may allow future generations to pursue a molecular genetic diagnosis with the aid of DNA obtained from a clearly affected individual.

With continued investigation into the molecular genetics of FDC and other familial forms of cardiomyopathy, improvements in the diagnosis of these conditions are inevitable. However, recognition of the responsible genetic mutations is just the beginning of efforts to understand the causes of these conditions, and to develop rational therapies based on molecular dissection of disease pathogenesis.

REFERENCES

1. Codd MB, Sugrue DD, Gersh BJ, Melton LJ, III. Epidemiology of idiopathic dilated and hypertrophic cardiomyopathy. a population-based study in Olmsted County, Minnesota, 1975–1984. Circulation 1989; 80:564–572.
2. Felker GM, Thompson RE, Hare JM, et al. Underlying causes and long-term survival in patients with initially unexplained cardiomyopathy. N Engl J Med 2000; 342:1077–1084.
3. Felker GM, Hu W, Hare JM, Hruban RH, Baughman KL, Kasper EK. The spectrum of dilated cardiomyopathy. The Johns Hopkins experience with 1278 patients. Medicine (Baltimore) 1999; 78:270–283.
4. Mestroni L, Maisch B, McKenna WJ, et al. Guidelines for the study of familial dilated cardiomyopathies. Collaborative research group of the european human and capital mobility project on familial dilated cardiomyopathy. Eur Heart J 1999; 20:93–102.
5. Michels VV, Moll PP, Miller FA, et al. The frequency of familial dilated cardiomyopathy in a series of patients with idiopathic dilated cardiomyopathy. N Engl J Med 1992; 326:77–82.
6. Goerss JB, Michels VV, Burnett J, et al. Frequency of familial dilated cardiomyopathy. Eur Heart J 1995; 16:2–4.
7. McKenna CJ, Codd MB, McCann HA, Sugrue DD. Idiopathic dilated cardiomyopathy: familial prevalence and HLA distribution. Heart 1997; 77:549–552.
8. Baig MK, Goldman JH, Caforio AL, Coonar AS, Keeling PJ, McKenna WJ. Familial dilated cardiomyopathy: cardiac abnormalities are common in asymptomatic relatives and may represent early disease. J Am Coll Cardiol 1998; 31:195–201.
9. Hunt SA, Baker DW, Chin MH, et al. ACC/AHA guidelines for the evaluation and management of chronic heart failure in the adult: executive summary. Circulation 2001; 104:2996–3007.
10. Dec GW, Fuster V. Idiopathic dilated cardiomyopathy. N Engl J Med 1994; 331:1564–1575.
11. Mestroni L, Rocco C, Gregori D, et al. Familial dilated cardiomyopathy: evidence for genetic and phenotypic heterogeneity. Heart muscle disease study group. J Am Coll Cardiol 1999; 34:181–190.
12. Kamisago M, Sharma SD, DePalma SR, et al. Mutations in sarcomere protein genes as a cause of dilated cardiomyopathy. N Engl J Med 2000; 343:1688–1696.
13. Meredith C, Herrmann R, Parry C, et al. Mutations in the slow skeletal muscle fiber myosin heavy chain gene (MYH7) cause laing early-onset distal myopathy (MPD1). Am J Hum Genet 2004; 75:703–708.
14. Hedera P, Petty EM, Bui MR, Blaivas M, Fink JK. The second kindred with autosomal dominant distal myopathy linked to chromosome 14q: genetic and clinical analysis. Arch Neurol 2003; 60:1321–1325.
15. Olson TM, Michels VV, Thibodeau SN, Tai YS, Keating MT. Actin mutations in dilated cardiomyopathy, a heritable form of heart failure. Science 1998; 280:750–752.
16. Olson TM, Kishimoto NY, Whitby FG, Michels VV. Mutations that alter the surface charge of alpha-tropomyosin are associated with dilated cardiomyopathy. J Mol Cell Cardiol 2001; 33:723–732.
17. Gerull B, Gramlich M, Atherton J, et al. Mutations of TTN, encoding the giant muscle filament titin, cause familial dilated cardiomyopathy. Nat Genet 2002; 30:201–204.

18. Daehmlow S, Erdmann J, Knueppel T, et al. Novel mutations in sarcomeric protein genes in dilated cardiomyopathy. Biochem Biophys Res Commun 2002; 298:116–120.
19. Murphy RT, Mogensen J, Shaw A, Kubo T, Hughes S, McKenna WJ. Novel mutation in cardiac troponin I in recessive idiopathic dilated cardiomyopathy. Lancet 2004; 363:371–372.
20. Hayashi T, Arimura T, Itoh-Satoh M, et al. Tcap gene mutations in hypertrophic cardiomyopathy and dilated cardiomyopathy. J Am College Cardiol 2004; 44:2192–2201.
21. Nigro V, Okazaki Y, Belsito A, et al. Identification of the Syrian hamster cardiomyopathy gene. Hum Mol Genet 1997; 6:601–607.
22. Coral-Vazquez R, Cohn RD, Moore SA, et al. Disruption of the sarcoglycan-sarcospan complex in vascular smooth muscle: a novel mechanism for cardiomyopathy and muscular dystrophy. Cell 1999; 98:465–474.
23. Fatkin D, Christe ME, Aristizabal O, et al. Neonatal cardiomyopathy in mice homozygous for the Arg403Gln mutation in the alpha cardiac myosin heavy chain gene. J Clin Invest 1999; 103:147–153.
24. Ho CY, Lever HM, DeSanctis R, Farver CF, Seidman JG, Seidman CE. Homozygous mutation in cardiac troponin T: implications for hypertrophic cardiomyopathy. Circulation 2000; 102:1950–1955.
25. Duggan DJ, Manchester D, Stears KP, Mathews DJ, Hart C, Hoffman EP. Mutations in the delta-sarcoglycan gene are a rare cause of autosomal recessive limb-girdle muscular dystrophy (LGMD2). Neurogenetics 1997; 1:49–58.
26. Tsubata S, Bowles KR, Vatta M, et al. Mutations in the human {delta}-sarcoglycan gene in familial and sporadic dilated cardiomyopathy. J Clin Invest 2000; 106:655–662.
27. Li D, Tapscoft T, Gonzalez O, et al. Desmin mutation responsible for idiopathic dilated cardiomyopathy. Circulation 1999; 100:461–464.
28. Goldfarb LG, Park KY, Cervenakova L, et al. Missense mutations in desmin associated with familial cardiac and skeletal myopathy. Nat Genet 1998; 19:402–403.
29. Olson TM, Illenberger S, Kishimoto NY, Huttelmaier S, Keating MT, Jockusch BM. Metavinculin mutations alter actin interaction in dilated cardiomyopathy. Circulation 2002; 105:431–437.
30. Bione S, Maestrini E, Rivella S, et al. Identification of a novel X-linked gene responsible for Emery-Dreifuss muscular dystrophy. Nat Genet 1994; 8:323–327.
31. Emery AE, Dreifuss FE. Unusual type of benign x-linked muscular dystrophy. J Neurol Neurosurg Psychiatry 1966; 29:338–342.
32. Buckley AE, Dean J, Mahy IR. Cardiac involvement in Emery Dreifuss muscular dystrophy: a case series. Heart 1999; 82:105–108.
33. Fishbein MC, Siegel RJ, Thompson CE, Hopkins LC. Sudden death of a carrier of X-Linked Emery-Dreifuss muscular dystrophy. Ann Intern Med 1993; 119:900–905.
34. Fatkin D, MacRae C, Sasaki T, et al. Missense mutations in the rod domain of the lamin A/C gene as causes of dilated cardiomyopathy and conduction-system disease. N Engl J Med 1999; 341:1715–1724.
35. Bonne G, Di Barletta MR, Varnous S, et al. Mutations in the gene encoding lamin A/C cause autosomal dominant Emery-Dreifuss muscular dystrophy. Nat Genet 1999; 21:285–288.
36. Eriksson M, Brown WT, Gordon LB, et al. Recurrent de novo point mutations in lamin A cause Hutchinson-Gilford progeria syndrome. Nature 2003; 423:293–298.
37. Cao H, Hegele RA. Nuclear lamin A/C R482Q mutation in canadian kindreds with Dunnigan-type familial partial lipodystrophy. Hum Mol Genet 2000; 9:109–112.
38. De Sandre-Giovannoli A, Chaouch M, Kozlov S, et al. Homozygous defects in LMNA, encoding lamin A/C nuclear-envelope proteins, cause autosomal recessive axonal neuropathy in human (Charcot-Marie-Tooth disorder type 2) and mouse. Am J Hum Genet 2002; 70:726–736.
39. Muchir A, Bonne G, van der Kooi AJ, et al. Identification of mutations in the gene encoding lamins A/C in autosomal dominant limb girdle muscular dystrophy with atrioventricular conduction disturbances (LGMD1B). Hum Mol Genet 2000; 9:1453–1459.

40. Chen L, Lee L, Kudlow BA, et al. LMNA mutations in atypical Werner's syndrome. Lancet 2003; 362:440–445.
41. Novelli G, Muchir A, Sangiuolo F, et al. Mandibuloacral dysplasia is caused by a mutation in LMNA-encoding lamin A/C. Am J Hum Genet 2002; 71:426–431.
42. Lammerding J, Schulze PC, Takahashi T, et al. Lamin A/C deficiency causes defective nuclear mechanics and mechanotransduction. J Clin Invest 2004; 113:370–378.
43. Nikolova V, Leimena C, McMahon AC, et al. Defects in nuclear structure and function promote dilated cardiomyopathy in lamin A/C-deficient mice. J Clin Invest 2004; 113:357–369.
44. Becane HM, Bonne G, Varnous S, et al. High incidence of sudden death with conduction system and myocardial disease due to lamins A and C gene mutation. Pacing Clin Electrophysiol 2000; 23:1661–1666.
45. Taylor MRG, Fain PR, Sinagra G, et al. Natural history of dilated cardiomyopathy due to lamin A/C gene mutations. J Am Coll Cardiol 2003; 41:771–780.
46. van Berlo JH, de Voogt WG, van der Kooi AJ, et al. Meta-analysis of clinical characteristics of 299 carriers of LMNA gene mutations: do lamin A/C mutations portend a high risk of sudden death? J Mol Med 2005; 83:79–83.
47. Schmitt JP, Kamisago M, Asahi M, et al. Dilated cardiomyopathy and heart failure caused by a mutation in phospholamban. Science 2003; 299:1410–1413.
48. Haghighi K, Kolokathis F, Pater L, et al. Human phospholamban null results in lethal dilated cardiomyopathy revealing a critical difference between mouse and human. J Clin Invest 2003; 111:869–876.
49. Minamisawa S, Hoshijima M, Chu G, et al. Chronic phospholamban-sarcoplasmic reticulum calcium ATPase interaction is the critical calcium cycling defect in dilated cardiomyopathy. Cell 1999; 99:313–322.
50. Bienengraeber M, Olson TM, Selivanov VA, et al. ABCC9 mutations identified in human dilated cardiomyopathy disrupt catalytic KATP channel gating. Nat Genet 2004; 36:382–387.
51. Wang Q, Shen J, Splawski I, et al. SCN5A mutations associated with an inherited cardiac arrhythmia, long QT syndrome. Cell 1995; 80:805–811.
52. McNair WP, Ku L, Taylor MRG, et al. SCN5A mutation associated with dilated cardiomyopathy, conduction disorder, and arrhythmia. Circulation 2004; 110:2163–2167.
53. Olson TM, Michels VV, Ballew JD, et al. Sodium channel mutations and susceptibility to heart failure and atrial fibrillation. JAMA 2005; 293:447–454.
54. Schonberger J, Levy H, Grunig E, et al. Dilated cardiomyopathy and sensorineural hearing loss: a heritable syndrome that maps to 6q23–24. Circulation 2000; 101:1812–1818.
55. Schonberger J, Wang L, Shin JT, et al. Mutation in the transcriptional coactivator EYA4 causes dilated cardiomyopathy and sensorineural hearing loss. Nat Genet 2005; 37:418–422.
56. Kelly DP, Strauss AW. Inherited Cardiomyopathies. N Engl J Med 1994; 330:913–919.
57. Muller T, Krasnianski M, Witthaut R, Deschauer M, Zierz S. Dilated cardiomyopathy may be an early sign of the C826A Fukutin-related protein mutation. Neuromuscul Disord 2005; 15:372–376.
58. Barth PG, Scholte HR, Berden JA, et al. An X-linked mitochondrial disease affecting cardiac muscle, skeletal muscle and neutrophil leucocytes. J Neurol Sci 1983; 62:327–355.
59. Kelley RI, Cheatham JP, Clark BJ, et al. X-linked dilated cardiomyopathy with neutropenia, growth retardation, and 3-methylglutaconic aciduria. J Pediatr 1991; 119:738–747.
60. Bione S, D'Adamo P, Maestrini E, Gedeon AK, Bolhuis PA, Toniolo D. A novel X-linked gene G4.5 is responsible for Barth syndrome, Nat Genet 1996; 12:385–389.
61. Watters DD, Nutter DO, Hopkins LC, Dorney ER. Cardiac features of an unusual X-linked humeroperoneal neuromuscular disease. N Engl J Med 1975; 293:1017–1022.
62. Koenig M, Hoffman EP, Bertelson CJ, Monaco AP, Feener C, Kunkel LM. Complete cloning of the Duchenne muscular dystrophy (DMD) cDNA and preliminary genomic organization of the DMD gene in normal and affected individuals. Cell 1987; 50:509–517.

63. Matsumura K, Burghes AH, Mora M, et al. Immunohistochemical analysis of dystrophin-associated proteins in Becker/Duchenne muscular dystrophy with huge in-frame deletions in the NH2-terminal and rod domains of dystrophin. J Clin Invest 1994; 93:99–105.
64. Muntoni F, Cau M, Ganau A, et al. Deletion of the Dystrophin muscle-promoter region associated with X-linked dilated cardiomyopathy. N Engl J Med 1993; 329:921–925.
65. Towbin JA, Hejtmancik JF, Brink P, et al. X-linked dilated cardiomyopathy. Molecular genetic evidence of linkage to the Duchenne muscular dystrophy (dystrophin) gene at the Xp21 locus. Circulation 1993; 87:1854–1865.
66. Malandrini A, Fabrizi GM, Truschi F, et al. Atypical McLeod syndrome manifested as X-linked chorea-acanthocytosis, neuromyopathy and dilated cardiomyopathy: report of a family. J Neurol Sci 1994; 124:89–94.
67. Ho M, Chelly J, Carter N, Danek A, Crocker P, Monaco AP. Isolation of the gene for McLeod syndrome that encodes a novel membrane transport protein. Cell 1994; 77:869–880.
68. Wallace DC. Mitochondrial defects in cardiomyopathy and neuromuscular disease. Am Heart J 2000; 139:S70–S85.
69. Wallace DC. Mitochondrial diseases in man and mouse. Science 1999; 283:1482–1488.
70. Mogensen J, Kubo T, Duque M, et al. Idiopathic restrictive cardiomyopathy is part of the clinical expression of cardiac troponin I mutations. J Clin Invest 2003; 111:209–216.
71. Dalakas MC, Park K-Y, Semino-Mora C, Lee HS, Sivakumar K, Goldfarb LG. Desmin myopathy, a skeletal myopathy with cardiomyopathy caused by mutations in the Desmin gene. N Engl J Med 2000; 342:770–780.
72. Zhang J, Kumar A, Kaplan L, Fricker FJ, Wallace MR. Genetic linkage of a novel autosomal dominant restrictive cardiomyopathy locus. J Med Genet 2005; 42:663–665.
73. Jacobson DR, Pastore RD, Yaghoubian R, et al. Variant-sequence transthyretin (isoleucine 122) in late-onset cardiac amyloidosis in Black Americans. N Engl J Med 1997; 336:466–473.
74. Marcus FI, Fontaine GH, Guiraudon G, et al. Right ventricular dysplasia: a report of 24 adult cases. Circulation 1982; 65:384–398.
75. McKenna WJ, Thiene G, Nava A, et al. Diagnosis of arrhythmogenic right ventricular dysplasia/cardiomyopathy. Task force of the working group Myocardial and pericardial disease of the European society of cardiology and of the scientific council on cardiomyopathies of the international society and federation of cardiology. Br Heart J 1994; 71:215–218.
76. Protonotarios N, Tsatsopoulou A, Patsourakos P, et al. Cardiac abnormalities in familial palmoplantar keratosis. Br Heart J 1986; 56:321–326.
77. McKoy G, Protonotarios N, Crosby A, et al. Identification of a deletion in plakoglobin in arrhythmogenic right ventricular cardiomyopathy with palmoplantar keratoderma and woolly hair (Naxos disease). Lancet 2000; 355:2119–2124.
78. Armstrong D, McKenna K, Purkis P, et al. Haploinsufficiency of desmoplakin causes a striate subtype of palmoplantar keratoderma. Hum Mol Genet 1999; 8:143–148 [published erratum appears in Hum Mol Genet May;8(5):943].
79. Norgett EE, Hatsell SJ, Carvajal-Huerta L, et al. Recessive mutation in desmoplakin disrupts desmoplakin-intermediate filament interactions and causes dilated cardiomyopathy, woolly hair and keratoderma. Hum Mol Genet 2000; 9:2761–2766.
80. Rampazzo A, Nava A, Malacrida S, et al. Mutation in human desmoplakin domain binding to plakoglobin causes a dominant form of arrhythmogenic right ventricular cardiomyopathy. Am J Hum Genet 2002; 71:1200–1206.
81. Bauce B, Basso C, Rampazzo A, et al. Clinical profile of four families with arrhythmogenic right ventricular cardiomyopathy caused by dominant desmoplakin mutations. Eur Heart J 2005; 26:1666–1675.
82. Gerull B, Heuser A, Wichter T, et al. Mutations in the desmosomal protein plakophilin-2 are common in arrhythmogenic right ventricular cardiomyopathy. Nat Genet 2004; 36:1162–1164.
83. Dalal D, Molin LH, Piccini JP, et al. Clinical features of arrhythmogenic right ventricular dysplasia/cardiomyopathy associated with mutations in plakophilin-2. Circulation 2006, in press.

84. Rampazzo A, Nava A, Miorin M, et al. ARVD4, a new locus for arrhythmogenic right ventricular cardiomyopathy, maps to chromosome 2 long arm. Genomics 1997; 45:259–263.
85. Tiso N, Stephan DA, Nava A, et al. Identification of mutations in the cardiac ryanodine receptor gene in families affected with arrhythmogenic right ventricular cardiomyopathy type 2 (ARVD2). Hum Mol Genet 2001; 10:189–194.
86. Priori SG, Napolitano C, Tiso N, et al. Mutations in the cardiac Ryanodine receptor gene (hRyR2) underlie Catecholaminergic Polymorphic Ventricular Tachycardia. Circulation 2001; 103:196–200.
87. Beffagna G, Occhi G, Nava A, et al. Regulatory mutations in transforming growth factor-[beta]3 gene cause arrhythmogenic right ventricular cardiomyopathy type 1. Cardiovas Res 2005; 65:366–373.

34
New Drugs for Heart Failure: Emerging Role of Oxidative Stress as a Target

Tania Chao and Wilson S. Colucci
Cardiovascular Section, Department of Medicine, Boston University Medical Center, Boston University School of Medicine, Boston, Massachusetts, U.S.A.

NEW THERAPEUTIC TARGETS IN HEART FAILURE

Heart failure is most often caused by a decrease in the mass and/or function of the myocardium, leading to impaired ability of the heart to function as a pump. This primary defect is often associated with and compounded by a variety of systemic alterations including the activation of neurohormonal pathways and vascular dysfunction, both of which further antagonize overall cardiovascular homeostasis. It is not surprising that the treatment of heart failure for many years focused on improving hemodynamic function through the development and use of agents that increase myocardial contractility and/or reduce vascular tone. However, despite the clinical testing of numerous potent positive inotropic and direct vasodilator agents, with rare exceptions these agents have not led to improved clinical outcomes. In contrast, the most successful agents have been those that inhibit neurohormonal pathways (e.g., beta-blockers and angiotensin system inhibitors). The clinical success of these agents can not be attributed to their direct hemodynamic actions, which in some cases are adverse (e.g., beta-blockers). Rather, the shared mode of action of neurohormonal antagonists appears to be the slowing of myocardial remodeling and disease progression.

MYOCYTE DEATH AND DYSFUNCTION IN HEART FAILURE

A common feature of both acute and chronic heart failure is a decrease in the number and/or function of cardiac myocytes. The loss of cardiac myocytes is best illustrated by myocardial infarction. However, it is now evident that cardiac myocytes may also be lost on a chronic basis via the process of apoptosis. Apoptotic myocyte death has been characterized in the chronic setting, but more recent studies suggest that accelerated myocyte loss may also contribute to the long-term outcome of patients being treated for acute decompensation. As a result, there is a rationale effort to discover and develop therapies that reduce myocyte loss. Myocardial dysfunction may also occur as a result of a decrease in the function of viable cardiac myocytes. Such alterations may be the result of alterations in proteins important in excitation-contraction coupling, and may involve changes in (1) the level of protein due to changes in gene expression or (2) protein function due to post-translational modifications.

OXIDATIVE STRESS IN HEART FAILURE

There is increasing evidence that oxidative stress is increased in heart failure and contributes to the pathophysiology of myocardial dysfunction. The discovery of effective clinical therapies has been paralleled by (1) the recognition that oxidative stress plays a fundamental role in regulating the growth, death and function of the cardiac myocyte, and (2) the further demonstration that most, if not all, of the stimuli implicated in the development of myocardial failure (e.g., mechanical strain, neurohormones, inflammatory cytokines) lead to increased oxidative stress in the cardiac myocyte. Oxidative stress may cause the death of cardiac myocytes by apoptosis, alter gene expression, and modify protein function via post-translational modifications.

This chapter focuses on two new pharmacologic approaches to the treatment of heart failure: the inhibition of xanthine oxidase and the activation of ATP-dependent potassium channels (K_{ATP}). While these therapies act by distinct pharmacologic mechanisms, both therapies mitigate the effects of oxidative stress.

REGULATION OF REACTIVE SPECIES IN THE MYOCARDIUM

Oxidative stress refers to any imbalance between the production of reactive oxygen species (ROS) and their removal by antioxidant defense mechanisms. Oxygen exists as a diradical, sharing two electrons in its outermost shell. Due to its structure, oxygen is able to accept up to four electrons in the process of reduction, to form water. However, should oxygen undergo a series of univalent reductions, partially reduced oxygen species, or free radicals are produced. The reduced forms of molecular oxygen include superoxide radical ($o_2^{\cdot -}$) formed when oxygen accepts one electron. Addition of a second electron results in hydrogen peroxide (H_2O_2). Addition of a third electron produces the hydroxyl radical ($^{\cdot}OH^{-}$) and a fourth electron produces water. The three intermediaries are extremely reactive and unstable. ROS have beneficial roles in the body (e.g., contributing to the oxidative burst in phagocytes in the protective immune response). On the other hand, when present in excessive levels ROS can react directly with lipids, proteins, and nucleic acids causing damage, impaired function and cell death. In addition, it is now appreciated that somewhat lower levels of ROS can activate signaling pathways that are involved in regulating numerous cellular functions including growth, gene expression, apoptosis, and protein function (1).

There are several sources of ROS in the heart and other tissues. Among these are the mitochondrial electron transport chain and several enzymes including xanthine oxidase, cyclooxygenases, lipoxygenase, nitric oxide synthases, peroxidases, and NADH oxidases. The ROS produced during normal metabolism are counterbalanced by antioxidants and naturally occurring free radical scavengers in the body. Non-enzymatic antioxidants include vitamins E, C, and beta-carotene. Among the best characterized cellular enzymes are superoxide dismutase, glutathione peroxidase, and catalase. Superoxide dismutases facilitate the formation of hydrogen peroxide (H_2O_2) from superoxide; catalase and glutathione peroxidase catalyze H_2O_2 to form water. Interestingly, these enzymes have been highly conserved during the process of evolution among aerobic organisms, emphasizing their crucial function in preventing oxidative stress.

OXIDATIVE STRESS IN MYOCARDIAL FAILURE

Heart failure is associated with elevated levels of oxidative stress which may be due to increased production of ROS, impaired free radical scavenging capability, or a combination of the two. There is increasing evidence that both mechanisms may play a role in the pathophysiology of the failing heart. Several animal models of heart failure, including models of pressure overload, surgical myocardial infarction, and pacing-induced heart failure demonstrate elevated levels of oxidative stress (1). Increased oxidative stress has also been observed in the transition from compensated hypertrophy to overt failure, and has been associated with decreased levels of antioxidant enzymes (1). Studies in humans likewise suggest that increased oxidative stress is present in patients with heart failure. Malondialdehyde and isoprostanes, both markers of lipid peroxidation, are significantly elevated in the plasma and pericardial fluid of heart failure patients (2). Oxidative stress correlates with severity of left ventricular dilation, and functional class and is elevated regardless of etiology, whether the cardiomyopathy is ischemic, valvular, or idiopathic in etiology.

Oxidative stress may act on the cardiac myocyte in several ways. At very high levels typical of ischemic reperfusion, there may be frank cellular necrosis due to direct damage to cellular components. However, at the levels typical of heart failure, the effects of oxidative stress are more subtle. Myocyte death at lower levels of ROS may be due to the activation of apoptotic pathways. In addition, myocyte dysfunction may occur due to alterations in the expression and/or function of proteins involved in excitation-contraction coupling.

MYOCYTE LOSS AND DYSFUNCTION IN HEART FAILURE

The two principal mechanisms by which myocytes in the heart may be lost are necrosis and apoptosis (3). Necrosis is an episodic process by which myocytes undergo loss of membrane integrity and total disruption of cellular function, followed by cell death, inflammation, and fibrosis. Clinically, the most common cause of necrosis is ischemia, resulting in myocardial infarction. A second, more recently recognized mechanism of cell death is apoptosis, which typically involves smaller numbers of cells, occurs over a more prolonged time course and may be present chronically, resulting in a substantial cumulative loss of cells. In contrast to necrosis, apoptosis is an energy-dependent process that is carried out by a highly organized biochemical cascade. Ischemia is also an important cause of apoptosis, and it is now recognized that apoptosis contributes significantly to myocyte loss in the setting of myocardial infarction. Importantly, additional apoptotic stimuli are now recognized, including oxidative stress, mechanical strain, and several neurohormones (e.g., norepinephrine and angiotensin).

While most attention has been paid to the loss of myocytes, it is now becoming clear that viable myocytes may be dysfunctional for a variety of reasons. Among these are transcriptional alterations in gene expression leading to changes in the amounts and/or isoforms of proteins that are involved in normal myocyte function (e.g., signaling proteins, contractile proteins). In addition, post-translational modifications of proteins can have an important effect on function. While much attention has focused on the phosphorylation of proteins, it now appears that oxidative modifications can have an important effect on protein function. Such oxidative modifications may be reversible and mediated by low levels of ROS, and under such conditions ROS may be viewed as signaling molecules.

The discovery that oxidative stress can act directly on the cardiac myocyte to cause apoptosis and contractile dysfunction has provided an important insight as to the success of neurohormonal antagonists in slowing disease progression in patients with chronic heart failure, and has stimulated a search for new ways to interfere with the production and/or actions of reactive oxygen species in the heart.

OXYPURINOL: AN ANTIOXIDANT FOR THE THERAPY FOR CHRONIC HEART FAILURE

Oxypurinol is the active metabolite of allopurinol, a xanthine oxidase inhibitor that is widely used for the treatment of gout. Xanthine oxidoreductase is an enzyme that degrades purines, metabolizing hypoxanthine to xanthine and subsequently to uric acid. It exists as two interconvertible forms: xanthine oxidase and xanthine dehydrogenase. Xanthine oxidase reduces oxygen to form superoxide and hydrogen peroxide, while xanthine dehydrogenase can reduce oxygen or NAD (and produce superoxide, hydrogen peroxide, and NADH). Several studies now suggest that xanthine oxidase is an important source of ROS in the cardiovascular system, and may serve as an important therapeutic target in the treatment of heart failure. Xanthine oxidase and its parent enzyme, xanthine dehydrogenase, are more abundant in failing explanted hearts than in controls (4).

Reactive oxygen species generated by xanthine oxidase may impair myocardial function in heart failure. In a rat heart failure model, perfusion with oxypurinol enhanced myocardial contractility in rats with or without myocardial failure. However, the fractional increase in contractility in the heart failure group was significantly higher (5). Myocardium from the heart failure group had a higher xanthine oxidase activity, leading to the suggestion that the magnitude of improved contractility was related to the level of xanthine oxidase activity (5). In mice treated with allopurinol after myocardial infarction, the xanthine oxidase activity was suppressed to levels comparable to that in sham-operated mice. Importantly, survival in the allopurinol-treated group was markedly improved, as was cardiac contractile function (6).

Intravenous allopurinol decreased myocardial oxygen consumption and increased myocardial efficiency in dogs with pacing-induced heart failure. As in the rat model, the increase in contractility was greater in the heart failure group (7). The antioxidant ascorbic acid had a similar effect, and allopurinol caused no further increase when infused after ascorbic acid, suggesting a similar mechanism of action. Inhibition of nitric oxide synthase abolished the effects of both allopurinol and ascorbic acid. These findings led to the suggestion that ROS, generated at least in part via xanthine oxidase, decreased the availability of nitric oxide (8).

Clinical Experience with Oxypurinol

There is limited clinical experience with oxypurinol in patients with heart failure. However, allopurinol has been shown to improve myocardial efficiency in patients with idiopathic dilated cardiomyopathy (4). Heart failure is characterized by mechanoenergetic uncoupling, a term used to describe the inefficient use of oxygen by the failing heart relative to the reduced left ventricular workload. Allopurinol infusion directly into the coronary arteries of cardiomyopathy patients resulted in a decrease in myocardial oxygen consumption but no change in left ventricular work, thus improving the efficiency of contraction (4). This finding is similar to that observed in a canine pacing-induced heart failure model, in which the improvements in myocardial efficiency were attributed to increased sensitivity of the myofilament to calcium (7). These findings suggest that xanthine oxidase and oxidative stress may in part be responsible for mechanoenergetic uncoupling (4).

OPT-CHF (A Phase II–III Prospective, Randomized, Double-Blind, Placebo-Controlled Efficacy and Safety Study of Oxypurinol Added to Standard Therapy in Patients with NYHA Class III–IV Congestive Heart Failure) is an ongoing clinical trial to determine whether oxypurinol improves clinical outcomes in patients with moderate heart failure. Four hundred clinically stable patients who were on standard therapy were randomized to receive oxypurinol in doses up to 600 mg per day versus placebo. The primary endpoint is a clinical composite including NYHA functional class and cardiovascular death.

NEW THERAPEUTIC TARGETS IN ACUTE DECOMPENSATED HEART FAILURE

Relatively few new agents have been developed for the acute (i.e., first line) management of decompensated heart failure, and treatment of such patients has continued to focus on improving hemodynamic function and alleviating symptoms through the use of diuretics, positive inotropes, and vasodilators. While the benefits of slowing disease progression have been most clear in the treatment of patients with chronic heart failure, there is emerging evidence that patients with acute decompensated heart failure may also be susceptible to progressive myocardial failure due to the accelerated loss of cardiac myocytes. In support of this thesis is the observation that circulating levels of cardiac troponins, indirect markers of myocyte death, are increased in the serum of patients with heart failure (9) and appear to increase further with episodes of decompensation despite the absence of ischemia (10). Likewise, there is evidence that elevated plasma troponin levels during an episode of decompensation predict worse survival independent of clinical ischemia, and that elevated troponin levels decline with successful hemodynamic interventions. These observations, though limited, have led to the suggestion that decompensated heart failure is associated with accelerated cardiac myocyte loss. As with chronic heart failure, myocyte loss during an episode of acute decompensated heart failure may occur via several potential mechanisms. Even in the absence of coronary artery disease, hemodynamic overload may lead to subendocardial ischemia and subsequent apoptosis and/or necrosis. In addition, several of the known stimuli for myocyte apoptosis, including norepinephrine, angiotensin, mechanical strain, and oxidative stress (1), are present in the myocardium during episodes of decompensated heart failure. Thus, there is reason to believe that myocyte loss may play an important role in the pathophysiology of acute, as well as chronic, heart failure.

CARDIOPROTECTION VIA ACTIVATION OF ATP-DEPENDENT POTASSIUM CHANNELS

It is now recognized that activation of mitochondrial K_{ATP} channels in cardiac myocytes is an important and potent cardioprotective mechanism (11). In this regard, agents that open mitochondrial K_{ATP} channels, including nicorandil, diazoxide, and pinacidil, have been shown to protect the myocardium against ischemia/reperfusion, myocardial infarction, and peri-operative ischemia. Recently, Marban and others have further demonstrated that the opening of mitochondrial K_{ATP} channels abrogates apoptosis in vitro (12). The anti-apoptotic effects K_{ATP} channel activation appear to be mediated via inhibition of the mitochondrial death pathway, and can be antagonized by agents that oppose K_{ATP} channel opening such as glibenclamide and 5-HD.

LEVOSIMENDAN: A NEW AGENT FOR THE TREATMENT OF DECOMPENSATED HEART FAILURE

Levosimendan is a new pharmacologic agent being evaluated for the treatment of decompensated heart failure. Levosimendan was developed through a molecular search for agents that increase myofilament sensitivity to calcium (13). Levosimendan is also a potent vascular smooth muscle vasodilator due to activation of K_{ATP} in the plasma membrane (14,15). The potent hemodynamic effects of levosimendan have been attributed to the combined effect of increased myocardial contractility and peripheral vasodilation, the latter leading to decreases in both preload and afterload. In addition to its well-described hemodynamic effects, levosimendan activates K_{ATP} channels in both the plasma membrane and the mitochondrial matrix of cardiac myocytes (16).

Direct Effects of Levosimendan on Cardiac Myocytes In Vitro

To determine if levosimendan causes opening of mitochondrial K_{ATP} channels in cardiac myocytes and thereby protects from apoptosis, we studied adult rat ventricular myocytes in culture. This is a well-characterized model system in which we and others have demonstrated the role of ROS in mediating myocyte apoptosis in response to beta-adrenergic stimulation (17–19). In this system, exposure to exogenous hydrogen peroxide (200 μM) for 24 hr leads to a marked increase in apoptosis. We found that pre-treatment with levosimendan for 30 min protects cardiac myocytes from H_2O_2-induced apoptosis as measured by TUNEL staining. This protective effect occurs at levosimendan concentrations as low as 10 nM, well below the therapeutic concentrations achieved in humans (20) and similar to the concentration range for activation of mitochondrial K_{ATP} channels. The anti-apoptotic effect of levosimendan was prevented by the K_{ATP} channel inhibitors 5-HD and glibenclamide, thereby implicating mitochondrial K_{ATP} activation as the protective mechanism of levosimendan. Furthermore, the anti-apoptotic effect of levosimendan was associated with a decrease in H_2O_2-induced cytochrome *c* release from the mitochondria. Thus, levosimendan appears to exert its anti-apoptotic effect, at least in part, by opening mitochondrial K_{ATP} channels that lead to inhibition of the mitochondrial apoptotic pathway.

Oxidative stress plays an important role in mediating myocyte apoptosis and progressive myocardial failure in response to hemodynamic overload and beta-adrenergic stimulation, two factors commonly present in patients with decompensated heart failure. Apoptosis also contributes to myocardial loss in response to ischemia. Preclinical studies have shown that levosimendan, acting in part via opening of mitochondrial K_{ATP} channels, decreases myocardial infarct size (21), thereby providing another potential mechanism by which activation of mitochondrial K_{ATP} by levosimendan might be beneficial in patients with decompensated heart failure.

The demonstration that levosimendan can oppose apoptosis via the activation of the mitochondrial K_{ATP} channel provides a potential mechanism by which levosimendan might protect cardiac myocytes during episodes of decompensated heart failure. These observations further provide a plausible explanation for how a short-term intervention in patients with decompensated heart failure could exert effects on long-term outcomes.

CLINICAL EFFECTS OF LEVOSIMENDAN

It is not known whether agents used in the acute management of decompensation exert significant effects on myocyte survival. However, there are robust circumstantial data to suggest that the choice of therapeutic agent may have an important effect on long-term clinical outcomes in such patients. In particular, several studies have suggested that long-term survival may be reduced after short-term treatment with dobutamine (22). Conversely, a growing body of data suggests that short-term treatment with levosimendan may improve long-term survival. For example, in the RUSSLAN trial, 504 patients with NYHA class III–IV heart failure were randomized to placebo or levosimendan in the setting of an acute myocardial infarction (23). At two weeks post-randomization, survival was significantly improved in the levosimendan group, a difference that persisted at 180 days. The LIDO trial compared levosimendan to dobutamine in 203 patients with decompensated heart failure requiring intravenous inotropic therapy. In this study, patients randomized to levosimendan had a significantly better survival at both 30 and 180 days (24). A meta-analysis of approximately 1000 patients who received levosimendan in four randomized trials, including RUSSLAN and LIDO, showed an almost 50% decrease in the risk of death as compared to either placebo or dobutamine (25). Recently, CASINO, a survival study comparing levosimendan to both placebo and dobutamine in patients with decompensated heart failure, was terminated prematurely after the randomization of only 227 patients because of a significant survival benefit of levosimendan over dobutamine and a similar trend versus placebo (26). Parissis et al. have demonstrated one possible mechanism by which levosimendan may improve survival in patients with decompensated heart failure. Among 27 patients admitted to the hospital with acutely decompensated heart failure and randomized to therapy with levosimendan or placebo, levosimendan therapy resulted in a significant decrease in the circulating levels of soluble Fas and Fas ligand, leading to the suggestion that the survival benefit observed with levosimendan may result from interference with the Fas-mediated apoptosis pathway (27).

Taken together, these observations with levosimendan present a striking degree of consistency that supports the thesis that levosimendan exerts a beneficial effect on survival. Since few of these studies were designed primarily to examine survival, and all were relatively small in size, final conclusions about the effects of levosimendan on survival must await the results of REVIVE and SURVIVE, two prospective survival studies comparing levosimendan to dobutamine in approximately 1300 patients with decompensated heart failure (28). Nevertheless, these data provide an intriguing suggestion that levosimendan exerts a favorable effect on survival. While the alleviation of symptoms should remain an important goal of therapy in such patients, it now appears possible that a therapeutic approach that includes a cardioprotective strategy can exert a clinically meaningful benefit on the progression of the underlying myocardial disease.

REFERENCES

1. Sawyer DB, Siwik DA, Xiao L, Pimentel DR, Singh K, Colucci WS. Role of oxidative stress in myocardial hypertrophy and failure. J Mol Cell Cardiol 2002; 34:379–388.
2. Keith M, Geranmayegan A, Sole MJ, et al. Increased oxidative stress in patients with congestive heart failure. J Am Coll Cardiol 1998; 31:1352–1356.

3. Olivetti G, Abbi R, Quaini F, et al. Apoptosis in the failing human heart. N Engl J Med 1997; 336:1131–1141.
4. Cappola TP, Kass DA, Nelson GS, et al. Allopurinol improves myocardial efficiency in patients with idiopathic dilated cardiomyopathy. Circulation 2001; 104:2407–2411.
5. Kogler H, Fraser H, McCune S, Altschuld R, Marban E. Disproportionate enhancement of myocardial contractility by the xanthine oxidase inhibitor oxypurinol in failing rat myocardium. Cardiovasc Res 2003; 59:582–592.
6. Stull LB, Leppo MK, Szweda L, Gao WD, Marban E. Chronic treatment with allopurinol boosts survival and cardiac contractility in murine postischemic cardiomyopathy. Circ Res 2004; 95:1005–1011.
7. Ekelund UE, Harrison RW, Shokek O, et al. Intravenous allopurinol decreases myocardial oxygen consumption and increases mechanical efficiency in dogs with pacing-induced heart failure. Circ Res 1999; 85:437–445.
8. Saavedra WF, Paolocci N, St John ME, et al. Imbalance between xanthine oxidase and nitric oxide synthase signaling pathways underlies mechanoenergetic uncoupling in the failing heart. Circ Res 2002; 90:297–304.
9. Missov E, Catzolari C, Pau B. Circulating cardiac Troponin I in severe congestive heart failure. Circulation 1997; 96:2953–2958.
10. Goto T, Takase H, Toriyama T, et al. Circulating concentrations of cardiac proteins indicate the severity of congestive heart failure. Heart 2003; 89:1303–1307.
11. O'Rourke B. Evidence for mitochondrial K+ channels and their role in cardioprotection. Circ Res 2004; 94:420–432.
12. Akao M, Ohler A, O'Rourke B, Marban E. Mitochondrial ATP-sensitive potassium channels inhibit apoptosis induced by oxidative stress in cardiac cells. Circ Res 2001; 88:1267–1275.
13. Edes I, Kiss E, Kitada Y, et al. Effects of Levosimendan, a cardiotonic agent targeted to troponin C, on cardiac function and on phosphorylation and Ca2+ sensitivity of cardiac myofibrils and sarcoplasmic reticulum in guinea pig heart. Circ Res 1995; 77:107–113.
14. Yokoshiki H, Katsube Y, Sunagawa M, Sperelakis N. The novel calcium sensitizer levosimendan activates the ATP-sensitive K+ channel in rat ventricular cells. J Pharmacol Exp Ther 1997; 283:375–383.
15. Yokoshiki H, Katsube Y, Sunagawa M, Sperelakis N. Levosimendan, a novel Ca2+ sensitizer, activates the glibenclamide-sensitive K+ channel in rat arterial myocytes. Eur J Pharmacol 1997; 333:249–259.
16. Kopustinskiene DM, Pollesello P, Saris NE. Levosimendan is a mitochondrial K(ATP) channel opener. Eur J Pharmacol 2001; 428:311–314.
17. Communal C, Singh K, Pimentel DR, Colucci WS. Norepinephrine stimulates apoptosis in adult rat ventricular myocytes by activation of the b-adrenergic pathway. Circulation 1998; 98:1329–1334.
18. Remondino A, Kwon SH, Communal C, et al. Beta-adrenergic receptor-stimulated apoptosis in cardiac myocytes is mediated by reactive oxygen species/c-Jun NH2-terminal kinase-dependent activation of the mitochondrial pathway. Circ Res 2003; 92:136–138.
19. Kwon SH, Pimentel DR, Remondino A, Sawyer DB, Colucci WS. H(2)O(2) regulates cardiac myocyte phenotype via concentration-dependent activation of distinct kinase pathways. J Mol Cell Cardiol 2003; 35:615–621.
20. Kivikko M, Antila S, Eha J, Lehtonen L, Pentikainen PJ. Pharmacodynamics and safety of a new calcium sensitizer, levosimendan, and its metabolites during an extended infusion in patients with severe heart failure. J Clin Pharmacol 2002; 42:43–51.
21. Kersten JR, Montgomery MW, Pagel PS, Warltier DC. Levosimendan, a new positive inotropic drug, decreases myocardial infarct size via activation of K(ATP) channels. Anesth Analg 2000; 90:5–11.
22. Massie BM. 15 years of heart-failure trials: what have we learned? Lancet 1998; 352:SI29–SI33.
23. Moiseyev VS, Poder P, Andrejevs N, et al. Safety and efficacy of a novel calcium sensitizer, levosimendan, in patients with left ventricular failure due to an acute myocardial infarction.

A randomized, placebo-controlled, double-blind study (RUSSLAN). Eur Heart J 2002; 23:1422–1432.
24. Follath F, Cleland JG, Just H, et al. Efficacy and safety of intravenous levosimendan compared with dobutamine in severe low-output heart failure (the LIDO study): a randomised double-blind trial. Lancet 2002; 360:196–202.
25. Cleland JG, Ghosh J, Freemantle N, et al. Clinical trials update and cumulative meta-analyses from the American College of Cardiology: WATCH, SCD-HeFT, DINAMIT, CASINO, INSPIRE, STRATUS-US, RIO-Lipids and cardiac resynchronisation therapy in heart failure. Eur J Heart Fail 2004; 6:501–508.
26. Zairis MN, Apostolatos C, Anastasiadis P, et al. The effect of a calcium sensitizer or an inotrope or none in chronic low output decompensated heart failure: results from the Calcium Sensitizer or Inotrope or None in Low Output Heart Failure Study (CASINO). J Am Coll Cardiol 2004; 43:206A (Abstract).
27. Parissis JT, Adamopoulos S, Antoniades C, et al. Effects of levosimendan on circulating pro-inflammatory cytokines and soluble apoptosis mediators in patients with decompensated advanced heart failure. Am J Cardiol 2004; 93:1309–1312.
28. Packer M, Colucci WS, Fisher L, et al. Development of a comprehensive new endpoint for the evaluation of new treatments for acute decompensated heart failure: results with levosimendan in the REVIVE I study. J Card Failure 2003; 9:S61 (Abstract).

35
New Surgery for Congestive Heart Failure

David D. Yuh
Division of Cardiac Surgery, The Johns Hopkins Hospital, Baltimore, Maryland, U.S.A.

INTRODUCTION

Improvements in the prevention and treatment of cardiovascular disease in young and middle-aged adults has extended the average life expectancy, resulting in a steadily increasing number of people with chronic cardiovascular disease. A large proportion of this population consists of individuals suffering from chronic congestive heart failure. In the United States, nearly five million persons suffer from heart failure, with almost 500,000 new patients diagnosed each year. While many of these patients achieve a reasonable quality of life with judicious medical management, a substantial segment experience severe congestive symptoms and profound debilitation that goes well beyond what current medical therapies can treat. A tiny fraction of these end-stage patients, about 3000 patients per year, undergo cardiac transplantation, relegating hundreds of thousands of heart failure patients to repeated inpatient admissions and death within several years of diagnosis. The perennial dearth of cardiac donors has driven the successful development of mechanical assist devices as a bridge to transplantation, however this strategy is limited to a selected group of patients who fit stringent cardiac transplant criteria. Most recently, "destination therapy" for medically-refractory heart failure patients who would not otherwise qualify for cardiac transplantation has been validated by the landmark REMATCH trial (1). However, although the quality of life among these patients was significantly improved with left ventricular assist devices (LVAD), long-term survival was quite limited by complications, with only 23% of LVAD patients surviving up to two years (2). The advent of newer generation LVADs brings modest promise of longer-term survival, however this has yet to be fully evaluated with multicenter trials. Furthermore, the relatively high health care costs associated with LVADs currently limits their broad short- and long-term use as a standard heart failure therapy.

Consequently, new alternative surgical strategies for the treatment of heart failure are being developed. Surgical ventricular remodeling and geometric mitral reconstruction represent two major strategies and are discussed elsewhere. The following chapter will briefly review other cardiac operations for heart failure patients, including minimally-invasive direct and transmyocardial revascularization, minimally-invasive biventricular epicardial lead placement, ablative operations for chronic and paroxysmal atrial fibrillation, and the ACORN cardiac support device.

ROBOT-ASSISTED, MINIMALLY INVASIVE CORONARY REVASCULARIZATION

Traditionally, coronary artery bypass grafting (CABG) is performed through a median sternotomy, providing optimal access to all cardiac structures and great vessels. The disfigurement and pain associated with this extensive incision has been a longstanding but heretofore acceptable consequence of cardiac surgery. Fueled largely by the advent of less invasive and traumatic laparoscopic and thoracoscopic techniques for non-cardiac operations and the rise of catheter-based interventions for myocardial revascularization, minimally-invasive approaches to cardiac surgery are being developed. However, clinical successes in minimally-invasive cardiac surgery have lagged behind those achieved with minimally-invasive laparoscopic surgery due to three primary issues. First, the rigidity and anatomy of the thoracic cage is not particularly amenable to the limited degrees of freedom provided by now-conventional endoscopic instruments. Consequently, the fine motions required in cardiac surgery are not easily achieved with these physical constraints. Second, the consequences of surgical errors or excessive delay in cardiac operations (e.g., vessel trauma, prolonged cardiopulmonary bypass) increase the potential for irreversible patient injury or even death. Third, results of conventional CABG have been overtly studied and have established exceptional "gold standard" outcomes, including 15–20 yr left internal mammary to left anterior descending (LAD) coronary artery graft patency rates of over 90%. Therefore, new minimally-invasive coronary revascularization strategies have employed technologically-advanced devices to project the surgeon's technical dexterity into a confined space through minimal incisions to achieve satisfactory outcomes.

The Intuitive da Vinci® Surgical System

Computerized robot-assisted surgery has enhanced the ability of surgeons to perform minimally-invasive procedures by placing a computer interface between the surgeon and dexterous instrument tips. A robotic minimally invasive surgical system in clinical use is the da Vinci® Surgical System (Intuitive Surgical, Sunnyvale, California, U.S.A.). This robotic system is comprised of three principal components: a surgeon "master" console, video cart, and "slave" tableside robot with two or three instrument arms and a stereoscopic endoscope (Fig. 1). The surgeon sits at the console and manipulates the instrument handles. These motions are relayed to a computer processor which digitizes the surgeon's hand motions and transmits them in real-time to robotic manipulators that actuate endoscopic instrument tips placed into the thoracic cavity via small ports (Fig. 2). The computer interface between the surgeon and the instrument tips permits the surgeon's digitized hand motions to be precisely manipulated and filtered by the system's control software. This interface enhances the surgeon's ability to perform minimally-invasive cardiac surgery in several ways. First, by filtering out high-frequency signals, surgical tremor is eliminated. Second, the computer interface allows for motion scaling, where comfortable macroscopic movements at the surgeon console are scaled down to a much smaller scale inside the patient, enhancing dexterity. Third, the computer interface permits the accurate translation of the surgeon's hand motions to a dexterous endoscopic "wrist" placed within the chest cavity, conferring much higher degrees of freedom than traditional manually actuated endoscopic instruments. Finally, a three-dimensional image of the surgical site is displayed to the surgeon sitting at the console, using stereoimages from the two-camera robotic endoscope.

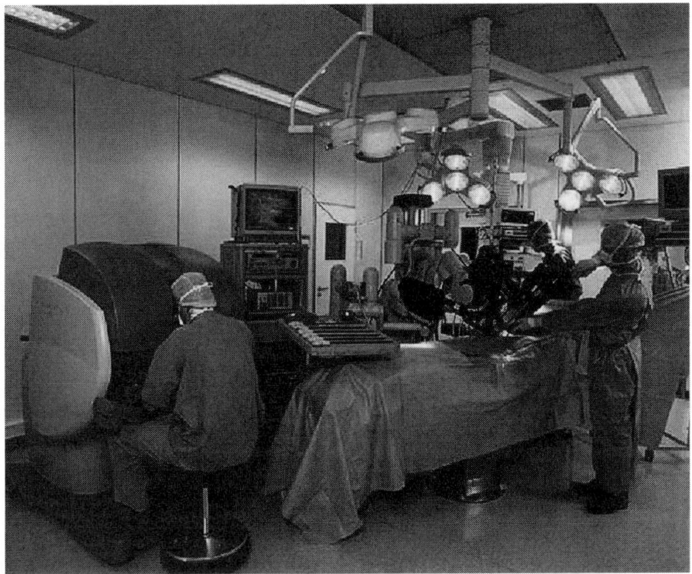

Figure 1 Components of the da Vinci® Surgical System. This system consists of a surgeon "master" console (*left*), video cart (*center*), and "slave" tableside robot with two or three instrument arms and a stereoscopic endoscope (*right*). *Source*: Photo courtesy of Intuitive Surgical, Sunnyvale, California, U.S.A.

Totally Endoscopic Coronary Artery Bypass Grafting

Early attempts to perform totally endoscopic coronary artery bypass grafting4 (TECAB) with conventional manually-operated thoracoscopic instruments proved difficult and often resulted in conversion of prohibitively long operative times (3). The advent of surgical robotic systems in the following years enabled the introduction of much more dextrous instrumentation through port-access and facilitated the development of endoscopic CABG. The first TECAB was performed by Loulmet and colleagues in 1998 (4).

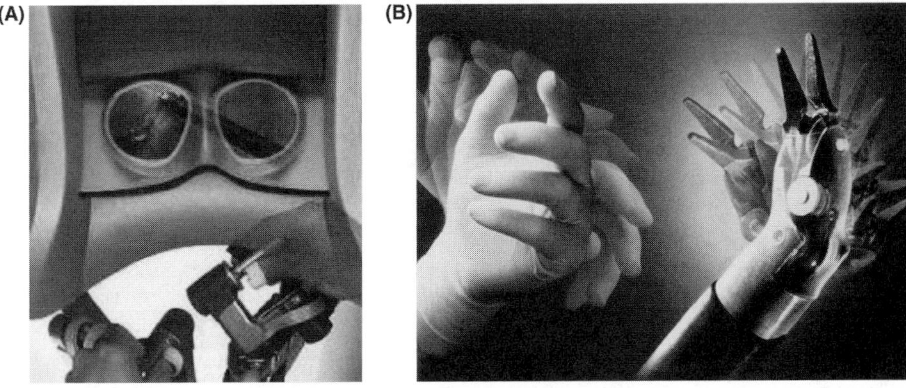

Figure 2 da Vinci® master console and endoscopic instrument tip. The master console at which the operating surgeon sits (**A**) provides a stereoscopic view of the operative field and instrument controls which actuate each of two (left and right) dexterous instrument tips (**B**) inserted into the chest via thoracoscopic ports. *Source*: Photos courtesy of Intuitive Surgical, Sunnyvale, California, U.S.A.

Subsequent efforts in Europe and the United States fostered the evolution of facilitating techniques for TECAB, including stabilizing devices, endovascular crossclamp and cardioplegia systems, and anastomotic devices.

TECAB methodologies are rapidly evolving; however, several general concepts are worth describing. Early successes with single-vessel TECAB, based upon the left internal mammary artery (LIMA) to LAD coronary artery anastomosis, were greatly facilitated with

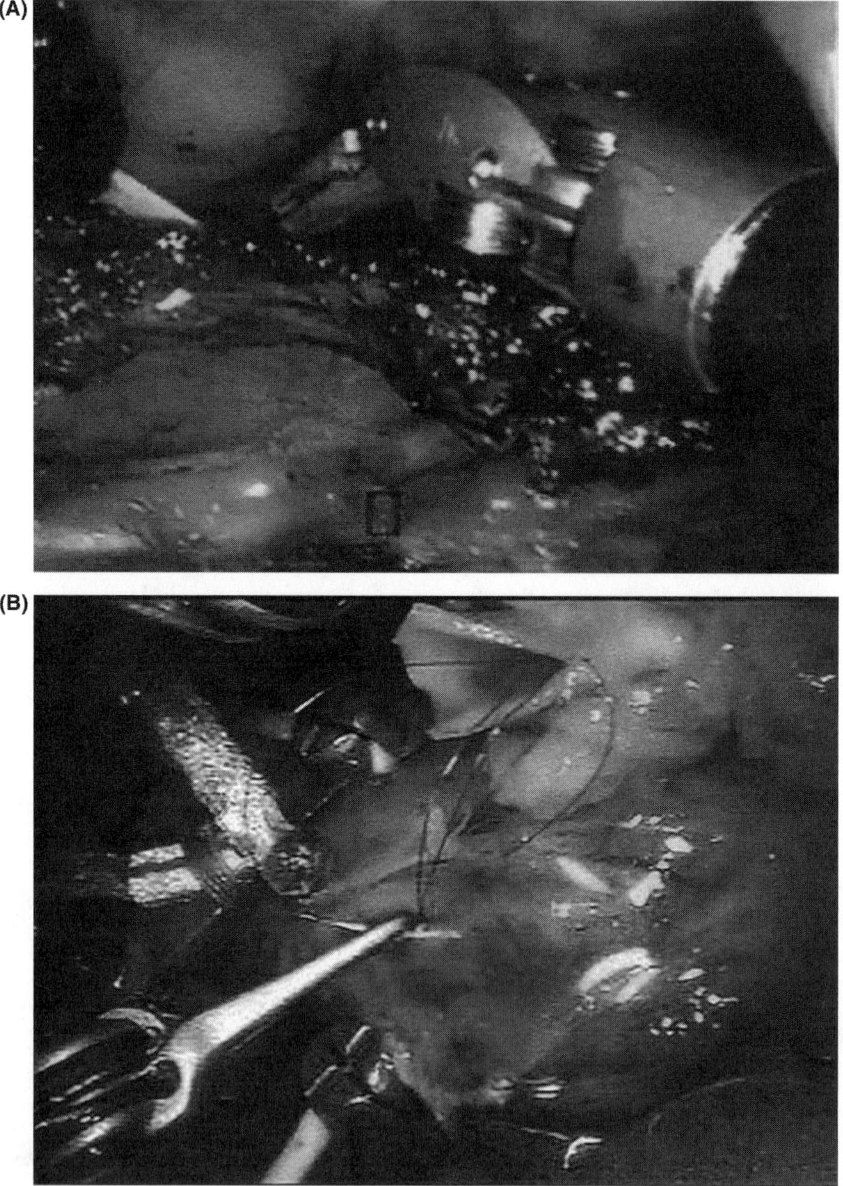

Figure 3 Totally endoscopic coronary artery bypass techniques. The left internal mammary artery (LIMA) is harvested as a pedicle by the da Vinci® robotic system (**A**). An anastomosis is created between the LIMA and the left anterior descending aorta (**B**) on the beating heart. Note the stabilization device. *Source*: From Ref. 5.

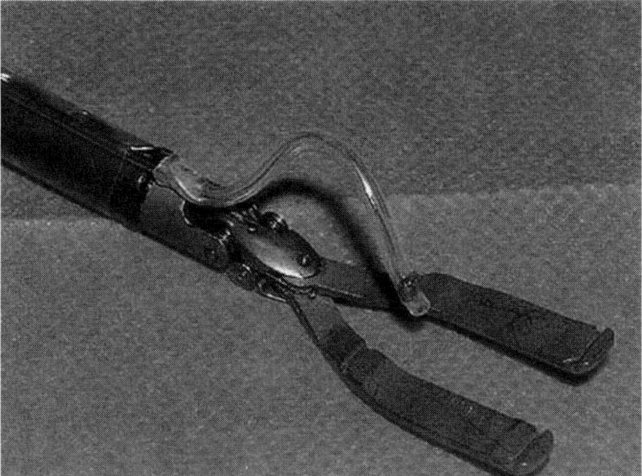

Figure 4 Endoscopic stabilization device.

cardiopulmonary bypass support delivered through femoral vessel cannulation in addition to the ability to arrest the heart with an ascending aortic occluding balloon or "endoclamp." The LIMA is detached from the left anterior chest wall and anastomosed to the LAD using the da Vinci Surgical System (Fig. 3). Mohr and colleagues describe their experience attempting TECAB in 35 patients (27 patients with arrested heart and 8 patients with beating heart) (5). TECAB was successfully completed in 22 of 27 of patients under arrested conditions with a 95.4% patency rate, as demonstrated by angiography at three months' follow-up. TECAB was successfully performed on the beating heart in 2 out of 8 patients, vusing an endoscopic stabilizer (Fig. 4).

The learning curve for TECAB is indeed steep, resulting in relatively long operative times and conversion rates; however, multiple studies have demonstrated steady reduction of these parameters with experience (6). Technical advances that will be required for widespread application of TECAB include improved target vessel identification modalities, stabilization devices, cardioplegia delivery systems, and distal/proximal anastomotic devices.

GEOMETRIC MITRAL RECONSTRUCTION

Functional mitral regurgitation frequently complicates and exacerbates end-stage dilated cardiomyopathy. It is associated with progressive ventricular dilatation, (Fig. 5) worsening congestive symptoms, and a deleterious impact upon survival rates. Historically, surgical correction of significant mitral insufficiency consisted of mitral valve replacement; however, in recent years the functional importance of maintaining the mitral subvalvular apparatus has resulted in the refinement and advocacy of mitral valve repair techniques.

MINIMALLY INVASIVE MITRAL VALVE REPAIR

The past decade has seen the evolution of minimally-invasive techniques for mitral valve repair. Cohn and colleagues (7) and Cosgrove and associates (8) developed and introduced

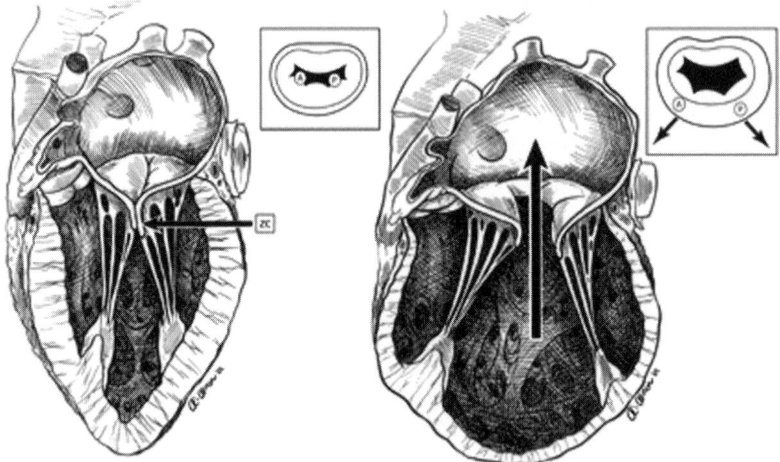

Figure 5 Geometric structural changes associated with failing, dilated left ventricle. Inadequate mitral leaflet coaptation results from mitral annular dilatation, papillary muscle displacement, increased leaflet tethering forces, and weakened leaflet closing forces. *Source*: From Badhwar V, Bolling SF. Nontransplant surgical options for heart failure. In: Cardiac Surgery in the Adult, 7th ed. New York: McGraw Hill, 2003:1515–1526.

minimally invasive mitral valve operations through attenuated or modified sternotomy incisions. Limited access and visibility and other technical challenges precluded widespread adoption of these approaches by many cardiac surgeons. Nevertheless, accumulating evidence with these minimally invasive approaches to valve repair has suggested improved clinical outcomes in terms of incisional pain, hospital stays, cosmesis, wound complications, and patient home recovery times (9). These incentives have powered the development of newer minimally-invasive approaches towards mitral valve repair. Two new successful strategies entail the use of the da Vinci robotic surgical platform (10,11) and specially-designed manually-actuated thoracoscopic instruments (12,13). These two approaches incorporate many common themes and are therefore described concomitantly.

The mitral valve can be approached via a right transpleural approach through a small right thoracotomy. In a modified left lateral decubitus position the right lung is deflated via selective lung ventilation. A small 4–5 cm mini-thoracotomy is created through the right fourth or fifth intercostal space and the pericardium is opened and suspended. The right (or left) femoral artery and vein are cannulated and, under hypothermic cardiopulmonary bypass, Sondergaard's interatrial groove is developed. A transthoracic aortic crossclamp or endovascular occluding balloon is then applied and the heart is arrested with antegrade cardioplegia. A standard transverse left atriotomy is then performed and a specially-designed atrial retractor is used to provide excellent exposure of the mitral valve. At this point one of two instrumentation strategies is employed.

In the robot-assisted approach, the da Vinci endoscope is placed through the minithoracotomy towards the mitral valve, providing excellent visualization. Two separate instrumentation ports are used to direct each of the robotic instrument arms into the left atriotomy. The mitral valve is repaired with standard techniques under videoscopic, robot-assisted guidance (Fig. 6). Once the valve is repaired, the robot is extracted from the patient, the left atriotomy closed, and the operation completed in the usual fashion. Another approach entails the use of manually-actuated extended

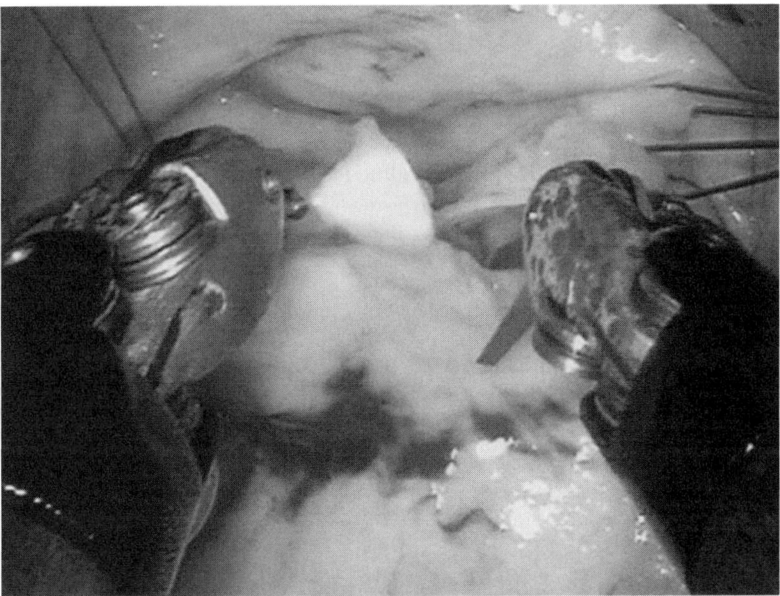

Figure 6 Posterior trapezoidal resection of mitral valve leaflet with the da Vinci® surgical robotic system. *Source*: From Ref. 10.

instruments to affect the same mitral repair under direct or videoscopic vision. Both approaches have been used with great success and have generally resulted in improved clinical outcomes. In a series of 25 patients undergoing robot-assisted mitral valve repair, Tatooles and colleagues describe the ability to extubate 21 patients (84%) in the operating room without the need for reintubation, permitting early ambulation and return of bowel function (9). Eight of these patients were successfully discharged home in less than 24 hr with an average length of stay of 2.7 days. Nifong and colleagues showed that robot-assisted mitral repair could be performed with similar operative times compared with standard techniques (11), although all groups describe a definite "learning curve" effect on operative times (Table 1). Long-term durability of these repairs is still under evaluation with accumulating experience; however, early results are encouraging.

Table 1 Inpatient Stays for Patients Undergoing Robot-Assisted Mitral Valve Repair (n=25)[a]

Variable	N(%)	Mean ± SD	Range
Extubated in OR	21(84%)		
ICH (hr)		35.4±18.5	18–72
LOS (days)		2.68±3.1	1–16
Discharged <24 hr	8(32%)		
Discharged <30 hr	12(48%)		
Pts requiring PRBCs	11(44%)		

[a]Postoperative data.

Abbreviations: ICU, intensive care units; LOS, length of stay; OR, operating room; PRBCs, packed red blood cells; Pts, patients; SD, standard deviation.

Source: From Ref. 9.

MINIMALLY INVASIVE, ROBOT-ASSISTED BIVENTRICULAR PACEMAKER LEAD PLACEMENT

Ventricular dysynchrony secondary to intraventricular conduction delay has been observed in up to 30% of heart failure patients (14). This discoordinate contraction pattern appears to contribute substantially to the already depressed cardiac contractility observed in patients with idiopathic and ischemic cardiomyopathies. Ventricular dysynchrony has been associated with mitral insufficiency and increased mortality rates (15,16). There is mounting evidence that ventricular resynchronization by way of biventricular pacing can, in selected heart failure patients, improve ventricular function, exercise capacity, and quality of life (17,18). Current biventricular systems rely upon intracardiac leads percutaneously implanted into the endocardial surfaces of the right atrium and right ventricle; the left ventricular lead is placed into the coronary sinus. Physiologic studies suggest that the most effective hemodynamic augmentation with resynchronization is achieved by pacing the posterobasal segment of the left ventricle, compared to the lateral or anterior segments. Achieving this nominal left ventricular lead position is often difficult with the percutaneous route for two reasons: (1) coronary sinus and venous anatomy precludes lead placement in 10–15% of cases and (2) it is often difficult to position the lead in the posterolateral vertical vein of the coronary sinus. Furthermore, in some cases, even adequate cannulation of the coronary sinus with the left ventricular lead results in intermittent or continuous left phrenic nerve stimulation which is often bothersome to the patient.

When the left ventricular lead cannot be placed by the usual percutaneous route, surgical epicardial placement of this lead is considered. Initially, surgical placement of this lead was conducted through a standard or mini-thoracotomy and, more recently, using standard handheld thoracoscopic instrumentation. Disadvantages with these approaches include fairly limited access to the entire left ventricular surface, including the nominal posterobasal surface of the left ventricle and the considerable postoperative pain associated with any thoracotomy. The recent use of minimally-invasive robot-assisted techniques to place the left ventricular epicardial pacing leads has reduced the morbidity associated with thoracotomy and provided much greater access to critical left ventricular surfaces not afforded with standard thoracoscopic methods. DeRose and colleagues described the first sustained experience with the robotic approach, reporting successful placement of epicardial leads in ten patients (19).

Methodology

We have used the intuitive da Vinci surgical robotic system to routinely place epicardial biventricular pacing leads which could not be placed in the catheterization laboratory or to replace leads that resulted in phrenic nerve stimulation. Although described robotic techniques vary slightly among different surgeons, there are many common themes which have evolved with collective experience.

After induction of general endotracheal anesthesia, selective right lung ventilation is achieved with insertion of a double-lumen endotracheal tube or bronchial blocker. We generally do not use intraoperative transesophageal echocardiography, although this may be useful for intraoperative hemodynamic management. The patient is then placed in a full right lateral decubitus position (i.e., right side down) and secured to the operating table. Cutaneous defibrillation pads are placed on the anterior and posterior chest wall. After the left lung is deflated, a 10 mm camera port is placed in the left seventh intercostal space just anterior to the scapular tip line and a 0° da Vinci videoscope is manually placed through this port to assure adequate lung isolation and anatomy of the left pleural space. To increase the working space between the heart and the lateral chest wall, 8–10 mm of CO_2 insufflation is instilled into the left chest, effectively shifting the mediastinum, including the heart away from the chest wall. One must be cautious during insufflation, since excessive mediastinal shift may result in varying degrees of hemodynamic compromise. Under videoscopic vision, two 5 mm da Vinci instrument ports are placed in the left fifth and ninth intercostal spaces along the scapular tip line. A 10 mm "working" port is placed in the seventh intercostal space approximately four centimeters posterior to the camera port for the introduction of the leads and any required suture materials. The da Vinci "slave" robot is moved toward the patient and docked to the camera and instrument ports. Forceps and electrocautery instruments are then carefully inserted into the left chest under videoscopic vision, taking care not to inadvertently puncture the lung or heart.

After any intrapleural adhesions are lysed, the pericardium is incised transversely 2 to 3 cm posterior to the course of the left phrenic nerve. At this point the circumflex marginal coronary branches are often identifiable as landmarks for epicardial lead placement. At times, temporary retraction sutures placed in the pericardial edges can facilitate exposure. The first epicardial lead is then placed into the left chest through the working port and grasped by the robotic forceps (Fig. 7), keeping the proximal end outside the chest. Either screw-in or suture-fixation (e.g., steroid eluting) leads may be utilized. We and others have found that the posterobasal region in proximity to the second and third obtuse marginal branches appears to be the optimal site for left ventricular lead placement (20). This nominal site can be identified using the coronary anatomy or by using a temporary pacing wire to map the ventricular electrogram, identifying the area of latest activation along the posterobasal ventricular surface in relation to the patient's intrinsic QRS complex. Once placed, the lead is tested for capture threshold and impedence, capped, and delivered entirely into the chest. Usually, a second "back-up" epicardial lead is placed in the vicinity of the first in an identical manner and the pericardium is loosely closed over both leads. The leads are then retrieved from the chest through the working or

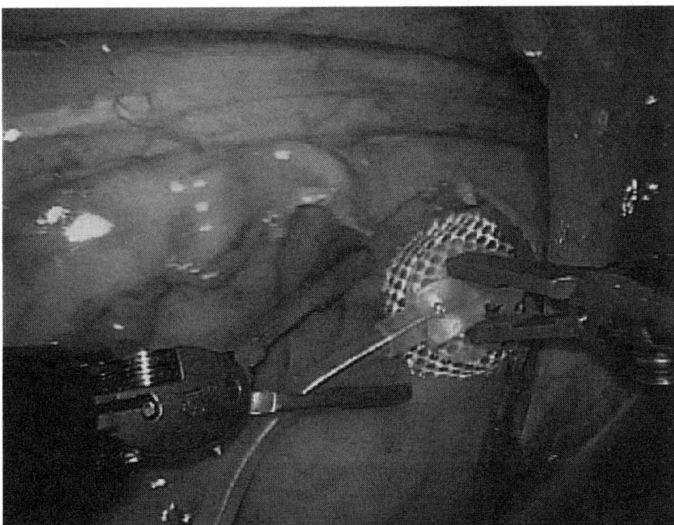

Figure 7 Robot-assisted epicardial biventricular lead placement as viewed by operating surgeon through da Vinci® master console. *Source*: From Ref. 19.

right instrument port and tunneled subcutaneously into a counter incision placed in the left axilla. A single soft 19 French Blake drain is placed into the left chest through the left instrument port under videoscopic guidance and all remaining ports are removed and incisions closed.

At this point, we reposition, reprep, and redrape the patient in a supine position. Usually, a biventricular generator has already been placed in a left subclavicular subcutaneous pocket. This pocket is reopened and the generator is temporarily extracted. The newly placed epicardial leads are then tunneled from the axillary counterincision to the generator pocket. Thresholds and impedances are retested and the best lead is connected to the device. The backup lead is capped and fixed to the pectoralis fascia using a fine monofilament suture. The device is then reinserted into the pocket which is subsequently closed. Finally, the device is interrogated and reprogrammed appropriately.

Often, the patient can be awakened and extubated in the operating room immediately after the procedure. As a precaution, we observe all of our patients in an intensive care unit setting for 24 hr prior to transfer to a monitored bed. The single pleural drain is usually removed on the first postoperative morning.

Clinical Results

The clinical series by DeRose reports a high degree of success with this robotic approach towards biventricular epicardial lead placement (19). The mean robotic operative time was 83 ± 53 min, with a clear reduction in operative times from an average of 108 min for the first five cases to an average of 50 min with the latter five cases; this is clearly a reflection of a learning curve. In our series (unreported data), we have achieved similar operative times. Although there have been no case-control studies to date, we and others have observed significantly reduced patient discomfort, hospitalization acuity, and inpatient stays using this minimally-invasive approach. Although this surgical approach carries the disadvantage of general anesthesia, compared to percutaneous methods, we and others have experienced surprisingly minimal hemodynamic difficulties during the intra- and postoperative periods. It remains to be seen whether this approach affords improved functional outcomes compared to standard percutaneous techniques.

MINIMALLY INVASIVE, ROBOT-ASSISTED TRANSMYOCARDIAL REVASCULARIZATION

Although CABG and percutaneous coronary interventions (PCI) are proven therapies for relief of angina stemming for ischemic heart disease, there exists a subset of "no-option" patients with intractable angina caused by diffuse, small-vessel coronary disease not amenable to these modalities. Transmyocardial laser revascularization (TMR) has shown some clinical promise in substantially reducing anginal symptoms in these patients either as sole therapy or in conjunction with CABG (21–25). Most recently, Allen and colleagues also demonstrated a significantly reduced risk of late death for no-option patients treated with sole therapy TMR compared to maximal medical therapy (26). TMR is currently delivered mainly via median sternotomy or left thoracotomy. We have recently developed a technique to combine the unique dexterity afforded by the da Vinci surgical robotic platform with a prototype flexible fiberoptic Holmium:Yttrium–Aluminum–Garnet (Ho:YAG) laser TMR device (CardioGenesis Corporation, Foothill Ranch, CA) to perform totally endoscopic off-pump TMR (27).

Methodology

The procedure is performed under general anesthesia with single-lung ventilation. The patient is placed in a full right lateral decubitus position. A left transpleural approach is taken, similar to that described for robot-assisted biventricular lead placement. Two transverse pericardiotomies are created approximately 2 cm medial and lateral to the left phrenic nerve in order to access all wall segments of the left ventricle. A prototype modification of the SoloGrip III TMR Ho:YAG laser handpiece (TMR2000; CardioGenesis Corporation, Foothill Ranch, CA) fitted with a 1.0 mm CardioGenesis CrystalFlex® fiberoptic probe (Fig. 8) is introduced into the left chest cavity through the working port and grasped by one of two da Vinci DeBakey forceps instruments under videoscopic guidance. Transmural channels are created through the anterior, anterolateral, apical, posterolateral, posterobasal, and/or inferior walls of the beating left ventricle at a density of approximately 1 channel/cm^2 (Fig. 9). The laser energy delivered to the myocardium consists of 7 Watt pulses at a 5 Hz repetition rate with a pulse width of 200 μsec (± 25%). The flexible probe is easily maneuverable by the da Vinci instrumentation and the cupped tip is gently placed upon each targeted area, oriented perpendicularly to the epicardial surface without deforming or compressing the left ventricle. Once the probe tip is seated on the epicardial surface, each channel is created by the tableside surgeon by advancing the CrystalFlex fiber, with the SoloGrip® handpiece, through the myocardium while discharging the laser pulses through it. Detection of transmural penetration is achieved with auditory feedback to the tableside surgeon. Early FDA safety trials evaluating this technique are underway.

SURGICAL TREATMENT OF ATRIAL FIBRILLATION

The surgical Maze III operation first performed and described by Cox in 1988 at Washington University Medical Center is the gold standard for the surgical treatment of atrial fibrillation (28,29). This operation consists of creating transmural isolating scars in atrial tissue, using a cut-and-sew technique, to interrupt aberrant conduction pathways responsible for atrial fibrillation. Long-term follow-up has demonstrated that over 90% of patients treated with the Maze III operation are free of atrial fibrillation, and that most of these patients are off of antiarrhythmic medications. However, this operation is a rather

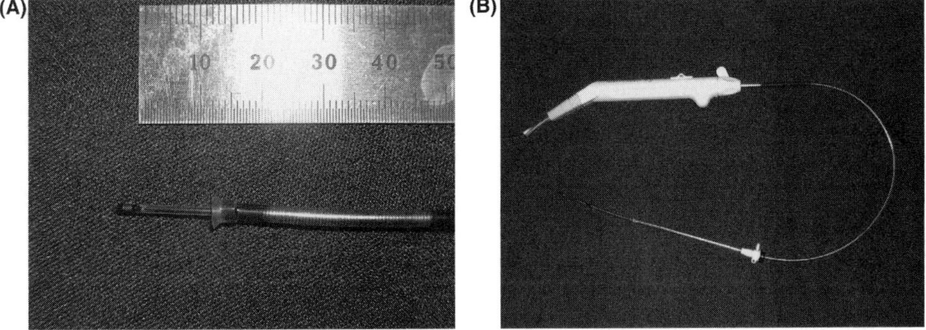

Figure 8 The prototype 1.0 mm Cardiogenesis CrystalFlex® fiberoptic probe (**A**) fitted to the commercially-available SoloGrip III® TMR Ho:YAG laser handpiece (**B**). *Source:* Photos courtesy of TMR2000; Cardiogenesis Corporation, Foothill Ranch, California, U.S.A.

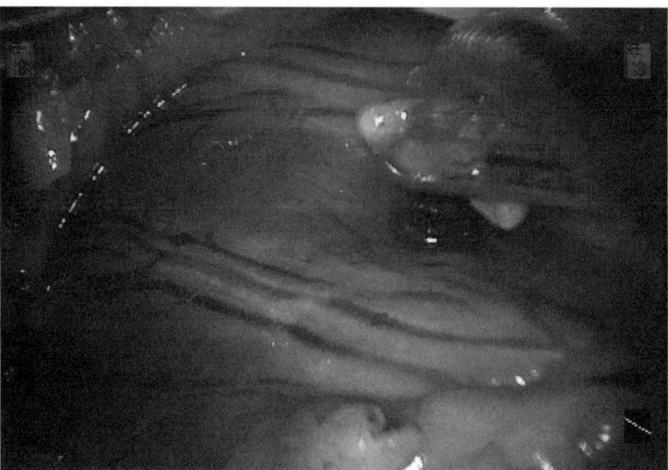

Figure 9 Surgeon's views through da Vinci® master console of robot-assisted, endoscopic transmyocardial revascularization. Transmural channels were created through the anterior (top), anterolateral, apical, posterolateral, posterobasal, and inferior (bottom) walls of the beating canine left ventricle. Note the preserved left phrenic nerve in the bottom of photo.

complex, extensive, and invasive operation and has consequently not been widely adopted.

In recent years, several different ablation devices using different forms of ablative energy have been devised, facilitating the creation of transmural linear lesion lines as a simpler substitute for the cut-and-sew techniques used with the original Cox Maze operations. Furthermore, simpler lesion patterns have been proposed to further simplify these ablative operations. Here we describe two devices representative of two different energy sources: the Guidant Flex-4™ and Flex-10™ microwave ablation devices and the Medtronic Cardioblate radiofrequency device.

Guidant Flex-4™ and Flex-10™ Microwave Ablation Devices

The microwave Guidant Flex-4 and Flex-10 devices (Guidant Corp., Fremont, CA) generate electromagnetic waves at delivered at high frequency (2450 MHz) by a malleable antenna probe (Fig. 10), provoking the vibration and rotation of water molecule dipoles in the targeted tissues and thereby creating friction and heat, creating necrotic lesions at a predictable depth. Shielding in the ablating tip inhibits microwave energy into non-targeted tissue (e.g., blood vessels). These flexible devices can be used to create both encircling and linear ablative lesions.

Several technical variations have been described using the Flex-4 and Flex-10 microwave ablation devices (30). An off-pump approach entails the encirclement of all four pulmonary veins by way of the transverse and oblique sinuses to create a continuous epicardial ablation line, often referred to as a "box" lesion, around the pulmonary veins (Fig.11). The same device is then manipulated to create a connecting lesion to the base of the left atrial appendage, which is then subsequently stapled off at its base.

Utilization of normothermic cardiopulmonary bypass and cardioplegic arrest affords the creation of additional endocardial lesion sets. Under cardiopulmonary bypass with the heart left beating and empty, the pulmonary vein box lesion is created as described above and the left atrial appendage is stapled off at its base. Endocardial right-sided lesions are

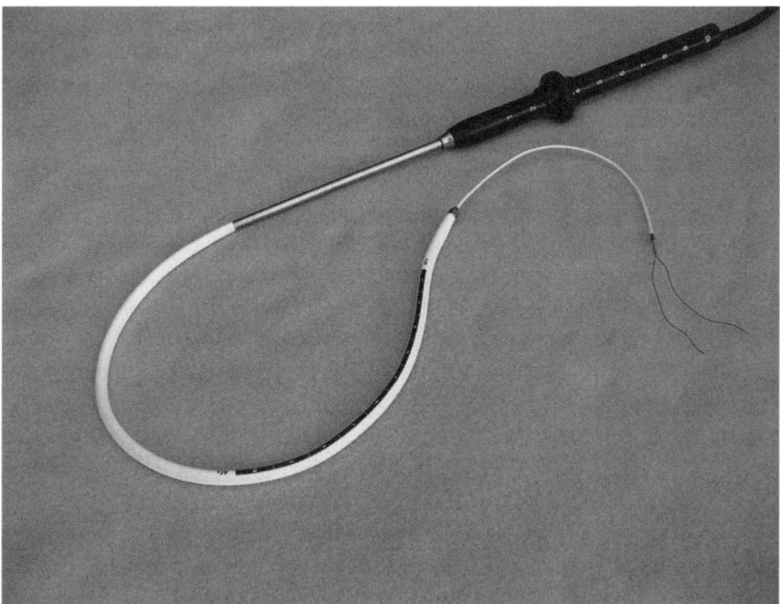

Figure 10 Flex-10™ microwave ablation device. *Source*: Photo courtesy of Guidant Corp., Fremont, California, U.S.A.

then created by amputating the right atrial appendage and creating a linear lesion from its base to the tricuspid valve annulus. Through a second lateral right atriotomy, additional lesions are created cranially into the superior vena cava and caudally into the inferior vena cava. Another lesion is drawn from the atriotomy to the posterior segment of the tricuspid valve annulus. Finally, a lesion line is created from the edge of the atriotomy, traversing the fossa ovalis and the isthmus into the coronary sinus and down into the inferior vena cava. Under cardioplegic arrest left-sided endocardial lesions are created via a transverse left atriotomy. These consist of a linear lesion connecting the base of the amputated left atrial appendage and the box lesion and another connecting lesion between the box lesion and mitral annulus near the P3 posterior leaflet segment.

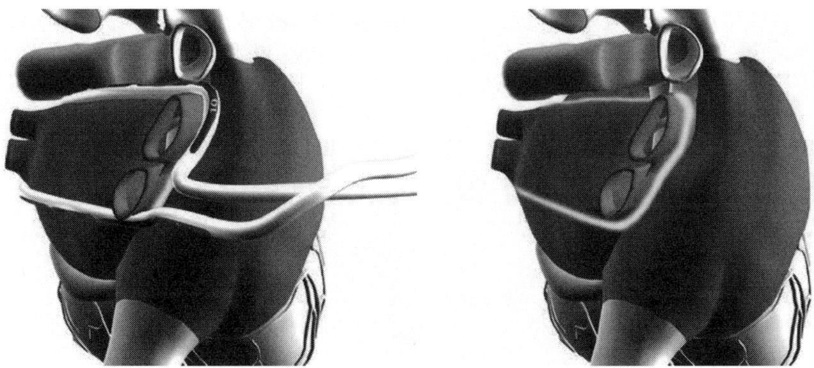

Figure 11 Creation of "box" lesion around pulmonary veins with the Flex-10™ microwave ablation device. *Source*: Photo courtesy of Guidant Corp., Fremont, California, U.S.A.

Most recently, the Guidant microwave ablation system has been used in the development of minimally-invasive approaches to atrial fibrillation ablation. Standard thoracoscopic- and robotic-based approaches are undergoing early trials.

Medtronic Cardioblate® Radiofrequency Ablation Device

The Medtronic Cardioblate® device (Medtronic, Minneapolis, MN) is based on a unipolar surgical ablation pen which is used to apply radiofrequency energy (484.2 kHz) to the endocardial surface. A grounding indifferent electrode is placed behind the right shoulder of the patient. Continuous saline irrigation is used to cool the surface of the treated endocardium. Lesions are created by repeated stroking (about 10 oscillations) of the endocardium with the pen. Both left- and right-sided lesions, as described above, can be created on the endocardial surface under cardiopulmonary bypass and cardioplegic arrest (30).

AtriCure Radiofrequency Ablation Device

The AtriCure ablation device (AtriCure Inc., Cincinnati, OH) delivers radiofrequency energy between two closely approximated 5 cm × 1 mm electrodes embedded in the jaws of a specially designed clamp (Fig. 12). A useful feature of this bipolar device is the ability to measure the drop in conduction of the tissue clamped between the two electrodes, confirming transmural ablation. Furthermore, the delivered energy is quite focused, resulting in discrete thin lesions (1 to 3 mm wide) with minimal collateral tissue injury. This characteristic may diminish the risk of extensive scarring which might otherwise lead to pulmonary vein stenosis or injury to other structures (e.g., valve leaflets, coronary sinus).

Damiano and colleagues have described the use of the AtriCure device in performing a modified Cox Maze atrial fibrillation ablation in conjunction with mitral valve surgery (31). Briefly, the technique is performed through a median sternotomy on normothermic cardiopulmonary bypass. With the heart empty and beating, the right and left pulmonary veins are each clamped with the AtriCure device and encircling lesions are created (Fig. 13). For the right-sided lesions, a small incision is made in the midpoint of the right atrial appendage and extended superiorly up to the atrioventricular groove. One jaw of the AtriCure device is placed through this incision and a lesion is created along the right atrial-free wall. A separate vertical right atriotomy is created approximately 2 cm from the

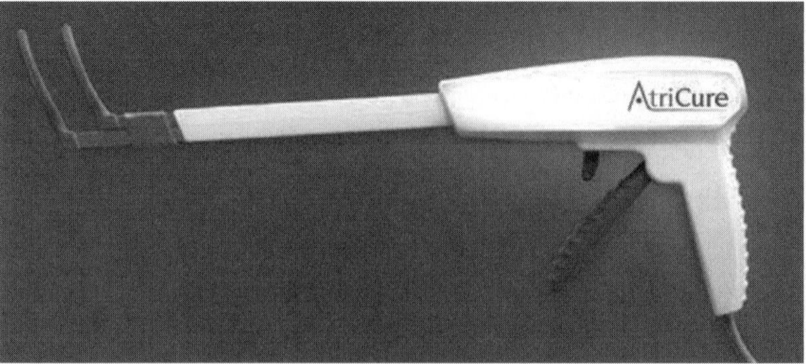

Figure 12 AtriCure radiofrequency ablation device. *Source*: Photo courtesy of AtriCure Inc., Cincinnati, Ohio, U.S.A.

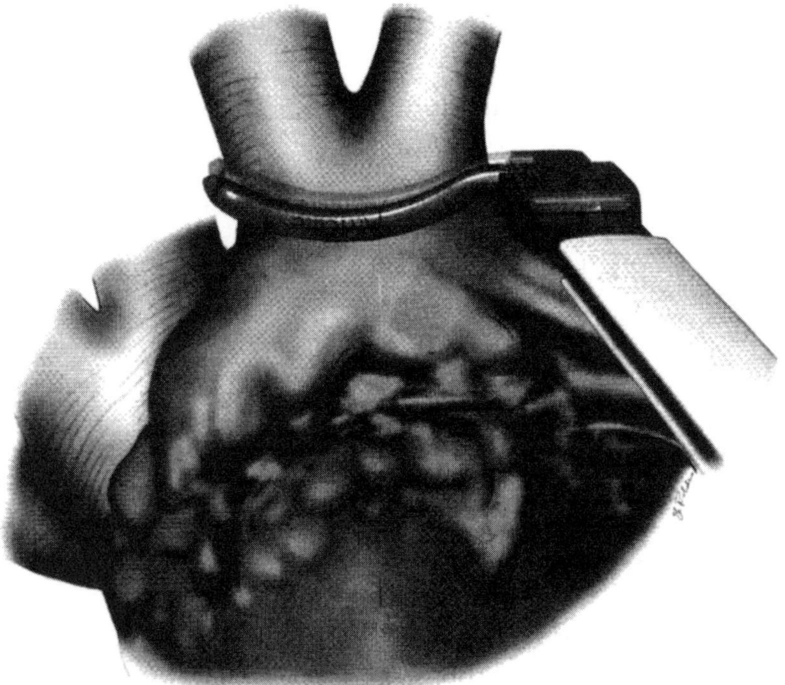

Figure 13 Left pulmonary vein isolation using the AtriCure bipolar radiofrequency ablation device. *Source*: From Ref. 31.

just created free wall ablation line and extended to the atrioventricular groove and inferiorly down toward the intraatrial septum. Four separate ablation lines are then created with the AtriCure device, with two extending to the tricuspid annulus, one extending towards the superior vena cava, and another one extending down towards the inferior vena cava. For the left-sided lesions, a standard transverse left atriotomy is created and a transseptal ablation line is created with the AtriCure device across the atrial septum onto the fossa ovalis. Another lesion is created extending from the atrioventricular groove to the mitral annulus. Mitral valve repair or replacement is then performed, the left atrial appendage is amputated, and a final left-sided lesion is created between the base of the appendage and the left superior pulmonary vein.

Wolf et al. at the University of Cincinnati have recently described an alternative off-pump ablative technique. Referred to as the Wolf "Mini-Maze," this technique is predicated on placing the AtriCure device around the right and left pulmonary veins through bilateral mini-thoracotomy incisions, guided by a videoscope placed through a separate thoracoport. The videoscope affords reasonable visualization, obviating the need to spread the ribs with a retractor; soft-tissue retractors are used instead. The left atrial appendage is also stapled off through the left mini-thoracotomy. Early results are promising with this attenuated approach.

Clinical Results

In a comparison of the Guidant and Medtronic ablation devices, Wisser et al. noted a similar successful conversion rate of around 80% when the devices were used to create biatrial Cox Maze III lesions in patients with chronic persistent atrial fibrillation (30). In all of these patients, ablation was performed in conjunction with valvular surgery. The authors noted an incidence of atrioventricular block of 13.6% and 10.5% with the Guidant and Medtronic devices, respectively, and postulated that this relatively high rate was due to lesion lines which ran close to the atrioventricular node.

In 43 cases using the AtriCure radiofrequency ablation device, Damiano et al. describe 91% of patients in sinus rhythm at six months with ten patients still on antiarrhythmics (31). Furthermore, follow-up MRI studies showed no evidence of pulmonary vein stenosis and preserved atrial contractility in all patients.

CARDIAC RESTRAINT DEVICES: THE ACORN CORCAP® DEVICE

Ventricular dilatation is a late manifestation of early compensatory structural changes encountered in heart failure. However, dilatation results in increased ventricular wall stress, myocyte overstretching, a less efficient spherical geometry and, in many cases, significant atrioventricular valve insufficiency which exacerbates volume overload. These macrostructural changes lead to debilitating congestive symptoms, are clearly associated with an increased mortality risk, and often are not adequately treated by medical therapies. The Acorn CorCap® cardiac support device (CSD; Acorn Cardiovascular Inc., St. Paul, MN) is an implantable passive mesh restraint that is surgically wrapped around the heart and fitted to provide circumferential diastolic support (Fig. 14). The CSD is designed to reduce end-diastolic ventricular wall stress and myocyte overstretching as well as volume overload dynamics. In doing so, it is thought that the compensatory remodeling processes leading to end-stage dilatation and dysfunction may be halted, ameliorated, or reversed.

The CSD consists of a polyester fabric mesh knitted in such a way to maximize flexibility, strength, and durability. Its bidirectional compliance profile is designed to emphasize circumferential versus apical-basal support to promote a more ellipsoid ventricular conformation. Patients appropriate for CSD implantation are adults suffering from systolic ventricular dysfunction and dilatation resulting in New York Heart Association (NYHA) functional class III or IV heart failure, despite optimal medical management.

Implantation

The CSD can be implanted with or without cardiopulmonary bypass, depending on whether concomitant cardiac procedures are anticipated. Through a sternotomy, the pericardium is opened and the left ventricular diameter is measured at the mid-papillary muscle level using transesophageal echocardiography. The heart's circumferential and base-to-apex dimensions are then measured and used to select one of six CSD sizes. The CSD is then wrapped around the ventricles, positioning the hemline of the device above or just below the atrioventricular groove. A series of interrupted 4–0 polypropylene sutures are used to secure the device around the base of the heart. A snug fit is desired, but not so much as to reduce the left ventricular diameter by more than 10%. This CSD sizing strategy is intended to relieve ventricular wall stress and myocyte stretching.

Clinical Results

Oz et al. describes a prospective case-control series of 48 patients with dilated ischemic or idiopathic dilated cardiomyopathy who underwent implantation of the CorCap device, of

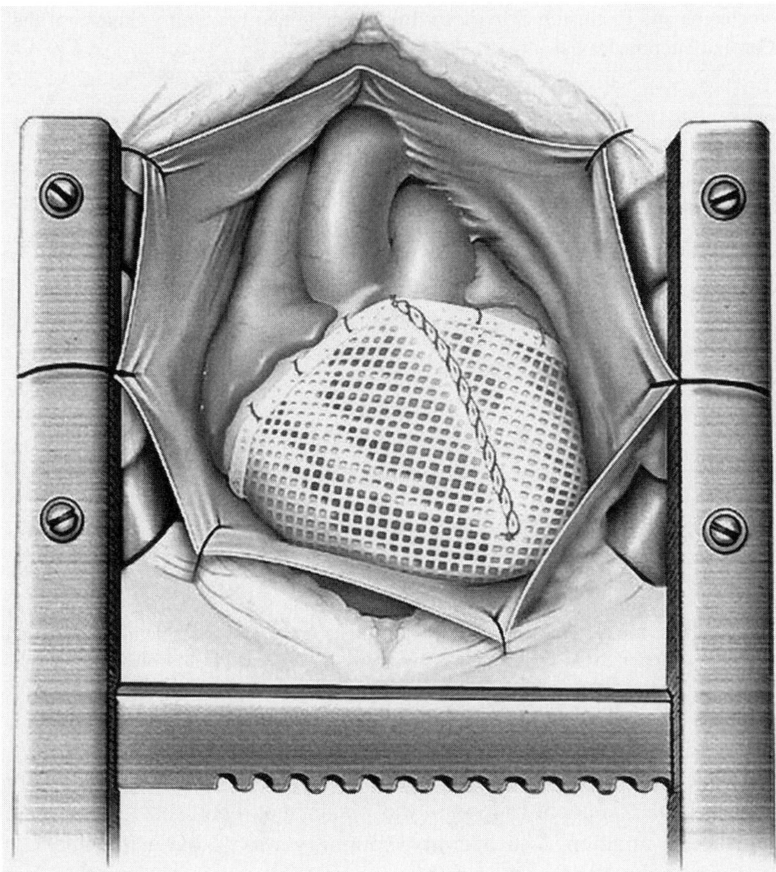

Figure 14 The Acorn CorCap® cardiac support device. The device is an implantable passive mesh restraint that is surgically wrapped around the heart and fitted to provide circumferential diastolic support. *Source*: From Ref. 32.

Table 2 Operative Times for Robot-Assisted Mitral Valve Repairs[a]

Variable	First 10 cases	Last 15 cases	*p* Value
Total OR time (min)	318.5	275.1	0.003
Procedure time (min)	209.9	192.2	0.345
CPB time (min)	137.2	119.5	0.093
Cross clamp time (min)	97.6	81.1	0.050
Leaflet repair (min)	26.2	15.6	0.001
Annuloplasty ring (min)	31.9	24.8	0.007
LOS (days)	4.2	1.67	0.043

Initial cases versus current experience. Note the reduced times over the last 15 cases versus the first 10 cases (n=25)

[a] Mean values.

Abbreviations: CPB, cardiopulmonary bypass; LOS, length of stay; OR, operating room.

Source: From Ref. 6.

Table 3 Major Inclusion and Exclusion Criteria for Initial Safety and Feasibility Studies of the Acorn CorCap® Cardiac Support Device

Inclusion	Exclusion
Dilated cardiomyopathy: ischemic or nonischemic	Current or anticipated need for LVAD or total artificial heart
Stable and optimal medical management	Likelihood of existing cardiothoracic adhesions preventing proper device placement
Adult (18–80 yr)	Patent CABG
Indexed LVEDD $\geq$30 mm/mm^2	NYHA IV dependent on intravenous inotropes
LVEF $\leq$35% or LVEF$\leq$45% for CSD valve surgery	NYHA IV dependent on intravenous inotropes
History of NYHA III or early stage IV	Late-stage heart failure with increased surgical risk
Acceptable renal function (creatinine $<$3.5 ml/dL), hepatic function (SGOT and SGPT $<2 \times$ normal), pulmonary function (FEV$_1$$>$1.5 L)	Acute myocardial infarction within 3 mo Hemodynamically unstable or uncontrolled arrhythmias Comorbid condition with life expectance $<$2 yr

Major inclusion and exclusion criteria.
Abbreviations: SGOT, aspartate aminotransferase; SGPT, alanine aminotransferase; FEV$_1$, forced expiratory volume in 1 sec; LVAD, left ventricular assist device; CABG, coronary artery bypass grafting; LVEF, left ventricular ejection fraction; NYHA, New York Heart Association; LVEDD, left ventricular end diastolic dimension.
Source: From Ref. 32.

whom 33 received concomitant cardiac surgery (32). Inclusion and exclusion criteria for this study are listed in Table 2. Patient follow-up was obtained at three, six, 12, and 18 to 24 months after CSD implantation. The operative mortality was 16.6% with nine late deaths including several not related to heart failure (i.e., malignancy in two patients and prosthetic valve thrombosis); other etiologies included pneumonia, ventricular arrhythmia, recurrent mitral insufficiency, and cerebral hemorrhage. Among the total of 17 deaths in the series, five occurred in patients with ischemic cardiomyopathy and 12 in patients with an idiopathic etiology. There were no intraoperative device-related complications.

In this study, the actuarial survival was 73% at 12 months and 68% at 24 months. In patients implanted with the CSD, ventricular chamber dimensions decreased and left ventricular ejection fraction and NYHA class were improved among patients receiving the CSD with or without concomitant cardiac operations). There was an observed trend towards increased left-ventricular end-diastolic pressure (LVEDP) in the untreated, control group and a decrease in LVEDP in the treatment group. There were no device-related adverse events or evidence of constrictive pathophysiology, and coronary artery flow reserve was maintained. More definitive clinical results with the CorCap device are still pending.

REFERENCES

1. Rose EA, Gelijns AC, Moskowitz AJ, et al. Long-term use of a left ventricular assist device for end-stage heart failure. NEJM 2001; 345:1435–1443.
2. Hunt SA. Comment—the REMATCH trial: Long-term use of a left ventricular assist device for end-stage heart failure. J Card Fail 2002; 8:59–60.

3. Stevens JH, Burdon TA, Siegel LC, et al. Port-access coronary artery bypass with cardioplegic arrest: acute and chronic canine studies. Ann Thorac Surg 1996; 62:435–440.
4. Loulmet D, Carpentier A, D'Attellis N, et al. Endoscopic coronary artery bypass grafting with the aid of robot-assisted instruments. J Thorac Cardiovasc Surg 1999; 118:4–10.
5. Mohr FW, Falk V, Diegeler A, et al. Computer-enhanced "robotic" cardiac surgery: experience in 148 patients. J Thorac Cardiovasc Surg 2001; 121:842–853.
6. Bonatti J, Schachner T, Bernecker O, et al. Robotic totally endoscopic coronary artery bypass: Program development and learning curve issues. JTCVS 127 2004; 127:504–510.
7. Cohn LH, Adams DH, Couper GS, et al. Minimally invasive cardiac valve surgery improves patient satisfaction while reducing costs of cardiac valve replacement and repair. Ann Thorac Surg 1997; 226:421–428.
8. Cosgrove DM, Sabik JF, Navis JL. Minimally invasive valve operations. Ann Thorac Surg 1998; 65:1535–1539.
9. Tatooles AJ, Pappas PS, Gordon PJ, Slaughter MS. Minimally invasive mitral valve repair using the da Vinci robotic system. Ann Thorac Surg 2004; 77:1978–1984.
10. Chitwood WR, Nifong LW, Elbeery JE, et al. Robotic mitral valve repair: trapezoidal resection and prosthetic annuloplasty with the da Vinci surgical system. J Thorac Cardiovasc Surg 2000; 120:1171–1172.
11. Nifong LW, Chu VF, Bailey BM, et al. Robotic mitral valve repair: experience with the da Vinci system. Ann Thorac Surg 2003; 75:438–443.
12. de Vaumas C, Philip I, Daccache G, et al. Comparison of minithoracotomy and conventional sternotomy approaches for valve surgery. J Cardiothorac Vasc Anesth 2003; 17:325–328.
13. Gulbins H, Pritisanac A, Hannekum A. Minimally invasive heart valve surgery: already established in clinical routine? Expert Rev Cardiovasc Ther 2004; 2:837–843.
14. Farwell D, Patel N, Hall A, Ralph S, Sulke A. How many people with heart failure are appropriate for biventricular resynchronization? Eur Heart J 2000; 21:1246–1250.
15. Shamim W, Francis DP, Yousufuddin M, et al. Intraventricular conduction delay: a prognostic marker in chronic heart failure. Int J Cardiol 1999; 70:171–178.
16. Littman L, Symanski JD. Hemodynamic implications of left bundle branch block. J Electrocardiol 2000; 33:113–121.
17. Abraham WT, Fischer WG, Smith AL. Cardiac resynchronization in chronic heart failure. NEJM 2002; 346:1845–1853.
18. Cazeau S, LeClerq C, Lavergne T, et al. Effects of multisite biventricular pacing in patients with heart failure and intraventricular conduction delay. NEJM 2001; 344:873–880.
19. DeRose JJ, Ashton RC, Belsley S, et al. Robotically assisted left ventricular epicardial lead implantation for biventricular pacing. JACC 2003; 41:1414–1419.
20. Butter C, Auricchio A, Stellbrink C, et al. Effect of resynchronization therapy stimulation site on the systolic function of heart failure patients. Circulation 2001; 104:3026–3029.
21. Burkhoff D, Schmidt S, Schulman SP, et al. Transmyocardial revascularization compared with continued medical therapy for treatment of refractory angina pectoris. Lancet 1999; 354:885–890.
22. Allen KB, Dowling RD, Fudge TL, et al. Comparison of transmyocardial revascularization with medical therapy in patients with refractory angina. NEJM 1999; 341:1029–1036.
23. Aaberge L, Nordstrand K, Dragsund M, et al. Transmyocardial revascularization with CO2 laser in patients with refractory angina pectoris. J Am Coll Cardiol 2000; 35:1170–1177.
24. Frazier OH, March RJ, Horvath KA. Transmyocardial revascularization with a carbon dioxide laser in patients with end-stage coronary disease. NEJM 1999; 341:1021–1028.
25. Schofeld PM, Sharples LD, Caine N, et al. Transmyocardial revascularization in patients with refractory angina: a randomized controlled trial. Lancet 1999; 353:519–524.
26. Allen KB, Dowling RD, Angell WW. Transmyocardial revascularization: 5-year follow-up of a prospective, randomized multicenter trial. Ann Thorac Surg 2004; 77:1228–1234.
27. Yuh, D.D., Simon, B.A., Fernandez, A., Ramey, N., Baumgartner, W.A., Totally endoscopic robot-assisted transmyocardial revascularization. J Thorac Cardiovasc Surg in press 2005; 130: 120–121.

28. Cox JL, Boineau JP, Schuessler RB, Kater KM, Lappas DG. Five-year experience with the Maze procedure for atrial fibrillation. Ann Thorac Surg 2005; 56:814–824.
29. Cox JL, Schuessler RB, Lappas DG, Boineau JP. An 8 1/2 year clinical experience with surgery for atrial fibrillation. Ann Surg 1996; 224:267–275.
30. Wisser W, Khazen C, Deviatko E, et al. Microwave and radiofrequency ablation ield similar success rates for treatment of chronic atrial fibrillation. Eur J Cardiothor Surg 2004; 25:1011–1025.
31. Damiano RJ, Gaynor SL. Atrial fibrillation ablation during mitral valve surgery using the Atricure device. Op Tech Thorac Cardiovasc Surg 2004; 9:24–33.
32. Oz M, Konertz WF, Kleber FX, et al. Global surgical experience with the Acorn cardiac support device. JTCVS 2003; 126:983–991.

36
Device and Alternative Therapies in Pediatric Heart Failure

Leslie B. Smoot and Ravi Thiagarajan
Department of Cardiology, Harvard Medical School, Children's Hospital, Boston, Massachusetts, U.S.A.

Jane E. Crosson
Pediatric Cardiology, The Johns Hopkins Hospital, Baltimore, Maryland, U.S.A.

INTRODUCTION

Unique aspects of end stage heart failure in children center around the diversity of underlying disease presenting in infancy and childhood, whether in the form of congenital cardiac malformation or cardiomyopathy. Device experience in children and young adults with advanced heart disease is less extensive than in adults, but a considerable knowledge base is developing nonetheless. Common to all these therapies are concerns about long-term effects in the growing and developing child, who may experience a many-fold increase in body size after therapy, and has a life expectancy significantly longer than the majority of adult patients receiving similar therapies. Challenges arise in attempting to "retrofit" adult therapies for pediatric patients who display important developmental differences in size, configuration, and physiologic response of the heart and vasculature. Etiologies of pediatric heart failure and cardiomyopathy also differ dramatically from those commonly encountered in adults. Therefore, some aspects of such therapy are unique to children and to those with congenital heart disease; these features will be the focus of this section.

UNIQUE ASPECTS OF PEDIATRIC HEART FAILURE AND DEVICE USE

Etiologies of myocardial failure in pediatric patients are primarily congenital heart disease with acute post-operative decompensation, acute or chronic congestive heart failure (CHF), and primary cardiomyopathy occurring at any age (1). In contrast, myocardial failure in the adult population often occurs in the setting of primary or secondary coronary vascular disease. There is a distinct paucity of coronary disease in pediatrics, the exceptions being Kawasaki Disease, anomalous origin of the left coronary artery arising from the pulmonary artery, dyslipidemias, and post-transplant coronary allograft vasculopathy (2).

Size differences in the pediatric patients provide the most obvious and predictable limitation to device utilization of all types, whether pacemaker, implantable defibrillator (ICD), ventricular assist devices (VADs), or extracorporeal membrane oxygenation (ECMO) machines. Limitations in miniaturizing of pulsatile flow devices for prolonged use in infants and small children affects the type and duration of support available to this group, and overall morbidity and mortality (3,4).

Cardiac malformations complicate treatment of myocardial dysfunction in approximately half of all pediatric patients with heart failure. Complex intracardiac disease, unusual vascular anatomy, and single ventricle physiology often influence treatment options in ways that are unique to this population and do not easily lend themselves to large randomized treatment protocols. Despite these limitations, there has been remarkable progress over the past decade, reflected in enhanced survival of children with acute and refractory myocardial failure.

Prognosis for ventricular failure in the pediatric age group is highly dependent on accurate diagnosis. It is especially important to identify potentially correctable anatomic factors in patients with congenital heart disease (CHD). Underlying genetic and metabolic abnormalities are often important in those with cardiomyopathy presenting in infancy or childhood (5). Potential for recovery of ventricular function is greatest in infants, independent of the underlying cause.

Implications and even definitions of success of heart failure therapies are often age dependent. Success in achieving "normal" quality of life may be dependent on both physical and psychological effects of therapeutic interventions, as well as the developmental stages at which interventions take place. Unlike interventions performed in older adults, success may not be defined by short-and medium-term results, due to unforeseen ramifications that may present decades later. For example, successful cardiac transplantation in childhood may offer excellent palliation through adolescence, but may entail significant morbidity and mortality in young adulthood (6).

ELECTROPHYSIOLOGY: CATHETER ABLATION AND DEVICE THERAPY

Rhythm disturbances occur primarily in the setting of complex congenital heart disease, either prior to or following surgical repair, or with primary myocardial diseases affecting the conduction system. Unlike the adult population, there are very few pediatric patients with typical findings of LV dysfunction with normal cardiac anatomy. The small size of pediatric patients significantly alters both the type and duration of virtually all therapeutic options including ablation, pacemakers, ICDs, and cardiac resynchronization therapy (CRT). Risk/benefit ratios take into account the possible need for open chest procedure for epicardial lead placement, and morbidity of implanted systems from pocket infection, lead placement compromising AV valve function or coronary sinus venous return, inappropriate defibrillation, and iatrogenic arrhythmia. Adult data cannot be applied directly to a heterogeneous pediatric population with unique cardiovascular anatomy and physiology. This heterogeneity also severely limits our ability to conduct large randomized trials to evaluate such therapies, a research tool which has dramatically altered management practices in the world of adult cardiology.

Catheter Ablation Therapy

The first reports of radiofrequency catheter ablation in pediatrics began to appear in 1991 (7). Early on, most ablations were performed for "medically-refractory" or life-threatening tachycardia, but as experience grew, less symptomatic patients began to choose ablation, according to data from the Pediatric Radiofrequency Catheter Ablation Registry (8). Although uncommon, ablation in tachycardia-induced cardiomyopathy remains an important indication. These ablations almost invariably are for atrial tachycardia or the so-called "permanent form of junctional reciprocating tachycardia" (PJRT), the primary causes of tachycardia-induced heart failure in children. It is not uncommon for such children to be referred for heart transplantation for cardiomyopathy, but once the causative role of the arrhythmia is recognized, ablative therapy can be performed and is curative in most cases. Walsh (9) reported an early ablation experience in 12 children with incessant ectopic atrial tachycardia and ventricular dysfunction. Ablation was successful in 11/12, with the 12th patient referred for surgery.

In the NASPE expert consensus conference on radiofrequency catheter ablation in children, supraventricular tachycardia associated with ventricular dysfunction is listed as one of the few Class I indications for catheter ablation (10). Success rates for atrial ectopic tachycardia in historical Registry cases were close to 90% regardless of age, and complication rates have been low at 2–4% (11). However, catheter ablation therapy has been limited in very young children by overall higher complication rates in patients under 4 yr old in the Registry data, and by animal data suggesting that lesion size can increase over time (12) and that coronary artery damage may be more likely in the immature heart (13).

Catheter ablative therapy has been applied for other pediatric heart failure indications, primarily to ablate the AV node in cases of intractable atrial tachycardia and for ablation of re-entry atrial tachycardia in patients with congenital heart disease. Results in the later category have been mixed, with long-term success rates of approximately 50% (14). Often multiple attempts are required. Some groups have had very good results with surgical maze procedures associated with revision of the Fontan pathway in selected patients with single ventricle physiology and atrial tachycardia. Mavroudis, et al (15) have shown significant improvement in functional class following this combined therapy.

Implantable Cardioverter Defibrillator Therapy

With the advent of smaller devices and better lead technology, and recognition of the life-saving abilities of the ICD, there has been increased utilization of these devices in pediatrics. Initial reports were limited to older children and teenagers being treated for secondary prevention (16), but currently therapy is being extended to younger patients, as well as for primary prevention in cardiomyopathy patients. Implantation of devices can be challenging in very small patients and those with complex heart disease (Fig. 1), often requiring a creative and/or combined transvenous and epicardial approach, and should only be performed in centers with extensive experience in such cases.

In the largest single-center pediatric study yet published, Alexander, et al (17) reported ICD implantation in 76 children and young adults, ages 1–30 yr old. Congenital heart disease was present in 42%, primary electrical disease in 33%, and hypertrophic or dilated cardiomyopathy in the remainder. Transvenous implantation

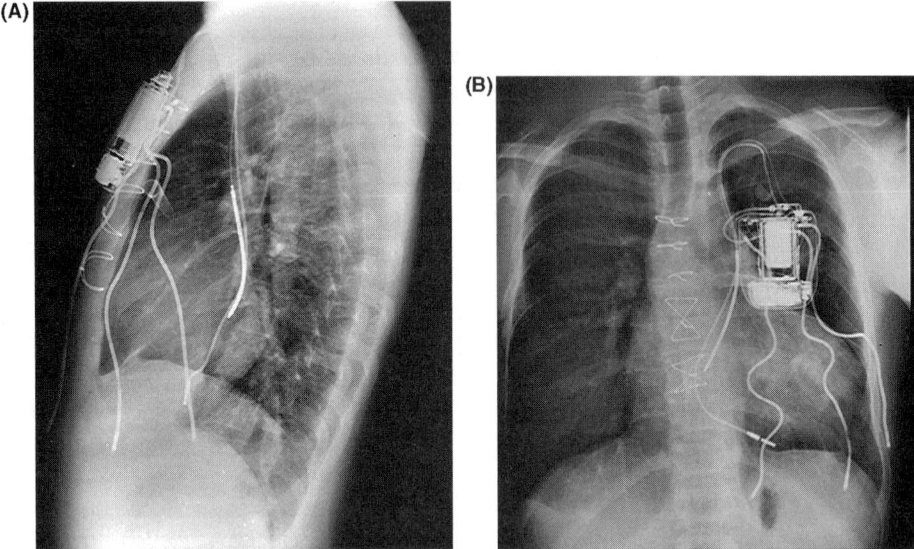

Figure 1 Novel lead configuration for an implantable cardioverter defibrillator. Anteroposterior (**A**) and lateral (**B**) chest roentgenograms of an 18-yr-old patient with tetralogy of Fallot and a prosthetic tricuspid valve, in whom a subcutaneous array and placement of the pace-sense lead in coronary sinus via the persistent left superior vena cava were utilized to avoid epicardial lead placement.

was accomplished in 93%; the remainder required either a subcutaneous array or epicardial patches. Appropriate therapy was delivered in 28% of patients overall, and in 33% of those with dilated cardiomyopathy. Of note were high rates of both lead failure (21%) and inappropriate therapy (25%), an experience widely shared in pediatric centers. In the 2004 study by Korte, et al. (18) even higher rates of both appropriate and inappropriate discharges were found. They reported 20 children with ICDs implanted for secondary prevention or syncope. Appropriate discharges occurred in 15 (75%) of the patients and inappropriate therapies in 10 (50%). Overall, there were 1.5 appropriate and 1.3 inappropriate therapies per patient-year of follow-up. Inappropriate therapies were primarily due to sinus or supraventricular tachycardia.

Although the current recommendations for prophylactic ICD placement in adult patients with heart failure are well-recognized, pediatric cardiologists have been slower to move in this direction due to this perceived increased morbidity of ICD therapy in children, technical difficulties, and lack of complete data on efficacy. The relatively high rate of appropriate therapy in the cardiomyopathy patients perhaps reflects greater utilization of defibrillator therapy for secondary rather than primary prevention in these patients.

Just as in adult patients, ICD implantation has been found to be a useful bridge to transplant. Dubin, et al (19) reported a multicenter study of 28 pediatric patients awaiting orthotopic heart transplantation who had an ICD. Age at implant ranged from 11 mo to 21 yr. Most ($n=22$) had cardiomyopathy; six had congenital heart disease. Only five patients received an ICD prophylactically with no documented arrhythmia, syncope or sudden death event. Thirteen patients (46%) had appropriate discharges at a mean of 7 mo after implant. Inappropriate discharges occurred in 25% of patients. Twenty-two patients had been transplanted by the conclusion of the study, while two had died, both of electromechanical dissociation.

Bradycardia Therapy

In this age of cardiac resynchronization, ventricular pacing for bradycardia increasingly is being recognized as a potential causative agent of heart failure. However, it must be acknowledged that many patients benefit greatly from the restoration of AV synchrony and maintenance of a normal heart rate. Most patients with congenital or surgically-acquired heart block do well for decades with dual-chamber or even single-chamber pacing.

This patient population does pose unique technical challenges, however. Even those with "uncomplicated" congenital heart block will require several pacing systems in their lifetimes, and will experience a many-fold increase in body size before they reach adulthood. Maintenance of venous access is essential, and necessitates careful consideration of when to convert from epicardial to transvenous systems, when to implant two leads, and when to extract existing leads. Increasingly novel approaches such as femoral access (20) are being explored.

Adding congenital heart disease to the equation injects further complexity into pacing decisions. Many of these patients, primarily those with single ventricles, must rely partially or exclusively on epicardial pacing. A recent study on adults with congenital heart disease requiring pacing revealed a high rate of lead-related complications (27%) and difficulty with venous access in 15% of patients (21). Long-term epicardial pacing has been made somewhat easier by the development of steroid-eluting leads, which have shown improved performance over nonsteroid leads (22). However, these suture-on leads can be difficult to implant in some patients due to pericardial thickening from previous cardiac surgery.

THERAPEUTIC CIRCULATORY SUPPORT MODALITIES

Factors influencing adequate circulatory support in the failing ventricle include those which: (1) enhance oxygen and nutrient delivery to the tissues and/or reduce metabolic demands of the body and (2) facilitate clearance of CO2, lactate, and other waste products (23). While primary efforts are directed at augmenting cardiac output in the patient with end-stage CHF, additional measures that reduce cardiac work or metabolic demands cannot be overlooked in management of the pediatric patient. Such measures may include hypothermia, continuous positive airway pressure (CPAP/BIPAP), or mechanical ventilation with appropriate sedation (24,25).

As with adults, acute cardiac failure or signs of inadequate circulation despite maximal medical therapy form the primary indications for direct mechanical circulatory support (1). These include progressive end-organ dysfunction, altered mental status, and rising lactate or metabolic acidosis despite maximal inotropic and indirect forms of cardiovascular support. In the pediatric population, primary indications for mechanical circulatory support vary significantly with age. Hypoxia is often associated with ventricular failure in neonatal and pediatric patients and, in combination with patient size and technical constraints, influence the type of support utilized (26).

Mechanical Cardiopulmonary Support

Extracorporeal Membrane Oxygenation

While an increasing variety of devices are being employed in pediatric patients, the primary modality used to date has been non-pulsatile flow support using ECMO. The ability of

ECMO to provide simultaneous cardiac and respiratory support in settings of refractory hypoxia, biventricular failure, pulmonary hypertension, or complex congenital heart disease accounts partially for its widespread use in pediatrics (27). Considerable experience was gained in its early use for primary neonatal and pediatric respiratory failure, followed by increasing utilization for pediatric (and adult) patients with primary cardiac failure (28,29). Additional factors leading to its widespread use in pediatrics include: the ability of ECMO to be employed rapidly following cardiac arrest, potential for peripheral cannulation, and its potential effectiveness in patients with complex intracardiac malformations and/or shunts (30). Today, ECMO is the most commonly used form of pediatric circulatory support, and is generally available in institutions with pediatric surgical and ICU familiarity with cardiac bypass.

Extracorporeal membrane oxygenation circuits are composed of an oxygenator, a pump, and a heat exchanger (23,31). Cannulation may be transthoracic (venous cannula in the right atrial appendage and arterial in the ascending aorta), or peripheral, utilizing the neck or femoral vessels. Intracardiac malformations and/or single ventricle physiology often require modifications of the standard approach to ensure adequate perfusion of the head, viscera, and extremities. Venous decompression is equally as important and often complicated in patients with congenital heart disease or prior vascular interventions. The importance of left atrial decompression has been recognized in ECMO patients with severe LV dysfunction who may not be able to eject even a small amount of blood returning from pulmonary veins. This often entails placement of an additional catheter in the left atrium (either surgically or via catheterization).

Limitations due to the need for small cannulae, small ventricular stroke volumes, and adequate anticoagulation issues (secondary to large artificial surface area to which blood is exposed), have had to be overcome in order to make ECMO feasible in a range of pediatric patients.

Extracorporeal membrane oxygenation is optimally used on a short term basis (<10–14 days) when there is potential for recovery of ventricular function or potential for bridging to transplantation.

In the Children's Hospital Boston (CHB) experience, recovery of cardiac function within 72 hr on ECMO support is an indicator of subsequent successful weaning from mechanical support.

ECMO as a Bridge to Transplant

As explained above, ECMO is currently the primary modality used to provide mechanical support in pediatric patients. Its ability to function in bridging to transplant those pediatric patients with irrecoverable ventricular dysfunction is limited by several factors including end-organ dysfunction, infection, coagulopathy associated with circuit, and central nervous system injury (32,33,34).

If long-term ventricular support is necessary, transition to a VAD may be attempted (28). Thiagarajan (35) reports 54% of patients receiving mechanical support underwent successful cardiac transplantation at Children's Hospital, Boston. Table 1 summarizes experience of multiple single pediatric centers involved in the utilization of ECMO in bridging patients to cardiac transplantation.

Patients under one year of age and patients with structural heart disease are less likely to be successfully bridged to cardiac transplantation (36). This may be due in part to the paucity of available ventricular support devices for patients weighing less than 15 kg. Regional differences in infant donor organ resources and thus wait times for this age

Table 1 Selected Single-Center Pediatric Experience in Transplantation from Extracorporeal Membrane Oxygenation

Center	Gajarski (32) Ann Arbor, MI	Kirshbom (2) Philadelphia, PA	Levi (29) UCLA[a], CA	Thiagarajan (35) Boston, MA
Period	1991–2001 (10 yr)	1994–2000 (6 yr)	1995–2001 (5 yr)	1992–2003 (11 yr)
Listed	21	31	17	39
Weaned	4 (20%)	6 (19%)	2 (17%)	5 (13%)
Transplanted	11 (57%)	11 (35%)	11 (58%)	19 (49%)
Survive to discharge	9 (82%)	11 (100%)	10 (91%)	15 (79%)

[a]UCLA, University of California, Los Angeles.

group may also account for poor success in the <1 yr age group. Strategies to optimize transplantation rates this group of patients includes using ABO-incompatible donors and/or continued development of ventricular support devices suitable for these patients.

In older children, transition from ECMO to a VAD support and subsequent successful transplantation is possible, more closely resembling outcomes in adults (27). In several centers, long-term survival outcomes are not different for patients receiving mechanical support prior to transplantation, as compared to those who did not (6).

VADs in Pediatrics

Utilization of VADs, including either single or biventricular assistance without oxygenation, has been limited by size and physiology in the pediatric age group. Intra-aortic balloon pumps (IABPs) and a variety of pulsatile ventricular support devices (VADs) have been successfully used in adults.

Intraortic balloon counterpulsation has been employed in a relatively small number of pediatric patients in recent decades. A variety of factors account for this, including difficulty obtaining and inserting appropriate balloon sizes, achieving optimal timing of device, and assessing effectiveness. Perhaps the single most cited drawback to use of IABP in children has been its diminished effectiveness due to increased aortic compliance and small aortic dimensions in young children as compared to adults (37,38).

Neither has the majority of pediatric patients in need been able to realize the benefits of long term VAD support enjoyed by their adult counterparts, whether extracorporeal or fully implantable, devices designed for adult use cannot be employed for individuals with BSA under 1.5 square meters or approximately 40 kg. Pulsatile devices such as the Heartmate/TCI are typically utilized for isolated left ventricular support with either pneumatic or electrically driven circuits, and implantable pumps with cannulation of the LV apex and ascending aorta. Characteristics limiting use in children include both size of the implantable pump, and minimal flows at >3 L/min. Physical constraints often prohibit abdominal implantation in pediatric patients despite adequate weight.

Recently, both single and biventricular support for pediatric patients has been expanded with the development of the Berlin heart, a pneumatically driven, paracorporeal device initially developed in 1992 (39). Its use in infants and children is made possible by the availability of pumps with a broad range of stroke volumes from 12 to 80 ml, and with pumping rates up to 140 bpm. Limited, though increasing, use of this device as a bridge to transplant in children with ventricular failure has been encouraging. Eventual decannulation after short-or medium-term therapy may also be possible.

PSYCHOSOCIAL ASPECTS OF ADVANCED HEART DISEASE IN PEDIATRICS

In all age groups there are expected but somewhat unpredictable psychosocial implications of aggressive support. These may be influenced by the duration of therapies, duration and type of any associated disability and the degree to which a "normal" quality of life can be achieved, with marked individuality of responses to adversity (40).

Non-cardiac pathology and natural history of underlying disease may significantly impact long term prognoses, and may be extremely difficult to identify or anticipate at early ages. Signs and symptoms of associated skeletal myopathy, metabolic or mitochondrial disease may be subtle or absent. Syndromic diagnosis with CHD may occur in settings of normal karyotype, and carry significant non-cardiac morbidity not yet clinically apparent.

Other issues that come into play in the psychosocial outcome of pediatric patients utilizing devices in the course of their treatment include the age and developmental stage of the patient, family dynamics, family and community resources, expectations of therapy, and short and long-term success of treatment (41).

There have been concerns about the potential for adverse psychological outcomes in children with ICDs. DeMaso, et al. (41) reported extensive psychological assessments of 20 children with ICDs and found that quality of life was experienced as lower than normal. However, the rate of depression was lower than in adult ICD patients, and no patient met the criteria for anxiety. No differences were found in this small group between patients who had experienced shocks and those who had not. A review of the available data on psychosocial adjustment of young ICD recipients, along with suggestions for intervention, has been provided by Sears et al. (42).

Challenges facing children and their families with end-stage heart failure are complex and continually evolve throughout the lifespan, with or without intervening cardiac transplantation (43). While descriptive data has been gathered for some aspects of pediatric experience in the setting of heart transplantation (44–47), collecting similar information on patients exhibiting a vast diversity of ages, developmental abilities, disease severity, acuity, diagnosis, and prognosis becomes even more difficult.

Defining measures to assess intangibles such as quality of life are further confounded by the fact that parents' perceptions of a child's health often has little correlation to either the child's perception of their disease or to more "objective" measures of disease severity (48). Further work in this area is expected to refine our understanding of these issues, and to assist in shaping treatment strategies that preserve both quantity and quality of life for pediatric heart failure patients.

REFERENCES

1. Duncan BW, et al. Mechanical circulatory support in children with cardiac disease. J Thorac Cardiovasc Surg 1999; 117:529–542.
2. Kirshbom PM, et al. Use of extracorporeal membrane oxygenation in pediatric thoracic organ transplantation. J Thorac Cardiovasc Surg 2002; 123:130–136.
3. Hansell DR. Extracorporeal membrane oxygenation for perinatal and pediatric patients. Respir Care 2003; 48:352–362 discussion 363–6.

4. Boettcher W, et al. Safe minimization of cardiopulmonary bypass circuit volume for complex cardiac surgery in a 3.7 kg neonate. Perfusion 2003; 18:377–379.
5. Schwartz ML, et al. Clinical approach to genetic cardiomyopathy in children. Circulation 1996; 94:2021–2038.
6. Fenton KN, et al. Long-term survival after pediatric cardiac transplantation and postoperative ECMO support. Ann Thorac Surg 2003; 76:843–846 (discussion 847).
7. Van Hare GF, et al. Percutaneous radiofrequency catheter ablation for supraventricular arrhythmias in children. J Am Coll Cardiol 1991; 17:1613–1620.
8. Kugler JD, et al. Radiofrequency catheter ablation for paroxysmal supraventricular tachycardia in children and adolescents without structural heart disease. Pediatric EP society, Radiofrequency catheter ablation registry. Am J Cardiol 1997; 80:1438–1443.
9. Walsh EP, et al. Transcatheter ablation of ectopic atrial tachycardia in young patients using radiofrequency current. Circulation 1992; 86:1138–1146.
10. Friedman RA, et al. NASPE Expert Consensus Conference: Radiofrequency catheter ablation in children with and without congenital heart disease. Report of the writing committee. North American Society of Pacing and Electrophysiology. Pacing Clin Electrophysiol 2002; 25:1000–1017.
11. Kugler JD, et al. Pediatric radiofrequency catheter ablation registry success, fluoroscopy time, and complication rate for supraventricular tachycardia: comparison of early and recent eras. J Cardiovasc Electrophysiol 2002; 13:336–341.
12. Saul JP, et al. Late enlargement of radiofrequency lesions in infant lambs. Implications for ablation procedures in small children. Circulation 1994; 90:492–499.
13. Paul T, et al. Coronary artery involvement early and late after radiofrequency current application in young pigs. Am Heart J 1997; 133:436–440.
14. Triedman JK, et al. Influence of patient factors and ablative technologies on outcomes of radiofrequency ablation of intra-atrial re-entrant tachycardia in patients with congenital heart disease. J Am Coll Cardiol 2002; 39:1827–1835.
15. Mavroudis C, Deal BJ, Backer CL. Surgery for arrhythmias in children. Int J Cardiol 2004; 97:39–51.
16. Kron J, et al. Preliminary experience with nonthoracotomy implantable cardioverter defibrillators in young patients. The medtronic transvene investigators. Pacing Clin Electrophysiol 1994; 17:26–30.
17. Alexander ME, et al. Implications of implantable cardioverter defibrillator therapy in congenital heart disease and pediatrics. J Cardiovasc Electrophysiol 2004; 15:72–76.
18. Korte T, et al. High incidence of appropriate and inappropriate ICD therapies in children and adolescents with implantable cardioverter defibrillator. Pacing Clin Electrophysiol 2004; 27:924–932.
19. Dubin AM, et al. The use of implantable cardioverter-defibrillators in pediatric patients awaiting heart transplantation. J Card Fail 2003; 9:375–379.
20. Costa R, et al. Transfemoral pediatric permanent pacing: long-term results. Pacing Clin Electrophysiol 2003; 26:487–491.
21. Walker F, et al. Long-term outcomes of cardiac pacing in adults with congenital heart disease. J Am Coll Cardiol 2004; 43:1894–1901.
22. Horenstein MS, Walters H, 3rd, Karpawich PP. Chronic performance of steroid-eluting epicardial leads in a growing pediatric population: a 10-year comparison. Pacing Clin Electrophysiol 2003; 26:1467–1471.
23. Boettcher W, Merkle F, Weitkemper HH. History of extracorporeal circulation: the conceptional and developmental period. J Extra Corpor Technol 2003; 35:172–183.
24. Nadar S, et al. Positive pressure ventilation in the management of acute and chronic cardiac failure: a systematic review and meta-analysis. Int J Cardiol 2005; 99:171–185.
25. Cleland JG, et al. Clinical trials update from the American College of Cardiology meeting: CARE-HF and the remission of heart failure. Women's Health Study, TNT, COMPASS-HF, VERITAS, CANPAP, PEECH and PREMIER. Eur J Heart Fail 2005; 7:931–936.

26. Deiwick M, et al. Heart failure in children—mechanical assistance. Thorac Cardiovasc Surg 2005; 53:S135–S140.
27. Kolovos NS, et al. Outcome of pediatric patients treated with extracorporeal life support after cardiac surgery. Ann Thorac Surg 2003; 76:1435–1441 discussion 1441–2.
28. Pagani FD, et al. Extracorporeal life support to left ventricular assist device bridge to heart transplant: A strategy to optimize survival and resource utilization. Circulation 1999; 100:II206–II210.
29. Levi D, et al. Use of assist devices and ECMO to bridge pediatric patients with cardiomyopathy to transplantation. J Heart Lung Transplant 2002; 21:760–770.
30. Booth KL, et al. Extracorporeal membrane oxygenation support of the Fontan and bidirectional Glenn circulations. Ann Thorac Surg 2004; 77:1341–1348.
31. Boettcher W, Merkle F, Weitkemper HH. History of extracorporeal circulation: the invention and modification of blood pumps. J Extra Corpor Technol 2003; 35:184–191.
32. Gajarski RJ, et al. Use of extracorporeal life support as a bridge to pediatric cardiac transplantation. J Heart Lung Transplant 2003; 22:28–34.
33. Fiser WP, et al. Pediatric arteriovenous extracorporeal membrane oxygenation (ECMO) as a bridge to cardiac transplantation. J Heart Lung Transplant 2003; 22:770–777.
34. Thiagarajan RR, Nelson DP. Should we be satisfied with current outcomes for cardiac extracorporeal life support? Pediatr Crit Care Med 2005; 6:89–90.
35. Thiagarajan RR, Blume ED, Roth SJ, del Nido PJ, Mayer JE, Laussen PC. Outcome of patients listed for heart transplantation on ECMO. Ped Crit Care Med 2003; 4:A99.
36. Morrow WR, et al. Outcome of listing for heart transplantation in infants younger than six months: predictors of death and interval to transplantation. The Pediatric Heart Transplantation Study Group. J Heart Lung Transplant 1997; 16:1255–1266.
37. Pollock JC, et al. Intraaortic balloon pumping in children. Ann Thorac Surg 1980; 29:522–528.
38. Park JK, Hsu DT, Gersony WM. Intraaortic balloon pump management of refractory congestive heart failure in children. Pediatr Cardiol 1993; 14:19–22.
39. Merkle F, et al. Pulsatile mechanical cardiac assistance in pediatric patients with the Berlin heart ventricular assist device. J Extra Corpor Technol 2003; 35:115–120.
40. Goldman AP, et al. The waiting game: bridging to paediatric heart transplantation. Lancet 2003; 362:1967–1970.
41. DeMaso DR, et al. Psychosocial factors and quality of life in children and adolescents with implantable cardioverter-defibrillators. Am J Cardiol 2004; 93:582–587.
42. Sears SF, Jr., et al. Young at heart: understanding the unique psychosocial adjustment of young implantable cardioverter defibrillator recipients. Pacing Clin Electrophysiol 2001; 24:1113–1117.
43. Bhat AH, Sahn DJ. Congenital heart disease never goes away, even when it has been 'treated': the adult with congenital heart disease. Curr Opin Pediatr 2004; 16:500–507.
44. Wray J, Radley-Smith R. Developmental and behavioral status of infants and young children awaiting heart or heart-lung transplantation. Pediatrics 2004; 113:488–495.
45. Uzark KC, et al. The psychosocial impact of pediatric heart transplantation. J Heart Lung Transplant 1992; 11:1160–1167.
46. Pollock-BarZiv SM, et al. Quality of life and function following cardiac transplantation in adolescents. Transplant Proc 2003; 35:2468–2470.
47. Hirshfeld AB, et al. Parent-reported health status after pediatric thoracic organ transplant. J Heart Lung Transplant 2004; 23:1111–1118.
48. Mussatto K. In: Shaddy RW, ed. Psychosocial Aspects of Acute and Chronic Heart Failure in Children, in Pediatric Heart Failure. Boca Raton: Taylor and Francis, 2005:833–868.

37
Surgical Management of Pediatric Heart Failure

Luca A. Vricella and Duke E. Cameron
Division of Cardiac Surgery, The Johns Hopkins Hospital, Baltimore, Maryland, U.S.A.

INTRODUCTION

The potential for clinical deterioration in medically-managed children with cardiomyopathy and myocarditis and the increase in complexity and volume of cardiac surgical procedures performed in neonates and infants have introduced the specific need and challenge of mechanically supporting the failing pediatric heart as a bridge to either recovery or transplantation (1–4). The first attempt to achieve post-operative myocardial recovery with veno-arterial bypass in a pediatric patient was reported by Spencer and coworkers in 1965 (5,6) and was followed by the first successful case of device-assistance by De Bakey in 1971 (7). Three decades following these initial reports, several devices are available as well-established treatment modality of refractory or irreversible cardiac failure in pediatric patients. Device selection is based on the particular indication for mechanical assistance (acute, chronic, or post-cardiotomy failure), the anticipated length of support and, most importantly, the size of the patient (1,8–11). For several years, extracorporeal membrane oxygenation (ECMO) and non-pulsatile centrifugal pumps have represented the mainstay of cardiac and pulmonary support in children (1,12). The limitations of these techniques and the introduction of other devices that allowed prolonged support in adults prompted their clinical application to larger pediatric patients with success (13–15). But adaptation of adult support systems to larger children excludes a substantial segment of the pediatric population that cannot accommodate larger devices. The field of pediatric circulatory support will therefore likely focus in the years to come on the development and refinement of ventricular assist devices (VADs) that are specifically designed for smaller patients, allowing for prolonged mechanical assistance in neonates, infants, and small children.

As the pathophysiology and medical management of pediatric heart failure is detailed elsewhere in this textbook, we will mainly focus on the indications for device implantation and outline the distinctive features and results of the different systems that are currently clinically available.

HEART FAILURE IN CHILDREN: SURGICAL INDICATIONS FOR DEVICE IMPLANTATION

Pediatric patients who require ventricular assistance (either in isolation or in association with the need for respiratory support) typically fall into one of three categories: (1) patients without structural congenital heart disease, (2) patients with cardiac malformations that require pre-operative recovery from respiratory or circulatory compromise related to their specific structural anomaly, and (3) patients who necessitate ventricular and/or respiratory support early or late after correction of cardiac malformations or staged palliation of congenital heart disease. These diagnostic categories are outlined in Table 1.

It is difficult to assess to what degree each of these diagnostic groups (cardiomyopathy and congenital heart disease) is represented in the cohort of children with heart failure that requires ventricular assistance as bridge to recovery or transplantation.

Patients with congenital heart disease who require VAD implantation are usually those who have undergone atrial switch operations for transposition of the great arteries, older children and young adults with congenitally corrected transposition, or patients who develop ventricular failure following staged palliation of univentricular heart disease. Aside from the first two morphologic sub-groups, it is fairly rare to develop heart failure and require transplantation in normally connected hearts with well-developed ventricles, except for acute, irreversible failure shortly after biventricular repair.

With regards to the other major diagnostic group, the actual incidence of pediatric cardiomyopathy (CM) is imprecisely defined because of variability in definition criteria and etiological heterogeneity. The Pediatric CM Registry reported in 2001 an incidence of 0.6 CM cases / 100,000 children (age <18 yr) (16). Among these patients, 52% were observed in patients of age <1 yr at the time of diagnosis (17).

The relative importance of the diagnostic group and age of pediatric patients requiring heart transplantation has been more recently analyzed by the International Society of Heart Lung Transplantation (18). When comparing age groups and the indications for transplantation, CM increases as an indication for transplant from 29% in neonates and infants to 62% in children between 11 and 18 yr of age. Conversely, the diagnosis of congenital heart disease decreases from 65% to 37%. This and other studies did not include those pediatric patients who expire while waiting for a suitable organ to become available, and may indeed benefit from timely VAD implantation as bridge to transplantation (19).

Table 1 Pediatric Cardiac Failure: Etiologic Groups (Acute and Chronic)

1. Cardiac failure in the absence of structural congenital heart disease
   a. Myocarditis (idiopathic, viral)
   b. Idiopathic cardiomyopathy (restrictive, dilated, hypertrophic)
   c. Non-idiopathic cardiomyopathy
      Inborn errors of metabolism
      Ischemic (Kawasaki's disease)
      Post cardiac arrest (ventricular dysfunction)
      Iatrogenic (chemotherapy, etc.)
      Nutritional
2. Preoperative
3. Postoperative
   a. Early (post-cardiotomy failure)
   b. Late (after complete intra-cardiac repair or palliation)

Aside from children who fail separation from cardio-pulmonary bypass, heart failure presents in children with signs and symptoms that are similar to those observed in adult patients. Dyspnea at rest or exertion is seen in the older pediatric population, while tachypnea, tachycardia, poor feeding, and failure to thrive are frequently present in neonates and infants. Prominent jugular veins, a gallop, hepato-splenomegaly, and peripheral edema are often evident on physical examination. Chest X-ray will usually disclose plethoric lung fields and an enlarged cardiac silhouette; imaging techniques, cardiac catheterization, and histologic findings on endomyocardial biopsy further help delineate etiology and severity of myocardial impairment (20).

Regardless of its underlying cause, progressive and/or untreated heart failure will lead to clinical deterioration and ultimately compromise end-organ perfusion. Metabolic acidosis, impaired mentation, and decreased urine output will then prelude to the downward spiral of multi-organ system failure secondary to persistent cardiogenic shock. Aggressive medical management with invasive monitoring and inotropic support is often capable of reversing this clinical situation, allowing for stabilization and possible bridging to recovery or transplantation. For those patients who fail to respond, availability of VADs represents, in the interim, the only hope for long-term survival (21).

Indications to proceed to device implantation are summarized in Table 2. Although for older pediatric patients indications are similar to those that have been established for adults, they still remain somewhat ill-defined in infants and small children. In the latter group, severe exacerbation of congestive heart failure, malignant arrhythmias, and acute hemodynamic decompensation should prompt aggressive attempts at hemodynamic stabilization and immediate consideration of VAD implantation. If at all possible, implantation should in fact be performed in a semi-elective setting rather than in an emergent clinical situation on a rapidly deteriorating patient. In case of rescue implantation in patients with profound hemodynamic compromise, the potential for meaningful neurologic recovery must also be kept in consideration.

Table 2 Indications for Ventricular Assist Device Implantation

1. Persistent CHF despite of maximized medical support $\pm$IABP
2. Hemodynamic parameters (older children/adolescents)
   a. SBP <90 mm Hg
   b. PCWP >20 mm Hg
   c. SVR >2000 dynes/sec/cm^2
   d. CI <1.8 L/min/m^2
3. End-organ dysfunction
   a. Decreased mentation
   b. Increase in creatinine levels and azotemia
   c. Progressive liver dysfunction
4. Inability to wean from cardio-pulmonary bypass after intra-cardiac repair
5. Recurrent malignant arrhythmias

Abbreviations: CHF, congestive heart failure; CI, cardiac index; IABP, intra-aortic balloon pump; PCWP, pulmonary capillary wedge pressure; SBP, systolic blood pressure; SVR, systemic vascular resistance.
Source: From Dunnington G, Pelletier M, Reitz BA. Ventricular assist devices in children. In Yuh DD, Vricella LA, Baumgartner WA, eds. The Johns Hopkins Manual of Cardiothoracic Surgery. New York: McGraw Hill.

CHOICE OF VENTRICULAR ASSIST DEVICE

When implanted in the acute phase, VADs should ideally accomplish several goals: separation from cardiopulmonary bypass and acute post-operative recovery, reversal of systemic or pulmonary hypoperfusion, and restoration of end-organ function. In the intermediate and long-term, ventricular assistance should be compatible with patient mobility, functional and psychological well-being, and minimization of late complications while waiting for myocardial recovery or a suitable allograft.

Currently available devices can be divided into three categories: (1) aortic counterpulsation devices (intra-aortic balloon pump, IABP), (2) non-pulsatile assist devices (ECMO, centrifugal and axial flow pumps), and (3) pulsatile assist devices.

Several factors must be kept in consideration when choosing which assist device should be utilized for the individual pediatric patient. The patient's clinical status (emergent or semi-elective, post-cardiotomy) certainly plays an important role. In the intra-operative setting, "acute type" modalities can be employed to bridge the patient to potential recovery of myocardial function. Centrifugal pumps or ECMO (in case of bi-ventricular failure or associated respiratory insufficiency) can be utilized in neonates, infants, and smaller children. In larger children with cardiac (non-respiratory) failure, a pulsatile device (i.e., Abiomed®) can be alternatively inserted in a single or biventricular support configuration. In the acute setting, consideration should also be given to intra-aortic counterpulsation as an additional form of myocardial support.

In cases in which chances of recovery appear remote and a prolonged wait on the transplant waiting list is likely, insertion of or post-operative conversion to a device designed for long-term support is indicated. For this purpose, a pneumatic positive displacement pump is most commonly utilized; in older children or adolescents, some centers have utilized axial flow pumps for bridging to transplantation as an alternative to pneumatic VADs. Device choice must not only focus on the clinical situation of the individual pediatric patient, but also on the level of expertise and experience of the center in which the child is cared for.

To follow is an overview of the currently available VADs. Certain devices which have been adapted to children with near-adult weight (such as Novacor® or Heartmate I®, for example) are discussed in detail elsewhere in this textbook. Figure 1 outlines a proposed decision-making algorithm for the pediatric patient who fails medical management.

SPECIFIC VENTRICULAR ASSIST DEVICES

Intra-aortic Balloon Counterpulsation

The IABP is the least invasive modality of ventricular assistance, with relative ease of device insertion and removal, and proven clinical efficacy in adults with cardiogenic shock (22). Although intra-aortic counterpulsation has been utilized with success in smaller children and infants, (23–28) its most prominent role is in larger children with post-cardiotomy or non-surgical heart failure. Neonates and infants will in fact usually suffer bi-ventricular and, often, concomitant respiratory failure. For this age group, ECMO is most typically indicated as first-line surgical support therapy.

The IABP device can be used as initial support system or as an adjunct to a VAD. The device is introduced via the femoral (most commonly), external iliac, or axillary artery. When inserted intra-operatively, the IABP can also be positioned in the proximal

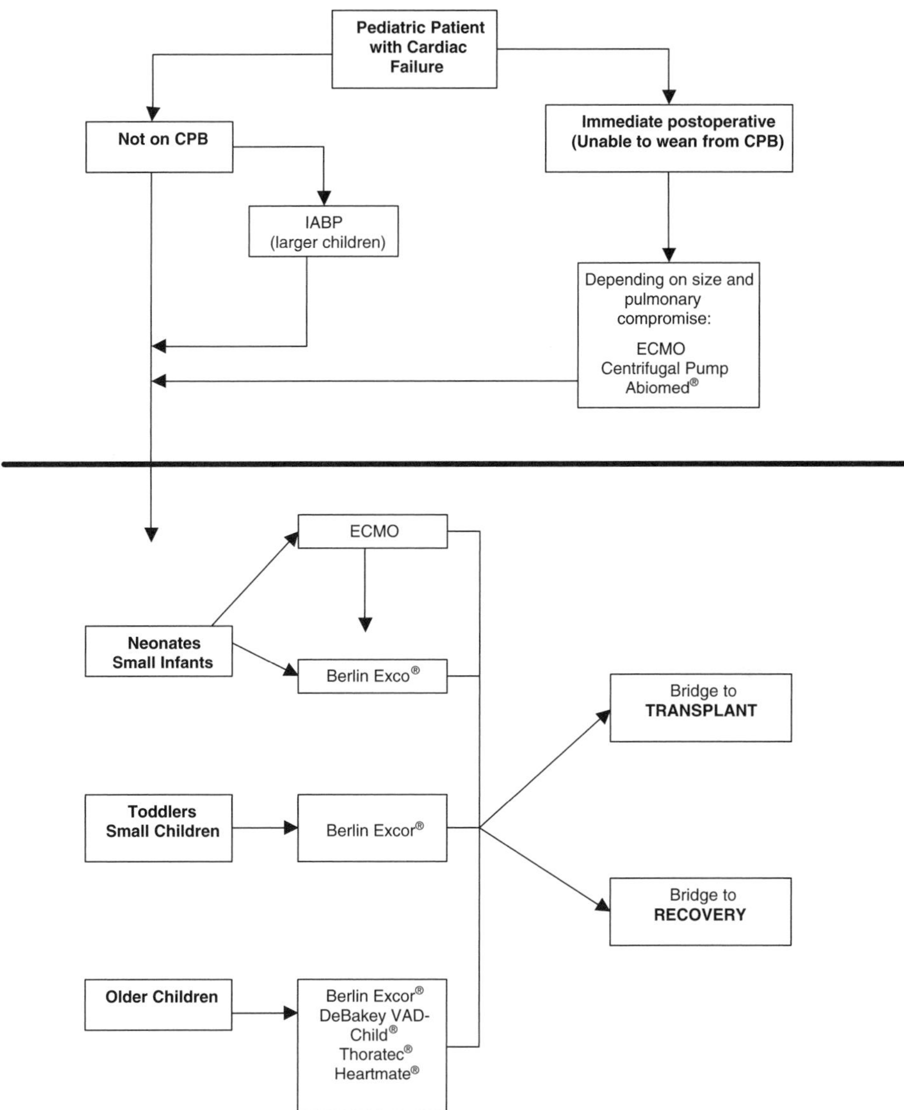

Figure 1 Decision-making algorithm for ventricular assist device implantation. *Abbreviations*: CPB, cardiopulmonary bypass; ECMO, extracorporeal membrane oxygenation; IABP, intra-aortic balloon pump.

descending aorta directly through the ascending aorta. The balloon should be placed above the diaphragm (Fig. 2) and is rhythmically deflated in diastole and inflated in diastole, timed either by the electrocardiogram (triggered by the patient's QRS complex) or by the arterial pressure tracing. During diastole, inflation of the balloon increases afterload, ameliorating diastolic coronary perfusion and myocardial oxygen delivery. In systole, deflation of the balloon creates a "vacuum effect" in the descending aorta that effectively lowers cardiac afterload, facilitating in turn left ventricular unloading and decreasing myocardial oxygen demand. Furthermore, the pulsatility derived from the inflation-deflation cycle provides improvement in splancnic perfusion (22,24,28,29). In cases of

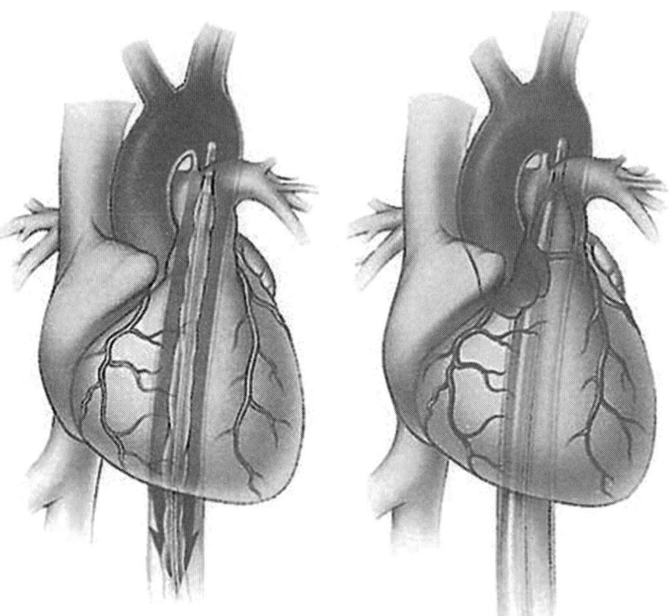

Figure 2 Intra-aortic balloon pump. The device is inserted in the proximal descending thoracic aorta and is deflated during systole (*left*) and inflated in diastole (*right*). *Source*: Image courtesy of Datascope®, New York, New York, U.S.A.

biventricular failure, IABP may be beneficial in improving right ventricular function by increasing right coronary artery perfusion, and by possibly reducing pulmonary vascular resistance (30).

Several limitations to the use of IABPs are readily evident in pediatric patients. The occurrence of femoral arterial complications must be carefully weighed against the rapid deterioration in the child's clinical condition and the need for ventricular support with counterpulsation. Diminished efficacy of diastolic pressure augmentation has been postulated as a consequence of the higher wall compliance of the pediatric aorta when compared to that observed in adults; (31) however, this concept has been challenged recently (28). The size and length of the balloon must also be considered. The balloon should be at least 50% of the stroke volume of the individual pediatric patient (approximately 0.5 cc/Kg of body weight) (32). Mesenteric, renal, and celiac arterial occlusion by the balloon have been reported, and the length of device should ideally span a distance between the left subclavian artery and the diaphragm (23). The smallest currently available devices are delivered with a 4.5 French catheter, increasing in diameter to 7.0 French. Balloon volumes range from 2.5 to 20 cc, with available length and diameter between 12.8 and 19.5 cm and 6 to 12 mm, respectively. Another technical limitation observed in pediatric patients with high heart rates is the difficulty in triggering of IABP inflation. For this reason, several centers are currently utilizing M-mode echocardiography for appropriate timing of device inflation (33,34).

Outcomes of pediatric balloon counterpulsation reflect the gravity of the underlying condition, with hospital survival below 60% in small series (23,27,28).

Non-pulsatile Devices

Centrifugal Pumps

In the absence of concomitant respiratory failure, perfusion can be sustained by a centrifugal pump. This is in fact one of the most common forms of support in cases of left (LVAD), right (RVAD), or biventricular (BVAD) failure; given the need for intra-thoracic cannulation, its role is almost always relegated to assistance in the immediate post-operative phase. Prior to institution of support with a centrifugal pump, correctable causes of post-operative severe ventricular dysfunction must be first thoroughly sought and addressed if present. Residual shunts, obstruction, and coronary inflow are some of the issues that, if unrecognized and not corrected, will make VAD implantation a futile effort. In the post-cardiotomy phase, aortic and right atrial cannulae utilized during the procedure can be simply connected to the circuit with minor technical modifications. In the intra-thoracic access LVAD configuration (Fig. 3), inflow is established from the left atrium, by cannulating either superior pulmonary vein, dome of the left atrium, or left atrial appendage. The return line is in the distal ascending aorta. For right ventricular assistance, similar cannulae connect the right atrium (via the right atrial appendage) to the main pulmonary artery. In case of biventricular failure, conversion from cardiopulmonary bypass to ECMO rather than to biventricular assistance might be simpler. In such instance, moving the cannulation site altogether in the cervical region (as typically done for

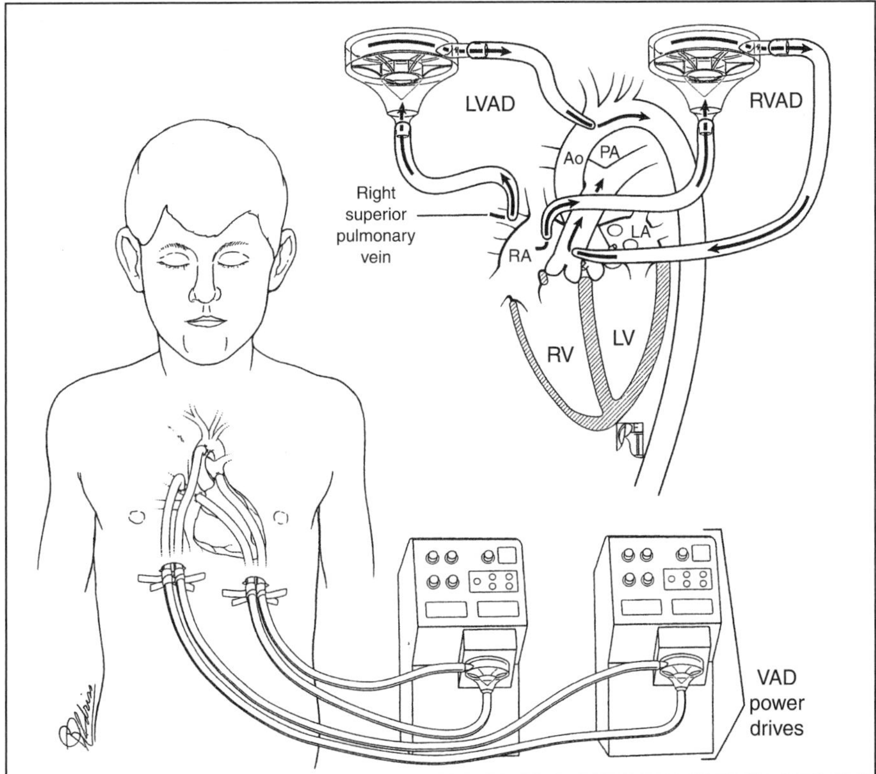

Figure 3 Biventricular support with centrifugal pumps (RVAD/LVAD). Left atrial drainage is achieved through the right superior pulmonary vein and arterial return is in the ascending aorta (LVAD). The right ventricular (RVAD) support system is interposed between right atrium and pulmonary artery. *Source*: From Ref. 32.

non-cardiac ECMO), allows for removal of the aortic and right atrial cannulae with the potential for better hemostasis and chest closure. ECMO requires, on the other hand, higher levels of anticoagulation, has been associated with less favorable long-term neurologic outcomes (35) and should be carefully considered as an alternative to centrifugal pumps in the coagulopathic patient. In comparison to roller-pumps (most commonly utilized in ECMO), centrifugal pumps are also less likely to cause significant hemolysis.

During centrifugal support, a left atrial pressure monitoring line should ideally be left in place to allow constant monitoring of the efficacy of decompression of the left-sided chambers. Evidence of recovery is manifested by ejection seen on arterial tracing upon weaning, coupled with amelioration of function and associated mitral regurgitation by trans-esophageal or trans-thoracic echocardiography. Isolated left ventricular assistance with centrifugal pumps has been utilized with success rates up to 70% after repair of anomalous origin of the left main coronary artery (36,37). Hospital survival rates for post-cardiotomy LVAD rescue of neonates and small infants (operative weight <6 Kg) are not very different, although survival at one year post-support has been reported to be as low as 30% (38).

Extracorporeal Membrane Oxygenation (ECMO)

Since its first reported successful clinical application in 1971, (39) ECMO has been utilized in children of all ages with excellent outcomes (40–42). This particular form of assistance is designed to either support respiratory function or cardiac failure with or without associated respiratory impairment. Severe respiratory failure represents the most frequent indication that leads to the institution of ECMO, with well-consolidated results in neonates and infants with meconium aspiration, (43) congenital diaphragmatic hernia, (44–46) primary neonatal pulmonary hypertension, and various other forms of isolated respiratory failure (40,47).

This particular type of non-pulsatile support is utilized also in pediatric patients with biventricular or combined cardiac and respiratory decompensation after cardiac surgical procedures, (48–50) as well as in infants and small children with primary cardiac failure, bridging to either recovery or transplantation (21,51,52).

In its most typical configuration for cardiac support (Fig. 4), the ECMO circuit incorporates a membrane oxygenator and utilizes veno-arterial bypass. Most commonly, venous return is provided by a cannula advanced into the right atrium from the right internal jugular vein. The arterial return line is placed into the right common carotid artery, positioning the tip of the cannula towards the innominate artery. Venous drainage is to a bladder-type reservoir, and propulsion across the membrane oxygenator is usually accomplished with a roller pump. In cases of preserved ventricular function and isolated respiratory insufficiency, veno-venous ECMO with a single dual-lumen cannula for both drainage and infusion can be utilized. A heat exchanger and, possibly, a hemodyalisis filter are interposed in the circuit as well. In acute post-cardiotomy failure, the right atrial and ascending aortic cannulae utilized during the surgical procedure can be directly connected to the ECMO circuit; consideration should also be given to decompression of the left cardiac chambers with a septostomy (53,54) or an additional left atrial vent line inserted in the circuit. An area of relative controversy in post-cardiotomy pediatric ECMO is that of shunt management in neonates and infants who have undergone placement of a systemic-to-pulmonary shunt as part of surgical palliation of congenital heart disease. Some authors (32) favor gradual release of shunt occlusion to limit the potential for pulmonary over-circulation, while others (55) maintain complete shunt

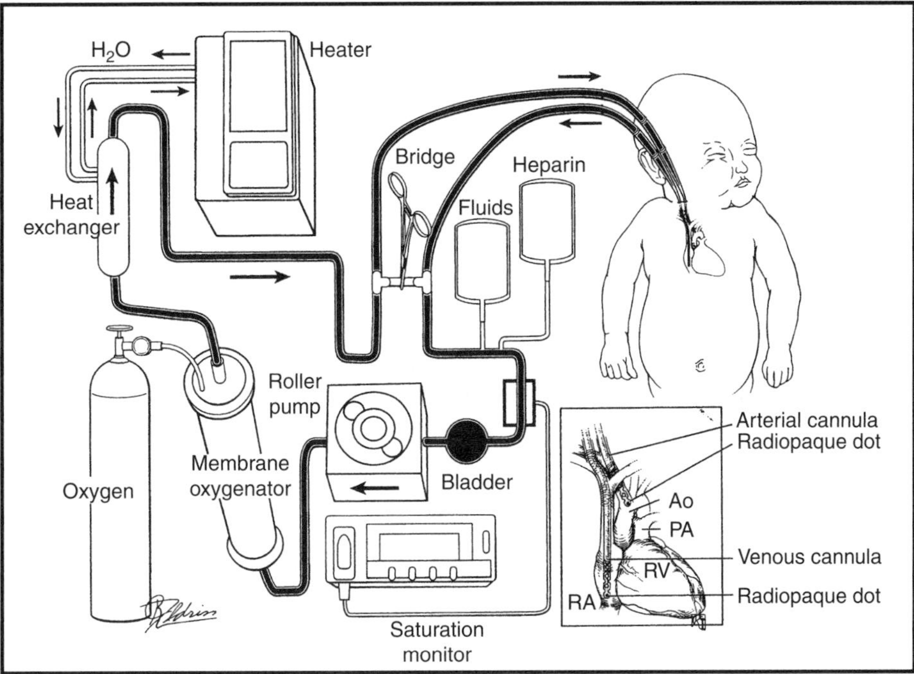

Figure 4 Infant support with veno-arterial extracorporeal membrane oxygenation. Cervical cannulation is illustrated. Intra-thoracic cannulation is alternatively used for post-cardiotomy patients. *Source*: From Ref. 32.

patency and increase perfusion flows to assure adequate systemic perfusion in spite of shunt runoff.

Although guidelines for anticoagulation vary between institutional protocols and with the patient's clinical condition and VAD flows, activated clotting time (ACT) is usually maintained between 180 and 200 sec during ECMO support. Other coagulation parameters (fibrinogen levels and prothrombin time) should be kept within normal range, and platelet count should be above 100,000/mL.

Outcomes of cardiac and/or respiratory support with ECMO differ according to indications and age group, rapidity of deployment of the system (56), and institutional experience. The Extracorporeal Life Support Organization registry report of 2004 included almost 29,000 patients (40). Of these, 66% were neonates with respiratory failure, with a 77% survival to hospital discharge. Hospital survival for children and adults requiring respiratory support with ECMO was lower (56 and 53%, respectively). Survival rates to discharge for patients with cardiac failure as an indication for mechanical support with ECMO were 38% and 43% for neonates and children. Clinical experience with ECMO for cardiac failure in adults has not been very promising thus far (57).

When ECMO is utilized in the post-operative phase after congenital heart surgery, survival as high as 67% has been reported (49). In this particular sub-group, better outcomes have been observed in patients who are not placed on ECMO from inability to wean from cardiopulmonary bypass, but rather in those in whom this support modality is instituted several hours after a period of meta-stability without hemodynamic collapse (58). This concept has nevertheless been recently challenged by Goldman and coworkers, who achieved a 64% hospital survival in patients identified as having reversible cardiac failure after satisfactory bi-ventricular repair, and in whom ECMO was instituted in the operating room (59). Better outcomes have been observed in patients with normally developed ventricles as opposed to those with univentricular heart disease (59,60). In a review of 74 patients who required ECMO support after surgical correction or palliation of congenital heart disease at the University of Michigan, (48) multivariate analysis identified functionally univentricular heart disease and need for hemofiltration on ECMO as significant predictors of adverse outcome.

Neurological complications, sepsis, and issues related to antigoagulation and thrombosis pose a significant threat to the early and long-term outlook of pediatric patients who require ECMO. Although the spectrum of possible neurologic outcome is quite broad and quantifying neuro-cognitive outcomes in neonates and infants is inherently challenging, the reported frequency of abnormal neuroimaging in pediatric patients on ECMO is between 28 and 52% (61). Incomplete neurological recovery has been observed in up to 10% of neonates and 30% of children at intermediate follow-up, (62) with early seizure activity recognized as a prognostic indicator of lower scoring on neuro-developmental testing at late follow-up (63).

Axial Flow Pumps

The two principal non-pulsatile devices that hold much promise in their application to pediatric patients are the DeBakey VAD®-*Child* (Micromed Technology, Houston, Tx) and the Jarvik 2000® system (Jarvik Research Inc., New York, NY). Axial flow impeller pumps are characterized by miniaturization, decrease in energy demand and excellent flow characteristics, features that are particularly attractive in the pediatric patient (64). Both

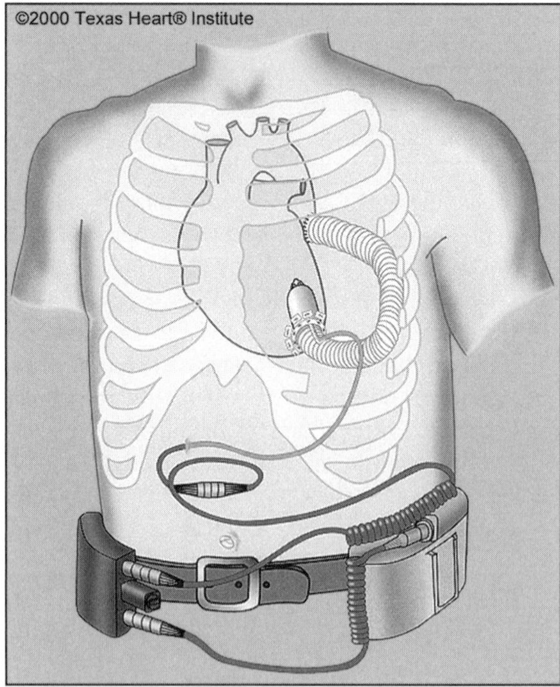

Figure 5 Jarvik 2000® ventricular assist device. In the schematic illustration, the system is inserted through a left thoracotomy between left ventricular apex and proximal descending aorta. *Source*: Image courtesy of the Texas Heart Institute, Houston, Texas, U.S.A.

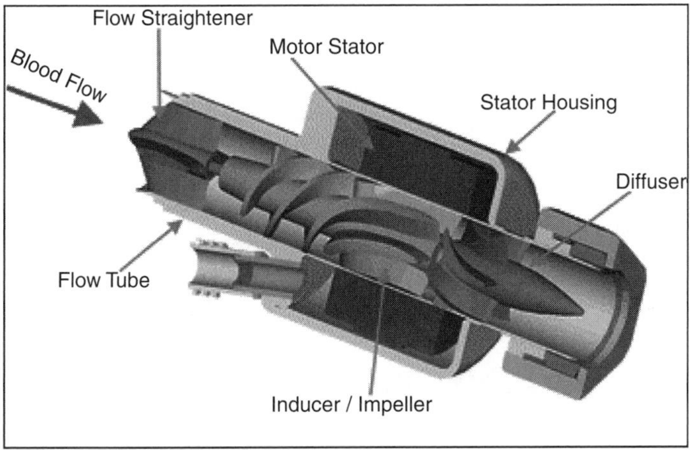

Figure 6 DeBakey VAD®-*Child* axial flow pump. *Source*: Image courtesy of Micromed Technology®, Houston, Texas, U.S.A.

devices are usually implanted in the LVAD configuration, either through a median sternotomy or via a left thoracotomy. In the former approach, the device is interposed between the left atrium or left ventricular apex and ascending aorta, while both systems can alternatively be inserted through the left chest (Fig. 5) between the left ventricle and descending aorta with or without the need for cardiopulmonary bypass (65). Implantable axial flow pumps result in substantial hemodynamic changes, with narrowing of pulse pressure and potential for peripheral vascular thrombosis, development of arterio-venous malformations and left ventricular or impeller thrombus formation, underscoring the need for very aggressive anti-coagulation (66,67).

The DeBakey VAD®-*Child* ventricular assist device measures 30 mm × 76 mm with a weight of 94 grams. In the VAD chamber, the inducer/impeller is driven by a direct-current magnetic motor stator that spins the impeller between 7500 and 12,500 RPM, with flows of up to 10 liters/min (Fig. 6). The wide range of flows and the size of its components (pump and inflow/outflow cannulae) make this device implantable in children with body surface area (BSA) greater than 0.7 m^2. The device is connected to a portable controller with a percutaneous driveline. Of the first 9 pediatric implants (mean age 14 yr and BSA of 1.64 m^2) reported by Morales et al. in 2004, 5 were successfully bridged to transplantation and the reminder died while waiting for a suitable donor (68).

The Jarvik 2000® VAD differs from other types of axial flow pumps in that the impeller is inserted within the left ventricle through its apex, rather than being interposed between inflow and outflow conduits. The device has been used with success in adult patients (66,69,70) and has shown promising results in rare reports of its utilization in pediatric patients (71). Retroauricolar power supply is currently being investigated as a future modification of this particular device (72).

Pulsatile Devices

The clinical use of pulsatile para-corporeal pumps in adults has been widely reported, and their utilization and success rates in children are increasing. These devices are typically inserted in LVAD and/or RVAD configuration via a median sternotomy. Although the Abiomed BVS 5000® VAD (Abiomed Inc., Danvers, MA) has been utilized for short-term

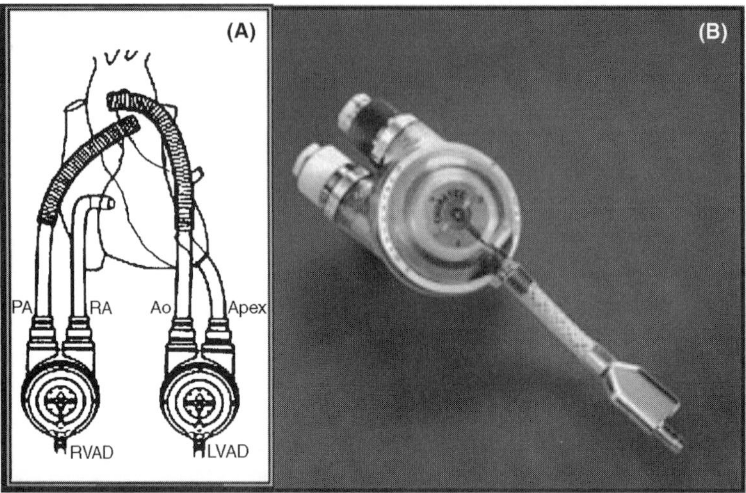

Figure 7 Thoratec® VAD. Schematic representation of Bi-VAD Thoratec® (**A**) and pneumatic pump head (**B**). *Source*: Image courtesy of Thoratec® Laboratories, Pleasanton, California, U.S.A.

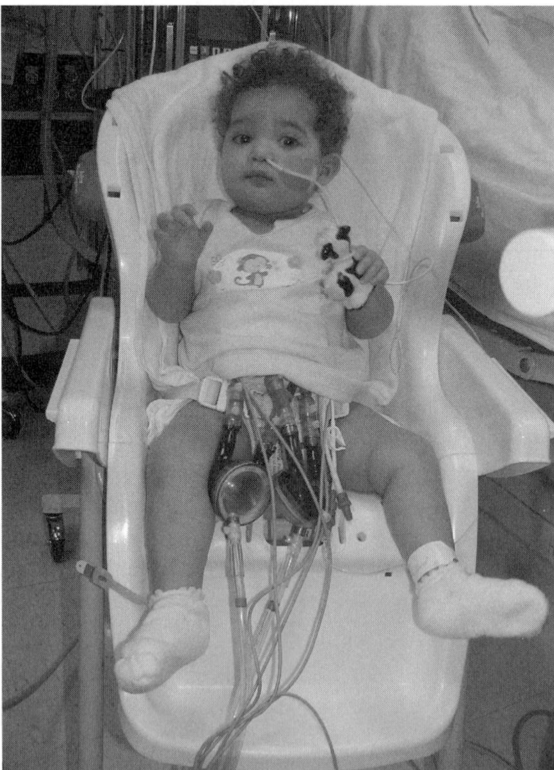

Figure 8 One-year-old child after implantation of biventricular Berlin Heart Excor® support system for restrictive cardiomyopathy. Bridged to heart transplantation 178 days after implant at The Johns Hopkins Hospital. *Source*: Photo courtesy of child's parents.

support in adults with good outcomes, it is not available in pediatric sizes, limiting its application mainly to the post-operative rescue of older children with inability to wean from cardiopulmonary bypass (71,73). This device is unique in that the para-corporeal component is divided into a reservoir that is filled by gravity and a pneumatic chamber that induces pulsatile device contractions. Similar size-related limitations apply to the Thoratec® VAD (Thoratec Laboratories, Pleasanton, CA), designed for long-term support (Fig. 7) (74). The largest reported study of pediatric patients (age <18) undergoing Thoratec® VAD implantation included 101 patients with the lowest operative weight of 17 Kg. Seventy-six children survived to either transplantation (66 patients) or recovery of myocardial function and device explantation (10 patients) (75).

Berlin Heart Excor®

The Berlin Heart Excor® (Berlin Heart, Berlin, Germany) paracorporeal pneumatic system is perhaps the most versatile unit for uni- or bi-ventricular support available for pediatric patients with cardiac failure. Its design is similar to that of the Thoratec® VAD, but is manufactured in sizes that can support patients ranging in size from neonates to adults (Fig. 8). The smallest pneumatic chambers have volume of 10 cc, making the device suitable for patients with weight as low as 2.2 Kg. Blood flow is directed by polyurethane tri-leaflet valves (Fig. 9), and anticoagulation is maintained with heparin or low-molecular weight heparin and transitioned to maintenance with warfarin and anti-aggregant therapy. Decrease in blood product transfusion requirements have been reported for this particular VAD when compared to ECMO (76). The device has been widely utilized in Europe, (77,78) and has been approved for compassionate use in the United States.

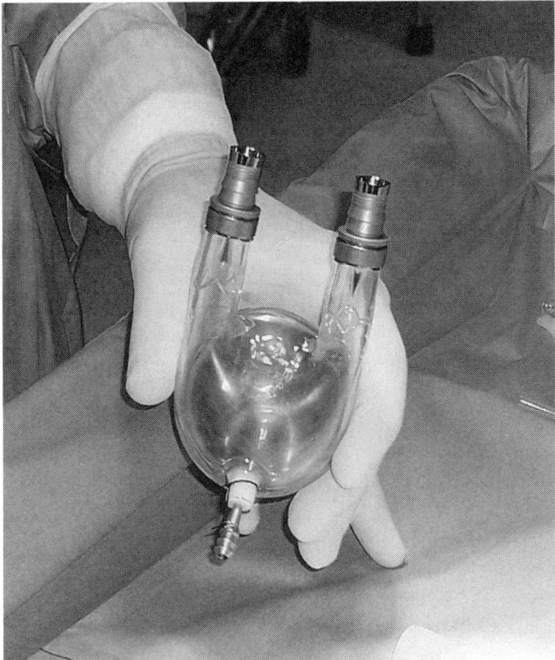

Figure 9 Berlin Heart Excor®. Pulsatile chamber (30 cc) after saline priming. Two polyurethane valves are seen below inflow and outflow cannulae.

Results in children undergoing support with the Berlin Heart Excor® VAD are similar to those obtained with other pulsatile devices in adults, with an overall survival to transplantation or recovery rates in excess of 70%, and with an 11% incidence of neurologic complications. As in most reported series of patients undergoing implantation of VADs, lower survival rates are observed in pediatric patients with diagnosis other than myocarditis and CM (75). In a subgroup analysis reported in 2005, an increase in survival to 70% has been reported in 18 patients younger than one year of age at device implantation (79).

Medos HIA-VAD®

The Medos HIA-VAD® ventricular assist device is a pneumatic para-corporeal unit with a design similar to that of the Berlin Heart Excor®, and has been utilized in limited series (71,80–82). The system utilizes left ventricular chambers of 10, 25, or 60 cc and right chambers of 9, 22.5 and 54 cc, making the device applicable to neonates as well as small children (80). In 2002, several centers reported the combined experience with this particular device, with a 36% overall survival rate in 64 pediatric cases (75).

CONCLUSIONS

In spite of the increase in complexity and number of cardiac surgical procedures and the prevalence of cardiomyopathy, ventricular assistance in infants and small children remains a major unaddressed need. Few devices are available for use in pediatric patients as bridge to cardiac transplantation or recovery, while donor organs are scarce in this age group. When irreversible cardiac failure occurs in children, prompt consideration should therefore be given to assist device implantation, with VAD choice largely guided by patient size, chance of myocardial recovery, and institutional expertise. Future efforts should be directed to the refinement of systems that are specifically designed for small patients, thereby limiting neurologic, infectious, and thrombotic complications.

REFERENCES

1. Levi D, Marelli D, Plunkett M, et al. Use of assist devices and ECMO to bridge pediatric patients with cardiomyopathy to transplantation. J Heart Lung Transplant 2002; 21:760–770.
2. Helman DN, Addonizio LJ, Morales DL, et al. Implantable left ventricular assist devices can successfully bridge adolescent patients to transplant. J Heart Lung Transplant 2000; 19:121–126.
3. Davies JE, Kirklin JK, Pearce FB, et al. Mechanical circulatory support for myocarditis: how much recovery should occur before device removal? J Heart Lung Transplant 2002; 21:1246–1249.
4. Grinda JM, Chevalier P, D'Attellis N, et al. Fulminant myocarditis in adults and children: bi-ventricular assist device for recovery. Eur J Cardiothor Surg 2004; 26:1169–1173.
5. Spencer FC, Eiseman B, Trinkle JK, et al. Assisted circulation for cardiac failure following intracardiac surgery with cardiopulmonary bypass. J Thorac Cradiovasc Surg 1965; 49:56–73.
6. Eiseman B, Spencer FC, Malette WG. Mechanical devices to assist or replace the failing heart. Annu Rev Med 1966; 17:463–472.
7. DeBakey ME. Left ventricular bypass pump for cardiac assistance. Clinical experience. Am J Cardiol 1971; 27:3–11.

8. Deiwick M, Hoffmeier A, Tjam TD, et al. Heart failure in children. Mechanical assistance. Thorac Cardiovasc Surg 2005; 53:S135–S140.
9. Chang AC, McKenzie ED, Mechanical cardiopulmonary support in children and young adults: extra-corporeal membrane oxygenation, ventricular assist devices, and long-term support devices. Pediatr Cardiol, 2005; 26:2–28.
10. Throckmorton AL, Allaire PE, Gutesell HP, et al. Pediatric circulatory support systems. ASAIO J 2002; 48:216–221.
11. Duncan BW. Mechanical circulatory support for infants and chidren with cardiac disease. Ann Thorac Surg 2002; 73:1670–1677.
12. Hines MH. ECMO and congenital heart disease. Semin Perinatol 2005; 29:34–39.
13. Pastuszko P, Gruber PJ, Wernovsky G, et al. Thoratec left ventricular assist device as a bridge to recovery in a child weighing 27 kilograms. J Thorac Cardiovasc Surg 2005; 127:1203–1204.
14. Reinhartz O, Copeland JG, Ferrar DJ. Thoratec ventricular assist devices in children with less than 1.3 m^2 of body surface area. ASAIO J 2003; 49:727–730.
15. Sadegi AM, Marelli D, Talamo M et al. Short-term bridge to transplant using the BVS 5000 in a 22-Kg child. Ann Thorac Surg 2000; 70:2151–2153.
16. Lipshultz SE, Sleeper LA, Towbin JA, et al. The incidence of pediatric cardiomyopathy: the prospective pediatric cardiomyopathy registry. J Am Coll Cardiol 2001; 37:465A–466A.
17. Feroncz C, Rubin JD, McCarter RJ, et al. Congenital heart disease: prevalence after birth. The Baltimore-Washington infant study. Am J Epidemiol 1985; 121:31–36.
18. Taylor DO, Edwards LB, Boucek MM et al. Registry of the International Society for Health and Lung Transplantation: twenty-second official adult heart transplant report - 2005, J Heart Lung Transplant 2005; 24:945–955.
19. Goldman AP, Cassidy J, de Leval M, et al. The waiting game: bridging to pediatric heart transplantation. Lancet 2003; 362:1948–1949.
20. Kay J, Colan S, Graham T, Jr. Congestive heart failure in pediatric patients. Am Heart J 2001; 142:923–928.
21. Reddy SL, Hasan A, Hamilton LR, et al. Mechanical versus medical bridge to transplantation in children. What is the best timing for mechanical bridge? Eur J Cardiothorac Surg 2004; 25:605–609.
22. Baskett RJ, Ghali WA, Maitland A, Hirsch GM. The intraaortic balloon pump in cardiac surgery. Ann Thorac Surg 2002; 74:1276–1287.
23. Veasy LG, Blalock RC, Orth JL, Bouceck MM. Intra-aortic balloon puming in infants and chidren. Circulation 1983; 68:1095–1100.
24. Pollock JC, Charlton MC, Williams WG, Edmonds JF, Trusler GA. Intraaortic balloon pumping in children. Ann Thorac Surg 1980; 29:522–528.
25. Del Nido PJ, Swan PR, Benson LN, et al. Successful use of intraaortic balloon pumping in a 2-kilogram infant. Ann Thorac Surg 1988; 46:474–476.
26. Pozzi M, Santoro G, Makundan S. Intraaortic balloon pump after treatment of anomalous origin of the left coronary artery. Ann Thorac Surg 1998; 65:555–557.
27. Pinkey KA, Minich LL, Tani LY, et al. Current results with intraaortic balloon pumping in infants and children. Ann Thorac Surg 2002; 73:887–891.
28. Akomea-Agyin C, Kejriwal NK, Franks R, Booker PD, Pozzi M. Intraaortic balloon pumping in children. Ann Thorac Surg 1999; 67:1415–1420.
29. Papaioannu TG, Stefanidis C. Basic principles of the intraaortic balloon pump and mechanisms affecting its performance. ASAIO J 2005; 51:296–300.
30. Nordhaug D, Steensrud T, Muller S, Husnes KV, Myrmel T. Intraaortic balloon pumping improves hemodynamics and right ventricular efficiency in acute ischemic right ventricular failure. Ann Thorac Surg 2004; 78:1426–1432.
31. Fischi MC, Tondato F, Adams R et al. Impact of intraaortic balloon counterpulsation on arterial blood flow in juvenile pigs with heart failure. J Invasive Cardiol, 2004;16:184.
32. Jacobs JP. Pediatric mechanical circulatory support. In: Mavroudis C, Backer C, eds. Pediatric Cardiac Surgery. 3rd ed. Chicago: Mosby, 2004:778–792.

33. Pantalos GM, Minich LL, Tani LY, McGough EC, Hawkins JA. Estimation of timing errors for the intraaortic balloon pump use in pediatric patients. ASAIO J 1999; 45:166–171.
34. Minch LL, Tani LY, McGough EC, Shaddy RE, Hawkins JA. A novel approach to pediatric intraaortic balloon pump timing using M-mode echocardiography. Am J Cardiol 1997; 80:367–369.
35. Ibrahim AE, Duncan BW, Blume ED, Jonas RA. Long-term follow-up of pediatric cardiac patients requiring mechanical circulatory support. Ann Thorac Surg 2000; 69:186–192.
36. del Nido PJ, Duncan BW, Mayer JE, Wessel DL, LaPierre RA, Jonas RA. Left ventricular assist device improves survival in children with left ventricular dysfunction after repair of anomalous origin of the left coronary artery from the pulmonary artery. Ann Thorac Surg 1999; 67:169–172.
37. Schwartz ML, Jonas RA, Colan SD. Anomalous origin of the left coronary artery from pulmonary artery: recovery of left ventricular function after dual coronary repair. J Am Coll Cardiol 1997; 30:547–553.
38. Thuys CA, Mullay RJ, Horton SB, et al. Centrifugal ventricular assist in children under 6 Kg. Eur J Cardiothorac Surg 1998; 13:130–134.
39. Wolfson PJ. The development and use of extracorporeal membrane oxygenation in neonates. Ann Thorac Surg 2003; 76:S2224–S2229.
40. Conrad SA, Rycus PT, Dalton H. Extracorporeal life support registry report 2004. ASAIO J 2005; 51:4–10.
41. Bennett CC, Johnson A, Field DJ, et al. UK collaborative randomized trial of neonatal extracorporeal membrane oxygenation: follow-up to age 4 years. Lancet 2001; 357:1094–1096.
42. Petrou S, Edwards L. Cost effectiveness analysis of neonatal extracorporeal membrane oxygenation based on four years results from the UK collaborative ECMO trial. Arch Dis Child Fetal Neonatal Ed 2004; 89:F263–F268.
43. Kugelman A, Gangitano E, Taschuk R, et al. Extracorporeal membrane oxygenation in infants with meconium aspiration syndrome: a decade of experience with venovenous ECMO. J Pediatr Surg 2005; 40:1082–1089.
44. Harrington KP, Goldman AP. The role of extracorporeal membrane oxygenation in congenital diaphragmatic hernia. Semin Pediatr Surg 2005; 14:72–76.
45. Davis PJ, Firmin RK, Manktelow B, et al. Long-term outcome following extracorporeal membrane oxygenation for congenital diaphragmatic hernia: the UK experience. J Pediatr 2004; 144:309–315.
46. Moya FR, Lally KP. Evidence-based management of infants with congenital diaphragmatic hernia. Semin Perinatol 2005; 29:112–117.
47. Bahrami KR, Van Meurs KP. ECMO for neonatal respiratory failure. Semin Perinatol 2005; 29:15–23.
48. Kolovos NS, Bratton SL, Moler FW, et al. Outcome of pediatric patients treated with extracorporeal life support after cardiac surgery. Ann Thorac Surg 2003; 76:1435–1442.
49. Alsoufi B, Shen I, Karamolou T, et al. Extracorporeal life support in neonates, infants and children after repair of congenital heart disease: modern era results at a single institution. Ann Thorac Surg 2005; 80:15–21.
50. Mahle WT, Forbess JM, Kirshbom PM, et al. Cost-utility analysis of salvage cardiac extracorporeal membrane oxygenation in children. J Thorac Cardiovasc Surg 2005; 129:1084–1090.
51. McMahon AM, van Doorn C, Burch M, et al. Improved early outcome for end-stage dilated cardiomyopathy in children. J Thorac Cardiovasc Surg 2004; 126:1781–1787.
52. Bae JO, Frischer JS, Waich M, Addonizio LJ, Lazar EL, Stolar CJ. Extracorporeal membrane oxygenation in pediatric cardiac transplantation. J Pediatr Surg 2005; 40:1051–1056.
53. Ward KE, Tuggle DW, Gessoroum MR, Overholt ED, Mantor PC. Transseptal decompression of the left heart during ECMO for severe myocarditis. Ann Thorac Surg 1995; 59:749–751.
54. Cheung MM, Goldman AP, Shekerdemian LS, et al. Percutaneous left ventricular "vent" insertion for left heart decompression during extracorporeal membrane oxygenation. Pediatr Crit Care Med 2003; 4:447–449.

55. Jaggers JJ, Forbess JM, Shah AS, et al. Extracorporeal membrane oxygenation for infant postcardiotomy support: significance of shunt management. Ann Thorac Surg 2000; 69:1476–1483.
56. Jacobs JP, Ojito JW, McConaghey TW, et al. Rapid cardiopulmonary support for children with complex congenital heart disease. Ann Thorac Surg 2000; 70:742–749.
57. Smedira NG, Moazami N, Golding CM, et al. Clinical experience with 202 adults receiving extracorporeal membrane oxygenation for cardiac failure: survival at 5 years. J Thorac Cardiovasc Surg 2001; 122:92–102.
58. Walters HL, III, Hakimi M, Rice MD, Lyons JM, Whittlesey GC, Klein MD. Pediatric cardiac surgery ECMO: multivariate analysis of risk factors for hospital death. Ann THorac Surg 1995; 60:329–336.
59. Chaturvedi RR, Macrae D, Brown KL, et al. Cardiac ECMO for biventricular hearts after pediatric open heart surgery. Heart 2004; 90:545–551.
60. Booth KL, Roth SJ, Thiagarajan RR, Almodovar MC, del Nido PJ, Laussen PC. Extracorporeal membrane oxygenation support of the fontan and bidirectional glenn circulations. Ann Thorac Surg 2004; 77:1341–1348.
61. Bulas D, Glass P. Neonatal ECMO neuroimaging and neurodevelopmental outcome. Semin Perinatol 2005; 29:58–65.
62. Amigoni A, Pettenazzo A, Biban P, et al. Neurologic outcome in children after extracorporeal membrane oxygenation: prognostic value of diagnostic tests. Pediatr Neurol 2005; 32:173–179.
63. Parish AP, Bunyapen C, Cohen MJ, Garrison T, Bhatia J. Seizures as a predictor of long-term neurodevelopmental outcome in survivors of neonatal extracorporeal membrane oxygenation (ECMO). J Child Neurol 2004; 19:930–934.
64. Duncan BW, Lorenz M, Kopcak MW, et al. The Pedipump: a new ventricular assist device for children. Artif Organs 2005; 29:527–530.
65. Frazier OH. Implantation of the Jarvik 2000 left ventricular assist device without the use of cardiopulmonary bypass. Ann Thorac Surg 2003; 75:1028–1030.
66. Frazier OH, Myers TJ, Westaby S, Gregoric ID. Clinical experience with an implantable, intracardiac, continuous flow circulatory support device: physiologic implications and their relationship to patient selection. Ann THorac Surg 2004; 77:133–142.
67. Delgado R, III, Frazier OH, Myers TJ, et al. Direct thrombolytic therapy for intraventricular thrombosis in patients with the Jarvik 2000 left ventricular assist device. J Heart Lung Transplant 2005; 24:231–233.
68. Morales DL, DiBardino DJ, McKenzie ED, et al. Lessons learned from the first application of the DeBakey VAD *Child*: an intracorporeal ventricular assist device for children. J Heart Lung Transplant 2005; 24:331–337.
69. Frazier OH, Myers TY, Gregoric ID, et al. Initial clinical experience with the Jarvik 2000 implantable axial-flow left ventricular assist system. Circulation 2002; 105:2855–2860.
70. Westaby S, Frazier OH, Beyersdorf F, et al. The Jarvik 2000 Heart. Clinical validation of the intraventricular position. Eur J Cardiothorac Surg 2002; 22:228–232.
71. Throckmorton AL, Allaire PE, Gutgesell HP, et al. Pediatric circulatory support systems. ASAIO J 2002; 48:216–221.
72. Hohlweg-Majert B, Gutwald R, Siegenthaler MP, Schmelzesein R. Implantation of the Jarvik 2000 left-ventricular-assist-device: role of the maxillofacial surgeon. Eur J Cardiothorac Surg 2005; 28:337–339.
73. Ashton RC, Oz MC, Michler RE, et al. Left ventricular assist device options in pediatric patients. ASAIO J 1995; 41:277–280.
74. Reinhartz O, Copeland JG, Farrar DJ. Thoratec ventricular assist device in children with less than 1.3 m^2 of body surface area. ASAIO J 2003; 49:727–730.
75. Reinhartz O, Stiller B, Eilers R, Farrar DJ. Current clinical status of pulsatile pediatric circulatory support. ASAIO J 2002; 48:455–459.
76. Stiller B, Lemmer J, Merkle F, et al. Consumption of blood products during mechanical circulatory support in children: comparison between ECMO and a pulsatile ventricular assist device. Intensive Care Med 2004; 30:1814–1820.

77. Merkle F, Boettcher W, Stiller B, Hetzer R. Pulsatile mechanical cardiac assistance in pediatric patients with the Berlin heart ventricular assist device. J Extra Corpor Technol 2003; 35:115–120.
78. Hetzer R, Loebe M, Potapov EV, et al. Circulatory support with pneumatic paracorporeal ventricular assist device in infants and children. Ann Thorac Surg 1998; 5:1498–1506.
79. Stiller B, Weng Y, Hubler M, et al. Pneumatic ventricular assist devices in children under 1 yr of age. Eur J Cardiothorac Surg 2005; 28:234–239.
80. Konertz W, Hotz H, Schneider M, Redlin M, Reul H. Clinical experience with the MEDOS HIA-VAD system in infants and children: a preliminary report. Ann Thorac Surg 1997; 63:1138–1144.
81. Grinda JM, Chevalier P, D'Attelis N, et al. Fulminant myocarditis in adults and children: bi-ventricualr assist device for recovery. Eur J Cardiothorac Surg 2004; 26:1169–1173.
82. Martin J, Sarai K, Schindler M, van de Loo A, Yoshitake M, Beyersdorf F. MEDOS HIA-VAD biventricular assist device for bridge to recovery in fulminant myocarditis. Ann Thorac Surg 1997; 63:1145–1146.

Index

AbioCor®
  background, 461
  clinical trials, 466–472
  description, 461–463
  future developments, 472
  operative technique, 464–466
  preoperative considerations, 463–464
  as total artificial heart, 461–472
ABIOMED AB 5000, 444–445
ABIOMED BVS 5000, 442–444
ACE inhibitors, 105
  rate control and, 174
Acid-base abnormalities, diuretics side effects and, 88
Acorn CorCap device, 635–637
Acute decompensated heart failure
  cardiac transplantation and, 493–494
  hydralazine, 103–104
  inotropic therapy and, 143–145
  nesiritide, 104
  nitrates, 103
  novel agents in treatment of, 104–105
  sodium nitroprusside, 102–103
  vasodilator therapy and, 101–105, 144–145
Acute heart failure, 203–221
  assessment of, 205–210
  causes, 205
  clinical evaluation, 206–210
  clinical history, 207
  diagnostic testing, 210
  future therapy, 218–220
  physical examination, 208
  pre-discharge goals, 220–221
  studies of, 210–212
  therapy for, 212–220
    angiotensin-converting enzyme inhibitors, 212–213
    beta-blockers, 213–214
[Acute heart failure]
    diuretics, 214
    inotropes, 216–218
    oxygen, 212
    vasodilators, 214–216
Adeno-associated virus, 577, 578
Adenosine antagonists, 90–91
Adenoviral vectors, 577–578
Adenovirus, 577
Adrenoceptors, beta-blockers and, 114
Advanced heart failure
  cardiac imaging, 24–27
  cardiomyopathy, 26–28
  causes and evaluation, 23–33
  endomyocardial biopsy, 27
  laboratory testing, 24–27
  patient evaluation, 23–27
Adverse drug interactions, diuretic side effects and, 89
Adverse effects, beta-blockers and, 128–129
Age
  cardiac transplantation and, 504
  chronic heart failure and, 8
  ventricular assist devices and, 429
Akt activation, long-term effects of, 583
Akt signaling, 582–583
Alcohol, heart failure and, 41
Aldosterone receptor antagonists,
  cardiac remodeling and, 76–77
  effect on mortality, 77–78
Allergic reactions, diuretics and, 89
Alpha receptors, beta-blockers and, 114–115
Ambulatory management, prognostic factors, 534–536
American College of Cardiology/American Heart Association consensus guideline, 495
Amiodarone toxicity, 501

Amiodarone, 193–194
Amlodipine, 109
Amplicons, 579
Amyloidosis, cardiac transplantation and, 504–505
Angina class, transmyocardial laser revascularization and, 390–391, 396
Angiotensin receptor blockers, 105–106
Angiotensin-converting enzyme inhibitors, 212–213
Antiarrhythmic drugs, 192–195
  beta-adrenergic blockers, 192–193
  Class I types, 193–195
  ICD interaction, 195
  sotalol, 195
  amiodarone, 193–194
  dofetilide, 194–195
Anti-fibrotic therapy, diastolic heart failure and, 244
Anti-ischemic therapy, diastolic heart treatment and, 242
Anxiety disorders, in transplant patients
  incidence of, 521
  manifestations of, 521–522
  treatment of, 522
Aortic regurgitation, 368
Aortic stenosis, 366
Aortic valve surgery, 366–367
  aortic regurgitation, 368
  aortic stenosis, 366
  low transvalvular gradient, 366–367
  LV dysfunction, 366–367
  severe, 366–367
Arginine vasopressin, 74–75
Arrhythmogenic right ventricular dysplasia, 186
Asymptomatic left ventricular dysfunction, 1–3
  prevalence of, 4
Aticure radiofrequency abalation device, 632–634
ATP-dependent potassium channels, heart failure drugs and, 613–614
Atrial arrhythmia, 167–176
  atrial fibrillation, 167–172
  atrial flutter, 174–176
  control of, 168–169, 172–174
  supraventricular arrhythmias, 176
Atrial fibrillation
  Aticure® radiofrequency abalation device, 632–634
  atrial arrhythmia and, 167–172
  clinical significance, 167
[Atrial fibrillation]
  Guidant® microwave ablation devices, 630–632
  heart failure, relationship of, 168
  management of, 168–169
  Medtronic® cardioblate radiofrequency ablation device, 632
  results, 634–635
  surgical treatment of, 630–635
Atrial flutter
  atrial arrhythmia and, 174–176
  heart failure, relationship between, 174–175
  management of, 175–176
  sinus rhythm, 175
Atrioventricular optimization, cardiac resynchronization therapy and, 282–285
Autologous mononuclear bone marrow cells (AMBMC), 559
Autosomal dominant familial dilated cardiomyopathy, 610–614

Bcl-2, 582
Beta adrenergic agonists, 139–141
  dobutamine, 141
  dopamine, 139–141
Beta receptors, beta-blockers and, 115–118
Beta-adrenergic blockers, antiarrhythmic drugs and, 192–192
Beta-blockers
  acute heart failure therapy and, 213–214
  adrenoceptors, 114
  alpha receptors, 114–115
  beta receptors, 115–118
  beta-adrenergic signaling, 114
  clinical guidelines, 125–129
  clinical trials, 118–125
  decompensation, 126–128
  heart failure and, 113–129
  inotrope use, 126–128
  pacer placement, 128
  rate control and, 172
  titration strategies, 126
Biomarkers, diastolic heart failure and, 239–240
Biventricular pacemaker lead placement, 625–628
Biventricular stimulation, 280–281
Blood pressure, diastolic heart failure and, 241–242
Blood-derived cells, 555–557
Body size, ventricular assist devices and, 429
Bone marrow cells, 552–555

Bradycardia therapy, 643
Brain natriuretic peptide (BNP), 536
Bridge to bridge devices, 447
Bridge to recovery system
  ABIOMED® AB 5000, 444–445
  ABIOMED® BVS 5000, 442–444
  centrifugal pumps, 445–446
  Levitronix Centrimag® blood pumping system, 446–447
  ventricular assist device types and, 442–447
Bridge to transplant devices
  first generation devices, 448–451
  second generation devices, 451–454
  ventricular assist devices and, 447–455
Bundle branch reentry VTs, 188–189

CABG, transmyocardial laser revascularization and, 393–394
Calcium handling, 584–585
Calcium sensitizers, levosimendan, 142–143
Cardiac catheterization
  cardiac transplantation and, 498
  myocardial viability and, 352–353
Cardiac contractile apparatus, heart failure and, 137–139
Cardiac gene therapy, vectors for, 576
Cardiac imaging, advanced heart failure and, 24–27
Cardiac MRI, myocardial viability and, 352
Cardiac myocyte, death and dysfunction, 609–610
Cardiac myosin binding protein C, 599
Cardiac regeneration repair, cell types involved in, 552–557
Cardiac remodeling
  aldosterone receptor antagonists, 76–77
  diuretics and, 76–77
  loop diuretics, 76
Cardiac restraint devices, Acorn CorCap® device, 635–637
Cardiac resynchronization therapy, 261–298
  clinical trials, 294
  defibrillation studies
    COMPANION, 297–298
    CONTAK CD, 297–298
    MIRACLE ICD, 297–298
  heart failure, 261
  implementation of, 268–277
    left ventricular lead placement, 268–269
  mechanisms of, 265–267
  pacemaker electrocardiography, 286–289
  pacing systems, 277–285
    biventricular stimulation, 280–281
[Cardiac resynchronization therapy]
    leads and electrodes, 277–278
    pulse generators, 279–280
    univentricular stimulation, 280–281
  patient selection, 289–294
  programming considerations, 281–285
  randomized trials, 295
Cardiac transplantation
  acute decompensation, 493–494
  candidate selection, 493–508
  chronic severe heart failure, 494
  contraindications to, 499–505
    age, 504
    amyloidosis, 504–505
    diabetes, 503
    hepatic dysfunction, 502–503
    malignancy, 504
    non-cardiac vascular disease, 502
    obesity, 503
    osteoporosis, 505
    pulmonary disease, 501–502
    renal dysfunction, 503
    social and cognitive factors, 505
  donor identification and management, 507–508
  general indications, 493–495
  infections, 500–501
    Chagas disease, 500–501
    cytomegalovirus, 501
    hepatitis C, 500–501
    Toxoplasma gondii, 501
    Trepoema pallidum, 501
    tuberculosis, 500–501
  obesity and, 51–52
  patient evaluation, 496–499
  TXP center, referral, 499, 506–507
  waitlist for TXP, outcomes, 506
Cardiac troponin I, 600
Cardiac α–myosin heavy chain, 599
Cardiac β–myosin heavy chain mutations, 599
Cardiomyocyte apoptosis, 581
Cardiomyocyte function, preservation of, 583
Cardiomyopathies
  advanced heart failure and, 26–28
  aortic valve surgery, 366–367
  autosomal dominant FDC, 610–614
  clinical implications, 618–619
  dilated, restrictive, right ventricular, 609–619
  famial restrictive, 615–616
  familial dilated (FDC), 609–615
  mitral valve surgery, 363–365
  reversible causes, 28–32

[Cardiomyopathies]
right ventricular, 616–618
statins, inflammation, 155–162
stress, 31–32
valvular surgery, 361–367
Cardiopulmonary exercise testing
cardiac transplantation and, 496–498
survival and, 497
Catheter ablation therapy, 641
Cell autonomous transgenes, 576
Cellular cardiomyoplasty, 549–585
Centrifugal pumps, ventricular assist devices and, 445–446
Cerclage technique. *See* multiple purse string
Chagas disease (*Trypanosoma cruzi*), 187–188, 500
Chronic heart failure
ACE inhibitors, 105
amlodipine, 109
angiotensin receptor blockers, 105–106
asymptomatic left ventricular dysfunction, 1–3
diagnosis of, 10–11
epidemiology of, 1–15
inotropic therapy and, 145–148
multivariate risk prediction, 8–9
nitrates and hydralazine, 106–109
prognosis of, 1–16
Resource Utilization Among Congestive Heart Failure Study (REACH), 15
risk factors, 3–8
special populations, 9–10
vasodilator therapy and, 105
Chronic intropic support, 147–148
Chronic obstructive pulmonary disease (COPD), 501
Chronic severe heart failure, cardiac transplantation and, 494
Class I antiarrhythmic drugs, 193–195
Combination therapy, loop diuretics, 85
Comorbidities, obesity and, 50–51
COMPANION study, 297–298
Congestive heart failure
diuretics and, 83–87
ischemic cardiomyopathy, 349
loop diuretics, 83–87
surgical techniques
atrial fibrillation, 630–635
cardiac restraint devices, 635–637
da Vinci® system, 621
geometric mitral reconstruction, 623
new minimally invasive mitral valve repair, 623–625
[Congestive heart failure]
robot-assisted biventricular pacemaker lead placement, 625–628
robot-assisted transmyocardial revascularization, 629–630
totally endoscopic coronary artery bypass grafting (TECAB), 621–623
revascularization and, 349
CONTAK CD®, 297–298
Continuous positive airway pressure, sleep apnea and, 338–343
COPD. *See* chronic obstructive pulmonary disease.
Coronary angiography, myocardial viability and, 352–353
Coronary heart disease, 5–7
Cytomegalovirus, 501

da Vinci® system, 621
DCM. *See* dilated cardiomyopathy.
Decompensated heart failure, drugs and, 613
beta-blockers and, 126–128
Defibrillation
cardiac resynchronization therapy, 294–297
COMPANION study, 297–298
CONTAK CD study, 297–298
MIRACLE ICD study, 297–298
Defibrillators, implantable, 305–324
Denervation, transmyocardial laser revascularization and, 395–396
Depression, in heart failure patients, 520–521
Destination therapy, inotropic therapy and, 146–147
Device therapy
continuous positive airway pressure, 338–343
enhanced external counterpulsation, 333–338
intra-aortic balloon counterpulsation, 329–333
Diabetes
cardiac transplantation and, 503
heart failure and, 8
obesity and, 50–51
Diastolic heart failure, 229–244
clinical assessment, 236–240
biomarkers, 239–240
exercise testing, 237–238
invasive testing, 239
noninvasive imaging, 236–237
definitions and classifications, 229–230
diagnostic criteria, 230
epidemiology, 230–232

[Diastolic heart failure]
future therapies, 243–244
pathophysiology, 232–236
vs. systolic heart failure, 232, 238
treatment, 240–243
anti-ischemic therapy, 242
blood pressure control, 241–242
exercise training, 243
fluid and sodium, 241
rate and rhythm control, 242–243
Diet, heart failure and, 37–52
alcohol, 41
fluid restriction, 40–41
sodium restriction, 40–41
Digoxin, 141–142
rate control and, 172–173
Dilated cardiomyopathy (DCM), cardiac resynchronization therapy and, 261
Dilated cardiomyopathy, 609–619
abnormal electrical timing, 263–264
Diltiazem, rate control and, 173
Diuretics, 71–91
acute heart failure and, 214
adenosine antagonists, 90–91
cardiac remodeling, 76–77
aldosterone receptor antagonists, 76–77
loop 76
congestive heart failure and-87
dopamine, 89
effects of, 71–72, 77–78
hemodynamic effects, 72
loop, neurohormonal effects of, 73
mechanisms of action, 78
natriuretic peptides, 90
pharmacodynamics, 82–83
pharmacokinetics, 80–82
pharmacology of, 78–83
resistance to, 83
side effects, 87–89
types of, 78, 89–91
vasopressin antagonists, 90
Dobutamine stress echocardiography, 351–352
Dobutamine, 141
Dofetilide, 194–195
Dopamine, 89, 139–141
DOR procedure. *See* endoventricular circular patch plasty.
Drug-induced cardiomyopathy, 33
Dying patient, managing, 542, 544
Dyslipidemia, obesity and, 51
Electrocardiography (EKG)
resting, 486
revascularization and, 350–351
secondary pulmonary hypertension and, 252
EKG. *See* electrocardiography.
Electrolyte abnormalities, diuretic side effects and, 87–88
Embryonic stem cells, 551, 557
Emphysema, 501
End of life
advance directives, 541
heart failure, 540–544
issues, 533–544
medication options, 543–544
Endarterectomy, 354–355
Endogenous cardiac stem cells, 549, 556–557
Endomyocardial biopsy, advanced heart failure and, 27
Endothelial function, statins and, 159–160
Endothelial progenitor cells, 551, 555–556
Endoventricular circular patch plasty, 374–376
Endpoints, transmyocardial laser revascularization and, 388–389
Enhanced external counterpulsation, 336
Ethnic minorities, chronic heart failure and, 10
Exercise
adherence to, 67
heart failure (HF) and, 56–67
heart failure normal ejection fraction (HFNEF), 66
safety of, 63
training, diastolic heart failure and, 52, 63–66, 243
Exercise capacity, prognostic factors, 535
Exercise stress testing
cardiopulmonary, 496–498
diastolic heart failure and, 237–238
revascularization and, 350–351
Exercise tolerance, transmyocardial laser revascularization and, 391
Exocytosis blockade, statins and, 160–161
Exogenous cells, 549

Familial restrictive cardiomyopathy, 615–616
genes associated with, 615
Familial dilated cardiomyopathy (FDC), 609–615
First generation ventricular assist devices, 448–451
Fluid restriction, heart failure and, 40–41
Furosemide-induced venodilation, 72–73

Gene therapy, heart failure and, 575–585
Genetics, hypertrophic cardiomyopathy and, 596
Geometric mitral reconstruction, 623
Glucocorticoid, 505
Grafting techniques, revascularization and, 354–355
Guidant microwave ablation device, 630–632

Health care system, barriers related to, 525–527
Health educational programs, 515–516
  evaluation of, 516
Health literacy tests, 514
Heart failure
  acute, 203–221
  acute decompensed, 101–105
  advanced. *See* advanced heart failure.
  atrial fibrillation and, 168
  atrial flutter and, 174–175
  beta-blockers, 113–129
  biological targets, 580–585
  cardiac contractile apparatus, 137–139
  cardiac resynchronization therapy and, 261
  chronic severe, 494–499
    vasodilator therapy and, 105
  congestive, diuretics and, 83–87
  device therapy for, 329, 333–338
  diabetes and, 50–51
  diastolic, 229–244
  diet, 37–52
  dilated cardiomyopathy (DCM), 261–265
  drugs, 609–615
  dyslipidemia and, 51
  end of life care, 540–544
  exercise, 59–67
  gene therapy for, 575–585
  heart, functional capacity, 59–61
  incidence of, 549
  inotropic therapy, 137–151
  levosimendan, 614
  management of, 99–109
  metabolic syndrome, 37–52
  myocyte death/dysfunction, 609–610
  obesity, 37–52
  oxidative stress in, 610
  oxypurinol, 612
  patient education program, 514, 517
  sleep apnea and, 51, 338–343
  vasoconstriction, 99–101
  venous thromboembolism and, 51
  ventricular arrhythmias and, 183–195
  weight gain and loss, 37–39
Heart failure clinics, 518
Heart failure management, goals of therapy, 538
Heart failure normal ejection fraction (HFNEF), 66
Heart failure patients, anxiety and, 521–522
Hematopoetic precursor cells, 555
Hematopoetic progenitor cells, 551
Hemopump. *See* transvalvular assist device.
Hepatic dysfunction, cardiac transplantation and, 502–503
Hepatitis C, 500–501
Herpes virus/amplicon, 577
Herpesvirus, 579
HF. *See* heart failure.
HFNEF. *See* heart failure normal ejection fraction.
Home-based monitoring, outpatient disease management, 519
Hospice care, 541–542
Hospital admission, transmyocardial laser revascularization and, 391
Hydralazine, 103–104
  chronic heart failure and, 106–109
Hypertension
  chronic heart failure and, 3–5
  pulmonary, cardiac transplantation and, 501
Hypertrophic cardiomyopathy (HCM), 591–605
  background of, 591–605
  cardiac troponin I, 600
  cardiac troponin T, 600
  diagnosis, 602–605
  genetic aspects, 596–599
  inherited, 600–602
  natural history, 594–596
  phenotype, 593–594
  screening strategy, 596
Hyperuricemia, diuretic side effects and, 88

ICD, antiarrhythmic drugs and, 195
Idiopathic VT, 189
Idopathic dilated cardiomyopathy, 161–162
Impella® system. 409–412
Implantable cardioverter defibrillator therapy, 641–642
Implantable defibrillators, 305–324
  complications of, 322
  device selection, 320–325
  guidelines for, 323
  patient selection, 308–324
  randomized trials, 309, 313–314
  sudden cardiac death, 305–308

[Implantable defibrillators]
prevention of, 308–320
Individual health care, barriers relating to, 526–527
Infections
cardiac transplantation and, 500–501
chagas disease, 500
cytomegalovirus, 501
hepatitis C, 500–501
Toxoplasma gondii, 501
Trepoema pallidum, 501
tuberculosis, 500–501
Inflammation
cardiomyopathy and, 155–162
statins, clinical trials and, 157–158
Inherited hypertrophic cardiomyopathy, 600–602
Inotropic therapy
acute decompensated 143–145
acute heart failure and, 216–218
beta-blockers and, 126–128
bridge to transplant, 145
chronic 145–148
destination therapy, 146–147
heart failure and, 137–151
mechanism of action, 139–143
risk and mortality of, 145
vs. vasodilators, acute decompensated 144–145
Inpatient management, prognostic factors, 534
Integrins, statins and, 158–159
Interventricular delay, dilated cardiomyopathy and, 263–264
Inter-ventricular timing, cardiac resynchronization therapy and, 285
Intra-aortic balloon counterpulsation, 652–654
complications of, 332
contraindications to, 332
indications for, 329–333
percutaneous left ventricular assist devices and, 405–406
Intramural delay, dilated cardiomyopathy and, 265
Intravascular ultrasound, myocardial viability and, 352–353
Intravenous infusion, loop diuretics and, 86
Intraventricular delay, dilated cardiomyopathy and, 263–265
Invasive testing, diastolic heart failure and, 239
Ischemic cardiomyopathy, revascularization and, 349, 357–358
Ischemic heart disease, 184

Laboratory testing
advanced heart failure and, 24–27
outpatient disease managemen, 519
Laser-tissue interactions, 394–395
Leads and electrodes, cardiac resynchronization therapy and, 277–278
Left atrial to femoral artery bypass, 406
Left heart disease, secondary pulmonary hypertension and, 253–255
Left ventricular dysfunction
revascularization and, 350
survival of, 350
Left ventricular ejection fraction (LVEF), prognostic factors, 535
Left ventricular hypertrophy and dilatation, 7–8
Left ventricular lead placement
cardiac resynchronization therapy and, 268–269
complicating factors, 269–271
optimal lead placement, 272–277
surgical approach, 271–272
Lentiviruses, 577–579
Levitronix Centrimag® blood pumping system, 446–447
Levosimendan
clinical effects, 615
heart failure and, 614
Lifestyle modifications, outpatient disease management, 519
Linear closure, septoplasty, 376
Loop diuretics
arginine vasopressin, 74–75
cardiac remodeling, 76
congestive heart failure and, 83–84
mortality and, 77
natriuretic peptides, 75–76
prostaglandins, 75
renin-angiotensin-aldosterone system (RASS), 73–74
resistance to, 85–87
sympathetic nervous system and, 74
LV dysfunction, aortic valve surgery and, 366–367

Malignancy, cardiac transplantation and, 504
Mechanical cardiopulmonary support, 643–645
Mechanism of action
beta adrenergic agonists, 139–141

[Mechanism of action]
calcium sensitizers, 142–143
inotropes, 139–143
phosphodiesterase inhibitors, 141
sodium-potassium aTPase pump inhibitors, 141–142
Mechanisms of harm, inotropic therapy, 143
Medicare program, 524
Medtronic Cardioblate® radiofrequency ablation device, 632
Mesenchymal stem cells, 551–555, 563
Metabolic syndrome
criteria for, 42
diuretics and, 88
heart failure and, 37–52
Micronutrient deficiency, heart failure and, 39
Milrinone, 141
Minimally invasive mitral valve repair, 623–625
MIRACLE ICD, 297–298
Mitral valve surgery, regurgitation, 363–365
Monomorphic ventricular tachycardia, 184–189
arrhythmogenic right ventricular dysplasia, 186
bundle branch reentry VTs, 188–189
Chagas'' disease, 187–188
evaluation and therapy, 189
idiopathic VT, 189
ischemic heart disease, 184
nonischemic dilated cardiomyopathy, 184–186
sarcoidosis, 186–187
Morbidity, transmyocardial laser revascularization and, 390
Mortality
loop diuretics and, 77
transmyocardial laser revascularization and, 389–390
Multiple purse string, 376
Multivariate risk prediction, chronic heart failure and, 8–9
Myocardial failure, oxidative stress, 611
Myocardial function, 391
Myocardial injection, 580
Myocardial perfusion, 392
Myocardial viability testing
cardiac catheterization, 352–353
cardiac MRI, 352
coronary angiography, 352–353
dobutamine stress echocardiography, 351–352
intravascular ultrasound, 352–353
positron emission tomography (PET), 351
[Myocardial viability testing]
revascularization and, 351–353
technetium scintigraphy, 351
thallium scintigraphy, 351
Myocarditis, cardiomyopathy and, 28–31
Myocardium
normal, 349–350
oxidative stress and, 610–611
Myocardium scarring, revascularization and, 349–350
Myocyte dysfunction, heart failure and, 611–612
Myocyte loss, heart failure and, 611–612
Myocyte necrosis, 550
Myosin light chains, hypertrophic cardiomyopathy, 599

Naked DNA, 576
Natriuretic peptides, 75–76, 90
Nesiritide, 104
Neurohormonal antagonist, heart failure and, 494
New York Heart Association classification scheme, 495
Nitrates, 103
chronic heart failure and, 106–109
Non-cardiac vascular disease, cardiac transplantation and, 502
Noninvasive imaging, diastolic heart failure and, 236–237
Nonischemic dilated cardiomyopathy, 184–186
Non-pulsatile devices, 655–659
percutaneous left ventricular assist device, 404–405
Nonresponders, pacemaker electrocardiography and, 287–289
Nonsustained ventriculary tachycardia, 191–192
Normal myocardium, 349–350

Obesity
cardiac transplant considerations, 51–52, 503
comorbidities, 50–51
diabetes, 50–51
dyslipidemia, 51
sleep apnea, 51
venous thromboembolism, 51
diagnostic considerations, 47–49
epidemiology and prognosis, 43–45
heart failure and, 37–52
pathophysiology, 45–47
treatment of, 49

Off-pump, revascularization and, 355
On-pump, revascularization and, 355
Osteoporosis
  cardiac transplantation and, 505
  cyclosporine, 505
  glucocorticoid, 505
Ototoxicity, diuretic side effects and, 89
Outpatient disease management, 516–519
  heart failure clinics, 518
  home-based monitoring, 519
  laboratory testing, 519
  lifestyle modifications, 519
  medications, 518–519
  strategies for, 518
  telemonitoring, 519
  transition from inpatient, 516–518
Oxidative stress, 609–615
  heart failure and, 610
  myocardial failure and, 610–611
Oxygen, acute heart failure therapy and, 212
Oxypurinol
  clinical experiences, 612–613
  heart failure and, 612

Pacemaker electrocardiography
  cardiac resynchronization therapy and, 286–289
  nonresponders, 287–289
  responders, 287–289
Pacer placement, beta-blockers and, 128
Pacing modes, cardiac resynchronization therapy and, 281
Pacing outputs, cardiac resynchronization therapy and, 285
Pacing systems
  biventricular stimulation, 280–281
  cardiac resynchronization therapy and, 277–285
  leads and electrodes, 277–278
  pulse generators, 279–280
  univentricular stimulation, 280–281
Palliative care, 541–542
PAR. *See* population risk factor.
Patent channels, transmyocardial laser revascularization and, 395
Pathophysiology
  diastolic heart failure, 232–236
  obesity, 45–47
Patient education, 513, 517
  challenges in, 514
  health literacy tests, 514
  learning strategies, 515
Patient evaluation, advanced heart failure and, 23–27
Patient management, ventricular assist devices and, 439–442
Patient selection
  cardiac resynchronization therapy and, 289–294
  ventricular assist devices and, 437–439
Pediatric aspects, 639–640
Pediatric catheter ablation therapy, 641
Pediatric device therapy
  bradycardia therapy, 643
  implantable cardioverter defibrillator, 641–642
Pediatric etiologic groups, 650
Pediatric psychosocial aspects, 646
Pediatric-specific ventricular assist devices, 652–662
Pediatric surgery
  indications for device implantation, 650–651
  management, 649–662
Pediatric ventricular assist device, choices of, 652
Percutaneous cardiopulmonary bypass, 406–407
Percutaneous left ventricular assist devices, 403–416
  benefits of, 405
  contemporary devices, 409–416
    Impella®system, 409–412
    TandemHeart®, 412–415
  history of, 405–409
    intra-aortic balloon pump, 405–406
    left atrial to femoral artery bypass, 406
    percutaneous cardiopulmonary bypass, 406–407
    transvalvular assist device, 407–409
  types, 404–405
Percutaneous myocardial laser revascularization, 396–397
Perfusion-based delivery, vectors, 580
Peripartum cardiomyopathy, 31
Pharmacodynamics, diuretics and, 82–83
Pharmacokinetics, diuretics and, 80–82
Phosphodiesterase inhibitors, milrinone, 141
Phosphoinositide 3–kinase, 582
Physical examination
  advanced heart failure and, 24
  secondary pulmonary hypertension and, 252
Plasmid DNA, 576
Plasmid DNA, 577
Population risk factor (PAR), 4

Positive lusitropes, diastolic heart failure and, 243–244
Positron emission tomography (PET), myocardial viability and, 351
Precursor cells, 549
Prognosis assessment, 533–544
Prognostic factors
  ambulatory management, 534–536
  clinical use of, 534–538
  exercise capacity as, 535
  left ventricular ejection fraction (LVEF), 535
  patient assessment, 536–537
  physical assessment, 536–537
Prolonged atrioventricular delay, dilated cardiomypathy and, 261–263
Prostaglandins, 75
Proteins, statins and, 159
Pulmonary disease
  cardiac transplantation and, 501–502
  chronic obstructive pulmonary disease (COPD), 501
  emphysema, 501
  pulmonary fibrosis, 501
Pulmonary fibrosis, 501
Pulmonary hypertension
  amiodarone toxicity, 501
  cardiac transplantation and, 501
  secondary, diagnosis and management of, 249–258
Pulsatile devices, 659–662
  percutaneous left ventricular assist type, 404–405
Pulse generators, cardiac resynchronization therapy and, 279–280

Quality of life, transmyocardial laser revascularization and, 391
Quality vs. quantity of life
  patient preference, 537–538
  transition point, 538–539

RASS. *See* renin-angiotensin-aldosterone system.
Rate and rhythm control, diastolic heart failure and, 242–243
  ACE inhibitors, 174
  atrial arrhythmia, 168–169, 172–174
  non-pharmacological, 173–174
  pharmacological, 172–173
    beta-blockers, 172
    digoxin, 172–173
    diltiazem, 173
REACH. *See* Resource Utilization Among Congestive Heart Failure Study.
Regenerative medicine, 549–585
Regurgitation, mitral valve surgery and, 363–365
Renal dysfunction, cardiac transplantations and, 503
Renin-angiotensin-aldosterone system (RASS),
Reoperations, revascularization and, 357
Repair mechanisms, 550–552
  paracrine factors, 550
  stem cell and myoctye fusion, 550
  stem cell differentiation, 550
Resource Utilization Among Congestive Heart Failure Study (REACH), 15
Responders, pacemaker electrocardiography and, 287–289
Resting echocardiography, 486
Restrictive cardiomyopathy, 609–619
Revascularization, 349–358
Revascularization
  congestive ischemic cardiomyopathy, 349
  coronary disease, 350
  investigational modalities, 350–351
    electrocardiography (EKG), 350–351
    exercise stress testing 350–351
  ischemic cardiomyopathy, management of, 357–358
  left ventricular dysfunction, 350
  myocardial viability, 351–353
  patient selection, 353
  principles of, 353–354
  stunned hibernating myocardium, 349–350
  technical considerations, 354–357
    endarterectomy, 354–355
    grafting techniques, 354–355
    off-pump, 355
    on-pump, 355
    reoperations, 357
Rhythm control
  atrial arrhythmia and, 168–172
  normal rhythm control maintenance, 170–172
  normal sinus rhythm, 169
Right heart catheterization, secondary pulmonary hypertension and, 253
Right ventricular cardiomyopathy, 609–619
  cardiomyopathies and, 616–618
  diagnostic criteria, 617
  genes associated with, 616
Right ventricular failure, ventricular assist devices and, 429–430

Robot-assisted biventricular pacemaker lead placement, 625–628
Robot-assisted transmyocardial revascularization, 629–630

Sarcoid cardiomyopathy, 32–33
Sarcoidosis, 186–187
Second generation devices, ventricular assist devices and, 451–454
Secondary pulmonary hypertension
basic science of, 250–251
clinical evaluation, 251–253
diagnosis and management of, 249–258
differential diagnosis, 252–253
echocardiography, 252
left heart disease, 253–255
management of, 253–258
pathology of, 250–251
pathophysiology of, 249–250
patient history in, 251–252
physical examination, 252
right heart catheterization, 253
surgical management, 257–258
systemic-to-pulmonary shunt, 255–257
Septoplasty, technique, 376–383
Side effects, diuretics and, 87–89
Sinus rhythm
atrial flutter and, 175
normal, rhythm control and, 169
Skeletal muscle-derived cells, 557
Skeletal myoblasts, 551, 559
Sleep apnea
continuous positive airway pressure and, 338–343
heart failure and, 338–343
obesity and, 51
prevalence in 340
Sleep-disordered breathing, 542
Sodium, diastolic treatment and, 241
Sodium nitroprusside, 102–103
Sodium restriction, heart failure and, 40–41
Sodium-potassium aTPase pump inhibitors, 141–142
Sole therapy transmyocardial laser revascularization, 386–388
Sotalol, 195
Statins
anti-cholesterol effects, 156–157
cardiomyopathy and, 155–162
clinical trials of, 157–158
discovery of, 155–156
endothelial function improvement, 159–160
exocytosis blockade, 160–161
[Statins]
idiopathic dilated cardiomyopathy, 161–162
integrin blockage, 158–159
leukocyte trafficking, 158–159
proteins, 159
vascular inflammation, 160–161
Stem cell therapy delivery routes, 557–558
Stem cell types, mechanisms and effects, 551
Stem cells
migration of, 558
potential complications, 563–564
Stress cardiomyopathy, 31–32
Sudden cardiac death, 305–306
indicators of, 306–308
primary prevention, with implantable defibrillators, 308–312
secondary prevention, with implantable defibrillators, 308–312
ventricular arrhythmias and, 183–192
Supraventricular tachycardias, atrial arrhythmia and, 176
Surgical ventricular remodeling, 371–383
approaches to, 373–374
contraindications, 374
endoventricular circular patch plasty, 374–376
history of, 372–373
indications for, 373
linear closure, 376
multiple purse string, 376
septoplasty technique, 376–383
Sustained polymorphic ventricular tachycardia, 189–191
Torsade de Pointes, 190–191
Sympathetic nervous system, loop diuretics and, 74
SynCardia CardioWest® total artificial heart, 475–491
clinical experience, 485–488
future applications, 489
indications for, 485
Syncope, ventricular arrhythmias and, 191
Systemic-to-pulmonary shunt, secondary pulmonary hypertension and, 255–257
Systolic vs. diastolic clinical features, 238
Systolic vs. diastolic mortality rate of, 232

Tachycardia-induced cardiomyopathy, 32
TandemHeart®, 409–412
Targeted gene expression, inotropic therapy and, 149
Technetium scintigraphy, 351
Telemonitoring, for outpatient disease management, 519

Tezosentan, 104–105
Thallium scintigraphy, 351
Therapeutic circulatory support modalities, 643–646
  mechanical cardiopulmonary support, 643–645
  ventricular support devices, 645–646
Third generation devices, ventricular assist devices and, 454–455
Titration guidelines, beta-blockers and, 126
Torsade de Pointes, 190–191
Total artificial heart
  AbioCor®, 461–472
  history of, 477–481
  rationale for, 476–488
  SynCardia CardioWest®, 475–491
Totally endoscopic coronary artery bypass grafting (TECAB), 621–623
Toxoplasma gondii, 501
Transmyocardial laser revascularization, 385–397
  angiogenesis, 396
  CABG, adjunct to, 393–394
  clinical trials, 385–386
  denervation, 395–396
  future of, 397
  history of, 385–386
  laser-tissue interactions, 394–395
  mechanisms, 394–396
  patent channels, 395
  percutaneous myocardial laser revascularization, 396–397
  results, 389–393
  sole therapy, 386–389
Transmyocardial revascularization, 629–630
Transplant status, ventricular assist devices and, 429
Transplants, inotropic therapy and, 145
Transvalvular assist device, 407–409
Trepoema pallidum, 501
Trypanosoma cruzi, 500
Tuberculosis, 500–501

United Network for Organ Sharing standards, 495, 505–506
Univentricular stimulation, cardiac resynchronization therapy and, 280–281

Valvular heart disease, 7
Valvular surgery, 361–367
  aortic valve surgery, 366–367
  mitral valve surgery, 363–365
  repair or replacement, 362–363
Vascular disease, non-cardiac, 502
Vascular inflammation, statins and decreasing of, 160–161
Vascular stiffness, diastolic heart failure and, 244
Vasoconstriction, heart failure and, 99–101
Vasodilator therapy
  ACE inhibitors, chronic 105
  acute decompensed 101–105
  acute heart failure and, 214–216
  amlodipine, 109
  angiotensin receptor blockers, 105–106
  heart failure management and, 99–109
  hydralazine, 103–104
  inotropic therapy, 144–145
  nesiritide, 104
  nitrates, 103, 106–109
  sodium nitroprusside, 102–103
Vasopressin antagonists, 90
Vectors
  delivery system, 579–580
  perfusion-based delivery, 580
Venous thromboembolism, obesity and, 51
Ventricular arrhythmias, 183–195
  antiarrhythmic drugs, 192–195
  monomorphic ventricular tachycardia, 184–189
  nonsustained ventriculary tachycardia, 191–192
  sudden cardiac death, 183–192
  sustained polymorphic ventricular tachycardia, 189–191
  syncope, 191
  ventricular ectopic activity, 191–192
Ventricular assist devices, 435–457
  bridge to transplant devices, 447–455
  contraindications of, 428–431
  destination therapy, 447–455
  future of, 455–456
  history, 435–436
  intra-aortic balloon counterpulsation, 652–654
  non-pulsatile devices, 655–659
  optimal medical therapy, 421–424
  outcome of, 455–456
  overview of, 436–437
  patient management, 439–442
  patient selection, 437–439
  pulsatile devices, 659–662
  right ventricular failure, 429–430
  survival benefit of, 424–428
  third generation devices, 454–455
  types, 442–455

Ventricular double-counting, cardiac resynchronization therapy and, 281–282
Ventricular ectropic activity, 191–192
Ventricular remodeling. *See* surgical ventricular remodeling.
Ventricular support devices, 645–646
Ventriculary tachycardia, nonsustained, 191–192

Vitamin deficiency, heart failure and, 39

Weight gain and loss
- heart failure and, 37–39
- micronutrient deficiency, 39
- vitamin deficiency, 39